# RADIOLOGY
# SECRETS PLUS

D1128782

7/27/18

$57.11

# RADIOLOGY SECRETS PLUS

## FOURTH EDITION

**DREW A. TORIGIAN, MD, MA, FSAR**
Associate Professor, Department of Radiology
Clinical Director, Medical Image Processing Group (MIPG)
Hospital of the University of Pennsylvania
Philadelphia, Pennsylvania

**PARVATI RAMCHANDANI, MD, FACR, FSAR**
Professor of Radiology and Surgery, Section Chief GU Radiology
Department of Radiology
Hospital of the University of Pennsylvania
Philadelphia, Pennsylvania

ELSEVIER

# ELSEVIER

1600 John F. Kennedy Blvd.
Ste 1800
Philadelphia, PA 19103-2899

RADIOLOGY SECRETS PLUS, FOURTH EDITION
ISBN: 978-0-323-28638-1

**Copyright © 2017 by Elsevier, Inc. All rights reserved.**

No part of this publication may be reproduced or transmitted in any form or by any means, electronic or mechanical, including photocopying, recording, or any information storage and retrieval system, without permission in writing from the publisher. Details on how to seek permission, further information about the Publisher's permissions policies and our arrangements with organizations such as the Copyright Clearance Center and the Copyright Licensing Agency, can be found at our website: www.elsevier.com/permissions.

This book and the individual contributions contained in it are protected under copyright by the Publisher (other than as may be noted herein).

---

### Notices

Knowledge and best practice in this field are constantly changing. As new research and experience broaden our understanding, changes in research methods, professional practices, or medical treatment may become necessary.

Practitioners and researchers must always rely on their own experience and knowledge in evaluating and using any information, methods, compounds, or experiments described herein. In using such information or methods they should be mindful of their own safety and the safety of others, including parties for whom they have a professional responsibility.

With respect to any drug or pharmaceutical products identified, readers are advised to check the most current information provided (i) on procedures featured or (ii) by the manufacturer of each product to be administered, to verify the recommended dose or formula, the method and duration of administration, and contraindications. It is the responsibility of practitioners, relying on their own experience and knowledge of their patients, to make diagnoses, to determine dosages and the best treatment for each individual patient, and to take all appropriate safety precautions.

To the fullest extent of the law, neither the Publisher nor the authors, contributors, or editors, assume any liability for any injury and/or damage to persons or property as a matter of products liability, negligence or otherwise, or from any use or operation of any methods, products, instructions, or ideas contained in the material herein.

---

Previous editions copyrighted 2011, 2006, and 1998.

**Library of Congress Cataloging-in-Publication Data**

Names: Torigian, Drew A., editor. | Ramchandani, Parvati, editor.
Title: Radiology secrets plus / [edited by] Drew A. Torigian, Parvati Ramchandani.
Description: Fourth edition. | Philadelphia, PA : Elsevier, Inc., [2017] | Preceded by: Radiology secrets plus / [edited by] E. Scott Pretorius, Jeffrey A. Solomon. 3rd ed. c2011. | Includes bibliographical references and index.
Identifiers: LCCN 2016020832 (print) | LCCN 2016022038 (ebook) |
    ISBN 9780323286381 (hardback : alk. paper) | ISBN 9780323315821 (E-Book)
Subjects: | MESH: Radiology | Examination Questions
Classification: LCC RC78 (print) | LCC RC78 (ebook) | NLM WN 18.2 | DDC
    616.07/57–dc23
LC record available at https://lccn.loc.gov/2016020832

*Executive Content Strategist:* James Merritt
*Content Development Specialist:* Lisa Barnes
*Publishing Services Manager:* Hemamalini Rajendrababu
*Senior Project Manager:* Beula Christopher
*Book Designer:* Ryan Cook
*Illustration Manager:* Emily Costantino
*Marketing Manager:* Melissa Darling

Printed in China

Last digit is the print number:   9   8   7   6   5   4   3   2   1

Working together
to grow libraries in
developing countries

www.elsevier.com • www.bookaid.org

*We would like to dedicate this book to our parents, who have supported us all the way and have made it possible for us to be where we are today; to our siblings, who have always encouraged us; to our spouses and children who bring joy and meaning to each day; and to all those who study and apply the art and science of radiology to do good for the patients entrusted to our care.*

# CONTRIBUTORS

**Chiemezie C. Amadi, MD, MA**
Assistant Professor of Radiology
Department of Radiology
Ohio State University
Columbus, Ohio

**Linda J. Bagley, MD**
Associate Professor
Department of Radiology
Perelman School of Medicine
University of Pennsylvania
Philadelphia, Pennsylvania

**Prashant T. Bakhru, MD**
Radiologist
Department of Radiology
Princeton Radiology
Princeton, New Jersey

**Richard D. Bellah, MD**
Associate Professor of Radiology and Pediatrics
Department of Radiology
The Children's Hospital of Philadelphia
University of Pennsylvania Perelman School of
    Medicine
Philadelphia, Pennsylvania

**Judy S. Blebea, MD**
Clinical Professor of Radiology
Department of Radiological Sciences
University of Oklahoma Health Science Center
Oklahoma City, Oklahoma

**William W. Boonn, MD**
Cardiovascular Radiologist
Department of Radiology
Hospital of the University of Pennsylvania
Philadelphia, Pennsylvania

**Kerry Bron, MD**
Attending Pediatric Radiologist
AI DuPont Hospital for Children
Wilmington, Delaware

**Anil Chauhan, MD**
Assistant Professor
Department of Radiology
University of Pennsylvania
Philadelphia, Pennsylvania

**Hailey H. Choi, MD**
Resident Physician
Department of Radiology
Medstar Georgetown University Hospital
Washington, District of Columbia

**Emily F. Conant, MD**
Professor of Radiology
Chief of Breast Imaging
Department of Radiology
University of Pennsylvania Perelman School of
    Medicine
Department of Radiology
Hospital of the University of Pennsylvania
Philadelphia, Pennsylvania

**Tessa Sundaram Cook, MD, PhD**
Assistant Professor of Radiology
Perelman School of Medicine;
Senior Fellow
Institute for Biomedical Informatics
University of Pennsylvania;
Director, 3-D and Advanced Imaging Laboratory
Department of Radiology;
Director, Center for Translational Imaging Informatics
Department of Radiology;
Fellowship Director, Imaging Informatics
Department of Radiology
Hospital of the University of Pennsylvania
Philadelphia, Pennsylvania

**Lu Anne Velayo Dinglasan, MD, MHS**
Assistant Professor of Radiology
Department of Radiology
University of Louisville
Louisville, Kentucky

**Michael L. Francavilla, MD**
Pediatric Radiologist
Children's Hospital of Philadelphia
Department of Radiology
Philadelphia, Pennsylvania

**Sara Chen Gavenonis, MD**
Christiana Care Health System
Department of Radiology
Newark, Delaware

**Barry Glenn Hansford, MD**
Department of Musculoskeletal Radiology
University of Michigan
Ann Arbor, Michigan

**Elizabeth M. Hecht, MD**
Associate Professor
Department of Radiology
Columbia University
New York, New York

**Steven C. Horii, MD, FACR, FSIIM**
Professor of Radiology, Department of Radiology
University of Pennsylvania Perelman School of
  Medicine;
Attending Radiologist, Department of Radiology
Hospital of the University of Pennsylvania;
Attending Radiologist, Center for Fetal Diagnosis and
  Therapy
Children's Hospital of Philadelphia;
Attending Radiologist, Department of Radiology
Penn Presbyterian Medical Center
Philadelphia, Pennsylvania

**Charles Intenzo, MD**
Professor Director, Nuclear Medicine
Department of Radiology
Thomas Jeffereson University Hospital
Philadelphia, Pennsylvania

**Ann K. Jay, MD**
Assistant Professor
Department of Radiology
MedStar Georgetown University Hospital
Washington, District of Columbia

**Saurabh Jha, MBBS, MRCS, MS**
Assistant Professor
Department of Radiology
Perelman School of Medicine;
Assistant Professor
Department of Radiology
Philadelphia, Pennsylvania

**Linda C. Kelahan, MD**
Resident Physician
Department of Radiology
Medstar Georgetown University Hospital
Washington, District of Columbia

**Sung Han Kim, MD**
Assistant Professor of Clinical Radiology
Department of Radiology
University of Pennsylvania
Philadelphia, Pennsylvania

**Woojin Kim, MD**
Director of Innovation
Montage Healthcare Solutions, Inc.
Philadelphia, Pennsylvania

**J. Bruce Kneeland, MD**
Chief, Musculoskeletal Imaging
Department of Radiology
Hospital of the University of Pennsylvania
Philadelphia, Pennsylvania

**Ana S. Kolansky, MD**
Clinical Associate Professor of Radiology
Department of Radiology
University of Pennsylvania
Philadelphia, Pennsylvania

**Ellie S. Kwak, MD**
Resident Physician
Department of Diagnostic Radiology
Columbia University Medical Center
New York, New York

**Sherelle L. Laifer-Narin, MD**
Associate Professor of Radiology
Director of Ultrasound and Fetal MRI
Columbia University/New York Presbyterian Hospital
New York, New York

**Bradley Lamprich, MD**
Clinical Assistant Professor
Department of Radiological Sciences
University of Oklahoma
Oklahoma City, Oklahoma

**Jill E. Langer, MD**
Professor
Department of Radiology
University of Pennsylvania School of Medicine
Philadelphia, Pennsylvania

**Charles T. Lau, MD, MBA**
Physician
Department of Radiology
VA Palo Alto Health Care System
Palo Alto, California

**Nam Ju Lee, MD, MMS**
Fellow
Department of Radiology
Perelman School of Medicine of the University of
  Pennsylvania
Philadelphia, Pennsylvania;
Faculty (current)
Department of Radiology
Staten Island University Hospital
Staten Island, New York

**Mindy Y. Licurse, MD**
Radiology Resident
Department of Radiology
Hospital of the University of Pennsylvania
Philadelphia, Pennsylvania

**Harold I. Litt, MD, PhD**
Associate Professor of Radiology and Medicine
Department of Radiology
Perelman School of Medicine of the University of
  Pennsylvania
Chief, Cardiovascular Imaging
Department of Radiology
Penn Medicine
Philadelphia, Pennsylvania

**Laurie A. Loevner, MD**
Professor and Chief
Division of Neuroradiology
University of Pennsylvania Health System
Philadelphia, Pennsylvania

**Angel J. Lopez-Garib, MD**
Assistant Professor
Department of Clinical Radiology
Musculoskeletal Division
University of Pennsylvania
Philadelphia, Pennsylvania

**Mesha L.D. Martinez, MD**
Pediatric Radiology Fellow
Department of Pediatric Radiology
Children's Hospital of Philadelphia
Philadelphia, Pennsylvania

**Elizabeth S. McDonald, MD, PhD**
Assistant Professor of Radiology
Department of Radiology
University of Pennsylvania
Philadelphia, Pennsylvania

**Wallace T. Miller, Jr., MD**
Professor of Radiology and Pulmonary Medicine
The Perelman School of Medicine
The University of Pennsylvania at The University of
    Pennsylvania University Medical Center
Philadelphia, Pennsylvania

**Jeffrey I. Mondschein, MD**
Associate Professor of Clinical Radiology and Surgery
Department of Radiology
Perelman School of Medicine at the University of
    Pennsylvania;
Attending Interventional Radiologist
Associate Professor of Clinical Radiology and Surgery
Department of Radiology
Hospital of the University of Pennsylvania–Penn
    Medicine
Philadelphia, Pennsylvania

**D. Andrew Mong, MD**
Assistant Professor of Clinical Radiology
Department of Radiology
The Children's Hospital of Philadelphia
Philadelphia, Pennsylvania

**Gul Moonis, MD**
Staff Radiologist
Department of Radiology
Columbia University Medical Center
New York, New York

**Eduardo Jose Mortani Barbosa, Jr., MD**
Assistant Professor of Radiology
Department of Radiology
University of Pennsylvania
Philadelphia, Pennsylvania

**Mohammed T. Nawas, MD**
Prosight Radiology Group
St. Luke's Hospital
Chesterfield, Missouri

**Andrew B. Newberg, MD**
Professor
Department of Radiology and Emergency Medicine
Thomas Jefferson University
Philadelphia, Pennsylvania

**Cuong Nguyen, MD**
Mecklenburg Radiology Associates
Interventional Neuroradiology
Charolotte, North Carolina

**Seong Cheol Oh, MD**
Associate
Department of Radiology
Geisinger Health System
Danville, Pennsylvania

**Avrum N. Pollock, MD**
Associate Professor of Radiology
Department of Radiology, Division of Neuroradiology
The Children's Hospital of Philadelphia
Philadelphia, Pennsylvania

**E. Scott Pretorius, MD**
Radiologist
US Teleradiology
Palm Springs, California

**Daniel A. Pryma, MD**
Associate Professor of Radiology and Radiation
    Oncology
Clinical Director, Nuclear Medicine and Molecular
    Imaging
Department of Radiology
University of Pennsylvania Perelman School of
    Medicine
Philadelphia, Pennsylvania

**Bryan Pukenas, MD**
Assistant Professor of Radiology and Neurosurgery
Department of Radiology
Perelman School of Medicine
University of Pennsylvania
Philadelphia, Pennsylvania

**Parvati Ramchandani, MD, FACR, FSAR**
Professor of Radiology and Surgery, Section Chief GU
    Radiology
Department of Radiology
Hospital of the University of Pennsylvania
Philadelphia, Pennsylvania

**Stephen E. Rubesin, MD**
Professor of Radiology
Hospital of the University of Pennsylvania
Philadelphia, Pennsylvania

**Alexander T. Ruutiainen, MD**
Staff Radiologist and Chief of Quality and Safety in
    Radiology
Department of Radiology
Veterans Administration Medical Center
Philadelphia, Pennsylvania

**Deepak Mavahalli Sampathu, MD, PhD**
Assistant Professor of Clinical Radiology
Department of Radiology
University of Pennsylvania
Philadelphia, Pennsylvania

**Mary H. Scanlon, MD, FACR**
Professor of Radiology
Vice Chair of Education
Department of Radiology
University of Pennsylvania
Philadelphia, Pennsylvania

**Scott Simpson, DO, MD**
Assistant Professor of Clinical Radiology
Lewis Katz School of Medicine
Temple University;
Attending Physician
Department of Radiology
Temple University Hospital
Philadelphia, Pennsylvania

**Jasmeet Singh, MD, MPHA**
Department of Radiology
University of Pennsylvania
Philadephia, Pennsylvania

**Jeffrey A. Solomon, MD, MBA**
Lecturer
Health Care Management
The Wharton School of Business
The University of Pennsylvania
Philadelphia, Pennsylvania

**S. William Stavropoulos, MD**
Professor of Radiology and Surgery
Vice Chair of Clinical Operations
Department of Radiology
Division of Interventional Radiology
Perelman School of Medicine at the University of
   Pennsylvania
Philadelphia, Pennsylvania

**Ting Yin Tao, MD, PhD**
Assistant Professor
Department of Radiology
St. Louis University School of Medicine;
Assistant Professor
Department of Radiology
Cardinal Glennon Children's Hospital
St. Louis, Missouri

**Elena Taratuta, MD**
Clinical Associate Professor of Radiology
Department of Radiology
Hospital of the University of Pennsylvania
Philadelphia, Pennsylvania

**Drew A. Torigian, MD, MA, FSAR**
Associate Professor, Department of Radiology
Clinical Director, Medical Image Processing Group
   (MIPG)
Hospital of the University of Pennsylvania
Philadelphia, Pennsylvania

**Jayaram K. Udupa, PhD**
Professor, Chief, Medical Image Processing Group
Department of Radiology
University of Pennsylvania
Philadelphia, Pennsylvania

**Susan P. Weinstein, MD**
Associate Professor
Department of Radiology
Perelman School of Medicine at the University of
   Pennsylvania
Philadelphia, Pennsylvania

**Andrew Spencer Wilmot, MD**
Fellow
Musculoskeletal Radiology
Hospital of the University of Pennsylvania
Philadelphia, Pennsylvania

**Courtney A. Woodfield, MD**
Department of Radiology
Clinical Director
Body Magnetic Resonance Imaging
Abington-Jefferson Health
Abington, Pennsylvania

**Corrie M. Yablon, MD**
Assistant Professor
Department of Radiology
University of Michigan
Ann Arbor, Michigan

**Hanna Zafar, MD, MHS**
Assistant Professor
Department of Radiology
University of Pennsylvania
Philadelphia, Pennsylvania

**Shaoxiong Zhang, MD, PhD**
Clinical Associate Professor of Radiology Section
Chief of Cardiothoracic Radiology
Hahnemann University Hospital
Drexel University College of Medicine
Philadelphia, Pennsylvania

# PREFACE

Radiology is an essential component of current medical practice, having assumed a central role in the evaluation and follow-up of many clinical problems, from the head to the toes. Becoming familiar with and knowledgeable about the indications and capabilities of various diagnostic and therapeutic procedures that are driven by imaging, across a wide range of clinical subspecialties and imaging modalities, is important for those who use radiology for any diagnostic and therapeutic purpose. We have endeavored to create a practical and interesting book that distills the essential aspects of imaging for each subspecialty of radiology.

Whether you are a trainee (medical student, resident, or fellow), a physician in practice (in radiology, nuclear medicine, or another medical specialty), or another type of health care provider, this book was written for you.

# ACKNOWLEDGMENT

We would like to thank our friends and colleagues E. Scott Pretorius, MD, and Jeffrey A. Solomon, MD, MBA, the two prior co-editors of *Radiology Secrets*, for the opportunity to serve as editors for the latest edition of this book. We would also like to thank all of the contributing authors for helping to make this book a reality; without their expertise, there would be no such book.

# CONTENTS

## XIII DIAGNOSTIC RADIOLOGY AS A PROFESSION

# TOP 100 RADIOLOGY SECRETS

1. Radiography is an imaging technique that uses x-rays to create images of a region of interest in the body; these images are projectional 2D images. Ultrasonography (US) is an imaging technique that uses high-frequency ultrasound waves to create images in real time. Computed tomography (CT) is an imaging technique that uses x-rays to create tomographic images. Magnetic resonance imaging (MRI) is an imaging technique that uses magnetism and radiofrequency waves to create tomographic images. Planar scintigraphy, single photon emission computed tomography (SPECT), and positron emission tomography (PET) are the nuclear medicine molecular imaging techniques available. They are used to image the distribution and accumulation of an administered radiotracer in organs/tissues of the body; the spatial distribution and amount of accumulation depend on the properties of the radiotracer and the disease states present in the involved organs.

2. Density, echogenicity, attenuation, and signal intensity are the descriptors of how bright or dark tissues are on radiography, US, CT, and MR images, respectively. Standardized uptake value (SUV) is a quantitative measure of PET radiotracer uptake in a tissue of interest.

3. If fluid has very high signal intensity on an MR image, then the image is likely T2-weighted. If fluid has low signal intensity on an MR image, then the image is likely T1-weighted. An easy reference organ is the signal intensity of cerebrospinal fluid on MR images; if it is bright, then the image is likely a T2-weighted image.

4. Quantitative radiology (QR) is the quantitative assessment of both normal and disease states using medical images in order to evaluate the severity, degree of change, and status of abnormal disease states relative to normal. This involves the development, standardization, and optimization of image acquisition protocols, computer-aided visualization and analysis (CAVA) methods, and reporting structures. CAVA provides quantitative information about objects of interest within digital images and involves use of image preprocessing, visualization, manipulation, and analysis.

5. A biomarker (biologic marker) is a characteristic that is objectively measured and evaluated as an indicator of normal biologic processes, pathogenic processes, or pharmacologic responses to a therapeutic intervention. Imaging biomarkers are obtained from image analysis.

6. Spatial resolution is the ability to display two separate but adjacent objects as distinct on an image. Contrast resolution is the ability to display tissues with different intensities as having distinct shades of gray on an image.

7. The picture archiving and communication system (PACS) is used to store and display medical images.

8. Distinguishing physiologic from allergic-like contrast reactions is important, as patients with physiologic reactions do not require future corticosteroid premedication, whereas those with allergic-like reactions may need future corticosteroid premedication.

9. Intravascular gadolinium-based contrast material is contraindicated for use in pregnant patients. However, iodinated contrast material can be administered to pregnant or potentially pregnant patients when needed for diagnostic purposes.

10. Dose optimization is often summarized as ALARA ("as low as reasonably achievable"), but it dictates that the radiologic examination should be tailored to the clinical question, patient size, and anatomy of interest.

11. Diagnostic mammography is indicated for women with a specific breast-related problem that needs to be evaluated. Screening mammography is indicated for asymptomatic patients.

12. Indications for breast MRI include evaluation for presence of breast cancer in the high-risk patient; evaluation of the extent of disease with a new breast cancer diagnosis; detection of an occult primary tumor in the presence of axillary disease; evaluation of silicone breast implant integrity; response monitoring of a known breast cancer to chemotherapy; and further diagnostic evaluation after an inconclusive mammographic and sonographic work-up.

13. On a frontal chest radiograph, the right atrium comprises the right heart border, whereas the aortic knob, main pulmonary artery, left atrial appendage, and left ventricle comprise the left heart border from superior to inferior. On a lateral chest radiograph, the left atrium comprises the posterior-superior heart border, whereas the right ventricle comprises the anterior heart border.

14. The most common cardiac or paracardiac mass is thrombus. The most common primary cardiac neoplasm is myxoma. The most common malignant neoplasm of the heart and pericardium is metastatic disease.

15. An aortic dissection is caused by a tear of the intima, creating a false channel or lumen within the wall of the aorta, which usually extends longitudinally within the aorta. Dissections involving the ascending aorta (Stanford type A and DeBakey types 1 and 2) are surgical emergencies, whereas descending aortic dissections are usually treated medically.

16. Cardiac CT provides not only accurate evaluation for coronary artery luminal stenosis with high sensitivity and specificity, but also valuable information about atherosclerotic plaque in the vessel wall.

17. An acute pulmonary embolus typically appears as a centrally located hypoattenuating filling defect within the pulmonary artery on CT. A chronic pulmonary embolus typically appears as an eccentrically located hypoattenuating filling defect within the pulmonary artery and may be associated with calcification, intraluminal bands or webs, decreased luminal caliber, or increased bronchial arterial collateral vessels.

18. Atherosclerosis is the most common cause of renal artery stenosis, most often occurs in older adults, and typically involves the proximal third of the renal artery. Fibromuscular dysplasia (FMD) is the second most common cause of renal artery stenosis, most often occurs in young or middle-aged women, and typically involves the distal third of the renal artery.

19. Be aware of the major blind spots on frontal chest radiography where nodules and masses are easily overlooked: the lung apices where the clavicles and ribs overlap, the hilar regions where vascular structures abound, the retrocardiac region, and the lung bases where there is superimposition with the upper abdominal soft tissue.

20. If you see lobar or segmental atelectasis on chest radiography, particularly without air bronchograms, be suspicious of an obstructive endobronchial lesion such as a lung cancer, and, at the minimum, get a short-term follow-up chest radiograph. If a pulmonary opacity does not resolve over time despite treatment with antimicrobial agents, be suspicious of a potential lung cancer.

21. Opacity is a nonspecific descriptor that implies a region that attenuates x-rays to a greater degree than surrounding tissues, and it can be due to any abnormality overlying or within the lung. Consolidation, however, specifically refers to an alveolar filling process, which opacifies the lung.

22. Imaging findings of reactivation tuberculosis (TB) may include upper lung zone predominant focal consolidation or nodular opacities, areas of cavitation, centrilobular, acinar, and/or tree-in-bud nodular opacities, interstitial miliary nodules, bronchiectasis, and thoracic lymphadenopathy (often with areas of central necrosis). When these findings are seen on imaging, alert the referring physician to the possibility of active TB.

23. Interstitial pulmonary edema, usually caused by congestive heart failure, is the most common interstitial abnormality encountered in daily practice.

24. Thymoma is the most common primary tumor of the anterior mediastinum and of the thymus. Neurogenic tumor is the most common mass of the posterior mediastinum.

25. If a pneumothorax is seen on chest radiography that is associated with contralateral mediastinal shift and inferior displacement of the ipsilateral hemidiaphragm, it is very worrisome for a tension pneumothorax. The physician caring for the patient must be notified immediately as emergent treatment is usually required to decompress the pneumothorax to prevent rapid death.

26. If a nasogastric tube, orogastric tube, or feeding tube is seen to extend into a distal bronchus, lung, or pleural space, the clinical staff should be notified immediately, and the radiologist should suggest that tube removal be performed only after a thoracostomy tube set is at the bedside in case a significant pneumothorax develops.

27. When air embolism is suspected during line placement or use, the patient should immediately be placed in the left lateral position to keep the air trapped in the right heart chambers, supplemental oxygen should be administered, and vital signs should be monitored.

28. Linear pneumatosis is highly suggestive of bowel ischemia.

29. Single-contrast gastrointestinal (GI) examinations use "thin barium" or water-soluble contrast material (no gas used) and are easier to perform in sick patients who cannot turn to detect bowel obstruction, perforation, or fistulas. Double-contrast GI examinations are more sensitive than single-contrast examinations for detecting mucosal abnormalities and use high-density barium and air/carbon dioxide, but they require patients to turn into different positions to coat the entire bowel, which can prove to be challenging for sick and debilitated patients.

30. Wall (mural) thickening is the hallmark of GI tract pathology. In general, the greater the degree of mural thickening, the more likely that malignancy is the underlying etiology. Asymmetric wall thickening and focal wall thickening are also features suggestive of malignancy.

31. The "target" sign, also known as mural stratification, is highly specific for the diagnosis of nonneoplastic disease when encountered in the small or large bowel. However, this specificity for nonneoplastic disease does not hold when it is encountered in the stomach.

32. Most hepatic lesions are hypointense relative to liver parenchyma on T1-weighted images. Lesion isointensity on T1-weighted images suggests that it is of hepatocellular origin.

33. On T2-weighted images, malignant hepatic lesions tend to have similar signal intensity as the spleen, whereas hepatic cysts and hemangiomas are hyperintense relative to the spleen and remain hyperintense on heavily T2-weighted images.

34. Metastatic disease to a cirrhotic liver is extremely rare. A focal hepatic lesion in a cirrhotic liver that either demonstrates arterial phase enhancement or isointensity to spleen on T2-weighted images is considered as hepatocellular carcinoma (HCC) until proven otherwise.

35. MRI has higher sensitivity than CT for the detection and localization of calculi within the gallbladder and biliary tree.

36. A splenic laceration is associated with a history of trauma, is irregular or branching in configuration, and is associated with adjacent areas of fluid, whereas a developmental splenic cleft is smooth without presence of surrounding fluid.

37. Pancreatic adenocarcinoma is generally unresectable when there is encasement of the mesenteric vasculature, invasion of organs other than the duodenum, or presence of distant metastatic disease.

38. Whenever you see visceral pelvic fat stranding on CT or MRI in a woman with an acute abdomen or pelvis, always consider the diagnosis of early pelvic inflammatory disease (PID) and notify the clinical team. This will allow them to definitively establish or exclude the diagnosis of PID and to implement therapy as needed to prevent future complications of PID.

39. Whenever you see findings of bowel obstruction on CT or MRI, always evaluate the etiology at the transition zone, and exclude the presence of a closed loop obstruction which constitutes a true surgical emergency.

40. If you visualize imaging findings of active arterial extravasation of contrast material, shock, or abdominal aortic aneurysm (AAA) rupture on CT or MRI, immediately check on the status of the patient, start resuscitative measures if needed, and get help from your clinical colleagues right away.

41. The anterior urethra in men is better evaluated on retrograde urethrography (RUG). The posterior urethra in men is better evaluated on voiding cystourethrography (VCUG).

42. An enhancing renal mass that does not contain macroscopic fat is considered to be secondary to renal cell carcinoma (RCC) until proven otherwise. Cystic renal lesions that contain thick or irregular walls, thick or irregular internal septations, or solid nodular components with enhancement are considered as suspicious for cystic RCC until proven otherwise. Presence of macroscopic fat within a renal mass is diagnostic of a renal angiomyolipoma (AML).

43. Most adrenal incidentalomas are benign in nature, and the most commonly detected incidental adrenal lesion is a nonhyperfunctional adrenal adenoma. Presence of microscopic lipid content within a small (≤3 cm in size) homogeneous adrenal gland nodule is essentially diagnostic of an adrenal adenoma. Presence of macroscopic fat within an adrenal gland nodule or mass is characteristic of an adrenal myelolipoma. Adrenal gland nodules/masses which have a large size (>4-5 cm), grow over time, are heterogeneous in appearance, or have irregular margins are more likely to be malignant in etiology.

44. Retroperitoneal tumors are usually malignant and are most commonly due to lymphoma, retroperitoneal sarcoma, and metastatic disease.

45. Septate uterus is the most common type of congenital uterine anomaly. Leiomyoma, or fibroid, is the most common neoplasm of the female genitourinary tract.

46. Most intratesticular masses are malignant, whereas most extratesticular scrotal masses are benign. Spermatoceles and epididymal cysts are the most common causes of a scrotal mass.

47. The imaging modality of choice for a patient with acute head trauma is an unenhanced brain CT scan.

48. Time is BRAIN. Rapid diagnosis of ischemic stroke and prompt initiation of treatment are critical for a good outcome. Diffusion-weighted imaging (DWI) is the most sensitive MRI sequence for detection of acute stroke.

49. An epidural hematoma has a biconvex lenticular shape, is contained by dural sutures, and is associated with temporal bone or other skull fractures. Large hematomas are treated promptly with clot evacuation to prevent brain herniation and associated complications. A subdural hematoma is crescentic in shape, is not contained by dural sutures but does not cross the falx or tentorium, and may or may not be associated with a skull fracture.

50. The most common primary intra-axial brain tumor in adults is glioblastoma multiforme. The most common posterior fossa/infratentorial neoplasm in adults is a metastasis. The most common extra-axial tumor in adults is meningioma.

51. MRI is the modality of choice for evaluating suprahyoid neck lesions, whereas infrahyoid neck lesions are imaged first with CT. CT is the imaging modality of choice for conductive hearing loss. MRI is the imaging modality of choice in adult-onset sensorineural hearing loss.

52. The most common cause of a cystic neck mass in an adult is metastatic lymphadenopathy.

53. The best predictor of acute sinusitis in the appropriate clinical setting (facial pain, nasal drainage, fever) is the presence of an air-fluid level on a CT scan.

54. Fatigue fractures are the result of abnormal stresses on normal bone, whereas insufficiency fractures are the result of normal stresses on abnormal bone.

55. The most common type of shoulder dislocation is anterior, whereas the most common type of hip dislocation is posterior.

56. A fat-fluid level seen in a joint space in the setting of trauma is due to a lipohemarthrosis and is indicative of an intraarticular fracture.

57. Osteoporosis is characterized by diminished bone density with otherwise normal bone architecture, whereas osteomalacia (in adults) and rickets (in children) are characterized by normal bone density in the setting of abnormal quality of bone. Both may manifest as osteopenia (i.e., diffusely increased lucency of bone) on radiography or CT.

58. Subperiosteal bone resorption is a pathognomonic radiographic sign of hyperparathyroidism. A Looser zone fracture is a pathognomonic radiographic sign of osteomalacia.

59. Metastatic calcification is due to alterations in calcium or phosphorus metabolism, whereas dystrophic calcification is due to tissue injury.

60. A large complex joint effusion with thick synovial enhancement and periarticular bone marrow edema raises suspicion for septic arthritis, particularly when only one joint is involved. Periarticular osteopenia, uniform joint space narrowing, osseous erosions, and soft tissue swelling are also suggestive imaging features of septic arthritis. However, whenever this diagnosis is suspected clinically, it should be confirmed or excluded by joint aspiration.

61. Necrotizing fasciitis is a surgical emergency, requiring prompt diagnosis and treatment. Its diagnosis, while primarily clinical, also rests in the identification of soft tissue emphysema. Other suggestive imaging features include fascial plane thickening, edema, or enhancement, as well as edema, phlegmon, or abscess formation in subjacent muscles.

62. Tennis elbow (lateral epicondylitis) and golfer's elbow (medial epicondylitis) are due to inflammation of the common extensor and common flexor tendons, respectively.

63. Ligament and tendon injuries are seen as full- or partial-thickness high signal intensity foci in the normally low signal structures on T2-weighted images.

64. MRI is the examination of choice for evaluation of suspected hip fractures when radiography fails to reveal the cause of hip pain, because it is a highly sensitive and specific modality for detection of radiographically occult fractures and is more sensitive than CT for detection of other possible causes of hip pain such as soft tissue injuries.

65. A meniscal tear is present when either abnormal signal intensity within a meniscus extending to the articular surface on two contiguous slices or abnormal meniscal morphology is visualized.

66. Ankle inversion occurs much more commonly than ankle eversion and results in injury to the anterior talofibular ligament, calcaneofibular ligament, and posterior talofibular ligament in sequence.

67. For a viable intrauterine gestation, an embryo should be visible sonographically by a mean gestational sac diameter of 25 mm, and an embryonic heart rate should be detected by a crown-rump length of 7 mm.

68. The most common sonographic finding of an ectopic pregnancy is an adnexal mass.

69. Sonographic features of thyroid nodules that are associated with a higher risk of malignancy include microcalcifications, coarse and dystrophic calcifications, marked hypoechogenicity, infiltrative and/or microlobulated margins, and taller-than-wide shape. Sonographic features associated with a very low risk of malignancy are a nearly entirely cystic nodule and a spongiform appearance in a nodule under 2 cm without marked vascularity, calcifications, or irregular margins.

70. Proper equipment and qualified personnel should be readily available prior to administration of conscious sedation to any patient.

71. The basic life support sequence of steps for patient resuscitation (C-A-B) includes assessment of **C**irculation (heart rate and blood pressure), establishment of an **A**irway, and assessment of **B**reathing (ventilation).

72. In most cases, inferior vena cava (IVC) filters should be placed below the lowest renal vein when possible.

73. AAA rupture is often fatal; AAAs must therefore be detected, monitored, and treated prior to rupture. Intervention is typically indicated when the aneurysm reaches 5.5 cm, although many clinicians treat at the 5 cm threshold.

74. Transarterial chemoembolization (TACE) is a liver-directed therapy for liver tumors, including HCC, hepatic metastases, and occasionally hepatic adenomas. Radiofrequency ablation (RFA) is a technique for generating heat and subsequent coagulation necrosis in living tissues through alternating electrical currents and is used to treat many conditions, including liver, kidney, bone, and lung tumors.

75. Embolization on both sides of a pseudoaneurysm, aneurysm, or arteriovenous fistula (AVF) is necessary to prevent reconstitution of flow via collaterals, which causes lesion recurrence.

76. An obstructed, infected biliary system constitutes a medical emergency.

77. Benign biliary strictures tend to taper gradually with smooth borders, whereas malignant biliary strictures tend to occur abruptly, often with irregular borders.

78. Urosepsis is an indication for emergent percutaneous nephrostomy (PCN).

79. $^{18}$F-fluoro-2-deoxy-2-D-glucose (FDG) PET imaging is useful for lesion characterization, tumor staging and pretreatment planning, clinical outcome prognostication, tumor response assessment, and tumor restaging. FDG PET changes management in up to 40% of patients with cancer, most often due to detection of distant metastases.

80. Focal FDG uptake in the uterus or adnexa of a postmenopausal woman, in the thyroid gland, or in the bowel is generally considered as suspicious for malignancy until proven otherwise. Lower levels of FDG uptake within tumors generally reflect a more indolent tumor biology and portend a more favorable clinical outcome. A reduction in tumor FDG uptake after therapy is more likely to be associated with a histopathologic response and improved patient survival than is a lack of change.

81. Any cause of increased bone turnover, including primary malignant bone tumors, osseous metastases, osteoid osteoma, osteomyelitis, trauma, degenerative change, metabolic bone disease, and Paget's disease, may lead to increased radiotracer uptake in bone on a bone scan or $^{18}$F-sodium fluoride ($^{18}$F-NaF) PET scan.

82. A "superscan" occurs when there is diffusely increased radiotracer uptake in the bones and is most commonly seen with widespread osseous metastatic disease, metabolic bone disease, or widespread Paget's disease.

83. Visualization of one or more wedge-shaped perfusion scan defects, segmental or subsegmental in distribution, unmatched to any finding on a ventilation scan or chest radiograph is suspicious for pulmonary embolism (PE).

84. Hot nodules on radioiodine thyroid scintigraphy are most often benign, whereas cold nodules may be due to thyroid cancer.

85. A GI bleeding scan is useful to detect and localize sites of active hemorrhage in the bowel and is considered as positive when there is a focus of growing radiotracer activity that moves through the bowel.

86. A reversible (or transient) defect on stress myocardial perfusion imaging (SMPI) occurs when there is a lack of myocardial perfusion during stress but normal myocardial perfusion during rest, and it implies coronary artery disease (CAD) with coronary artery stenosis of at least 70%. A nonreversible (or fixed) defect on SMPI occurs when there is a lack of myocardial perfusion during both stress and rest, and it implies scarring, such as from prior myocardial infarction, or chronically ischemic but viable hibernating myocardium.

87. Symmetric hypometabolism in the bilateral temporoparietal regions of the brain is a classic finding observed on FDG PET imaging in patients with Alzheimer's disease.

88. Seizure foci have increased perfusion and metabolism on ictal cerebral blood flow (CBF) and FDG PET brain scans, respectively, whereas decreased perfusion and metabolism may be observed on interictal scans.

89. The dose-limiting toxicity of most radiopharmaceutical therapies is bone marrow suppression.

90. The epiglottis should be triangular or flat in configuration on lateral neck radiography. Recognition of a bulbous or thumblike appearance of the epiglottis indicates acute epiglottitis, which is a medical emergency.

91. Croup, or acute laryngotracheobronchitis, is characterized by symmetric subglottic narrowing on frontal neck radiography leading to the "steeple" sign due to edema of the subglottic tissues.

92. Tetralogy of Fallot is the most common cyanotic congenital heart disease (CHD) of childhood and has four characteristic features: right ventricular outflow tract obstruction, an overriding aorta, a ventricular septal defect (VSD), and right ventricular hypertrophy.

93. A malignant or "interarterial" course of an anomalous coronary artery between the aortic root and pulmonary arterial trunk may lead to extrinsic compression of the artery, potentially resulting in sudden death.

94. Necrotizing enterocolitis (NEC) predominantly occurs in premature infants and may manifest as diffuse gaseous distention of bowel, loss of the normal symmetric bowel gas pattern, persistent focal dilation of bowel, ascites, pneumatosis intestinalis, portal venous gas, or pneumoperitoneum on abdominal radiography. When pneumoperitoneum develops, this is a definite sign of bowel perforation, necessitating surgical intervention.

95. An ingested coin in the esophagus is typically visualized en face on a frontal chest radiograph, whereas an aspirated coin in the trachea is typically visualized end-on on a frontal chest radiograph.

96. When there is complete duplication of the kidney, the Weigert-Meyer rule states that the lower pole ureter inserts normally into the bladder at the trigone, whereas the upper pole ureter inserts ectopically into the bladder medial and caudal to the lower pole ureteral insertion site.

97. The most common solid renal mass in infants is fetal renal hamartoma, also known as mesoblastic nephroma, and the most common childhood abdominal malignancy is Wilms tumor. The most common primary pediatric bone tumors are Ewing sarcoma and osteosarcoma.

98. The usual sequence of ossification of the secondary ossification centers of the elbow can be remembered by the mnemonic CRITOE: **C**apitellum (1 year), **R**adial head (3 years), **I**nternal (medial) epicondyle (5 years), **T**rochlea (7 years), **O**lecranon (9 years), and **E**xternal (lateral) epicondyle (11 years).

99. Metaphyseal corner fractures or bucket-handle fractures have high specificity for child abuse. Posterior rib fractures, fractures of the scapula, spinous process, or sternum, vertebral compression fractures, complex skull fractures, and multiple fractures of different ages are suggestive of child abuse as well. Subdural hematomas, particularly when interhemispheric or seen in the posterior fossa/tentorial locations, are suspicious for head trauma related to shaken infant syndrome.

100. The legal requirements for a finding of malpractice are establishment of physician-patient relationship; breach of the duty of care, or negligence; adverse outcome with injury or harm; and direct causality between negligence and outcome. The most common reasons that radiologists are sued are failure to diagnose; failure to communicate findings in an appropriate and timely manner; and failure to suggest the next appropriate procedure.

# I

# INTRODUCTION TO
# IMAGING MODALITIES

# CHAPTER 1

# INTRODUCTION TO RADIOGRAPHY, FLUOROSCOPY, AND TOMOSYNTHESIS

*Drew A. Torigian, MD, MA, FSAR*

## RADIOGRAPHY

1. What is radiography?

   Radiography is an imaging technique that uses x-rays to create projectional (2D) images of a region of interest in the body. It is performed by shining x-rays on a film or other image detector with a patient placed in front of it in a certain orientation. Different types of tissues in the patient attenuate x-rays to different degrees, leading to formation of a composite of x-ray shadows that will ultimately create the radiographic image. It is most commonly used to evaluate the bones and joints, the chest (especially the lungs), the abdomen and pelvis (especially the bowel), and the breasts (in which case it is called mammography).

2. When were x-rays discovered?

   Wilhelm Conrad Roentgen is credited with the discovery of x-rays in 1895, and was the first to systematically study them. He was also the first to obtain an x-ray photograph of part of the human body, his wife's hand, discovering its potential medical use. In 1901, he received the first Nobel Prize in physics. X-rays are sometimes referred to as Roentgen rays.

3. How do x-rays differ from other types of electromagnetic radiation?

   X-rays have higher energies, higher frequencies, and shorter wavelengths in the electromagnetic spectrum than ultraviolet light, visible light, infrared light, microwaves, and radio waves, and lower energies, lower frequencies, and longer wavelengths than gamma rays. Diagnostic x-rays typically have energies between 20 and 150 keV.

4. How do x-rays interact with matter?

   X-rays may either pass through matter unaffected, may be absorbed, or may be scattered (the latter of which leads to decreased image quality). Key factors that influence which interactions occur include the incident x-ray photon energy and the physical density, thickness, and atomic number of the material being imaged.

5. What is an x-ray tube?

   An x-ray tube is a device that is used to create x-rays for diagnostic imaging. It contains a negatively charged cathode that contains a filament (usually made of coiled tungsten wire) to produce electrons. The electrons are accelerated toward a positively charged anode that contains a target (usually made of tungsten or made of molybdenum and rhodium in mammography) where x-rays are produced. Both the cathode and anode are housed within a vacuum tube.

6. How are x-rays for diagnostic imaging produced?

   In the x-ray tube, about 90% of x-rays are created when electrons emitted from the cathode pass close to positively charged atomic nuclei within the anode target and change direction, resulting in a loss of energy in the form of x-ray photons known as bremsstrahlung ("braking") x-rays. An additional 10% of x-rays are produced when inner shell atomic electrons of the anode target are ejected by incident electrons, followed by relaxation of outer shell atomic electrons to fill the inner shell vacancies, leading to emission of energy in the form of x-ray photons known as characteristic x-rays.

7. What is a focal spot?

   A focal spot is the apparent source of x-rays in an x-ray tube. Smaller focal spots (such as those used in mammography) produce sharper images, whereas larger focal spots (such as those used in fluoroscopy) tolerate greater amounts of heat.

8. What is a collimator?

   A collimator is a device used to narrow the x-ray beam as it leaves the x-ray tube prior to entering the patient, reducing x-ray scatter and improving image contrast.

9. What happens to most of the energy entering the x-ray tube?

   Most (99%) of the energy is converted to heat, whereas about 1% is converted to x-rays.

10. What key input parameters may be adjusted when generating x-rays?

    The key parameters are the voltage applied across the x-ray tube (measured in kilovolts [kV]), the current flowing through the x-ray tube (measured in milliamperes [mA]), and the exposure time (measured in milliseconds [ms]). The

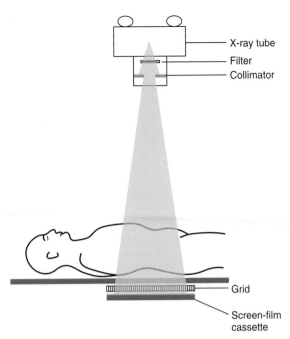

**Figure 1-1.** Schematic for apparatus used in screen film radiography.

product of tube current (in mA) and exposure time (in s) can be expressed in milliampere-seconds (mAs), which is directly proportional to x-ray tube output.

11. **What are the effects of increasing kV?**
X-ray peak and mean energies increase, penetration power increases, radiograph exposure increases, and image contrast (which primarily depends on kV) decreases.

12. **What are the effects of increasing mAs?**
X-ray exposure of a radiograph increases radiograph exposure. X-ray peak energy, mean energy, and penetration power do not change.

13. **What is screen film radiography?**
In screen film radiography (Figure 1-1), a sheet of film coated with a light-sensitive silver halide emulsion is placed in a light-tight cassette between two intensifying screens. The screens convert incident x-rays into visible light which then expose the film. The exposed film is then removed from the cassette, developed, and fixed to create a hardcopy radiograph.

14. **What is computed radiography (CR)?**
In CR, a photostimulable storage phosphor plate is used to transiently store a latent image following an x-ray exposure in the form of electrons trapped within the phosphor. This latent image is then extracted offline by a separate laser-based device that scans the plate to create a softcopy digital radiographic image that is stored electronically. CR eliminates the need to store hardcopy radiographic film and improves the ability to adjust the brightness and contrast of the digital image as needed.

15. **What is digital radiography (DR)?**
In DR (Figure 1-2), x-ray exposures upon a flat panel image detector are automatically processed into digital radiographic images in a fully integrated device without further user interaction.

16. **What is dual energy radiography?**
In dual energy radiography, two radiographic images of a patient are (nearly) simultaneously acquired at two different mean x-ray beam energies. These images are then combined to create a subtraction image to highlight either soft tissue or bone components present in the patient, as these components differentially attenuate the x-rays at different energies.

17. **What is an anti-scatter grid?**
An anti-scatter grid is a device, typically composed of narrow parallel strips of lead, that is placed between the patient and the image detector. It blocks scattered x-rays from reaching the film but allows nonscattered x-rays that pass from the x-ray tube and through the patient to reach the film, improving image contrast. The grid moves during the x-ray exposure, so that the grid is not visible on the radiographic image.

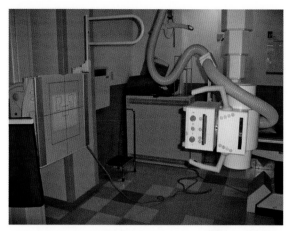

**Figure 1-2.** Typical DR unit with x-ray tube located on right and anti-scatter grid and flat panel detector located on left.

18. What is the inverse square law?
    The x-ray beam intensity decreases with the square of the distance from the x-ray source. Thus, if the distance between oneself and an x-ray source is doubled, the x-ray exposure decreases by fourfold.

19. What is the difference between a posteroanterior (PA) and an anteroposterior (AP) radiograph?
    These differ based on the direction of the x-ray beam passing through a patient. A PA radiograph occurs when the x-ray beam enters from the posterior aspect of the patient and exits anteriorly to reach the x-ray detector. An AP radiograph occurs when the x-ray beam enters from the anterior aspect of the patient and exits posteriorly to reach the x-ray detector.

20. What are the five basic densities seen on a radiograph?
    These include air, fat, soft tissue, bone, and metal. Air appears black on a radiograph, because it minimally attenuates the x-ray beam. Bone appears white and metal appears even more white on a radiograph, because they both markedly attenuate the x-ray beam. Fat and soft tissue attenuate intermediate amounts of the x-ray beam and appear dark gray and brighter gray, respectively.

21. How does mammographic technique differ from that performed in chest and abdominal radiography?
    A lower kV (for higher image contrast) and a higher mA (for a shorter exposure time) are used in mammography compared to those in radiography of the chest and abdomen.

## FLUOROSCOPY

22. What is fluoroscopy?
    Fluoroscopy is a projectional (2D) imaging technique that uses continuously emitted x-rays to perform real-time imaging of a patient. An x-ray tube in the fluoroscope (Figure 1-3) emits an x-ray beam that passes through the patient and falls upon an image intensifier. The image intensifier converts the x-ray radiation into visible light images and amplifies them. These images are then displayed on a monitor and can be viewed or recorded.

23. What are some clinical applications of fluoroscopy?
    Fluoroscopy is commonly used to evaluate the gastrointestinal tract with esophagography, an upper gastrointestinal examination (to evaluate the stomach), a small bowel follow-through, or a barium enema (to evaluate the large bowel). It is also commonly used in interventional procedures such as arthrography, myelography, and angiography.

24. What general types of contrast agents are used in gastrointestinal fluoroscopic studies?
    Barium sulfate is the standard oral contrast agent used for routine gastrointestinal fluoroscopic studies. More viscous suspensions are used for double-contrast (air and oral contrast) studies, whereas less viscous suspensions are used for single-contrast (oral contrast only) studies. When gastrointestinal tract perforation is suspected, a water-soluble contrast agent such as Gastrografin is instead utilized to prevent barium peritonitis, although it is contraindicated when there is a risk of aspiration because it may induce acute pulmonary edema.

25. What is digital subtraction angiography (DSA)?
    DSA is a fluoroscopic imaging technique in which a precontrast digital mask image is subtracted from images acquired after intravascular contrast administration. This results in improved image contrast between contrast-enhanced vessels and background, because background structures such as bone and soft tissue do not enhance and are removed from the image.

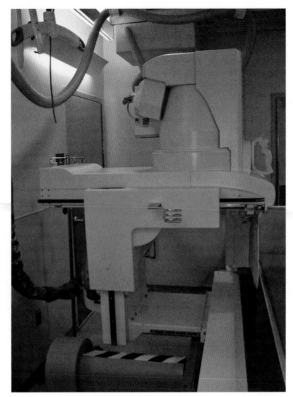

**Figure 1-3.** Typical fluoroscope with x-ray tube located on top.

## TOMOSYNTHESIS

26. What is tomosynthesis, and how does it work?

Tomosynthesis is an x-ray-based imaging technique that is used to create high-resolution tomographic (cross-sectional) images of a region of interest in the body. It works by first acquiring multiple x-ray images of a patient from various angles with a digital flat panel detector and then using computer algorithms to reconstruct the data into tomographic images.

27. What are some clinical applications of tomosynthesis?

Tomosynthesis can be used to potentially improve the detection of breast cancer (particularly in women with dense breast tissue) compared to mammography and to improve the detection of small lung nodules in the chest compared to chest radiography.

### KEY POINTS

- Radiography is an imaging technique that uses x-rays to create projectional (2D) images of a region of interest in the body.
- Fluoroscopy is a projectional (2D) imaging technique that uses continuously emitted x-rays to perform real-time imaging of a patient.
- Digital tomosynthesis is an x-ray-based imaging technique that is used to create high-resolution tomographic (cross-sectional) images of a region of interest in the body.
- Increasing kV increases the peak energy, mean energy, and penetration power of x-rays, increases radiograph exposure, and decreases image contrast.
- Increasing mAs increases the amount of x-rays produced, does not change x-ray energy or penetration power, and increases radiograph exposure.

**BIBLIOGRAPHY**

Nickoloff EL. AAPM/RSNA physics tutorial for residents: physics of flat-panel fluoroscopy systems. Survey of modern fluoroscopy imaging: flat-panel detectors versus image intensifiers and more. *Radiographics*. 2011;31(2):591-602.
Tingberg A. X-ray tomosynthesis: a review of its use for breast and chest imaging. *Radiat Prot Dosimetry*. 2010;139(1-3):100-107.

Cowen AR, Kengyelics SM, Davies AG. Solid-state, flat-panel, digital radiography detectors and their physical imaging characteristics. *Clin Radiol.* 2008;63(5):487-498.

Dobbins JT 3rd, McAdams HP, Godfrey DJ, et al. Digital tomosynthesis of the chest. *J Thorac Imaging.* 2008;23(2):86-92.

Rowlands JA. The physics of computed radiography. *Phys Med Biol.* 2002;47(23):R123-R166.

Pooley RA, McKinney JM, Miller DA. The AAPM/RSNA physics tutorial for residents: digital fluoroscopy. *Radiographics.* 2001;21(2):521-534.

Schueler BA. The AAPM/RSNA physics tutorial for residents: general overview of fluoroscopic imaging. *Radiographics.* 2000;20(4):1115-1126.

Wang J, Blackburn TJ. The AAPM/RSNA physics tutorial for residents: X-ray image intensifiers for fluoroscopy. *Radiographics.* 2000;20(5):1471-1477.

Chotas HG, Dobbins JT 3rd, Ravin CE. Principles of digital radiography with large-area, electronically readable detectors: a review of the basics. *Radiology.* 1999;210(3):595-599.

Bushberg JT. The AAPM/RSNA physics tutorial for residents. X-ray interactions. *Radiographics.* 1998;18(2):457-468.

McKetty MH. The AAPM/RSNA physics tutorial for residents. X-ray attenuation. *Radiographics.* 1998;18(1):151-163, quiz 49.

McCollough CH. The AAPM/RSNA physics tutorial for residents. X-ray production. *Radiographics.* 1997;17(4):967-984.

Seibert JA. The AAPM/RSNA physics tutorial for residents. X-ray generators. *Radiographics.* 1997;17(6):1533-1557.

Ritenour ER. Physics overview of screen-film radiography. *Radiographics.* 1996;16(4):903-916.

# CHAPTER 2

# INTRODUCTION TO ULTRASONOGRAPHY, CT, AND MRI

*Drew A. Torigian, MD, MA, FSAR*

## ULTRASONOGRAPHY (US)

1. **What is ultrasonography (US), and how does it work?**
   US is a structural imaging technique that uses high-frequency mechanical ultrasound waves (with frequencies greater than audible sound waves) to create real-time tomographic (cross-sectional) images. A hand-held transducer is applied to a part of the body to transmit ultrasound waves into the patient. Reflected ultrasound waves (echoes) are then detected by the transducer and processed by a computer to create digital images that can be viewed or recorded (Figure 2-1).

2. **When was US first used for clinical diagnostic purposes?**
   US was first used as a clinical diagnostic imaging technique in 1942 by Karl Dussik to locate brain tumors and the cerebral ventricles.

3. **What are some common clinical applications of US?**
   US is often used for initial evaluation of the abdominal organs (e.g., to evaluate for acute cholecystitis and choledocholithiasis), the pelvic organs (e.g., to evaluate for uterine leiomyomas, ovarian torsion, ectopic pregnancy, endometrial abnormalities, prostate cancer, and testicular torsion), the vessels (e.g., to evaluate for carotid artery stenosis and femoral vein deep venous thrombosis), the thyroid and parathyroid glands (e.g., to assess for thyroid nodules and parathyroid adenomas), and the joints (e.g., to assess for rotator cuff tears) and to serve as a real-time imaging guide during percutaneous biopsies. As US does not involve the use of ionizing radiation, it is also used during pregnancy (e.g., to evaluate the embryo/fetus for congenital anomalies) and in the pediatric setting (e.g., to evaluate the brain and hip joints in infants).

4. **Why is gel used in US?**
   Gel is applied between the transducer and skin to displace air and minimize large reflections that would interfere with ultrasound transmission from the transducer into the patient and vice versa. Reflections tend to occur at tissue interfaces where there are large differences in the speed of propagation of ultrasound waves, such as at air/soft tissue and bone/soft tissue interfaces. Gel decreases such reflections at the skin surface by matching the acoustic impedances of the transducer surface and skin surface.

5. **What is a transducer, and what types are available for US?**
   A transducer (Figure 2-2) is an electronic device that is used to produce ultrasound waves for transmission into the patient and to receive reflected ultrasound waves (echoes) to create digital images. Lower-frequency ultrasound transducers have a greater depth of tissue penetration, whereas higher-frequency ultrasound transducers have a higher spatial resolution. For general abdominal US, which requires sufficient depth of penetration to image the liver, spleen, and pancreas, a 3- to 5-MHz transducer may be utilized. For US of superficial structures such as the thyroid gland or scrotum, a 10-MHz transducer is often used. Endovaginal transducers are commonly used for gynecologic and early pregnancy examinations, whereas endorectal probes are available for prostate gland examinations.

6. **What is echogenicity?**
   Echogenicity is the descriptor of how bright or dark a tissue is on a US image, which depends on whether ultrasound waves are reflected, refracted, attenuated, or transmitted by the tissue. Hyperechoic or echogenic tissues (including air and bone) appear bright, hypoechoic tissues appear dark gray, and anechoic tissues (such as fluid) appear black.

7. **What is posterior acoustic enhancement?**
   This is the appearance of increased echogenicity beyond a tissue due to the increased transmission of ultrasound waves, and it is most commonly seen with fluid-filled structures such as cysts or the gallbladder.

8. **What is posterior acoustic shadowing?**
   This is the appearance of markedly decreased echogenicity beyond a highly reflecting or absorbing tissue due to the lack of ultrasound wave transmission. This is most commonly due to air, bone, or calcification such as in gallstones. For this reason, US is not used to image air-filled or osseous structures.

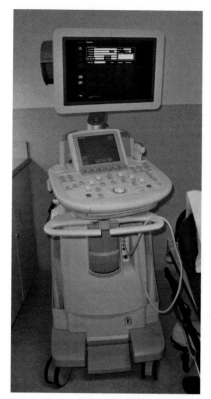

**Figure 2-1.** Typical mobile US unit with control panel and display monitor.

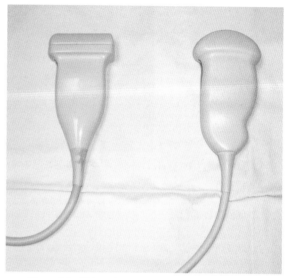

**Figure 2-2.** US transducers (linear on left, curved on right).

9. **What is Doppler US?**

Doppler US allows the imaging and quantification of blood flow velocity in vessels. It is based on the Doppler effect, which refers to the change in sound wave frequency and wavelength that occurs whenever the source of reflected waves (e.g., blood) is moving with respect to the detector (e.g., a transducer). Echoes from blood flowing toward a transducer will have higher frequencies and shorter wavelengths than blood flowing away from a transducer.

## COMPUTED TOMOGRAPHY (CT)

10. **What is computed tomography (CT), and how does it work?**

CT is a structural imaging technique that uses x-rays to create tomographic (cross-sectional) images. A patient is placed onto a scanner table and passes through the CT gantry, which contains an x-ray tube and an oppositely located array of x-ray detectors that rotate together about the patient (Figure 2-3). A large number of x-ray projections are obtained from multiple angles at each slice position in the patient, each of which contains data regarding the differential attenuation of x-rays by different tissue types in the patient. These projections are then used by a computer to reconstruct CT images.

11. **When was CT developed?**

CT was developed in the late 1960s and early 1970s by Sir Godfrey Hounsfield in the United Kingdom at EMI Central Research Laboratories, and the first patient brain CT scan was obtained in 1971. Hounsfield, along with Allan Cormack, received the Nobel Prize in Physiology or Medicine in 1979.

12. **What are some common clinical applications of CT?**

CT is commonly used to evaluate patients with neoplastic, infectious, noninfectious inflammatory, and traumatic disorders and as a problem-solving tool to further characterize abnormalities detected on radiography or US. It is especially useful for evaluation of the lungs, airways, bowel, cortical bone, urothelial system, and vasculature.

13. **What is multislice CT (MSCT)?**

MSCT, also known as multidetector row CT (MDCT), uses x-ray detector arrays that have multiple rows of detector elements to acquire multiple simultaneous channels of data per x-ray beam rotation. This offers many advantages compared to single slice CT (SSCT), including faster scan times and the ability to generate CT images with submillimeter thickness, providing high-resolution images that are isotropic (i.e., composed of voxels that are cubic in

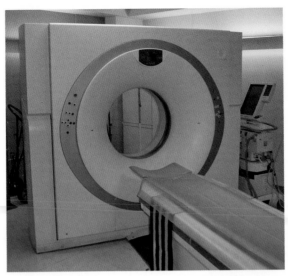

**Figure 2-3.** Typical MSCT scanner with CT gantry (which contains x-ray tube) and patient table.

shape). In essence, volumetric CT image data from a patient can now be acquired, and can then be reconstructed into 2D images in any plane of section and with any slice thickness desired. All modern CT scanners are MSCT scanners.

14. **What is dual-source CT (DSCT)?**

In DSCT, two x-ray tubes and two detector arrays located at 90-degree angles from one another are used in the CT gantry to acquire CT images. This improves the temporal resolution (i.e., acquisition speed) of the scanner and is mainly used in coronary CT studies to overcome cardiac motion artifacts during image acquisition.

15. **What is dual-energy CT (DECT)?**

In DECT, two sets of CT images are (nearly) simultaneously acquired at two different (low and high kilovoltage) mean x-ray beam energies. These images are then combined to create new images that highlight or suppress certain tissues of interest based on differential attenuation of the x-rays at different energies. For example, although iodine in contrast material and calcium in bone have similar high attenuation on standard CT images, the attenuation of iodine increases more markedly than calcium on low kilovoltage images relative to high kilovoltage images. Thus, new CT images demonstrating the contrast-enhanced vessels while suppressing surrounding bones can be created.

16. **What is the difference between sequential and helical CT acquisition?**

Sequential (or axial) CT acquisition is a step-and-shoot mode in which the patient table does not move during image acquisition of one or several slices at a time through the patient. Subsequently, the table advances and the process is repeated until the entire body region has been scanned. Helical (or spiral) CT acquisition is faster and involves continuous image acquisition while the patient table moves through the CT gantry. In this mode, the x-ray tube traces a helical trajectory around the patient. All modern CT scanners are helical scanners but can acquire images in sequential mode if desired.

17. **What is attenuation?**

Attenuation describes how bright or dark a tissue is on a CT image and is based on how much a tissue blocks (i.e., attenuates) the x-ray beam before reaching the x-ray detector. Attenuation of a tissue is predominantly determined by its atomic number (electron density) and physical density, although x-ray tube voltage also affects tissue attenuation. Every pixel (or voxel) on a CT image is assigned a gray scale value according to the mean attenuation of the tissue it corresponds to, which is called the CT number or relative attenuation coefficient. This is measured in Hounsfield units (HU), where pure water is the reference standard with an assigned CT number of 0 HU. Gas (−1000 HU) appears black, fat (−20 to −150 HU) appears dark gray, fluid (0 to 20 HU) appears gray, soft tissue (≈20 to 80 HU) appears bright gray, and bone, calcification, metal, and concentrated iodinated contrast material (≈150 to 1000 HU) appear white.

## MAGNETIC RESONANCE IMAGING (MRI)

18. **What is magnetic resonance imaging (MRI), and how does it work?**

MRI is a structural and functional imaging technique that uses magnetism and radiofrequency (RF) waves to create tomographic (cross-sectional) images. A patient is placed into a scanner that contains a magnet that generates a very strong magnetic field (Figure 2-4). Atomic nuclei in the body, such as of hydrogen atoms, have a net magnetic moment and act like tiny magnets, aligning themselves with the main magnetic field. RF waves are turned on to knock the nuclear magnetic moments out of alignment. When the RF waves are then turned off, the nuclei realign themselves

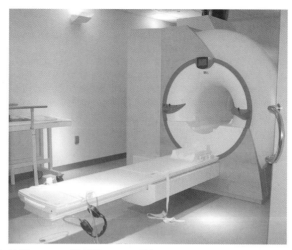

**Figure 2-4.** Typical MRI scanner with MRI gantry (which contains superconducting magnet) and patient table.

(i.e., relax) in the direction of the main magnetic field although at differential rates in different tissues. These differential relaxation rates lead to different signal properties of tissues that are detected by an RF coil placed around the patient. Magnetic gradients, controlled linear alterations of the magnetic field over distance in prespecified directions, are utilized to spatially localize the tissue signals so that MR images can be created. The process by which atomic nuclei undergo absorption or emission of RF energy is known as nuclear magnetic resonance (NMR).

19. When was MRI developed?

Isidor Rabi discovered the phenomenon of nuclear magnetic resonance in 1938 and received the Nobel Prize in Physics in 1944. Raymond Damadian discovered that the NMR signals of cancers appear different from those of normal tissues in 1971, proposed the concept of (and filed a patent for) the use of NMR for detecting cancer in the human body in 1972, and was the first to perform a human body MRI scan with the first full-body MRI scanner in 1977. In 1973, Paul Lauterbur produced the first tomographic MR image, and in 1976, Sir Peter Mansfield produced the first tomographic MR image of a human's finger. Lauterbur and Mansfield received the Nobel Prize in Physiology or Medicine in 2003.

20. What are some common clinical applications of MRI?

MRI is commonly used to evaluate patients with neoplastic, infectious, and noninfectious inflammatory disorders and as a problem-solving tool to further characterize abnormalities detected on radiography, US, CT, or PET/CT. It is especially useful for evaluation of the brain and spinal cord, breasts, heart and vasculature, abdominal and pelvic organs, and musculoskeletal soft tissue structures including the bone marrow, as it provides excellent soft tissue contrast. Because MRI does not involve the use of ionizing radiation, it is also used during pregnancy and in the pediatric setting.

21. What are some contraindications to the use of MRI?

In general, presence of metallic or electronic objects in the body such as orbital metallic foreign bodies, cerebral aneurysm clips, transvenous pacemakers, implantable cardioverter defibrillators, neurostimulators, and cochlear implants are contraindications for MRI, due to risks of device malfunction, device movement with tissue injury, or device heating with tissue injury. However, some patients with newer MRI-compatible versions of implanted metallic or electronic devices may be able to undergo MRI. A comprehensive website that provides updated information regarding the MRI safety of implants and devices is found at www.mrisafety.com. Claustrophobia is also a relative contraindication to MRI but can be alleviated by using patient sedation, a wide bore short length scanner, or an open field scanner. Pregnancy is not a contraindication to MRI, but it is a contraindication for use of gadolinium-based contrast material.

22. What is the typical field strength of magnets used in clinical MRI?

Magnetic field strengths of 0.5 to 3 Tesla (equivalent to 10,000 to 60,000 times the magnetic field strength of the Earth) are typically used in clinical MRI scanners, most often created by a superconducting magnet. Higher field strengths are desirable, as image signal-to-noise ratio (SNR) increases linearly with field strength, although there is a limit because the rate of energy deposition in tissue also increases with the square of field strength.

23. What are T1 and T2?

T1, the longitudinal relaxation time, is a measure of how long it takes atomic nuclei to realign longitudinally with the main magnetic field after they have been knocked over by an RF pulse. T2, the transverse relaxation time, is a measure of how long it takes a group of atomic nuclei that have been knocked over by an RF pulse to become maximally disordered in the transverse plane. Different tissues have different T1 and T2 times (usually on the order of milliseconds [ms]), which form the basis for T1-weighted and T2-weighted MR image contrast, respectively. The T2 of a tissue is always less than its T1.

24. What is a pulse sequence?

A pulse sequence is a preprogrammed sequence of instructions regarding the timing, strength, and duration of RF pulses and magnetic gradients that are to be applied by the MRI scanner to create specific types of MR images. For example, pulse sequences can be created so that images are acquired slice by slice (2D) or volumetrically (3D) or are acquired during certain portions of the respiratory or cardiac cycles if desired. Image slice orientation, thickness, and spatial resolution can be adjusted, tissues of interest (such as fat or water) can be suppressed, and image contrast (or weighting) can be altered to accentuate other tissues of interest.

25. What is k space?

k space is a 2D graphical depiction of the digitized MR signal data required to create an MR image. Every point in k space contains information about every voxel in the MR image, and the inverse Fourier transform of k space creates the MR image.

26. What are TR and TE?

The repetition time (TR), the time to complete one full iteration of a pulse sequence, and the echo time (TE), the time between the start of a pulse sequence and the acquisition of data, are two parameters (usually reported in milliseconds [ms]) that are adjusted in a pulse sequence to change image contrast. TE is always shorter than TR.

27. What is a spin echo (SE) pulse sequence?

An SE pulse sequence begins with a 90-degree RF pulse (i.e., an RF pulse that flips atomic nuclei by 90 degrees), followed by a 180-degree RF pulse, leading to formation of an MRI signal called a spin echo. The pulse sequence is then repeated until enough spin echoes have been acquired to create MR images.

28. What is a fast spin echo (FSE) pulse sequence?

An FSE pulse sequence begins with a 90-degree RF pulse, followed by a series of 180-degree RF pulses, leading to formation of multiple spin echoes. Since multiple spin echoes are obtained at a time, fewer repetitions of the pulse sequences are required to create MR images, leading to faster image acquisition times. This pulse sequence is commonly used to obtain T2-weighted images and sometimes T1-weighted images.

29. What is a gradient recalled echo (GRE) pulse sequence?

A GRE pulse sequence begins with a <90-degree RF pulse, followed by application of a magnetic field gradient, leading to formation of an MRI signal called a gradient recalled echo. The pulse sequence is then repeated until enough gradient recalled echoes have been acquired to create MR images. The TR and TE are short, leading to rapid acquisition times. As such, this pulse sequence is commonly used to obtain precontrast and postcontrast T1-weighted images.

In addition, in-phase T1-weighted GRE images (where signals from fat and water protons in the same voxel add to each other) are used to detect iron deposition, metal, and gas in tissues as manifested by a loss of signal intensity relative to out-of-phase T1-weighted images, whereas out-of-phase T1-weighted GRE images (where signals from fat and water protons in the same voxel cancel each other) are used to detect presence of microscopic lipid within tissues as manifested by a loss of signal intensity relative to in-phase T1-weighted images.

30. What is signal intensity (SI)?

SI is the descriptor of how bright or dark a tissue is on an MR image. As SI is not calibrated to a standard, it is important to describe SI of a tissue of interest in comparison to another reference tissue such as skeletal muscle or liver.

31. What are T1-weighted images?

T1-weighted images are MR images that display SIs of tissues based on their T1 properties and are typically acquired using short TR and TE values.

32. What are T2-weighted images?

T2-weighted images are MR images that display SIs of tissues based on their T2 properties and are typically acquired using long TR and TE values.

33. What typically has high SI on T1-weighted images?

Fat, proteinaceous fluid, subacute hemorrhage, paramagnetic substances such as melanin, and gadolinium-based contrast material have high T1-weighted SI relative to skeletal muscle. Note that fat may alternatively have low SI on T1-weighted images if fat suppression is applied.

34. What typically has high SI on T2-weighted images?

Fat (on T2-weighted FSE images), simple fluid, fluid-filled organs, cysts, and hemangiomas have high T2-weighted SI relative to skeletal muscle. In general, if fluid (such as in the cerebrospinal fluid, gallbladder, or bladder) is seen to have very high SI on an MR image, then it is likely T2-weighted, whereas if it has low SI, then it is likely T1-weighted.

35. What typically has low SI on both T1-weighted and T2-weighted images?

Gas, cortical bone, fibrous tissue (such as in ligaments and tendons), chronic hemorrhage, iron, metal, and fast flow in blood vessels have low T1-weighted and T2-weighted SI relative to skeletal muscle.

36. Why is it important to acquire precontrast and postcontrast images with the same imaging parameters?

Tissue SIs will change from precontrast to postcontrast images if the imaging parameters are changed but will also change if tissue enhancement following intravenous contrast administration is present. Thus, if the imaging parameters differ between precontrast and postcontrast image acquisitions, it would not be possible to determine whether an observed increase in tissue SI on postcontrast images is due to true enhancement or is artifactual in nature.

37. What is diffusion-weighted imaging (DWI)?

DWI is a functional MR imaging technique that provides information about tissue structure, water content, and cellularity by measurement of the average diffusivity of water molecules due to Brownian motion within a tissue of interest. DWI is useful to detect acute cerebral infarction and also to detect and characterize malignant lesions in the body.

38. What is diffusion-tensor imaging (DTI)?

DTI is a functional MR imaging technique that provides information about tissue microstructure through measurement of the direction-specific diffusivities of water molecules within a tissue of interest. DTI is particularly useful to assess the white matter tracts of the brain for pretreatment planning in patients with brain tumors.

39. What is magnetic resonance spectroscopy (MRS)?

MRS is a functional technique that provides quantitative information about the endogenous molecular composition of a tissue of interest. The data are typically displayed as a spectrum of chemical compound abundances, most often based on the magnetic properties of the hydrogen atom nuclei. MRS is most commonly used clinically to characterize brain lesions.

---

### KEY POINTS

- US is a structural imaging technique that uses high-frequency mechanical ultrasound waves to create real-time tomographic images.
- CT is a structural imaging technique that uses x-rays to create tomographic images.
- MRI is a structural and functional imaging technique that uses magnetism and RF waves to create tomographic images.
- Echogenicity, attenuation, and signal intensity are the descriptors of how bright or dark tissues are on US, CT, and MR images, respectively.
- If fluid has very high SI on an MR image, then it is likely T2-weighted, whereas if it has low SI, then it is likely T1-weighted.

---

**BIBLIOGRAPHY**

Coltrera MD. Ultrasound physics in a nutshell. *Otolaryngol Clin N Am*. 2010;43(6):1149-1159, v.

Wells PN. Ultrasound imaging. *Phys Med Biol*. 2006;51(13):R83-R98.

Boote EJ. AAPM/RSNA physics tutorial for residents: topics in US: Doppler US techniques: concepts of blood flow detection and flow dynamics. *Radiographics*. 2003;23(5):1315-1327.

Hangiandreou NJ. AAPM/RSNA physics tutorial for residents. Topics in US: B-mode US: basic concepts and new technology. *Radiographics*. 2003;23(4):1019-1033.

Dussik KT. On the possibility of using ultrasound waves as a diagnostic aid. *Neurol Psychiat*. 1942;174:153-168.

Kaza RK, Platt JF, Cohan RH, et al. Dual-energy CT with single- and dual-source scanners: current applications in evaluating the genitourinary tract. *Radiographics*. 2012;32(2):353-369.

Coursey CA, Nelson RC, Boll DT, et al. Dual-energy multidetector CT: how does it work, what can it tell us, and when can we use it in abdominopelvic imaging? *Radiographics*. 2010;30(4):1037-1055.

Goldman LW. Principles of CT: multislice CT. *J Nucl Med Technol*. 2008;36(2):57-68, quiz 75-6.

Beckmann EC. CT scanning the early days. *Br J Radiol*. 2006;79(937):5-8.

Prokop M. General principles of MDCT. *Eur J Radiol*. 2003;45(suppl 1):S4-S10.

Cody DD. AAPM/RSNA physics tutorial for residents: topics in CT. Image processing in CT. *Radiographics*. 2002;22(5):1255-1268.

Hounsfield GN. Computerized transverse axial scanning (tomography). 1. Description of system. *Br J Radiol*. 1973;46(552):1016-1022.

Kwee TC, Basu S, Saboury B, et al. Functional oncoimaging techniques with potential clinical applications. *Front Biosci (Elite Ed)*. 2012;4:1081-1096.

Plewes DB, Kucharczyk W. Physics of MRI: a primer. *J Magn Reson Imaging*. 2012;35(5):1038-1054.

Ridgway JP. Cardiovascular magnetic resonance physics for clinicians: part I. *J Cardiovasc Magn Reson*. 2010;12:71.

Pooley RA. AAPM/RSNA physics tutorial for residents: fundamental physics of MR imaging. *Radiographics*. 2005;25(4):1087-1099.

Mansfield P, Maudsley AA. Medical imaging by NMR. *Br J Radiol*. 1977;50(591):188-194.

Lauterbur PC. Image formation by induced local interactions: examples employing nuclear magnetic resonance. *Nature*. 1973;242:190-191.

Damadian R. Tumor detection by nuclear magnetic resonance. *Science*. 1971;171(3976):1151-1153.

Rabi II, Zacharias JR, Millman S, et al. A new method of measuring nuclear magnetic moment. *Phys Rev J1 - PR*. 1938;53(4):318-327.

# CHAPTER 3

# INTRODUCTION TO NUCLEAR MEDICINE AND MOLECULAR IMAGING

*Drew A. Torigian, MD, MA, FSAR, and Andrew B. Newberg, MD*

1. **What is molecular imaging?**
   Molecular imaging is the visualization, characterization, and measurement of biologic processes at the molecular and cellular levels in humans and other living systems. It is essentially a noninvasive means to study in vivo biochemistry and cell biology and is useful to optimize diagnosis and therapy of disease in individualized patients. Nuclear medicine techniques and optical imaging techniques are most commonly used to perform molecular imaging, the former predominantly in humans and the latter predominantly in small animals for preclinical research.

2. **What is nuclear medicine, and how is a nuclear medicine test performed?**
   A radioactive compound (i.e., a radiotracer) that targets a molecular process, cellular process, or disease of interest is administered to a patient. Photons are emitted from the radiotracer in the patient, and an imaging detector is used to detect the distribution of the radiotracer. Images are then created by a computer system. The main nuclear medicine imaging techniques include planar scintigraphy, single photon emission computed tomography (SPECT), and positron emission tomography (PET). Nuclear medicine techniques are used not only for diagnostic purposes, but also less commonly to treat cancer, in which case the radiotracers used accumulate in tumor sites and also emit charged particles that promote cancer cell death.

3. **How does molecular imaging differ from structural imaging?**
   Molecular imaging allows for the noninvasive functional and molecular characterization of normal tissues and disease processes of interest, even when morphologic changes in tissues have not yet occurred. Structural imaging (such as with radiography, computed tomography [CT], magnetic resonance imaging [MRI], and ultrasonography [US]) allows for the noninvasive anatomic assessment of normal tissues and disease conditions based on morphologic and gross functional alterations that occur. Molecular imaging techniques typically have higher contrast resolution (i.e., the ability to distinguish between differences in image intensity) and lower spatial resolution (i.e., the ability to distinguish two adjacent structures as being separate) compared to structural imaging techniques. As such, molecular imaging and structural imaging techniques are complementary.

4. **What is the difference between x-rays used in radiography and CT and gamma rays used in nuclear medicine techniques?**
   X-rays and gamma rays are both types of ionizing electromagnetic radiation (i.e., they are photons that are energetic enough to remove electrons from other atoms or molecules) with wavelengths shorter than those of visible light. X-rays are emitted by electrons located outside of the nucleus of an atom, whereas gamma rays are emitted by unstable nuclei within atoms and have higher energies than x-rays. Diagnostic x-ray imaging is referred to as transmission imaging, since images are formed by the transmission of x-ray photons from an external source (outside the patient) through the patient to external detectors. Nuclear medicine imaging is referred to as emission imaging because images are formed by the emission of gamma ray photons from an internal source (inside the patient) through the patient to external detectors.

5. **What is radioactivity, and when was it discovered?**
   Radioactivity (i.e., radioactive decay) is the process by which unstable atoms that do not have sufficient binding energy to hold their nuclei together emit ionizing radiation, and it occurs in exponential fashion. Alpha decay occurs when an alpha particle (identical to a helium nucleus) is emitted. Beta decay occurs when a beta particle (such as a positron) is emitted. Gamma decay occurs when a gamma ray is emitted during transition of an atomic nucleus to a lower energy state. Henri Becquerel discovered spontaneous radioactivity from uranium in 1896, and Pierre and Marie Curie discovered radium and polonium in 1898. As a result, all three received the Nobel Prize in Physics in 1903.

6. **When was the positron discovered?**
   Carl Anderson discovered the positron (the "positive electron") in 1932 and subsequently received the Nobel Prize in Physics in 1936. Positron emission by certain radioisotopes makes PET imaging feasible.

7. **How are radioisotopes and radiotracers created?**
   Generators are devices that contain a radioactive parent radioisotope with a relatively long half-life that decays to a short-lived daughter radioisotope, which is then used for diagnostic imaging or therapy. The most commonly used one is the technetium-99m ($^{99m}$Tc) generator, which has molybdenum-99 ($^{99}$Mo) as the parent radioisotope. As decay of

**Table 3-1.** Commonly Used Radioisotopes in Diagnostic Nuclear Medicine

| NAME | PHYSICAL HALF-LIFE | USED WITH |
|---|---|---|
| Technetium-99m ($^{99m}$Tc) | 6 hours | Planar scintigraphy, SPECT |
| Iodine-123 ($^{123}$I) | 13.2 hours | Planar scintigraphy, SPECT |
| Indium-111 ($^{111}$In) | 67 hours | Planar scintigraphy, SPECT |
| Thalium-201 ($^{201}$Tl) | 73.1 hours | Planar scintigraphy, SPECT |
| Gallium-67 ($^{67}$Ga) | 78.3 hours | Planar scintigraphy, SPECT |
| Xenon-133 ($^{133}$Xe) | 5.3 days | Planar scintigraphy, SPECT |
| Rubidium-82 ($^{82}$Rb) | 1.3 minutes | PET |
| Oxygen-15 ($^{15}$O) | 2 minutes | PET |
| Nitrogen-13 ($^{13}$N) | 10 minutes | PET |
| Carbon-11 ($^{11}$C) | 20 minutes | PET |
| Gallium-68 ($^{68}$Ga) | 68 minutes | PET |
| Fluorine-18 ($^{18}$F) | 110 minutes | PET |
| Copper-64 ($^{64}$Cu) | 12.7 hours | PET |
| Iodine-124 ($^{124}$I) | 4.2 days | PET |

$^{99}$Mo occurs, $^{99m}$Tc is formed and can then be eluted for use with various molecules to obtain scans of different physiologic processes. Cyclotrons are circular devices in which charged particles are accelerated and deflected into a target to create radioisotopes such as carbon-11 ($^{11}$C) and fluorine-18 ($^{18}$F). Medical grade nuclear reactors are sometimes used to create other isotopes.

8. What are some commonly used radioisotopes in diagnostic nuclear medicine?
   See Table 3-1. Such radioisotopes are often used to label specific molecular compounds that target a molecular process, cellular process, or disease of interest which may then be imaged.

9. What is the physical half-life of a radioisotope?
   The physical half-life of a radioisotope is the average amount of time it takes for half of the original radioactive compound to have undergone radioactive decay. After 5 half-lives, approximately 97% of the original radioactivity of the compound will have decayed. Note that it is not possible to predict when exactly an individual radioisotope atom in the compound will decay.

10. What units are used to measure radioactivity?
    To measure the dose of radioactivity, the becquerel (Bq) is equal to 1 disintegration per second (dps) and is the SI unit of radioactivity. The curie (Ci) is equal to $3.7 \times 10^{10}$ dps, or 37 MBq, which is approximately equal to the radioactivity of 1 gram of radium-226 ($^{226}$Ra), and is the non-SI unit of radioactivity. The effect of ionizing radiation on the body is typically measured by the Sievert (Sv), the SI unit, or the rem (roentgen equivalent in man), the non-SI unit, where 1 Sv = 100 rem. One Sv is defined as the biologic effect of depositing one joule of radiation energy in one kilogram of human tissue.

11. What is a dose calibrator?
    A dose calibrator is a device that is used in nuclear medicine to measure the amount of radioactivity in a radiotracer before it is administered to a patient.

12. How are nuclear medicine imaging tests generally performed?
    A radiotracer is administered to a patient (most commonly intravenously, although oral or inhalational routes are also possible). After waiting for a certain delay time to allow for biodistribution of the radiotracer, the patient is then placed into the scanner. For planar scintigraphy and SPECT, gamma rays are emitted by the radioactive isotopes in the radiotracers. For PET, positrons that are emitted by the radioactive isotopes in the radiotracer molecules travel several millimeters within tissue before annihilating with electrons that are encountered, leading to emission of two gamma rays in opposite directions. The gamma rays leave the body, pass through a collimator (in planar scintigraphy and SPECT), and are detected by one or more scintillation crystals in detectors surrounding the patient. The light signals created by the scintillation crystals are then detected by photomultiplier tubes (PMT), which lead to creation of voltage signals that are digitized for computers to process. Ultimately, when enough signals are detected, the computer reconstructs images that reflect the spatial distribution and amount of accumulation of the radiotracer in organs/

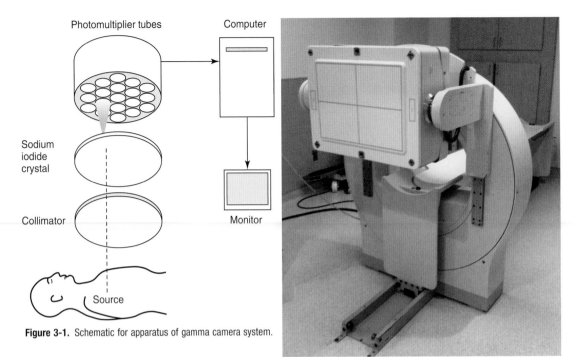

**Figure 3-1.** Schematic for apparatus of gamma camera system.

**Figure 3-2.** Typical single head gamma camera system used in planar scintigraphy.

tissues of the body (which depend on the properties of the administered radiotracer and the disease states present in the patient).

13. What is planar scintigraphy?
    Planar scintigraphy is a nuclear medicine technique in which non-tomographic (2D) planar images of the spatial distribution and amount of accumulation of a radiotracer in the body are created. This is performed using a gamma camera system (Figures 3-1 and 3-2), including a collimator made of perforated or folded lead to absorb most emitted radiation from the radiotracer except that arriving perpendicular to the detector face, and a thallium-doped sodium iodine scintillation crystal. Unfortunately, the collimator wastes > 99% of the emitted signal and is rate-limiting. Planar images can be obtained either statically or dynamically over time to create a video of a particular physiological process of interest.

14. What are some examples of common clinical applications of planar scintigraphy?
    - A ventilation-perfusion (V/Q) scan is useful to assess for acute pulmonary embolism.
    - A three-phase bone scan is useful to determine if osteomyelitis is present.
    - A thyroid scan is useful to determine if a thyroid nodule is benign or malignant.
    - A hepatobiliary scan is useful to assess for acute cholecystitis, bile duct obstruction, or biliary leak.
    - A bleeding scan is useful to localize sites of lower gastrointestinal hemorrhage.

15. What is SPECT?
    SPECT is a nuclear medicine technique in which tomographic (cross-sectional) images of the spatial distribution and amount of accumulation of a single gamma ray emitting radiotracer in the body are created. It also requires the use of a collimator, which generally results in lower sensitivity and poorer image quality compared to PET. Furthermore, SPECT requires the use of radioisotopes that emit single gamma rays, which are usually metallic elements that are difficult to incorporate into biologically important compounds. SPECT/CT scanners (Figure 3-3) are most often employed for SPECT imaging to provide coregistered molecular and structural images.

16. What are some examples of common clinical applications of SPECT/CT?
    - $^{111}$In-octreotide SPECT/CT is useful to assess neuroendocrine tumors before and after treatment.
    - $^{99m}$Tc-sestamibi SPECT/CT is useful to preoperatively localize parathyroid adenomas, particularly when ectopic in location.
    - $^{201}$Tl SPECT/CT is useful to detect and evaluate the effects of coronary artery disease on myocardial perfusion.

17. What is PET?
    PET is a nuclear medicine technique in which tomographic (cross-sectional) images of the spatial distribution and amount of accumulation of a positron emitting radiotracer in the body are created. Collimators are not required in PET

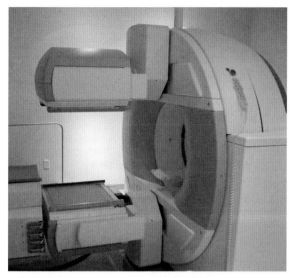

**Figure 3-3.** Typical dual head gamma camera SPECT/CT scanner.

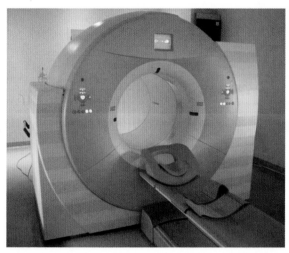

**Figure 3-4.** Typical PET/CT scanner with gantry (which contains x-ray tube for CT and scintillation crystals for PET) and patient table.

because pairs of colinear gamma ray photons emitted in opposite directions from areas of positron annihilation are used to localize sites of radiotracer uptake in the body. This is performed by a process known as coincidence detection, where only photons with the correct energy that are detected simultaneously by detectors located 180 degrees from each other are registered as true events and used to create images. Today, PET/CT scanners (Figure 3-4) are most commonly used for PET imaging to provide coregistered molecular and structural images, improving image quality, anatomic localization of sites of radiotracer uptake, and diagnostic performance. PET/MRI scanners have recently become available for clinical use, providing the additional advantages of decreased radiation dose and improved soft tissue contrast resolution afforded by MRI, but they are much more expensive, require additional safety measures and personnel training for implementation, and require longer image acquisition times compared to those for PET/CT.

18. What are some examples of common clinical applications of PET/CT?
- $^{18}$F-fluorodeoxyglucose (FDG) PET/CT is useful to stage cancers at baseline, to guide treatment, and to assess tumor response following therapeutic intervention.
- FDG PET/CT is also useful to localize seizure foci in the brain, to assess patients with cognitive impairment, and to evaluate for brain tumor recurrence.
- $^{82}$Rb PET/CT is useful to detect and evaluate the effects of coronary artery disease on myocardial perfusion.

- $^{18}$F-sodium fluoride (NaF) PET/CT is useful to detect and evaluate osteoblastic metastatic disease in patients with cancer.
- $^{11}$C-acetate PET/CT is useful to detect the presence and location of recurrent prostate cancer in men with biochemical recurrence following treatment.

19. What is a standardized uptake value (SUV)?

An SUV is a quantitative measure of PET radiotracer uptake in a tissue of interest and is a unitless value. It is calculated as the ratio of tissue radiotracer activity concentration (i.e., accumulated radiotracer dose in a tissue of interest/volume of the tissue of interest) compared to whole body radiotracer activity concentration (i.e., injected radiotracer dose/body weight [where one assumes that 1 g of body weight = 1 ml volume]). If the distribution of an injected radiotracer were uniform throughout the body, then the SUV would be measured as 1 everywhere. Maximum SUV (SUVmax) is the SUV of the hottest voxel within a lesion. Mean SUV (SUVmean) is the average of the SUVs of all voxels within a lesion. Peak SUV (SUVpeak) is the average of the SUVs of a subset of voxels centered about the hottest voxel within a lesion.

20. What is total lesional glycolysis (TLG)?

TLG (also called metabolic volumetric product [MVP]) is a global measure of disease burden in the body and is derived by first calculating the product of SUV and volume for each lesion and then summing these products over all lesions encountered in the body. TLG measurements are generally useful to prognosticate patient outcome and to quantitatively assess treatment response.

21. What is optical imaging, and how does it work?

Optical imaging utilizes nonionizing electromagnetic radiation near or within the visible light spectrum to create images and is often used in conjunction with a variety of fluorescent or bioluminescent compounds that target a molecular process, cellular process, or disease of interest. It has a very high sensitivity of detection, but it suffers from a limited depth of penetration of light into tissues and also from light scattering. As a result, optical imaging is predominantly used in preclinical small animal research to study the biodistribution, pharmacokinetics, or pharmacodynamics of new therapeutics that are being developed.

22. What is the difference between fluorescence and bioluminescence?

Fluorescence occurs when a molecule absorbs light from an outside source and then emits light due to the excitation and relaxation of electrons within the molecule, respectively. An example of a fluorescent compound is green fluorescent protein (GFP). Bioluminescence describes light creation by living organisms via chemical reactions between molecules without requiring the absorption of light from an outside source. For example, enzymes called luciferases act on pigment molecules called luciferins to create bioluminescence in insects such as fireflies, marine organisms, and some fungi and bacteria. Fluorescent and bioluminescent molecular compounds are commonly used in conjunction with optical imaging in preclinical research studies.

23. What is Cherenkov radiation?

Cherenkov radiation was discovered and characterized by Pavel Cherenkov in 1934 (for which he received a Nobel Prize in Physics in 1958 along with Ilya Frank and Igor Tamm) and is observed as a faint blue glow such as may be seen in the water surrounding nuclear reactors. It is the equivalent of the sonic boom for light, and it occurs when a charged particle moves through a medium at a speed greater than the speed of light in that medium (which is less than the speed of light in a vacuum), leading to emission of visible light photons. Optical imaging techniques based on detection of Cherenkov radiation along with Cherenkov specific contrast agents are currently being utilized in preclinical research studies.

## KEY POINTS

- Molecular imaging is complementary with structural imaging.
- Nuclear medicine techniques are predominantly used in the clinical setting for molecular imaging, whereas optical imaging techniques are predominantly used in preclinical research.
- Planar scintigraphy, SPECT, and PET imaging are the primary nuclear medicine molecular imaging techniques available. They are used to image the spatial distribution and amount of accumulation of an administered radiotracer in organs/tissues of the body (which depend on the properties of the radiotracer and the disease states present).
- SUV is a quantitative measure of PET radiotracer uptake in a tissue of interest.

**BIBLIOGRAPHY**

Kwee TC, Torigian DA, Alavi A. Overview of positron emission tomography, hybrid positron emission tomography instrumentation, and positron emission tomography quantification. *J Thorac Imaging*. 2013;28(1):4-10.

Torigian DA, Zaidi H, Kwee TC, et al. PET/MR imaging: technical aspects and potential clinical applications. *Radiology*. 2013;267(1):26-44.

Zanzonico P. Principles of nuclear medicine imaging: planar, SPECT, PET, multi-modality, and autoradiography systems. *Radiat Res*. 2012;177(4):349-364.

Alavi A, Yakir S, Newberg AB. Positron emission tomography in seizure disorders. *Ann N Y Acad Sci*. 2011;1228:E1-E12.

Peterson TE, Furenlid LR. SPECT detectors: the Anger Camera and beyond. *Phys Med Biol.* 2011;56(17):R145-R182.

Xu Y, Liu H, Cheng Z. Harnessing the power of radionuclides for optical imaging: Cerenkov luminescence imaging. *J Nucl Med.* 2011;52(12):2009-2018.

Delbeke D, Schöder H, Martin WH, et al. Hybrid imaging (SPECT/CT and PET/CT): improving therapeutic decisions. *Semin Nucl Med.* 2009;39(5):308-340.

Luker GD, Luker KE. Optical imaging: current applications and future directions. *J Nucl Med.* 2008;49(1):1-4.

Basu S, Zaidi H, Houseni M, et al. Novel quantitative techniques for assessing regional and global function and structure based on modern imaging modalities: implications for normal variation, aging and diseased states. *Sem Nucl Med.* 2007;37(3):223-239.

Margolis DJ, Hoffman JM, Herfkens RJ, et al. Molecular imaging techniques in body imaging. *Radiology.* 2007;245(2):333-356.

Torigian DA, Huang SS, Houseni M, et al. Functional imaging of cancer with emphasis on molecular techniques. *CA Cancer J Clin.* 2007;57(4):206-224.

Huang SC. Anatomy of SUV. Standardized uptake value. *Nucl Med Biol.* 2000;27(7):643-646.

# CHAPTER 4

# INTRODUCTION TO IMAGE PROCESSING, VISUALIZATION, AND ANALYSIS

*Drew A. Torigian, MD, MA, FSAR, and Jayaram K. Udupa, PhD*

1. What is a digital image?
   A digital image is an image discretized in spatial coordinates and in brightness. It can be represented by a multidimensional array of integers.

2. What is the difference between a pixel and a voxel?
   A pixel, or picture element, is the smallest element of a 2D digital image that can be individually processed, whereas a voxel, or volume element, is the smallest element of a 3D digital image that can be individually processed. A voxel that is the same length in all three dimensions is called an isotropic voxel.

3. What is image reconstruction?
   Image reconstruction is a mathematical technique implemented in computers within scanners to reconstruct tomographic or volumetric images from acquired projectional data of a patient. For example, filtered back projection (FBP) and iterative reconstruction (IR) methods are commonly used to create tomographic images in CT.

4. What is the field of view (FOV) of an image?
   FOV is the width of an image, which tends to represent the width of the body region that is imaged by the scanner.

5. What is the matrix size of an image?
   Matrix size is the number of pixels along the length and width of a digital image. This can be the same in both directions (e.g., 512 × 512 in CT) or can differ between the two directions (e.g., 256 × 192 in MRI).

6. What is signal-to-noise ratio (SNR)?
   SNR is the ratio of the mean intensity (i.e., signal) of an object on an image to the standard deviation of the background noise on an image and is a rough measure of image quality.

7. What is contrast-to-noise ratio (CNR)?
   CNR is the difference in SNR between two objects or tissue regions on an image that are adjacent to one another and is another commonly used measure of image quality to indicate the measureable contrast between the two regions.

8. What is spatial resolution?
   Spatial resolution is the ability to portray two separate but adjacent objects as distinct on an image. It is a function of pixel (or voxel) size, is calculated as FOV/matrix size, and is typically measured in line pairs per millimeter (lp/mm), referring to the ability of an imaging technique to distinguish two closely placed line objects as separate.

9. What is contrast resolution?
   Contrast resolution is the ability to portray tissues with different intensities in different shades of gray on an image.

10. What is temporal resolution?
    Temporal resolution is the ability to acquire multiple images in a short amount of time. This factor becomes important when imaging moving objects such as the heart, lungs, and joints.

11. What is a modulation transfer function (MTF)?
    An MTF is a measure of the resolution capability of an imaging system. It is calculated as the ratio of output contrast to input contrast in an imaging system. It indicates the imaging system's ability to retain sharpness or its blurring characteristics.

12. What is quantitative radiology (QR)?
    QR is the quantitative assessment of medical images to evaluate normal states and the severity, degree of change, or status of abnormal disease states relative to normal. This involves the development, standardization, and optimization of image acquisition protocols, computer-aided visualization and analysis (CAVA) methods, and reporting structures. QR is increasingly becoming an integral part of clinical radiology practice.

13. What is the purpose of computer-aided visualization and analysis (CAVA)?
    The purpose of CAVA is to produce quantitative and improved qualitative information about one or more objects of interest within digital images through the use of a computer. The four major operations used in CAVA are preprocessing, visualization, manipulation, and analysis.

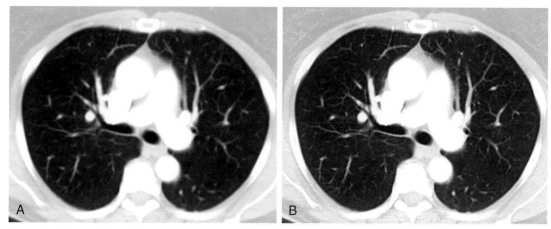

**Figure 4-1.** Filtering. **A,** Chest CT image reconstructed with a suppressing filter. Note smoother appearance of lungs. **B,** Same chest CT image reconstructed with an enhancing filter. Note sharper appearance of lungs.

14. What is image preprocessing?

Image preprocessing is a set of computer-based techniques used to prepare an image dataset to facilitate subsequent visualization, manipulation, and analysis. Some commonly used preprocessing techniques include volume of interest (VOI) restriction, filtering, interpolation, registration, segmentation, and image algebraic operations (e.g., addition, subtraction, etc.).

15. What is VOI restriction?

This is a preprocessing technique used to reduce the amount of unneeded data in an image dataset. For example, one may delete some image slices at the upper and lower portions of a stack of contiguous axial tomographic images, crop slices to reduce the length and width of each slice, or remove certain unwanted objects such as the scanner table from the image slices.

16. What is filtering?

Filtering is a preprocessing technique used to enhance wanted (object) information and suppress unwanted (noise, artifact, or background) information in an image dataset. The most commonly used enhancing filter is an edge enhancing operation, leading to sharper image quality, whereas the most commonly used suppressing filter is a smoothing operation, leading to smoother image quality (Figure 4-1).

17. What is interpolation?

Interpolation is a preprocessing technique used to change the level of discretization (pixel or voxel size) in an image. For example, one may reslice a volumetric image dataset into a set of tomographic slices of a prespecified thickness and orientation.

18. What is registration?

Registration is a preprocessing technique used to match two image datasets or objects within images as closely as possible. This can be performed with a rigid transformation (using translation and rotation operations) or with a non-rigid transformation (also using deformation operations). For example, one may register PET and CT image datasets acquired from a patient to create hybrid PET/CT images. As another example, one may register MRI scans acquired from a patient on two separate occasions to aid in detection of disease change over time.

19. What is segmentation?

Segmentation is a preprocessing technique used to recognize and delineate objects in an image dataset. Recognition is the determination of an object's approximate whereabouts in an image, which is a high-level task in which humans typically outperform computers. Delineation is the determination of an object's precise spatial extent and composition in an image, which is a low-level task in which computers typically outperform humans. For example, one may segment the lungs from the thorax on a chest CT study and then segment areas of lung emphysema (Figure 4-2).

20. What is thresholding?

Thresholding is a commonly used and the simplest segmentation technique in which a gray scale threshold value range or interval is applied to an image dataset. All pixels (or voxels) with gray scale values lying in the threshold range are included in the segmented region, whereas the others are not.

21. What is the purpose of image visualization?

Image visualization is used to create visual renditions of objects of interest in an image dataset to enhance one's understanding about such objects.

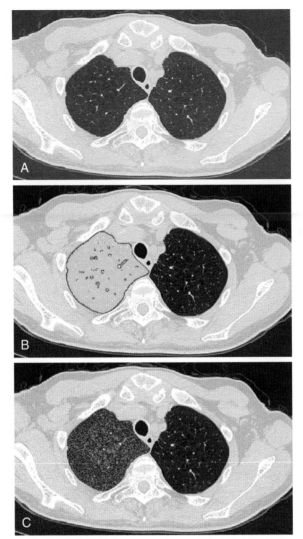

**Figure 4-2.** Segmentation. **A,** Chest CT image in patient with mild emphysema. **B,** Same chest CT image with segmented right lung (orange color overlay). **C,** Same chest CT image with segmented emphysema in right lung (green color overlay).

22. What are some ways to visualize tomographic images?

In section mode, images can be visualized as axial, sagittal, coronal, or oblique sections, or even as curved sections (also known as multiplanar reformations [MPRs]). Curved MPRs are commonly used to analyze vascular structures on CT or MR angiography.

In volume mode, images can be visualized with the following renderings (Figure 4-3):

- Maximum intensity projection (MIP): A 2D rendered image is displayed in which the gray scale intensity assigned to each pixel is the maximum of the intensities of all voxels encountered along the projection axis. This is most commonly used when objects of interest are the brightest in the image (e.g., enhancing vessels and osseous or calcified structures).
- Minimum intensity projection (MinIP): A 2D rendered image is displayed in which the gray scale intensity assigned to each pixel is the minimum of the intensities of all voxels encountered along the projection axis. This is most commonly used when objects of interest are the darkest in the image (e.g., lungs, air-filled tracheobronchial tree, and air-filled bowel).
- Surface-shaded display (SSD): A 2D rendered image of an object surface is displayed. This is infrequently used given the availability of volume rendering techniques.
- Volume-rendered (VR): A 2D rendered image of an object volume is displayed in which each voxel is assigned a brightness level or color and an opacity value ranging from 0% to 100%, which can be adjusted interactively as desired. The viewpoint is often external to the object of interest, although it can also be located internal to the

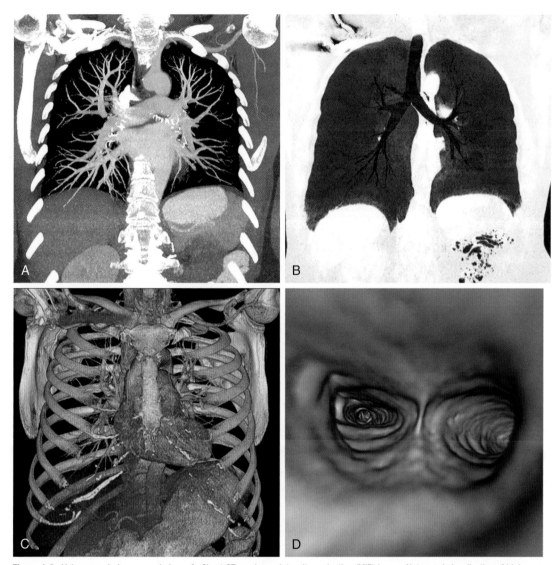

**Figure 4-3.** Volume mode image renderings. **A,** Chest CT maximum intensity projection (MIP) image. Note good visualization of high attenuation contrast-enhanced pulmonary vascular structures. **B,** Chest CT minimum intensity projection (MinIP) image. Note good visualization of very low attenuation structures such as gas-filled lungs, tracheobronchial tree, and upper abdominal bowel loops. **C,** Chest CT volume-rendered (VR) image from external viewpoint. Note good visualization of 3D spatial relationships of thoracic skeleton, heart, and upper abdominal organs. **D,** Virtual endoscopic chest CT VR image within trachea. Note normal appearing tracheal bifurcation and proximal mainstem bronchi.

object of interest to create virtual endoscopic (also called endoluminal or "fly through") images. Virtual endoscopy is commonly used in virtual CT colonoscopy to visualize the large bowel and also in virtual CT bronchoscopy to visualize the tracheobronchial tree.

23. What is the difference between window level and window width?
    Window level is the gray scale value that is selected to be displayed as the midlevel intensity on an image and determines the displayed image brightness. Window width is the range of gray scale values that is selected to be displayed in image voxels as shades of gray around the selected window level and determines the displayed image contrast. For gray scale values above or below this selected range, image voxels are displayed white and black, respectively. A narrow window width provides high contrast. Preset window level and width combinations are commonly used to optimally display certain tissue types on digital images.

24. What is the purpose of image manipulation?
    Image manipulation is used to interactively change visual renditions of objects of interest in an image dataset to enhance one's understanding about such objects. For example, one may simulate performance of a surgical procedure

on a patient using an image dataset acquired from the patient or may use image datasets from multiple patients to develop new interventional techniques to treat various disease conditions.

25. What is the purpose of image analysis?

Image analysis is used to extract quantitative information about one or more objects of interest from image datasets. For example, one may quantify the morphological features of objects, such as size, curvature, area, volume, shape, position, boundary characteristics, and interobject spatial relationships, or the change in these parameters with motion, in the case of dynamic objects. Alternatively, one may quantify the intensity features of objects, such as histogram-based intensity properties (mean, maximum, minimum, skewness, kurtosis) or texture-based intensity properties (contrast, homogeneity, energy, entropy), or the change in these parameters with motion, in the case of dynamic objects.

26. What is the purpose of computer-aided diagnosis (CAD)?

CAD is used for automatic detection and characterization (i.e., diagnosis) of lesions of interest on image datasets. Typically, CAD is used to improve the diagnostic accuracy and efficiency of image interpretation by a radiologist or nuclear medicine physician. For example, CAD can be used to aid in the detection and characterization of lung nodules on chest CT, of colon polyps and masses on virtual CT colonoscopy, and of breast cancers on mammography.

27. What is a biomarker?

A biomarker (biologic marker) is a characteristic that is objectively measured and evaluated as an indicator of normal biologic processes, pathogenic processes, or pharmacologic responses to a therapeutic intervention. Imaging biomarkers are obtained from image analysis.

28. What is a clinical endpoint?

A clinical endpoint is a characteristic that reflects how a patient feels, functions, or survives and is typically considered as the primary endpoint in clinical research studies. For example, survival and improvement in quality of life are clinical endpoints.

29. What is a surrogate endpoint?

A surrogate endpoint is a biomarker that may be used in place of a clinical endpoint so that a clinical research study can be practically conducted or completed more quickly. For example, disease response seen on imaging or on laboratory testing following therapy is a surrogate endpoint. Please note that not all biomarkers are surrogate endpoints.

30. What is radiomics?

Radiomics is a field of study in QR that involves the high-throughput extraction of large numbers of quantitative features from diagnostic images. The purpose is to develop new quantitative imaging biomarkers that may be clinically useful to improve the diagnostic accuracy of disease detection, staging, or phenotyping (e.g., characterization of specific disease histopathology, prediction of disease response to therapy, prognostication of patient outcome).

31. What is radiogenomics?

Radiogenomics is a field of study in QR and the basic sciences that is focused on defining associations between image-based phenotypes and molecular phenotypes of disease. This may be useful to better understand the biologic significance of certain image-based features encountered on diagnostic imaging or to develop and validate new imaging biomarkers to address unanswered clinical questions.

## KEY POINTS

- Quantitative radiology (QR) is the quantitative assessment of medical images to evaluate normal states and the severity, degree of change, or status of abnormal disease states relative to normal. This involves the development, standardization, and optimization of image acquisition protocols, computer-aided visualization and analysis (CAVA) methods, and reporting structures.
- CAVA provides quantitative information about objects of interest within digital images and involves the use of image preprocessing, visualization, manipulation, and analysis.
- A biomarker (biologic marker) is a characteristic that is objectively measured and evaluated as an indicator of normal biologic processes, pathogenic processes, or pharmacologic responses to a therapeutic intervention. Imaging biomarkers are obtained from image analysis.
- Spatial resolution is the ability to display two separate but adjacent objects as distinct on an image.
- Contrast resolution is the ability to display tissues with different intensities as having distinct shades of gray on an image.

**BIBLIOGRAPHY**

Kuo MD, Jamshidi N. Behind the numbers: decoding molecular phenotypes with radiogenomics—guiding principles and technical considerations. *Radiology.* 2014;270(2):320-325.

Gatenby RA, Grove O, Gillies RJ. Quantitative imaging in cancer evolution and ecology. *Radiology.* 2013;269(1):8-14.

Lambin P, Rios-Velazquez E, Leijenaar R, et al. Radiomics: extracting more information from medical images using advanced feature analysis. *Eur J Cancer.* 2012;48(4):441-446.

Strimbu K, Tavel JA. What are biomarkers? *Current Opin HIV AIDS.* 2010;5(6):463-466.

Giger ML, Chan HP, Boone J. Anniversary paper: history and status of CAD and quantitative image analysis: the role of medical physics and AAPM. *Med Phys.* 2008;35(12):5799-5820.

Cody DD. AAPM/RSNA physics tutorial for residents: topics in CT. Image processing in CT. *Radiographics.* 2002;22(5):1255-1268.

Udupa JK, Herman GT. Medical image reconstruction, processing, visualization, and analysis: the MIPG perspective. Medical Image Processing Group. *IEEE Trans Med Imaging.* 2002;21(4):281-295.

Biomarkers Definitions Working Group. Biomarkers and surrogate endpoints: preferred definitions and conceptual framework. *Clin Pharmacol Ther.* 2001;69(3):89-95.

Udupa JK, Herman GT. 3D imaging in medicine. 2nd ed. Boca Raton, FL: CRC Press; 2000.

# CHAPTER 5

# COMPUTERS IN RADIOLOGY

*Mindy Y. Licurse, MD, and William W. Boonn, MD*

1. **What is PACS?**
   PACS stands for Picture Archiving and Communication System. On the most basic level, PACS integrates image acquisition modalities, workstation displays, the image archiving system, and the underlying network.

2. **How are PACS images stored?**
   The PACS archive traditionally has been composed of short-term and long-term storage. Short-term storage is usually composed of redundant arrays of inexpensive (or independent) discs (RAID) arrays that provide quick access to image data. After a certain amount of time (3 to 30 days, depending on the size of the short-term archive), images from the short-term archive are moved to the long-term archive, which is usually composed of magnetic tape or magneto-optical media. Images cannot be viewed directly from the long-term archive. Instead, images need to be "fetched" from the long-term archive and copied back to the short-term archive before being viewed on a workstation. This compromise was made because of the high cost of RAID storage. The cost of RAID storage has decreased enough more recently so that several PACS archives are now being designed as "always online" systems. These new systems are composed only of RAID arrays, which essentially place all images in the short-term archive and eliminate the need for fetching.

3. **What is image compression?**
   Image compression is the process of reducing image file size using various mathematical algorithms. Compression is usually expressed as a ratio (e.g., 10:1). A 10-megabyte (MB) file that is compressed at a ratio of 10:1 would have a final size of 1 MB. Generally, as compression ratios increase, file sizes decrease. However, a price is inevitably paid in decreased image fidelity.

4. **What is the difference between "lossy" and "lossless" compression?**
   Encoding an image is a process that converts a raw image (e.g., the original radiograph) into a more compact coded file. Decoding converts the coded file to a decoded image. If the raw image and the decoded image are the same, the compression method is considered lossless. If there is a difference between the raw image and the decoded image, the method of encoding and decoding is considered lossy. Lossless compression can usually achieve ratios of 2:1 or 3:1. Lossy compression can achieve much higher compression ratios; however, overcompression may destroy fine detail, making the image unacceptable for diagnostic purposes.

5. **What is RIS?**
   RIS stands for Radiology Information System. RIS is the core system responsible for managing workflow within a radiology department. Tasks include patient scheduling and tracking, examination performance tracking, examination interpretation, billing, and handling of radiology reports including result distribution. RIS must work optimally with the PACS to properly enable information sharing. Over the past several years, with the evolution of radiology to filmless environments, RIS capabilities have increased tremendously in addition to merging of RIS/PACS interdependent functionality.

6. **What is HIS?**
   HIS stands for Hospital Information System. HIS manages patient demographics; insurance and billing; and often other clinical information systems, including laboratory results, physician orders, and electronic medical records.

7. **What is DICOM?**
   DICOM stands for Digital Imaging and Communications in Medicine. It is a standard that establishes rules that allow medical images and associated information to be exchanged between imaging equipment from different vendors, computers, and hospitals. A computed tomography (CT) scanner produced by vendor A and a magnetic resonance imaging (MRI) scanner produced by vendor B can send images to a PACS from vendor C using DICOM as a common language. In addition to storing image information, other DICOM standard services include query/retrieve, print management, scheduling of acquisition and notification of completion, and security profiles.

8. **What determines image storage size?**
   Image size, generally expressed in megabytes, is determined by spatial resolution and bit depth. Spatial resolution for a two-dimensional (2D) image is defined by a matrix of horizontal and vertical pixels. A single image in a typical CT

scan is composed of a matrix of 512 vertical pixels × 512 horizontal pixels, whereas a chest radiograph image might have a matrix size of 2500 vertical pixels × 2000 horizontal pixels. For a given anatomic area of interest, images with a larger matrix size have greater spatial resolution.

Bit depth is defined by the number of shades of gray within the image, where $2^n$ equals shades of gray and $n$ equals bit depth. An image with a bit depth of 1 has 2 shades of gray (pure black and pure white). A 6-bit image contains 64 shades of gray; 7-bit, 128 shades; 8-bit, 256 shades; and 12-bit, 4096 shades. Most diagnostic-quality digital images in CT, MRI, and computed radiography/digital radiography are displayed in 10 or 12 bits.

The file size of an imaging study also depends on the number of images in that study. A chest radiograph may have 2 images (posteroanterior and lateral), whereas a CT scan of the abdomen may have 50 images. With the advent of multidetector row CT scanners, it is now possible to acquire thinner slices in much less time, often resulting in much larger studies. This capability also allows images to be reconstructed in different planes. All of this contributes to an increased number of images and, overall, larger study sizes for storage. A CT angiogram may contain 500 to 1000 images or more.

9. How large are these studies?

Table 5-1 shows approximate matrix and file sizes for various imaging modalities. These values vary depending on bit depth, number of images acquired, and compression technique.

10. What is teleradiology?

Teleradiology is the process of sending digital radiology images over a computer network to a remote location (across town or across the globe) for viewing and interpretation. The American College of Radiology publishes a set of guidelines and standards for teleradiology that include minimal display requirements, security and privacy provisions, and documentation standards.

11. What is IHE?

Integrating the Healthcare Enterprise (IHE) is an initiative undertaken by medical specialists and other care providers, administrators, information technology professionals, and industry professionals to improve the way computer systems in health care share information. IHE promotes coordinated use of established communications standards such as DICOM and HL7 (see question 12) to address specific clinical needs that support optimal patient care. Systems developed in accordance with IHE communicate with one another better, are easier to implement, and enable care providers to use information more effectively.

12. What is HL7?

Health Level 7 (HL7) is the standard used by most RIS and HIS to exchange information between systems. It was designed for sending notifications about events in a health system (e.g., a patient is admitted) and transmitting information (e.g., laboratory data and radiology reports). It was not designed to handle image information, because that role is primarily served by DICOM.

13. How are conventional radiographs integrated into an all-digital PACS?

There are three methods. The first method is to obtain a conventional radiograph on film and digitize the image using a scanner. In fully digital environments, this method is usually reserved for digitizing "outside" films or films from settings where digital acquisition has not yet been implemented, such as in the operating room. The second and third methods for acquiring digital radiographs are computed radiography (CR) and digital radiography (DR).

**Table 5-1.** Approximate Matrix and File Sizes for Various Imaging Studies

| | Image Matrix | | Images | | File Size (in MB) | |
|---|---|---|---|---|---|---|
| MODALITY | X | Y | AVERAGE | RANGE | AVERAGE | RANGE |
| CR | 2000 | 2500 | 3 | 2-5 | 30 | 20-50 |
| DR | 3000 | 3000 | 3 | 2-5 | 54 | 40-90 |
| Digital mammography | 3000 | 3000 | 6 | 4-8 | 100 | 75-150 |
| Multidetector row CT | 512 | 512 | 500 | 200-1000 | 250 | 100-600 |
| MRI | 256 | 256 | 200 | 80-1000 | 25 | 10-150 |
| Ultrasonography | 640 | 480 | 30 | 20-60 | 20 | 10-40 |
| Nuclear medicine | 256 | 256 | 10 | 4-30 | 1 | 0.5-4 |
| Digital fluoroscopy (without digital subtraction angiography [DSA]) | 1024 | 1024 | 20 | 10-50 | 20 | 10-50 |
| Digital fluoroscopy (with DSA) | 1024 | 1024 | 150 | 120-240 | 450 | 360-720 |

14. What is voice recognition (or speech recognition)?

Voice recognition is the process by which a computer system recognizes spoken words and converts them into text. Comprehending human languages falls under a different field of computer science called natural language processing. Early systems required that the speaker speak slowly and distinctly, separating each word with a short pause. These systems were called discrete speech systems. More recently, continuous speech systems have become available that allow the user to speak more naturally.

15. What are the advantages and disadvantages of voice or speech recognition relative to conventional dictation/transcription?

There are several advantages to voice recognition over conventional dictation for radiology reporting. Report turnaround time is vastly reduced, overall cost is decreased (because transcriptionists are no longer required), and users who take advantage of text macros can dictate standard reports in less time.

The disadvantages include erroneous reports because of poor recognition of the speech of certain individuals (sometimes because of lack of training) and difficulty in recognizing similar sounding words (e.g., "hypointense" vs. "hyperintense"). Poor recognition and inefficient use of macros often result in increased dictation time and frustration on the part of the radiologist, which is usually remedied with better training and support.

16. What is structured reporting?

Structured reporting enables the capture of radiology report information so that it can be retrieved later and reused. A key feature of a structured report is consistent organization. A report of an abdominal CT study might follow subheadings that describe each of the anatomic areas listed in the report, such as the liver, spleen, pancreas, and kidneys. This feature of structured reporting is sometimes called "itemized reporting" or "standardized reporting" and is preferred by referring physicians, presumably because specific information can be found more easily than in a narrative report. There are no reliable data on the frequency with which reports of this type are currently used. Structured reports also use standard language.

When defined terms from a standard lexicon are associated with imaging reports, the information in the report becomes more accessible and reusable. For many years, mammography has fostered the use of structured reporting as strictly defined—choosing from a limited set of options, such as the six Breast Imaging Reporting and Data System (BI-RADS) categories, to express the likelihood of cancer on a mammogram. BI-RADS reduces the variability and improves the clarity of communication among physicians. Correlation of the recorded structured data items to histopathologic findings (often performed automatically) provides regular feedback to radiologists on their strengths and weaknesses, improving the overall quality of mammographic interpretation.

17. What is RadLex?

RadLex is a comprehensive lexicon for the indexing and retrieval of online radiology resources developed by the Radiological Society of North America (RSNA) and other radiology organizations, including the American College of Radiology (ACR). It has been designed to satisfy the needs of software developers, system vendors, and radiology users by adopting the best features of existing terminology systems, while producing new terms to fill critical gaps. RadLex also provides a comprehensive and technology-friendly replacement for the ACR Index for Radiological Diagnoses. Rather than "reinventing the wheel," RadLex unifies and supplements other lexicons and standards, such as SNOMED-CT and DICOM.

18. What is CADe?

CADe stands for computer-aided detection, a computerized system that identifies portions of an image that may correlate to abnormalities, utilized to decrease perception error and reduce false negative rates. The FDA has approved the use of CADe for mammography, chest radiography, chest CT, and CT colonography. This is not to be confused with CADx (or CAD), which is computer-aided diagnosis. CADe of a finding requires validation by a radiologist, whereas CADx presumes independent clinical diagnosis of a disease.

19. What is BI-RADS?

Breast Imaging Reporting and Data System (BI-RADS) is a standard lexicon developed by the ACR used for reporting mammography findings in addition to breast ultrasonography and MRI findings.

20. What types of injuries can result from working at a PACS workstation, and what are some potential remedies?

Repetitive stress symptoms have been reported in the literature as being highly prevalent among radiologists working in PACS-based environments. Compared to film reading environments, PACS-based environments and electronic workstations have important factors that directly affect comfort and, therefore, performance, including seating, heat, noise, and light. For example, cubital tunnel syndrome may result from compression of the ulnar nerve at the medial elbow due to prolonged elbow flexion or extrinsic pressure. Having a padded chair arm rest and a hands-free dictation microphone can help prevent this syndrome. Additional interventions including use of an ergonomic mouse, adjustable chairs, workstation tables, and educational training have resulted in improved symptoms. With the advent of filmless interpretation, growing concerns regarding repetitive stress symptoms have prompted some radiology departments to implement ergonomic solutions.

21. What is image sharing?

Image sharing refers to the electronic exchange of patient medical images between hospitals, physicians, and patients. While past image sharing has depended largely on physical media, predominantly compact discs (CDs), there has been a recent push from the National Institutes of Health (NIH) to develop an image exchange method without relying on physical media. In response, the RSNA has developed an Image Share Network (ISN) based on the XDS.I.b profile of IHE. The ISN is essentially a secure web-based network that has been piloted to several institutions nationwide and allows for both physician and patient access to medical images.

Image sharing has become increasingly important. Benefits of image sharing include potentially improved interpretative quality given the availability of a prior imaging study for comparison, decreased numbers of inappropriately ordered or duplicated exams with associated decreased radiation exposure, shared diagnostic information for improved patient care by multiple care providers for the same patient, and timely availability of images or results at the point of care.

Challenges to optimal image sharing include concerns regarding privacy and security, given the use of protected health information, in addition to competitive concerns by health care institutions across the board. Having a high-security Health Insurance Portability and Accountability Act (HIPAA)-compliant data hosting center is necessary, and strict standards must be met to be HIPAA certified. Features that are secure and compliant include proper ability for identification and authentication, authorized privileges, access control, confidentiality, integrity of data, and accountability with audit trails. Other challenges include bandwidth requirements necessary for the image sharing network, which requires significant investment.

22. What is XDS?

XDS, which stands for cross-enterprise document sharing, helps manage access of patient electronic health records across health enterprises, by creating a standard set of specifications to enable sharing of medical documents between enterprises. XDS assumes that enterprises belong to an XDS affinity domain, which is a group of health care enterprises with shared policies usually bound through legal agreements. Four systems for mediating sharing of data within the XDS profile include the document repository, document registry, document source, and document consumer. Exchange of data itself takes place through XDS transactions. Key transactions include a provider/register document set, a registry stored query, and retrieval of the document set. XDS-I is an extended profile with new specifications optimized specifically for medical imaging.

23. What is Imaging 3.0?

Imaging 3.0 is a model framework for the evolution of radiology, created by the ACR, for the purpose of optimally equipping radiologists for value-based health care and a more active role in patient care. Imaging 3.0 principles are suggested at every decision making point in the delivery of imaging care, including steps prior to and following interpretation, by utilizing proper information technology systems and processes. Principles of Imaging 3.0 affect security and privacy, workflow processes, business intelligence analytics, clinical decision support, dose and safety, education and training qualifications, image acquisition, archiving and retrieval, image display, reporting and communication, transmission and communication, RIS/EMR integration, and communication with mobile devices.

24. What factors are important to consider when choosing a mobile device for use in radiology departments?

Mobile devices have become integral to everyday life. To operate within a secure and optimal environment within radiology, multiple aspects must be considered. The main factors include:

- Security: Access to the device, communication with other devices via Wi-Fi or cellular networks, and HIPAA compliance.
- Bandwidth: Important for data transfer speeds.
- Screen resolution: Radiographs are usually the largest images in terms of pixel number, with the exception of mammograms, for which a full-resolution image ranges from 4 to 12 megapixels (MPs).
- Display size: Typical desktop PACS displays are about 21 inches diagonally, tablet displays are about 10 inches, and phone displays are about 3.5 inches. Display size of a phone is currently too small to adequately view a radiographic image. For CT, MR, ultrasonographic, and nuclear medicine images, the smartphone display is likely adequate for an on-call scenario, although daily use is not likely practical at this time.
- Pixel pitch: Length of one side of a square pixel, which ranges from 270 microns for low-resolution desktop displays to 78 microns for the latest iPhones with "retina display." Increased pixels lead to increased information in a fixed area, but pixels must at least be at the threshold of human perception.
- Luminance: Brightness, which affects ability to discriminate contrast in radiologic images. Mobile devices have output luminances currently of 400 to 500 cd/m2, on par with desktop medical displays. Given the automated power management features on many mobile devices to dim the display in certain settings, display dimming must be checked for and prevented on the viewing application.

25. Can I interpret radiology images on a tablet device?

Many radiology applications for image viewing are labeled "not for diagnostic interpretation." However, there are FDA-approved applications for interpreting images on a mobile device "when no dedicated workstation is available." Under the FDA, "a mobile application that displays radiological images for diagnosis transforms the mobile platform into a class II Picture Archiving and Communications Systems (PACS)." These are subjected to regulatory oversight and considered regulated medical devices which must comply with device classifications associated with the transformed platforms.

26. What are the display requirements for diagnostic interpretation of radiology images?
Display requirements include luminance response, pixel pitch, and display size.
- Luminance response: Brightness and contrast of gray scale medical images result from luminance related to image gray level values.
- Maximum luminance: Perceived contrast of image depends on ratio of luminance (LR) for maximum gray value ($L_{max}$) to luminance of lowest gray value ($L_{min}$). Note that this is different from the contrast ratio often reported by monitor manufacturers. All display devices in one facility should have the same LR.
- $L_{max}$ of diagnostic monitors should be at least 350 cd/m$^2$, although monitors for interpretation of mammograms should have $L_{max}$ of at least 420 cd/m$^2$. Monitors for other purposes should have $L_{max}$ of at least 250 cd/m$^2$.
- DICOM gray scale display function (GSDF) should be used to set intermediate gray values with similar response functions among all monitors in a facility.
- Calibration: Luminance response, LR, and GSDF can be selected using the monitor on-screen display controls, although some devices may require software from the monitor manufacturer to set luminances of each gray level.
- Quality control: Display devices should be periodically checked to verify the luminance response. Both basic and advanced verification tests may be utilized. Contrast response of monitors for diagnostic interpretation should be within 10% of the GSDF over the full LR and the contrast response should be within 20% of the GSDF over the full LR for other purposes.
- Pixel pitch: Spacing of pixel structures, which determines amount of detail that can be presented. Determines maximum spatial frequency that can be presented in an image. The maximum spatial frequency that can be described by digital signals with a constant pitch $P$ is 1/(2P) cycles/mm. Optimal pixel pitch should be small to present all spatial frequencies within human visual perception. The pixel pitch should be about 0.200 mm but not larger than 0.210 mm for diagnostic interpretation.
- Display size: Visualization of the full scene is optimal when the diagonal display distance is about 80% of the viewing distance, which corresponds to approximately 21 inches (53 cm) when there is an arm's length viewing distance of about 60 cm. An aspect ratio (width to height) of 3:4 or 4:5 works well for presentation of radiographic images.

27. Where can I learn more about imaging informatics? Are there formal training programs and certifications available?
- The Society for Imaging Informatics in Medicine (SIIM) is a health care organization involved in advancing the field of imaging informatics, with the overarching goal to improve quality and delivery of patient care. SIIM has a plethora of online resources (http://siim.org) and online educational content for both newcomers and veterans in the field of informatics.
- Fellowships are available and growing for those interested in advancing their informatics skills. A list of current imaging informatics fellowship programs is available at http://siim.org/about/fellows/imaging-informatics-fellowships.
- The RSNA has information about informatics (http://www.rsna.org/Informatics.aspx) with links to IHE, the RSNA Teaching File System, RSNA Image Share, and RadLex in addition to information about Meaningful Use, reporting templates, and more.
- The ACR has online resources about informatics including in-depth reference guides created by the Information Technology (IT) and Informatics Committee in collaboration with the Quality and Safety Commission (http://www.acr.org/Advocacy/Informatics).
- The American Board of Imaging Informatics (https://www.abii.org) is a nonprofit organization that sets the professional certification standards for candidates interested in becoming a Certified Imaging Informatics Professional (CIIP) through a formal training pathway. The American Medical Informatics Association (AMIA) is an organization for leading informatics professionals throughout all of medicine and the health care industry (http://www.amia.org).
- The Healthcare Information and Management Systems Society (HIMSS) is a nonprofit organization for health through information technology (http://www.himss.org).

## KEY POINTS

- Image storage size is determined by spatial resolution and bit depth, and storage size of an imaging examination is determined by image storage size and the total number of images.
- The Digital Imaging and Communications in Medicine (DICOM) standard is currently used to allow medical images and associated information to be exchanged between imaging equipment from different vendors, computers, and hospitals.
- The picture archiving and communication system (PACS) is used to store and display medical images.

## BIBLIOGRAPHY

Langer SG, Tellis W, Carr C, et al. The RSNA Image Sharing Network. *J Digit Imaging.* 2015;28(1):53-61.

Freiherr G. HIMSS 2014: The challenge of image sharing [Internet]. Place unknown: Carestream. Available from: <http://www.carestream.com/blog/2014/02/05/himss-2014-the-challenge-of-image-sharing/>. Accessed on 01.09.14.

Thompson AC, Kremer Prill MJ, Biswal S, et al. Factors associated with repetitive strain, and strategies to reduce injury among breast-imaging radiologists. *J Am Coll Radiol.* 2014;11(11):1074-1079.

FDA issues final guidance on mobile medical apps. FDA News Release [Internet]. Available from <http://www.fda.gov/newsevents/newsroom/pressannouncements/ucm369431.htm>. September 23, 2013. Accessed on 01.09.14.

Hirschorn DS, Choudhri AF, Shih G, et al. Mobile devices. In: ACR reference guide in information technology for the practicing radiologist. Reston, VA: ACR; 2013:1-15.

McEnery KW. Radiology information systems and electronic medical records. In: ACR reference guide in information technology for the practicing radiologist. Reston, VA: ACR; 2013:1-14.

McGinty GB, Allen B Jr, Wald C. Imaging 3.0. In: ACR reference guide in information technology for the practicing radiologist. Reston, VA: ACR; 2013:1-11.

Mendelson DS, Erickson BJ, Choy G. Image sharing. In: ACR reference guide in information technology for the practicing radiologist. Reston, VA: ACR; 2013:1-15.

Norweck JT, Seibert JA, Andriole KP, et al. ACR-AAPM-SIIM technical standard for electronic practice of medical imaging. *J Digit Imaging.* 2013;26(1):38-52.

Ridley EL. FDA mobile medical apps guidance includes radiology apps [Internet]. [Place unknown]: AuntMinnie.com. Available from: <http://www.auntminnie.com/index.aspx?sec=ser&sub=def&pag=dis&ItemID=104542>. September 23, 2013. Accessed on 01.09.14.

Boiselle PM, Levine D, Horwich PJ, et al. Repetitive stress symptoms in radiology: prevalence and response to ergonomic interventions. *J Am Coll Radiol.* 2008;5(8):919-923.

Weiss DL, Langlotz CP. Structured reporting: patient care enhancement or productivity nightmare? *Radiology.* 2008;249(3):739-747.

Dreyer KJ, Hirschorn DS, Thrall JH, et al. PACS: a guide to the digital revolution. 2nd ed. New York: Springer; 2006.

Langlotz CP. RadLex: a new method for indexing online educational materials. *Radiographics.* 2006;26(6):1595-1597.

Horii SC, Horii HN, Mun SK, et al. Environmental designs for reading from imaging workstations: ergonomic and architectural features. *J Digit Imaging.* 2003;16(1):124-131, discussion 3.

Liu BJ, Cao F, Zhou MZ, et al. Trends in PACS image storage and archive. *Comput Med Imaging Graph.* 2003;27(2-3):165-174.

Ratib O, Ligier Y, Bandon D, et al. Update on digital image management and PACS. *Abdom Imaging.* 2000;25(4):333-340.

Siegel EL, Kolodner RM. Filmless radiology. New York: Springer; 1999.

Horii SC. Primer on computers and information technology. Part four: A nontechnical introduction to DICOM. *Radiographics.* 1997;17(5):1297-1309.

# CHAPTER 6

# INTRODUCTION TO CONTRAST AGENTS

*Drew A. Torigian, MD, MA, FSAR, and Parvati Ramchandani, MD, FACR, FSAR*

1. **What is a radiographic contrast agent?**

   A radiographic contrast agent is a substance that is administered to a patient during an imaging examination to improve its diagnostic performance. Contrast agents are most often administered via the intravenous (IV) and oral routes for computed tomography (CT) and magnetic resonance imaging (MRI) examinations. However, other routes of contrast administration may be utilized, depending on the particular imaging study to be performed. For example, arteriography requires the intraarterial (IA) administration of contrast material, while arthrography requires the intraarticular injection of contrast material directly into a joint. Intrathecal contrast administration is required for myelography.

   A catheter is used to inject the contrast material in some procedures. In hysterosalpingography, a catheter or cannula is placed into the external cervical os to opacify the uterine cavity. In retrograde urethrography, a Foley catheter is placed at the urethral meatus in a male to inject contrast material to evaluate the urethra. In cystography, injection of contrast material is performed through a catheter placed in the urinary bladder. In retrograde pyelography, contrast material is administered through catheters placed into the renal collecting systems with cystoscopic guidance to evaluate the pyelocalyceal systems and ureters in patients who cannot receive intravenous contrast material.

   The administration of radiographic contrast agents by the various routes mentioned above is widely used in clinical practice, and is usually not associated with any adverse effects. However, prior to administering contrast material, attention must be given to the clinical indication for the procedure, and to the clinical status of the patient in order to minimize adverse side effects and to maximize diagnostic yield. It is essential that in a facility where contrast material is routinely administered for imaging studies, trained personnel along with appropriate equipment and medications be available on site to manage a contrast reaction, should one occur.

2. **What types of contrast agents are available for intravascular use?**

   Iodinated contrast agents are used in all studies where x-rays are utilized, such as CT, intravenous urography (IVU), and all fluoroscopic studies. These can be broadly classified based on osmolality (high, low, or iso-), ionicity (ionic or nonionic), and the number of benzene rings in the chemical structure (monomeric or dimeric). Nonionic contrast agents are associated with less discomfort during intravascular administration and fewer adverse reactions compared to ionic contrast agents. Therefore, nonionic low osmolal or iso-osmolal contrast agents are almost exclusively used in current clinical practice for intravascular injections, particularly in developed countries.

   Gadolinium-based contrast agents are used in MRI studies and can be classified based on ionicity (ionic or nonionic), the chelating ligand (macrocyclic or linear), and the pharmacokinetics (extracellular or organ specific). Ionic and nonionic agents have relatively little or no difference in acute reactions and discomfort.

   There are other types of intravascular contrast agents, such as iron oxide–based contrast agents that are used in MRI studies and microbubble contrast agents that are used in ultrasonography (US) studies; these will not be discussed because they are beyond the scope of this chapter.

3. **How common are acute adverse reactions to intravascular contrast material?**

   Acute adverse events occur in up to 0.7% of patients who receive intravascular low or iso-osmolality iodinated contrast material, and in up to 0.04% of patients who receive gadolinium-based contrast material.

   Most adverse reactions to contrast agents are mild and not life-threatening, usually requiring only observation, reassurance, and/or supportive measures. Severe and potentially life-threatening adverse events occur rarely and unpredictably, most often within the first 20 minutes following contrast administration.

4. **What are the categories of acute adverse reaction to contrast agents?**

   Allergic-like reactions, rather than true allergies, are seen with radiographic contrast administration and are referred to as anaphylactoid reactions. These are not true hypersensitivity reactions, and immunoglobulin E (IgE) antibodies are not involved. The clinical manifestations may be similar to allergic reactions (such as hives or bronchospasm), but these reactions are often idiosyncratic and prior sensitization is not required, unlike with true allergies. These reactions are independent of the dose and concentration of the contrast agent. A history of prior allergic-like contrast reaction may indicate the need for corticosteroid premedication prior to future contrast-enhanced studies that utilize a similar contrast agent.

   Physiologic reactions to contrast agents are associated with the dose, molecular toxicity, and physical and chemical characteristics of the contrast agent. A history of a prior physiologic contrast reaction does not indicate the need for future corticosteroid premedication.

   For a detailed classification of acute adverse reactions to contrast agents, see Table 6-1.

**Table 6-1.** Classification of Acute Contrast Reactions

| SEVERITY | ALLERGIC-LIKE | PHYSIOLOGIC |
|---|---|---|
| Mild: self-limited symptoms and signs | Limited urticaria/pruritus<br>Limited cutaneous edema<br>Limited "itchy"/"scratchy" throat<br>Nasal congestion<br>Sneezing/conjunctivitis/rhinorrhea | Limited nausea/vomiting<br>Transient flushing/warmth/chills<br>Headache/dizziness/anxiety/altered taste<br>Mild hypertension<br>Vasovagal reaction that resolves spontaneously |
| Moderate: more pronounced symptoms and signs, potentially becoming severe if untreated | Diffuse urticaria/pruritus<br>Diffuse erythema, stable vital signs<br>Facial edema without dyspnea<br>Throat tightness or hoarseness without dyspnea<br>Wheezing/bronchospasm, mild or no hypoxia | Protracted nausea/vomiting<br>Hypertensive urgency<br>Isolated chest pain<br>Vasovagal reaction that requires and is responsive to treatment |
| Severe: often life-threatening, potentially resulting in permanent morbidity or death if not managed appropriately | Diffuse edema, or facial edema with dyspnea<br>Diffuse erythema with hypotension<br>Laryngeal edema with stridor and/or hypoxia<br>Wheezing/bronchospasm, significant hypoxia<br>Anaphylactic shock (hypotension and tachycardia)<br>Pulmonary edema<br>Cardiopulmonary arrest | Vasovagal reaction resistant to treatment<br>Arrhythmia<br>Convulsions, seizures<br>Hypertensive emergency<br>Pulmonary edema<br>Cardiopulmonary arrest |

5. What are the 5 important immediate assessments that should be made when evaluating a patient for a potential contrast reaction?
   1. How does the patient look (e.g., level of consciousness and appearance of the skin)?
   2. How does the patient's voice sound? Can the patient speak?
   3. How is the patient's breathing?
   4. What is the patient's pulse strength and rate?
   5. What is the patient's blood pressure?
      For full details regarding the treatment algorithms for acute contrast reactions, which are beyond the scope of this chapter, please see the American College of Radiology (ACR) Manual on Contrast Media (http://www.acr.org/quality-safety/resources/contrast-manual).

6. What are some risk factors that predispose patients to acute adverse contrast reactions?
   • Prior allergic-like reaction to contrast material. (Patients with a history of prior severe contrast reaction have an ≈5- to 6-fold increased risk of a future contrast reaction.)
   • History of severe allergies or reactions to other agents (food or medications), especially when to multiple agents.
   • History of asthma, bronchospasm, or atopy.
   • History of cardiac or renal disease.

7. When do adverse reactions to intravascular iodinated contrast material usually occur?
   Most reactions to intravascular iodinated contrast occur within 1 hour of intravenous administration. However, delayed adverse reactions may occasionally occur between 1 hour and 1 week following contrast administration. Such delayed reactions are seen more commonly in young adults, women, and patients with a history of allergy, are most commonly cutaneous (e.g., urticaria, rash, or angioedema), and are typically mild to moderate in severity and self-limited. The incidence of delayed allergic-like reactions has been reported to range from 0.5% to 14% and may occur more commonly with iso-osmolal dimeric contrast agents.

8. What is iodine "mumps"?
   Iodine "mumps" is sialoadenopathy or salivary gland swelling that may rarely occur in delayed fashion following iodinated contrast administration.

9. When is premedication indicated prior to contrast administration?
   The primary indication for premedication prior to contrast-enhanced imaging is the pretreatment of patients at increased risk for an acute allergic-like reaction to contrast material. Premedication generally involves the administration of corticosteroids, sometimes in conjunction with H1 blockers.
      At our institution, indications for premedication include:
   • Prior moderate or severe allergic-like reaction to contrast material.
   • Prior intravenous contrast reaction requiring administration of epinephrine.
   • Prior life-threatening reaction to any allergen or medication.

- Presence of asthma with active wheezing.
- Presence of asthma requiring intubation in the last 3 months.

10. **What is a breakthrough reaction?**

    A breakthrough reaction is a repeat contrast reaction that occurs in a premedicated patient. Breakthrough reactions are most often similar to the index reaction in terms of severity and clinical presentation. Presence of severe allergies to any other substance, more than four allergies, any drug allergy, and chronic use of oral corticosteroids are associated with a higher risk of a moderate or severe breakthrough reaction.

11. **Is there a specific association between presence of a shellfish allergy and an increased allergy to iodinated contrast material?**

    It is an incorrectly held perception in clinical practice that shellfish allergy specially predisposes patients to contrast reaction. An allergy to shellfish does not increase the risk for an adverse reaction to iodinated contrast material any more than do other allergies.

12. **Is there a specific association between presence of an allergy to iodinated contrast material and having a future reaction to gadolinium-based contrast material?**

    Although there is no cross-reactivity between iodinated and gadolinium-based contrast agents, patients with a history of previous reaction to iodinated contrast material have an increased risk of acute reaction to gadolinium-based contrast material.

13. **How often does extravasation of intravenous contrast material occur?**

    Extravasation of intravenous contrast material (i.e., when administered contrast material escapes the vascular lumen and infiltrates the interstitial tissue at the site of injection) may occur in up to 0.9% of patients following intravenous administration of iodinated contrast material. Extravasation is less commonly encountered following intravenous gadolinium-based contrast administration, because the injected contrast volumes are much lower (typically <20 ml) compared to those studies utilizing iodinated contrast material (typically 100 ml). Most extravasations are limited to the superficial (skin and subcutaneous) soft tissues, and may either be asymptomatic or associated with soft tissue swelling, tightness, pain, or tenderness. However, most contrast extravasations resolve without incident following conservative management with elevation of the extremity and application of warm or cold compresses.

14. **What is the most common severe injury that may occur following extravasation of intravenous contrast material?**

    Acute compartment syndrome is the most common severe injury following intravenous contrast extravasation. This is an extremely rare complication, which occurs when the tissue pressure within a closed muscle compartment exceeds the perfusion pressure secondary to the increased fluid content, leading to muscle and nerve ischemia. It is more likely to occur after the extravasation of a large volume of contrast material, particularly when located in less capacious/distensible areas of the extremity such as the hand, wrist, or forearm.

    If there is clinical evidence for a severe extravasation injury such as progressive swelling or pain, altered tissue perfusion as manifested by a decreased capillary refill, change in sensation in the affected limb, or skin ulceration or blistering, then immediate surgical consultation is indicated. Compartment syndrome is typically treated with decompressive fasciotomy.

15. **What is contrast-induced nephropathy (CIN)?**

    CIN is a deterioration in renal function that is caused by intravascular iodinated contrast administration. It occurs uncommonly, and its exact pathophysiology is not understood. CIN is most commonly defined as either an absolute ($\geq$0.5 mg/dL) or relative ($\geq$25%) increase in serum creatinine levels compared to baseline levels within 48 to 72 hours following the intravascular administration of iodinated contrast material, which is not attributable to other causes. Serum creatinine usually begins to increase within 24 hours of contrast administration, peaks within 4 days, and often returns to baseline within 7 to 10 days.

16. **What are the major risk factors for CIN?**

    Preexisting severe renal insufficiency is the most important risk factor. Other risk factors may include advanced age, dehydration, diabetes mellitus, hypertension, cardiovascular disease, multiple myeloma, hyperuricemia, and administration of multiple doses of iodinated contrast material within a 24-hour period.

17. **What is the best way to prevent CIN?**

    Patient hydration is the simplest and most effective action to prevent CIN in patients who will receive intravascular iodinated contrast material. Otherwise, the simplest and most effective action is to avoid administration of intravascular iodinated contrast material.

18. **Does metformin increase the risk of CIN?**

    No. Metformin, an oral antihyperglycemic drug often used to treat non-insulin-dependent diabetes mellitus, does not confer an increased risk of CIN. However, patients taking metformin who develop renal insufficiency following intravascular iodinated contrast administration may be at increased risk to develop lactic acidosis. Therefore, metformin is temporarily discontinued prior to contrast administration, withheld for 48 hours after contrast administration, and reinstituted only after renal function has been reassessed and found to be normal.

19. Which factors require assessment of patient renal function prior to administration of intravascular contrast material?
    - Patient age >60
    - History of renal disease, including:
      - Dialysis
      - Renal transplant
      - Single kidney
      - Renal cancer
      - Renal surgery
    - History of hypertension requiring medical therapy
    - History of diabetes mellitus
    - Metformin or metformin-containing drug combinations (for iodinated contrast material administration only)
         At our institution, when the serum creatinine level is ≤1.4 mg/dL, iodinated contrast material can be administered, assuming that there are no other contraindications. When the serum creatinine level is between 1.5 and 1.9 mg/dL or rising, iodinated contrast material can still be administered, but only after a conversation with the referring physician has taken place to discuss the risks and benefits of administering contrast material and possible diagnostic test alternatives. When the serum creatinine level is ≥2.0 mg/dL, iodinated contrast material is generally not administered unless there is an urgent medical necessity.

20. What are the major contraindications to the administration of intravascular contrast material?
    - Patient refuses to receive intravascular contrast material.
    - Patient did not receive premedication, when indicated, prior to scheduled contrast administration.
    - Patient has renal insufficiency.
    - Patient has thyroid disease that will be treated with systemic [131]I radiotherapy. This contraindication applies for iodinated, not gadolinium-based, contrast material only. The reason is that iodinated contrast material transiently decreases [131]I radiotracer uptake in the thyroid gland, potentially decreasing the effectiveness of subsequent radioiodide therapy.
    - Patient is pregnant. This contraindication particularly applies for the intravascular administration of gadolinium-based contrast material.

21. Can intravascular iodinated contrast material be safely administered to anuric patients with end-stage renal disease who are on dialysis?
    Yes, patients with anuric end-stage chronic renal disease who do not have a functioning renal transplant can receive intravascular iodinated contrast material without risk of further renal damage, given that the kidneys are no longer functioning. Early postprocedural dialysis is not supported by expert guidelines; the volume of intravenous contrast material may add to fluid overload and should be included in the fluid intake of such patients.
         However, there is a potential risk of converting an oliguric patient on dialysis to an anuric patient on dialysis following contrast administration, although this is somewhat speculative.

22. What is nephrogenic systemic fibrosis (NSF), and who is at risk for developing this complication?
    NSF is a rare systemic fibrotic disorder that primarily involves the skin and subcutaneous tissues, but it can also affect other organs including the lungs, pleura, pericardium, skeletal muscle, and internal organs. It occurs in patients with severe acute or chronic renal dysfunction, including patients who are receiving dialysis of any form, and in many cases is believed to be secondary to the release of free gadolinium ($Gd^{3+}$) ions from the chelates that constitute gadolinium-based contrast agents, with subsequent deposition of insoluble gadolinium phosphate precipitates in bodily tissues. As the contrast agents are metabolized through the renal system, they have a prolonged half-life in patients with decreased renal function, increasing the likelihood that gadolinium release and deposition in tissues will occur. However, NSF can occur without exposure to gadolinium-based contrast agents.
         When NSF is associated with gadolinium-based contrast agents, it usually manifests within 2 to 10 weeks following contrast administration. The risk of NSF may be related to the specific type of contrast agent, the cumulative dose, and the residual renal function of the patient. Macrocyclic gadolinium-based contrast agents are the most stable ones and are associated with the lowest risk of NSF, followed by linear ionic and linear nonionic agents in order of decreasing stability and associated increased risk of NSF.
         NSF has a high morbidity and mortality rate and has no known uniformly effective treatment. Therefore, patients who are planning to undergo MRI with gadolinium-based contrast agents must be carefully screened for renal dysfunction. When the estimated glomerular filtration rate (eGFR) is ≥60 mL/min/1.73m², gadolinium-based contrast material can be administered as indicated, assuming there are no other contraindications. When the eGFR is 30 to 59 mL/min/1.73m², a macrocyclic gadolinium-based contrast material can be administered using the lowest possible dose. When the eGFR is <30 mL/min/1.73m², gadolinium-based contrast material is generally not administered unless there is an urgent medical necessity.

23. Is intravascular iodinated contrast material contraindicated for use in pregnant women?
    No. Even though iodinated contrast material crosses the blood-placental barrier and enters the fetus, there have been no reports of neonatal hypothyroidism or teratogenic effects following maternal intravascular administration of iodinated contrast material.

Because there are no available data to suggest any potential harm to the fetus from exposure to intravascular iodinated contrast administration, iodinated contrast material can be administered to pregnant or potentially pregnant patients when needed for diagnostic purposes. A more important consideration in pregnancy is the risk of radiation exposure to the fetus from imaging studies.

24. **Is intravascular gadolinium-based contrast material contraindicated for use in pregnant women?**
Yes. Gadolinium-based contrast material is assumed to cross the blood-placental barrier and enter the fetus. Although there have been no known adverse effects to fetuses following maternal intravascular gadolinium-based contrast administration, no well-controlled studies of the teratogenic effects of gadolinium-based contrast material in pregnant women have been performed. Yet, teratogenic effects have been shown in animal studies following intravascular administration of high and repeated doses of gadolinium-based contrast material. Furthermore, gadolinium chelates may accumulate in the amniotic fluid with potential for release of free gadolinium ($Gd^{3+}$) ions, potentially conferring a risk for the development of NSF in the mother or fetus.
     Because it is unclear how gadolinium-based contrast material will affect the fetus, gadolinium-based contrast material is contraindicated for use in pregnant women, and it is used only with extreme caution in rare cases following informed patient consent when there is a potential significant benefit to the patient or fetus that outweighs the possible but unknown risk to the fetus.

25. **Is intravascular contrast material safe for use in women who are breast-feeding?**
Yes. Less than 1% of administered iodinated contrast material or gadolinium-based contrast material is excreted in breast milk, and <1% of the contrast material ingested by infants through breast-feeding is absorbed through the gastrointestinal tract. Furthermore, direct toxicity or allergic sensitization or reaction in infants to absorbed contrast material has not been reported. If the mother has concerns about any potential ill effects to her infant, she may express and discard breast milk for 12 to 24 hours after having received contrast material. In anticipation of this, the mother may use a breast pump to obtain and save breast milk during the 24 hours prior to receiving contrast material.

26. **What major types of enteric contrast agent are available?**
Barium sulfate enteric contrast agents (predominantly used in gastrointestinal fluoroscopic and CT studies) are utilized for distention and opacification of the gastrointestinal tract and may be administered by mouth, per rectum, via an ostomy, or via an indwelling bowel catheter. Iodinated enteric contrast agents can alternatively be utilized to distend and opacify the bowel.

27. **What are the major complications of barium sulfate enteric contrast material?**
Leakage of barium sulfate enteric contrast material from the bowel into the mediastinum or peritoneal cavity can lead to mediastinitis or peritonitis, respectively. As such, when bowel perforation is suspected or known to exist, iodinated water-soluble enteric contrast material, rather than barium sulfate enteric contrast material, is administered.
     Aspiration of large volumes of barium sulfate contrast material can lead to acute respiratory distress or pneumonia.
     Adverse reactions to barium sulfate enteric contrast material can occur but are rare and are almost always mild.

28. **What are the major complications of iodinated contrast material when used as an oral contrast agent?**
Aspiration of high-osmolality iodinated oral contrast material can lead to life-threatening pulmonary edema. As such, in patients at high risk for aspiration, this can be mitigated or prevented by use of low or iso-osmolal iodinated oral contrast material or by use of barium sulfate enteric contrast material.
     Approximately 1% to 2% of iodinated enteric contrast material is absorbed and subsequently excreted into the urinary tract. Adverse reactions to iodinated enteric contrast material are rare but can be moderate or severe, particularly in patients with a history of prior reaction to intravascular contrast material, as well as in those with active inflammatory bowel disease, where there may be increased enteric absorption of contrast material.

## KEY POINTS

- A history of a previous severe reaction to a contrast agent increases the overall risk for a subsequent contrast reaction by ≈5- to 6-fold.
- Distinguishing physiologic from allergic-like contrast reactions is important because patients with physiologic reactions do not require future corticosteroid premedication, whereas those with allergic-like reactions may need future corticosteroid premedication.
- Patient hydration is the simplest and most effective action to prevent CIN in patients who will receive intravascular iodinated contrast material.
- If there is clinical evidence for a severe extravasation injury, then immediate surgical consultation is indicated.
- Intravascular gadolinium-based contrast material is contraindicated for use in pregnant patients. However, iodinated contrast material can be administered to pregnant or potentially pregnant patients when needed for diagnostic purposes.

## BIBLIOGRAPHY

Nicola R, Shaqdan KW, Aran S, et al. Contrast media extravasation of computed tomography and magnetic resonance imaging: management guidelines for the radiologist. *Curr Probl Diagn Radiol.* 2016;45(3):161-164.

ACR Manual on Contrast Media, Version 10.1. Available at: <http://www.acr.org/quality-safety/resources/contrast-manual>: ACR Committee on Drugs and Contrast Media, 2015;1-129.

Azzalini L, Spagnoli V, Ly HQ. Contrast-Induced nephropathy: from pathophysiology to preventive strategies. *Can J Cardiol.* 2015.

Beckett KR, Moriarity AK, Langer JM. Safe use of contrast media: what the radiologist needs to know. *Radiographics.* 2015;35(6):1738-1750.

Davenport MS, Cohan RH, Ellis JH. Contrast media controversies in 2015: imaging patients with renal impairment or risk of contrast reaction. *AJR Am J Roentgenol.* 2015;204(6):1174-1181.

Davis PL. Anaphylactoid reactions to the nonvascular administration of water-soluble iodinated contrast media. *AJR Am J Roentgenol.* 2015;204(6):1140-1145.

Lee SY, Rhee CM, Leung AM, et al. A review: radiographic iodinated contrast media-induced thyroid dysfunction. *J Clin Endocrinol Metab.* 2015;100(2):376-383.

Nicola R, Shaqdan KW, Aran K, et al. Contrast-induced nephropathy: identifying the risks, choosing the right agent, and reviewing effective prevention and management methods. *Curr Probl Diagn Radiol.* 2015;44(6):501-504.

Pomara C, Pascale N, Maglietta F, et al. Use of contrast media in diagnostic imaging: medico-legal considerations. *Radiol Med.* 2015;120(9):802-809.

Rose TA Jr, Choi JW. Intravenous imaging contrast media complications: the basics that every clinician needs to know. *Am J Med.* 2015;128(9):943-949.

Tirada N, Dreizin D, Khati NJ, et al. Imaging pregnant and lactating patients. *Radiographics.* 2015;35(6):1751-1765.

Davenport MS, Cohan RH, Khalatbari S, et al. The challenges in assessing contrast-induced nephropathy: where are we now? *AJR Am J Roentgenol.* 2014;202(4):784-789.

Thomsen H, Webb JAW. Contrast media: safety issues and ESUR guidelines. 3rd ed. New York: Springer; 2014.

Kaewlai R, Abujudeh H. Nephrogenic systemic fibrosis. *AJR Am J Roentgenol.* 2012;199(1):W17-W23.

Tremblay E, Therasse E, Thomassin-Naggara I, et al. Quality initiatives: guidelines for use of medical imaging during pregnancy and lactation. *Radiographics.* 2012;32(3):897-911.

Wang PI, Chong ST, Kielar AZ, et al. Imaging of pregnant and lactating patients: part 1, evidence-based review and recommendations. *AJR Am J Roentgenol.* 2012;198(4):778-784.

Prince MR, Zhang H, Zou Z, et al. Incidence of immediate gadolinium contrast media reactions. *AJR Am J Roentgenol.* 2011;196(2):W138-W143.

Hunt CH, Hartman RP, Hesley GK. Frequency and severity of adverse effects of iodinated and gadolinium contrast materials: retrospective review of 456,930 doses. *AJR Am J Roentgenol.* 2009;193(4):1124-1127.

Wiginton CD, Kelly B, Oto A, et al. Gadolinium-based contrast exposure, nephrogenic systemic fibrosis, and gadolinium detection in tissue. *AJR Am J Roentgenol.* 2008;190(4):1060-1068.

Wang CL, Cohan RH, Ellis JH, et al. Frequency, management, and outcome of extravasation of nonionic iodinated contrast medium in 69,657 intravenous injections. *Radiology.* 2007;243(1):80-87.

# CHAPTER 7

# RADIATION DOSE AND SAFETY CONSIDERATIONS IN IMAGING

*Tessa Sundaram Cook, MD, PhD*

1. What is the terminology for radiation dose?

Absorbed dose, equivalent dose, and effective dose are all used to describe the effects of radiation on tissue. Absorbed dose specifically refers to the energy transferred to a quantity of tissue by ionizing radiation. Equivalent dose can be derived from absorbed dose by applying a weighting factor that describes the type of radiation, in order to account for the different biological effects of different types of radiation. X-rays, gamma rays, and beta particles, some types of radiation used in medical imaging, are assigned a weighting factor of 1.

Effective dose is the weighted sum of the equivalent doses for all the tissues of the body. The tissue weighting factors are determined by the International Commission on Radiological Protection (ICRP) and periodically updated. ICRP Publication 103 was the most recent update of the tissue weighting factors, which was released in 2007 [1]. Effective dose is meant to confer an estimate of risk of adverse effects due to exposure to ionizing radiation; it does not describe the actual amount of radiation imparted to or absorbed by the body.

2. In what units is radiation dose expressed?

The modern International System of Units (SI) unit for absorbed radiation dose is the gray (Gy), where 1 Gy = 1 Joule (J)/kilogram (kg) = 100 rad. The sievert (Sv) is the SI unit for equivalent dose, which describes the risk of stochastic biological adverse events, such as cancer and genetic damage, when tissue is irradiated. For ionizing radiation used in diagnostic imaging (x-rays, gamma rays), 1 Sv = 100 rem = 1 Gy. Absorbed dose from a medical imaging test is typically on the order of milligrays (mGy), and the associated biological risk is therefore on the order of millisieverts (mSv). The Sv is also the unit for effective dose, which takes into account the different sensitivities of different types of tissue to ionizing radiation.

3. What organizations make recommendations or monitor the use of ionizing radiation in medical imaging?

The International Commission on Radiological Protection (ICRP) is a not-for-profit, volunteer effort based in the United Kingdom. It is responsible for maintaining the International System of Radiological Protection. The ICRP studies and reports on many aspects of radiation protection, including radiation effects and protection of individuals who are exposed to ionizing radiation in the course of their medical care. The ICRP collaborates with the International Commission on Radiation Units and Measurements (ICRU), a standards body that establishes the units of ionizing radiation and the quantities they represent. The National Council on Radiation Protection and Measurements (NCRP) was chartered by the United States Congress. In conjunction with other organizations such as the ICRP and ICRU, it aims to publish information about radiation protection and radiation units. The Nuclear Regulatory Commission (NRC) is a United States government agency responsible for the safe use of nuclear materials, including those used in medical imaging. The International Atomic Energy Agency (IAEA) is an international organization affiliated with the United Nations. Its mission is to promote the safe and responsible use of nuclear energy. The National Electrical Manufacturers Association (NEMA) was involved in the original development of the Digital Imaging and Communications in Medicine (DICOM) standard used for the creation, storage, and transfer of medical images. The Medical Imaging & Technology Alliance (MITA) of NEMA represents manufacturers of medical imaging equipment and recently introduced the computed tomography (CT) Dose Check initiative for alerts and notifications intended to decrease the risk of exposing patients to excess radiation during CT imaging. The Joint Commission (JC) is currently developing standards for diagnostic imaging and educates the public about medical imaging tests. In 2011, they introduced a Sentinel Event Alert regarding the risks associated with radiation exposure from diagnostic imaging, and requiring reporting of adverse events.

4. What are the recommended annual dose limits for radiation exposure?

Annual dose limits for radiation exposure are established by the NRC in the Code of Federal Regulations [2]. Radiation workers may not receive more than 50 mSv per year to the whole body or 500 mSv to an individual organ or to the skin. A lower annual limit of 150 mSv is prescribed for the lens of the eye, because of the increased risk of cataracts. Radiation workers are required to wear thermoluminescent dosimeters (typically embedded within badges or rings) so that their exposure can be monitored. Radiation workers who exceed annual limits will be prevented from continuing in their occupations for the rest of the year if they exceed the annual limit. Members of the general public are limited to 1 mSv per year. In the United States, this does not apply to individuals who are exposed to ionizing radiation from

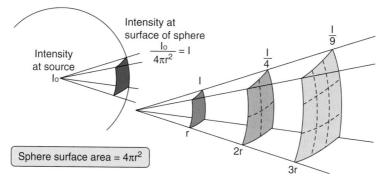

**Figure 7-1.** The inverse square law states that the exposure to radiation from a point source decreases in intensity by $1/r^2$, where $r$ is the distance from the source. *(From http://www.cyberphysics.co.uk/general_pages/inverse_square/inverse_square.htm.)*

medical imaging, and at present there are no limits on the annual exposure of an individual patient. However, many European countries have established diagnostic reference levels (DRLs), which provide recommended limits on radiation dose indices for diagnostic and interventional radiology examinations as well as nuclear medicine studies.

5. **What is the ALARA principle?**
   ALARA stands for "As Low as Reasonably Achievable" [2]. It is the principle that is intended to guide the use of ionizing radiation in medical imaging. According to ICRP Publication 105, there are two principles of radiation safety: justification and dose optimization. Justification indicates that the benefit of the imaging procedure outweighs the risk associated with exposing the patient to a small amount of ionizing radiation. Dose optimization is often summarized as ALARA, but it dictates that the exam should be tailored to the clinical question, patient size, and the anatomy of interest. Furthermore, it also describes the need for proper equipment maintenance and testing, to assure that the amount of radiation to which a patient is exposed is appropriate for the study type.

6. **What is the inverse square law?**
   The inverse square law is a geometric relationship (Figure 7-1) that expresses the intensity of energy emitted by a point source as a function of the distance from that source. It assumes that energy dissipates equally in all directions and that its intensity is inversely proportional to the square of the distance $r$ from the source (i.e., $1/r^2$). The inverse square law is applicable to different types of electromagnetic radiation, including radio waves, light, x-rays, and gamma rays. For this reason, it is a tenet of radiation safety for radiation workers who use fluoroscopy: by doubling one's distance from the x-ray tube of the fluoroscope, one's radiation exposure is decreased by 75%.

7. **What are stochastic and nonstochastic effects of radiation exposure?**
   There are two types of adverse effects from radiation exposure: nonstochastic (also known as deterministic) and stochastic (also known as probabilistic). Nonstochastic effects are nonprobabilistic. They have a known minimum threshold of radiation exposure. If this threshold is not exceeded, it is extremely rare for deterministic effects to occur. However, if the threshold is exceeded, the severity of the deterministic effect will depend on the dose of radiation to which the individual has been exposed. This is commonly described as a dose-related response. Examples of deterministic effects include erythema, epilation (hair loss), cataracts, and, at sufficiently high doses, death. By comparison, stochastic effects are probabilistic. The probability of the occurrence of a stochastic effect is greater at higher doses of radiation exposure, but the severity of the effect is similar whether it occurs from exposure to more or less radiation. The two categories of stochastic effects include cancer induction and genetic mutation. Stochastic effects are not presently believed to have a specific exposure threshold, although this is a subject of debate.

8. **What is the BEIR VII report?**
   The Biological Effects of Ionizing Radiation (BEIR) VII report was issued by the National Research Council in 2006. It describes the relationship between low doses of radiation exposure and the associated risk of solid cancers [3]. Data from Japanese atomic bomb survivors, Chernobyl survivors, patients who underwent radiation therapy for lung and breast cancers, radiation workers (including pilots, medical professionals, and nuclear workers), and individuals living at high altitudes were reviewed in developing the model. The data from the radiation workers showed a protective effect, while the individuals living at high altitudes did not show an increased cancer incidence; data from the former were not included in the model. The report states that "At doses less than . . . 100 mSv, statistical limitations make it difficult to evaluate cancer risk in humans," and the committee felt that the safest conclusion was that the risk would continue linearly toward zero. This resulted in the so-called *linear no-threshold model* for cancer risk estimation.

9. **What is the linear no-threshold model?**
   The linear no-threshold (LNT) model (Figure 7-2) effectively states that there is no safe level of exposure to ionizing radiation, and that cancer risk can be increased at any level of exposure. It was the primary conclusion of the BEIR VII report. Alternative models include a linear model with threshold, a super-linear model, and radiation hormesis. These models were not felt to be supported by the data analyzed for the BEIR VII report. There has been much confusion and

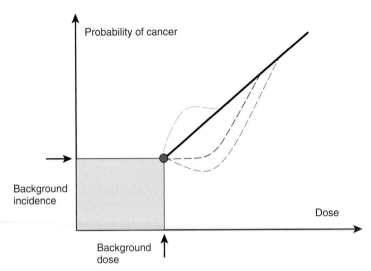

**Figure 7-2.** Models that describe the risk of cancer from exposure to ionizing radiation. The solid black line represents the linear no-threshold model, the dashed black line represents a linear model with a threshold, the dashed blue line represents a super-linear model, and the dashed red line represents hormesis. *(From [23].)*

controversy about deriving cancer risk based on radiation exposure since the introduction of the LNT model [4]. In addition, the appropriateness of the LNT model continues to be questioned, while the lifetime attributable cancer risks based on the BEIR VII report are often incorrectly quoted as scientific fact rather than as "subjective confidence intervals" that incorporate opinion in addition to numerical analysis.

10. **What is radiation hormesis?**
   Radiation hormesis is a hypothesis that suggests that exposure to low levels of radiation expxosure is actually beneficial to biological tissues by stimulating their innate protective mechanisms [5]. In this context, low levels of exposure are defined as those similar to background radiation exposure. The protective mechanisms include: detoxification of reactive oxygen species, repair of DNA damage, induction of apoptosis, increased immune-mediated cell death, induction of terminal differentiation, and increased expression of "stress response" genes. The hypothesis is that exposure to low levels of ionizing radiation stimulates the housekeeping functions of the immune system and persists for hours to days after the exposure. There continues to be a great deal of controversy surrounding this hypothesis, as it is contrary to the LNT hypothesis that was previously introduced. At present, there is no conclusive evidence for either hypothesis.

11. **What are the biological effects of radiation exposure?**
   Radiation exposure causes direct and indirect damage to biological tissues at the cellular level [6]. If the energy of a radiation particle is absorbed by the nucleus of a cell, it has the potential to damage the cell's DNA or an organelle critical for survival. This is considered a direct effect. If the cellular injury is severe enough or interferes with mitosis, the cell will be marked for apoptosis. Alternatively, if the water within the cell absorbs the energy of the radiation particle, reactive oxygen species (also known as free radicals) can be produced via the radiolysis of water. This is considered an indirect effect and can result in damage to the DNA of the originally radiated cell or to other (even distant) cells in the body. Cells that are more mitotically active (i.e., dividing more often) are more sensitive to direct damage from radiation. DNA damage can occur in the form of single-strand or double-strand breaks, single-base alterations, or abnormal cross-linking between DNA strands or between DNA strands and proteins. If the damage is not severe enough to result in cell death, it can be propagated to subsequent generations of cells.

12. **What are the typical sources and annual levels of background radiation exposure?**
   Annual background radiation has been increasing due to the dramatic rise in medical imaging over the past two decades. In the early 1980s, the total annual background radiation exposure was approximately 3.2 mSv, of which only 15% was from medical imaging. Two decades later, the total annual background exposure is approximately 6.2 mSv, with nearly 50% attributed to medical imaging. Figure 7-3 illustrates the breakdown of annual background radiation, comparing the 1980s to 2006. The largest exposure from medical imaging is due to CT.

13. **What are the typical levels of radiation exposure caused by various imaging tests?**
   The actual radiation dose to a patient depends on many factors, including age, gender, body habitus, the type of imaging study, and the parts of the body being radiated. Skin dose is typically higher than organ dose, because the subcutaneous tissues absorb some radiation. Recall that effective dose is not a representation of actual radiation dose to the patient, but rather a metric intended to express the risk of adverse events as a result of the exposure. Mettler et al. provided a detailed catalog of effective doses for diagnostic, interventional, and nuclear medicine procedures in

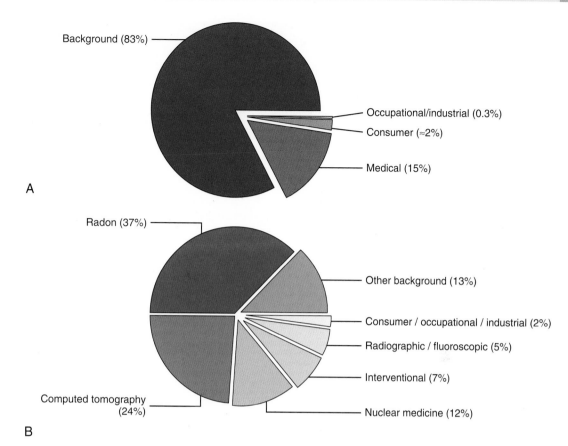

**Figure 7-3.** Annual background radiation in the 1980s (**A**) as compared to 2006 (**B**). Not only has the total annual exposure increased, but so has the proportion attributed to medical imaging. *(From [24].)*

2008, some of which are summarized in Table 7-1 [7]. As a result of the adoption of a variety of dose reduction measures, these reported values are higher than those currently used in clinical practice.

14. **What tools are used to measure radiation exposure in diagnostic imaging?**
    For radiography and CT, phantoms are used to measure and calibrate the output of the x-ray tube [8]. Radiography phantoms are typically geometric structures composed of different materials, such as a combination of acrylic, aluminum, and Lucite. Some radiography phantoms also contain an air gap to simulate air-filled anatomic structures. Mammographic phantoms are composed of acrylic and designed to simulate specific compositions of breast tissue at particular compressed thicknesses. Cylinders of poly(methyl methacrylate) at specific diameters (10 cm, 16 cm, and 32 cm) are used for CT calibration; the different sizes are designed to simulate different body parts (16 cm for head; 32 cm for body) or patient sizes (10 cm and 16 cm for pediatric patients; 32 cm for adult patients). The CT phantoms have holes into which pencil ionization chambers can be inserted to measure $CTDI_{100}$. Dose calibrators, special types of ionization chambers are used in nuclear medicine to measure the amount of radioactivity in a sample of isotope before it is administered to patients. Thermoluminescent dosimeters are incorporated into badges and rings and worn by all radiation workers to track occupational exposure. No devices exist to measure actual absorbed patient dose, and there are no means to directly measure internal organ dose. Monte Carlo simulations, computationally intensive mathematical models that simulate the patient and the type of radiation exposure, can be used to estimate organ doses. However, these estimates are dependent on assumptions made about the scanning equipment and the patient [9]. Some organ dose calculations use mathematical models of a hermaphrodite phantom, while others use anthropomorphic phantoms. This is an ongoing area of research as to development of more patient-specific models that can be used for organ dose calculation. As new imaging equipment is designed, the modeling of the scanner is updated to incorporate this information.

15. **What is CTDI?**
    The computed tomography dose index (CTDI) represents a set of radiation dose descriptors developed to explain the radiation dose to a phantom from a series of rotations of the x-ray tube [10]. $CTDI_{100}$ represents the radiation exposure to a 100-mm pencil ionization chamber. When this chamber is placed at the center or near the periphery of a cylindrical CT phantom, the $CTDI_w$ can be calculated as a weighted average, giving twice as much weight to the

**Table 7-1.** Effective Doses for Common Diagnostic Radiology Examinations (Summarized from [7])

| EXAMINATION/PROCEDURE | AVERAGE EFFECTIVE DOSE (MSV) | RANGE OF EFFECTIVE DOSES IN THE LITERATURE (MSV) |
|---|---|---|
| **Radiography** | | |
| Posteroanterior chest | 0.02 | 0.007-0.050 |
| Posteroanterior and lateral chest | 0.1 | 0.05-0.24 |
| Lumbar spine | 1.5 | 0.5-1.8 |
| Knee | 0.005 | N/A |
| **Fluoroscopy** | | |
| Upper gastrointestinal series | 6 | 1.5-12.0 |
| Barium enema | 8 | 2.0-18.0 |
| **CT** | | |
| Head | 2 | 0.9-4.0 |
| Chest | 7 | 4.0-18.0 |
| Abdomen | 8 | 3.5-25.0 |
| Pelvis | 6 | 3.3-10.0 |
| **Interventional** | | |
| Head and/or neck angiography | 5 | 0.8-19.6 |
| Coronary angiography (diagnostic) | 7 | 2.0-15.8 |
| Abdominal angiography or aortography | 12 | 4.0-48.0 |
| Transjugular intrahepatic portosystemic shunt (TIPS) placement | 70 | 20-180 |
| **Dental Radiography** | | |
| Intraoral radiography | 0.005 | 0.0002-0.0010 |
| Panoramic radiography | 0.1 | 0.007-0.090 |
| Dental CT | 0.2 | N/A |

peripheral measurement as to the central one. This weighted average can then be adapted for axial or helical scanning to produce the volume CTDI, denoted as $CTDI_{vol}$. The $CTDI_{vol}$ is typically used to compare CT protocols on different scanner equipment and as a cutoff for accreditation. However, because it is a phantom-based calculation, it does not incorporate features of the patient, such as size, age, gender, and the anatomic region of interest, which can cause significant variation in actual absorbed patient dose. It is critical to remember that none of the CTDI descriptors represents actual dose absorbed by the patient as a result of a CT examination.

16. What is SSDE?

The size-specific dose estimate (SSDE) was introduced by AAPM Task Group 204 to address the difficulty in comparing CT dose indices between protocols and scanners [11]. The SSDE was derived using computer models designed to simulate CT scanning of patients of different age, gender, and size, because these factors strongly influence the radiation dose received. The SSDE is calculated by multiplying the $CTDI_{vol}$ by a conversion factor that depends on patient diameter at the center of the scan region. It helps to provide a better estimate of the $CTDI_{vol}$ that accounts for patient size. It is designed to be used for pediatric patients and adult patients up to a specific diameter. Using the SSDE to compare protocols across scanners or patients is more accurate than using an uncorrected $CTDI_{vol}$ or DLP, although the SSDE is also not a measurement of actual patient absorbed dose [12].

17. What is DLP, and how is it calculated?

The dose-length product (DLP) is another type of CT radiation dose parameter. It represents the product of $CTDI_{vol}$ and the craniocaudal (head to toe) dimension of the scan region and is reported in units of mGy-cm [10]. For a specific CT imaging protocol, the DLP can vary from one patient to the next because taller patients may require a longer scan region than shorter patients. As with CTDI, DLP does not represent actual dose absorbed by the patient. In addition, SSDE cannot be multiplied by scan length to produce a modified DLP.

18. What is effective dose, and how is it calculated?

Effective dose is defined as "the mean absorbed dose from a uniform whole-body irradiation that results in the same total radiation detriment as from the nonuniform, partial-body irradiation in question" [13]. It was introduced in 1975 to provide a means by which the "detriment," or underlying risk of biological injury, could be normalized for exposures of different parts of the body to different types of radiation at different levels. Numerically speaking, effective dose is the weighted sum of the absorbed organ and tissue doses; the weighting factors are designed to convey the radiation detriment associated with each organ or tissue. However, organ and tissue doses are impossible to measure and can only be calculated with a large number of assumptions. The concept of effective dose was originally intended for use at the population level for the general population or the population of radiation workers. It was never intended to describe the radiation exposure to an individual patient, even though conversion factors exist for calculating effective dose estimates from DLP. Effective dose continues to be used as a surrogate for radiation exposure in the absence of more appropriate and accurate metrics. Effective dose is not actual patient dose and should not be reported as such or used to determine if a patient has had "too much" radiation that would preclude another imaging examination.

19. **What approaches are available to reduce exposure to imaging radiation dose?**

Many simple modifications can decrease unnecessary radiation exposure to patients. The first and most important consideration is: Does the study need to be done? If there is a modality that does not require ionizing radiation (such as ultrasonography [US] or magnetic resonance imaging [MRI]) that would provide equivalent or better diagnostic information, it should be performed instead. Each modality—radiography, fluoroscopy, CT, and nuclear medicine techniques—has unique dose reduction techniques. In radiography, dose reduction is best achieved by properly configuring the imaging study: correctly positioning the patient, aligning the x-ray tube with the detector, adding or removing the grid as appropriate, and using collimation. Dose reduction in fluoroscopy can be achieved by using the "last image hold" feature, which retains the last low-dose exposure on the display screen after the x-ray tube has been turned off. If there is a finding of interest on this exposure, a full-dose image can be acquired. In addition, only turning on the x-ray tube incrementally rather than leaving it on continuously significantly reduces patient radiation exposure. Minimizing the distance between the x-ray tube, patient, and image intensifier can also decrease radiation exposure. For long interventional procedures, periodically readjusting the angle of the x-ray tube can decrease the risk of skin injury. In CT, simple adjustments like centering the patient in the scanner bore, setting the scan region to not include anatomy beyond the region of interest, minimizing the number of image acquisitions, and adjusting the scan parameters for patient size can all decrease radiation exposure. Recent technological advancements such as x-ray tube current modulation, x-ray tube voltage optimization, iterative reconstruction (an alternative to filtered back-projection for reconstructing images from the raw CT data), dual-energy scanning, larger detectors, and more powerful x-ray tubes have also enabled dramatic decreases in the amount of radiation used to image patients [14]. The most technologically advanced CT scanners currently available can perform chest CT examinations at effective doses only slightly higher than those of a frontal and lateral chest radiographic examination. In nuclear medicine studies, using only as much radiotracer as is necessary for diagnosis can help decrease radiation exposure. One salient example of this is perfusion-only scintigraphy, which is sometimes performed in pregnant patients with suspected pulmonary embolism. The extra radiation exposure from a second dose of radiotracer used for a ventilation scan is eliminated, and a decreased dose of radiotracer is used for the perfusion scan. All the techniques described above can be implemented in adult and pediatric patients. However, it is also critical when imaging pediatric patients to use pediatric protocols instead of adult protocols.

20. **What is the American College of Radiology (ACR) Dose Index Registry (DIR)?**

The ACR DIR is an international effort to collect CT radiation dose indices and provide comparison data to participating facilities. Facilities are able to transmit their dose indices to the ACR electronically, either directly from the CT scanner on which the study was performed or from an auxiliary computer at the facility. The ACR provides each facility with a web-based dashboard on which they can access summary reports of their submitted parameters, as well as comparisons to equivalent facilities in their region and at the national level (Figure 7-4). For example, a small community hospital is compared to other similar hospitals, rather than to a large academic medical center. In order to perform these head-to-head comparisons, each participating facility must map their unique exam codes and descriptions to a set of standard exam codes and descriptions called the RadLex Playbook. More information about the DIR is available online at http://www.acr.org/Quality-Safety/National-Radiology-Data-Registry/Dose-Index-Registry.

21. **What is Image Wisely?**

The Image Wisely campaign is a collaboration between the ACR, the Radiological Society of North America (RSNA), the American Association of Physicists in Medicine (AAPM), and the American Society of Radiologic Technologists (ASRT). Its goal is to decrease the amount of radiation used in medical imaging procedures and to decrease the number of unnecessary imaging examinations performed. The Image Wisely website (http://www.imagewisely.org) offers a variety of resources for radiologists, medical physicists, technologists, medical professionals, and patients to learn more about imaging modalities, equipment, and radiation safety.

22. **What is Image Gently$^{SM}$?**

The Alliance for Radiation Safety in Pediatric Imaging, also known as the Image Gently$^{SM}$ alliance, was launched in 2007 to increase awareness and provide education about radiation safety in pediatric imaging. It is a collaborative effort of the Society of Pediatric Radiology (SPR), the ACR, the AAPM, and the ASRT. The Image Gently$^{SM}$ website (http://www.imagegently.org) provides resources for parents, imaging technologists, physicists, radiologists, and referring providers. It also offers information about different imaging modalities and particular considerations when imaging children of different ages.

23. **What is the Mammography Quality Standards Act (MQSA)?**

The Mammography Quality Standards Act of 1992 is a federal mandate to ensure high quality in performance and reporting of mammography in the United States. All aspects of mammography practice are highly regulated, including

| Category | Number of Facilities | Mean | Std Dev | Min | 25th %ile | 50th %ile | 75th %ile | Max |
|---|---|---|---|---|---|---|---|---|
| DIR | 463 | 14 | 5 | 3 | 10 | 13 | 16 | 41 |
| Suburban | 187 | 14 | 5 | 5 | 10 | 13 | 16 | 38 |
| Middle Atlantic | 106 | 14 | 6 | 5 | 10 | 13 | 16 | 38 |
| Community Hospital | 212 | 15 | 6 | 5 | 11 | 14 | 18 | 41 |

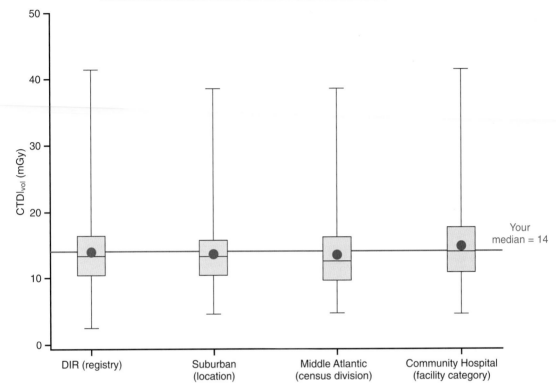

**Figure 7-4.** The ACR's Dose Index Registry (DIR) provides enrolled facilities with comparison CT dose indices from other comparable facilities, in an effort to guide protocol modifications to reduce unnecessary radiation exposure and ultimately develop international benchmarks for radiation exposure for various CT examinations. CTDI$_{vol}$ = volume computed tomography dose index. *(From http://www.acr.org/~/media/ACR/Documents/PDF/QualitySafety/NRDR/DIR/DIRSampleReport.pdf.)*

the accreditation of facilities that perform mammography; the initial and continued training of technologists who perform mammography, radiologists who interpret it, and medical physicists who manage it; and the performance of quality control testing (including test type, schedule, and responsible individuals). MQSA has been updated as clinical practice transitioned from screen-film mammography to full-field digital mammography and after digital breast tomosynthesis (DBT) was introduced. The ACR is a Food and Drug Administration (FDA)-approved accreditation body for full-field digital mammography and DBT.

24. What are the risks of radiation to the fetus?

The risks associated with fetal radiation exposure depend on the gestational age of the fetus and the radiation dose absorbed [15]. During the first week after conception, there is an all-or-nothing effect for which the threshold radiation exposure is unknown in humans but ranges from 50 to 100 mGy preimplantation and 250 mGy postimplantation in animals. If the fetus survives this radiation exposure, the pregnancy will progress normally. After the first week of gestation, there is a risk of growth retardation with exposures above 200 mGy, organ malformation with exposures above 250 mGy, or severe mental retardation or decreased IQ with exposures above 100 mGy. All these effects were observed during the first trimester. The risk of childhood cancer increases by less than 1% with 100 mGy of exposure, while the risk of a birth defect increases by approximately 0.2% for the same exposure. As a reference, most imaging procedures result in substantially less than 50 mGy of absorbed dose to the fetus, which is well under the thresholds for the deterministic effects described above. A 50 mGy fetal exposure is associated with a 0.42% increase in the probability of childhood cancer and a 0.1% increase in the probability of birth defects.

25. **What types of imaging are permissible in the setting of pregnancy?**

    A variety of imaging modalities, including those that use ionizing radiation and those that do not, can be used in pregnant patients. Pregnant patients are consented for possible risks to themselves and their unborn children before the imaging is performed. MRI and US are generally considered as safe in pregnancy. Radiography, CT, and fluoroscopy, although delivering ionizing radiation, can be used judiciously when the potential diagnostic benefits outweigh the potential risks of radiation exposure. The gravid abdomen can be shielded with lead drapes for imaging of the chest, and in early pregnancy the pelvis can be shielded if abdominal imaging is required. Nuclear medicine examinations are used only if absolutely necessary and are customized to administer decreased doses of radiotracer. The use of intravenous contrast is limited in pregnancy, as both gadolinium-based MRI contrast agents and iodinated CT contrast agents cross the placenta [16]. Gadolinium-based MRI contrast agents are typically not administered to pregnant patients as they are excreted by the fetal kidneys into the amniotic fluid and can remain there for an unspecified period of time. Animal studies have shown teratogenic effects from gadolinium exposure, but evidence in humans is limited and has shown no adverse effects. If necessary, iodinated CT contrast is used as it can be excreted by the maternal kidneys. However, free iodine that enters the fetal circulation can affect fetal thyroid function. Neonates of mothers who have received iodinated contrast media during pregnancy undergo thyroid function testing during the first week of life to identify any potential issues.

26. **What are the potential safety hazards of US, and how are they avoided?**

    Diagnostic US is an extremely safe modality that is regularly used in a variety of patients. Because it uses high-frequency sound rather than ionizing radiation, it is safe in pregnant patients and children of all ages. In fact, US is the preferred imaging modality in children, and it is even used in neonates (typically for brain imaging). Pulsed Doppler imaging, a high-power ultrasound mode, is used sparingly during the first trimester, a vulnerable period for the developing fetus, because there is evidence of adverse effects in animal studies [17].

27. **How is a radioactive spill managed?**

    Spills of radioactive material are typically classified into major and minor types. Classification as a major or minor spill depends on the radiotracer. For example, a major spill is considered to have occurred with only 1 mCi of $^{131}$I, but with greater than 100 mCi of $^{99m}$Tc, $^{201}$Tl, or $^{67}$Ga. The approach to cleaning up a radioactive spill is summarized in Box 7-1 [18]. For both major and minor spills, individuals in the surrounding area should be warned, and the spill should be covered in an attempt to prevent further spread. Minor spills can be cleaned with soap and water, but major spills should be contained and cleanup should proceed under the direction of the radiation safety officer. Contaminated materials (e.g., clothing, paper towels, gloves, etc.) should be collected and either isolated for the appropriate period of time based on the radiotracer's half-life or disposed of appropriately for that particular radiotracer.

28. **What are the potential safety hazards of MRI, and how are they avoided?**

    The greatest safety hazard of MRI is related to the very powerful magnet within the scanner. Any ferromagnetic materials within the scanner room have the potential to become projectiles and become attached to the outer housing of the scanner or embedded in the scanner bore. This applies to nonmedical objects (e.g., keys, jewelry/piercings, watches, hair accessories, hearing aids, pagers/mobile phones, computers, scissors, weapons, etc.) as well as equipment commonly found in the hospital (e.g., wheelchairs, stretchers, oxygen canisters, laryngoscopes, etc.). If this occurs while a patient is on the scanner table, drastic—even fatal—consequences may result. For this reason, patients are screened for ferromagnetic materials before entering the MRI scanner room, and medical staff are required to complete MRI safety training before being allowed to enter the scanner room. In addition, there are a number of contraindications to MRI that are discussed below.

29. **What are some contraindications to performing MRI?**

    There are numerous contraindications to MRI for which patients should be screened prior to imaging [19, 20]. Absolute contraindications have historically included pacemakers/defibrillators, metallic foreign bodies in the eyes, deep brain stimulators, cerebral aneurysm clips, cochlear implants, Swan-Ganz catheters, and bullet fragments. The risks of performing MRI when these devices or implants are present include tissue heating, device movement, or device damage resulting in malfunction or necessitating replacement. Relative contraindications exist when certain types of implants, such as cardiac prosthetic valves, have been acutely implanted (e.g., less than 4 to 6 weeks). More recently,

---

**Box 7-1.** Procedure for Managing a Radioactive Spill (from [18])

1. Notify all persons in the area that a spill has occurred.
2. Prevent the spread of contamination by isolating the area and covering the spill (absorbent paper).
3. If clothing is contaminated, remove and place in plastic bag.
4. If an individual is contaminated, rinse contaminated region with lukewarm water and wash with soap.
5. Notify the radiation safety officer.
6. Wear gloves, disposable laboratory coat, and booties to clean up spill with absorbent paper.
7. Put all contaminated absorbent paper in labeled radioactive waste container.
8. Check the area or contaminated individual with appropriate radiation survey meter.

it has become possible for patients with pacemakers/defibrillators to undergo MRI in a controlled setting [21]. New devices are continuously being developed that are MRI-safe or MRI-compatible (safe under specific scanner settings and configurations). http://www.mrisafety.com provides a regularly updated comprehensive database regarding which devices are MRI-safe or MRI-compatible.

30. **What is specific absorption rate (SAR), and what are the mandated limits?**
The specific absorption rate (SAR) is defined as the rate at which energy is absorbed by tissue when exposed to a radiofrequency pulse, such as during MRI or therapeutic US. It is described in units of watts per kilogram (W/kg). For example, 1 W/kg would increase the temperature of a slab of tissue by 1° C/hr. SAR is proportional to the square of the magnetic field strength, so it increases by a factor of 4 when switching from a 1.5-T scanner to a 3-T scanner. For MRI, SAR limits are defined for the whole body, local anatomy, or extremities. Different limits are specified by the FDA and the International Electrotechnical Commission (IEC) [22].

31. **What is quenching?**
Quenching is the rapid release of the liquid cryogens used to maintain the magnet of an MRI scanner in its superconducting state. Liquid cryogens are gases kept in their liquid state at very low temperatures. For MRI scanners, helium is typically used and allows the superconducting magnets to operate at a very low level of energy consumption. When the magnet quenches, the liquid helium evaporates and is vented out of the building, and the release is typically accompanied by a loud bang or hissing. The magnetic coils then change from being superconductive to resistive, and the magnetic field strength drops significantly (though not always completely to zero). Quenching may be spontaneous or intentional (i.e., by pressing the scanner's STOP button); both causes are extremely rare. Spontaneous quenching may occur due to magnet malfunction, severe vibration, or insufficient or impure cryogens. Intentional quenching may be necessary if the magnet is resulting in injury to a patient or medical personnel, or in the event of a fire or other event that requires emergent access to the MRI scanner room.

## KEY POINTS

- Dose optimization is often summarized as ALARA ("as low as reasonably achievable"), but it dictates that the radiologic examination should be tailored to the clinical question, patient size, and anatomy of interest.
- A variety of imaging modalities, including those that use ionizing radiation and those that do not, can be utilized in the pregnant patient, as long as they are adjusted to minimize fetal and maternal exposure while still yielding diagnostic information.
- Many resources exist to assist radiologists and ordering providers to minimize unnecessary radiation exposure to patients; these include the Image Wisely and Image Gently[SM] initiatives, as well as the American College of Radiology's Dose Index Registry.

**BIBLIOGRAPHY**

1. The 2007 Recommendations of the International Commission on Radiological Protection. ICRP publication 103. *Annals ICRP.* 2007;37(2-4):1-332.
2. NRC. 10 CFR Part 20: Standards for protection against radiation [Internet]. Available at <www.nrc.gov/reading-rm/doc-collections/cfr/part020/full-text.html>. 1991.
3. National Research Council of the National Academies. Health risks from exposure to low levels of ionizing radiation: BEIR VII Phase 2. Washington, D.C.: The National Academies Press; 2006.
4. Hendee WR, O'Connor MK. Radiation risks of medical imaging: separating fact from fantasy. *Radiology.* 2012;264(2):312-321.
5. Feinendegen LE. Evidence for beneficial low level radiation effects and radiation hormesis. *Br J Radiol.* 2005;78(925):3-7.
6. Morgan WF, Day JP, Kaplan MI, et al. Genomic instability induced by ionizing radiation. *Radiat Res.* 1996;146(3):247-258.
7. Mettler FA Jr, Huda W, Yoshizumi TT, et al. Effective doses in radiology and diagnostic nuclear medicine: a catalog. *Radiology.* 2008;248(1):254-263.
8. AAPM. Standardized methods for measuring diagnostic x-ray exposure (Report #31) [Internet]. Available at <www.aapm.org/pubs/reports/rpt_8.pdf>. 1990.
9. Lee C, Kim KP, Long D, et al. Organ doses for reference adult male and female undergoing computed tomography estimated by Monte Carlo simulations. *Med Phys.* 2011;38(3):1196-1206.
10. McNitt-Gray MF. AAPM/RSNA physics tutorial for residents: topics in CT. Radiation dose in CT. *Radiographics.* 2002;22(6):1541-1553.
11. AAPM. Size-specific dose estimates (SSDE) in pediatric and adult body CT examinations (Report #204) [Internet]. Available at <www.aapm.org/pubs/reports/rpt_204.pdf>. 2011.
12. Seibert JA, Boone JM, Wootton-Gorges SL, et al. Dose is not always what it seems: where very misleading values can result from volume CT dose index and dose length product. *J Am Coll Radiol.* 2014;11(3):233-237.
13. McCollough CH, Schueler BA. Calculation of effective dose. *Med Phys.* 2000;27(5):828-837.
14. McCollough CH, Primak AN, Braun N, et al. Strategies for reducing radiation dose in CT. *Radiol Clin North Am.* 2009;47(1):27-40.
15. McCollough CH, Schueler BA, Atwell TD, et al. Radiation exposure and pregnancy: when should we be concerned? *Radiographics.* 2007;27(4):909-917, discussion 17-8.
16. Webb JA, Thomsen HS, Morcos SK. The use of iodinated and gadolinium contrast media during pregnancy and lactation. *Eur Radiol.* 2005;15(6):1234-1240.
17. Salvesen KA, Lees C, Abramowicz J, et al. Safe use of Doppler ultrasound during the 11 to 13 + 6-week scan: is it possible? *Ultrasound Obstet Gynecol.* 2011;37(6):625-628.

18. Ziessman HA, O'Malley JP, Thrall JH, et al. Nuclear medicine: the requisites. 4th ed. Philadelphia, PA: Elsevier Saunders; 2014.
19. Shellock FG, Crues JV. MR procedures: biologic effects, safety, and patient care. *Radiology*. 2004;232(3):635-652.
20. Dill T. Contraindications to magnetic resonance imaging: non-invasive imaging. *Heart*. 2008;94(7):943-948.
21. Zikria JF, Machnicki S, Rhim E, et al. MRI of patients with cardiac pacemakers: a review of the medical literature. *AJR Am J Roentgenol*. 2011;196(2):390-401.
22. Bottomley PA. Turning up the heat on MRI. *J Am Coll Radiol*. 2008;5(7):853-855.
23. Fahey FH, Treves ST, Adelstein SJ. Minimizing and communicating radiation risk in pediatric nuclear medicine. *J Nucl Med Technol*. 2012;40(1):13-24.
24. NCRP. Ionizing radiation exposure of the population of the United States (Report #160) [Internet]. Available at <http://www.ncrponline.org/Publications/Press_Releases/160press.html>. 2009.

# II
# BREAST IMAGING

# CHAPTER 8

# SCREENING MAMMOGRAPHY

*Susan P. Weinstein, MD*

1. **What is a screening mammogram?**

   A screening mammogram is a radiographic examination of the breasts performed to detect clinically occult breast cancer in asymptomatic women.

2. **When should an average woman start getting mammograms?**

   This is currently a topic of debate. The American College of Radiology (ACR) recommends that a woman get a baseline mammogram at age 40 and annual screening mammograms thereafter. The American Cancer Society (ACS) recommends that women with an average risk of breast cancer should undergo screening mammography starting at age 45 (annually in women of age 45-54 and either annually or biennially in women age 55 and older), although they should have the opportunity to begin annual screening between ages 40-44. The United States Preventative Services Task Force (USPSTF) recommends that women of ages 50-74 undergo biennial screening mammography, although biennial screening may be started in women of age 40-49 on an individual basis.

3. **Are there instances when screening should start earlier than 40?**

   Women who have been treated for Hodgkin lymphoma should begin screening 10 years after chest wall/mediastinal radiation. Patients who received radiation therapy during puberty are at greatest risk for breast cancer, whereas those who received radiation therapy after age 30 have a minimally increased risk over the general population. For patients with a history of a first-degree relative with breast cancer, screening should begin 10 years before the age at which the relative was diagnosed. If the relative was diagnosed after age 50, there would be no impact on the screening recommendation. If the relative was diagnosed before age 50, the woman should begin screening before the age of 40. Women with genetic mutations also begin screening at an earlier age. These include *BRCA1* and *BRCA2* mutation carriers as well as women with *PTEN* mutations. Also included are women and their first-degree relatives with the following syndromes: Li-Fraumeni, Cowden, and Bannayan-Riley-Ruvalcaba.

4. **How many views are obtained for a routine mammogram?**

   Four views are obtained for a routine mammogram. Mediolateral oblique (MLO) and craniocaudal (CC) views of each breast are obtained (Figure 8-1). In some patients, more than four images may be needed to visualize all of the breast parenchyma adequately.

5. **Which view visualizes the most breast tissue?**

   MLO view visualizes the most breast tissue.

6. **Which portion of the breast is better visualized on the CC view than on the MLO view?**

   The medial breast is better visualized on the CC view.

7. **What if there are comparison studies elsewhere? Do we need to get them?**

   If the mammogram is negative, no. Research has shown that it is not cost-effective and does not improve patient care to obtain comparison studies for examinations that are normal. If there is an abnormal finding, an attempt should be made to get the prior studies from the outside institution. If they cannot be obtained, the patient should be recalled for additional evaluation.

8. **What is the incidence of screening-detected breast cancer?**

   In a population that has never been screened, the incidence is about 6 to 10 per 1000. In a population that is routinely screened, the incidence decreases to about 2 to 4 per 1000 women screened.

9. **What is the reported sensitivity of screening mammography?**

   False-negative interpretation (mammograms that are interpreted as negative although a cancer is present) is reported to occur in 15% to 20%. The sensitivity decreases as the glandularity of the breast tissue increases. The sensitivity of mammography in women with dense breast tissue is about 50%. With fatty breast tissue, the sensitivity of mammography is quite high, in the high 90s percentile.

10. **What is the difference between a screening mammogram and a diagnostic mammogram?**

    A screening mammogram is performed as part of routine annual surveillance. A diagnostic mammogram is performed when the patient has a history of breast cancer or presents with a breast-related complaint or symptom such as a breast lump, abscess, or nipple discharge.

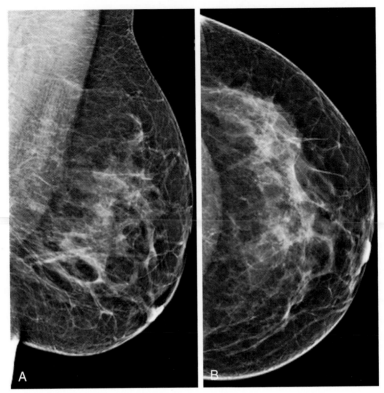

**Figure 8-1. A,** Normal MLO view of a breast. **B,** Normal CC view of a breast.

11. Are there other types of breast cancer screening modalities? Which modalities are used in everyday clinical practice?

Digital mammography is the standard today. Film screen mammography is slowly being phased out in clinical practice. Based on the digital platform, digital breast tomosynthesis (DBT) imaging can also be performed. In DBT imaging, multiple images are acquired through the breast over a range of angles resulting in reconstruction of 9 to 25 images. Instead of one image, multiple images are generated for each mammographic view. Studies to date have demonstrated improved lesion conspicuity for suspicious masses and architectural distortion across all breast densities with DBT.

Screening breast ultrasonography (US) consists of examination of both breasts in asymptomatic women. The largest prospective study to date was sponsored by the American College of Radiology Imaging Network (ACRIN). The goal of the prospective, multicenter trial was to compare the diagnostic yield of screening mammography plus US versus screening mammography alone in high-risk women. Although screening US examinations found additional breast cancers, there were also some false-positive results.

Screening magnetic resonance imaging (MRI) is not likely to be used in everyday clinical practice for the average risk woman because of the lack of availability, high cost, and potential for false-positive interpretations. However, MRI screening is used to screen very high-risk patients. The average woman has approximately 12% lifetime risk of being diagnosed with breast cancer. The American Cancer Society guidelines recommend MRI screening in women with a greater than 20% to 25% lifetime risk for breast cancer. The screening groups include women who are carriers of the *BRCA* mutations or untested women with a first-degree relative who is a known carrier; women with a history of mantle field radiation before age 30; and women with Li-Fraumeni, Cowden, and Bannayan-Riley-Ruvalcaba syndromes. MRI screening cancer yield in high-risk patients has consistently been 2% to 3%.

12. Is digital mammography better than film screen mammography in detecting breast cancer?

The largest prospective multicenter trial comparing digital mammography with film screen mammography is the Digital Mammographic Imaging Screening Trial (DMIST) sponsored by ACRIN. The study recruited more than 49,000 women. Overall, in the general population, the study showed that the accuracy of digital mammography was similar to film screen mammography. However, digital mammography was superior to film screen mammography in certain subpopulations, including women younger than age 50 years, women with heterogeneously or extremely dense breasts, and premenopausal or perimenopausal women.

13. **Is there an age at which breast cancer screening should stop?**
    In the United States, there are no guidelines for when screening should stop. In other countries, the recommended age at which screening should stop ranges from 59 to 74 years.

14. **What are some risk factors for developing breast cancer?**
    Perhaps the greatest risk factor is being a female. Men get breast cancer, but male breast cancer accounts for less than 1% of all breast cancers diagnosed annually. Other risk factors include presence of a genetic mutation (*BRCA1* and *BRCA2*) carrier status, prior mantle field radiation, having a first-degree relative with breast cancer, personal history of breast cancer, history of breast atypia such as atypical ductal hyperplasia and lobular carcinoma in situ on biopsy, early menarche, late menopause, nulliparous status, late first-term pregnancy (>30 years old), and advancing age.

15. **True or false: Most breast cancers occur in women with a family history of breast cancer.**
    False. About 20% of breast cancers occur in patients with a positive family history. About 75% to 80% of breast cancers are sporadic.

16. **True or false: The incidence of breast cancer is currently rising.**
    False. The incidence of breast cancer steadily increased from the 1980s until the 1990s. The increased incidence in the 1980s has been partly attributed to early detection due to increased breast cancer screening with mammography during this time period. The incidence leveled off in the 1990s, began to decline starting about 1999 until 2003, and now has plateaued according to the National Cancer Institute Surveillance Epidemiology and End Results (SEER) data. The reason for this decreased incidence is unclear and may only become evident over time. According to the SEER data, it is projected that 246,660 women will be diagnosed with breast cancer in 2016, representing 15% of all cancer, and that 40,450 women will die of cancer from breast cancer.

17. **It has been said that one in eight women has a risk of developing breast cancer. Does a 40-year-old woman have the same risk as an 80-year-old woman?**
    No. The one-in-eight risk of developing breast cancer refers to an overall lifetime risk if the woman lives to age 85. Given identical circumstances, an average 40-year-old woman has a much lower risk than an 80-year-old woman.

18. **What are *BRCA1* and *BRCA2* genes?**
    *BRCA1* and *BRCA2* are tumor suppressor genes which have autosomal dominant expression and may be inherited from the maternal or paternal side. Women who carry a *BRCA1* or *BRCA2* gene mutation have an increased risk of developing cancer, with breast and ovarian cancers being the two most common types. With regards to breast cancer, women who have the genetic mutation tend to develop breast cancer at an earlier age than the general population and are more likely to develop bilateral breast cancer. Men with *BRCA1* and *BRCA2* mutations are at increased risk of developing prostate cancer. Men who carry the *BRCA1* mutation are also at increased risk for breast cancer. Approximately 65% of *BRCA1* mutation carriers and 45% of *BRCA2* mutation carriers will be diagnosed with breast cancer by age 70.

19. **How much radiation does a woman receive from a routine screening mammogram?**
    The amount of radiation for a digital mammogram is typically 3 to 5 mGy for a two-view digital examination. Although there is radiation exposure, the amount is considered small and is believed to be outweighed by the benefits of early breast cancer detection from screening.

20. **What is the call-back rate? What should the call-back rate be for a radiologist?**
    The call-back rate is the percentage of the screening cases that the radiologist recommends for additional imaging evaluations. The call-back rate should be 10% or less.

21. **Is the breast a modified skin gland, fatty tissue, muscle, or lymphatic structure?**
    The breast tissue is derived from ectodermal origin and is a modified skin gland.

22. **How does accessory breast tissue form? Where is it most commonly located?**
    Breast tissue development begins at about 6 weeks of gestation and originates from ectodermal elements. The "milk line" extends from the groin region to the axillary region. Most of the potential breast tissue atrophies except in the fourth intercostal region, where "normal" mammary tissue eventually develops. The lack of appropriate regression results in accessory breasts anywhere along the "milk line."

## KEY POINTS

- Mammography is still the best screening test to detect subclinical breast cancer.
- The sensitivity of mammography is in the range of 85%.
- Most breast cancers occur in women with no family history of the disease.

## BIBLIOGRAPHY

Siu AL. U.S. Preventive Services Task Force. Screening for Breast Cancer: U.S. Preventive Services Task Force Recommendation Statement. *Ann Intern Med.* 2016;164(4):279-296.

Oeffinger KC, Fontham ET, Etzioni R, et al. American Cancer Society. Breast Cancer Screening for Women at Average Risk: 2015 Guideline Update From the American Cancer Society. *JAMA.* 2015;314(15):1599-1614.

Kopans DB. Digital breast tomosynthesis from concept to clinical care. *AJR Am J Roentgenol.* 2014;202(2):299-308.

Berg WA, Blume JD, Cormack JB, et al. Combined screening with ultrasound and mammography vs mammography alone in women at elevated risk of breast cancer. *JAMA.* 2008;299(18):2151-2163.

Lehman CD, Isaacs C, Schnall MD, et al. Cancer yield of mammography, MR, and US in high-risk women: prospective multi-institution breast cancer screening study. *Radiology.* 2007;244(2):381-388.

Saslow D, Boetes C, Burke W, et al. American Cancer Society guidelines for breast screening with MRI as an adjunct to mammography. *CA Cancer J Clin.* 2007;57(2):75-89.

Pisano ED, Gatsonis C, Hendrick E, et al. Diagnostic performance of digital versus film mammography for breast-cancer screening. *N Engl J Med.* 2005;353(17):1773-1783.

Shapiro S, Coleman EA, Broeders M, et al. Breast cancer screening programmes in 22 countries: current policies, administration and guidelines. International Breast Cancer Screening Network (IBSN) and the European Network of Pilot Projects for Breast Cancer Screening. *Int J Epidemiol.* 1998;27(5):735-742.

# CHAPTER 9

# DIAGNOSTIC MAMMOGRAPHY

*Susan P. Weinstein, MD*

1. **What are the indications for a diagnostic mammogram?**
   Some indications for a diagnostic mammogram include a history of breast cancer, breast lump, nipple discharge, focal breast pain, breast implants, history of breast biopsy, history of an abnormal mammogram, and follow-up for a previously evaluated mammographic finding (BI-RADS category 3 lesion).

2. **What views are performed for diagnostic mammography? How are patients who have undergone diagnostic mammography informed of results?**
   Routine views are performed with additional views as needed. Routine views include bilateral craniocaudal (CC) and mediolateral oblique (MLO) views. Additional views may include spot compression views, magnification views, exaggerated views, and rolled views. Ultrasonography (US) may also be performed if indicated. US evaluation may be performed to further evaluate a mammographic finding, such as a mass, or may be performed to further evaluate clinical symptoms, most commonly a clinically palpable breast mass. The imaging evaluation is completed while the patient is present at the imaging center, and the patient is informed of the results before he or she leaves. At our institution, the physician discusses the results with the patient.

3. **What is BI-RADS?**
   The Breast Imaging Reporting and Data System (BI-RADS) lexicon was developed by the American College of Radiology (ACR) to provide a clear, concise way to report mammographic results. A BI-RADS category is reported at the end of every mammogram report and summarizes the findings of the mammogram (Table 9-1).

4. **What types of mammographic changes may be seen after breast conservation?**
   Surgical therapy and radiation therapy often result in tissue distortion and edema. Other findings include skin thickening and trabecular thickening. The first mammogram after completion of therapy serves as a baseline study for the patient. Post-therapy changes, such as the degree of skin thickening and distortion, should remain stable or improve over time. If the post-treatment findings worsen, then there should be concern for recurrent disease and further evaluation is needed.

5. **Does mammography have high sensitivity in detecting recurrent breast cancer after breast conservation?**
   The sensitivity of mammography in detecting recurrent tumor is limited by the post-therapy changes present on the mammogram: edema, distortion, and trabecular thickening. Overall, studies suggest that mammography does not detect tumor recurrence about one third of the time. Recurrence presenting as calcifications is easier to detect than that presenting as a mass after breast conservation therapy. Physical examination also plays an important complementary role in evaluating patients after breast conservation. There is new literature suggesting that breast magnetic resonance imaging (MRI) may detect additional cancers.

6. **What is the incidence of recurrent breast cancer in a patient after breast conservation?**
   Recent literature suggests that recurrence rates are fairly low after breast conservation therapy, less than 1% per year.

7. **True or false: In patients who develop recurrence after breast conservation, survival rates are about the same as for patients who had a mastectomy as the initial treatment.**
   True. Recurrence after breast conservation does not seem to affect the overall survival rate for patients with breast cancer. Survival depends on the size of the recurrence, however.

8. **What are some contraindications to breast conservation?**
   - Multicentric cancer (i.e., the presence of breast cancer in different quadrants of the breast) is a contraindication. If there is multifocal tumor, however (i.e., more than one focus of cancer localized to the same quadrant of the breast), breast conservation therapy is feasible.
   - Size of the cancer relative to the breast size is a relative contraindication. Some clinicians use 5 cm as a cutoff; however, others use a relative measurement as a size cutoff. A 6-cm cancer in a large breast may result in acceptable cosmesis, whereas in a small breast, it would result in unacceptable cosmetic results.
   - First-trimester or second-trimester pregnancy.
   - History of prior radiation therapy to the chest or mediastinum.
   - Active collagen vascular disease.

| Table 9-1. BI-RADS Lexicon | |
|---|---|
| **BI-RADS CATEGORY** | **DEFINITION** |
| 1 | Normal mammogram. The patient should return in 1 year for annual mammography. |
| 2 | Benign finding on mammogram. The patient should return in 1 year for annual mammography. |
| 3 | There is a high likelihood of benignity (>98%). A short-term follow-up is recommended in 6 months. The follow-up is performed over a total of 2-3 years. |
| 4 | A biopsy is warranted: >2% but <95% likelihood of malignancy. |
| 4a | Low likelihood of malignancy. |
| 4b | Intermediate likelihood of malignancy. |
| 4c | Moderate likelihood of malignancy. |
| 5 | A biopsy is recommended. There is a high likelihood of malignancy (≥95%). |
| 6 | Confirmed malignancy. |
| 0 | The imaging evaluation is incomplete. Additional evaluation or prior studies are needed for comparison. |

9. In a patient who is planning to have breast conservation, when is it necessary to obtain a postbiopsy mammogram shortly after a successful excisional biopsy?

If the malignancy was associated with calcifications on the mammogram, a postbiopsy mammogram should be obtained to ensure that all the suspicious microcalcifications have been removed. If there are residual calcifications, the likelihood that there is residual disease is quite high. The inverse is not true. If there are no residual calcifications, this does not indicate that there is no residual disease. There may be portions of the cancer that are not calcified. The decision to re-excise is also based on histopathologic margin status.

For breast cancers that manifest as a mass on the mammogram, a postbiopsy mammogram is not needed. The decision to re-excise should be based on the histopathologic margins. Due to the postbiopsy changes in the surgical bed, it would be difficult to differentiate between postbiopsy changes and residual tumor.

10. True or false: In a patient with a history of breast cancer, it is beneficial to get a mammogram more frequently than once a year.

False. No studies have shown a benefit of an increased frequency of screening. Annual mammography is recommended even in women who have a history of breast cancer.

11. What is a 6-month follow-up? How long is the follow-up performed for BI-RADS category 3 lesions?

Six-month follow-up is performed for BI-RADS category 3 lesions (after an appropriate imaging workup). The follow-up is performed for a total of 2 to 3 years at 6-month intervals. For lesions that fit the "probably benign" criteria, less than 2% of the lesions should be malignant. That is, greater than 98% of the lesions should be benign.

12. How is the mastectomy bed evaluated?

We do not recommend routine imaging evaluation of the mastectomy bed. No studies have shown the benefit of routine imaging evaluation of the surgical bed. Instead, clinical evaluation is recommended. If there is a palpable area of concern on the physical examination, US should be performed as the next step of evaluation.

13. What types of surgical reconstruction are available after a mastectomy?

There are various types of tissue flaps, such as transverse rectus abdominis musculocutaneous flaps and latissimus dorsi flaps. Alternatively, silicone or saline implants may be used for reconstruction, or a combination of both.

14. True or false: After a benign breast biopsy, significant residual changes are usually visible on a mammogram.

False. After a benign breast biopsy, the breast tissue usually heals with few residual changes. Infrequently, distortion and postbiopsy changes may persist.

15. For all breast biopsies, approximately what percentage of the pathology results should be malignant?

The positive predictive value for all breast biopsies should be approximately 20% to 25%. This means that 75% to 80% of the biopsies that are performed will yield benign results.

16. A 47-year-old woman presents with a newly palpable breast mass and has a negative mammogram. What should be done next?

The next step in the evaluation should be a directed US evaluation of the area of palpable concern.

17. If US results are negative, what should be done next? What percentage of the time can a cancer be missed on US and mammography?

If US and mammography results are negative, clinical management is advised. This may include clinically following the patient or performing a biopsy if the palpable area is clinically suspicious. Based on the literature, the negative predictive value of combined mammography and US is 95% to 100%. That is, if both studies are negative, a cancer may be missed 5% of the time or less.

18. What types of nipple discharge are considered suspicious and warrant additional imaging evaluation? What imaging workup is recommended for suspicious nipple discharge?

Nipple discharge that is spontaneous, bloody, clear, or serosanguineous is considered suspicious. The first step in the evaluation should be mammography. The mammogram results may be normal or show a finding. At our institution, we also perform US to look for any suspicious lesions that may be causing the discharge. Typically, we look in the subareolar and periareolar regions.

If the mammogram and US are normal, the next step may be a galactogram. The involved ductal orifice is cannulated with a thin catheter. A small amount of contrast material, typically less than 5 cc, is injected into the ductal system until resistance is felt. A mammogram is then obtained to look for filling defects that may be the cause of the discharge (Figure 9-1). If there is a filling defect, the defect may be due to various causes, such as debris, a papilloma, or a malignancy.

MRI may also have a role in the evaluation of nipple discharge. Ultimately, if there is clinically suspicious discharge with no clear explanation, surgical duct exploration may be performed.

19. What types of nipple discharge are associated with benign etiologies?

The typical benign discharge may be greenish, brownish, or milky in color. Bilaterality and discharge arising from multiple ductal orifices are also benign characteristics.

20. In a patient with a suspicious type of nipple discharge, what is the likelihood that the discharge is due to cancer?

The likelihood is about 10%.

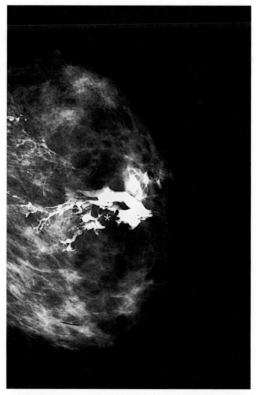

**Figure 9-1.** Papilloma on galactogram. Mammographic image obtained after contrast material injection into breast duct shows contrast material within ductal system. Note lobulated filling defect (*) in ductal system surrounded by contrast material. This patient had presented with bloody nipple discharge.

21. What is the most common etiology for bloody nipple discharge?

    Benign solitary papillomas are the most common etiology of bloody nipple discharge. Solitary papillomas arise within the ducts close to the nipple and are benign tumors composed of glandular and fibrous elements. Solitary papillomas do not increase a woman's risk for breast cancer.

    Papillomatosis is a condition in which there are multiple papillomas arising in the peripheral ducts. Papillomatosis typically does not cause nipple discharge. There is an increased risk of breast cancer associated with papillomatosis.

22. What are the most common histologic types of breast cancer?

    The most common histologic types of breast cancer are invasive ductal carcinoma, intraductal (ductal carcinoma in situ [DCIS]) carcinoma, and invasive lobular carcinoma. Subtypes of invasive ductal carcinoma include medullary, mucinous, papillary, cribriform, metaplastic, micropapillary, and tubular. Less common histologic types of breast cancer include sarcoma and lymphoma. Metastasis to the breast is rare but may occur.

    Inflammatory breast carcinoma is a rare, aggressive form of breast cancer that describes a clinical presentation of breast cancer rather than a histologic diagnosis, although most of these cancers are of ductal origin. Patients present with a red, warm, swollen breast with skin dimpling (peau d'orange) mimicking the skin of an orange. Inflammatory breast cancer represents less than 5% of breast cancers.

    Paget disease of the breast is a rare form of breast cancer involving the areola. It is a clinical diagnosis where patients present with itching, scaling, and redness around the nipple area. Clinically, it may be confused with dermatitis or eczema. There may be associated DCIS or invasive carcinoma, along with the nipple changes.

23. Is lobular carcinoma in situ (LCIS) a form of cancer? What is the significance of LCIS?

    LCIS has no clinical or mammographic correlate. It is a histologic diagnosis. LCIS is not a cancer or a premalignant lesion but is a marker that identifies women who may be at increased risk for developing breast cancer. In a patient previously diagnosed with LCIS, the risk of developing breast cancer in either breast is about 33%.

24. What is the differential diagnosis for a red swollen breast?

    The differential diagnosis includes infection, inflammatory breast cancer, history of prior radiation, and lymphatic or vascular obstruction. The history of prior radiation should be easy to corroborate with the patient. Patients with infection and inflammatory breast cancer can present with similar histories: a red, swollen, tender breast. Imaging should be performed to exclude a mass or an abscess. If the patient's symptoms do not improve with antibiotic treatment, inflammatory breast cancer should be excluded. The skin appears red and swollen in inflammatory carcinoma because the dermal lymphatics are infiltrated with tumor cells. Typically, a punch biopsy of the skin confirms the diagnosis, although occasionally, punch biopsy results may be falsely negative.

25. Is there such a thing as a mammographic emergency?

    Probably the only breast imaging–related emergency is an abscess that needs to be drained, but this problem can usually be managed clinically. If a fluctuant mass is present, it can be drained by palpation. Otherwise, if there is clinical concern of an abscess, the patient can be treated symptomatically. Patients are usually in too much pain to get a mammogram; if they undergo imaging, US is usually performed to look for a collection.

26. How many views are obtained in a patient with breast augmentation?

    At our institution, four routine views (CC and MLO views) and four implant-displacement views are obtained. (At some institutions, an implant-displacement mediolateral view may also be obtained.) On the four routine views, the breast implant is imaged. The glandular tissue is not well compressed on these views. The implant-displacement views are obtained with the implant pushed back so that the breast tissue can be compressed. Usually the presence of the breast implants limits visualization of the posterior breast tissue.

27. Where can the implants be placed in the breast?

    They can be placed in the retropectoral position, behind the pectoralis muscle. Alternatively, they can be placed in the retroglandular position, in front of the pectoralis muscle.

28. What types of implants are available?

    Currently, saline and silicone implants are available. In the past, silicone implants were available only for breast reconstruction in patients with a history of breast cancer. Silicone implants are available now for cosmetic augmentation as well. In 2006, the Food and Drug Administration (FDA) approved silicone implants for cosmetic surgery after taking them off the market in 1992 because of a controversy regarding silicone implants and a possible association with connective tissue disease. No studies to date have definitively associated silicone implants with connective tissue disease.

29. What is the most sensitive imaging evaluation for implant rupture?

    MRI is the reference standard. US may be used to evaluate for rupture as well, but the examination is operator dependent. Rupture may be contained within the fibrous capsule surrounding the implant shell (intracapsular) or may extend outside the fibrous capsule (extracapsular). Although mammography detects extracapsular rupture, it is limited in the evaluation of intracapsular rupture, the more common form of rupture. MRI findings of implant rupture include the "linguine" sign (the most reliable finding) where serpentine low signal intensity foci representing the deflated implant shell are seen within a background of high signal intensity silicone; and the "keyhole" or "noose" signs where a small amount of silicone is seen between a nondeflated implant shell and the fibrous capsule.

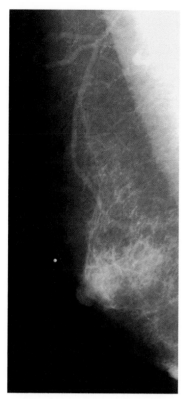

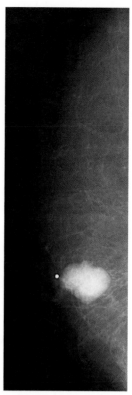

**Figure 9-2.** Gynecomastia on mammogram. MLO view of breast shows glandular tissue in subareolar region in male patient who presented with breast pain.

**Figure 9-3.** Invasive breast cancer on mammogram. MLO view of breast reveals lobulated circumscribed mass in subareolar region in male patient who presented with breast lump. This mass is definitely masslike, in contrast to changes of gynecomastia seen in Figure 9-2.

30. A man presents with a breast lump. How should the patient be imaged? What is the most common etiology for a breast lump in a man?

    For a man presenting with a breast lump, we usually recommend bilateral mammography. Sometimes, US may be needed if there is dense tissue in the area of the breast lump on the mammogram. The most common etiology for a breast lump in a man is gynecomastia. Usually this is bilateral, although it may be asymmetric (Figure 9-2). A clinical workup should be recommended to evaluate for the etiology of the gynecomastia.

31. What is the etiology of gynecomastia?

    There is a long differential diagnosis for gynecomastia. In infants and in teenagers, it is most commonly due to hormonal influences. Transplacental maternal hormones are responsible in infants. In teenagers, the hormonal fluctuations of adolescence are thought to be responsible. Other pathologic processes should be excluded, however. A few common etiologies for gynecomastia are marijuana use, certain types of medications, liver dysfunction, androgen deficiency, or any condition that causes an imbalance of estrogen relative to testosterone. Finally, hormone-secreting tumors should be excluded.

32. Do men get breast cancer? What is the frequency?

    Yes, but male breast cancers are rare, accounting for less than 1% of all breast cancers (Figure 9-3). Male breast cancer is most commonly diagnosed between 60 and 70 years of age. The most common clinical sign is a painless mass. Other signs include skin dimpling or retraction, and occasionally discharge. Men are often treated with mastectomy. Breast conservation therapy is uncommon in men. In addition, male patients may receive radiation therapy or chemotherapy or both depending on stage, lymph node status, and final surgical margins. Overall, stage or stage, the prognosis for male breast cancer is similar to that for female breast cancer. In the past, it was thought that male breast cancer had a worse prognosis than female breast cancer; however, this was due to the later stage at which the disease was diagnosed in men, as they do not undergo screening.

33. True or false: Breast cancer can manifest in the following ways: calcifications, masses, architectural distortion, and density.

    True for all of the above. Benign lesions may also manifest in the same ways, but the morphology of the lesions will be different.

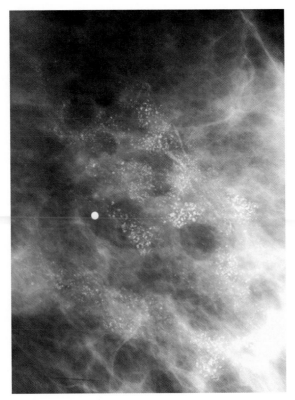

**Figure 9-4.** Malignant breast calcifications on mammogram.

34. Classify the following terms commonly used to describe breast calcifications as indicative of benign, indeterminate, or malignant patterns.
    a. Popcorn
    b. Rim
    c. Amorphous
    d. Heterogeneous
    e. Indistinct
    f. Round
    g. Milk of calcium
    h. Linear, branching
    i. Rodlike
    j. Dystrophic
    k. Pleomorphic
       Benign: a, b, f, g, i, j; indeterminate: c, e; malignant: d, h, k.

35. Figures 9-4 through 9-9 show images of breast calcifications. Classify them as benign or malignant patterns of calcification.
    Figures 9-4 and 9-5 display malignant calcifications. Figures 9-6, 9-7, 9-8, and 9-9 show different types of benign calcifications.

36. What is a triple-negative breast cancer, and what is its significance?
    A breast cancer is termed triple-negative when it does not express receptors for estrogen, progesterone, and human epidermal growth factor receptor-2. Triple-negative cancers tend to be more aggressive, with a higher rate of recurrence than other subtypes. Studies have shown that triple-negative cancers also disproportionately affect premenopausal African American women and are more common in carriers of the *BRCA1* mutation.

37. A patient presents with a palpable breast mass and a stable mammogram. The mass in Figure 9-10 is seen on US. What should be the radiologist's recommendation?
    Although the mammogram was considered stable, the next step in the evaluation of the patient should include a targeted US examination. The mass is very hypoechoic but does not have any features that would suggest that it is a cyst. The indistinct margins also make the mass suspicious. In this case, core needle biopsy was performed under US, revealing a diagnosis of invasive ductal carcinoma.

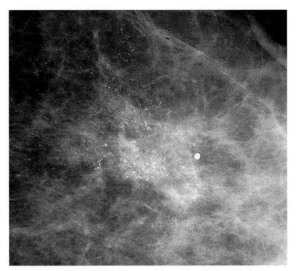

**Figure 9-5.** Malignant breast calcifications on mammogram.

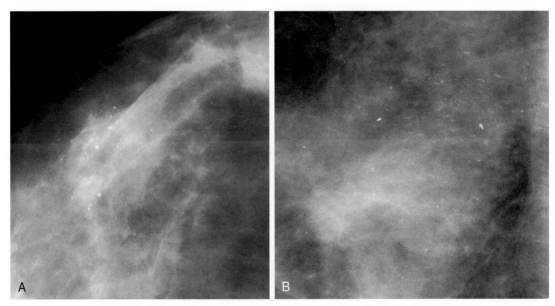

**Figure 9-6.** Benign (milk of calcium) calcifications on mammogram. **A,** CC view. **B,** MLO view.

38. **What is the difference between multifocal and multicentric breast cancer?**
    Multifocal breast cancer indicates the presence of 2 or more foci of breast cancer in the same breast quadrant, while multicentric breast cancer indicates the presence of 2 or more foci in different quadrants of the breast. Usually patients with multicentric cancer are not eligible for breast conservation therapy given that the tumors are in separate quadrants.

39. **Are radial scars associated with prior surgery?**
    No, radial scars are not associated with prior surgery. A radial scar is a benign proliferative lesion. If it is larger than 1 cm, it is called a complex sclerosing lesion. The classic appearance of a radial scar is that of an area of architectural distortion with central lucency. If a radial scar is seen on a core needle biopsy, excisional biopsy is recommended for further evaluation, because it can be difficult to exclude presence of breast carcinoma on the core biopsy results alone.

40. **What is a fibroadenoma?**
    Fibroadenomas are common breast lesions that are composed of stromal and epithelial elements. They are typically diagnosed in young women in their 20s and 30s and present as firm, mobile palpable breast masses. The classic US

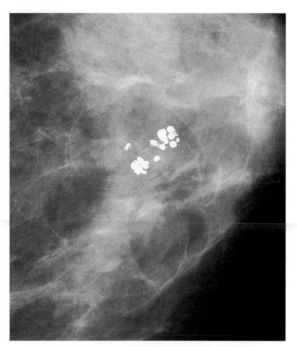

**Figure 9-7.** Benign round calcifications on mammogram.

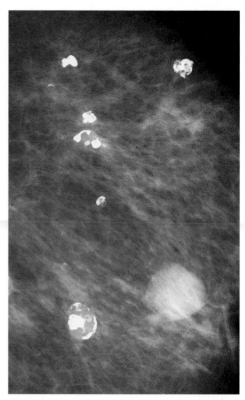

**Figure 9-8.** Benign popcorn calcifications on mammogram.

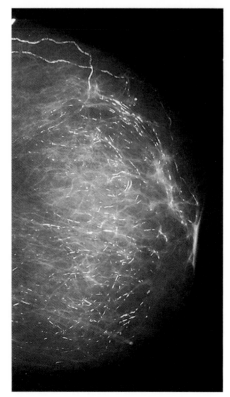

**Figure 9-9.** Benign secretory calcifications on mammogram.

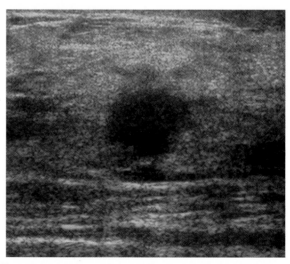

**Figure 9-10.** Invasive ductal breast cancer on US. Note hypoechoic mass in breast without posterior through-transmission.

appearance is a circumscribed oval hypoechoic mass. Fibroadenomas that are larger than 10 cm are called giant fibroadenomas.

### 41. What is a phylloides tumor?

Phylloides tumors are uncommon breast tumors, accounting for less than 1% of breast tumors. They most commonly occur in women in their 30s and 40s. Phylloides tumors are composed of stromal and epithelial elements, similar to fibroadenomas, but can be locally aggressive and demonstrate rapid growth. Wide excision is the treatment of choice with close clinical follow-up, because these lesions can recur if adequate margins are not obtained. On US, these lesions may look similar to fibroadenomas or may demonstrate lobulated or irregular margins.

### 42. What is Mondor's disease?

Mondor's disease is a superficial thrombophlebitis involving the breast. It classically presents as a superficial painful cord and is a self-limiting condition that will resolve in 1 to 2 weeks with supportive care. It has been associated with prior surgery, trauma, biopsy, inflammatory processes, and breast cancer. On US, a tubular structure with no flow is seen that is firm to palpation, representing a thrombosed breast vein.

## KEY POINTS

- The BI-RADS categories are essential for reporting results of diagnostic mammography.
- Diagnostic mammography is indicated for women with a specific breast-related problem that needs to be evaluated. Screening mammography is indicated for asymptomatic patients.
- In patients who have had breast conservation, postbiopsy changes may limit the sensitivity of mammography.
- In a patient presenting with a palpable breast mass, if the mammogram results are negative, the imaging evaluation should not stop at that point. Directed US evaluation is necessary to complete the evaluation.

## BIBLIOGRAPHY

Gweon HM, Cho N, Han W, et al. Breast MR imaging screening in women with a history of breast conservation therapy. *Radiology.* 2014;272(2):366-373.

Margolis NE, Morley C, Lotfi P, et al. Update on imaging of the postsurgical breast. *Radiographics.* 2014;34(3):642-660.

Nguyen C, Kettler MD, Swirsky ME, et al. Male breast disease: pictorial review with radiologic-pathologic correlation. *Radiographics.* 2013;33(3):763-779.

Yeh ED, Jacene HA, Bellon JR, et al. What radiologists need to know about diagnosis and treatment of inflammatory breast cancer: a multidisciplinary approach. *Radiographics.* 2013;33(7):2003-2017.

Trop I, Dugas A, David J, et al. Breast abscesses: evidence-based algorithms for diagnosis, management, and follow-up. *Radiographics.* 2011;31(6):1683-1699.

Irshad A, Ackerman SJ, Pope TL, et al. Rare breast lesions: correlation of imaging and histologic features with WHO classification. *Radiographics.* 2008;28(5):1399-1414.

Nakahara H, Namba K, Watanabe R, et al. A comparison of MR imaging, galactography and ultrasonography in patients with nipple discharge. *Breast Cancer.* 2003;10(4):320-329.

Dershaw DD. Breast imaging and the conservative treatment of breast cancer. *Radiol Clin North Am.* 2002;40(3):501-516.

Kaiser JS, Helvie MA, Blacklaw RL, et al. Palpable breast thickening: role of mammography and US in cancer detection. *Radiology.* 2002;223(3):839-844.

Dennis MA, Parker SH, Klaus AJ, et al. Breast biopsy avoidance: the value of normal mammograms and normal sonograms in the setting of a palpable lump. *Radiology.* 2001;219(1):186-191.

Soo MS, Rosen EL, Baker JA, et al. Negative predictive value of sonography with mammography in patients with palpable breast lesions. *AJR Am J Roentgenol.* 2001;177(5):1167-1170.

Bassett LW. Imaging of breast masses. *Radiol Clin North Am.* 2000;38(4):669-691, vii-viii.

Orel SG, Dougherty CS, Reynolds C, et al. MR imaging in patients with nipple discharge: initial experience. *Radiology.* 2000;216(1):248-254.

# CHAPTER 10

# BREAST ULTRASONOGRAPHY (US) AND BREAST PROCEDURES

*Susan P. Weinstein, MD*

1. What are the labeled structures on the ultrasound image in Figure 10-1?
   The structures are skin (A), subcutaneous fat (B), glandular tissue (C), fat (D), muscle (E), and rib (F).

2. What type of transducer should be used to perform breast US?
   A linear array transducer should be used. It should ideally have a frequency of 10 MHz or greater.

3. List the indications for targeted breast US after a mammographic evaluation.
   - To evaluate a palpable abnormality further. In patients presenting with palpable breast masses, even if the mammogram results are negative, a targeted sonographic evaluation of the palpable area is a necessary part of the evaluation.
   - To characterize a mammographic finding or abnormality. For example, if there is a new or enlarging mass seen on mammography, sonography is needed to characterize the mass. If the mass is demonstrated to be a cyst on sonography, nothing further needs to be done. But, if there is an enlarging or new solid mass, a biopsy is needed. As the mass is visible on sonography, the biopsy may be performed under ultrasound guidance.

4. When would breast US be indicated without obtaining a mammogram first?
   - In patients who are younger than 30 and in pregnant patients, it is recommended to start with breast US. For other patients presenting with palpable masses, mammography should be obtained first, with the following exceptions. At our institution, a mammogram is obtained first in women who are older than 30. To evaluate the palpable abnormality further, US follows mammography. If the patient is younger than 30, US is performed first. Age 30 is an arbitrary number; different institutions may have a different cutoff age.
   - In patients who have had a mastectomy, there is not enough tissue to obtain a mammogram. If there is a palpable area, sonographic evaluation should be performed.
   - In women who are lactating, sonography may be performed first.

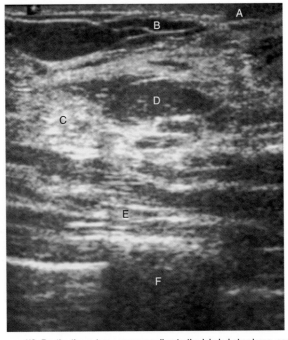

**Figure 10-1.** Normal breast tissue on US. For the tissue types corresponding to the labeled structures, see the answer to question 10-1 above.

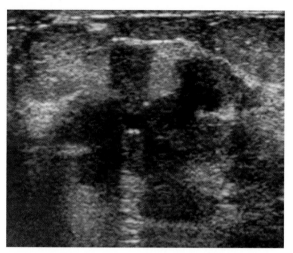

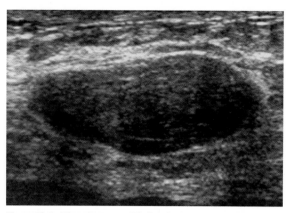

**Figure 10-3.** Fibroadenoma on US. Note benign-appearing well-circumscribed oval mass in breast of another woman who presented with palpable breast mass.

**Figure 10-2.** Invasive breast cancer on US. Note highly suspicious hypoechoic lobulated solid mass with irregular margins in breast of woman who presented with palpable breast mass.

5. What are some suspicious lesion features for malignancy on US?

Suspicious features on US include a markedly hypoechoic appearance, posterior acoustic shadowing, angular or irregular margins, spiculations, microlobulations, a mass that is taller than it is wide, and ductal extension (Figure 10-2). Although these features are usually seen in malignant lesions, benign masses may also exhibit some of these findings.

6. What are some benign lesion features on US?

Benign features on US include absence of malignant features, well-circumscribed mass, ellipsoid shape that is wider than it is tall, and hyperechogenicity (Figure 10-3). Although these features are typically seen in benign lesions, some malignant masses may exhibit some of these features. Some carcinomas can be well circumscribed, including invasive ductal carcinoma (not otherwise specified) as well as medullary, papillary, and colloid subtypes of ductal carcinoma.

7. What types of biopsy procedures may be performed to evaluate breast lesions?

*Fine needle aspiration (FNA)* is readily available and needs no special equipment. Overall, it is less traumatic than core biopsy or excisional biopsy. However, as only cells are aspirated, the results may be inconclusive. In addition, it is often difficult to evaluate tumor receptor expression on FNA specimens.

*Core needle biopsy* is a minimally invasive percutaneous procedure that can be performed under US guidance or stereotactic mammographic guidance. A wide range of needles is available on the market in terms of needle gauge and vacuum versus nonvacuum assistance. Which type of needle is used tends to be based on personal preferences, although stereotactic biopsies are almost always done with vacuum assistance to maximize the retrieval of calcifications. Biopsies performed under US tend to be easier and faster to perform than stereotactic biopsies, partly because of the real-time imaging available with US guidance. At our institution, the stereotactic method is used to biopsy calcifications, although biopsy of solid masses may also be obtained using this method. Percutaneous core biopsies are less expensive, are faster to perform, and are less traumatic than surgical biopsies. The false-negative rates are similar to open biopsies.

There are limitations to performing stereotactic core needle biopsies. Lesions that are in the far posterior breast or behind the nipple may be difficult to access. In addition, the minimum compression thickness of the breast required to perform a stereotactic biopsy is 25 to 30 mm, depending on the needle used.

For both core needle biopsy and FNA, the radiologist reviews the pathology results to confirm that the pathology results are concordant with the imaging findings. If core needle biopsy of a category 5 BI-RADS lesion, or a highly suspicious mass, yields benign pathology results, this may be considered "discordant." Excisional biopsy may then be needed for further evaluation if there is discordance between the pathology results and the imaging appearance.

*Needle localization followed by excisional biopsy* has traditionally been the reference standard. The area of concern is localized with mammography on the day of surgery, and then the patient goes to outpatient surgery. To confirm removal of the localized lesion, a specimen radiograph is obtained. At our institution, we image the specimen while the patient is still in the operating room, and the findings are called in to the surgeon.

8. What are the relative disadvantages of FNA, core needle biopsy, and needle localization/excision?

*FNA:* The results depend on the skill of the individual performing the procedure and the cytopathologist. There can be a high percentage of unsatisfactory aspirates (20% to 30% of cases). Invasive versus in situ cancer cannot be differentiated on FNA. The false-negative rate for image-guided FNA is unknown.

*Core needle biopsy:* Tissue displacement may occur during the biopsy procedure, resulting in misinterpretation of intraductal carcinoma as invasive carcinoma. Inversely, cancer can occasionally be understaged on core needle biopsy. That is, due to sampling, only DCIS may be biopsied and the invasive portion may not be sampled on a core biopsy.

*Needle localization with excisional biopsy:* This is the most expensive and most traumatic of all the biopsy procedures.

9. How can one be certain that the lesion of interest was actually what was sampled during core needle biopsy?

After a stereotactic biopsy, a specimen radiograph is used to confirm that representative calcifications are in the specimen. Dynamic imaging and needle placement under direct visualization are used to confirm that the target was sampled during a US-guided biopsy.

10. What is the lesion depth, or the *z* axis, calculated on a stereotactic biopsy?

Stereotaxis is a technique used to localize breast lesions for biopsy. A digital image of the lesion, the scout image, is taken on the stereotactic machine. This image is obtained at 0 degrees. Two views are taken at ±15 degrees from the original 0-degree scout image. From the three views, the machine calculates the *z* axis, which is the depth the needle needs to be placed to obtain a biopsy sample of the lesion. The *x* and *y* axes of the target are obtained from the original scout image.

11. In what circumstances would a stereotactic biopsy be difficult to perform?
- Subareolar lesion location. Lesions in the subareolar region are difficult to access due to the location and thickness of the tissue.
- Thin breast tissue. Compression thickness of less than 2.5 to 3.0 cm may make biopsy sampling difficult depending on the type of needle utilized.
- Very posterior lesion location. It is difficult to access and target lesions that are very posterior in the breast.
- Lesions that are difficult to see. The calcifications or lesions should be easily visible for targeting.

12. In what circumstances would US-guided biopsy be difficult to perform?
- Lesions that are close to the skin surface.
- Lesions that are behind the nipple.
- Lesions that are close to the chest wall.
- Presence of very thin tissue.

13. What is a discordant pathology result?

When a percutaneous breast biopsy is performed, one of the radiologist's roles is to ensure the histopathologic diagnosis is concordant, or makes sense in light of the imaging appearance. If the imaging appearance is highly suspicious and the histopathologic results are benign, this may suggest a discordance. If there is discordance, the radiologist may suggest excisional biopsy for further evaluation.

14. In what situations or histopathologic diagnoses should an excisional biopsy be recommended after a percutaneous breast biopsy?

When there is histopathologic-imaging discordance, excisional biopsy should be recommended. When a high-risk lesion such as atypical ductal hyperplasia is present on histopathologic evaluation, excisional biopsy should also be recommended. When atypical ductal hyperplasia is present on percutaneous breast biopsy, cancer is present on excisional biopsy in up to 56% of cases. Other histopathologic diagnoses that should be considered for excisional biopsy include papillary lesions, radial scars, atypical lobular hyperplasia, and lobular carcinoma in situ.

---

## KEY POINTS

- For optimal imaging evaluation, a US transducer with a frequency of at least 10 MHz should be used to perform a breast US examination.
- In addition to performing percutaneous breast biopsies, the radiologist's role includes evaluating the pathology results for concordance with the imaging findings.
- If atypical ductal hyperplasia is present on histopathologic evaluation of a percutaneous biopsy specimen, excisional biopsy should be recommended because there is a high frequency of coexistent breast cancer.

**BIBLIOGRAPHY**

Sung JS. High-quality breast ultrasonography. *Radiol Clin North Am.* 2014;52(3):519-526.
Hooley RJ, Scoutt LM, Philpotts LE. Breast ultrasonography: state of the art. *Radiology.* 2013;268(3):642-659.
Mahoney MC, Newell MS. Breast intervention: how I do it. *Radiology.* 2013;268(1):12-24.
Hashimoto BE. New sonographic breast technologies. *Semin Roentgenol.* 2011;46(4):292-301.
Cardenosa G. *Breast imaging companion.* 3rd ed. Philadelphia, PA: Lippincott Williams & Wilkins; 2008.
Kopans DB. *Breast imaging.* 3rd ed. Philadelphia, PA: Lippincott Williams & Wilkins; 2006.
Liberman L. Percutaneous image-guided core breast biopsy. *Radiol Clin North Am.* 2002;40(3):483-500, vi.

# CHAPTER 11

# BREAST MRI

*Elizabeth S. McDonald, MD, PhD, and Emily F. Conant, MD*

1. **What are the indications for breast magnetic resonance imaging (MRI)?**
   General indications for breast MRI include:
   - Establish the extent of disease in the setting of a newly diagnosed breast cancer.
   - Further evaluate an imaging finding that is incompletely characterized by diagnostic mammography and/or breast ultrasonography (US).
   - Evaluate for residual disease in the setting of positive margins after lumpectomy or other operative procedure.
   - Evaluate a patient with metastatic adenocarcinoma to the axilla of unknown primary.
   - Evaluate for silicone breast implant rupture.
   - Presence of a hereditary gene or syndrome known to predispose to breast cancer (BRCA1/2 carrier, Li-Fraumeni syndrome, Cowden syndrome, Bannayan-Riley-Ruvalcaba syndrome) or a first-degree relative affected by one of these.
   - An estimated lifetime risk of breast cancer greater than 20% to 25%.
   - History of prior thoracic radiation therapy between the ages of 10 and 30.
   - Monitor the response of a known breast cancer to neoadjuvant chemotherapy.

2. **What are the contraindications for breast MRI?**
   Pregnancy is a contraindication for breast MRI because it is not known if the contrast agent used is safe during pregnancy. Other contraindications are those that apply to any MRI examination, such as presence of a pacemaker; a metallic foreign body in the eye, brain, or near other vital structures; a cochlear implant; or a drug infusion device, to name a few. A patient completes a detailed questionnaire about possible contraindications and is checked with a metal detector before being brought into the MRI suite.

3. **What are the risks of breast MRI?**
   The main risks are a reaction to the contrast agent used during the examination and false-positive results, resulting in unnecessary medical tests and procedures.

4. **How sensitive is breast MRI at finding breast cancer?**
   A large meta-analysis of fourteen studies in high-risk women between 2000 and 2011 found that breast MRI had a sensitivity of 84.6% for detecting cancer versus 38.6% for mammography and 39.6% for US. MRI can detect cancer that is occult on mammography, US, and physical examination [1].

5. **If a biopsy is performed based on an abnormal MRI finding, how likely will this be cancer?**
   One analysis evaluating 10 studies using breast MRI for screening women at high risk for breast cancer found that the positive predictive value (PPV) for malignancy among patients who had a biopsy varied from 17% to 89% (mean of 45%) [2]. Approximate benchmarks in the current BI-RADS atlas for biopsies performed as a result of screening breast MRI are that 20%-50% of biopsies for high risk women should be positive for cancer [3].

6. **What are the typical sequences used in a breast MRI?**
   Breast MRI is usually performed in the axial or sagittal plane on a 1.5- or 3-Tesla (T) magnet. We perform breast MRI in the sagittal plane on a 1.5-T magnet and use T1-weighted spin echo, fat-suppressed T2-weighted fast spin echo, and fat-suppressed three-dimensional T1-weighted spoiled gradient-recalled echo sequences. After intravenous contrast administration, the breast is usually scanned three times approximately 90 seconds apart to obtain dynamic postcontrast images. These sequential images provide information for kinetic analysis that can help to characterize lesions as benign or malignant. Delayed phase axial T1-weighted fat-suppressed images are then obtained to visualize the axillae and chest wall, and to allow for multiplanar correlation. Subtraction images are created by subtracting the precontrast images from the postcontrast images to aid with identification of areas of abnormal enhancement. These images are easily degraded by patient motion between sequences and so it is important to assess for motion before using these images for diagnostic interpretation. Both spatial (morphology) and temporal (kinetic) information is acquired in every case unless the examination is performed without contrast material to evaluate the integrity of silicone implants.

7. **Which is more helpful to characterize a lesion as malignant, morphology on postcontrast images or kinetic analysis features?**
   Lesion morphology is a more accurate predictor of malignancy and should be given priority over lesion kinetic analysis.

8. What are the ACR recommended morphologic descriptors for abnormal enhancement on breast MRI?

The ACR has developed a Breast Imaging-Reporting and Data System (BI-RADS) Atlas for mammography, US, and MRI reporting. According to the Atlas, each lesion should be characterized based on size, location (breast quadrant), and affected breast (right or left). Additional morphologic descriptors depend on whether the lesion is discrete with convex borders (mass) or not discrete with concave or unclear borders (nonmass). A mass is additionally characterized according to shape (oval, round, irregular), margin (circumscribed, irregular, spiculated), and internal enhancement (homogeneous, heterogeneous, rim, dark internal septations). Nonmass enhancement is usually described according to the distribution (focal, linear, segmental, regional, multiple regions, diffuse) and internal enhancement pattern (homogeneous, heterogeneous, clumped, clustered ring). If a lesion is too small to be characterized (≤4 mm) and the radiologist would like to call attention to it, it can be called a focus.

9. What kinds of enhancement kinetics are seen?

At least three postcontrast sequences are generally acquired to determine whether the initial enhancement gradually increases (persistent enhancement), stays the same (plateau enhancement), or decreases (washout enhancement). This information can help to characterize a lesion as benign or malignant. A washout curve is generally regarded as the most suspicious, but some benign masses, such as lymph nodes, also demonstrate this kinetic enhancement pattern.

10. What are the typical morphologic and kinetic features of a benign mass on breast MRI?

Features that are suggestive of a benign lesion are a round or oval shape, circumscribed margin, and homogeneous internal enhancement or dark nonenhancing internal septations. Additionally, the T2-weighted images can be used for lesion characterization. A round or oval mass with homogeneous high T2-weighted signal intensity that is greater than that of normal fibroglandular tissue and circumscribed margins has a very high likelihood of being benign.

11. What are some commonly observed benign masses?

One commonly observed mass is a normal intramammary lymph node (Figure 11-1). This will commonly present as a round or oval mass less than 1 cm in size with circumscribed margins. Lymph nodes will also generally have high T2-weighted signal intensity and washout enhancement kinetics. Careful assessment of the non-fat-suppressed T1-weighted images may demonstrate bright central fatty hila. The corresponding areas will have low signal intensity on the fat-suppressed T1-weighted images.

Another commonly observed benign mass is a fibroadenoma (Figure 11-2). This will commonly present as an oval mass with circumscribed margins and homogeneous enhancement. Fibroadenomas will also generally have homogeneous high T2-weighted signal intensity and persistent enhancement kinetics.

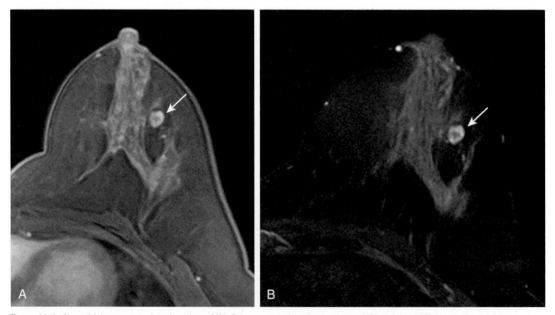

**Figure 11-1.** Normal intramammary lymph node on MRI. Fat-suppressed contrast-enhanced T1-weighted MR image (**A**) and fat-suppressed T2-weighted MR image (**B**) through breast are shown. A mass is noted with oval shape and circumscribed margins, with heterogeneous internal enhancement (arrow, **A**). The mass also has high T2-weighted signal intensity (arrow, **B**). The center of this mass does not enhance and has low signal intensity on fat-suppressed T1-weighted and T2-weighted images due to fatty hilum.

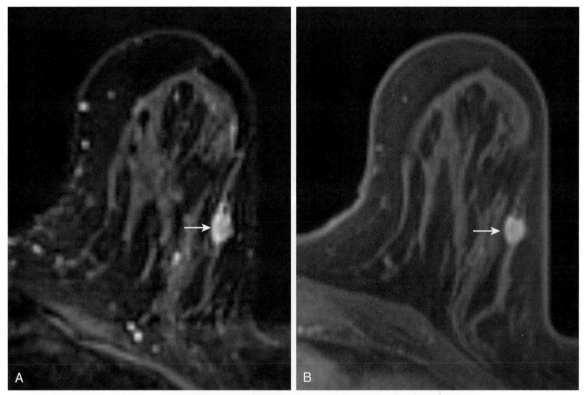

**Figure 11-2.** Benign fibroadenoma on MRI. Fat-suppressed contrast-enhanced T1-weighted subtraction MR image (**A**) and fat-suppressed T2-weighted MR image (**B**) are shown. A mass is noted with oval shape, circumscribed margins, and homogeneous internal enhancement (arrow, **A**). The mass also has homogeneous high T2-weighted signal intensity (arrow, **B**).

12. What are the typical features of a malignant mass on breast MRI?

    Features typical of malignancy include an irregular shape, irregular or spiculated margins, and heterogeneous internal enhancement. The T2-weighted signal intensity may also be heterogeneous. An example of a malignant mass (invasive ductal carcinoma) is shown in Figure 11-3.

13. Are there associated findings that may increase the probability that a breast mass is malignant?

    Additional findings associated with breast malignancy include nipple or skin retraction, abnormal pectoralis muscle enhancement, skin thickening and enhancement (Figure 11-4), and lymphadenopathy (Figure 11-5).

14. What are the typical features of malignant nonmass enhancement?

    Suspicious distributions for nonmass enhancement are linear and segmental (Figures 11-6 and 11-7). Suspicious internal enhancement patterns are heterogeneous (Figure 11-6), clumped, and clustered ring (Figure 11-7). Unlike masses, there is no definitive benign appearance for nonmass enhancement.

15. How should a breast MRI report be organized?

    The ACR recommends that the report be organized in the following fashion:
    1. Indication for examination.
    2. MRI technique.
    3. Succinct description of overall breast composition.
    4. Clear description of any important findings.
    5. Comparison to previous examinations.
    6. BI-RADS assessment.
    7. Management recommendation.

16. What are the BI-RADS assessment categories used to indicate management recommendations?

    There are seven assessment categories used in the BI-RADS Atlas used to indicate management recommendations (see Table 11-1).

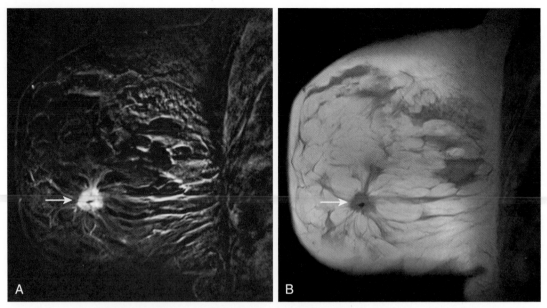

**Figure 11-3.** Invasive ductal carcinoma of breast on MRI. Fat-suppressed contrast-enhanced T1-weighted subtraction MR image (**A**) and non-fat-suppressed noncontrast T1-weighted MR image (**B**) are shown. A mass is noted with irregular shape, spiculated margins, and heterogeneous internal enhancement (arrow, **A**). Also note very low signal intensity biopsy clip located within mass (arrow, **B**).

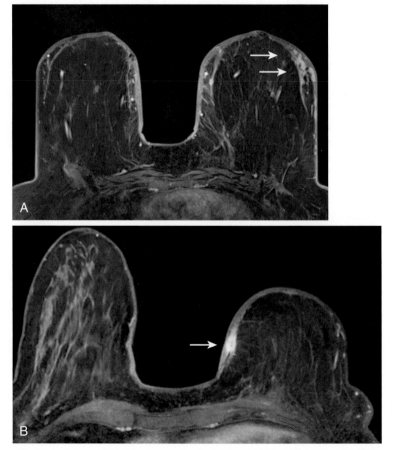

**Figure 11-4.** Recurrent breast carcinoma on MRI. Fat-suppressed contrast-enhanced T1-weighted subtraction MR image in patient status post bilateral mastectomy and breast reconstruction (**A**) demonstrates skin thickening and abnormal enhancement (arrows). Recurrent breast carcinoma on MRI. Fat-suppressed contrast-enhanced T1-weighted subtraction MR image in another patient status post left mastectomy and breast reconstruction (**B**) shows skin thickening and abnormal enhancement (arrow).

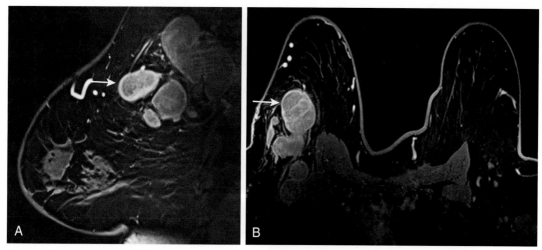

**Figure 11-5.** Metastatic axillary lymphadenopathy on MRI. Sagittal (**A**) and axial (**B**) fat-suppressed contrast-enhanced T1-weighted subtraction MR images demonstrate massively enlarged axillary lymph nodes (arrows).

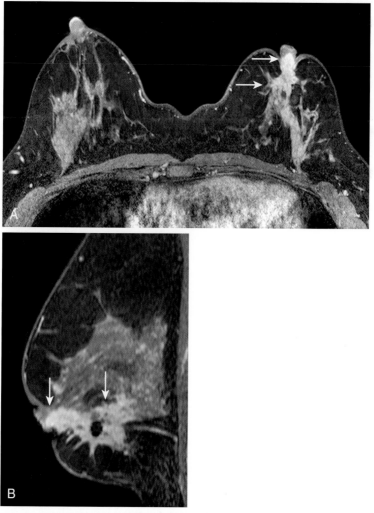

**Figure 11-6.** Breast ductal carcinoma in situ (DCIS) on MRI. Fat-suppressed contrast-enhanced axial (**A**) and sagittal (**B**) T1-weighted subtraction MR images show segmentally distributed nonmass enhancement with heterogeneous internal enhancement extending posterior from and involving nipple, resulting in nipple retraction. Signal void from biopsy clip is present at posterior aspect of disease on this sagittal image.

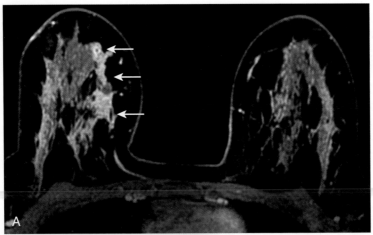

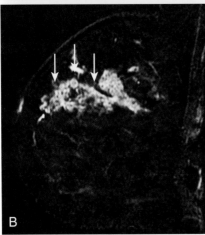

**Figure 11-7.** Breast DCIS. Fat-suppressed contrast-enhanced axial (**A**) and sagittal (**B**) T1-weighted subtraction MR images demonstrate segmentally distributed nonmass enhancement with clustered ring internal enhancement pattern. Extensive DCIS was confirmed on MRI-guided biopsy, and was not suggested by concurrent mammography and US.

**Table 11-1.** BI-RADS Assessment Categories and Recommended Management

| | |
|---|---|
| Assessment 0, Incomplete. | Management: Need additional imaging. |
| Assessment 1, Negative. | Management: Routine follow-up. |
| Assessment 2, Benign. | Management: Routine follow-up. |
| Assessment 3, Probably benign. <2% chance of malignancy | Management: Short interval follow-up imaging (usually 6 months). |
| Assessment 4, Suspicious. 2% to 94% chance of malignancy | Management: Needs a tissue diagnosis. |
| Assessment 5, Highly suspicious. ≥95% chance of malignancy | Management: Needs a tissue diagnosis. |
| Assessment 6, Known malignancy. | Management: Surgical and/or oncological. |

17. Does breast MRI have to be performed with contrast material?

Currently, all breast MRI is performed with intravenous contrast material unless the indication is only to evaluate for breast implant rupture. Examination techniques, such as diffusion-weighted imaging (DWI), are being developed to screen for malignancy without use of a contrast agent [4,5].

18. Should breast MRI generally be ordered as a unilateral or bilateral examination?

Breast MRI should generally be ordered as a bilateral examination so that the parenchymal enhancement can be evaluated for symmetry with the opposite side [6]. Asymmetric parenchymal enhancement can be a sign of breast malignancy.

19. What are the next steps after characterizing abnormal enhancement on breast MRI?

Indeterminate enhancement requires follow-up (BI-RADS 3) or tissue diagnosis (BI-RADS 4). The criteria for follow-up are beyond the scope of this chapter. If tissue diagnosis is needed, careful attention should be paid to any concurrent imaging study such as a mammogram to see if the biopsy can be performed with another modality to reduce costs to the patient and also eliminate the need for a contrast injection. Masses often warrant MRI-directed US to see if the biopsy can be performed under ultrasound guidance. If neither of these other approaches is possible, then MRI-guided percutaneous core biopsy or wire localization for surgical excision is indicated.

20. What is MRI-directed US?

MRI-directed US is an examination performed after an abnormal finding on breast MRI to evaluate the sonographic characteristics of the finding and to determine whether the finding can be sampled using ultrasound guidance. US is a less expensive and more comfortable option for the patient and also does not require an injection of contrast.

21. How is breast MRI biopsy performed?

Breast MRI biopsy is generally performed with a specialized breast MRI coil that allows access to the breast for biopsy with a vacuum assisted 9 or 10 gauge core needle. The lesion is localized following a contrast injection, and after tissue sampling, a small MRI-compatible clip is placed to mark the biopsy site in case further intervention is needed. The details of MRI-guided breast biopsy are beyond the scope of this chapter but have been reported elsewhere [7].

22. Is there any recommended follow-up after a benign breast biopsy?

There is no standard of care for MRI follow-up after benign biopsy, so this decision is left to the discretion of the treating radiologist and will depend on the confidence level that the appropriate lesion was sampled, given the pathologic results and imaging features.

23. What are the signs of breast implant rupture?

MRI can be used to determine whether a silicone implant is intact [8]. A normal implant is oval or ellipsoid in shape. Mammography is usually sufficient to determine whether a saline implant is intact. The body normally creates a fibrous capsule around a silicone gel implant, closely abutting the silicone elastomer shell of the intact implant. An intracapsular, or contained, rupture describes a rupture where the silicone has migrated beyond the ruptured implant elastomer but remains contained within the fibrous capsule. An extracapsular, or free, rupture describes when the silicone from the ruptured implant migrates freely beyond the fibrous capsule into the surrounding breast tissues.

On noncontrast breast MRI, an intracapsular rupture can be identified as low signal intensity wavy lines inside the fibrous capsule, known as the "linguine" sign (Figure 11-8). The appearance of silicone on both sides of the implant radial folds is known as the "keyhole" sign or "teardrop" sign, which also suggests intracapsular rupture.

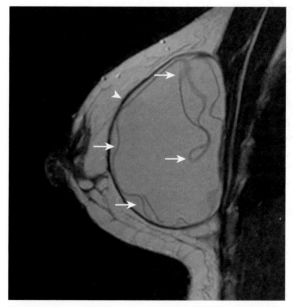

**Figure 11-8.** Intracapsular breast implant rupture on MRI. Noncontrast T2-weighted MR image without fat suppression shows multiple wavy low signal intensity lines within a silicone breast implant, representing the "linguine" sign, characteristic of intracapsular rupture (arrows). The wavy lines are due to portions of elastomer shell of implant floating in free silicone that are still contained by a fibrous capsule, seen as a thin black line around the silicone collection (arrowhead).

## KEY POINTS

- The optimal indications for breast MRI are currently still being determined, but include evaluation for presence of breast cancer in the high-risk patient; evaluation of the extent of disease with a new breast cancer diagnosis; detection of an occult primary tumor in the presence of axillary disease; evaluation of silicone breast implant integrity; response monitoring of a known breast cancer to chemotherapy; and further diagnostic evaluation after an inconclusive mammographic and sonographic work-up.
- MRI features suggestive of a benign breast mass include a round or oval shape, circumscribed margin, homogeneous high T2-weighted signal intensity, and dark nonenhancing internal septations, whereas MRI features suggestive of a malignant breast mass include an irregular shape, irregular or spiculated margins, and heterogeneous signal intensity or internal enhancement.
- Linear and segmental distributions of nonmass breast enhancement, and heterogeneous, clumped, and clustered ring internal enhancement patterns of nonmass breast enhancement are suspicious for breast malignancy.

**BIBLIOGRAPHY**

1. Lehman CD. Clinical indications: what is the evidence? *Eur J Radiol.* 2012;81(suppl 1):S82-S84.
2. DeMartini W, Lehman C. A review of current evidence-based clinical applications for breast magnetic resonance imaging. *Top Magn Reson Imaging.* 2008;19(3):143-150.
3. American College of Radiology. *Breast imaging reporting and data system (BI-RADS).* 5th ed. Reston, VA: American College of Radiology; 2013.
4. Partridge SC, McDonald ES. Diffusion weighted magnetic resonance imaging of the breast: protocol optimization, interpretation, and clinical applications. *Magn Reson Imaging Clin N Am.* 2013;21(3):601-624.
5. McDonald ES, Hammersley JA, Chou S-H, et al. Performance of diffusion-weighted magnetic resonance imaging as a rapid, non-contrast technique for detecting mammographically occult breast cancer in elevated-risk women with dense breasts. AJR Am J Roentgenol. In press.
6. Friedman PD, Swaminathan SV, Herman K, et al. Breast MRI: the importance of bilateral imaging. *AJR Am J Roentgenol.* 2006;187(2):345-349.
7. Price ER. Magnetic resonance imaging-guided biopsy of the breast: fundamentals and finer points. *Magn Reson Imaging Clin N Am.* 2013;21(3):571-581.
8. Middleton MS. MR evaluation of breast implants. *Radiol Clin North Am.* 2014;52(3):591-608.

# III
# NONINVASIVE CARDIAC AND VASCULAR IMAGING

# CHAPTER 12

# CARDIAC AND PERICARDIAC IMAGING

*Nam Ju Lee, MD, MMS, and Harold I. Litt, MD, PhD*

1. **What forms the borders of the heart on the frontal posteroanterior (PA) or anteroposterior (AP) chest radiograph?**
   The chest radiograph represents an important first step in the imaging workup of cardiovascular disease. On a PA frontal view of the chest, a cardiothoracic ratio (cardiac width : thoracic width) of less than 1 : 2 is considered normal in adults. Analysis of the cardiac silhouette can yield valuable information about chamber enlargement. The right atrium comprises the right heart border. This border becomes bulbous when the right atrium is enlarged. Superiorly, three convexities (called the "three moguls") comprise the left heart border, which, from superior to inferior, are the aortic knob, main pulmonary artery, and left atrial appendage. Inferiorly, the left ventricle (lateral wall and apex) comprises the left heart border.

2. **What forms the borders of the heart on the lateral chest radiograph?**
   Superiorly, the left atrium comprises the posterior heart border. Inferiorly, the left ventricle comprises the posterior heart border. The right ventricle comprises the anterior heart border; inferiorly, this abuts the posterior aspect of the sternum (Figure 12-1).

3. **What are the signs of left atrial enlargement on the chest radiograph?**
   Cardiac chamber enlargement can generally be identified by increased prominence of convexity of the corresponding heart border. In particular, left atrial enlargement causes a posterior bulging of the superoposterior heart border. On the frontal chest radiograph, signs of left atrial enlargement include enlargement of the left atrial appendage, "splaying" of the carina and elevation of the left main stem bronchus, and a "double density" projecting over the central portions of the heart, sometimes extending toward the right (Figure 12-2).

4. **What are the signs of right ventricular enlargement on the chest radiograph?**
   On the frontal chest radiograph, right ventricular enlargement can cause rounding of the left heart border (obscuring the normal shadow created by the left ventricle) and uplifting of the cardiac apex. On the lateral chest radiograph, right ventricular enlargement can displace normal retrosternal aerated lung (filling in the "anterior clear space"), although this is an unreliable finding (Figure 12-3).

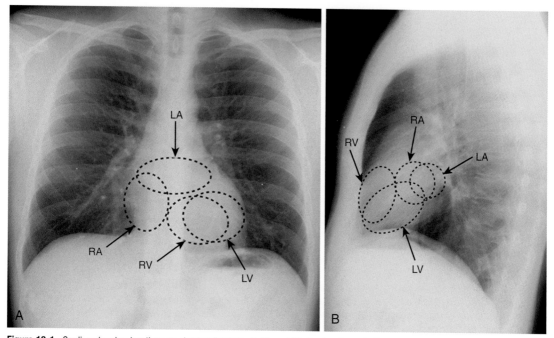

**Figure 12-1.** Cardiac chamber locations on chest radiograph. **A,** Normal PA chest radiograph. **B,** Normal lateral chest radiograph. Locations of cardiac chambers are outlined. *RA* = right atrium, *LA* = left atrium, *RV* = right ventricle, *LV* = left ventricle.

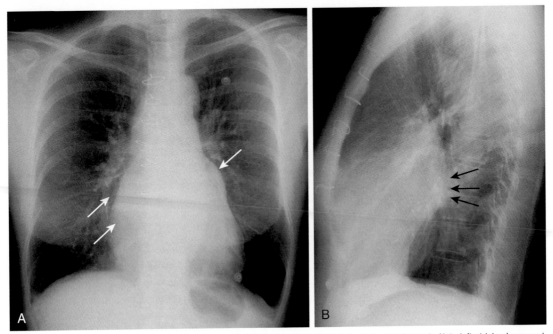

**Figure 12-2.** Left atrial enlargement on chest radiograph. **A,** PA chest radiograph. **B,** Lateral chest radiograph. Note left atrial enlargement (*arrows*) seen as "double density" projecting over right heart, enlarged left atrial appendage ("third mogul"), and convexity of superoposterior heart border.

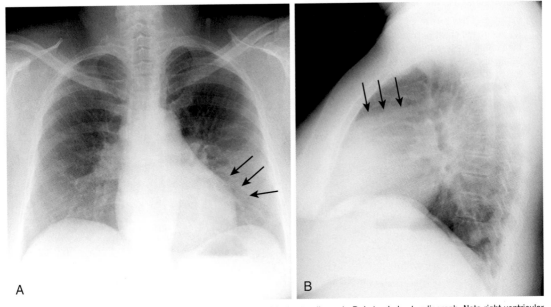

**Figure 12-3.** Right ventricular enlargement on chest radiograph. **A,** PA chest radiograph. **B,** Lateral chest radiograph. Note right ventricular enlargement (*arrows*) seen as rounded uplifted left heart border and extra density in retrosternal clear space.

5. What is Eisenmenger syndrome?

Small left-to-right shunts, such as with an atrial septal defect (ASD) or ventricular septal defect (VSD), are commonly asymptomatic early in life and may go undetected. Over time, the right side of the cardiopulmonary circulation responds to the increased volume with pulmonary arterial hyperplasia. This hyperplasia ultimately leads to elevated pulmonary vascular resistance and an increase in right-sided pressures (pulmonary hypertension). When right-sided pressures exceed left-sided pressures, the left-to-right shunt switches to become a right-to-left shunt. Dyspnea, fatigue, and cyanosis develop. This syndrome usually manifests in young adulthood.

6. What are the advantages of MRI for imaging the heart?

Magnetic resonance imaging (MRI) does not use ionizing radiation, and therefore may be a more appropriate modality for radiation-sensitive populations such as children and pregnant women. The contrast material used for MRI, which contains gadolinium rather than iodine used for computed tomography (CT), is associated with fewer allergic reactions and a lower incidence of contrast-induced nephropathy. MRI can also be used for functional evaluation, with a temporal resolution that is superior to CT, although not as good as that of echocardiography. Unlike echocardiography, MRI provides more operator-independent image quality, without interference from bone and air, and allows superior visualization of the right ventricle as well as measurement of blood flow. MRI has much higher soft tissue contrast compared to other imaging modalities, allowing for visualization of edema and scar tissue.

7. What are the disadvantages of MRI?

MRI examinations of the heart are lengthy, taking up to one hour, compared to minutes for CT. The examination also requires a good deal of patient cooperation with many breath holds of 15 to 20 seconds each. Claustrophobic patients may not be able to undergo the examination. MRI is costly and is generally not performed in patients with pacemakers or defibrillators, which limits its usage for many cardiac diseases. Also, CT has better spatial resolution than magnetic resonance angiography (MRA) in noninvasive coronary artery imaging, allowing for visualization of both calcified and noncalcified plaques as well as luminal obstruction. Furthermore, CT allows for simultaneous assessment of the lung parenchyma, which is more limited on MRI.

8. What are the indications for cardiac MRI?

Indications for cardiac MRI presently include evaluation of known or suspected coronary artery disease, cardiac masses and thrombi, pericardial abnormalities, valvular heart disease, cardiomyopathy, congenital cardiac disease, dysrhythmia, and aortic disease.

9. What are the contraindications to performing cardiac MRI?

Cardiac MRI is contraindicated in most patients with intracranial or intraocular metal or shrapnel, cochlear implants, most pacemakers or defibrillators, and some older prosthetic valves. Pregnancy is a relative contraindication, although it may still be performed when the benefit to the mother is greater than the unknown risk to the fetus. However, gadolinium-containing contrast material is contraindicated in pregnancy.

10. What are the standard planes for cross-sectional cardiac imaging?

The oblique orientation of the heart with respect to the body axis requires special planes of imaging. The four-chamber view of the heart captures all four cardiac chambers in a single image and includes the tricuspid and mitral valves. The short-axis view of the heart is perpendicular to the four-chamber view and allows accurate measurement of septal thickness and ventricular free wall thickness. In the short-axis view, the left ventricle is depicted in cross section and appears almost circular. Standard axial images also are commonly used. Coronal images are sometimes used to evaluate the diaphragmatic surface of the heart (Figure 12-4).

11. How is bright blood MRI accomplished, and why is it used?

As its name implies, bright blood imaging is an MRI technique whereby flowing blood has high signal intensity compared with tissue. This technique is accomplished through the use of gradient echo MR imaging. Bright blood imaging techniques are useful because they are fast and have high spatial resolution; they are commonly used for depicting blood vessels, cardiac chambers, and valve leaflets. Turbulent blood flow causes dark "jets" in bright blood images, allowing the detection of valvular stenosis or incompetence.

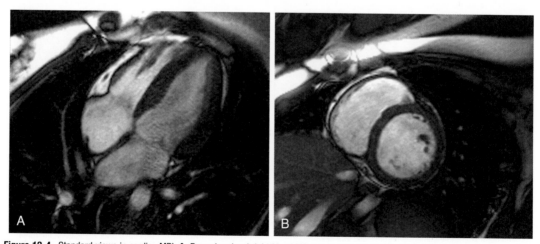

**Figure 12-4.** Standard views in cardiac MRI. **A,** Four-chamber bright blood MR image of heart. **B,** Short-axis bright blood MR image of heart.

12. **How is dark blood MRI accomplished, and why is it used?**

Dark blood imaging is an MRI technique whereby the blood signal intensity is suppressed; this can be done with spin echo or inversion recovery imaging. By reducing the signal from blood, myocardial tissue and vessel walls stand out from the background and can be seen in great detail. Dark blood imaging techniques are useful for detailed analysis of myocardial morphology and composition, cardiac anatomy, and vascular anatomy.

13. **How is cine imaging accomplished, and why is it used?**

Cine imaging portrays the heart in motion. Images are acquired during all phases of the cardiac cycle which requires synchronization with the electrocardiogram (ECG) signal. In MRI, this is accomplished with bright blood gradient echo imaging. The most common sequence used for cine imaging is steady state free precession (SSFP), also called balanced fast field echo (FFE), fast imaging employing steady state acquisition (FIESTA), or true fast imaging with steady state precession (FISP) imaging by different MRI vendors. Cine imaging is necessary to evaluate cardiac function and can be used to detect wall motion abnormalities, calculate ejection fraction (where ejection fraction = [(end diastolic volume − end systolic volume) / (end diastolic volume)] × 100%), and study the motion of valve leaflets.

14. **How are late gadolinium enhancement (LGE) images obtained, and how are they used?**

LGE images are obtained 10 to 15 minutes after intravenous injection of gadolinium-based contrast. Inversion recovery pulses are used to null the signal from normal myocardium to accentuate the bright signal from abnormal myocardium. When an appropriate inversion time (TI) is used, normal myocardium is dark. Myocardial late (or delayed) enhancement is present when there is myocardial fibrosis or scarring. Subendocardial or transmural late enhancement is usually related to prior myocardial infarction, while midmyocardial or epicardial late enhancement is related to nonischemic heart disease (Figure 12-5).

15. **What are some diseases that affect valvular function, and how can they be diagnosed with imaging?**

The aortic, pulmonic, mitral, and tricuspid valves can become stenotic, incompetent, or both. A chamber draining through a stenotic valve experiences a pressure load; if this chamber is a ventricle, it responds with muscular hypertrophy. If this chamber is an atrium, however, it responds with enlargement. A chamber draining through an incompetent (regurgitant) valve experiences a volume load (Figure 12-6) and responds with enlargement (whether it is an atrium or a ventricle). Echocardiography and MRI can measure chamber size and velocity and direction of blood flow across a valve orifice, detecting and quantifying valvular disease.

16. **How is phase contrast imaging accomplished, and why is it used?**

Moving protons (of blood) in a magnetic field gradient produce a phase shift proportional to their velocity and direction, while stationary protons (of tissue) produce no phase shift. This produces a signal that is proportional to the velocity of blood moving through the slice. Phase contrast cine gradient echo images (i.e., velocity-encoded images) exploit this property to quantify the velocity of blood moving through a stenotic valve in order to estimate the pressure gradient across the valve. To calculate the pressure gradient across a stenosis, the modified Bernoulli equation is used (where

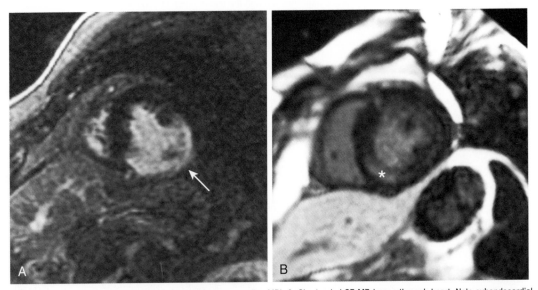

**Figure 12-5.** Ischemic versus nonischemic heart disease on cardiac MRI. **A,** Short-axis LGE MR image through heart. Note subendocardial and transmural late enhancement in inferior and lateral walls (*arrow*) of left ventricular myocardium reflecting prior myocardial infarction. **B,** Short-axis LGE MR image in different patient. Note area of midmyocardial late enhancement in noncoronary distribution (*) typical of nonischemic cardiomyopathy in this patient with sarcoidosis.

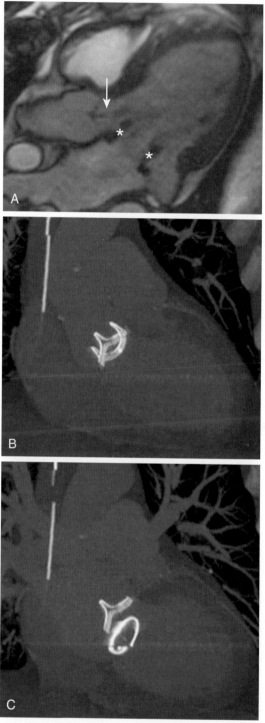

**Figure 12-6.** Valvular disease and prosthetic valves on MRI and CT. **A,** Bright blood cine acquisition MR image shows inferiorly directed signal void from aortic valve in diastole suggesting aortic regurgitation (*arrow*); left ventricle is mildly dilated. Note prosthetic mitral valve (⋆). **B** and **C,** Maximum intensity projection (MIP) CT images through heart demonstrate three-pronged bioprosthetic aortic valve (Carpentier-Edwards) with blood flow direction into aortic outflow tract. Note C-shaped mitral annular ring that is more inferior and to left of aortic valve prosthesis.

pressure gradient [in mm Hg] $= 4 \times v_{max}^2$ and $v_{max}$ is the maximum velocity [in m/sec]). Phase contrast images are also useful to evaluate regurgitant fraction, flow through an intracardiac shunt, flow velocity, and collateral flow.

17. **Why is Qp/Qs important, and how is it measured on MRI?**
In patients with intracardiac shunting, the evaluation of the ratio of pulmonic to systemic blood flow (Qp/Qs) is important because it often determines subsequent therapy. A Qp/Qs of <1.5 is usually managed conservatively in asymptomatic patients. A Qp/Qs of >1.5 in a patient whose pulmonary vascular resistance is not markedly elevated is usually referred for surgical correction. Velocity-encoded images are used to measure left-to-right shunting by comparing the flow in the proximal main pulmonary artery with the flow in the proximal aorta.

18. **What is the normal imaging appearance of the pericardium?**
The normal pericardium is seen as a thin (≤2 mm) curvilinear structure surrounding the heart on cross-sectional images.

19. **What imaging features may be seen with congenital absence of the pericardium?**
Congenital absence of the pericardium is rare, may be partial (most commonly) or complete, and is associated with other congenital abnormalities (mostly cardiopulmonary) in 30% to 50% of patients. Partial absence most commonly occurs on the left. Imaging studies may show lucency between the aorta and main pulmonary artery in the aorticopulmonary window due to herniated lung parenchyma as well as nonvisualization of the pericardium. Focal bulging of the left atrial appendage through a pericardial defect may also be seen with partial pericardial absence. With complete pericardial absence, the heart may rotate up and to the left with associated straightening and elongation of the left cardiac border.

20. **What are the imaging findings of a pericardial effusion?**
Small pericardial effusions can be difficult to detect with chest radiography. The cardiac silhouette may show a globular "water bottle" configuration as the pericardial effusion increases. Pericardial effusion may lead to the "Oreo cookie" sign, which refers to an opaque band of fluid between the lucent pericardial fat and subpericardial fat on a lateral chest radiograph. Although the sign is specific, the sensitivity is limited. Hemorrhagic pericardial fluid or nodularity of the pericardium can be seen on CT or MRI, which are features more suggestive of a malignant effusion.

21. **What are the imaging findings of acute pericarditis?**
Pericardial thickening and enhancement are imaging features of acute pericarditis on CT and MRI. Sometimes, pericardial effusion and inflammatory infiltration of the surrounding fat may be seen.

22. **What are some imaging findings of chronic (constrictive) pericarditis?**
Chronic (constrictive) pericarditis can be caused by cardiac surgery, radiation, or tuberculosis; however, most cases are idiopathic. Patients commonly present with right heart failure. Imaging findings include pericardial thickening, pericardial calcification, and abnormal motion of the interventricular septum (Figure 12-7). None of these findings is pathognomonic. In the appropriate clinical setting, and with invasive or noninvasive hemodynamic findings suggesting constrictive or restrictive physiology, a thickened pericardium seen on CT or MRI is sufficient to make the diagnosis of constrictive pericarditis.

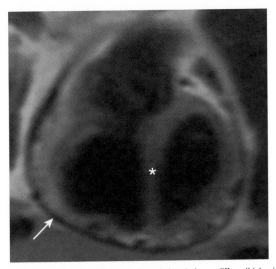

**Figure 12-7.** Constrictive pericarditis on MRI. Dark blood MR image through heart shows diffuse thickening of pericardium (*arrow*). Note flattening of interventricular septum (*) indicating pressure equalization between two ventricles.

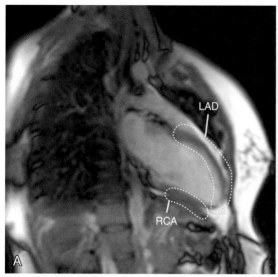 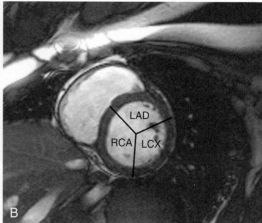

**Figure 12-8.** Coronary vascular territories on MRI. **A,** Vertical long-axis bright blood MR image through heart. **B,** Short-axis bright blood MR image through heart. Coronary vascular territories are delineated. *LAD* = left anterior descending (artery), *RCA* = right coronary artery, *LCX* = left circumflex (artery).

23. What portions of the heart are supplied by the right coronary, left anterior descending, and left circumflex arteries?

    The left anterior descending artery supplies the left ventricular apex and the anterior portion of the interventricular septum. The right coronary artery supplies the posteroinferior wall of the left ventricle and the posterior portion of the interventricular septum. The left circumflex artery supplies the lateral wall of the left ventricle (Figure 12-8).

24. What are noninvasive methods of coronary artery imaging?

    Imaging of the coronary arteries is a major part of evaluating ischemic heart disease. Traditionally, this imaging has been performed through cardiac catheterization, an invasive procedure that requires arterial puncture. Newer technologies promise noninvasive, cross-sectional imaging of coronary artery patency and can offer the potential to characterize coronary artery plaque. MRI, using bright blood, dark blood, and gadolinium-enhanced images, can be used to assess vessel patency and determine lipid content in coronary plaques. Coronary CT angiography can image vessel patency, potentially with a higher spatial resolution than MRI, and measure coronary calcification.

25. What is the most sensitive imaging technique for the detection of myocardial infarction?

    Cardiac MRI with delayed phase postcontrast images (i.e., a "viability study") is the most sensitive imaging technique. Echocardiography can detect areas of myocardial wall thinning or abnormal myocardial contraction. Cardiac single photon emission computed tomography (SPECT) can detect areas of nonviable myocardium. MRI has greater specificity than echocardiography, however, and greater spatial resolution and sensitivity than SPECT. Acute or chronic myocardial infarction shows accumulation of gadolinium-based contrast material in a delayed fashion (10 to 15 minutes after contrast administration), probably owing to a combination of increased vascular permeability and enlargement of the extracellular space. The percentage of the myocardial thickness showing delayed phase enhancement correlates inversely with the likelihood of return of function of that segment of myocardium after a revascularization procedure.

26. How long after myocardial infarction does a ventricular aneurysm develop?

    A ventricular aneurysm develops in the setting of remote prior myocardial infarction. Areas of the heart muscle that have undergone infarction ultimately become thin and fibrotic; these weak areas of myocardium can balloon out over time because of chronic exposure to systemic blood pressure. True ventricular aneurysms usually have a wide mouth, are most commonly anteriorly located, and may undergo mural calcification, resulting in a characteristic curvilinear density on chest radiographs (Figure 12-9).

27. How long after myocardial infarction does a ventricular pseudoaneurysm develop?

    Infarcted myocardial tissue undergoes a predictable sequence of histologic changes. As the tissue undergoes necrosis, it becomes mechanically weak and is prone to rupture. This most commonly occurs approximately 3 to 7 days after the infarction. Myocardial rupture most often occurs in the ventricular free wall but can also occur in the interventricular septum (causing a left-to-right shunt) or in a papillary muscle (causing mitral regurgitation). If the myocardial rupture is contained, a ventricular pseudoaneurysm forms. These pseudoaneurysms characteristically have a narrow mouth because they essentially represent rupture through a small hole in the myocardium, and they are

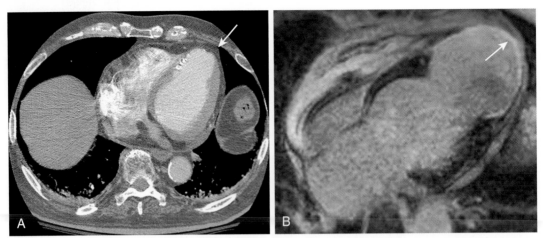

**Figure 12-9.** True ventricular aneurysm on CT and MRI. **A,** Axial contrast-enhanced CT image through heart shows ballooning and marked wall thinning (*arrow*) of myocardium at left ventricular apex. Anterior location is characteristic for true ventricular aneurysm. **B,** LGE MR image through heart also demonstrates marked myocardial thinning at left ventricular apex as well as transmural late enhancement due to prior myocardial infarct (*arrow*).

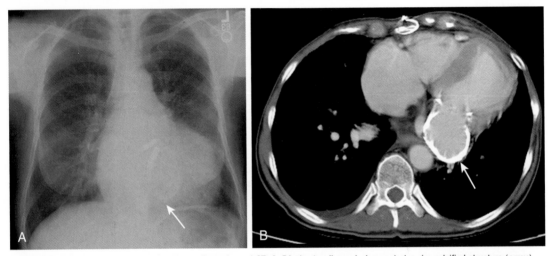

**Figure 12-10.** Ventricular pseudoaneurysm on radiography and CT. **A,** PA chest radiograph demonstrates rim calcified structure (*arrow*) overlying left heart. **B,** Axial contrast-enhanced CT image through heart shows outpouching (*arrow*) arising from posteroinferior portion of left ventricle with extensive mural calcification (indicating chronicity). Posterior or inferior location is characteristic for ventricular pseudoaneurysm.

more commonly posteriorly or inferiorly located. Myocardial pseudoaneurysms are generally considered to be unstable because they themselves may rupture (Figure 12-10).

28. **What is the differential diagnosis of a regional wall motion abnormality?**
    A wall motion abnormality indicates a portion of myocardium that has abnormally reduced contractility. This reduced contractility usually occurs on the basis of previous or ongoing ischemia and suggests heart muscle that is acutely ischemic, infarcted, stunned, or hibernating. Acutely ischemic myocardium cannot contract properly because of inadequate blood flow and poor energy supply. Infarcted myocardium is nonviable, does not contract, and may eventually exhibit "paradoxical" motion with ballooning out during systole instead of thickening. When a portion of heart muscle remains viable after a temporary episode of acute ischemia, it can become "stunned," where wall motion abnormality persists because of chemical changes in the myocardium that resolve over time. Finally, chronically ischemic myocardium can down-regulate its own contractility to match its energy demands with energy supply; this is termed "hibernating" and may signify tissue at risk for future infarction.

29. **What are some causes of dilated cardiomyopathy and restrictive cardiomyopathy?**
    Cardiomyopathies are diseases that involve primary dysfunction of the heart muscle. This broad collection of diseases can be divided on a pathophysiologic basis into dilated, hypertrophic, and restrictive subtypes, with some overlap

occurring between these categories. A few causes of dilated cardiomyopathy include previous myocarditis related to viral infection (especially by coxsackievirus B and cytomegalovirus), and toxic exposure (e.g., cocaine, alcohol, and doxorubicin). Causes of restrictive cardiomyopathy include infiltrative systemic disorders such as sarcoidosis, amyloidosis, eosinophilic cardiomyopathy (Löffler syndrome), and Fabry disease. On MRI, nonischemic cardiomyopathy may show midmyocardial or subepicardial delayed enhancement not corresponding to a coronary artery distribution.

30. **What are the findings of hypertrophic cardiomyopathy on MRI?**

    Hypertrophic cardiomyopathy is inherited as an autosomal dominant trait with variable penetrance. Genotype positive patients may be asymptomatic or have atrial fibrillation, heart failure, syncope, or even sudden cardiac death. Asymmetric hypertrophy of the ventricular wall can occur anywhere with variable phenotype. Systolic anterior motion of the mitral valve and left ventricular outflow tract obstruction can also be seen. MRI is useful for diagnosis and treatment planning by identifying the distribution of the thickened myocardium, maximum wall thickness, and late enhancement, and for quantifying the subaortic pressure gradient (Figure 12-11). LGE is helpful to predict prognosis as well as to differentiate this condition from other disorders that may cause abnormal myocardial wall thickening.

31. **How does a patient with myocarditis present clinically, and what are the findings on MRI?**

    Myocarditis has been reported in up to 12% of young adults presenting with sudden death. MRI is indicated in patients with current or persistent symptoms, evidence for significant myocardial injury, and a suspected viral etiology. MRI is of potential use in patients with chest pain, elevated troponin levels, and normal coronary arteries, where it can identify myocarditis in more than 30% of patients. Findings on MRI include increased myocardial signal intensity on T2-weighted images resulting from intracellular and interstitial edema, arterial phase enhancement from hyperemia and capillary leak, and LGE from fibrosis.

32. **In a patient with an abnormal ECG finding and a family history of sudden death, cardiac MRI shows a dilated right ventricle with abnormal wall motion and a normal left ventricle. What is the most likely diagnosis?**

    Arrhythmogenic right ventricular dysplasia or cardiomyopathy (ARVD/C) is the most likely diagnosis. This is a disease of unknown etiology, characterized by fatty or fibrous infiltration of the myocardium. It is a common cause of sudden death and may be familial. Diagnosis is made through a combination of clinical, imaging, ECG, and pathologic findings. MRI is a useful test for evaluating right ventricular morphology, composition, and function, and the diagnostic criteria for ARVD/C include specific thresholds for right ventricular size and function. Suggestive findings on MRI include dysfunction, dilation, or thinning of the right ventricular wall; aneurysms of the right ventricle; and fatty infiltration of the right ventricular wall. Treatment consists of placement of an implantable cardioverter defibrillator. The diagnosis of ARVD/C should not be made on the basis of imaging findings alone.

33. **What is myocardial noncompaction, and how does it appear on MRI?**

    Noncompacted myocardium is a congenital abnormality in the structure of ventricular tissue due to a morphogenetic defect during embryogenesis. It seems to occur as a result of an arrest in endomyocardial morphogenesis. A family history of dilated cardiomyopathy is not uncommon. It manifests in early childhood, often associated with other cardiac and extracardiac anomalies. Clinical presentation includes ventricular dysrhythmias, thromboembolism, and progressive systolic heart failure, diastolic heart failure, or both. Myocardial noncompaction may be suggested when the ratio of the maximum thickness of the myocardial trabecular layer to compacted layer is ≥2.3 in end-diastole with a decreased ejection fraction in the absence of other types of structural heart disease.

34. **What happens when a ventricle becomes dilated?**

    When a ventricle becomes dilated, according to Laplace's law, parietal stress (i.e., the force against arterial tissue) increases, inducing further mechanical disadvantage due to the increased oxygen demand and subsequent worsening of the ventricular systolic performance. Hence, myocardial dysfunction leads to more myocardial dysfunction in a vicious cycle causing adverse ventricular remodeling.

35. **What are common cardiac or paracardiac masses?**

    The most common cardiac or paracardiac mass is thrombus (Figure 12-12, *A*). Patients with indwelling central venous catheters are at risk for developing right atrial thrombus, and patients with atrial fibrillation are at increased risk for developing left atrial thrombus. Deep venous thrombi of the extremities can migrate to the right atrium before causing a pulmonary embolism. Other causes of thrombus in the atria include hypercoagulable states and tumors that invade the inferior vena cava and propagate as tumor thrombus into the right atrium (e.g., renal cell carcinoma, adrenal carcinoma, and hepatocellular carcinoma). The most common primary cardiac neoplasm is a myxoma (Figure 12-12, *B* and *C*). Most myxomas are found in the left atrium and originate from the atrial septum. Myxomas may prolapse and cause valvular regurgitation.

36. **How can you differentiate tumor from thrombus?**

    MRI is the most accurate imaging examination for differentiation of tumor from thrombus. On gradient echo MR images, thrombus shows low signal intensity without enhancement after contrast administration, whereas neoplasms enhance.

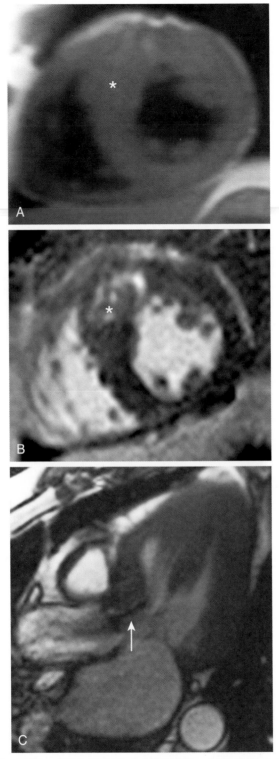

**Figure 12-11.** Hypertrophic cardiomyopathy on MRI. **A,** Short-axis dark blood MR image through heart shows asymmetric wall thickening (∗) in anteroseptal left ventricular myocardium. **B,** Short-axis LGE MR image through heart demonstrates heterogeneous intramural late enhancement in same region. **C,** Bright blood MR image through heart shows signal void in left ventricular outflow tract (*arrow*) reflecting elevated blood flow velocities from outflow tract obstruction caused by hypertrophic septum.

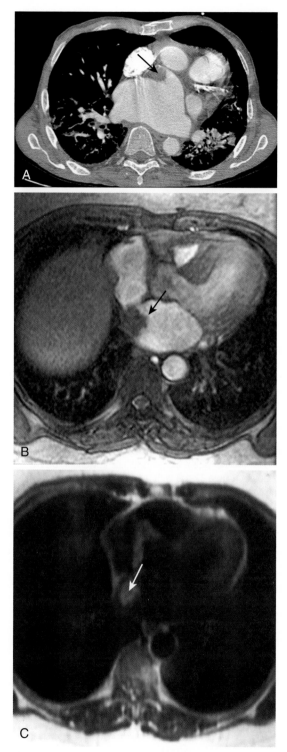

**Figure 12-12.** Intraatrial lesions on CT and MRI. **A,** Axial contrast-enhanced CT image through heart shows low attenuation filling defect (*arrow*) in anterior aspect of markedly dilated left atrium representing thrombus. This patient had undergone heart transplantation. **B,** Axial bright blood and **C,** Axial T2-weighted MR images through heart in different patient show mass (*arrows*) in left atrium that is hyperintense on T2-weighted images due to myxoma.

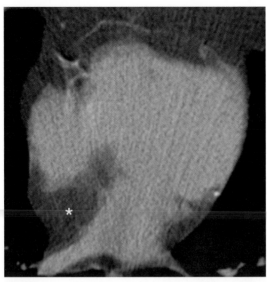

**Figure 12-13.** Lipomatous hypertrophy of interatrial septum on CT. Unenhanced CT image through heart shows fat attenuation thickening of interatrial septum (*).

37. What is the most common malignancy of the heart and pericardium?

Metastatic disease is the most common malignancy of the heart and pericardium. Lung cancer, lymphoma, breast cancer, and melanoma all can involve the heart or pericardium. Lung cancer is the most common primary tumor of patients with cardiac metastases; however, melanoma is the most likely tumor to spread to the heart. Primary tumors of the heart are rare, and primary malignant tumors of the heart are exceedingly rare.

38. What does lipomatous hypertrophy of the interatrial septum (LHIS) look like on imaging studies?

LHIS is characterized by benign fatty infiltration of the interatrial septum and is usually discovered incidentally. It most commonly occurs in older, obese people, with a higher incidence in women. On CT, LHIS appears as fat attenuation thickening of the interatrial septum (Figure 12-13) with relative sparing of the fossa ovalis. On MRI, LHIS shows homogeneous high signal intensity similar to fat on all imaging sequences.

## KEY POINTS

- On a frontal chest radiograph, the right atrium comprises the right heart border, whereas the aortic knob, main pulmonary artery, left atrial appendage, and left ventricle comprise the left heart border from superior to inferior. On a lateral chest radiograph, the left atrium comprises the posterior-superior heart border, whereas the right ventricle comprises the anterior heart border.
- Subendocardial or transmural LGE is usually related to prior myocardial infarction, while midmyocardial or epicardial LGE is related to nonischemic heart disease.
- True ventricular aneurysms usually have a wide mouth and are most commonly anteriorly located, whereas ventricular pseudoaneurysms characteristically have a narrow mouth and are more commonly posteriorly or inferiorly located.
- The most common cardiac or paracardiac mass is thrombus. The most common primary cardiac neoplasm is myxoma. The most common malignant neoplasm of the heart and pericardium is metastatic disease.

**BIBLIOGRAPHY**

Jimenez Juan L, Crean AM, Wintersperger BJ. Late gadolinium enhancement imaging in assessment of myocardial viability: techniques and clinical applications. *Radiol Clin North Am.* 2015;53(2):397-411.

Lin K, Carr JC. MR Imaging of the coronary vasculature: imaging the lumen, wall, and beyond. *Radiol Clin North Am.* 2015;53(2):345-353.

Tavano A, Maurel B, Gaubert JY, et al. MR imaging of arrhythmogenic right ventricular dysplasia: What the radiologist needs to know. *Diagn Interv Imaging.* 2015;96(5):449-460.

Bogaert J, Olivotto I. MR imaging in hypertrophic cardiomyopathy: from magnet to bedside. *Radiology.* 2014;273(2):329-348.

de Roos A, Higgins CB. Cardiac radiology: centenary review. *Radiology.* 2014;273(2 suppl):S142-S159.

Leong DP, Joseph MX, Selvanayagam JB. The evolving role of multimodality imaging in valvular heart disease. *Heart.* 2014;100(4):336-346.

Motwani M, Kidambi A, Greenwood JP, et al. Advances in cardiovascular magnetic resonance in ischaemic heart disease and non-ischaemic cardiomyopathies. *Heart.* 2014;100(21):1722-1733.

Orwat S, Diller GP, Baumgartner H. Imaging of congenital heart disease in adults: choice of modalities. *Eur Heart J Cardiovasc Imaging.* 2014;15(1):6-17.

Gunaratnam K, Wong LH, Nasis A, et al. Review of cardiomyopathy imaging. *Eur J Radiol.* 2013;82(10):1763-1775.

Verde F, Johnson PT, Jha S, et al. Congenital absence of the pericardium and its mimics. *J Cardiovasc Comput Tomogr.* 2013;7(1):11-17.

Manning WJ, Pennell DJ. *Cardiovascular magnetic resonance.* 2nd ed. Philadelphia: Saunders Elsevier; 2010.

Yared K, Baggish AL, Picard MH, et al. Multimodality imaging of pericardial diseases. *JACC Cardiovasc Imaging.* 2010;3(6):650-660.

Friedrich MG, Sechtem U, Schulz-Menger J, et al. Cardiovascular magnetic resonance in myocarditis: A JACC White Paper. *J Am Coll Cardiol.* 2009;53(17):1475-1487.

Jeudy J, White CS. Cardiac magnetic resonance imaging: techniques and principles. *Semin Roentgenol.* 2008;43(3):173-182.

O'Sullivan PJ, Gladish GW. Cardiac tumors. *Semin Roentgenol.* 2008;43(3):223-233.

Sparrow PJ, Kurian JB, Jones TR, et al. MR imaging of cardiac tumors. *Radiographics.* 2005;25(5):1255-1276.

Troughton RW, Asher CR, Klein AL. Pericarditis. *Lancet.* 2004;363(9410):717-727.

Wang ZJ, Reddy GP, Gotway MB, et al. CT and MR imaging of pericardial disease. *Radiographics.* 2003;23(Spec No):S167-S180.

Grebenc ML, Rosado-de-Christenson ML, Green CE, et al. Cardiac myxoma: imaging features in 83 patients. *Radiographics.* 2002;22(3):673-689.

Chiles C, Woodard PK, Gutierrez FR, et al. Metastatic involvement of the heart and pericardium: CT and MR imaging. *Radiographics.* 2001;21(2):439-449.

Grebenc ML, Rosado de Christenson ML, Burke AP, et al. Primary cardiac and pericardial neoplasms: radiologic-pathologic correlation. *Radiographics.* 2000;20(4):1073-1103, quiz 110-111, 112.

# CHAPTER 13

# AORTIC IMAGING

*Jasmeet Singh, MD, MPHA, and Harold I. Litt, MD, PhD*

1. What is the normal imaging appearance of the aorta on computed tomography (CT) and magnetic resonance imaging (MRI)?

   The normal aorta on imaging can be divided into the following five parts: the aortic root, the ascending aorta, the proximal (anterior) aortic arch, the distal (posterior) aortic arch, and the descending thoracic aorta. The proximal segment of the ascending aorta is the aortic root, which begins at the upper part of the left ventricle and is approximately 3 cm in diameter in adults. The aortic root and most of the ascending aorta (approximately 5 cm long) is contained within the pericardium. The aortic root has three cusps, which define three spaces called the sinuses of Valsalva: the right, left, and noncoronary sinuses. The right coronary artery normally arises from the right cusp, and the left coronary artery arises from the left cusp. The ascending aorta is located along the right mediastinal border and becomes the aortic arch at the origin of the innominate artery. The aortic arch also gives rise to the left common carotid and left subclavian arteries.

   The descending aorta begins where the aortic arch ends, immediately beyond the origin of the left subclavian artery. The aorta descends within the thorax adjacent to the vertebral column after crossing superiorly and then posteriorly over the root of the left lung. After crossing the diaphragmatic hiatus, it becomes the abdominal aorta, which is approximately 2 cm in diameter. Eventually, the abdominal aorta ends by dividing into right and left common iliac arteries, slightly to the left of the midplane at the lower border of the fourth lumbar vertebra. The descending aorta is the most posterior structure adjacent to the spine.

   On CT or MRI, the normal aortic lumen will appear round in cross-section with a thin wall.

2. What typical CT and MRI protocols/techniques are used to image the aorta?

   Computed tomographic angiography (CTA) is performed to assess diseases of the aorta and has established itself as the principal diagnostic test for aortic pathology.

   Many CTA examinations include a nonenhanced acquisition from the supra-aortic vessels to the iliac and femoral arteries. The noncontrast scan can be useful for detection of aortic calcification, allowing for discrimination between calcification and contrast enhancement, as well as detection of high-attenuation intramural hematoma. This is then followed by a contrast-enhanced scan, acquired during the time when contrast enhancement is highest in the aorta (usually about 20 to 25 seconds after beginning an intravenous injection). Delayed phase imaging may be performed 1 to 5 minutes later in some cases to detect endoleaks in patients with stent-grafts, to evaluate the venous system, and to detect slow contrast extravasation. CTA scans are performed preferably using contrast agents with higher iodine concentrations in order to obtain high levels of vascular enhancement. Scanning protocols may differ from one institution to another depending on the type of scanner, data storage capacity, and resources available for patient monitoring.

   CTA data acquisition can also be synchronized to the electrocardiogram (ECG) signal, allowing for effective freezing of the motion of the heart at various parts of the cardiac cycle. Two main techniques for ECG-synchronized imaging are prospective triggering and retrospective gating. Prospective triggering acquires data during only a prespecified portion of the cardiac cycle, while retrospective gating acquires data throughout the cardiac cycle. Retrospective gating allows evaluation of cardiac and valvular motion, but at the cost of increased radiation dose compared to prospective triggering.

   Magnetic resonance angiography (MRA) is usually performed to include a combination of bright blood and dark blood images before and after contrast administration. As in CTA, ECG-synchronized acquisitions can be performed with prospective triggering or retrospective gating. Prospectively triggered dark blood T1-weighted or inversion recovery sequences performed in axial and oblique sagittal planes are useful for evaluating the aortic wall to look for atherosclerotic plaque and wall thickening in vasculitis.

   A contrast-enhanced MR angiogram is then usually performed with a three-dimensional gradient echo acquisition obtained during a breath hold. The imaging plane and slice thickness are optimized to the anatomy of interest (e.g., an oblique sagittal acquisition for the thoracic aorta or a coronal acquisition for the abdominal aorta). Because there is no radiation dose, multiple acquisitions can be obtained at various phases of contrast enhancement as needed.

   In patients with renal disease, contrast allergy, or poor venous access, noncontrast MRA techniques can be used, although image quality may not be as good as that with contrast MRA. Commonly used sequences for this approach are time-of-flight (TOF) and steady state free precession (SSFP) techniques. Additionally, phase-contrast (PC) MRA allows measurement of blood flow and can supplement the other techniques listed above.

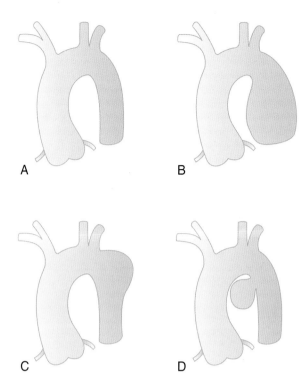

**Figure 13-1.** Types of aortic aneurysms. **A,** Normal configuration of thoracic aorta. **B,** Fusiform aneurysmal dilation of descending thoracic aorta. Fusiform aneurysms are common in atherosclerosis. **C,** Eccentric, or saccular, aneurysm of descending thoracic aorta, such as caused by infection. **D,** Pseudoaneurysm, a contained rupture. In true aneurysms, all three layers of the vessel wall are intact. In pseudoaneurysms, the intima or media or both have been disrupted, only leaving intact adventitia.

3. What are aneurysms and pseudoaneurysms, and how do they differ?
   An aneurysm (also known as a true aneurysm) is dilation of a vessel in which all three layers of the vessel wall remain intact. A pseudoaneurysm (also known as a false aneurysm) is a contained rupture and implies disruption of at least part of the aortic wall (i.e., the intima, media, or both), with intact adventitia. Pseudoaneurysms are potentially highly unstable lesions. They are often post-traumatic or iatrogenic in nature (Figure 13-1).

4. What is a mycotic aneurysm? Which imaging findings help suggest the diagnosis?
   One might think mycotic means "related to fungus," but mycotic aneurysm refers to an aneurysm caused by any type of infection, usually bacterial. Imaging features that may suggest the diagnosis are rapid change in size, adjacent inflammation, perivascular gas, eccentric or saccular configuration, or lack of atherosclerotic calcification.

5. What is an inflammatory abdominal aortic aneurysm (AAA)?
   Inflammatory AAAs are aortic aneurysms associated with retroperitoneal fibrosis. These aneurysms are surrounded by extensive inflammation and fibrosis that often lead to complications such as ureteral obstruction. Some authorities believe that the surrounding fibrosis is a result of microscopic leakage of the aneurysm causing a severe secondary inflammatory response, whereas others espouse a viral or immune reaction–related etiology. Inflammatory aneurysms are much less common than atherosclerotic aneurysms.

6. What are aortoenteric and aortocaval fistulas, and how are they diagnosed?
   Aortic aneurysms, usually when inflamed or infected, can erode into adjacent structures, such as bowel or the inferior vena cava, leading to connections between the aortic lumen and the lumina of these structures. The transverse portion of the duodenum and the inferior vena cava (IVC) are common locations for such fistulas as the expanding aneurysmal abdominal aorta exerts pressure on these adjacent structures. An aortoenteric fistula is suggested when there is a loss of fat plane between the enlarged aorta and the involved bowel loop, with inflammatory stranding in that region. Sometimes, air can be seen in the aortic lumen. If an aortoenteric or aortocaval fistula is suspected, imaging should first be performed without oral or intravenous contrast material, so that high attenuation in the affected bowel or IVC lumen on postcontrast scans can be correctly attributed to the fistula rather than from normal opacification by the administered contrast material (Figure 13-2).

7. What is an aortic dissection, and how is it different from aortic transection?
   Aortic dissection is caused by a tear of the intima, creating a false channel or lumen within the wall of the aorta. Flowing blood dissects along the course of the aorta, extending the false lumen longitudinally and into branch vessels. The classic clinical presentation is "ripping" back or chest pain.

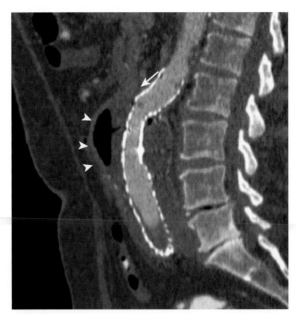

**Figure 13-2.** Aortoenteric fistula on CTA. Sagittal multiplanar reformatted CTA image demonstrates large amount of gas within abdominal aortic aneurysm sac (*arrowheads*) and loss of fat plane between duodenum and aortic aneurysm (*arrow*). Indwelling endovascular stent-graft is also seen within abdominal aorta.

Aortic transection (perhaps better referred to as traumatic aortic injury) occurs in trauma patients. The entire aortic wall is injured or transected, leading to hemorrhage or pseudoaneurysm formation. Transection is usually a focal injury, usually in the chest. Dissections extend for some distance and require more extensive imaging of the entire aorta and its branch vessels.

8. **In the setting of blunt trauma, where do aortic injuries most commonly occur?**
   Most injuries seen by radiologists occur at the aortic isthmus, which is just distal to the takeoff of the left subclavian artery. Most authorities believe this is due to asymmetric aortic fixation at this location, leading to shear stress. Radiologists less commonly see injuries to the ascending aorta because many patients with this type of injury die before reaching the hospital.

9. **How are traumatic aortic injuries diagnosed?**
   Clinical suspicion or chest radiographic findings should be enough to send a patient with an unstable condition to surgery. If the patient's condition is relatively stable, most authorities now recommend CTA, preferably with a multidetector computed tomography (MDCT) scanner. Catheter angiography, previously the mainstay of diagnosis, is now most useful for problem solving when CTA is nondiagnostic or equivocal.

10. **Name the chest radiographic findings that are suggestive of thoracic aortic pathology.**
    Primary signs include an enlarged or enlarging aorta, an indistinct aortic contour, or displacement of intimal atherosclerotic calcifications (in aortic dissection). Secondary signs, indicating mass effect from an aneurysm or hematoma, include mediastinal widening; displacement of adjacent structures such as the trachea, the left main stem bronchus, or a nasogastric tube in the esophagus; an "apical cap," or mediastinal hematoma extending above the lung apex; or pleural or pericardial effusion (which can be hemorrhagic, but is more commonly due to exudative fluid secondary to the adjacent acute aortic process). Many of these findings are not specific for aortic pathologic conditions. Even mediastinal hematoma in the setting of trauma is not specific because it may be secondary to venous rather than arterial injury.

11. **What are the two classification schemes for aortic dissection?**
    The Stanford classification categorizes dissections into those involving the ascending aorta regardless of involvement of the descending aorta, and those involving the descending aorta only:
    - Type A: Ascending aorta involved with or without descending aorta.
    - Type B: Descending aorta only.
      The DeBakey classification denotes three categories of aortic dissection: involvement of the ascending aorta alone, descending aorta alone, or both. A mnemonic for this system is BAD:
    - Type 1: Both ascending and descending aorta.
    - Type 2: Ascending aorta only.
    - Type 3: Descending aorta only.

Remember that the descending aorta is defined as that portion of the aorta distal to the takeoff of the left subclavian artery.

12. **How are dissections that involve the ascending aorta managed differently from those that involve the descending aorta only?**

Dissections involving the ascending aorta (Stanford type A and DeBakey types 1 and 2) are surgical emergencies because mortality is significantly greater in medically managed patients (approximately 90% in the first 3 months) compared with surgically treated patients. This high mortality rate is mostly due to hemopericardium causing cardiac tamponade, acute aortic regurgitation, or involvement of coronary artery origins with acute myocardial infarction. Descending aortic dissections are usually treated medically (with antihypertensive agents) because morbidity and mortality are greater with surgery than with medical management. Complicated descending aortic dissections may require surgical or endovascular intervention, however.

13. **Which lumen is usually larger in aortic dissection—the true or false lumen?**

Approximately 90% of the time, the false lumen is larger in caliber than the true lumen.

14. **Describe other acute aortic syndromes that are often called variants of aortic dissection.**

Penetrating atherosclerotic ulcer is a focal tear of the intima caused by ruptured plaque, leading to ulceration into the aortic wall. It is different from a dissection because a dissection is not focal, but rather propagates along the length of the vessel.

Intramural hematoma is a hemorrhage into the wall of the vessel, generally between the inner and outer layers of the media. Intramural hematoma may occur without an intimal tear, such as secondary to rupture of the vasa vasorum (small blood vessels in the wall of the aorta); this is usually secondary to hypertension but can be caused by trauma. Alternatively, it may be associated with an intimal tear, such as secondary to a penetrating aortic ulcer (Figure 13-3).

A recently described entity, known as a limited intimal tear, is diagnosed when there is a shallow tear of the intima, without extension of the tear to form a false lumen.

**Warning**: These terms can become extremely confusing because one form of an aortic pathologic condition can lead to another. In part because of this confusion in terminology, there are numerous controversies in the surgical literature regarding prognosis and management of the "dissection variants."

15. **What is the best imaging modality for diagnosing each of these conditions?**

CT and MRI are the two best modalities for evaluating these conditions. CT is generally preferred because it is faster (important in patients with an unstable condition) and has better spatial resolution. MRI is often used for problem solving in patients with a stable condition or in patients with an iodinated contrast allergy. For patients with renal disease on permanent dialysis, CT is performed because of the risk of nephrogenic systemic fibrosis related to gadolinium-based MRI contrast agents. For patients with renal disease who are not on permanent dialysis, noncontrast MRA techniques can be used. Although these techniques generally have lower spatial resolution and take longer to acquire than contrast-enhanced MRA, they are usually sufficient to exclude an acute aortic syndrome. Ultrasonography (US) also has been used, but it cannot visualize the entire aorta and misses the extent of disease or associated complications. At this time, the main indication for use of catheter angiography for these conditions is treatment of complications.

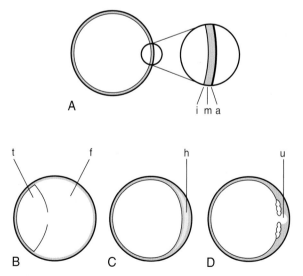

**Figure 13-3.** Aortic wall anatomy and pathologic conditions. **A,** Layers of the aortic wall. *i* = intima, *m* = media, *a* = adventitia. **B,** Aortic dissection, between the intima and media. *t* = true lumen, *f* = false lumen. **C,** *h* = intramural hematoma. **D,** *u* = penetrating atherosclerotic ulcer.

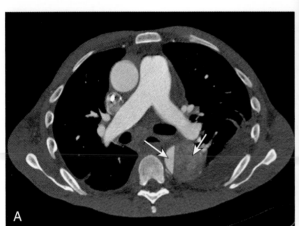

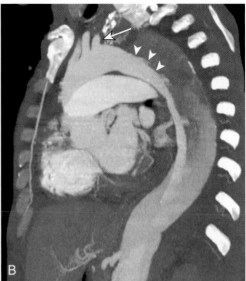

**Figure 13-4.** Aortic dissection on CTA. **A,** Axial CT image shows enhancement of true lumen (*long arrow*) and minimal enhancement of larger false lumen (*short arrow*) of aorta with separation of both lumina by linear dissection flap. **B,** Oblique sagittal maximum intensity projection (MIP) reformatted CT image reveals that aortic dissection is of type B, as it begins just distal to takeoff of left subclavian artery (*arrow*). The dissection flap is indicated by arrowheads.

16. How can these conditions be distinguished on axial CT or MR images?

    A dissection flap most often appears as a linear or curvilinear focus across the vessel, separating the true lumen from the false lumen (Figure 13-4), which may be calcified. Intramural hematomas usually appear as a crescentic region of high attenuation or high T1-weighted signal intensity with smooth borders. The presence of an irregular luminal border with peripheral low attenuation may reflect ulcerated atherosclerotic plaque or thrombus. A limited intimal tear most often appears as a subtle contour abnormality of the aortic wall without history of trauma or presence of an intimal flap or intramural hematoma.

17. What is the utility of precontrast imaging when performing CTA or MRA of the aorta?

    Subacute hemorrhage has higher attenuation than flowing blood on noncontrast CT and high signal intensity on precontrast T1-weighted MRI. These findings can be easily obscured in the presence of an intravenous contrast material. Precontrast imaging is mandatory to detect the presence of intramural hematoma. Noncontrast CT images are also useful to detect the presence, location, and amount of atherosclerotic calcification. Calcification is generally difficult to visualize on MR images.

18. How large must the thoracic and abdominal aortas be to be called aneurysmal?

    Any artery dilated by more than 50% of its normal caliber is called aneurysmal. Most authorities define an aortic aneurysm as an aorta that is greater than or equal to 4 cm in diameter in the thoracic aorta and 3 cm in diameter in the abdomen. The aorta should normally decrease in size as it extends distally, and any focal dilation should be considered abnormal.

19. When is an AAA usually repaired?

    Surgical repair of an AAA is generally considered for aortas larger than 5 cm in caliber or for aortas that are symptomatic or display rapid growth.

20. What is Laplace's law, and how is it relevant to aortic aneurysms?

    Laplace's law states that the larger the radius of a sphere, the greater the wall stress. With regard to aneurysms, this means that as an aneurysm increases in size, the stress on the aortic wall also increases. Therefore, the aneurysm becomes more prone to rupture with increasing size.

21. Can the overall size of an aortic aneurysm be determined by catheter angiography?

    No. Often there is an extensive mural thrombus in an aneurysm, and a large aneurysm can have a normal-sized lumen. Only the lumen is opacified by catheter angiography, and the outer size of the aneurysm cannot be determined by this method.

22. How is the size of the aorta most accurately measured on CT or MRI?

    Drawing a line perpendicular to the course of the aorta is required for accurate measurement of the aortic diameter. This is often different than the cross-section of the aorta commonly seen on axial CT and MR images because these

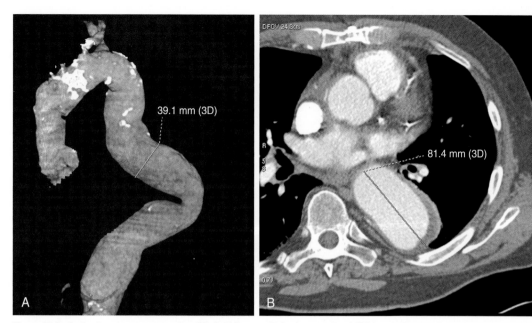

**Figure 13-5.** Aortic diameter measurement on CT. **A,** Oblique sagittal volume-rendered CTA image of tortuous aorta shows proper way to measure diameter of tortuous aorta. Imaginary line is drawn down center of long axis of vessel, and transverse diameter is measured perpendicular to that line. Measurements such as this must be made using multiplanar or three-dimensional reformatting to compensate for vessel tortuosity. **B,** Axial CT image from same study shows how reliance on axial images can result in overestimation of aortic size. At this level, tortuous aorta is coursing roughly in axial plane and appears much more dilated than it actually is.

images are axial to the patient's body, not axial relative to the course of the aorta. Accurate measurement, especially of a tortuous vessel, often requires multiplanar or three-dimensional reformatting (Figure 13-5).

23. **Name two methods of repairing aneurysms, and compare their advantages and disadvantages.**
Surgical repair and endovascular stent-graft repair are two methods of repairing aneurysms. Surgical repair is a more definitive treatment, requiring no imaging follow-up, and has known long-term durability. Endovascular repair is newer, and long-term data are unavailable. Because of potential complications of endovascular repair, follow-up imaging and reintervention often are required. Many patients with aortic aneurysm are not surgical candidates, however, because of comorbidities such as cardiopulmonary disease; endovascular repair is preferred for these patients. More recent large studies have shown lower operative mortality and short-term morbidity, but an increase in repeat procedures for endovascular repair compared with open surgical repair of AAAs. Thoracic aortic endovascular repair is a newer procedure, with fewer outcomes studies at present.

24. **What criteria are used to determine whether an aortic aneurysm can be treated by endovascular technique?**
    • The relationship of the aneurysm to the origins of other vessels: In the abdomen, the relationship of the aneurysm to the renal arteries is of paramount importance because the angiographer would not want to occlude the origin of these arteries with a stent-graft. In the chest, it is preferable not to cover the origin of the left subclavian artery with the stent, but this can be done if needed, with placement of a carotid-subclavian arterial bypass graft.
    • The luminal size of the common and external iliac arteries: Because the stent-graft is delivered to the aorta via a femoral artery approach, the angiographer needs a vessel large enough to accommodate the size of the delivery system (currently 6 to 8 mm).
    • The length of the aneurysm and whether it extends into the iliac arteries: This determines the size and type of stent-graft used.

25. **Why is follow-up imaging of stent-grafts needed?**
Follow-up imaging is performed to look for complications and to reevaluate the size of the aneurysm after endovascular repair. Ideally, the aneurysm sac gradually decreases in size after repair. Complications include migration of the stent-graft, hemorrhage, infection, and endoleak.

26. **What is the expected CT and MR imaging appearance of the aorta after stent-graft repair?**
CT is used postoperatively to assess for stent placement (location, stent patency, aorta size, and any associated complications). In particular, it is of utmost importance to document any increase or decrease in the size of the aorta, including the proximal and distal aortic necks. Following stent-graft repair, a follow-up CT is performed at 1st and 4th week followed by a 6-month scan, a 1-year scan, and then scans annually thereafter. Periaortic changes (aortic wall

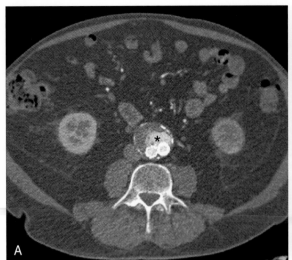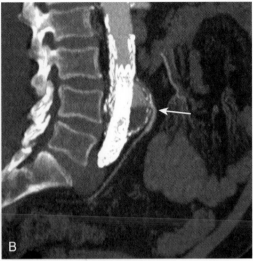

**Figure 13-6.** Type II endoleak on CTA. **A,** Axial CT image shows contrast material within AAA sac outside of stent lumen indicating endoleak (*). **B,** Oblique sagittal MIP CT image demonstrates endoleak communicating with inferior mesenteric artery (*arrow*).

thickening, atherosclerosis, and effusion), perigraft leak, and/or aortic dissection may be seen immediately following the procedure.

MRI is usually not performed after stent placement because the artifacts caused by stainless steel stents will generally obscure the aneurysm sac. However, stent-grafts composed of nitinol or elgiloy do not cause appreciable artifact, and for these patients, contrast-enhanced MRA has a higher sensitivity for endoleak detection compared to CTA. With respect to the MRI findings following stent-graft repair, the early normal postoperative changes are characterized by a perigraft collar of low-intermediate T1-weighted signal intensity and high T2-weighted signal intensity consistent with the perigraft fluid. Two to three months postoperatively, the perigraft collar is characterized by low signal intensity fibrotic tissue.

27. What are endoleaks, and what imaging technique is used to find them?
    An endoleak is defined as residual blood flow in the "aneurysm sac" (in other words, between the native aortic wall and the wall of the stent-graft). This complication is subcategorized into 5 types based on the origin of the blood flow to the aneurysm sac. Type II endoleaks are the most common and are related to reversed flow into the aneurysm sac from collateral vessels such as the inferior mesenteric artery or lumbar arteries (Figure 13-6). Screening for endoleaks is usually performed with CTA or MRA. An appropriate protocol requires precontrast images and postcontrast arterial phase and delayed phase images because endoleaks may sometimes be identified only on delayed phase images. CT and MRI cannot always delineate the type of endoleak, and catheter angiography may be required to define the type of endoleak. Many endoleaks can be repaired percutaneously with coil or glue embolization.

28. What other types of aortic procedures can be performed through an endovascular approach?
    Newer endovascular aortic procedures include treatment of aortic coarctation using stents and placement of percutaneous aortic valves for patients with severe aortic stenosis who are not surgical candidates. Both of these procedures require appropriate iliac artery access vessels, similar to endovascular aneurysm repair.

29. How do aortic coarctation and pseudocoarctation differ?
    Aortic coarctation is a hemodynamically significant stenosis of the aorta, most commonly seen just distal to the takeoff of the left subclavian artery. Pseudocoarctation mimics coarctation because there is an apparent focal narrowing of the proximal descending aorta. This narrowing is due to buckling of a tortuous aorta, however, and does not result in a hemodynamically significant pressure gradient across the area of narrowing. Rib notching, owing to collateral intercostal arteries, is seen in true coarctation but not in pseudocoarctation.

30. What measurements are required for planning of transcatheter aortic valve replacement (TAVR)?
    Determination of eligibility for and planning of TAVR requires knowledge of both aortic root geometry and suitability of the access route for the valve. Measurements of the aortic annulus diameter, area, and perimeter are obtained from systolic phase ECG-gated acquisitions to determine which (if any) of the available prostheses will fit in the patient's aortic root (Figure 13-7). Coronary occlusion by the prosthesis is a rare but devastating complication of TAVR, and therefore the distance from the aortic annulus to the coronary artery ostia is measured to make sure that there is adequate clearance. The femoral artery is the preferred access route, and therefore femoral, iliac, and aortic minimal luminal diameters are measured; the presence of a large amount of calcified or noncalcified plaque in any of these

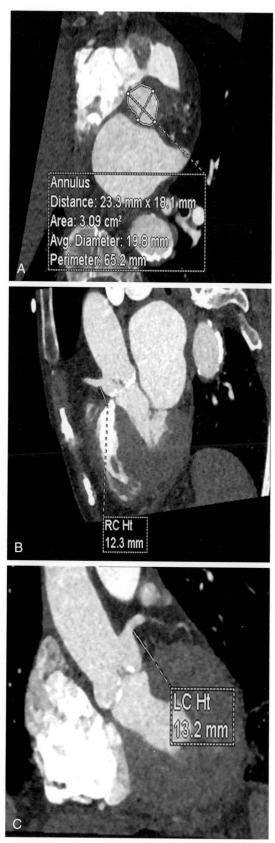

**Figure 13-7.** Multiplanar reformatted views from systolic reconstruction of ECG-gated CTA study of aortic root demonstrating aortic annulus measurements needed for planning of TAVR including: **A,** Aortic annular diameter, area, and perimeter. **B,** Right coronary artery distance from aortic annular plane. **C,** Left coronary artery distance from aortic annular plane.

vessels is also noted. If the transfemoral access route is not adequate, the prosthesis can be implanted through the subclavian artery, the ascending aorta, or the left ventricular apex. The use of CTA for TAVR planning has been demonstrated to reduce postprocedural complications such as perivalvular leak and aortic root rupture.

31. What is a bovine aortic arch?

Most people have three large arteries originating from the aortic arch: the innominate artery (right brachiocephalic artery), the left common carotid artery, and the left subclavian artery. The most common variant of aortic arch anatomy is termed a bovine arch, in which there are two vessels that arise from the aorta. The more proximal of these is a common trunk of the innominate artery and left common carotid artery. The more distal vessel is the left subclavian artery. This anatomic variant is of no clinical significance except when planning aortic surgery.

## KEY POINTS

- An aneurysm (or true aneurysm) is dilation of a vessel in which all three layers of the vessel wall remain intact. Any artery dilated by more than 50% of its normal caliber is called aneurysmal.
- A pseudoaneurysm (or false aneurysm) is a contained rupture and implies disruption of at least part of the aortic wall with intact adventitia. Pseudoaneurysms are potentially highly unstable lesions.
- An aortic dissection is caused by a tear of the intima, creating a false channel or lumen within the wall of the aorta, and usually extends longitudinally within the aorta.
- Dissections involving the ascending aorta (Stanford type A and DeBakey types 1 and 2) are surgical emergencies, whereas descending aortic dissections are usually treated medically.
- An aortic transection is caused by traumatic injury or transection of the aorta, leading to hemorrhage or pseudoaneurysm formation, and is usually focal.

**BIBLIOGRAPHY**

Stein E, Mueller GC, Sundaram B. Thoracic aorta (multidetector computed tomography and magnetic resonance evaluation). *Radiol Clin North Am.* 2014;52(1):195-217.

Blanke P, Schoepf UJ, Leipsic JA. CT in transcatheter aortic valve replacement. *Radiology.* 2013;269(3):650-669.

Shin JH, Angle JF, Park AW, et al. CT imaging findings and their relevance to the clinical outcomes after stent graft repair of penetrating aortic ulcers: six-year, single-center experience. *Cardiovasc Intervent Radiol.* 2012;35(6):1301-1307.

Ueda T, Chin A, Petrovitch I, et al. A pictorial review of acute aortic syndrome: discriminating and overlapping features as revealed by ECG-gated multidetector-row CT angiography. *Insights Imaging.* 2012;3(6):561-571.

Manning WJ, Pennell DJ. *Cardiovascular magnetic resonance.* 2nd ed. Philadelphia, PA: Saunders Elsevier; 2010.

Sakamoto I, Sueyoshi E, Uetani M. MR imaging of the aorta. *Magn Reson Imaging Clin N Am.* 2010;18(1):43-55.

Vu QD, Menias CO, Bhalla S, et al. Aortoenteric fistulas: CT features and potential mimics. *Radiographics.* 2009;29(1):197-209.

Bean MJ, Johnson PT, Roseborough GS, et al. Thoracic aortic stent-grafts: utility of multidetector CT for pre- and postprocedure evaluation. *Radiographics.* 2008;28(7):1835-1851.

Ueda T, Fleischmann D, Rubin GD, et al. Imaging of the thoracic aorta before and after stent-graft repair of aneurysms and dissections. *Semin Thorac Cardiovasc Surg.* 2008;20(4):348-357.

Chirillo F, Salvador L, Bacchion F, et al. Clinical and anatomical characteristics of subtle-discrete dissection of the ascending aorta. *Am J Cardiol.* 2007;100(8):1314-1319.

Stavropoulos SW, Charagundla SR. Imaging techniques for detection and management of endoleaks after endovascular aortic aneurysm repair. *Radiology.* 2007;243(3):641-655.

Yu T, Zhu X, Tang L, et al. Review of CT angiography of aorta. *Radiol Clin North Am.* 2007;45(3):461-483, viii.

Macedo TA, Stanson AW, Oderich GS, et al. Infected aortic aneurysms: imaging findings. *Radiology.* 2004;231(1):250-257.

Macura KJ, Corl FM, Fishman EK, et al. Pathogenesis in acute aortic syndromes: aortic dissection, intramural hematoma, and penetrating atherosclerotic aortic ulcer. *AJR Am J Roentgenol.* 2003;181(2):309-316.

LePage MA, Quint LE, Sonnad SS, et al. Aortic dissection: CT features that distinguish true lumen from false lumen. *AJR Am J Roentgenol.* 2001;177(1):207-211.

Coady MA, Rizzo JA, Goldstein LJ, et al. Natural history, pathogenesis, and etiology of thoracic aortic aneurysms and dissections. *Cardiol Clin.* 1999;17(4):615-635, vii.

Dyer DS, Moore EE, Mestek MF, et al. Can chest CT be used to exclude aortic injury? *Radiology.* 1999;213(1):195-202.

Creasy JD, Chiles C, Routh WD, et al. Overview of traumatic injury of the thoracic aorta. *Radiographics.* 1997;17(1):27-45.

Auffermann W, Olofsson PA, Rabahie GN, et al. Incorporation versus infection of retroperitoneal aortic grafts: MR imaging features. *Radiology.* 1989;172(2):359-362.

DeBakey ME, McCollum CH, Crawford ES, et al. Dissection and dissecting aneurysms of the aorta: twenty-year follow-up of five hundred twenty-seven patients treated surgically. *Surgery.* 1982;92(6):1118-1134.

# CHAPTER 14

# CORONARY ARTERIAL IMAGING

*Shaoxiong Zhang, MD, PhD, and Harold I. Litt, MD, PhD*

1. **What are some noninvasive methods of coronary artery imaging?**

   Imaging the coronary arteries is an important part of evaluating ischemic heart disease. Traditionally, this imaging has been performed using cardiac catheterization, an invasive procedure that requires arterial puncture. Newer technologies promise noninvasive, cross-sectional imaging of coronary artery patency and offer the potential to characterize coronary artery plaque. Coronary magnetic resonance imaging (MRI), using bright blood, dark blood, and contrast-enhanced techniques, can image vessel anatomy and vessel patency and determine lipid content in coronary plaques. Coronary computed tomography angiography (CTA) can image vessel anatomy and vessel patency, potentially with a higher spatial resolution than MRI, and measure coronary arterial calcification.

2. **What is coronary CTA, and how does it differ from routine chest CT?**

   Coronary CTA is a contrast-enhanced CT study optimized for visualization of the coronary arteries (Figure 14-1). On a regular CT scan of the chest, the heart appears blurred because of its motion, so coronary CT requires synchronization of image acquisition to the electrocardiogram (ECG) signal. The challenge of imaging the coronary arteries is compounded by the fact that these vessels are very small and move a large amount in every cardiac cycle. The left main coronary artery measures a maximum of 5 mm in diameter, and for much of their course the other arteries are only about 2 mm in diameter; therefore the resolution of the CT scanner must be in the submillimeter range. The right coronary artery can move up to 5 cm in each cardiac cycle—imaging a 2 mm structure that moves 5 cm in each direction every second is challenging. To acquire high-quality images, the following techniques are employed: ECG gating, multidetector image acquisition, fast gantry rotation, and, in some scanners, dual x-ray tubes.

3. **How long does a cardiac CT acquisition take?**

   To acquire an image, the gantry of the CT scanner must rotate 180 degrees around the patient. With a rotation speed of 330 msec, a modern scanner acquires enough data to make an image in 165 msec, which is the temporal resolution. Some scanners have two x-ray tubes, which permit image acquisition using only 90 degrees of gantry rotation, improving the temporal resolution to 83 msec. This temporal resolution, however, is still quite slow compared to digital subtraction angiography (DSA), which has a temporal resolution of 7 to 10 msec, and therefore gating is still required. The total acquisition time will depend on the width of the CT scanner detector; wide detector (e.g., 320 slice) machines can acquire images of the entire heart during a single heartbeat, while smaller (e.g., 64 slice) detector scanners will take 4 to 5 heartbeats.

4. **What is gating?**

   Gating is the process of synchronizing the CT acquisition to the cardiac cycle. ECG leads are placed on the patient and connected to the scanner. Images can be acquired either prospectively or retrospectively. The aim is to leverage the temporal resolution of the scanner to maximal advantage by acquiring data during phases in the cardiac cycle when cardiac motion is least; this is usually in late diastole.

   In **retrospective gating**, the patient is scanned in a continuous helical fashion. The x-ray tube is on throughout the cardiac cycle, although tube current modulation may be used to decrease the radiation dose during phases of the cardiac cycle where motion is most prominent (e.g., systole). Images are then reconstructed from data acquired during specific portions of the cardiac cycle. Advantages include the ability to reconstruct images from any phase of the cardiac cycle, which may help in evaluation of a coronary artery segment that is blurred during the preferred late diastolic phase. In addition, if images are generated from all phases of the cardiac cycle, functional information is available regarding ejection fraction, valve motion, and wall motion. Retrospective gating is, however, accompanied by a relative radiation dose penalty compared with prospective gating of about 2 to 3 : 1.

   In **prospective gating** (also called prospective triggering), the x-ray tube is turned on only during a specific phase of the cardiac cycle, usually in late diastole when cardiac motion is at a minimum. During the remainder of the cycle, the table moves, and the patient is repositioned for the next set of images, which are taken during the same phase of the next heartbeat. Prospective gating exposes the patient to a lower radiation dose than retrospective gating. Strict heart rate control is required for a prospective scan, however, because if there is motion blur on an image, there are no data available from other points in the cardiac cycle to attempt reconstruction at a different phase.

5. **Can coronary CT imaging be performed at any heart rate?**

   To minimize motion and acquire images of diagnostic quality, a slow rate and regular cardiac rhythm are highly desirable. A rate of 60 beats/minute or less is ideal because it allows for effective use of prospective gating, minimizing radiation dose. Administration of oral beta-blockers is a safe method of achieving this heart rate in most

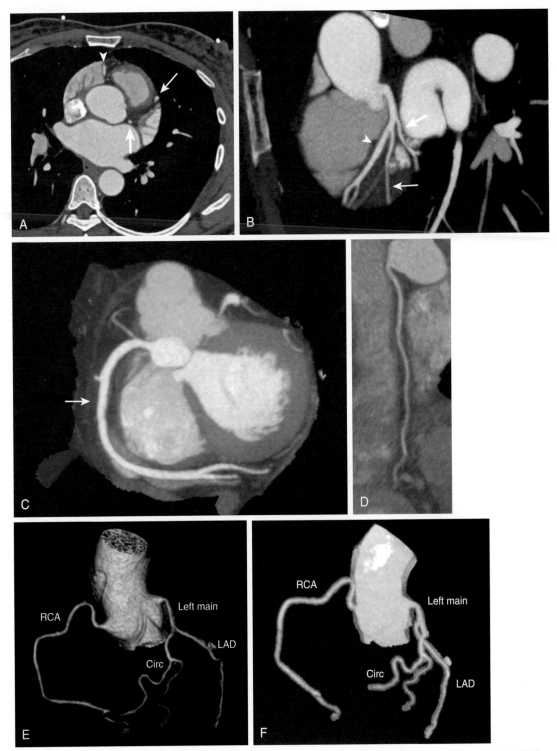

**Figure 14-1.** Normal coronary arteries on CT. **A,** Axial image shows right coronary (*arrowhead*), LAD (*thin arrow*), and circumflex (*thick arrow*) arteries. **B,** Maximum intensity projection (MIP) image shows left main artery branching into LAD (*arrowhead*), first diagonal (*thin arrow*), and circumflex (*thick arrow*) arteries. **C,** Additional MIP image shows RCA (*thin arrow*). **D,** Curved planar reformatted image of RCA allows evaluation of entire vessel on single image. **E,** Volume-rendered (VR) image with subtraction of heart permits evaluation of entire arterial tree with 3D perspective. **F,** Wide-slab MIP with heart subtraction shows vessels with less 3D perspective. *RCA* = right coronary artery; *Circ* = circumflex (artery); *LAD* = left anterior descending (artery).

patients. Contraindications include severe asthma or congestive obstructive pulmonary disease, heart failure, and heart block. In the setting of acute chest pain, cocaine use is also a contraindication. As technology continues to advance, CT scanners with improved temporal resolution and motion reduction postprocessing have increased the upper heart rate limit for a quality study.

6. **What are the indications for CT coronary calcium scoring, and how is it performed?**
CT for coronary calcium scoring is appropriate for asymptomatic intermediate coronary artery disease (CAD) risk patients, and for the specific subset of low-risk patients in whom a family history of premature CAD is present. Intermediate risk is defined as a 10-year risk of cardiovascular events between 10% and 20% using Framingham risk factors.
　　Coronary calcium scoring is performed using a noncontrast, prospectively ECG-gated CT scan of the heart. It is a very safe test because no contrast material is required and radiation doses are negligible (around 1 mSv, compared to an average annual background radiation dose of 3 mSv).

7. **What is the diagnostic performance of CT coronary calcium scoring?**
Coronary calcium scoring allows for detection and quantification of subclinical coronary atherosclerosis. It has been shown to identify at-risk patients with a higher predictive accuracy than conventional risk factor assessment. Moreover, the Multi-Ethnic Study of Atherosclerosis (MESA) trial of 6809 patients demonstrated that coronary calcium score was the most accurate tool for predicting long-term cardiac events. Compared to patients with no coronary calcium, hard event rates in patients with scores from 101 to 300 were increased 7.73-fold, and 9.67-fold among those with a score above 300. Three other large trials have confirmed the benefits of imaging subclinical coronary atherosclerosis for improved risk prediction, including in elderly patients.

8. **What are the indications, contraindications, typical scanning protocols, advantages, and disadvantages for coronary CTA versus magnetic resonance angiography (MRA)? Which patients can benefit from coronary CTA?**
The largest group of referrals for coronary CTA is patients with atypical or low-risk chest pain. In these patients, a negative study prevents a chain of cardiac investigations such as stress tests and cardiac catheterization. These patients may present to the emergency department or may be scanned on an outpatient basis. Chest pain patients with a high risk of acute coronary syndrome are not typically evaluated by coronary CTA because the probability of requiring intervention is high enough to justify catheterization in many cases. Evaluation for aberrant coronary artery origin and course is also a good indication for coronary CTA, as is further evaluation of a patient with an equivocal stress test. In addition, evaluation of coronary bypass graft patency is a common indication. General contraindications for CTA are allergy to iodinated contrast media, renal insufficiency, and pregnancy; specific contraindications to coronary CTA would also include dysrhythmia and tachycardia, particularly if the patient is unable to receive beta-blockers because of a history of asthma or recent cocaine use.
　　The advantages of coronary CTA over coronary MRA include lower cost, ability to identify calcified versus noncalcified plaque, and higher spatial resolution which can be obtained in isotropic fashion and a much shorter scan time. The main disadvantages are the use of ionizing radiation and iodinated contrast material. A typical protocol for coronary CTA utilizes prospective ECG triggering during a dual-phase injection of 60 to 100 ml of iodinated contrast.
　　The most common indication for coronary MRA is for evaluation of coronary artery anomalies. The utility of coronary MRA in assessing coronary artery stenosis is limited. Although software techniques and hardware have substantially changed over the years, MRI systems have not been able to match results from the various generations of CT systems, except in cases with high coronary calcium score in which coronary CTA may be of limited use. On the other hand, coronary MRA has the advantage of no exposure to ionizing radiation or potentially nephrotoxic contrast agents. Contraindications to MRA include claustrophobia and presence of implanted medical devices such as pacemakers. Typically, coronary MRA is obtained during free breathing using respiratory navigator gating. Coronary MRA at 1.5 T is generally performed without gadolinium-based contrast material using a steady state free precession technique, while 3T protocols typically use a nonbalanced gradient echo technique after contrast administration.

9. **What is the normal CT and MR imaging appearance of the coronary arteries?**
On unenhanced CT images, a normal coronary artery is a tubular structure demonstrating similar attenuation to the myocardium and blood pool. Due to the presence of surrounding fat, the coronary artery can usually be clearly identified on nonenhanced CT images; however, the lumen of the coronary artery is not distinguishable from the vessel wall. Coronary CTA, however, is able to highlight the lumen with the use of intravenous contrast material. The coronary artery is then identified as a tubular structure with similar attenuation to the ventricular cavity. The vessel wall is visible but to a much lesser degree.
　　Coronary MRA can be performed without or with intravenous contrast material. Unenhanced MR images of the coronary artery may be obtained by a dark blood technique with intermediate or T2-weighting, which is useful for depicting the vessel wall, or by bright blood technique, typically with the use of navigator respiratory gating technique. Contrast-enhanced coronary MRA may also be performed to improve the visualization of coronary artery anatomy and pathology. On dark blood images, the coronary arterial wall is visualized while the lumen of the vessel is dark. On bright blood images, the coronary artery lumen appears bright, similar to that on CTA images.

10. **What is the normal coronary arterial anatomy, and what is the frequency and significance of anatomic variants?**

    The left main coronary artery originates from the left sinus of Valsalva and then typically bifurcates into the circumflex and left anterior descending (LAD) branches, or trifurcates with an additional intermediate ramus branch in about one third of cases. The LAD coronary artery usually descends in the anterior interventricular groove. Diagonal branches arise from the LAD coronary artery and descend toward the lateral margin of the left ventricular wall. The circumflex branch enters the left atrioventricular groove to supply obtuse marginal branches to the lateral and posterolateral walls of the left ventricle.

    The right coronary artery (RCA) originates from the right coronary sinus of Valsalva at a slightly lower level than the origin of the left main coronary artery. The RCA descends in the anterior right atrioventricular groove. It usually gives off the conus branch as its first branch and then two or three large right ventricular wall branches. The acute marginal branch is the first large branch, which occasionally continues to the apex.

    In 70% of patients, the RCA is dominant, passing down the atrioventricular groove to the crux of the heart, where it gives off the posterior descending artery and posterior left ventricular branches. Approximately 20% of patients have a co-dominant supply, in which the posterior descending artery originates from the RCA, but branches from the circumflex artery also supply this territory. In left coronary dominant patients (10%), the circumflex branch travels all the way around the ventricle, supplying both the posterior descending coronary artery and the posterior left ventricular branches.

11. **Can I use nitroglycerin to dilate the coronary arteries and obtain better images?**

    Yes, use of a nitroglycerin spray or tablet at the beginning of the scan is effective in dilating the coronary arteries and improving visualization of coronary branches. Nitroglycerin is contraindicated in the setting of hypotension and phosphodiesterase inhibitor use.

12. **How much radiation exposure is there for a patient undergoing coronary CTA?**

    Radiation exposure is a perennial issue for all CT studies. Opponents of coronary CTA have touted high radiation dose from the study as a reason to choose the more established catheter angiography or nuclear stress test. Prospective gating results in an average dose of 4 mSv; however newer techniques with lower tube voltage can reduce the dose to 1 to 2 mSv in some cases. In comparison, diagnostic catheterization results in an average dose of 5 to 7 mSv, with considerable operator-dependent variation. A nuclear medicine study using sestamibi with stress and rest phases provides a radiation dose of about 15 mSv. Regardless, all efforts should be made to reduce dose and to consider which organs are exposed. It is prudent to be especially conscious of radiation dose in young women because of the relatively high breast dose from coronary CTA.

13. **What are the advantages and disadvantages of coronary CTA versus catheter angiography?**

    Coronary CTA is less invasive than catheter angiography and avoids the potential complications of groin hematoma, pseudoaneurysm, retroperitoneal hematoma, dissection, and sedation-related complications. In addition to showing the lumen of the vessel, coronary CTA depicts the vessel wall and plaque or other pathology within it (Figure 14-2), which can only be inferred from catheter angiography. Analysis of plaque composition is also possible. Coronary CTA shows anatomic abnormalities such as aberrant course or origin of the arteries (Figure 14-3) and coronary artery fistulas, both of which are difficult to evaluate at catheterization. Coronary CTA depicts bypass grafts easily (Figure 14-4)—another challenge for catheter angiography. Coronary CTA also depicts other causes of chest pain, such as pulmonary embolus, aortic dissection, or pneumonia. In the presence of a coronary artery stent (Figure 14-5), stent patency versus obstruction is usually determinable by CTA, although evaluation of the degree of patency or extent of in-stent stenosis is limited by beam hardening artifact from the stent. The presence of a very large amount of coronary calcium also complicates the evaluation of the degree of stenosis. Catheter angiography also permits diagnosis and intervention in one procedure, and in a patient for whom intervention is considered a likely outcome of the diagnostic procedure, catheter angiography should be used (Table 14-1).

14. **Can I use coronary CTA as a single study for a patient with chest pain to exclude cardiac ischemia, aortic dissection, and pulmonary embolus?**

    Extending the range of coronary CTA to include the entire chest for additional indications is possible. However, it involves increasing both the radiation dose and the dose of intravenous contrast material required for simultaneous opacification of the pulmonary arteries, coronary arteries, and aorta. The application of clinical acumen to focus the workup more narrowly whenever possible is preferable. If this "triple rule out" scan is to be attempted, prospective gating would be advantageous in minimizing the radiation dose.

15. **Are there uses for cardiac CT other than coronary artery evaluation?**

    Cardiac CT can be used for multiple purposes beyond coronary artery evaluation. For example, another common indication is pretreatment evaluation of pulmonary vein ostia and anatomy in patients with atrial fibrillation who will undergo electrophysiologic assessment and potential ablation therapy. Cardiac masses and valvular pathology may also be evaluated by CT, although echocardiography and magnetic resonance imaging (MRI) may be more definitive. One advantage of CT is its ability to depict calcium accurately, which may be helpful to characterize certain masses and may affect treatment strategies for valvular disease.

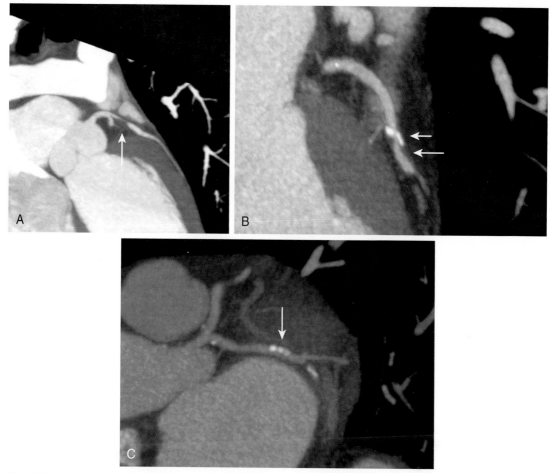

**Figure 14-2.** Coronary atherosclerotic plaque on CTA. **A,** MIP image shows noncalcified plaque (*arrow*) in proximal LAD coronary artery causing 90% stenosis. **B,** MIP image demonstrates mixed plaque in LAD coronary artery composed of calcified (*thick arrow*) and noncalcified (*thin arrow*) components causing 70% stenosis. **C,** MIP image shows calcified plaque (*thin arrow*) in circumflex artery causing mild stenosis.

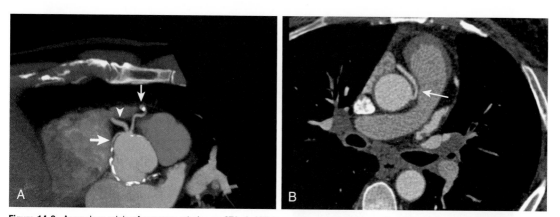

**Figure 14-3.** Anomalous origin of coronary arteries on CTA. **A,** MIP image shows LAD (*thin arrow*), right coronary (*arrowhead*), and circumflex (*thick arrow*) arteries all arising from right cusp. LAD artery and circumflex artery course anterior to pulmonary artery and ascending aorta, respectively. **B,** Axial image in different patient demonstrates RCA (*arrow*) arising from left cusp and passing between aorta and pulmonary artery (interarterial course), susceptible to compression between these two great arteries.

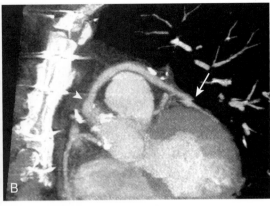

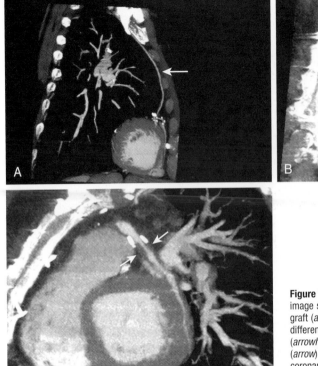

**Figure 14-4.** Coronary artery bypass grafts on CTA. **A,** MIP image shows patent left internal mammary artery (LIMA) bypass graft (*arrow*) extending to LAD artery territory. **B,** MIP image in different patient demonstrates patent saphenous vein bypass (*arrowhead*) extending from ascending aorta to LAD artery (*arrow*) territory. Note wide caliber of vein graft relative to native coronary artery. **C,** MIP image shows noncalcified plaque causing stenosis (*arrows*) of vein graft.

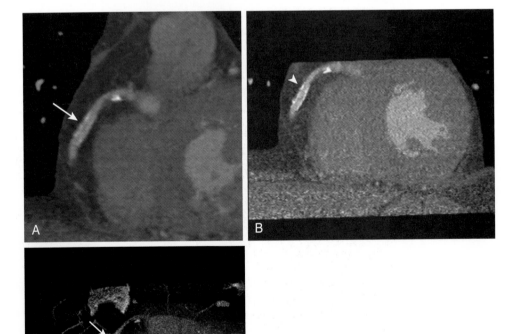

**Figure 14-5.** Coronary artery stent patency evaluation on CTA. **A,** Oblique image reveals RCA stent (*arrow*) although indistinct in appearance. **B,** Oblique image with sharper reconstruction kernel more clearly shows stent patency (*arrowhead*) at cost of increased noise in remainder of image. **C,** VR image gives overview as to stent location (*arrow*).

**Table 14-1.** Utility of Coronary CTA versus Catheter Angiography

|  | CORONARY CTA | CATHETER ANGIOGRAPHY |
|---|:---:|:---:|
| Vessel stenosis | + | ++ |
| Plaque composition | + | − |
| Aberrant course | + | +/− |
| Graft evaluation | + | +/− |
| Stent evaluation | +/− | + |
| Extracardiac findings | + | − |
| Ability to intervene | − | + |
| Risk of complication | Very low | Intermediate |

16. **How is a coronary CTA examination reviewed?**
Initially, the noncontrast images are reviewed for lung and mediastinal pathology. A coronary calcium score is calculated. Then, the coronary CTA images are reviewed. From the raw data of the CTA data acquisition, multiple reconstructions may be generated in various phases of the cardiac cycle (if retrospective gating was used). The reconstructed images are typically reviewed at a dedicated workstation in the axial plane and via multiplanar reformatted (MPR) images generated by the interpreting physician to best depict the arteries. The myocardium, cardiac valves, pericardium, and extracardiac structures are also thoroughly evaluated. More advanced workstation functions, such as curved planar reformation of the coronary arteries, may be used as an aid to interpretation but are not used to replace analysis of the entire dataset by the radiologist. Finally, if retrospective gating was employed, a cine sequence of the heart is reconstructed to evaluate cardiac wall motion and to calculate ejection fraction.

17. **How are coronary artery stenoses reported?**
Coronary artery plaques are described by:
- The vessel and the vessel segment.
- Plaque composition (i.e., calcified, mixed, or noncalcified).
- Plaque length.
- Degree of stenosis.
    Degree of stenosis is best characterized by percentage values (e.g., "50%" stenosis). A percentage is more specific than qualitative descriptors such as "moderate," although the precision with which stenoses can be measured will depend on study quality.

18. **What are the CT and MR imaging (and relevant clinical) features of some common coronary arterial pathologies?**
Coronary CT is the reference standard for evaluation of coronary calcification in vivo. Coronary calcification is defined by a lesion with attenuation greater than 130 Hounsfield units. The calcium score can be obtained either by conventional Agatston score or a volumetric score, with the Agatston being the most common methodology. The score is obtained by multiplying a factor related to the peak Hounsfield unit value in the plaque by the area of the plaque and summing the calcification score from all of the plaques in each of the vessels—namely left main artery, LAD artery, circumflex artery, and RCA.
    A coronary arteriovenous fistula (AVF) is visualized as an abnormal communication between the coronary artery and coronary venous system, typically showing dilation of tortuous vessels with drainage most commonly to the coronary sinus. This can be identified either by coronary CTA or MRA (Figure 14-6, *A*).
    Coronary artery aneurysms and coronary anomalies can be assessed by coronary CTA or MRA and are discussed individually below (Figure 14-6, *B*).

19. **Which congenital coronary artery anomalies can cause sudden death?**
Normally, the right and left main coronary arteries arise from the aorta at the right and left sinuses of Valsalva, respectively. Anomalous origin of the coronary arteries occurs rarely (seen in about 1% of cardiac catheterizations) (see Figure 14-3). Sudden death is associated with the left main coronary artery arising from the right sinus (particularly when the artery courses between the aorta and the pulmonary artery, known as an interarterial course), the RCA arising from the left sinus with an interarterial course, or a single coronary artery. The left main coronary artery may also arise from the pulmonary trunk; this anomaly tends to manifest earlier, with congestive heart failure or sudden death.

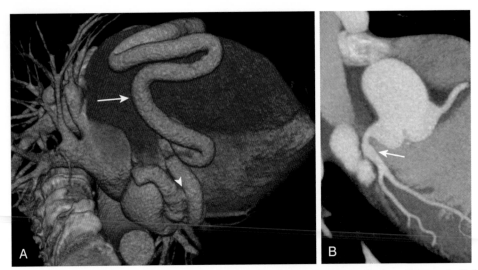

**Figure 14-6.** Coronary AVF and coronary aneurysm on CTA. **A,** VR image shows massively dilated and tortuous RCA (*arrow*) with fistulous connection to coronary sinus (*arrowhead*) due to AVF. **B,** MIP image demonstrates fusiform dilation of proximal LAD coronary artery (*arrow*) due to aneurysm.

20. **What is the usefulness of CT in imaging atherosclerosis?**

    Atherosclerosis is the leading cause of death in the United States. Cardiac CT plays an important role in evaluating atherosclerotic disease. Nonenhanced coronary CT for calcium scoring can assess overall atherosclerotic plaque burden, and coronary CTA can directly visualize the plaque itself in addition to evaluating the degree of luminal stenosis. There are two particularly important concepts for plaque imaging with coronary CTA: the Glagov phenomenon and plaque components.

    The Glagov phenomenon (positive remodeling) is outward remodeling of the coronary arteries in the earlier stages of atherosclerosis. Although there is significant atherosclerotic plaque present in the vessel wall, the lumen remains patent without significant narrowing due to this phenomenon.

    Coronary CTA can detect different atherosclerotic plaque components: noncalcified plaque = plaque with lower attenuation compared with the contrast-enhanced vessel lumen without any calcification; calcified plaque = plaque that is predominantly calcified; or mixed plaque = plaque with both calcified and noncalcified portions.

    Recent studies have demonstrated the utility of coronary CTA in assessing vulnerable plaque which can be seen in some noncalcified plaques; features thought to demonstrate vulnerability of the plaque include positive remodeling, low attenuation plaque, and the so-called "napkin-ring" sign where a low attenuation lipid-rich necrotic plaque core is surrounded by a peripheral area of higher attenuation fibrous plaque tissue.

21. **What is myocardial bridging, and is it important?**

    The coronary arteries are located in the epicardial fat, which is a fat layer deep to the pericardium but superficial to the myocardium. Myocardial bridging is present if a coronary artery courses into the myocardium and is surrounded by muscle for part of its course (Figure 14-7). The significance of myocardial bridging is that, theoretically, an artery surrounded by myocardium may be compressed when the myocardium contracts during systole (systolic compression), limiting blood supply and causing myocardial ischemia. Catheter angiography has difficulty in identifying myocardial bridging unless there is associated systolic compression since the myocardium is not depicted. Until more recently, myocardial bridging was rarely diagnosed. Coronary CTA shows myocardial bridging in 25% to 40% of patients, most commonly in the LAD coronary artery. If multiphase data are available, the vessel should be viewed in systole to ensure that there is no systolic compression. Myocardial bridging in the absence of systolic compression is almost always an incidental finding without clinical significance. Systolic compression may be more likely in cases in which the bridged arterial segment is relatively long and is located deep within the myocardium.

22. **What is a coronary artery aneurysm?**

    A coronary artery aneurysm is defined as a 50% or greater increase in coronary artery diameter compared with adjacent arterial segments. Coronary artery aneurysms are uncommon lesions, with an overall incidence of 1.6%; incidence among individuals imaged with angiography is as high as 5%. Most commonly, these aneurysms involve the RCA, followed by the LAD artery or circumflex artery. Coronary angiography has been considered as the standard reference technique for diagnosing coronary aneurysms, but it is invasive and expensive. However, if the aneurysm contains substantial thrombus, its true size may be underestimated on catheter angiography. ECG-gated CTA allows a more rapid and accurate delineation of the size and shape of coronary artery aneurysms.

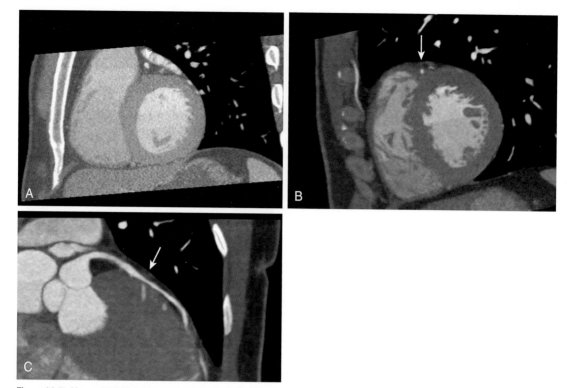

**Figure 14-7.** Myocardial bridging on CTA. **A,** Oblique image shows normal proximal LAD artery (*arrowhead*) located in and surrounded by epicardial fat. **B** and **C,** Oblique and MIP images demonstrate bridged LAD artery (*arrows*) surrounded by myocardium for short segment.

23. **What are the CT and MR imaging features of coronary arterial stents and bypass grafts (including various types)?**

    Coronary arterial stents can be easily visualized on CT images as high-attenuation metallic mesh foci with the presence of stent struts. Different reconstruction algorithms (e.g., sharp kernels) can be used to improve the visualization of coronary stents. In the future, with improvements in spatial resolution and image noise reduction, the evaluation of in-stent restenosis will be more feasible. A sensitivity of 85% to 95% and specificity of 86% to 95% are achievable for detection of in-stent stenosis by CT compared to catheter angiography by using a sharper reconstruction kernel. The factors that affect the visualization of in-stent restenosis include motion artifacts, blooming artifacts, stent diameter, stent composition (less dense metals such as stainless steel provide better images than stents with denser metals such as tantalum), and the presence of coronary calcifications.

    CT has been utilized to evaluate the patency of bypass grafts since the development of electron beam computed tomography (EBCT) in the 1980s. However, with the development of multidetector computed tomography (MDCT), coronary CTA can be utilized to evaluate the patency of bypass grafts more efficiently due to its superior spatial resolution. Specifically, anastomotic patency can now be better assessed compared to EBCT given better image quality and improved visualization software with curved planar reformats and 3D reconstructions.

    Saphenous venous grafts can be effectively evaluated by CT, including jump grafts that have a side-to-side anastomosis (i.e., a diagonal branch) first and then continue to an anastomosis with a second vessel more distally (i.e., an obtuse marginal branch). Evaluation of arterial bypass grafts such as internal mammary graft and radial artery graft may be limited by the presence of multiple surgical clips associated with these grafts, which may produce extensive artifacts. However, the overall patency can usually be adequately assessed. Bypass graft stenosis, occlusion, and aneurysm formation can be identified by CTA.

    Coronary MRA has been studied to evaluate the patency of coronary bypass grafts and may be an alternative modality for assessing bypass graft patency when coronary CTA is contraindicated. The evaluation of coronary artery stent patency by MRA is not yet clinically feasible given artifacts caused by the metal in stents.

24. **Have clinical trials shown an advantage to using coronary CTA in place of catheter angiograms or nuclear stress tests?**

    Early coronary CTA studies performed on 4- and 16-slice MDCT scanners raised doubt as to the accuracy of coronary CTA. Newer studies performed on 40- and 64-slice MDCT scanners, using catheter angiography as the reference standard, show coronary CTA to have a sensitivity of 96% to 99% for stenoses of greater than 50% on a per-patient level, with a specificity of 88% to 93%. Other studies have compared the use of coronary CTA in low-risk chest pain patients in the emergency department in place of serial cardiac enzymes and nuclear stress testing. These studies show quicker discharge, lower cost, and no missed cardiac events (for follow-up periods of 1 year) for the coronary CTA group, and support the use of coronary CTA as accurate and cost-effective in low-risk chest pain patients. In addition, coronary CTA provides a large amount of data that are mostly unobtainable by catheter angiography and nuclear stress testing, such as plaque composition, extent of vessel remodeling, extracardiac findings, aberrant coronary artery course, and numerous other pathologies.

## KEY POINTS

- Cardiac CT provides not only accurate evaluation for coronary artery luminal stenosis with high sensitivity and specificity but also valuable information about atherosclerotic plaque in the vessel wall.
- With the development of new technologies including improved scanners and improved prospective gating and image reconstruction algorithms, coronary CTA can be performed at very low radiation doses of about 1 mSv.
- Cardiac CT can be used for multiple other purposes beyond coronary artery evaluation such as electrophysiologic planning for potential ablation therapy in the setting of atrial fibrillation and evaluation of cardiac masses and valvular pathology.

## BIBLIOGRAPHY

Lin K, Carr JC. MR Imaging of the coronary vasculature: imaging the lumen, wall, and beyond. *Radiol Clin North Am.* 2015;53(2):345-353.

Corban MT, Hung OY, Eshtehardi P, et al. Myocardial bridging: contemporary understanding of pathophysiology with implications for diagnostic and therapeutic strategies. *J Am Coll Cardiol.* 2014;63(22):2346-2355.

Heye T, Kauczor HU, Szabo G, et al. Computed tomography angiography of coronary artery bypass grafts: robustness in emergency and clinical routine settings. *Acta Radiol.* 2014;55(2):161-170.

Maurovich-Horvat P, Ferencik M, Voros S, et al. Comprehensive plaque assessment by coronary CT angiography. *Nature Reviews Cardiol.* 2014;11(7):390-402.

Otsuka K, Fukuda S, Tanaka A, et al. Prognosis of vulnerable plaque on computed tomographic coronary angiography with normal myocardial perfusion image. *Eur Heart J Cardiovasc Imaging.* 2014;15(3):332-340.

Staniak HL, Bittencourt MS, Pickett C, et al. Coronary CT angiography for acute chest pain in the emergency department. *J Cardiovasc Computed Tomography.* 2014;8(5):359-367.

Wong DT, Soh SY, Ko BS, et al. Superior CT coronary angiography image quality at lower radiation exposure with second generation 320-detector row CT in patients with elevated heart rate: a comparison with first generation 320-detector row CT. *Cardiovasc Diagnosis Ther.* 2014;4(4):299-306.

Stojanovska J, Garg A, Patel S, et al. Congenital and hereditary causes of sudden cardiac death in young adults: diagnosis, differential diagnosis, and risk stratification. *Radiographics.* 2013;33(7):1977-2001.

Hamilton-Craig CR, Friedman D, Achenbach S. Cardiac computed tomography—evidence, limitations and clinical application. *Heart Lung Circ.* 2012;21(2):70-81.

Nasir K, Clouse M. Role of nonenhanced multidetector CT coronary artery calcium testing in asymptomatic and symptomatic individuals. *Radiology.* 2012;264(3):637-649.

Rinehart S, Qian Z, Vazquez G, et al. Demonstration of the Glagov phenomenon in vivo by CT coronary angiography in subjects with elevated Framingham risk. *Int J Cardiovasc Imaging.* 2012;28(6):1589-1599.

Malago R, Pezzato A, Barbiani C, et al. Coronary artery anatomy and variants. *Pediatr Radiol.* 2011;41(12):1505-1515.

Sakuma H. Coronary CT versus MR angiography: the role of MR angiography. *Radiology.* 2011;258(2):340-349.

Taylor AJ, Cerqueira M, Hodgson JM, et al. ACCF/SCCT/ACR/AHA/ASE/ASNC/NASCI/SCAI/SCMR 2010 Appropriate Use Criteria for Cardiac Computed Tomography. A Report of the American College of Cardiology Foundation Appropriate Use Criteria Task Force, the Society of Cardiovascular Computed Tomography, the American College of Radiology, the American Heart Association, the American Society of Echocardiography, the American Society of Nuclear Cardiology, the North American Society for Cardiovascular Imaging, the Society for Cardiovascular Angiography and Interventions, and the Society for Cardiovascular Magnetic Resonance. *J Cardiovasc Computed Tomography.* 2010;4(6):407 e1-407 e33.

Diaz-Zamudio M, Bacilio-Perez U, Herrera-Zarza MC, et al. Coronary artery aneurysms and ectasia: role of coronary CT angiography. *Radiographics.* 2009;29(7):1939-1954.

Zenooz NA, Habibi R, Mammen L, et al. Coronary artery fistulas: CT findings. *Radiographics.* 2009;29(3):781-789.

O'Brien JP, Srichai MB, Hecht EM, et al. Anatomy of the heart at multidetector CT: what the radiologist needs to know. *Radiographics.* 2007;27(6):1569-1582.

# CHAPTER 15

# PULMONARY VASCULAR IMAGING

*Eduardo Jose Mortani Barbosa, Jr., MD, and Chiemezie C. Amadi, MD, MA*

1. **What is the normal appearance of the pulmonary vessels on computed tomography (CT) and magnetic resonance imaging (MRI)?**

   The main pulmonary artery originates from the right ventricular outflow tract, anterior and to the left of the aortic root, and serves as a conduit for blood from the right ventricle to the pulmonary circulation. It bifurcates into the right and left pulmonary arteries. The right pulmonary artery passes horizontally through the mediastinum anterior to the major bronchi before bifurcating into the truncus arteriosus and right interlobar arteries, whereas the left pulmonary artery arches more superiorly to pass over the left mainstem bronchus before descending posterior to the major bronchi as the left interlobar artery. The pulmonary arteries then branch into lobar, segmental, and subsegmental pulmonary arterial branches.

   The pulmonary veins, typically numbering four in total (right superior, right inferior, left superior, and left inferior), drain into the left atrium. However, common pulmonary venous trunks and accessory pulmonary veins are not uncommonly encountered.

   On contrast-enhanced CT and MRI, the pulmonary arteries and veins will generally enhance to a degree similar to that of the right ventricle and left atrium, respectively, which will vary depending on the timing of image acquisition relative to the start of intravenous contrast administration. Other than the pulmonary valve leaflets at the origin of the main pulmonary artery, no filling defects are normally seen within the lumina of these vessels. The segmental pulmonary arteries are always located adjacent to bronchi, which are on average of similar caliber, whereas the pulmonary veins are located separately.

2. **What are the indications for computed tomography angiography (CTA) versus magnetic resonance angiography (MRA) for pulmonary vascular imaging?**

   Both CTA and MRA demonstrate high sensitivity and specificity for diagnosis of pulmonary vascular diseases including acute and chronic pulmonary embolism (PE), pulmonary hypertension, pulmonary arterial aneurysm, pulmonary arteriovenous malformation (AVM), and partial or total anomalous pulmonary venous return.

   Unlike catheter angiography or echocardiography, CTA is noninvasive and is not limited by body habitus, air, or bone in terms of obtaining an acoustic window. MRA does not utilize iodinated contrast material and does not involve ionizing radiation. Thus, MRA is especially suitable for imaging children, women of childbearing age, or patients with allergies or other contraindications to iodinated contrast material.

3. **What are the typical CTA and MRA pulmonary vascular imaging protocols?**

   On modern multidetector computed tomography (MDCT) scanners, CTA for pulmonary arterial evaluation utilizes a high rate of iodinated contrast material injection (4 to 6 ml/sec) via a peripheral vein. Scanning is timed to obtain optimal contrast opacification of the pulmonary arteries. Thin-section axial and multiplanar CT images of 1 mm thickness are then reconstructed through the chest. With the latest generation CT scanners, image acquisition times can be less than 5 seconds, providing high-quality images even in patients who are unable to breath hold.

   Bright blood MRA utilizing steady state free precession (SSFP) gradient echo sequences and 2D time of flight (TOF) techniques may be performed without gadolinium-based intravenous contrast material. 3D contrast-enhanced MRA is an additional technique used to image the pulmonary vasculature with greater detail. Similar to CTA, the image data can be reformatted on a computer workstation to obtain multiplanar views for optimal evaluation.

4. **What is the role of chest radiography in the diagnosis of pulmonary embolism (PE)?**

   Chest radiography is usually the first imaging modality used on a patient with suspected PE. It is neither sensitive nor specific for PE but may demonstrate suggestive ancillary findings such as a pleural effusion, a dome-shaped peripheral opacity referred to as a Hampton hump that reflects a pulmonary infarct, a prominent central artery known as the Fleischner sign, or an area of apparent pulmonary lucency resulting from decreased lung perfusion termed the Westermark sign. It may alternatively demonstrate other findings that are diagnostic of other disease conditions.

5. **What are advantages of CTA for assessment of PE?**

   CTA is the current reference standard for PE evaluation. One important advantage of CTA over catheter pulmonary arteriography and pulmonary scintigraphy is that it may be used to diagnose other causes of the patient's symptoms, such as pleural effusion, pneumonia, atelectasis, or malignancy. Moreover, in contrast to conventional pulmonary arteriography, CTA is noninvasive, safer, faster to perform, and more widely available. CTA has several advantages over pulmonary scintigraphy. It is less dependent on patient cooperation and is faster to perform. In addition, pulmonary scintigraphy may have a 60% to 70% indeterminate rate, especially in patients with underlying lung disease or other comorbidities, limiting diagnostic accuracy.

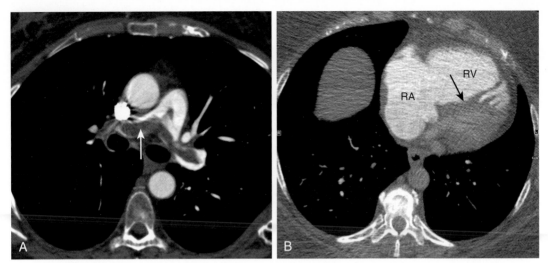

**Figure 15-1.** Acute saddle PE and right heart strain on CT. **A,** Axial CT image shows centrally located hypoattenuating filling defect (*arrow*) in main pulmonary artery and straddling right and left pulmonary arteries. **B,** Axial CT image reveals right atrial (*RA*) dilation and right ventricular (*RV*) dilation with leftward bowing of interventricular septum (*arrow*) indicating right heart strain.

6. What are the direct CTA findings of PE?

   The most specific finding of PE is a partial or complete hypoattenuating intraluminal filling defect within a pulmonary artery. It should be present on at least two contiguous images (Figure 15-1, *A*).

7. What are the indirect CTA findings of PE?

   A pulmonary artery with an acute embolus may be slightly enlarged, whereas one with a chronic embolus may be decreased in caliber. Parenchymal findings, such as wedge-shaped peripheral opacities denoting areas of pulmonary infarction, can sometimes be seen as well. Areas of decreased pulmonary perfusion can manifest as wedge-shaped areas of subtle peripheral hypoenhancement. A pleural effusion can sometimes be seen. Signs of right heart strain including right heart dilation and flattening or leftward deviation of the interventricular septum may also be present (Figure 15-1, *B*), and generally portend a worse clinical outcome.

8. How can acute PE be distinguished from chronic PE on CTA?

   It may sometimes be difficult to differentiate acute from chronic PE, and chronic PE may be present with superimposed acute PE. However, an acute pulmonary embolus typically appears as a centrally located hypoattenuating filling defect within the artery and is often occlusive, whereas a chronic pulmonary embolus will typically be eccentrically located within the artery. Sometimes intraluminal linear or curvilinear hypoattenuating bands or webs may be seen in chronic PE. This can be conceptually understood because the appearance of chronic PE is due to progressive but incomplete recanalization of a prior acute PE. Chronic PE can also calcify, whereas acute PE does not, and may lead to diminution in pulmonary arterial caliber or luminal obliteration. Long-standing PEs are more likely than acute emboli to cause pulmonary hypertension, leading to right heart enlargement and enlargement of the central pulmonary arteries. Mosaic attenuation of the lungs, seen as sharply demarcated regions of decreased and increased attenuation in the lungs related to areas of hypoperfusion, blood redistribution, and associated pulmonary air trapping, may also be seen with chronic PE. Lastly, increased bronchial arterial collateral vessels can be seen in some cases of chronic PE (Figure 15-2).

9. What are other uses for CT in the setting of PE?

   CT also can be used to evaluate the lower extremity venous system for thrombosis, using the same contrast bolus, by imaging the lower extremities shortly after the thoracic scan has been performed. Lower extremity ultrasonography (US) is generally used to evaluate the lower extremity veins for deep venous thrombosis (DVT), but CT has several advantages. One is that it is operator independent, in contrast to US. CT can also be used to evaluate for DVT in areas that are inaccessible to US or difficult to evaluate. This includes the deep pelvic veins (a common source of thrombus that may embolize to the lungs) and the region near the adductor canal. Furthermore, US is more limited in patients who are obese or who have had recent surgery.

10. What is pulmonary hypertension, and what CT and MRI findings are suggestive?

    Pulmonary hypertension is comprised of a heterogeneous group of disorders that cause abnormal elevation of pressure in the pulmonary circulation, with a mean pulmonary artery pressure higher than 25 mm Hg, regardless of the underlying mechanism. There are 5 World Health Organization (WHO) classifications of pulmonary hypertension, which can be broadly categorized into precapillary (wedge pressure <15 mm Hg) and postcapillary (wedge pressure >15 mm

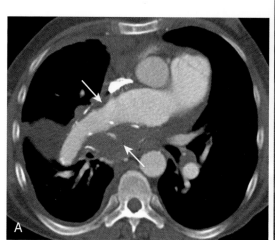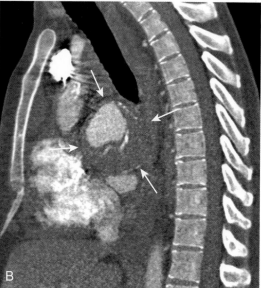

**Figure 15-2.** Chronic PE and pulmonary artery aneurysm on CT. **A,** Axial CT image demonstrates eccentric hypoattenuating filling defects (*arrows*) in aneurysmal right pulmonary artery with calcifications. **B,** Sagittal CT image shows aneurysm of right pulmonary artery (*arrows*) with extensive eccentric hypoattenuating filling defect with calcifications.

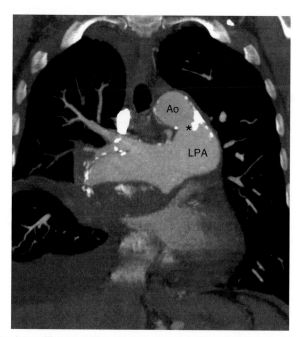

**Figure 15-3.** Pulmonary hypertension on CT. Coronal CT image demonstrates dilation and peripheral calcification of central pulmonary arteries. Note patent ductus arteriosus (*) between aorta (*Ao*) and left pulmonary artery (*LPA*) as underlying etiology.

Hg) etiologies. CT and MRI findings in pulmonary hypertension may vary depending on the underlying etiology, but typical findings may include (Figure 15-3):
- Main pulmonary artery caliber >29 mm.
- Main pulmonary artery diameter greater than that of the ascending aorta.
- Enlargement of segmental pulmonary arteries relative to the adjacent segmental bronchi.
- Right ventricular hypertrophy.
- Right ventricular and right atrial dilation.
- Straightening or leftward bowing of the interventricular septum.

- Delayed phase contrast enhancement with a midwall distribution at the right ventricular septal insertion that points into the interventricular septum, more prominent at the base of the heart (only on MRI).
- Dilation of the inferior vena cava and hepatic veins.
- Mosaic attenuation of the lungs (only on CT).
- Centrilobular ground glass attenuation nodules (due to cholesterol granulomas or pulmonary capillary hemangiomatosis, only on CT).

11. What is a pulmonary artery aneurysm, and what is the major differential diagnosis?

A pulmonary artery aneurysm is defined as focal dilation of the pulmonary artery, involving all 3 layers of the arterial wall, to a diameter greater than 50% than that of the normal arterial caliber. Pulmonary artery aneurysms are rare, and etiologies may be congenital or acquired.

Among acquired causes, pulmonary artery aneurysms can be idiopathic, mycotic (i.e., infectious), or related to vasculitis (including Behçet's syndrome, Hughes-Stovin syndrome, Marfan's syndrome, Takayasu's arteritis, or giant cell arteritis). Occasionally, chronic PE (see Figure 15-2) or severe pulmonary hypertension may lead to pulmonary arterial aneurysms.

Major differential diagnostic considerations include a pulmonary artery pseudoaneurysm (i.e., a contained rupture that involves less than all 3 arterial wall layers), and a pulmonary AVM. Pulmonary artery pseudoaneurysms are most often post-traumatic (particularly due to penetrating trauma), iatrogenic (such as from Swan-Ganz catheter placement), or mycotic in nature. A pulmonary artery pseudoaneurysm in the setting of pulmonary tuberculosis is called a Rasmussen aneurysm and is typically located adjacent to a chronic pulmonary parenchymal site of disease or adjacent to an area of pulmonary cavitation.

12. What is a pulmonary AVM, and what is the clinical presentation?

A pulmonary AVM is an abnormal communication between a pulmonary artery and a draining pulmonary vein, causing blood to bypass the pulmonary capillary bed before returning to the left heart. Pulmonary AVMs may be asymptomatic but can manifest with a wide range of clinical symptoms. Paradoxic emboli to the systemic arterial circulation may occur, leading to stroke, brain abscess, myocardial infarction, or acute limb ischemia, due to loss of the filter effect of the lung such that systemic venous clots are able to access the systemic arterial circulation. Pulmonary AVMs may cause vague symptoms and signs, such as chest pain and dyspnea on exertion, because of right-to-left shunting of deoxygenated blood. With severe shunting, high-output cardiac failure can result. One sign that may suggest pulmonary AVM is orthodeoxia, indicating oxygen desaturation in the upright position. Most pulmonary AVMs occur in the lower lobes of the lungs, and therefore shunting of blood and oxygen desaturation are maximal when blood flow to the lung bases is greatest (i.e., in the upright position).

13. With what hereditary disorder are pulmonary AVMs associated?

Although pulmonary AVMs are often isolated, they can be associated with hereditary hemorrhagic telangiectasia (HHT), also known as Osler-Weber-Rendu syndrome. HHT is an autosomal dominant genetic disorder that causes vascular malformations that can lead to multiple pulmonary AVMs. It is characterized by telangiectasias of the skin and mucosal linings and AVMs in internal organs including the lungs, liver, and brain. It is wise to screen family members of patients who present with pulmonary AVMs so that they can be properly diagnosed and receive treatment.

14. You are asked to start a peripheral intravenous line in a patient with a known pulmonary AVM. What special precautions should you take?

Patients with pulmonary AVMs lack the filter function performed by the pulmonary capillary bed. This situation predisposes patients to paradoxic emboli from endogenous and exogenous sources. Air or other material accidentally introduced into the venous system could pass through the shunt and cause a stroke. Care must be taken that all venous lines are free of air and that filters are used to prevent paradoxic emboli.

15. What are the imaging characteristics of a pulmonary AVM on radiography, CT, and MRI?

On a chest radiograph, pulmonary AVMs appear as serpentine or nodular densities in the lungs that may appear to connect to the hilum. On CT and MRI, they appear as serpentine, tubular, or nodular foci in the lungs that have vascular connections with a feeding pulmonary artery and a draining pulmonary vein, and which enhance to a degree similar to that of other pulmonary arteries. On dynamic contrast-enhanced images, one may see enhancement in a sequential manner from the feeding pulmonary artery, to the AVM, to the draining pulmonary vein (Figure 15-4).

16. What is partial anomalous pulmonary venous return (PAPVR)?

PAPVR occurs when part of the pulmonary venous system drains directly into the systemic venous circulation, creating a left-to-right shunt. It can occur in isolation or be associated with either an atrial septal defect (ASD) or a hypogenetic lung. When PAPVR is associated with an ASD (usually a sinus venosus defect), the right upper lobe pulmonary vein drains into the superior vena cava (SVC). When PAPVR occurs with a hypogenetic lung, it is a component of scimitar syndrome (Figure 15-5).

17. What is scimitar syndrome, and what are its associated imaging findings?

Scimitar syndrome, or hypogenetic lung or pulmonary venolobar syndrome, is a rare disorder characterized by a hypoplastic lung (almost exclusively on the right) in association with an anomalous pulmonary vein. This anomalous pulmonary vein can drain into many structures, including the infradiaphragmatic inferior vena cava (IVC), suprahepatic

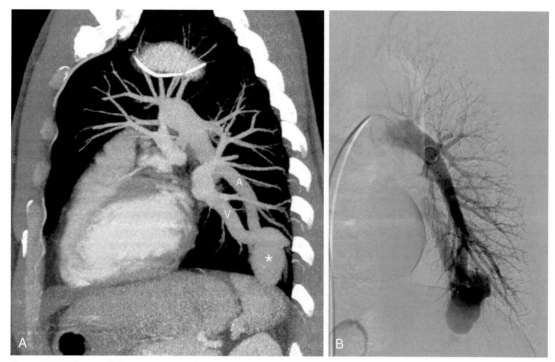

**Figure 15-4.** Pulmonary AVM on CT and catheter pulmonary angiography. **A,** Oblique maximum intensity projection (MIP) CT image shows serpentine nodular enhancing lesion (*) in left lower lobe of lung that connects to feeding pulmonary artery (*A*) and draining pulmonary vein (*V*). **B,** Oblique fluoroscopic image during catheter pulmonary angiography shows similar findings.

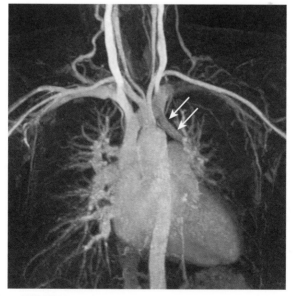

**Figure 15-5.** PAPVR on MRA. Coronal MIP MRA image shows anomalous left superior pulmonary vein (*arrows*) draining into left brachiocephalic vein.

IVC, portal vein, or right atrium. The chest radiograph typically shows a small right lung with a curvilinear tubular opacity paralleling the right heart border (the "scimitar" sign) due to an anomalous right pulmonary vein. Cardiac dextroposition, pulmonary artery hypoplasia/aplasia, or systemic arterial collateral supply to the ipsilateral lung may also be seen. On CT and MRI, the course and anatomy of the anomalous vasculature can be well visualized.

18. What is the most common primary neoplasm of the pulmonary artery?

Neoplasms associated with the pulmonary vascular system are exceedingly rare. Angiosarcoma is the most common primary neoplasm of the pulmonary artery. Pulmonary artery angiosarcomas can sometimes be difficult to distinguish from occlusive PE on CT and MRI because both may fill the lumen of the pulmonary artery. However, angiosarcomas frequently span the entire luminal diameter of the main or proximal pulmonary arteries, may enhance, may contain internal vascularity, may have metabolic activity on [18]F-fluorodeoxyglucose (FDG) positron emission tomography (PET), and may be associated with extension into the mediastinum or lung. These imaging findings are not seen with bland PE. The diagnosis can be confirmed by endovascular biopsy if necessary.

## KEY POINTS

- An acute pulmonary embolus typically appears as a centrally located hypoattenuating filling defect within a pulmonary artery on CT and MRI.
- A chronic pulmonary embolus typically appears as an eccentrically located hypoattenuating filling defect within a pulmonary artery and may be associated with calcification, intraluminal bands or webs, decreased luminal caliber, or increased bronchial arterial collateral vessels.
- In the setting of acute PE, findings of right heart strain including right heart dilation and flattening or leftward deviation of the interventricular septum may be present and generally portend a worse clinical outcome.
- Central pulmonary artery dilation is the major imaging finding that suggests presence of pulmonary hypertension.
- When multiple pulmonary AVMs are encountered, the patient may have hereditary hemorrhagic telangiectasia (i.e., Osler-Weber-Rendu syndrome).

**BIBLIOGRAPHY**

Gill SS, Roddie ME, Shovlin CL, et al. Pulmonary arteriovenous malformations and their mimics. *Clin Radiol.* 2015;70(1):96-110.

Carter BW, Lichtenberger JP 3rd, Wu CC. Congenital abnormalities of the pulmonary arteries in adults. *AJR Am J Roentgenol.* 2014;202(4):W308-W313.

Swift AJ, Wild JM, Nagle SK, et al. Quantitative magnetic resonance imaging of pulmonary hypertension: a practical approach to the current state of the art. *J Thorac Imaging.* 2014;29(2):68-79.

Lacombe P, Lacout A, Marcy PY, et al. Diagnosis and treatment of pulmonary arteriovenous malformations in hereditary hemorrhagic telangiectasia: an overview. *Diagnostic Interven Imag.* 2013;94(9):835-848.

Porres DV, Morenza OP, Pallisa E, et al. Learning from the pulmonary veins. *Radiographics.* 2013;33(4):999-1022.

Schiebler ML, Bhalla S, Runo J, et al. Magnetic resonance and computed tomography imaging of the structural and functional changes of pulmonary arterial hypertension. *J Thorac Imaging.* 2013;28(3):178-193.

Araoz PA, Haramati LB, Mayo JR, et al. Panel discussion: pulmonary embolism imaging and outcomes. *AJR Am J Roentgenol.* 2012;198(6):1313-1319.

Barbosa EJ Jr, Gupta NK, Torigian DA, et al. Current role of imaging in the diagnosis and management of pulmonary hypertension. *AJR Am J Roentgenol.* 2012;198(6):1320-1331.

Junqueira FP, Lima CM, Coutinho AC Jr, et al. Pulmonary arterial hypertension: an imaging review comparing MR pulmonary angiography and perfusion with multidetector CT angiography. *Br J Radiol.* 2012;85(1019):1446-1456.

Katre R, Burns SK, Murillo H, et al. Anomalous pulmonary venous connections. *Semin Ultrasound CT MR.* 2012;33(6):485-499.

Murillo H, Cutalo MJ, Jones RP, et al. Pulmonary circulation imaging: embryology and normal anatomy. *Semin Ultrasound CT MR.* 2012;33(6):473-484.

Pena E, Dennie C, Veinot J, et al. Pulmonary hypertension: how the radiologist can help. *Radiographics.* 2012;32(1):9-32.

Restrepo CS, Betancourt SL, Martinez-Jimenez S, et al. Tumors of the pulmonary artery and veins. *Semin Ultrasound CT MR.* 2012;33(6):580-590.

Restrepo CS, Carswell AP. Aneurysms and pseudoaneurysms of the pulmonary vasculature. *Semin Ultrasound CT MR.* 2012;33(6):552-566.

Castaner E, Gallardo X, Ballesteros E, et al. CT diagnosis of chronic pulmonary thromboembolism. *Radiographics.* 2009;29(1):31-50, discussion-3.

Dillman JR, Yarram SG, Hernandez RJ. Imaging of pulmonary venous developmental anomalies. *AJR Am J Roentgenol.* 2009;192(5):1272-1285.

Nguyen ET, Silva CI, Seely JM, et al. Pulmonary artery aneurysms and pseudoaneurysms in adults: findings at CT and radiography. *AJR Am J Roentgenol.* 2007;188(2):W126-W134.

Remy-Jardin M, Pistolesi M, Goodman LR, et al. Management of suspected acute pulmonary embolism in the era of CT angiography: a statement from the Fleischner Society. *Radiology.* 2007;245(2):315-329.

Castaner E, Gallardo X, Rimola J, et al. Congenital and acquired pulmonary artery anomalies in the adult: radiologic overview. *Radiographics.* 2006;26(2):349-371.

Wittram C, Maher MM, Yoo AJ, et al. CT angiography of pulmonary embolism: diagnostic criteria and causes of misdiagnosis. *Radiographics.* 2004;24(5):1219-1238.

Frazier AA, Galvin JR, Franks TJ, et al. From the archives of the AFIP: pulmonary vasculature: hypertension and infarction. *Radiographics.* 2000;20(2):491-524, quiz 30-1, 32.

# CHAPTER 16

# CT ANGIOGRAPHY AND MR ANGIOGRAPHY OF THE PERIPHERAL AND VISCERAL VASCULATURE

*Saurabh Jha, MBBS, MRCS, MS, and Drew A. Torigian, MD, MA, FSAR*

1. **What are the clinical indications for computed tomography angiography (CTA) and magnetic resonance angiography (MRA) of the peripheral and visceral arteries?**
   CTA and MRA are noninvasive methods of assessing the arteries and veins, which have all but replaced catheter angiography. The clinical indications for these examinations can be thought of in the following broad areas:
   - Ischemia.
   - Aneurysm/dissection.
   - Compression syndromes.
   - Traumatic injury.

2. **What is the most important principle for performing contrast-enhanced CTA and MRA?**
   The most important principle in performing contrast-enhanced vascular imaging is the timing of the image acquisition. The images must be acquired when the opacification of the vessel (artery or vein) of interest is as high as possible. This requires careful synchronization of image acquisition with the injection of contrast material.

3. **How is the image acquisition timed following contrast administration in a CTA?**
   The image acquisition can be timed in one of three ways:
   - Empirical delay.
   - Bolus tracking.
   - Test bolus.

   When using an empirical delay, the images are acquired after a preset delay from the time of contrast administration. This is the method generally used for imaging of the veins. The time delay depends on the vein of interest. To assess the infrarenal inferior vena cava (IVC) and the iliac veins, a delay of 140 seconds from the time of contrast injection is used. To assess the portal veins and the renal veins, the delay is typically 70 to 90 seconds. For assessment of the central veins of the chest and upper extremities, a delay of 90 seconds is used.

   Imaging of the arteries requires more nuance because the window for optimal enhancement of the arteries is short. This is most often achieved by tracking the bolus of injected contrast material. A cursor is placed in a region of interest (ROI), which is the aortic segment most proximal to the artery of interest. For example, if the artery of interest is the celiac artery, then the ROI can be the descending thoracic aorta or abdominal aorta. After a specified time delay, known as the monitoring delay, low dose single slice images are obtained through the ROI every 1 to 2 seconds, while simultaneously tracking the attenuation of the aorta. When its attenuation exceeds a predetermined threshold, typically 130 HU, the scan commences after another time delay known as the scan delay.

   When using a test bolus, a small volume of contrast material, typically 20 ml, is injected at the same rate as the main injection. An ROI is placed in the aorta and low dose single slice images are obtained. The attenuation of the artery is then measured on each image at different points in time, and the time to peak maximal enhancement (PME) is calculated. The image acquisition for the diagnostic scan is then timed by using the time to PME plus a few extra seconds because a larger contrast volume is administered.

   Note that these techniques of image acquisition timing can also be utilized with MRA.

4. **When should a test bolus be used?**
   There may be local preferences, but in general, a test bolus is used in the following circumstances:
   - The aorta is diseased by atherosclerosis, or there is aortic dissection. In both situations, the ROI may inadvertently be placed in a segment of the aorta which does not opacify following contrast administration as much as it should.
   - The patient has a depressed ejection fraction (typically a left ventricular ejection fraction of less than 20%).
   - The volume of administered contrast material is reduced because of renal impairment.

5. **Describe a typical computed tomography (CT) protocol for assessing the arteries.**
   Unenhanced precontrast images are often, but not always, obtained. Some indications for obtaining unenhanced precontrast images include: suspected hemorrhage, penetrating trauma, evaluation of the aorta following stent or surgical repair, and suspected acute aortic syndrome.

Arterial phase images are obtained after the injection of 100 ml of iodinated contrast material mixed with saline at a rate of 4 to 5 ml per second, using bolus tracking, with a monitoring delay of 12 seconds and a scan delay of 6 seconds.

Venous phase images are not routinely obtained. Some indications for venous phase imaging include: suspected mesenteric ischemia, suspected hemorrhage, evaluation of an indwelling stent graft to detect an endoleak, and suspected venous thrombus.

6. **Is the quality of evaluation of the arteries of the lower extremities better with a wide-detector multidetector row CT (MDCT) scanner?**

   Asked differently, is a 256-detector MDCT scanner better than a 64-detector MDCT scanner to assess the lower extremity arteries? Not necessarily. The acquisition time of wide-detector MDCT scanners is shorter and could lead to outrunning of the contrast bolus. That is, the scan could reach the lower extremities before the contrast material has arrived in this location.

7. **How can we mitigate outrunning of the contrast bolus when using a wide-detector MDCT scanner?**

   Wide-detector MDCT scanners can be slowed by slowing the gantry rotation time, using narrower detector coverage where offered, and by reducing the pitch. Additionally, the threshold attenuation for triggering the scan during bolus tracking can be increased, and the scan delay can also be increased. These measures will ensure that the scan starts later with less chance of outrunning the contrast bolus. Finally, it is prudent to acquire, immediately, a second set of images through the most peripheral part of the peripheral circulation (i.e., through the anatomic region the contrast takes the longest amount of time to reach). For assessment of the arteries of the lower legs, this means a second image acquisition from the knees to the toes.

8. **What is the most important consideration when imaging the arteries of the upper extremities?**

   The most important consideration is laterality. It is important to inject contrast material on the side opposite the side of pathology. Otherwise, concentrated contrast material passing through the upper extremity veins will lead to streak artifact (on CT) or susceptibility artifact (on MRI) that may obscure the adjacent arteries of interest.

9. **How is MRA image acquisition timed?**

   The arterial phase of MRA can be timed by visualization of the contrast material entering the arterial tree of interest. The alternative is to obtain multiple acquisitions (multiphasic imaging) through the anatomic region of interest after contrast administration. Because MRA does not involve ionizing radiation, there is no penalty in terms of radiation exposure with multiphasic imaging.

   Multiphasic imaging is typically used to assess the temporal filling pattern of vascular lesions. This is also utilized when the arteries of interest are confined to an extremity, such as in the hand or calf.

10. **Describe a typical MRA protocol.**

    The specific protocol will vary depending on the particular artery or vein of interest, and the clinical indication. However, imaging sequences that are usually obtained include:
    - **Multiplanar heavily T2-weighted images:** These are useful to assess the nonvascular structures in the anatomic region of interest and to detect fluid collections.
    - **Unenhanced precontrast T1-weighted images:** These are useful to detect subacute hemorrhage, which has high T1-weighted signal intensity, and to serve as a baseline of comparison with contrast-enhanced images to assess for presence of enhancement.
    - **3D T1-weighted contrast-enhanced MRA images acquired during the arterial and venous phases of enhancement:** These are useful to assess the arteries and, to a lesser extent, the veins in high detail.
    - **2D axial delayed phase contrast-enhanced T1-weighted images:** These are useful to assess the veins.

11. **What are the options if the patient cannot receive intravenous gadolinium-based or iodinated contrast material?**

    This depends on the clinical question. Unenhanced CT can still be useful to detect ruptured aortic pathology, intramural hematoma, and stigmata of mesenteric ischemia in the bowel. However, it cannot generally detect an aortic dissection, and it cannot assess vessel patency, vessel wall abnormalities, or vascular graft dehiscence.

    On magnetic resonance imaging (MRI), vascular assessment without intravenous contrast material is still possible using one or more of the following image sequences:
    - Time of flight (TOF) images.
    - Phase contrast (PC) images.
    - Arterial spin labeled (ASL) images.
    - Balanced steady state free precession images.

12. **What must you tell the MRI technologists when performing a TOF MRA?**

    There are three important points to communicate. First, you must decide if you want to use a saturation band and, if so, the direction of the saturation band. A saturation band removes signal from a vessel depending on the direction of its blood flow. For example, if you want the lower extremity arteries not to have signal, apply a superior saturation band to nullify the craniocaudal arterial flow of blood. Conversely, if it is signal in the veins that you want to remove, then apply an inferior saturation band to nullify the caudocranial venous flow of blood. Generally, when assessing the arteries, the signal in the veins is removed, and vice versa. However, you may elect not to use a saturation band.

Second, it is important to specify the plane of the sequence. The image acquisition must be perpendicular to the long axis of the vessel of interest, or as close to the perpendicular as possible. For example, to assess the arteries of the calf, the axial plane is used. To assess the renal arteries, the sagittal plane is used.

Third, decide whether the TOF image acquisition should be gated to the cardiac or respiratory cycle. For assessment of the arteries in the calf and foot, gating may help to improve image quality.

13. **What is the advantage of TOF MRA?**
    This approach can determine the directionality of blood flow, which is useful to distinguish between antegrade and retrograde flow.

14. **What are the disadvantages of TOF MRA?**
    The sequence is limited for assessment of vessels that have a tortuous course, such as the splenic artery, and is also limited for assessment of vessels that do not run perpendicular to the plane of section. It is not as good for assessing veins, because blood flow in veins is slower. Furthermore, it does not distinguish high-grade stenosis from moderate-grade stenosis as well as contrast-enhanced MRA.

15. **Is CTA or contrast-enhanced MRA better?**
    It depends on local preferences and expertise. CTA is quicker than MRA, and therefore is generally preferred for evaluation of potentially unstable or claustrophobic patients, but it exposes patients to ionizing radiation. CTA is superior when there are indwelling metallic stents in the artery. Stents, particularly stainless steel stents, lead to blooming artifact on MRA. CTA is also useful to assess the burden of atherosclerotic calcification, which is useful, for example, for preoperative planning of abdominal aortic aneurysm (AAA). Paradoxically, MRA is better for evaluating heavily calcified arteries that are also small, such as arteries of the calf. This is because it is difficult to distinguish between heavy calcification and iodinated contrast material on CTA, particularly when an artery is heavily calcified.

    The spatial resolution of CTA can be as small as 0.6 mm, whereas MRA is typically on the order of 1 mm. MRA is more amenable to postprocessing because it is easier to subtract background structures. Both CTA and MRA can offer a snapshot of organ perfusion, but MRA offers more dynamic information without radiation exposure.

    MRA allows image acquisition in any plane, whereas CTA provides only for image acquisition in the axial plane. However, multiplanar reconstructions and reformations can subsequently be created in any plane of interest.

16. **When performing a contrast-enhanced MRA, what must you communicate to the technologists?**
    The plane of section in which you want to reconstruct 2D images from the acquired 3D MRA images. The technologists may call this "the plane of injection." Put simply, this is the plane that allows for full coverage of the artery of interest while using the thinnest depth of the 3D volume of image acquisition to minimize acquisition time. For the renal arteries, it is either the coronal or axial plane, but not the sagittal plane. For the celiac arterial tree, it is the axial plane. For the superior mesenteric artery (SMA), it is the sagittal plane. For the lower extremity arteries, it is the coronal plane.

17. **Is CTA or MRA preferred for assessment of the renal arteries?**
    Both work well. If MRA is used, then a tight field of view (FOV) should be prescribed (i.e., a tight "plane of injection") around the renal arteries and abdominal aorta to derive a spatial resolution comparable to CTA. CTA is preferred to assess the patency of an indwelling renal artery stent.

18. **Is CTA or MRA preferred for assessment of the iliac arteries for percutaneous access?**
    CTA is preferred, although MRA may also be used. CTA gives a better indication of the amount of atherosclerotic calcification in the arteries, which affects management.

19. **Is CTA or MRA preferred for assessment of the calf and foot vessels?**
    Both have strengths and weaknesses. CTA ensures reasonable temporal uniformity of arterial opacification, so long as the contrast bolus is not outrun. Multistation MRA may be so delayed as to lead to venous opacification in the calves, making it difficult to distinguish between artery and vein. However, MRA is preferred when heavily calcified arteries are present.

20. **Is CTA or MRA preferred for assessment of arteriovenous malformations?**
    MRA is preferred because multiphasic imaging is feasible and provides information about the vascular abnormality. This helps to distinguish between high and low flow vascular lesions. Also, MRI gives better information about the surrounding soft tissues secondary to superior soft tissue contrast.

21. **Is CTA or MRA preferred for assessment of mesenteric ischemia?**
    Both assess the mesenteric arteries and veins well. However, CT may better depict some stigmata of acute bowel ischemia/infarction such as pneumatosis, portal venous gas, and pneumoperitoneum. Furthermore, CTA is much faster to perform compared to MRA, which is an advantage for the evaluation of potentially unstable patients.

22. **Is CTA or MRA preferred for assessment of arterial trauma following penetrating trauma?**
    CTA is preferred. Metallic shrapnel causes susceptibility artifact on MRA, which can obscure the arteries. Active arterial extravasation of contrast material is well depicted on CTA as extraluminal contrast material which does not conform to a known vascular structure. Again, CTA is much faster to perform compared to MRA, which is an advantage for evaluation of potentially unstable patients.

23. **Is CTA or MRA preferred for assessment of endoleaks following stent graft repair of an aneurysm?**
    CTA is preferred because the stent graft causes susceptibility artifact on MRA. Embolization coils, when present, also cause susceptibility artifacts. These can obscure portions of the aneurysm, limiting evaluation.

24. **Is CTA or MRA preferred for assessment of entrapment syndromes?**
    MRA is preferred for assessment of entrapment vasculopathies such as popliteal entrapment syndrome or thoracic outlet syndrome (TOS) because MRA also allows for assessment of soft tissue structures such as muscles and tendons, which often lead to the compression of the artery of interest.

25. **Is CTA or MRA preferred for assessment of venous thrombosis?**
    MRA is more robust in the sense that one can use contrast-enhanced MRA techniques as well as noncontrast techniques to improve the sensitivity for detection of venous thrombosis. If the vein of interest displays a flow void on a spin echo MRI sequence, then the presence of acute thrombus is unlikely.

26. **How are CT and MR angiographic images visualized?**
    To diagnose vessel pathology, an image is created in a plane that allows the long axis of the vessel to be viewed. To view vessels in this perspective, images are transferred to a dedicated 3D workstation where the physician or a specially trained technologist performs reconstructions. There are several modes of image presentation that may be utilized for CTA and MRA, including multiplanar reformation (MPR), curved MPR, maximum intensity projection (MIP), surface-shaded display (SSD), and volume rendering (VR). These are described in more detail in Chapter 4.

27. **What is a hemodynamically significant artery stenosis?**
    Different arterial distributions can tolerate different degrees of stenosis, depending on the metabolic activity of the target organ and the availability of collateral blood supply. On CTA and MRA, most authors define "significant stenosis" as a diameter reduction of >70%, although a more conservative definition is >50%. Pressure gradients cannot be measured on CTA and MRA. Although quantitative measurements of the degree of stenosis are important, the presence of clinical symptoms should be the major determinant in the decision to treat an arterial lesion. Sequential subcritical stenoses result in a pressure decrease that approximates the sum of each stenosis. Additional signs of hemodynamically significant stenosis are poststenotic dilation of a vessel and delayed enhancement of the target organ.

28. **How do we measure stenosis?**
    The most accepted way is to calculate the ratio of the luminal diameter of the stenotic vessel segment to the luminal diameter of a normal-appearing vessel segment. This method was adopted from conventional angiography. Although well established, this method may lack precision because it uses a 2D representation of a 3D object to estimate a stenosis. It also relies on the ability to select a normal segment of vessel for use as a reference. This may be problematic because even normal vessels taper distally, and it may be difficult to find an area adjacent to a stenosis that is not aneurysmal or affected by poststenotic dilation. CTA and MRA offer the unique opportunity to evaluate the stenosis precisely, by measurement of the decrease in luminal cross-sectional area. With the development of more automated vessel analysis tools, measurements of luminal cross-sectional areas are expected to become the reference standard.

29. **What are the major branches of the celiac artery, superior mesenteric artery (SMA), and inferior mesenteric artery (IMA)?**
    The celiac artery gives rise to the splenic, left gastric, and common hepatic arteries (CHA). The CHA gives rise to the right gastric, proper hepatic, and gastroduodenal arteries (GDA). The GDA gives rise to the right gastroepiploic, anterior superior pancreaticoduodenal, and posterior superior pancreaticoduodenal arteries. The splenic artery gives rise to the short gastric, dorsal pancreatic, great pancreatic (arteria pancreatica magna), and left gastroepiploic arteries. The transverse pancreatic artery arises from the dorsal pancreatic artery. The proper hepatic artery gives rise to cystic, right hepatic, and left hepatic arteries.
    The SMA gives rise to the inferior pancreaticoduodenal, jejunal, ileal, ileocolic, right colic, and middle colic arteries.
    The IMA gives rise to the left colic artery and sigmoid arterial branches, and then terminates as the superior hemorrhoidal (rectal) artery.
    See Figure 16-1 for normal abdominal arterial anatomy on CTA.

30. **What is the most common variant of the celiac axis?**
    Conventional hepatic arterial anatomy is seen in only 55% of the population. The most common variant is replacement of the hepatic artery: a replaced left hepatic artery arising from the left gastric artery (20%) and a replaced right hepatic artery arising from the SMA (20%) (Figure 16-2).

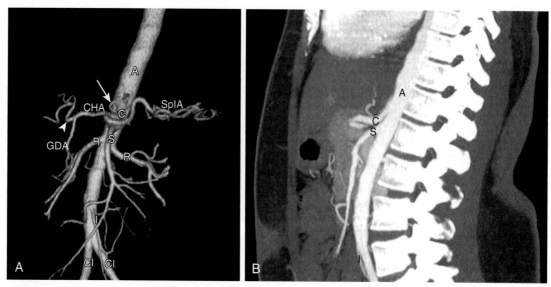

**Figure 16-1.** Normal abdominal arterial anatomy on CTA. **A,** Oblique coronal contrast-enhanced CTA volume-rendered (VR) image obtained through abdomen shows celiac artery (*C*), superior mesenteric artery (*S*), inferior mesenteric artery (*I*), and bilateral renal arteries (*R*) arising from abdominal aorta (*A*). Left gastric artery (*arrow*) arises from superior aspect of celiac artery. Common hepatic artery (*CHA*) and splenic artery (*SplA*) also arise from celiac artery. Gastroduodenal artery (*GDA*) and proper hepatic artery (*arrowhead*) arise from CHA. Abdominal aorta bifurcates distally into common iliac arteries (*CI*). **B,** Sagittal CTA maximum intensity projection (MIP) image through abdomen again demonstrates celiac artery (*C*), superior mesenteric artery (*S*), and inferior mesenteric artery (*I*) arising from abdominal aorta (*A*).

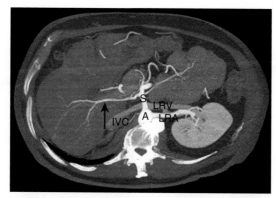

**Figure 16-2.** Variant hepatic arterial anatomy on CTA. Axial contrast-enhanced CTA MIP image through abdomen reveals right hepatic artery (*arrow*) arising from superior mesenteric artery (*S*) instead of from celiac artery and extending to right hepatic lobe, in keeping with replaced right hepatic artery. Note abdominal aorta (*A*), left renal artery (*LRA*), inferior vena cava (*IVC*), and left renal vein (*LRV*).

31. What are the major collateral pathways in the abdomen?
    Collateral pathways become important in arterial occlusion. The mesenteric vascular bed is rich in collaterals.
    - **Pancreaticoduodenal arcade:** between the superior and inferior pancreaticoduodenal arteries.
    - **Arc of Buhler:** between the proximal celiac artery and proximal SMA.
    - **Arch of Barkow:** between the right and left gastroepiploic arteries.
    - **Arc of Riolan:** between the proximal SMA and proximal IMA.
    - **Marginal artery of Drummond:** between the distal SMA and distal IMA.

32. What is the meandering mesenteric artery?
    This is another name for the Arc of Riolan. This is also known as the central anastomotic artery.

33. What artery is often occluded during open or endovascular repair of an AAA?
    The IMA.

34. Why are angiographic studies performed on potential renal donors?
    Donor kidney harvesting is often performed laparoscopically. The surgeon's field of view is limited, so precise information concerning the location, size, and number of renal arteries and veins is required before surgery. This is extremely important because of the variability of the renal vasculature in humans.

35. What is the prevalence of accessory renal arteries in the general population?

Approximately 30% of people have accessory renal arteries, which is the most common clinically relevant renal vascular variant (Figure 16-3). Significant post-transplant complications may result if even a small vessel that supplies the ureter is accidentally sacrificed. Larger arteries that supply the renal pelvis or significant portions of renal parenchyma must be preserved, sometimes necessitating complicated reconstructive surgery.

36. What is the most common left renal vein anatomic variant?

Generally, renal veins have more consistent anatomy than renal arteries. Knowledge of the venous anatomy before laparoscopic surgery is important to prevent vascular injury and bleeding. The left renal vein is longer than the right renal vein, which is one reason that the left kidney is preferred for transplantation.

The most common left renal vein anatomic variant is a circumaortic left renal vein, which occurs in up to 10% of the population. With this anatomic variant, the left renal vein forms a ring around the aorta. The anterior segment of the ring connects with the inferior vena cava at the expected level of the left renal vein, and the posterior segment connects with the inferior vena cava below the insertion of the anterior segment. A retroaortic left renal vein is less common and occurs in up to 3% of the population. Multiple renal veins constitute the most common renal vein variant overall, occurring in 15% to 30% of the population.

37. What are the major normal variants of the IVC?
- Double IVC (Figure 16-4).
- Left (transposed) IVC.
- Azygos continuation of the IVC.

38. What segment is missing in azygos continuation of the IVC?

The hepatic segment of the IVC is absent, and the azygos vein is enlarged. This variant is associated with heterotaxia syndrome and polysplenia.

39. What anatomic structure is used as a reference for the parts of the subclavian artery?

The anterior scalene muscle is the key anatomic landmark. The first part of the subclavian artery is medial to this muscle, the second part is posterior to this muscle, and the third part is lateral to this muscle.

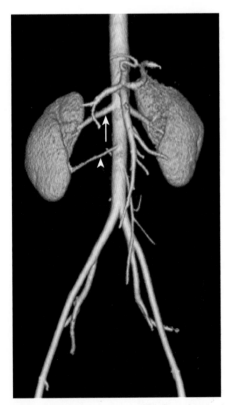

**Figure 16-3.** Accessory renal artery on CTA. Coronal contrast-enhanced CTA VR image through abdomen shows inferior accessory right renal artery (*arrowhead*) with smaller caliber relative to main right renal artery (*arrow*).

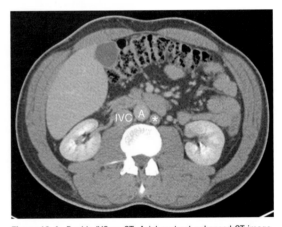

**Figure 16-4.** Double IVC on CT. Axial contrast-enhanced CT image through abdomen demonstrates inferior vena cava (*IVC*) to right of abdominal aorta (*A*) and additional inferior vena cava (*\**) to left of abdominal aorta.

40. At what point does the subclavian artery become the axillary artery?

The subclavian artery becomes the axillary artery when it crosses the outer edge of the first rib.

41. What are the major branches of the upper extremity arterial tree?

The brachial artery gives rise to the deep brachial (profunda brachii), ulnar collateral, radial, and ulnar arteries. The ulnar artery gives rise to the common interosseous artery and predominantly supplies the superficial palmar arch. The radial artery is smaller than the ulnar artery and predominantly supplies the deep palmar arch.

42. What structures separate the superficial femoral artery (SFA) from the popliteal artery and the external iliac artery from the common femoral artery (CFA)?

The SFA becomes the popliteal artery after entering the adductor (Hunter's) canal. The external iliac artery becomes the CFA when it crosses the inguinal ligament, which is approximated by the origins of the deep circumflex iliac and inferior epigastric arteries from the distal external iliac artery.

43. On an anterior projection, which thigh vessel takes a more medial course: the SFA or the deep femoral (profunda femoris) artery (DFA)?

The normal course of the SFA is medial to that of the DFA (Figure 16-5).

44. What is meant by "single-vessel," "two-vessel," or "three-vessel" runoff?

There are three infrapopliteal arteries: anterior tibial, posterior tibial, and peroneal arteries (see Figure 16-5). The number of these calf vessels that are continuously patent from the origin to the ankle defines the number of runoff vessels (Figure 16-6). A higher number usually corresponds to a better prognosis after surgery or endovascular procedures.

45. What is the distribution of peripheral vascular disease in different age groups?

Generally, young smokers have more proximal disease involving the iliac vessels. Older patients, especially patients with diabetes mellitus, have more distal disease involving the infrapopliteal vessels. This difference is important

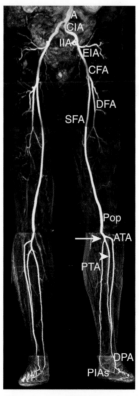

**Figure 16-5.** Normal pelvic and lower extremity arterial anatomy on MRA. Coronal contrast-enhanced MRA MIP image through pelvis and lower extremities reveals distal abdominal aorta (*A*), common iliac artery (*CIA*) which bifurcates into external iliac artery (*EIA*) and internal iliac artery (*IIA*), common femoral artery (*CFA*) which bifurcates into superficial femoral artery (*SFA*) and deep femoral artery (*DFA*), popliteal artery (*Pop*), anterior tibial artery (*ATA*) which arises from popliteal artery (located anteriorly and laterally) and extends into dorsal aspect of foot as dorsalis pedis artery (*DPA*), tibioperoneal trunk (*arrow*) which arises from popliteal artery and bifurcates into peroneal artery (*arrowhead*) (located posteriorly and laterally) and posterior tibial artery (*PTA*) (located posteriorly and medially), and medial and lateral plantar arches (*PIAs*) which arise from posterior tibial artery in plantar aspect of foot. Patency of three infrapopliteal arteries to level of ankle indicates three-vessel runoff.

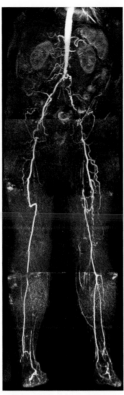

**Figure 16-6.** Peripheral vascular disease on MRA. Coronal contrast-enhanced MRA MIP image through pelvic and lower extremities shows multiple chronically occluded segments of pelvic and lower extremity arterial system with collateral formation secondary to atherosclerotic disease. On left, common iliac, external iliac, superficial femoral, and anterior tibial arteries are affected with two-vessel runoff via peroneal and posterior tibial arteries remaining. On right, superficial femoral, popliteal, anterior tibial, and posterior tibial arteries are affected with one-vessel runoff via peroneal artery remaining.

because patency rates after treatment of proximal disease using endovascular and surgical methods are significantly greater.

46. What compressive disorders may involve the popliteal artery?
    Cystic adventitial disease and popliteal entrapment syndrome.

47. How does one assess for popliteal entrapment syndrome?
    Popliteal entrapment syndrome is an uncommon condition that typically affects young athletic men who present with calf claudication.
    On imaging, popliteal artery patency is assessed in both stress and rest positions, where stress is achieved by dorsiflexion or plantar flexion. Entrapment of the popliteal artery is usually, but not always, a result of an abnormal anatomic relationship with the medial head of the gastrocnemius muscle, in which the popliteal artery is more medially located than it should be. In some cases, the popliteal artery is normally positioned but is entrapped by a hypertrophied gastrocnemius muscle (Figure 16-7).
    In patients with suspected popliteal entrapment syndrome, MRA is preferred to CTA. Both lower extremities are imaged because the condition is bilateral in ≈25% of cases.

48. What are the causes of venous contamination?
    Venous contamination is contrast opacification of the crural veins during arterial opacification. The causes are:
    • Delayed image acquisition through the calf. This is more likely to be encountered during MRA than CTA.
    • Inflammation such as by cellulitis or osteomyelitis.
    • Arteriovenous shunting.

49. A 40-year-old heavy smoker has pain in the foot at rest. Should one be thinking about atherosclerosis as the underlying etiology?
    Atherosclerosis is certainly a diagnostic consideration. However, Buerger's disease (thromboangiitis obliterans), a rare inflammatory vasculitis, should also be a differential diagnostic consideration.
    Buerger's disease involves small- and medium-sized vessels, leading to arterial narrowing and occlusion, and most often affects young to middle-age patients who use tobacco. It is characterized by presence of multiple vascular

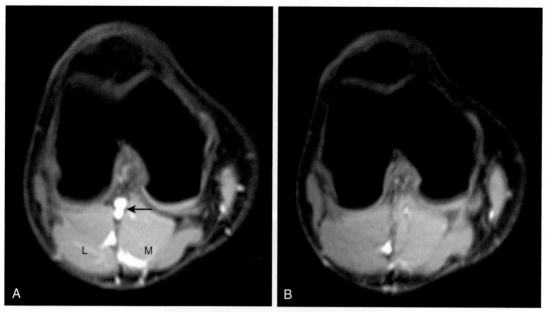

**Figure 16-7.** Popliteal entrapment syndrome on MRA. **A,** Axial postcontrast fat-suppressed T1-weighted MR image through knee during rest demonstrates patent popliteal vessels (*arrow*) and surrounded by hypertrophied medial (*M*) and lateral (*L*) heads of gastrocnemius muscle. **B,** Axial postcontrast fat-suppressed T1-weighted MR image through knee in same patient during plantar flexion now reveals marked compression of popliteal vessels by hypertrophied gastrocnemius muscle.

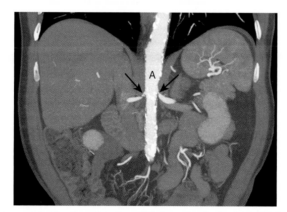

**Figure 16-8.** Renal artery stenosis secondary to atherosclerosis on CTA. Coronal contrast-enhanced CTA image through proximal renal arteries shows marked narrowing of ostial portions of renal arteries (*arrows*) with poststenotic dilation along with extensive atherosclerotic calcification of abdominal aorta (*A*).

stenoses and/or occlusions with "corkscrew" collaterals on imaging, and it rarely involves vessels proximal to the popliteal and brachial arteries.

50. How may renal arterial steno-occlusive disease present clinically?
    - Refractory hypertension.
    - Renal insufficiency or failure.
    - Acute flank pain (when acute).
    - Hematuria (when acute).

51. What are the common causes of renal artery stenosis?
    - Atherosclerosis (most common cause) (Figure 16-8).
    - Fibromuscular dysplasia (FMD) (second most common cause).
    - Vasculitis.
    - Radiation therapy.

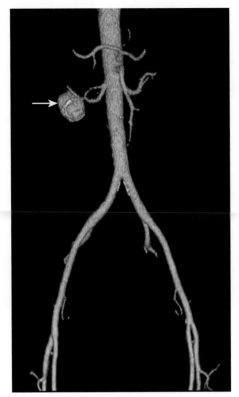

**Figure 16-9.** Renal artery aneurysm on CTA. Oblique coronal contrast-enhanced CTA VR image obtained through abdomen demonstrates large aneurysm (*arrow*) of right renal artery.

52. What are the common causes of renal artery aneurysms/pseudoaneurysms?
    - Atherosclerosis (Figure 16-9).
    - FMD.
    - Vasculitis such as by polyarteritis nodosa (PAN).
    - Infection such as by tuberculosis.
    - Connective tissue disease such as Ehlers-Danlos syndrome.
    - Trauma.

53. What are the common causes of renal artery dissection?
    - Extension from aortic dissection.
    - Atherosclerosis.
    - FMD.
    - Connective tissue disease such as Ehlers-Danlos syndrome.
    - Segmental arterial mediolysis (SAM).

54. How is FMD classified?
    - Intimal.
    - Medial.
    - Adventitial.
      The medial type of FMD is the most common, accounting for ≈80% of cases.

55. How does FMD present?
    FMD is an idiopathic noninflammatory arterial wall disease that typically involves small- to medium-sized vessels. It may be discovered incidentally, but it most commonly presents with hypertension, most often affecting young or middle-aged women.

    On CTA and MRA, FMD classically resembles a "string of beads" with alternating areas of luminal narrowing and dilation, and it affects the renal arteries bilaterally in ≈40% of cases. FMD typically involves the mid or distal portions of the main renal artery, whereas atherosclerosis typically involves the proximal or ostial portions of the main renal artery and usually affects older patients. The stenotic lesions in FMD that lead to hypertension respond favorably to angioplasty.

56. **Does a normal CTA or MRA exclude presence of polyarteritis nodosa (PAN)?**

PAN is an uncommon vasculitis which affects the kidneys in 90% of cases and leads to arterial wall thickening and microaneurysms. It affects medium-sized arteries, such as the intrarenal renal arteries, which are just within the resolution of CTA and MRA. The abnormalities may or may not be seen on CTA and MRA, which do not have the spatial resolution to confidently exclude PAN.

57. **What is the median arcuate ligament, and what is its significance?**

The median arcuate ligament is an archlike fibrous band formed from fibers derived from the medial edges of the left and right diaphragmatic crura during their ascent anterosuperiorly. The median arcuate ligament may occasionally cause a stenosis of the proximal celiac artery because of extrinsic compression. The clinical significance of such a stenosis is frequently uncertain, as it is often detected incidentally on imaging in asymptomatic patients. Severe celiac stenosis and even celiac arterial occlusion are often well tolerated.

The diagnosis of median arcuate ligament syndrome (also known as celiac artery compression syndrome) can be suggested by imaging findings seen on CTA and MRA acquired during inspiration and expiration. The characteristic imaging appearance is narrowing of the nonostial proximal celiac artery during end inspiration, which is best seen in the sagittal plane. Other associated imaging findings may include poststenotic dilation, upward hooking of the celiac artery, and a prominent pancreaticoduodenal arcade. The degree of stenosis depends on the phase of the respiratory cycle, often becoming more pronounced during end expiration, because the aorta and celiac artery move superiorly during expiration.

58. **Can ostial celiac artery or SMA occlusion result in mesenteric ischemia?**

Because of the extensive collaterals between the three main mesenteric vessels, occlusion of just one of these three vessels usually does not cause symptoms or signs of mesenteric ischemia. Severe stenosis of at least two of the vessels is generally necessary for symptomatic mesenteric ischemia. The state of the celiac artery and SMA is important to determine during preoperative planning for stent graft repair of an AAA. The reason is that the IMA is occluded during the placement of a stent graft, and the IMA may be the sole supply of blood to the gut.

Acute mesenteric ischemia is most commonly secondary to arterial embolic disease (in 40% to 50%) followed by arterial thrombosis (in 20% to 30%), whereas chronic mesenteric ischemia is most commonly secondary to atherosclerotic disease. The causes of bowel ischemia/infarction are described in more detail in Chapter 32.

59. **What is SMA syndrome?**

SMA syndrome is a condition secondary to compression of the third portion of the duodenum between the abdominal aorta and the SMA. Patients may present with abdominal pain, early satiety, nausea, and vomiting. This is a rare condition which typically occurs in people who have rapidly lost weight, such as in patients hospitalized with burns or who suffer from anorexia nervosa, and most commonly affects young women.

The normal aortomesenteric distance (AMD) between the abdominal aorta and SMA is 10 to 28 mm. The normal aortomesenteric angle (AMA) between the abdominal aorta and SMA is 25° to 60°. Compression of the duodenum is typically seen when the AMD is ≤8 mm and when the AMA is ≤22°. Upstream dilation of the proximal duodenum and stomach is also typically seen in this condition.

60. **What is nutcracker syndrome?**

Nutcracker syndrome is secondary to compression of the left renal vein as it passes between the abdominal aorta and SMA, resulting in outflow obstruction and left renal vein hypertension (Figure 16-10). Patients may present with left flank pain and hematuria. Associated left perirenal or periureteral varices, a left varicocele in men, or left pelvic and vulvar varices in women may be encountered.

61. **Which vein is compressed in May-Thurner syndrome?**

In May-Thurner syndrome, the left common iliac vein is compressed by the right common iliac artery, leading to left lower extremity swelling, with or without thrombosis of the left iliac and femoral veins (Figure 16-11). This condition may be treated with thrombolysis and stent placement in the iliac veins.

62. **Is CT or MRI the preferred imaging modality to assess for acute lower extremity deep vein thrombosis (DVT)?**

Neither. The first line imaging test used to assess for acute lower extremity DVT is ultrasonography (US). CT or MRI is useful for assessment of extension of femoral vein thrombus into the iliac veins, presence of acute DVT in the iliac veins, and presence of chronic thrombus and the degree of collateral vessels.

Acute DVT typically appears as a central nonenhancing luminal filling defect within a vein or as segmental nonopacification of a vein on contrast-enhanced CT and MRI, often with increased venous caliber. High attenuation on unenhanced CT, loss of a normal flow void on unenhanced MRI, infiltration of the surrounding fat, and edema and enlargement of the ipsilateral extremity soft tissue may also be visualized (Figure 16-12).

Chronic DVT typically appears as a vein with decreased caliber or luminal obliteration, sometimes with an eccentrically located nonenhancing luminal filling defect or with linear/curvilinear fibrotic bands on contrast-enhanced CT and MRI. Associated collateral veins and ipsilateral muscle enlargement are commonly seen as well.

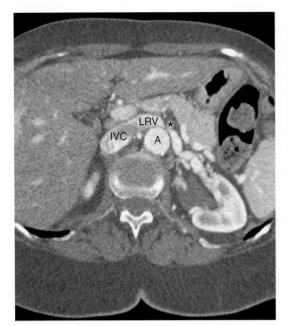

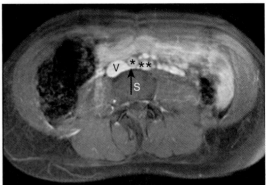

**Figure 16-11.** May-Thurner syndrome on MRI. Axial postcontrast fat-suppressed T1-weighted MR image through lower abdomen shows marked compression of proximal left common iliac vein (*arrow*) between right common iliac artery (*) and lumbar spine (*S*). Note proximal right common iliac vein (*V*) and left common iliac artery (**).

**Figure 16-10.** Nutcracker syndrome on CT. Axial contrast-enhanced CT image through abdomen reveals marked compression of left renal vein (*LRV*) between superior mesenteric artery (*) and abdominal aorta (*A*). Note inferior vena cava (*IVC*) to right of abdominal aorta.

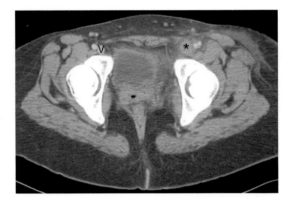

**Figure 16-12.** Acute DVT on CT. Axial contrast-enhanced CT image through pelvis demonstrates central nonenhancing luminal filling defect (*) within expanded left common femoral vein along with infiltration of surrounding fat. Note patent contralateral common femoral vein (*V*) for comparison.

63. **What is pelvic congestion syndrome?**

Pelvic congestion syndrome is a condition characterized by chronic dull pelvic pain, pressure, and heaviness that persists for >6 months' duration, secondary to congested pelvic veins. It usually affects multiparous women of reproductive age.

On CTA and MRA, imaging findings may include dilated gonadal veins (>6 mm in caliber), prominent (>4 mm) serpentine periuterine or periovarian veins, perineal varices, retrograde flow of contrast material into the gonadal veins, or reversal of blood flow in the gonadal veins on TOF MRA. Associated findings of nutcracker syndrome may also be present.

It is important to note that dilated gonadal and periuterine veins are commonly seen in asymptomatic parous women, and therefore in isolation (i.e., without associated clinical symptoms or signs) do not indicate presence of pelvic congestion syndrome.

64. **How do patients with thoracic outlet syndrome (TOS) present?**

The clinical presentation is secondary to compression of the subclavian artery, subclavian vein, and/or brachial plexus as these structures traverse the thoracic outlet. Patients may present with symptoms and signs of upper extremity tingling, weakness, swelling, heaviness, numbness, or hand claudication, which are typically reproduced or exacerbated by elevation or sustained use of the upper extremities. Young women are most commonly affected.

Major causes of TOS include osseous abnormalities (including a cervical rib, or excess callus, exostosis, or tumor of the first rib or clavicle) as well as soft tissue abnormalities (including a fibrous band, congenital and acquired muscle abnormalities, and soft tissue scarring).

65. List some useful tips regarding imaging assessment of patients with suspected TOS.
   - Obtain cervical spine and chest radiographs first to exclude osseous abnormalities in these locations.
   - Administer intravenous contrast material for CTA or MRA via an upper extremity vein contralateral to the symptomatic side, in order to eliminate artifacts secondary to concentrated contrast material within the veins that may obscure the arterial structures of interest.
   - Perform biphasic image acquisition, first with the arm by the side, and second with the arm elevated. This enables visualization of compression of the subclavian artery, subclavian vein, and/or brachial plexus, which may sometimes only be detected during arm elevation.
   - MRA is generally preferred because the soft tissue structures can be delineated.
   - Sagittal images are very useful to assess for compression of anatomic structures in the thoracic outlet.

66. Is CTA or MRA better to assess for subclavian steal syndrome?
   Subclavian steal syndrome is a clinical diagnosis. This syndrome occurs in the setting of a high grade stenosis or occlusion of the subclavian artery proximal to the origin of the vertebral artery, most commonly on the left side. In this situation, there is reversal of blood flow in the ipsilateral vertebral artery, diverting blood flow from the posterior circulation of the brain to the upper extremity. As such, the patient experiences symptoms, such as syncope, from reduced blood flow in the vertebrobasilar arterial system.

   CTA and MRA can both depict stenosis or occlusion of the proximal subclavian artery. TOF MRA can also demonstrate a characteristic reversal of the direction of blood flow in the ipsilateral vertebral artery (Figure 16-13).

67. List some principles regarding CTA and MRA assessment of the vasculature of a transplanted kidney.
   - Do not confuse anastomotic narrowing for a true renal arterial stenosis.
   - Perform biphasic image acquisition following intravenous contrast administration if renal artery stenosis and renal vein thrombosis are suspected.
   - Ensure that the plane of injection during MRA covers the renal vasculature. You may need to supervise this personally, given the off-axis plane of the transplanted kidney.
   - Do not forget to assess the iliac arterial inflow for presence of stenoses.
   - Do not forget to look for nonvascular complications such as hematoma, lymphocele, hydronephrosis, and post-transplant lymphoproliferative disorder (PTLD).

68. What is the main clinical indication for pancreatic transplantation?
   The pancreas is usually transplanted in patients with type I diabetes mellitus. This is most often performed in conjunction with transplantation of the kidney, which is known as simultaneous pancreas-kidney transplantation.

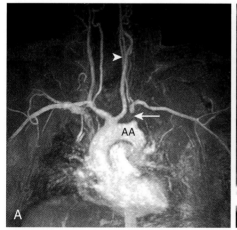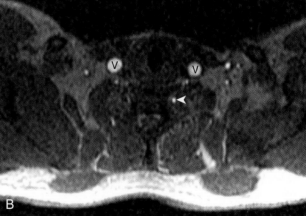

**Figure 16-13.** Subclavian steal syndrome on MRA. **A,** Coronal contrast-enhanced MRA MIP image through thorax and lower neck reveals segmental occlusion of proximal left subclavian artery (*arrow*). Note patent left vertebral artery (*arrowhead*) and aortic arch (*AA*). **B,** Axial TOF MRA image obtained through neck during application of saturation band to suppress signal from vessels with caudocranial blood flow shows high signal intensity within internal jugular veins (*V*) as well as within left vertebral artery (*arrowhead*). This latter finding indicates reversal of blood flow in left vertebral artery from caudocranial direction normally to craniocaudal direction.

69. What is the vascular anatomy of the pancreatic transplant?

The donor SMA and splenic artery are anastomosed to a donor iliac artery Y-graft (composed of the common iliac artery and the proximal internal and external iliac arteries). The donor common iliac artery is then anastomosed to the recipient common iliac artery or external iliac artery. The SMA supplies the head of the pancreatic transplant, whereas the splenic artery supplies the body and tail of the pancreatic transplant. The donor portal vein is attached to the recipient superior mesenteric vein (SMV), iliac vein, or IVC and receives venous blood flow from the donor SMV and splenic vein.

---

## KEY POINTS

- The most important principle for performing contrast-enhanced CTA and MRA is the timing of the image acquisition.
- When evaluating the arteries of the upper extremities via contrast-enhanced CTA or MRA, administer the intravenous contrast material on the side contralateral to the side of suspected pathology to eliminate venous contrast-related artifacts that may obscure the adjacent arteries.
- Accessory renal arteries are the most common clinically relevant renal vascular variant.
- Atherosclerosis is the most common cause of renal artery stenosis, most often occurs in older adults, and typically involves the proximal third of the renal artery.
- FMD is the second most common cause of renal artery stenosis, most often occurs in young or middle-aged women, and typically involves the distal third of the renal artery.

---

**BIBLIOGRAPHY**

Knuttinen MG, Xie K, Jani A, et al. Pelvic venous insufficiency: imaging diagnosis, treatment approaches, and therapeutic issues. *AJR Am J Roentgenol.* 2015;204(2):448-458.

Smillie RP, Shetty M, Boyer AC, et al. Imaging evaluation of the inferior vena cava. *Radiographics.* 2015;35(2):578-592.

Tolat PP, Foley WD, Johnson C, et al. Pancreas transplant imaging: how I do it. *Radiology.* 2015;275(1):14-27.

White RD, Weir-McCall JR, Sullivan CM, et al. The celiac axis revisited: anatomic variants, pathologic features, and implications for modern endovascular management. *Radiographics.* 2015;35(3):879-898.

Lamba R, Tanner DT, Sekhon S, et al. Multidetector CT of vascular compression syndromes in the abdomen and pelvis. *Radiographics.* 2014;34(1):93-115.

Pillai AK, Iqbal SI, Liu RW, et al. Segmental arterial mediolysis. *Cardiovasc Intervent Radiol.* 2014;37(3):604-612.

AbuRahma AF, Yacoub M. Renal imaging: duplex ultrasound, computed tomography angiography, magnetic resonance angiography, and angiography. *Semin Vasc Surg.* 2013;26(4):134-143.

Bozlar U, Ogur T, Khaja MS, et al. CT angiography of the upper extremity arterial system: Part 2—Clinical applications beyond trauma patients. *AJR Am J Roentgenol.* 2013;201(4):753-763.

Bozlar U, Ogur T, Norton PT, et al. CT angiography of the upper extremity arterial system: Part 1—Anatomy, technique, and use in trauma patients. *AJR Am J Roentgenol.* 2013;201(4):745-752.

Jens S, Koelemay MJ, Reekers JA, et al. Diagnostic performance of computed tomography angiography and contrast-enhanced magnetic resonance angiography in patients with critical limb ischaemia and intermittent claudication: systematic review and meta-analysis. *Eur Radiol.* 2013;23(11):3104-3114.

Jesinger RA, Thoreson AA, Lamba R. Abdominal and pelvic aneurysms and pseudoaneurysms: imaging review with clinical, radiologic, and treatment correlation. *Radiographics.* 2013;33(3):E71-E96.

Mousa AY, Gill G. Renal fibromuscular dysplasia. *Semin Vasc Surg.* 2013;26(4):213-218.

Wu W, Chaer RA. Nonarteriosclerotic vascular disease. *Surg Clin North Am.* 2013;93(4):833-875, viii.

Dimmick SJ, Goh AC, Cauzza E, et al. Imaging appearances of Buerger's disease complications in the upper and lower limbs. *Clin Radiol.* 2012;67(12):1207-1211.

Osiro S, Zurada A, Gielecki J, et al. A review of subclavian steal syndrome with clinical correlation. *Med Sci Monit.* 2012;18(5):RA57-RA63.

Wheaton AJ, Miyazaki M. Non-contrast enhanced MR angiography: physical principles. *J Magn Reson Imaging.* 2012;36(2):286-304.

Colyer WR, Eltahawy E, Cooper CJ. Renal artery stenosis: optimizing diagnosis and treatment. *Prog Cardiovasc Dis.* 2011;54(1):29-35.

Napoli A, Anzidei M, Zaccagna F, et al. Peripheral arterial occlusive disease: diagnostic performance and effect on therapeutic management of 64-section CT angiography. *Radiology.* 2011;261(3):976-986.

Meaney JF, Fagan AJ, Beddy P. Magnetic resonance angiography of abdominal vessels at 3 T. *Top Magn Reson Imaging.* 2010;21(3):189-197.

Okahara M, Mori H, Kiyosue H, et al. Arterial supply to the pancreas; variations and cross-sectional anatomy. *Abdom Imaging.* 2010;35(2):134-142.

Sebastia C, Peri L, Salvador R, et al. Multidetector CT of living renal donors: lessons learned from surgeons. *Radiographics.* 2010;30(7):1875-1890.

Furukawa A, Kanasaki S, Kono N, et al. CT diagnosis of acute mesenteric ischemia from various causes. *AJR Am J Roentgenol.* 2009;192(2):408-416.

Hazirolan T, Metin Y, Karaosmanoglu AD, et al. Mesenteric arterial variations detected at MDCT angiography of abdominal aorta. *AJR Am J Roentgenol.* 2009;192(4):1097-1102.

Ersoy H, Rybicki FJ. MR angiography of the lower extremities. *AJR Am J Roentgenol.* 2008;190(6):1675-1684.

Hai Z, Guangrui S, Yuan Z, et al. CT angiography and MRI in patients with popliteal artery entrapment syndrome. *AJR Am J Roentgenol.* 2008;191(6):1760-1766.

Das CJ, Neyaz Z, Thapa P, et al. Fibromuscular dysplasia of the renal arteries: a radiological review. *Int Urol Nephrol.* 2007;39(1):233-238.

Shih MC, Hagspiel KD. CTA and MRA in mesenteric ischemia: part 1, Role in diagnosis and differential diagnosis. *AJR Am J Roentgenol.* 2007;188(2):452-461.

Demondion X, Herbinet P, Van Sint Jan S, et al. Imaging assessment of thoracic outlet syndrome. *Radiographics.* 2006;26(6):1735-1750.

Sheehy N, MacNally S, Smith CS, et al. Contrast-enhanced MR angiography of subclavian steal syndrome: value of the 2D time-of-flight "localizer" sign. *AJR Am J Roentgenol.* 2005;185(4):1069-1073.

Urban BA, Ratner LE, Fishman EK. Three-dimensional volume-rendered CT angiography of the renal arteries and veins: normal anatomy, variants, and clinical applications. *Radiographics.* 2001;21(2):373-386, questionnaire 549-55.

# IV
# THORACIC IMAGING

# CHAPTER 17

# IMAGING OF LUNG NODULES AND MASSES

*Drew A. Torigian, MD, MA, FSAR, and Charles T. Lau, MD, MBA*

1. **What is a solitary pulmonary nodule (SPN)?**

   An SPN is a solitary focal lesion in the lung that measures 3 cm or less. A solitary focal lesion that is greater than 3 cm is considered to be a mass, and most masses are malignant. Approximately 150,000 SPNs are detected annually in the United States, often incidentally on imaging. A goal of radiologic evaluation of SPN is to noninvasively assess the likelihood of malignancy within the nodule. SPN is the initial radiographic finding in 30% of patients with lung cancer, and the prognosis depends partly on the stage at presentation.

2. **List some causes of pulmonary nodules.**

   Primary lung cancer and solitary metastasis from extrapulmonary malignancies are common causes of SPNs detected on chest radiography. Pulmonary granuloma and pulmonary hamartoma are other common causes. Box 17-1 provides a more complete list. Many other entities can cause SPNs or multiple pulmonary nodules, including malignancy (e.g., metastatic disease), infections, vasculitis, and inflammatory diseases (e.g., sarcoidosis, rheumatoid arthritis, or inhalational lung disease). Be careful about a "confluence of shadows" or overlap of normal vascular and skeletal structures that can mimic a nodule on a chest radiograph. Nipple shadows can also mimic nodules but often appear bilaterally and symmetrically.

3. **What is the general approach to the evaluation of SPN?**

   The initial step is to determine whether a "nodule" identified on chest radiography is truly a pulmonary nodule or a pseudolesion that mimics a nodule (some of the causes of a pseudolesion are listed in Box 17-1). If a "nodule" is actually a pseudolesion caused by a skeletal finding, such as a rib fracture, it exhibits the same anatomic relationship to its apparent bone of origin on multiple radiographic projections. A true pulmonary nodule that overlaps with skeletal structures on one radiographic projection would appear to move away from its apparent bone of origin on other radiographic projections. Radiopaque nipple markers are sometimes helpful in distinguishing nipples from true pulmonary nodules. When a true lung nodule has been confirmed, a more detailed investigation begins.

4. **What further diagnostic steps may be implemented in the workup of indeterminate pulmonary nodules?**

   Comparison with prior imaging studies is the first step, as long-term stability is suggestive of benignity. Thin-section unenhanced computed tomography (CT) is the next most common step for further evaluation of indeterminate pulmonary nodules and is useful for identifying the presence of fat or specific patterns of calcification within a nodule that indicate benignancy. Fluorodeoxyglucose (FDG) positron emission tomography (PET), follow-up chest CT, and tissue sampling are some other options available for the workup of indeterminate pulmonary nodules. The choice is based on multiple factors, including the pretest probability of malignancy, the morphologic features of the nodules, and the patient's clinical history and current status. Although CT nodule densitometry and MRI may also be useful to characterize lung nodules as benign or malignant, they are uncommonly used for this purpose in clinical practice.

5. **What are the Fleischner Society guidelines?**

   The Fleischner Society guidelines provide general recommendations regarding what diagnostic tests should be performed next to evaluate incidentally detected lung nodules on CT. Different guidelines apply depending on whether the nodule is solid or subsolid in attenuation. Exclusion criteria from these guidelines, such as a personal history of prior malignancy, also exist.

6. **What are some potential blind spots on chest radiography and CT when trying to detect pulmonary nodules?**

   On chest radiography, potential blind spots include the lung apices where the clavicles and ribs overlap, the hila and retrocardiac region where superimposed cardiovascular structures are located, and within the lung bases below the level of the anterior portions of the hemidiaphragms where abdominal soft tissue overlaps.

   On CT, potential blind spots include the central portions of the lungs (e.g., the hilar regions and the azygoesophageal recess) and the endoluminal portions of the trachea and bronchi.

7. **List some morphologic imaging features of nodules assessed on CT.**
   - Location
   - Shape
   - Size/volume
   - Margins
   - Attenuation

**Box 17-1.** Differential Diagnosis of Causes of Solitary Pulmonary Nodule (SPN)

**Neoplastic**

Primary lung cancer (No. 1 cause of SPN detected on chest radiography)
Metastasis
Lymphoma/post-transplant lymphoproliferative disorder
Carcinoid tumor
Primary lung sarcoma
Hamartoma (No. 3 cause of SPN detected on chest radiography, No. 2 cause of benign SPN)

**Infections**

Granuloma (No. 2 cause of SPN detected on chest radiography, No. 1 cause of benign SPN)
Bacterial infection
Viral infection
Fungal infection
Mycobacterial infection
Parasitic infection
Septic emboli (often multiple, peripheral, and cavitary)

**Vascular**

Pulmonary infarction (often peripheral and wedge-shaped, associated with pulmonary embolism)
Vasculitis
Arteriovenous malformation
Pulmonary venous varix (tubular and avidly enhancing on CT)
Pulmonary artery aneurysm

**Inflammatory**

Sarcoidosis
Inhalational lung disease
Hypersensitivity pneumonitis
Organizing pneumonia
Bronchiolitis

Langerhans cell histiocytosis (associated with upper lobe predominant cystic interstitial lung disease in smokers)
Rheumatoid (necrobiotic) nodule
Inflammatory pseudotumor

**Congenital**

Intrapulmonary lymph node
Pulmonary sequestration (solid or cystic opacity most often in lower lobes)
Bronchial atresia

**Traumatic**

Radiation therapy (typically has linear margins and known history of prior radiation therapy)
Pulmonary contusion (associated with traumatic injury to the chest)

**Pseudonodules**

Rounded atelectasis ("folded lung," typically a subpleural opacity associated with pleural thickening or effusion and "comet-tail" sign of swirling bronchovascular structures central to opacity)
Pulmonary scarring
Mucoid impaction
Fluid in interlobar fissure (often lenticular in shape on lateral chest radiograph in the location of a fissure)
Healing rib fracture
Bone island
Spinal osteophyte
Skin lesion
Nipple shadow
Pleural lesion
Mediastinal lesion
Overlap of vascular and osseous structures

- Presence of fat
- Presence and pattern of calcification
- Presence of enhancement
- Change in features over time

8. Describe morphologic imaging findings that are suggestive of a benign SPN.

Small size and smooth, well-defined margins suggest a benign SPN, although 15% and 40% of malignant nodules are less than 1 cm and 2 cm in diameter, respectively, and 20% of malignant nodules have well-defined margins. Intranodular fat is a reliable indicator of a hamartoma, which is a benign lesion (Figure 17-1). Central, diffusely solid, laminated, and "popcorn-like" patterns of nodule calcification are indicative of benignancy, with the first three typically seen in calcified granulomas and the last in a pulmonary hamartoma (Figure 17-2). Indeterminate patterns of calcification exist, and 15% of lung cancers may contain amorphous, stippled, or punctate and eccentric patterns of calcification. Avidly enhancing serpentine or tubular feeding arteries and a dilated draining vein associated with an enhancing nodular lung opacity are pathognomonic of an arteriovenous malformation (Figure 17-3). Small satellite nodules adjacent to a smooth dominant nodule strongly suggest a granulomatous infection. Ground glass opacity surrounding a nodule ("CT halo" sign) may be seen with angioinvasive opportunistic infection, such as by aspergillosis, particularly in the setting of neutropenia (Figure 17-4). Similarly, gas in a crescentic shape along the margin of a nodule (the "air crescent" sign) can be seen in the setting of an angioinvasive fungal infection. A three-dimensional ratio of the nodule's largest axial diameter to the largest craniocaudal diameter greater than 1.78:1 (i.e., a flattened configuration) is highly suggestive of benignancy. A peripheral rim of enhancement or the "enhancing rim" sign of a nodule may also suggest a benign SPN.

9. Describe morphologic imaging findings that are suggestive of a malignant SPN.

Size greater than 1 cm is more suggestive of malignancy. Lobulated or spiculated margins with distortion of adjacent vessels and lung architecture can also be associated with malignancy, although a lobulated or spiculated margin is

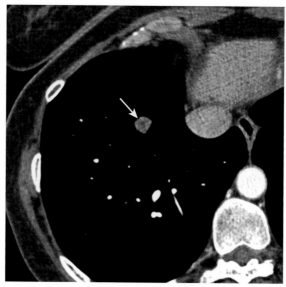

**Figure 17-1.** Pulmonary hamartoma on CT. Note smoothly marginated round nodule (*arrow*) that contains low-attenuation fat pathognomonic for hamartoma.

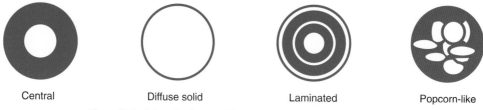

| Central | Diffuse solid | Laminated | Popcorn-like |

**Figure 17-2.** Schematic diagram of four benign patterns of nodule calcification.

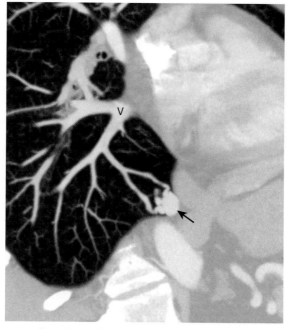

**Figure 17-3.** Pulmonary arteriovenous malformation on CT. Note tubular nodular nidus in right lung (*arrow*) that has draining veins leading to pulmonary vein (*V*). Other images show enhancing feeding pulmonary artery to nidus (not shown).

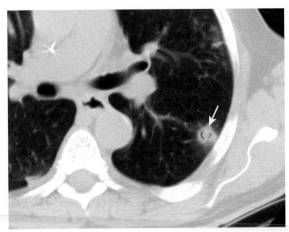

**Figure 17-4.** Invasive aspergillosis with "CT halo" sign and "air crescent" sign on CT. Note partially cavitary pulmonary nodule (*arrow*) surrounded by faint ground glass opacity secondary to pulmonary hemorrhage, along with peripheral crescentic areas of internal gas.

seen in 25% and 10% of benign nodules. The "corona radiata" sign consists of very fine linear strands extending outward from a nodule and is strongly suggestive of malignancy. Partially solid nodules (i.e., nodules composed of ground glass and solid components) tend to be malignant and are most often due to lung adenocarcinoma. Internal inhomogeneity, particularly caused by cystic/bubbly lucencies or pseudocavitation, strongly suggests malignancy, most often from adenocarcinoma in situ (AIS) or minimally invasive adenocarcinoma (MIA). Cavitary nodules with maximal wall thickness greater than 15 mm and wall irregularity tend to be malignant, whereas nodules with wall thickness 4 mm or less tend to be benign.

10. **How does measurement of the doubling time of nodules aid in the determination of a benign SPN?**
Doubling time, the time required for a nodule to double in volume (equivalent to an increase of about 26% in diameter), for most malignant nodules is 1 to 15 months. Nodules that double in volume more rapidly or more slowly than this tend to be benign. Generally, lack of growth of a nodule over a 2-year period is strongly suggestive of benignancy, although some malignant nodules, such as nodules secondary to AIS, MIA, bronchial carcinoid, or some pulmonary metastases, may take longer to grow. Initial follow-up CT scans for indeterminate pulmonary nodules generally are performed 3 to 12 months after the initial CT scan to assess for interval growth depending on the size and appearance of the nodule and the presence of risk factors for malignancy, such as a patient history of tobacco use.

11. **How does the degree of enhancement of pulmonary nodules on CT aid in the determination of benignancy?**
The degree of enhancement of pulmonary nodules is directly related to the likelihood of malignancy and the vascularity of the nodules, and may be determined through CT nodule densitometry. Nodule enhancement of less than 15 HU (a measure of attenuation) on CT after intravenous contrast administration is strongly predictive of benignancy, whereas enhancement of more than 15 HU may indicate either malignancy or active inflammation. False-negative enhancement studies may occur occasionally when central necrosis, cavitation, or abundant mucin is present within a pulmonary nodule or if a pulmonary nodule is very small.

12. **How does FDG PET aid in the differentiation of benign and malignant lung nodules?**
Malignant pulmonary nodules generally have increased glucose metabolism with increased uptake, trapping, and accumulation of FDG, a radioisotopic glucose analogue that can be detected on PET imaging. However, active inflammatory granulomatous pulmonary nodules may also show increased uptake of FDG. Lack of FDG uptake in a pulmonary nodule measuring 10 mm or more suggests benignancy, although malignant nodules that are due to AIS, MIA, or bronchial carcinoid or that are less than 10 mm may have low or absent FDG uptake. Dual-time-point FDG PET with early and delayed imaging can characterize pulmonary nodules further because malignant nodules tend to accumulate radiotracer over time, and benign nodules tend to wash out radiotracer gradually. In general, FDG PET/CT is useful for characterizing lung nodules, and it is currently recommended when a solid indeterminate lung nodule >8-10 mm in diameter is present in the setting of a low-moderate pretest probability of malignancy or when a persistent part-solid indeterminate nodule >8–10 mm in diameter is present.

13. **Describe some clinical features that suggest whether SPN is more likely to be malignant and whether it is more likely to be due to lung cancer or a pulmonary metastasis.**
Older patient age (>35 years old), history of prior malignancy, presence of symptoms and signs of malignancy such as hemoptysis, and history of tobacco use all increase the likelihood that an SPN is malignant rather than benign. In

patients with a history of extrapulmonary malignancy, lung cancer tends to be a more frequent cause of SPN than pulmonary metastasis or a benign lesion. However, this can vary depending on the type of extrapulmonary malignancy. For example, a solitary metastasis is a more common cause of SPN than lung cancer in patients with melanoma, sarcoma, and testicular cancer. Multiplicity of pulmonary nodules also favors metastases over lung cancer. Finally, primary lung cancer occurs more commonly in the upper lung fields, whereas pulmonary metastases occur more commonly in the lower lung fields. There are no imaging criteria, however, that can definitively distinguish a solitary pulmonary metastasis from a primary lung cancer.

14. What minimally invasive procedures may be used to obtain tissue samples from SPN?

Image-guided transthoracic needle biopsy is the procedure of choice for definitive characterization of peripheral pulmonary nodules, whereas conventional bronchoscopic needle biopsy is typically used for the characterization of nodules that involve the central airways and lungs. Electromagnetic navigational bronchoscopy (ENB) is a rapidly growing technique that permits bronchoscopists to biopsy peripheral lung nodules as well.

15. What are the potential complications of transthoracic needle biopsy?

Pneumothorax is the most common complication, which may occur in up to 25% of cases, particularly when severe emphysema is present. Nondiagnostic or false-negative biopsy results, hemoptysis, hemorrhage, pain, infection, air embolus, and tumor seeding are less common complications. Avoidance of crossing pulmonary fissures with the biopsy needle decreases the incidence of pneumothorax.

16. How important is lung cancer as a public health issue?

Lung cancer is the most common cause of cancer-related death in men and women, and it is the second most common cause of cancer after prostate cancer in men and breast cancer in women. Tobacco use is the top risk factor for lung cancer, and 85% of lung cancer deaths are due to smoking. The risk of developing lung cancer is proportional to the number of pack-years of smoking. Synchronous primary lung cancers occur in <5% of patients with lung cancer, but metachronous primary lung cancers may occur in 15%, with a latency of about 4 to 5 years. Overall, survival rates for patients with lung cancer are poor (<15% at 5 years), although patients with treated early-stage disease or with AIS or MIA tumor subtypes tend to have much better survival.

17. What are the major histologic types and subtypes of lung cancer?

Histologically, 75% are non–small cell lung cancers (NSCLC), for which the prognosis primarily depends on surgical stage at diagnosis, and 25% are small cell lung cancers (SCLC), which behave aggressively with early and wide dissemination. NSCLC may be subdivided into adenocarcinoma, squamous cell carcinoma, and large cell carcinoma subtypes, in order of decreasing frequency. AIS and MIA are less aggressive subtypes of adenocarcinoma.

18. Summarize some of the different features of the various histologic types and subtypes of lung cancer.

**Adenocarcinoma** is the subtype that occurs most frequently in nonsmokers, although the vast majority of adenocarcinomas occur in smokers. Adenocarcinomas tend to develop in the lung periphery. **Squamous cell carcinoma** is even more strongly associated with tobacco use, tends to develop centrally, and may cavitate.

    **Large cell carcinoma** is a histologic diagnosis of exclusion among the subtypes of lung cancer, is strongly associated with tobacco use, and often manifests as a large peripheral lung mass. **Small cell lung carcinoma** usually arises centrally within the chest with extensive metastatic lymphadenopathy involving the hila and mediastinum and only rarely cavitates, but it may manifest in a more limited form in one hemithorax or as an SPN.

19. What is a superior sulcus tumor?

**Superior sulcus tumor** (or **Pancoast tumor**) usually refers to a primary lung cancer that is located in the lung apex and often involves the adjacent pleura, chest wall, brachial plexus, or subclavian vessels (Figure 17-5). Superior sulcus tumors can manifest clinically as chest, shoulder, and arm pain with paresthesias, along with Horner syndrome (ipsilateral ptosis, miosis, and anhidrosis) caused by invasion of the stellate ganglion. Squamous cell carcinoma is the most common subtype responsible, and adenocarcinoma is the second most common.

20. Describe the major imaging findings related to lung cancer.

Findings include a pulmonary or endobronchial nodule or mass associated with obstructive (or resorptive) atelectasis or pneumonitis; thoracic lymphadenopathy; pleural, mediastinal, or chest wall involvement; or distant metastatic disease (Figure 17-6).

    Sometimes, obstructive segmental or lobar atelectasis may be the only sign of lung cancer on chest radiography, particularly if no air bronchograms are present. When a peripheral concavity caused by obstructive atelectasis coexists with an associated focal central convexity caused by a central mass, an S-shaped smooth fissural margin results, which is known as the "S sign of Golden" (Figure 17-7).

    Unilateral hilar lymphadenopathy; unilateral pleural effusion (particularly when present on the left); abrupt occlusion of a bronchus (the "bronchial cutoff" sign); and obscuration of a hilar, mediastinal, or diaphragmatic structure (the "silhouette" sign) are other chest radiographic findings of pulmonary malignancy. Adenocarcinoma spectrum lesions may appear as a solitary nodule; subsolid pulmonary nodules; or solitary, multiple, or diffuse foci of chronic pulmonary consolidation. Cavitation or cystic change may be present (Figure 17-8).

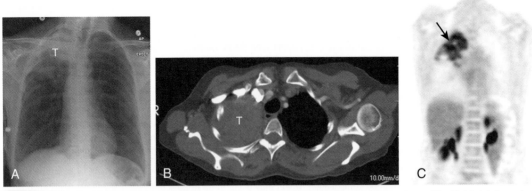

**Figure 17-5. A,** Pancoast tumor secondary to NSCLC on chest radiograph. Note right apical pulmonary tumor (*T*) with lobulated margins. **B,** Pancoast tumor secondary to NSCLC on CT. Note soft tissue attenuation right apical pulmonary tumor (*T*). **C,** Pancoast tumor secondary to NSCLC on FDG PET. Note avid FDG uptake in right apical pulmonary tumor (*arrow*).

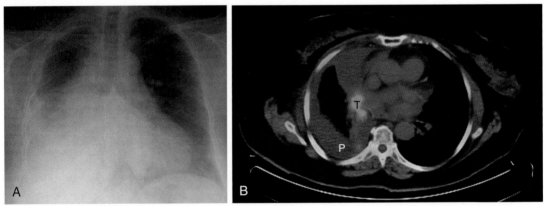

**Figure 17-6. A,** Unresectable NSCLC associated with malignant pleural effusion on chest radiograph. Note soft tissue fullness in right hilum along with obscuration of right hemidiaphragm owing to large right pleural effusion. **B,** Unresectable NSCLC associated with malignant pleural effusion on FDG PET/CT. Note soft tissue tumor (*T*) in right hilum along with large loculated right pleural effusion (*P*) that has areas of FDG uptake.

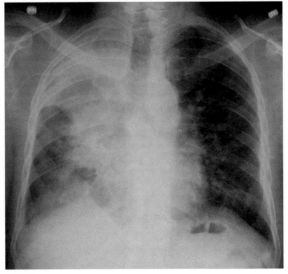

**Figure 17-7.** NSCLC causing lobar atelectasis with "(reverse) S sign of Golden" on chest radiograph. Note right upper lobe obstructive atelectasis with S-shaped fissural margin with focal convexity centrally owing to central mass and concavity more distally. Note lack of air bronchograms typical of obstructive atelectasis.

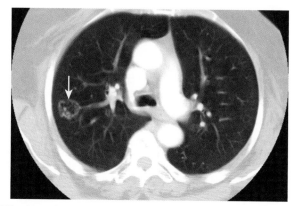

**Figure 17-8.** MIA subtype of NSCLC on CT. Note SPN (*arrow*) in right lung with cystic or cavitary change.

---

**Box 17-2.** AJCC TNM Staging System of Lung Cancer

*T = Primary Tumor*

| | |
|---|---|
| T0 | No evidence of primary tumor |
| T1 | ≤3 cm, surrounded by lung/visceral pleura, and no invasion of mainstem bronchus |
| T1a | ≤2cm |
| T1b | >2 cm and ≤3 cm |
| T2 | >3 cm and ≤7 cm, involvement of mainstem bronchus ≥2 cm from carina, invasion of visceral pleura, or obstructive atelectasis of part of lung |
| T2a | >3 cm and ≤5 cm |
| T2b | >5 cm and ≤7 cm |
| T3 | >7 cm, invasion of chest wall, mediastinal pleura, diaphragm, parietal pericardium, mainstem bronchus <2 cm from carina, obstructive atelectasis of entire lung, or presence of separate tumor nodules in same lobe of lung |
| T4 | Invasion of mediastinal structures, or presence of separate tumor nodules in different ipsilateral lobe of lung |

*N = Regional Lymph Nodes*

| | |
|---|---|
| N0 | No regional lymph node metastases |
| N1 | Ipsilateral hilar, peribronchial, or intrapulmonary lymphadenopathy |
| N2 | Ipsilateral mediastinal or subcarinal lymphadenopathy |
| N3 | Supraclavicular, scalene, contralateral mediastinal, or contralateral hilar lymphadenopathy |

*M = Distant Metastasis*

| | |
|---|---|
| M0 | No distant metastasis |
| M1 | Distant metastasis |
| M1a | Presence of separate tumor nodules in contralateral lung or metastatic involvement of pleura |
| M1b | Presence of distant metastases |

*Stage*

| | |
|---|---|
| 0 | Carcinoma in situ |
| IA | T1 N0 M0 |
| IB | T2a N0 M0 |
| IIA | T1-2a N1 M0, T2b N0 M0 |
| IIB | T2b N1 M0, T3 N0 M0 |
| IIIA | T1-2 N2 M0, T3 N1-2 M0, T4 N0-1 M0 |
| IIIB | T4 N2 M0, Any T N3 M0 |
| IV | Any T Any N M1 |

*Note*: Any T4 or N2 lesion is at least stage IIIA, any N3 lesion is at least stage IIIB, and any M1 lesion is stage IV. Patients with stage 0 to IIIA lesions are generally treated with surgery, whereas patients with stage IIIB and IV lesions are generally treated with medical therapy.

---

21. **Summarize the American Joint Committee on Cancer (AJCC) tumor node metastasis (TNM) staging system for lung cancer.**
    For the answer, see Box 17-2.

22. **Are there any other staging systems used in patients with SCLC?**
    The Veterans Administration Lung Study Group (VALSG) system is also used, and it classifies SCLC as either limited stage disease (LD) or extensive stage disease (ED). With LD, cancer is confined to one hemithorax and may be present in regional lymph nodes or ipsilateral supraclavicular nodes, all of which can be encompassed in a safe radiotherapy field. Otherwise, ED is present. This system is used as the majority of patients with SCLC undergo nonsurgical treatment.

23. **When is NSCLC generally considered unresectable?**
    When NSCLC is stage IIIB (i.e., with the presence of invasion of vital mediastinal structures or unresectable lymphadenopathy) or stage IV (i.e., with the presence of metastases involving the pleura, contralateral lung, or distant sites), it is generally considered unresectable. Symptoms and signs are rarely present until the disease is advanced in stage and more likely to be unresectable.

24. **Are there any reliable screening tests for lung cancer? What is the National Lung Screening Trial (NLST)?**

Yes, low dose chest CT (LDCT) is the only diagnostic test that has been shown to decrease lung cancer specific mortality rates in individuals at high risk for lung cancer. This was shown by the NLST, a large multicenter prospective trial that compared screening with frontal chest radiography to screening with thin-section LDCT, in participants of age 55 to 74 with ≥30 pack-year smoking history and history of smoking within the past 15 years. The NLST was the largest and most expensive (>$200M) randomized clinical trial of a single screening test in the history of medicine in the United States.

25. **Are there any risks of LDCT screening for lung cancer?**

Yes, there is a high false-positive rate of LDCT screening, as a substantial number of LDCT screening scans are positive (i.e., noncalcified nodules ≥4 mm or other findings suspicious for lung cancer), requiring follow-up imaging or invasive tissue sampling, although 96% of detected lung nodules turn out to be benign. The NLST showed that ≈320 high-risk people must be screened to prevent 1 death from lung cancer. Fortunately, the risk of adverse events following LDCT screening is <2%. Research is ongoing in the search for laboratory biomarkers to improve the specificity of LDCT screening and reduce false-positive results.

26. **Name some treatment options for lung cancer.**

Surgical resection (typically lobectomy or pneumonectomy with lymph node resection), chemotherapy, and radiation therapy may be used depending on the stage of disease and the histology of the tumor. Cessation of tobacco use is also part of treatment. Techniques such as percutaneous ablation of focal lung or bronchial tumors as well as stereotactic body radiation therapy (SBRT) are also available.

27. **Describe the imaging findings of pulmonary metastases.**

Solitary or multiple pulmonary and endobronchial nodules or masses are often seen (Figure 17-9), which may be ill-defined or well-circumscribed, ground glass or solid in attenuation, and often associated with metastases at other thoracic or extrathoracic anatomic locations. Depending on the underlying primary malignancy, the lesions may be homogeneous or heterogeneous with cystic, necrotic, calcific, or hemorrhagic change, and they may vary in size from very small (miliary) nodules to very large "cannonball" masses. Pneumothorax is often associated with pulmonary metastatic disease from osteogenic sarcoma. Overall, the lungs are an extremely common site of metastatic disease.

28. **What is lymphangitic carcinomatosis?**

Lymphangitic carcinomatosis is the spread of metastatic disease along the lung interstitium with subsequent lymphatic obstruction, interstitial edema, and fibrosis. Primary tumors of the breast, lung, stomach, pancreas, ovary, and cervix are often associated with lymphangitic carcinomatosis. On chest radiography, the lungs may appear clear or they may show a central linear pattern of interstitial thickening that is commonly bilateral but asymmetric in distribution between the lungs. On CT, typical smooth or nodular thickening of the interlobular septa is seen often with peribronchovascular thickening and asymmetric involvement of the lungs (Figure 17-10).

29. **What are pulmonary carcinoid tumors?**

These are rare neuroendocrine neoplasms that range from low-grade typical carcinoids to more aggressive atypical carcinoids. They are not related to tobacco use and occur slightly more commonly in women. Most arise centrally in an endobronchial location and are commonly associated with segmental or lobar obstructive atelectasis or pneumonitis, whereas the remainder appear as well-circumscribed peripheral pulmonary nodules or masses. These lesions typically show avid enhancement, and 40% may be associated with internal calcification. Carcinoid syndrome is rarely associated with pulmonary carcinoid tumors.

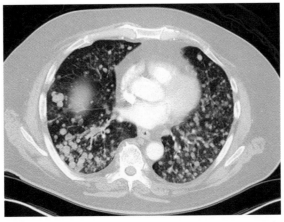

**Figure 17-9.** Pulmonary metastases on CT. Note multiple, variably sized, smoothly marginated nodules throughout lungs.

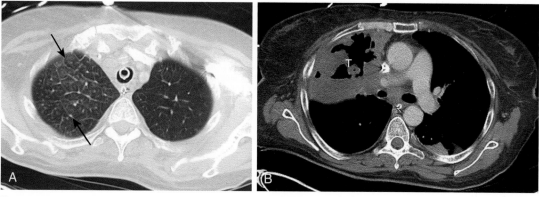

**Figure 17-10. A,** Lymphangitic carcinomatosis in NSCLC on CT. Note smooth asymmetric thickening of interlobular septa (*arrows*) in right upper lobe of lung. **B,** Lymphangitic carcinomatosis in NSCLC on CT. Note large cavitary tumor (*T*) in right upper lobe of lung more inferiorly secondary to lung cancer.

30. **What is a pulmonary hamartoma?**
    Pulmonary hamartoma is the most common benign neoplasm of the lung and typically manifests as an asymptomatic well-circumscribed SPN, during the fourth through seventh decades of life. Pathologically, these are mesenchymal tumors that have foci of mature cartilage separated by islands of fat and bronchial epithelium, often with fibrosis, calcification, or ossification. Typical CT findings include a smoothly marginated SPN that often contains visible fat or dense foci of calcification or ossification or both.

31. **What is congenital bronchial atresia?**
    Congenital bronchial atresia is due to atresia or stenosis of a bronchus at or near its origin, most often seen in the apicoposterior segment of the left upper lobe. Imaging findings include hyperlucency with air trapping and decreased vascularity to the portion of lung supplied by the involved bronchus, along with a nonenhancing hilar mass (bronchocele) or nonenhancing branching soft tissue opacities, usually with bronchial dilation owing to mucoid impaction. Congenital bronchial atresia can appear as an SPN on chest radiography.

## KEY POINTS

- Be aware of the major blind spots on frontal chest radiography: the lung apices where the clavicles and ribs overlap, the hilar regions where vascular structures abound, the retrocardiac region, and the lung bases where there is superimposition with the upper abdominal soft tissue.
- If you see lobar or segmental atelectasis on chest radiography, particularly without air bronchograms, be suspicious of an obstructive endobronchial lesion such as a lung cancer, and, at the minimum, get a short-term follow-up chest radiograph.
- If a pulmonary opacity does not resolve over time despite treatment with antimicrobial agents, be suspicious of a potential lung cancer.
- The best way to prevent lung cancer is through prevention (i.e., by not smoking or by quitting smoking).
- Although mucoid impaction of a bronchus may mimic a pulmonary nodule on chest radiography, one should exclude an endobronchial lesion as the cause for mucus retention in a bronchus if resolution is not seen on follow-up imaging.

**BIBLIOGRAPHY**

Siegel R, Ma J, Zou Z, et al. Cancer statistics, 2014. *CA Cancer J Clin.* 2014;64(1):9-29.
Vilstrup MH, Torigian DA. FDG PET in thoracic malignancies. *PET Clin.* 2014;9(4):391-420.
Gould MK, Donington J, Lynch WR, et al. Evaluation of individuals with pulmonary nodules: when is it lung cancer? Diagnosis and management of lung cancer, 3rd ed: American College of Chest Physicians evidence-based clinical practice guidelines. *Chest.* 2013;143(5 suppl):e93S-120S.
Kanne JP, Jensen LE, Mohammed TL, et al. ACR Appropriateness Criteria Radiographically Detected Solitary Pulmonary Nodule. *J Thorac Imaging.* 2013;28(1):W1-W3.
Kwee TC, Torigian DA, Alavi A. Oncological applications of positron emission tomography for evaluation of the thorax. *J Thorac Imaging.* 2013;28(1):11-24.
Naidich DP, Bankier AA, MacMahon H, et al. Recommendations for the management of subsolid pulmonary nodules detected at CT: a statement from the Fleischner Society. *Radiology.* 2013;266(1):304-317.
Bach PB, Mirkin JN, Oliver TK, et al. Benefits and harms of CT screening for lung cancer: a systematic review. *JAMA.* 2012;307(22):2418-2429.
Houseni M, Chamroonrat W, Zhuang H, et al. Multimodality imaging assessment of pulmonary nodules. *PET Clin.* 2011;6(3):231-250.

National Lung Screening Trial Research Team, Aberle DR, Adams AM, et al. Reduced lung-cancer mortality with low-dose computed tomographic screening. *N Engl J Med.* 2011;365(5):395-409.

Edge SB, Byrd DR, Compton CC, et al. Lung. In: *AJCC Cancer Staging Manual.* New York: Springer; 2010:253-270.

Ravenel JG, Mohammed TL, Movsas B, et al. ACR Appropriateness Criteria noninvasive clinical staging of bronchogenic carcinoma. *J Thorac Imaging.* 2010;25(4):W107-W111.

Hansell DM, Bankier AA, MacMahon H, et al. Fleischner Society: glossary of terms for thoracic imaging. *Radiology.* 2008;246(3):697-722.

MacMahon H, Austin JH, Gamsu G, et al. Guidelines for management of small pulmonary nodules detected on CT scans: a statement from the Fleischner Society. *Radiology.* 2005;237(2):395-400.

# IMAGING OF AIRSPACE LUNG DISEASE

Scott Simpson, DO, MD, Wallace T. Miller, Jr., MD, and Drew A. Torigian, MD, MA, FSAR

1. **What is the difference between a pulmonary acinus and a secondary pulmonary lobule?**
   The acinus (Latin for "berry") is a structural unit of the lung distal to a terminal bronchiole, supplied by first-order respiratory bronchioles, which contains alveolar ducts and alveoli. It is 0.6 to 1 cm in size and is the largest unit in which all airways participate in gas exchange.
   
   The secondary pulmonary lobule contains up to 25 acini, is 1 to 2.5 cm in size, is polyhedral in shape, and is the smallest unit of the lung that is surrounded by connective tissue septa. Its centrilobular, or core, structures include bronchioles, pulmonary arterioles, and lymphatic vessels, whereas the peripheral interlobular septa contain pulmonary veins and lymphatic vessels.

2. **When a patient is suspected of having airspace lung disease, what is the first imaging method of evaluation that is utilized?**
   Chest radiography. Although the sensitivity and specificity are not as high as in chest computed tomography (CT), the cost and radiation dose are significantly less, and the results are often diagnostic.

3. **When is chest CT used to assess airspace lung disease?**
   Chest CT for assessment of airspace lung disease is usually not necessary because common causes (e.g., pulmonary edema and pneumonia) will resolve with appropriate therapy. Chest CT is utilized when airspace disease persists despite intervention or when a patient's clinical picture does not align with the radiographic imaging appearance.

4. **True or false: Referring to an "opacity" on chest radiography or CT implies airspace disease.**
   False. The term **opacity** is a nonspecific descriptor that implies a region that attenuates x-rays to a greater degree than surrounding tissues. This can be due to any abnormality overlying or within the lung such as skin thickening, a mass, a pleural effusion, or airspace disease.

5. **What is the definition of consolidation?**
   Consolidation specifically refers to an alveolar filling process, which renders the lung opacified (Figure 18-1). This appears as a homogeneous increase in lung attenuation that obscures vessels and airway walls, and may be focal, multifocal, or diffuse in distribution.

6. **What is the "silhouette" sign?**
   The majority of structures visible on chest radiographs are due to the attenuation difference with air in the adjacent lung. Thus, the heart and mediastinal borders, the borders of the chest wall, and the vessels within the lungs are all seen because they attenuate x-rays to a greater extent than the adjacent air-filled lung. If the lung adjacent to one of these structures is consolidated, then there is no longer an attenuation difference between the lung and the structure, and so the structure and the normally visualized border disappear. This phenomenon has been termed the "silhouette" sign and is a specific marker of airspace lung disease (see Figure 18-1).
   
   This sign is useful to help localize sites of lung disease. For instance, if the diaphragm is obscured, this implies lower lobe lung involvement. If the right heart border is obscured, this denotes a right middle lobe lung involvement. If the left heart border is obscured, this implies left upper lobe (lingular) lung involvement. If the aortic knob or right paratracheal stripe is obscured, this implies upper lobe lung involvement.

7. **What is an air bronchogram?**
   In a normal chest radiograph, the air-filled bronchi are not distinguishable from the surrounding air-filled alveoli. If the alveoli become consolidated, then there is an attenuation difference between the air-filled bronchi and the surrounding fluid-filled alveoli. As a result, one or more bronchi become visible as dark branching lines within the opacified lung. This phenomenon is termed an "air bronchogram." The presence of an air bronchogram is a specific marker of airspace lung disease (see Figure 18-1).

8. **What is the difference between an acinar opacity and an air alveologram?**
   An acinar opacity refers to an ill-defined nodular opacity in the lung measuring 0.5 to 1 cm due to opacification of an acinus with surrounding aerated lung. Acinar opacities may coalesce and lead to larger areas of consolidation.
   
   An air alveologram is the converse and refers to a small rounded lucency in the lung when a normally aerated acinus is surrounded by opacified lung parenchyma. Both are signs of airspace lung disease.

9. **What is the definition of ground glass opacity?**
   The term *ground glass opacity* was first described on CT of the chest and refers to an increase in lung attenuation that does not obscure the pulmonary vasculature (Figure 18-2). This is in contrast to consolidation which obscures

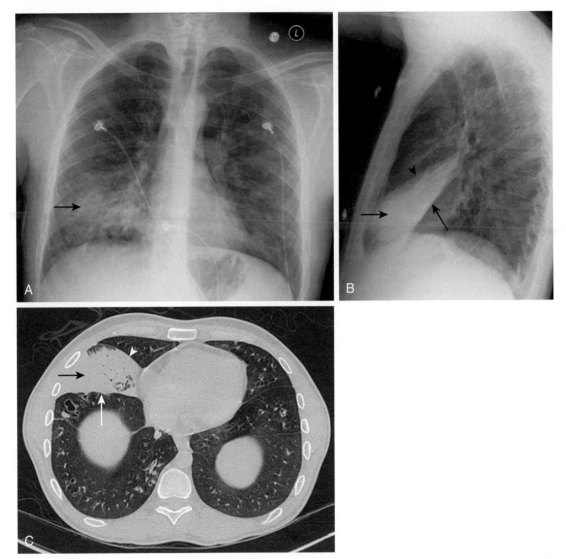

**Figure 18-1.** Pulmonary consolidation, "silhouette" sign, and air bronchograms due to bacterial lobar pneumonia on chest radiograph and CT. **A,** Frontal chest radiograph shows focal consolidation (*arrow*) in right lung base with obscuration of right heart border ("silhouette" sign) indicating right middle lobe involvement. **B,** Lateral chest radiograph redemonstrates focal consolidation (*short arrow*) in right middle lobe. Note anterosuperiorly located minor fissure (*arrowhead*) and posteroinferiorly located major fissure (*long arrow*) confirming location in right middle lobe. **C,** Axial CT image through lung bases reveals focal consolidation (*black arrow*) in right middle lobe. Small rounded and linear gas-filled lucencies caused by unopacified bronchi are also seen within opacified lung, representing air bronchograms that specifically indicate presence of surrounding airspace lung disease. Note anteriorly located minor fissure (*arrowhead*) and posteriorly located major fissure (*white arrow*) confirming location in right middle lobe.

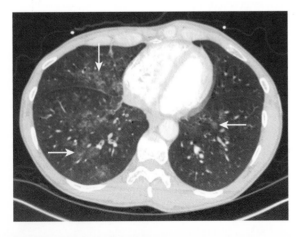

**Figure 18-2.** Ground glass opacities due to DAH on CT. Note faint multifocal patchy opacities (*arrows*) in lungs that do not obscure underlying pulmonary vasculature.

underlying bronchovascular anatomy and appears much more opaque. Like consolidation, ground glass opacity can be focal, multifocal, or diffuse and can be seen in acute or chronic conditions. It can be caused by partial filling of airspaces, interstitial thickening, decreased lung aeration, and/or an increase in capillary blood volume. There is no direct correlate of ground glass opacity on chest radiographs. Paradoxically, some patients with ground glass opacity on CT examination will have chest radiographs that appear normal, whereas others will appear as consolidation and yet others will appear as a faint increased opacification of the lungs.

10. What is the crazy paving pattern?

This is a CT-related term that refers to presence of pulmonary ground glass opacity with superimposed interlobular septal thickening and intralobular lines, resembling irregularly shaped paving stones (Figure 18-3). The crazy paving pattern was originally associated with pulmonary alveolar proteinosis (PAP), but it can be seen in a wide variety of disease conditions including infection, hemorrhage, pulmonary edema, and some chronic disorders.

11. What are centrilobular nodules and tree-in-bud opacities?

Centrilobular nodules are small (less than 1 cm) focal opacities located in the centers of secondary pulmonary lobules on CT, which spare pleural and fissural surfaces and are often ill-defined. These are due to pathologies that affect the bronchioles, pulmonary arterioles, and lymphatic vessels found in the central portions of secondary pulmonary lobules. Although seen in various disease conditions, their presence usually indicates infectious or inflammatory small airways disease such as by hypersensitivity pneumonitis, respiratory (smoking-related) bronchiolitis, and endobronchial spread of infection.

Tree-in-bud opacities appear as tiny centrilobular branching structures on CT, most often in the lung periphery, which resemble budding trees (Figure 18-4). These are due to filling of the distal bronchioles and involvement of the adjacent alveoli, most often caused by infectious bronchiolitis, bronchitis, and aspiration.

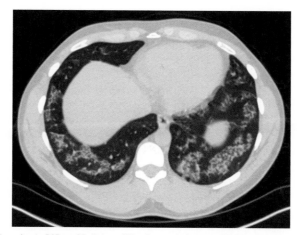

**Figure 18-3.** Crazy paving pattern due to PAP on CT. Note multifocal ground glass opacities in lungs with superimposed linear radiodense foci caused by thickened interlobular and intralobular septa, resembling irregularly shaped paving stones.

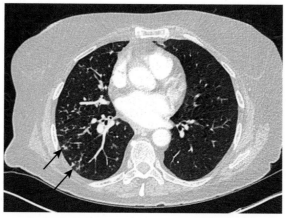

**Figure 18-4.** Tree-in-bud opacities due to infectious bronchiolitis on CT. Note tiny branching structures (*arrows*) in lung periphery resembling budding trees, caused by filling of distal bronchioles and involvement of adjacent alveoli.

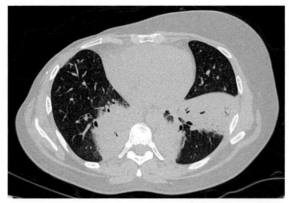

**Figure 18-5.** Chronic airspace disease due to pulmonary mucosa associated lymphoid tissue (MALT) lymphoma on CT. Note multifocal pulmonary consolidation in lower lobes with associated air bronchograms. This appearance was unchanged compared to prior CT examinations (*not shown*), indicating chronicity.

12. True or false: Consolidation and ground glass opacities indicate pneumonia.

    False. While consolidation and ground glass opacities usually indicate an acute reversible process, they can be seen in a wide variety of conditions, including some malignancies.

13. True or false: Consolidation and ground glass opacity can be seen in acute and chronic conditions.

    True. Although these abnormalities are more commonly associated with acute illnesses, chronic inflammatory and neoplastic disorders can also present as airspace disease.

14. What are some causes of acute airspace disease?

    Blood (such as from trauma or vasculitis), pus (from pneumonia or aspiration), or water (due to cardiogenic or noncardiogenic pulmonary edema) filling the alveoli.

15. What are some causes of chronic airspace disease?

    Malignancy (lymphoma, bronchoalveolar subtype lung cancer) (Figure 18-5), organizing pneumonia, mycobacterial and fungal infections, chronic eosinophilic pneumonia, and PAP.

16. What are some causes of diffuse airspace disease?

    Cardiogenic and noncardiogenic pulmonary edema, adult respiratory distress syndrome (ARDS), *Pneumocystis jiroveci* (formerly *carinii*) pneumonia (PCP), inhalational lung injury, pulmonary hemorrhage, and PAP.

17. What are some causes of multifocal or patchy airspace disease?

    Pneumonia, aspiration, pulmonary contusion, and pulmonary hemorrhage when acute. Organizing pneumonia, mycobacterial infection, fungal infection, chronic eosinophilic pneumonia, PAP, vasculitis, and malignancy (lymphoma, lung cancer, and pulmonary metastasis) when chronic.

18. What are some causes of focal airspace disease?

    Pneumonia, aspiration, pulmonary contusion, and pulmonary infarction when acute. Malignancy (lymphoma, lung cancer, and pulmonary metastasis), organizing pneumonia, and lipoid pneumonia when chronic.

19. What are some causes of peripheral airspace disease?

    Pneumonia, pulmonary infarction, and pulmonary contusion when acute. Organizing pneumonia, chronic eosinophilic pneumonia, and vasculitis when chronic.

20. What is atelectasis?

    Atelectasis is reduced inflation of part or all of the lung and may be subsegmental, segmental, lobar, or whole lung in extent. Whereas subsegmental atelectasis is usually not clinically significant (despite being very common, particularly in the inpatient setting and after surgery), larger amounts of atelectasis can result in significantly decreased pulmonary gas exchange.

21. What types of atelectasis may occur?

    Atelectasis can be passive, compressive, resorptive, cicatricial, or discoid.

    Passive atelectasis occurs when the lung is allowed to retract (e.g., due to presence of a pneumothorax).

    Compressive atelectasis results from extrinsic compression of the lung by a space occupying process (e.g., a bulla or lung mass).

    Resorptive (or obstructive) atelectasis occurs due to airway obstruction (e.g., from mucus plugging or endobronchial tumor) that results in peripheral alveolar gas resorption.

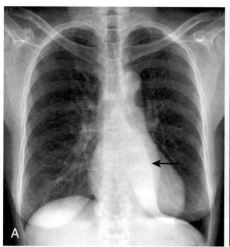
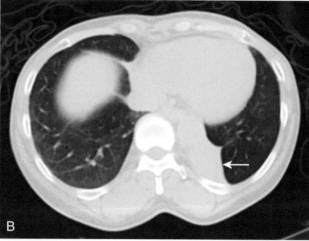

**Figure 18-6.** Tight left lower lobe atelectasis on chest radiograph and CT. **A,** Frontal chest radiograph shows triangular consolidation within inferomedial aspect of left lung with extra curvilinear edge seen along its lateral border (*arrow*) representing deviated major fissure. Also note subtle decreased width of left lung relative to right lung. **B,** Axial CT image through lung bases shows consolidation within left lower lobe with volume loss. Note associated posteromedial shift of major fissure (*arrow*) from its expected normal position.

Cicatricial atelectasis results from lung fibrosis (e.g., from prior mycobacterial infection or radiation therapy). Discoid (or platelike) atelectasis is a form of adhesive atelectasis due to hypoventilation, and it has a bandlike or linear configuration, most often seen in the lung bases.

22. What are the imaging features of atelectasis?

Atelectasis typically appears as a well-defined homogeneous area of lung opacification, sometimes with air bronchograms, that is often confined to a pulmonary segment or lobe, although it can range from a minimal linear opacity to complete lung opacification (Figure 18-6). This is frequently associated with decreased lung volume as well as abnormal shift of pleural fissures, bronchi, and pulmonary vessels toward the atelectatic lung parenchyma. As atelectasis represents normal but nonaerated lung tissue, it will enhance uniformly on CT or magnetic resonance imaging (MRI) after intravenous contrast administration. This is in contrast to other airspace opacities such as by pneumonia and tumors which tend to have more heterogenous and variable enhancement. Indirect signs of atelectasis may include ipsilateral diaphragmatic or cardiomediastinal shift toward the atelectatic lung parenchyma, ipsilateral rib space narrowing, and compensatory hyperinflation of unaffected portions of the lungs.

23. What is rounded atelectasis, and what is the "comet tail" sign?

Rounded atelectasis is a form of chronic atelectasis that occurs next to sites of pleural fibrosis and is the result of retraction of visceral pleural scar. Over time, this results in infolding of the lung, which eventually develops a rounded masslike appearance. To confidently establish the diagnosis of rounded atelectasis, one must see a rounded subpleural area of opacity with an adjacent pleural thickening, and curvilinear bronchovascular structures extending into the margin of the opacity (the latter of which is known as the "comet tail" sign) (Figure 18-7).

24. What is the "Luftsichel" sign?

The "Luftsichel" (air sickle) sign represents a small curvilinear lucency that parallels the left upper mediastinum on a frontal chest radiograph. This occurs in the setting of left upper lobe atelectasis due to interposition of the superior segment of the left lower lobe between the medially displaced and collapsed left upper lobe and aortic arch.

25. What is the "juxtaphrenic peak" sign?

The "juxtaphrenic peak" sign refers to a peaked or tented appearance of either hemidiaphragm, most often occurring in the setting of upper lobe atelectasis (Figure 18-8). It is the result of traction upon an inferior accessory fissure being pulled superiorly toward the atelectatic upper lobe.

26. What is the "S sign of Golden"?

With upper lobe atelectasis, the major fissure is pulled superomedially and appears as a straight or concave line on a frontal chest radiograph. However, when the atelectasis is secondary to a central obstructing mass, the central portion of the major fissure will appear convex due to the mass, whereas the peripheral fissure will appear concave as the peripheral lung atelectasis. Thus, on a frontal chest radiograph, the fissure will have an S shape (on the left) or a reverse S shape (on the right). This "S sign of Golden" (first described by Golden in 1925) therefore signifies presence of a central obstructing mass with associated resorptive upper lobe atelectasis.

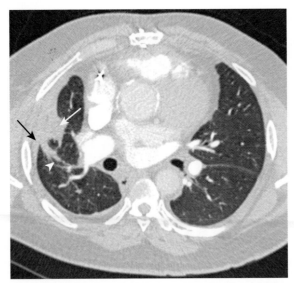

**Figure 18-7.** "Comet tail" sign due to rounded atelectasis on CT. Note rounded subpleural focal opacity (*white arrow*) in right lung base adjacent to pleural thickening (*black arrow*) with associated curvilinear bronchovascular structures (*arrowhead*) extending into margin of opacity.

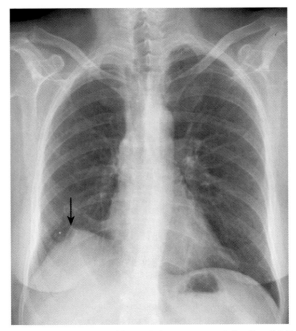

**Figure 18-8.** "Juxtaphrenic peak" sign on chest radiograph. Note tented appearance and elevation of right hemidiaphragm. This patient was status post right upper lobectomy.

27. What is right middle lobe syndrome?
    Right middle lobe syndrome represents chronic nonobstructive collapse of the right middle lobe, often with bronchiectasis, and is most commonly seen in the elderly. Contributing factors include chronic inflammation (particularly atypical mycobacterial infection), poor collateral ventilation, and a relatively narrow bronchial ostium.

28. What are the different types of pulmonary edema, and what are some common causes of each?
    Pulmonary edema can result from increased hydrostatic pressures and increased capillary permeability from endothelial injury. Cardiogenic pulmonary edema is secondary to elevated pulmonary venous pressures and is typically the result of congestive heart failure, but it can also be seen after acute myocardial infarction, volume overload, and acute renal failure.

Noncardiogenic pulmonary edema is most commonly associated with ARDS. ARDS is a serious and common disorder with a high mortality rate due to diffuse alveolar damage and can be caused by a wide spectrum of both intrathoracic and extrathoracic disorders. Some additional causes of noncardiogenic pulmonary edema include chronic renal failure, anaphylaxis, drug toxicity, severe upper airway obstruction, neurogenic disorders, inhalational or burn injury, near-drowning, amniotic fluid embolism (during delivery), and fat embolism (after fracture).

29. True or false: A normal sized heart on a chest radiograph excludes the presence of pulmonary edema.

    False. A normal sized heart usually excludes cardiogenic edema but can be seen in the setting of noncardiogenic pulmonary edema.

30. True or false: The radiographic appearance of hydrostatic pulmonary edema correlates well with left atrial pressures.

    True. There is a fairly consistent relationship between left atrial pressures and chest radiograph findings in the setting of cardiogenic pulmonary edema.

31. What is cephalization?

    Normally, on a frontal upright chest radiograph, vessels in the lower lung zones are larger than vessels in the upper lung zones as a result of gravity. However, when vessels in the upper lung zones appear larger than those in the lower lung zones, this is known as cephalization. This occurs when pulmonary venous pressure is elevated, typically in patients with chronic left ventricular failure, and reflects a redistribution of blood flow to the upper lung zones.

32. What is alveolar edema?

    Alveolar edema reflects transudative fluid filling the alveolar sacs. This is seen when pulmonary capillary wedge pressure exceeds 25 mm Hg. This often appears as hazy central airspace opacities on chest radiographs and ground glass opacities on CT.

    Mimickers of this pattern include certain infections such as PCP or viral pneumonia, pulmonary hemorrhage, inhalational exposures, or diffuse alveolar damage.

33. What is "bat wing" pulmonary edema, and is this the most common radiographic pattern of pulmonary edema?

    A "bat wing" pattern (also called a "butterfly" pattern) of pulmonary edema appears as extensive perihilar mid and upper lung zone airspace opacities. This is a less common pattern of pulmonary edema and is seen only 10% to 15% of the time.

34. True or false: Pleural effusions can be unilateral in congestive heart failure.

    True. However, it would be unusual to have a large unilateral pleural effusion in this setting. A unilateral pleural effusion in the setting of heart failure is usually small in size and more commonly seen on the right. Typically, pleural effusions in congestive heart failure are bilateral and fairly symmetric.

35. True or false: Pulmonary edema can be unilateral.

    True. In the vast majority of cases, pulmonary edema is a bilateral process. However, it can rarely occur as a unilateral process. The only common cause of unilateral pulmonary edema is the phenomenon known as "re-expansion" pulmonary edema. This is a moderately common complication of high-volume thoracentesis, which paradoxically results in worsening, rather than improvement, of hypoxemia as a result of ventilation-perfusion mismatch. Other uncommon causes of unilateral pulmonary edema include diseases that reduce contralateral lung perfusion (such as with a central pulmonary embolus, hypoplastic pulmonary artery, or severe unilateral lung disease of any cause).

36. How does pulmonary edema appear on CT?

    Initially, pulmonary edema will appear as areas of smooth bilateral interlobular septal thickening, most often in the dependent portions of the lung. As the pulmonary edema worsens, fluid extends from the interstitium into the alveolar spaces. When this occurs, one will begin to see hazy ground glass opacities, often centrally located and symmetric (Figure 18-9). In very severe cases, pulmonary edema will show symmetric consolidation of the lungs. Asymmetric consolidation is relatively uncommon in pulmonary edema and will usually indicate the presence of a superimposed process such as pneumonia.

    Additional findings that suggest pulmonary edema is present include the presence of cardiomegaly and pleural effusions.

37. What are the definitions of acute lung injury (ALI) and acute respiratory distress syndrome (ARDS)?

    ALI and ARDS both reflect permeability pulmonary edema secondary to an insult to the alveolar-capillary unit. The inciting insult is more typically at the level of the vascular endothelium and is mediated via a neutrophil-dependent inflammatory cascade. There is a long list of causes that includes both intrathoracic (e.g., pneumonia, inhalational injury) and extrathoracic (e.g., pancreatitis, sepsis) etiologies.

    From a clinical standpoint, ALI is defined as an acute lung disease with bilateral pulmonary opacities on a chest radiograph, a pulmonary wedge pressure of 18 mm Hg or less, and a ratio of arterial oxygen to the fraction of inspired

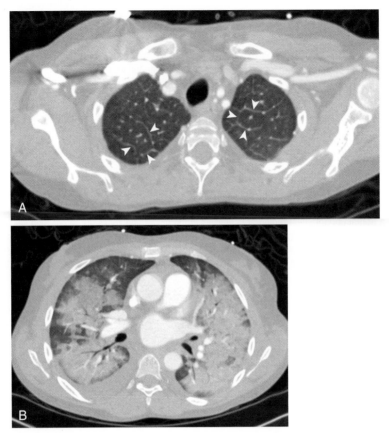

**Figure 18-9.** Pulmonary edema on CT. **A,** Axial CT image through lung apices shows bilateral smooth interlobular septal thickening (*arrowheads*) conforming to polygonal shapes of secondary pulmonary lobules. **B,** Axial CT image through mid lung zone demonstrates symmetric pulmonary consolidation with air bronchograms and surrounding areas of ground glass opacity. This patient had end-stage renal disease.

oxygen ($PaO_2/FiO_2$) of 300 mm Hg or less. ARDS is a more severe form of ALI and is defined by a $PaO_2/FiO_2$ ratio of 200 mm Hg or less.

38. What are the pathophysiological phases of ARDS, and how do these manifest on imaging?
    The first phase of ARDS is known as the acute or exudative phase. This begins 1 to 7 days after the initial insult and is characterized by interstitial and alveolar protein-rich (exudative) pulmonary edema with the accumulation of neutrophils, macrophages, and red blood cells. Endothelial and epithelial injury are present with denuding of the alveolar epithelium, reducing surfactant production and leading to areas of atelectasis. Prominent hyaline membranes are present.
    The subacute or proliferative phase begins around 7 to 14 days after the insult. At this point, some edema has been reabsorbed and the body is now attempting to repair the alveolar-capillary unit via proliferating type II pneumocytes. The inflammatory response begins to decrease and one may begin to see infiltration of fibroblasts and collage deposition.
    The chronic or fibrotic phase is seen after around day 14. The inflammatory cells present in the first two phases are no longer seen. Areas of fibrosis may be present, although not all cases of ARDS result in fulminant regions of pulmonary fibrosis.
    As noted above, within the first few hours there may be no radiographic evidence of ARDS. During the acute phase, one will typically see a rapid appearance of widespread, usually symmetric, pulmonary airspace opacities which can mimic cardiogenic pulmonary edema. Uniform bilateral airspace opacity is more often seen with ARDS than with cardiogenic pulmonary edema and tends to fluctuate less from day to day on chest radiographs when due to ARDS. Air bronchograms may be seen in ARDS but are almost never seen in cardiogenic pulmonary edema. Furthermore, most patients with ARDS are intubated, so that absence of an endotracheal tube makes ARDS less likely.
    During the subacute phase, the opacities begin to appear more coarse and sharply defined. In later stages, one can see varying degrees of fibrotic change ranging from none to multifocal areas of scarring. Interestingly, the scarring can occur in areas that were unaffected by the airspace process, namely the anterior or nondependent portions of

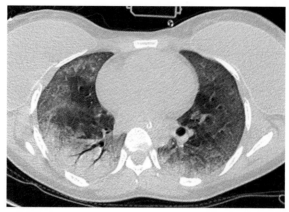

**Figure 18-10.** ARDS on CT. Note consolidation in posterior (dependent) lungs with associated air bronchograms and ground glass opacity in more anterior (nondependent) lungs forming uniform gradient of decreasing pulmonary opacification from posterior to anterior, characteristic of extrathoracic cause of ARDS. This patient had silicone embolism syndrome following illicit silicone buttock injections.

lung. This is the result of ventilator-associated lung injury, related to oxygen toxicity and barotrauma, whereas the consolidated lung is more protected from this phenomenon.

39. True or false: Causes of ARDS can be intrathoracic or extrathoracic, and this distinction can be inferred on CT imaging.

True. Causes of ARDS include both intrathoracic and extrathoracic etiologies. Sometimes, this distinction can be made on CT. One should suspect an extrathoracic cause of ARDS when there is uniform consolidation and ground glass opacity in the lungs with a posterior to anterior gradient of decreasing severity (Figure 18-10). That is, the lungs are densely consolidated in their dependent (posterior) portions, centrally less opacified by ground glass opacity, and normally aerated anteriorly. If the pattern is asymmetric and patchy, one should rather consider an intrathoracic etiology such as pneumonia.

40. What are some chronic CT findings of ARDS?

Not all cases of ARDS progress to fibrosis. When fibrosis ensues, it is typically confined to areas of lung that remained aerated and thus sustained oxygen toxicity and barotrauma during intubation. This most commonly occurs in the anterior portions of the lungs but can be seen in any region previously affected by ARDS.

41. What is aspiration, what are some of its common underlying causes, and what is its radiographic appearance?

Aspiration describes a multitude of situations where solid or liquid material enters the airways and lungs, and it is the most common cause of widespread pneumonia in hospitalized patients. This can be the result of any neurological impairment (e.g., stroke, impaired mental status) or functional (e.g., achalasia, scleroderma) or mechanical (e.g., esophageal obstruction, tracheoesophageal fistula) disturbance of the pharynx and/or esophagus.

Typically, aspiration leads to multifocal airspace opacities in the lower lobes of the lungs, as they are the most gravitationally dependent. Opacities in the anterior aspects of the lungs or more extensive opacification of the lungs can also be seen but is less common. In the acute setting, one can see associated findings of bronchitis (bronchial wall thickening), bronchiolitis (tree-in-bud opacities), and airspace filling (consolidation and/or ground glass opacities). Significant aspiration of gastric contents can lead to fulminant ARDS, also known as Mendelson's syndrome. Superimposed infection can then ensue in the form of bronchopneumonia, lung abscess, or empyema.

In the chronic setting, one may see bronchiectasis, chronic bronchial wall thickening, and pulmonary scarring.

42. What is pneumonia, and what are some of its associated complications?

Pneumonia is an infection of the lung, which can be of a bacterial, viral, fungal, mycobacterial, or parasitic etiology.

Thoracic complications of pneumonia may include parapneumonic pleural effusion, lung abscess, bronchopleural fistula, empyema, and mediastinal abscess. Some infections can also invade the chest wall and lead to soft tissue abscess formation and osteomyelitis.

43. What are some clinical questions one may ask the referring physician when evaluating imaging studies in a patient with suspected pneumonia?

When assessing a radiographic abnormality suspicious for pneumonia, it is important to touch base with the referring physician. In particular, one should establish that the abnormality is in line with clinical suspicion. Not all pulmonary opacities on chest radiographs are due to pneumonia, and so patients should have some clinical evidence of infection such as fever, sputum production, or leukocytosis to make pneumonia the most likely diagnosis. A short-term follow-up chest radiograph after treatment is useful to confirm interval resolution of a suspected pneumonia after treatment.

It is also helpful to identify where the patient may have acquired the infection. Was it in the community, a hospital, a nursing home, or in a foreign country? The statistical likelihoods of different types of infection will vary in these different settings.

Lastly, one of the most important questions to ask is whether the patient is immunocompromised (e.g., if the patient has known cancer, has recently received chemotherapy, has undergone prior solid organ or bone marrow transplantation with associated immunosuppressive therapy, or has human immunodeficiency virus [HIV] infection). These patients are at a much greater risk for opportunistic infections, and this therefore would alter the major differential diagnostic considerations for the type of infection that may be present.

44. **What are the common causes and imaging appearances of: Bacterial pneumonia? Viral pneumonias? Fungal pneumonias? Mycobacterial pneumonias? Pneumocystis pneumonia?**
    Bacterial pneumonias such as those caused by *Streptococcus pneumoniae* usually present with a pattern of bronchiolitis, bronchopneumonia, or lobar pneumonia. Thus, one will see varying degrees of tree-in-bud opacities, ground glass opacity, and pulmonary consolidation. Bronchopneumonia tends to be multifocal, patchy, and peribronchial, reflecting endobronchial spread of infection. Lobar pneumonia is largely confined to one lobe of the lung and tends to start in the lung periphery with consolidation and associated air bronchograms (see Figure 18-1). It should be noted that some viral, fungal, and mycobacterial pneumonias can appear identical on imaging to bacterial pneumonias.

    Many individuals with viral infection and lower respiratory tract symptoms (cough, dyspnea, wheezing) will have normal imaging exams. When abnormal, imaging will most often appear as a bronchiolitis (tree-in-bud opacities on CT or subtle perivascular interstitial opacities on chest radiographs), a bronchopneumonia (tree-in-bud opacities and patchy regions of consolidation on CT or multifocal areas of consolidation on chest radiographs), or as multifocal pneumonia (multifocal areas of consolidation on CT and chest radiographs) (Figure 18-11).

    Fungal pneumonias, with the exception of PCP, typically result in mass-forming areas of consolidation with or without cavitation (Figure 18-12). Miliary nodules (i.e., profuse ≤3 mm discrete uniformly sized nodules) may also be seen with fungal pneumonias.

    Mycobacterial pneumonias, in particular those caused by *Mycobacterium tuberculosis* (TB), classically result in upper lobe predominant nodules, bronchiolitis, and cavitary lung disease (Figure 18-13). Nontuberculous mycobacterial infections in the lung will most often appear as scattered regions of bronchiectasis, bronchial wall thickening, and tree-in-bud opacities on CT and as irregular linear and nodular opacities on chest radiographs.

    PCP characteristically appears as uniform diffuse ground glass opacity on CT and may appear as a very faint haze on chest radiographs. Some opportunistic viral infections, including those caused by cytomegalovirus (CMV) and herpes simplex virus (HSV), can also appear as diffuse ground glass opacities.

    It should be noted that imaging features of pneumonia demonstrate significant overlap, and oftentimes one cannot definitively determine the category of causative pathogen based on imaging features alone.

45. **In the setting of pulmonary consolidation, what are some additional CT findings that are helpful to predict whether the underlying etiology is infectious or noninfectious?**
    As already discussed, pulmonary consolidation is a nonspecific imaging feature with a wide variety of causes. However, consolidation in the presence of tree-in-bud opacities is almost always due to infection.

46. **True or false: Cavitation is a nonspecific imaging feature.**
    True. Cavitation is a nonspecific imaging finding that can be seen in a wide array of pathologies including multiple types of infection, vasculitis, traumatic injury, congenital lung disease, and pulmonary malignancy.

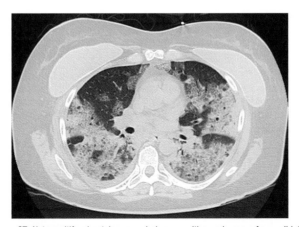

**Figure 18-11.** Viral pneumonia on CT. Note multifocal patchy ground glass opacities and areas of consolidation in lungs with air bronchograms. This patient had infection by H1N1 influenza virus.

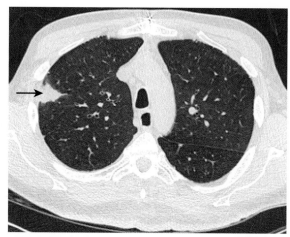

**Figure 18-12.** Fungal pneumonia on CT. Note focal masslike area of consolidation (*arrow*) in right upper lobe with surrounding ground glass opacity ("halo" sign). This patient, who was status post prior cardiac transplantation and therefore immunosuppressed, had invasive *Aspergillus fumigatus* infection.

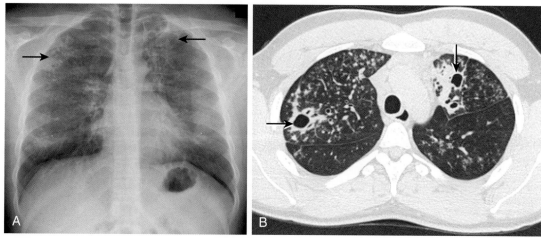

**Figure 18-13.** Active postprimary (reactivation) TB pneumonia on chest radiograph and CT. **A,** Frontal chest radiograph shows upper lung zone predominant areas of focal pulmonary consolidation with lucent areas of cavitation (*arrows*). Multiple ill-defined pulmonary nodular opacities are seen as well. **B,** Axial CT image through upper lung zones demonstrates cavitation (*arrows*) within focal areas of consolidation in upper lobes. Multiple centrilobular lung nodules are also seen, many of which are clustered and some of which have tree-in-bud configuration. These findings suggest that this patient has active infection, is highly infectious, and therefore should be isolated.

47. **What are some common infections that cavitate?**
Infectious cavitary lung disease can be related to either pneumonia or septic emboli. Septic emboli are the result of hematogenous dissemination of infection. The source is usually extrathoracic with common locations including infected cardiac valves or indwelling venous catheters. The appearance of septic emboli is usually of multiple cavitating and noncavitating nodules, typically 1 to 3 cm in size, often peripheral in location. These nodules may demonstrate the "feeding vessel" sign, where one can see a pulmonary arterial branch extend to the lesion. Septic emboli, like thrombotic emboli, can lead to areas of pulmonary infarction. Radiographically, pulmonary infarcts appear as peripheral wedge-shaped areas of opacity, which may have areas of central clearing.
    Pneumonias that cavitate are usually bacterial, fungal, or mycobacterial in etiology. Some common bacterial pneumonias include *Staphylococcus aureus*, *Klebsiella pneumoniae*, and polymicrobial infections from oropharyngeal aspiration.

48. **What are the "halo" and "air crescent" signs, and what infection is classically associated with these signs?**
Both signs are classically associated with angioinvasive aspergillosis, an opportunistic fungal infection commonly seen in the setting of bone or solid organ transplantation where the absolute neutrophil count is severely reduced. As the name implies, this infection affects blood vessels leading to areas of pulmonary infarction and hemorrhage. The typical

imaging appearance is that of a nodule or masslike area of consolidation with a surrounding "halo" of ground glass opacity (see Figures 18-12 and 18-14). In this setting, the halo represents pulmonary hemorrhage. Should the neutrophil count recover, the necrotic lung will begin to contract as part of the healing process, leaving a "crescent" of air. This is an important prognostic sign as it implies neutrophil recovery (see Figure 18-14).

In the setting of **neutropenia and fever**, these radiographic signs are nearly specific for fungal infection, in particular angioinvasive *Aspergillus*, the most common offending organism. However, other processes can result in similar imaging appearances. The "halo" sign can be seen in other infections such as TB, pulmonary malignancies, and vasculitis.

49. **What is a fungus ball, and if it is suspected, what imaging-based maneuver can be performed to confirm the suspicion?**
    A fungus ball is a discrete mass of intertwined fungal hyphae mixed with mucus, cellular debris, and fibrin and is also known as an aspergilloma (because it is typically due to *Aspergillus fumigatus*) or a mycetoma. It represents a noninvasive form of infection that occurs in structurally abnormal lungs, usually a preexisting cavity, in an immunocompetent host. One will see an air cyst, cavity, or bronchiectatic segment in the lung containing a dependent nodule that represents the clumped fungus (Figure 18-15). The nodule is typically not adherent to the surrounding

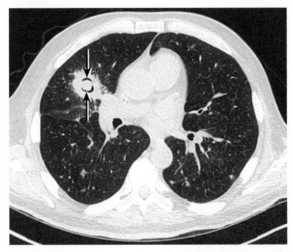

**Figure 18-14.** "Air crescent" sign and "halo" sign due to invasive *Aspergillus fumigatus* infection on CT. Note nodule in right upper lobe that contains crescentic foci of very low attenuation gas (*arrows*) representing "air crescent" sign. Also note surrounding mild ground glass opacity indicating "halo" sign. This patient had history of acute myelogenous leukemia.

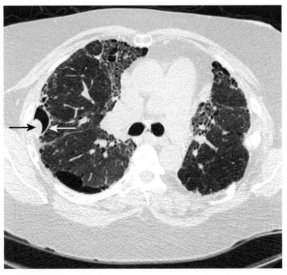

**Figure 18-15.** Fungus ball on CT. Note gas-filled cyst in right upper lobe (*white arrow*) that contains dependent nodule (*black arrow*) due to aspergilloma. Also note peribronchovascular and subpleural regions of ground glass opacity and traction bronchiectasis due to fibrotic lung disease caused by sarcoidosis.

wall, which is in contradistinction to a lung cancer that could develop in a preexisting cystic space. One could therefore image the patient in the supine and prone positions to verify that the nodular filling defect is mobile, which would confirm a fungus ball.

50. **What is the "Monad" sign?**

Sometimes, the fungus ball almost completely fills the cavity, leaving only a thin crescent of air. This thin crescent of air is known as the "Monad" sign and is different from the "air crescent" sign seen in the setting of angioinvasive aspergillosis.

51. **What is allergic bronchopulmonary aspergillosis (ABPA)?**

ABPA is a noninvasive form of pulmonary aspergillosis that occurs almost exclusively in asthmatics, usually younger than 40 years of age. Patients often will have peripheral eosinophilia and IgE specific antibodies against *Aspergillus*.

ABPA is the result of an IgE mediated hypersensitivity reaction to *Aspergillus* within the bronchial lumen. Repeated episodes of inflammation lead to bronchial wall breakdown and eventually bronchiectasis. Secretions, containing eosinophils and fungal hyphae, fill and can obstruct the affected airways.

This manifests radiographically as central and upper lobe predominant bronchiectasis, bronchial wall thickening, and mucoid impaction, findings that could mimic cystic fibrosis. The mucoid impactions on CT can sometimes have high attenuation, which is a suggestive sign of ABPA.

52. **What is a bronchocele, and what is the "finger-in-glove" sign?**

A bronchocele occurs when a dilated bronchus is filled with secretions. When large enough, bronchoceles can appear on imaging as tubular or branching Y- or V-shaped structures, similar in configuration to fingers within a glove (Figure 18-16). Although characteristic for ABPA, the "finger-in-glove" sign can be seen in cystic fibrosis as well as in any other disorder that causes a bronchocele to form, such as bronchial atresia or an obstructive endobronchial lesion.

53. **What is the radiographic appearance of primary TB?**

Primary TB can occur anywhere in the lung. Most cases are asymptomatic and are thus not seen by imaging in the acute stages. Primary TB typically appears as a focal area of consolidation. Cavitation is not a common feature. An associated pleural effusion may be visualized. Rarely, primary TB can result in hematogenous dissemination, marked by multiple tiny randomly distributed miliary pulmonary nodules.

54. **What is a Ghon complex, a Ghon focus, and a Ranke complex, and how do these appear on imaging?**

A Ghon complex indicates acute TB infection in both the lung and ipsilateral hilar lymph nodes. Acutely, the lymphadenopathy characteristically appears centrally low in attenuation, reflecting necrosis. When the primary site of

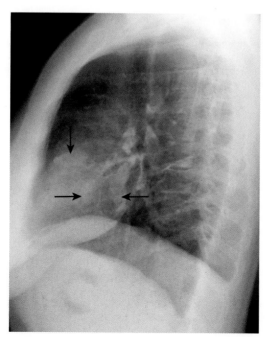

**Figure 18-16.** "Finger-in-glove" sign due to ABPA on lateral chest radiograph. Note tubular densities in right middle lobe superimposed upon heart with configuration similar to gloved fingers caused by dilated opacified bronchi. This patient had history of asthma.

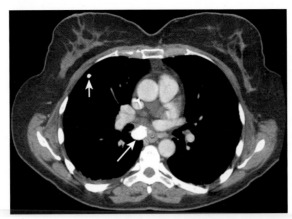

**Figure 18-17.** Ghon focus and Ranke complex due to healed TB on CT. Note calcified pulmonary granuloma (Ghon focus) (*short arrow*). Also note calcified subcarinal mediastinal lymph node (*long arrow*). Together, these findings comprise Ranke complex.

pulmonary infection heals, a calcified granuloma will often form, termed a Ghon focus (Figure 18-17). If the affected lymph nodes calcify, the presence of both a pulmonary granuloma and calcified lymph nodes indicates a Ranke complex (see Figure 18-17).

55. **What are the imaging findings associated with postprimary (reactivation) TB?**
Postprimary or reactivation TB most often affects the apical or posterior segments of the upper lobes and less commonly the superior segments of the lower lobes. Imaging findings may include focal consolidation or nodular opacities, areas of cavitation, centrilobular, acinar, and/or tree-in-bud nodular opacities (due to endobronchial spread of infection), interstitial miliary nodules (due to hematogenous spread of infection), bronchiectasis, and thoracic lymphadenopathy (often with areas of central hypoattenuation due to necrosis on CT) (see Figure 18-13). When these findings are seen on imaging, one should alert the referring physician to the possibility of active TB.

56. **True or false: A miliary appearance on imaging is specific for TB.**
False. Miliary disease may be due to hematogenous dissemination of infection (TB, fungi), metastatic disease (e.g., from renal cell carcinoma, thyroid cancer, melanoma), sarcoidosis, or inhalational lung disease (e.g., silicosis).

57. **True or false: Typical (TB) and atypical mycobacterial infections are easily distinguished on imaging.**
False. Reactivation TB and the classic appearance of atypical mycobacteria may be indistinguishable by imaging.

58. **What is Lady Windermere syndrome?**
Lady Windermere syndrome represents the nonclassical form of atypical mycobacterial infection and most commonly occurs in elderly women. Typical imaging features include right middle lobe and lingula predominant scarring, nodules, bronchiectasis, bronchitis, and bronchiolitis. Cavitary nodules as seen in TB and the classical form of atypical mycobacterial infection are not present.

59. **What infectious organism(s) should you suspect in the setting of: HIV infection and perihilar ground glass opacities on CT? Heart transplantation and a solitary cavitary mass? Chest wall invasion?**
• PCP (with HIV infection and perihilar ground glass opacities).
• Fungal, *Nocardia*, or *Actinomyces* infection (with heart transplantation and a solitary cavitary mass).
• Actinomycosis, mucormycosis, blastomycosis, *Streptococcus anginosus*, and TB (with chest wall invasion).

60. **What are the pulmonary manifestations of drug toxicity on imaging?**
Pharmacologic therapies that can result in pulmonary toxicity are vast. Common culprit drugs include chemotherapeutic agents such as methotrexate, bleomycin, busulfan, and cyclophosphamide. Additional commonly used drugs such as nitrofurantoin and amiodarone have also been linked to pulmonary toxicity.
The patterns of drug toxicity are usually in the form of noncardiogenic pulmonary edema, diffuse alveolar damage, pulmonary hemorrhage, organizing pneumonia, pulmonary eosinophilic syndromes, or chronic interstitial pneumonias such as usual interstitial pneumonia (UIP) or nonspecific interstitial pneumonia (NSIP). Thus, the imaging manifestations are quite varied.

61. **What drug can result in high attenuation pulmonary consolidation on CT?**
Amiodarone is an antiarrhythmic agent commonly used to treat supraventricular and ventricular arrhythmias. NSIP is the most common pulmonary manifestation of amiodarone toxicity. An additional but distinctive feature of amiodarone-related pulmonary toxicity is high attenuation pulmonary consolidation. The increased attenuation is the result of amiodarone, an iodine-containing compound, which accumulates within type II pneumocytes. Similarly, increased

hepatic attenuation may also be seen due to deposition in the liver. Rarely, amiodarone can result in life-threatening ARDS.

62. What drug used to treat patients with acute myelogenous leukemia can result in pulmonary hemorrhage?

All-trans-retinoic acid (ATRA) is a therapy specifically used to treat patients with acute promyelocytic leukemia. Alveolar hemorrhage is a well-known side effect. As in other causes of alveolar hemorrhage, one sees widespread ground glass opacities and areas of pulmonary consolidation.

63. What is diffuse alveolar hemorrhage (DAH), and what is its imaging appearance?

DAH is a potentially life-threatening condition that occurs when blood products fill the alveolar spaces. Clinically, patients will often present with hemoptysis, although this will not be present in up to one third of patients. In the absence of hemoptysis, bronchoscopy or biopsy may be required to establish the diagnosis. Nonspecific laboratory markers include anemia and thrombocytopenia.

Major causes of DAH include vasculitis (such as granulomatosis with polyangiitis), systemic lupus erythematosus, Goodpasture's syndrome, and bleeding diatheses (such as with hematologic malignancies [leukemia, lymphoma], coagulopathy, or disseminated intravascular coagulation).

DAH typically manifests as widespread ground glass opacities with or without areas of consolidation that tend to spare the lung apices and periphery. Sometimes, the ground glass opacities can appear nodular and centrilobular in distribution. Intermixed areas of septal thickening, or a crazy paving pattern, may also be present. Despite the name, DAH can be localized or multifocal rather than diffuse in distribution (see Figure 18-2). When diffuse, DAH is often radiographically indistinguishable from pulmonary edema or ARDS.

64. What disease condition should you consider to be present in a patient with renal failure, sinonasal disease, and pulmonary alveolar hemorrhage?

Granulomatosis with polyangiitis (GPA), previously known as Wegener's granulomatosis.

65. What is the imaging appearance of pulmonary contusions and lacerations?

Pulmonary contusions usually manifest as peripheral consolidations with or without ground glass opacities near or at a site of penetrating or blunt trauma. Contusions often clear within a couple days.

Pulmonary lacerations are the result of pulmonary parenchymal tearing and can be direct as in the setting of a stabbing or gunshot injury or indirect from shear forces. Initially, lacerations may not be evident because they may be masked by surrounding pulmonary contusion or be filled with hemorrhage. When seen, they are typically linear or stellate in configuration, and they may be filled with gas, fluid, and/or hemorrhage (Figure 18-18). Unlike pulmonary contusions, lacerations persist for a much longer period of time.

66. What is pulmonary alveolar proteinosis (PAP), and what is the difference between primary and secondary PAP?

PAP is a rare lung disease characterized by the accumulation of an abnormal surfactant-like material within the alveoli. PAP can be primary (idiopathic) or secondary. The primary form is more common and is seen in young and

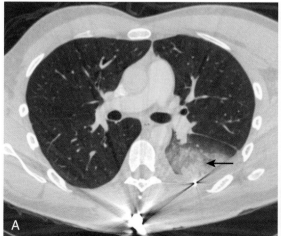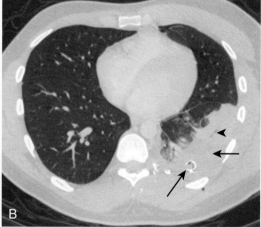

**Figure 18-18.** Pulmonary contusion and laceration on CT. **A,** Axial CT image through mid lung zone shows patchy ground glass opacity and consolidation (*arrow*) in left lower lobe due to pulmonary contusion. Note very high attenuation foci in posterior chest wall with associated streak artifacts due to metallic bullet fragments. **B,** Axial CT image more inferiorly demonstrates obliquely oriented consolidation (*short arrow*) in left lower lobe with internal linear gas-filled lucency (*arrowhead*) indicating pulmonary laceration with surrounding contusion. Left chest tube is present (*long arrow*) in left pleural space. This patient recently suffered thoracic gunshot injury.

middle-aged adults, whereas the secondary form is seen in the setting of hematologic malignancy, inhalational lung disease, or immunodeficiency states. Patients with PAP have subacute or chronic symptoms and can even be asymptomatic.

67. What is the classic CT appearance of PAP?

PAP is characterized by bilateral fairly symmetric and geographic areas of crazy paving (see Figure 18-3). Although the crazy paving pattern has classically been associated with PAP, a multitude of disease conditions can result in a crazy paving pattern.

68. What entity can result in fat (or near fat) low attenuation pulmonary opacities on CT?

Lipoid pneumonia. This occurs after aspiration of fatty substances such as those that contain mineral oil or petroleum jelly and is often asymptomatic, although sometimes it is associated with cough or dyspnea. On imaging, focal or multifocal alveolar opacities are seen, most often in the lower lobes, often perihilar in distribution. Sometimes, they may appear masslike with irregular margins, potentially mimicking lung cancer, and may be surrounded by ground glass opacities. Characteristic fat (or near fat) low attenuation components, when present, are highly suggestive of the diagnosis.

69. What is organizing pneumonia, and what are some common causes?

Organizing pneumonia is a nonspecific pulmonary reactive process characterized by alveolar inflammation with plugs of granulation tissue filling the small airways. It can result from a wide array of disease processes but is most commonly due to infection, drug toxicity, and systemic illnesses.

70. What is meant by the term *cryptogenic organizing pneumonia* (COP), and what are its imaging features?

The term COP is applied when organizing pneumonia is present without a clear etiology. Clinically, COP is characterized by months of low-grade fevers, cough, and malaise. Symptoms and imaging features typically rapidly improve with corticosteroid administration, although relapses can occur in 50% of cases.

COP has a wide variety of imaging manifestations, but it is most often characterized by chronic waxing and waning patchy lower lobe predominant airspace opacities, which are frequently peripheral and peribronchovascular in distribution. Ground glass opacities and nodules are common accompanying features. The appearance and clinical presentation can be confused with those of pneumonia, often leading to months of delayed appropriate management.

71. What is the "reversed halo" sign or "atoll" sign?

The "reversed halo" sign is characterized by ring-shaped or crescentic peripheral consolidation and central ground glass opacity. The appearance has been likened to an atoll, a ring-shaped coral reef that encompasses a central lagoon, with the peripheral land representing the consolidation and the central body of water representing the ground glass opacity.

It should be noted that the imaging appearance of organizing pneumonia is quite protean and can manifest as multiple or solitary nodules mimicking malignancy, ground glass opacities, or a crazy paving pattern.

72. How can one distinguish between chronic eosinophilic pneumonia and COP on imaging?

Chronic eosinophilic pneumonia and COP share some similar imaging features. Both are characterized by consolidations which can wax and wane. COP tends to be more peribronchovascular in distribution and is more often associated with nodules and a lower lobe predominance. In contradistinction, chronic eosinophilic pneumonia is classically confined to the subpleural region with an upper lung zone predominance (Figure 18-19).

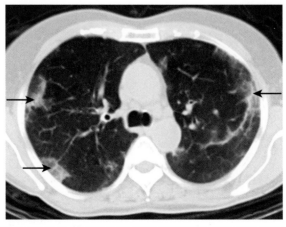

**Figure 18-19.** Chronic eosinophilic pneumonia on CT. Note upper lung zone predominant opacities in lungs with predominantly subpleural distribution (*arrows*). This patient had history of asthma, fever, and eosinophilia.

73. **What should one clinically suspect in a patient with persistent pulmonary consolidation and bronchorrhea?**

Invasive mucinous lung adenocarcinoma, formerly known as mucinous bronchioloalveolar cell lung carcinoma. Note that comparison with prior imaging studies is of utmost importance to establish that an underlying etiology of pulmonary consolidation is chronic, as this prolonged time course would in general not be expected with other etiologies such as pneumonia or aspiration that typically have a more acute time course of evolution.

---

## KEY POINTS

- Opacity is a nonspecific descriptor that implies a region that attenuates x-rays to a greater degree than surrounding tissues, and it can be due to any abnormality overlying or within the lung. Consolidation, however, specifically refers to an alveolar filling process, which renders the lung opacified.
- Air bronchograms and the "silhouette" sign are specific findings of airspace disease.
- Comparison with prior imaging studies is essential to determine whether airspace disease is acute or chronic in nature. This distinction is important because etiologies such as alveolar edema, bacterial or viral infection, aspiration, or hemorrhage are more likely in the acute setting, whereas other etiologies such as malignancy, fungal or mycobacterial infection, organizing pneumonia, and PAP are more likely in the chronic setting.
- Tree-in-bud opacities appear as tiny centrilobular branching structures on CT, most often in the lung periphery, resembling budding trees. These are indicators of small airways disease and are most often caused by infectious bronchiolitis and aspiration.
- Imaging findings of reactivation TB may include upper lung zone predominant focal consolidation or nodular opacities, areas of cavitation, centrilobular, acinar, and/or tree-in-bud nodular opacities, interstitial miliary nodules, bronchiectasis, and thoracic lymphadenopathy (often with areas of central necrosis). When these findings are seen on imaging, one should alert the referring physician to the possibility of active TB.

---

### BIBLIOGRAPHY

Ketai L, Jordan K, Busby KH. Imaging Infection. *Clin Chest Med*. 2015;36(2):197-217.

El-Sherief AH, Gilman MD, Healey TT, et al. Clear vision through the haze: a practical approach to ground-glass opacity. *Curr Probl Diagn Radiol*. 2014;43(3):140-158.

Lichtenberger JP 3rd, Digumarthy SR, Abbott GF, et al. Diffuse pulmonary hemorrhage: clues to the diagnosis. *Curr Probl Diagn Radiol*. 2014;43(3):128-139.

Nambu A, Ozawa K, Kobayashi N, et al. Imaging of community-acquired pneumonia: roles of imaging examinations, imaging diagnosis of specific pathogens and discrimination from noninfectious diseases. *World J Radiol*. 2014;6(10):779-793.

Prather AD, Smith TR, Poletto DM, et al. Aspiration-related lung diseases. *J Thorac Imaging*. 2014;29(5):304-309.

Zompatori M, Ciccarese F, Fasano L. Overview of current lung imaging in acute respiratory distress syndrome. *European Resp Rev*. 2014;23(134):519-530.

Miller WT Jr, Panosian JS. Causes and imaging patterns of tree-in-bud opacities. *Chest*. 2013;144(6):1883-1892.

Miller WT Jr, Barbosa E Jr, Mickus TJ, et al. Chest computed tomographic imaging characteristics of viral acute lower respiratory tract illnesses: a case-control study. *J Comput Assist Tomogr*. 2011;35(4):524-530.

Frazier AA, Franks TJ, Cooke EO, et al. From the archives of the AFIP: pulmonary alveolar proteinosis. *Radiographics*. 2008;28(3):883-899, quiz 915.

Hansell DM, Bankier AA, MacMahon H, et al. Fleischner Society: glossary of terms for thoracic imaging. *Radiology*. 2008;246(3):697-722.

Jeong YJ, Lee KS. Pulmonary tuberculosis: up-to-date imaging and management. *AJR Am J Roentgenol*. 2008;191(3):834-844.

Martinez S, Heyneman LE, McAdams HP, et al. Mucoid impactions: finger-in-glove sign and other CT and radiographic features. *Radiographics*. 2008;28(5):1369-1382.

Martinez S, McAdams HP, Batchu CS. The many faces of pulmonary nontuberculous mycobacterial infection. *AJR Am J Roentgenol*. 2007;189(1):177-186.

Washington L, Palacio D. Imaging of bacterial pulmonary infection in the immunocompetent patient. *Semin Roentgenol*. 2007;42(2):122-145.

Chong S, Lee KS, Yi CA, et al. Pulmonary fungal infection: imaging findings in immunocompetent and immunocompromised patients. *Eur J Radiol*. 2006;59(3):371-383.

Waite S, Jeudy J, White CS. Acute lung infections in normal and immunocompromised hosts. *Radiol Clin North Am*. 2006;44(2):295-315, ix.

Webb WR. Thin-section CT of the secondary pulmonary lobule: anatomy and the image—the 2004 Fleischner lecture. *Radiology*. 2006;239(2):322-338.

Franquet T, Gimenez A, Hidalgo A. Imaging of opportunistic fungal infections in immunocompromised patient. *Eur J Radiol*. 2004;51(2):130-138.

Goo JM, Im JG. CT of tuberculosis and nontuberculous mycobacterial infections. *Radiol Clin North Am*. 2002;40(1):73-87, viii.

Franquet T, Muller NL, Gimenez A, et al. Spectrum of pulmonary aspergillosis: histologic, clinical, and radiologic findings. *Radiographics*. 2001;21(4):825-837.

Gluecker T, Capasso P, Schnyder P, et al. Clinical and radiologic features of pulmonary edema. *Radiographics*. 1999;19(6):1507-1531, discussion 32-33.

# CHAPTER 19

# RADIOGRAPHY OF INTERSTITIAL LUNG DISEASE

*Wallace T. Miller, Jr., MD, and Drew A. Torigian, MD, MA, FSAR*

1. **What radiographic features distinguish interstitial diseases from airspace diseases?**
   Two primary characteristics radiographically distinguish interstitial diseases from airspace diseases. First, interstitial diseases displace little of the air within the lung, whereas airspace diseases displace large amounts of air. Interstitial diseases change the overall opacity of the lung very little, whereas airspace diseases in most cases dramatically increase the opacity (whiteness) of the lung on chest radiography. Second, interstitial diseases appear as increases in small nodules (generally <5 mm in diameter) or thin lines (<5 mm in width) (or both) within the lung, whereas airspace diseases appear as indistinctly marginated patches of opacity. See Figure 19-1 for the normal appearance of the lungs on frontal chest radiography.

2. **What factors influence the likelihood of one interstitial disease over another interstitial disease?**
   Three primary factors affect the likelihood of a given interstitial disease:
   1. The relative incidence of a given disease in the general population. Typical presentations of common diseases are most likely, followed by atypical presentations of common diseases, typical presentations of uncommon diseases, and atypical presentations of uncommon diseases.
   2. The clinical history of the patient.
   3. The radiographic pattern of the interstitial disease.

3. **What is the most common interstitial abnormality identified on chest radiography?**
   Interstitial pulmonary edema, usually caused by congestive heart failure, is the most common interstitial abnormality encountered in daily practice. A diagnosis of interstitial pulmonary edema should be considered in all cases of interstitial abnormality detected on a chest radiograph. In many cases, it might be advisable to diurese the patient and repeat the chest radiograph as the first diagnostic test.

4. **Name the most common interstitial abnormalities other than interstitial pulmonary edema.**
   Idiopathic pulmonary fibrosis and sarcoidosis are the most common chronic interstitial disorders in the United States and should be among the first diagnoses considered when encountering a chest radiograph with an interstitial abnormality.

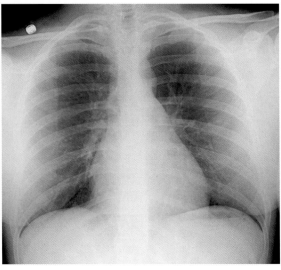

**Figure 19-1.** Normal lungs on frontal chest radiograph. Note normal sharp delineation of branching vessels from bilateral hila outward.

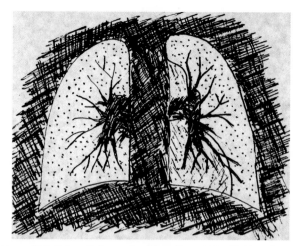

**Figure 19-2.** Schematic image of nodular pattern of interstitial lung disease.

5. **What radiographic characteristics help determine the diagnosis of interstitial disorders?**
   Interstitial abnormalities may be roughly subdivided into abnormalities that produce small round opacities (*nodular interstitial diseases*) and abnormalities that produce small networks of holes (*reticular interstitial diseases*). In this chapter, we describe one nodular pattern of interstitial disease and the three following reticular patterns of interstitial disease: the peripheral reticular pattern, the linear pattern, and the cystic pattern.

6. **What is the appearance of a nodular interstitial pattern on chest radiography?**
   A normal chest radiograph typically shows many small nodular opacities that represent normal blood vessels end on. In most cases, these small nodules can be recognized as blood vessels because they overlap with a small line of similar diameter, which represents an adjacent branch of the pulmonary vascular tree. The nodular pattern of interstitial lung disease appears as increased numbers of small nodular opacities (<10 mm in diameter) that are randomly distributed throughout the lung parenchyma. These small nodules do not overlap with the normal vascular lines of the lung (Figures 19-2 and 19-3).

7. **What disorders cause nodular interstitial diseases?**
   Four broad groups of disorders cause nodular interstitial diseases:
   - Granulomatous lung diseases
   - Nodular pneumoconioses
   - Small metastases
   - Smoking-related lung diseases

8. **Discuss granulomatous lung diseases that cause nodular interstitial disease.**
   Sarcoidosis is the most common granulomatous interstitial lung disease to cause a micronodular pattern. This idiopathic disorder typically manifests in middle-aged individuals, especially African Americans. Miliary infections also cause a small nodular pattern and are typified by miliary tuberculosis but also include miliary spread of histoplasmosis, cryptococcosis, coccidioidomycosis, and blastomycosis. These infections typically affect immunocompromised individuals, such as patients with human immunodeficiency virus (HIV) infection, patients who have undergone organ transplantation, or patients with a history of long-term corticosteroid use. Extrinsic allergic alveolitis or hypersensitivity pneumonitis not only causes a granulomatous interstitial fibrosis, but may also produce an interstitial nodular pattern of lung disease.

9. **Discuss pneumoconioses and tumors that lead to nodular interstitial lung disease.**
   Pneumoconioses that may produce a micronodular interstitial pattern are silicosis, coal workers' pneumoconiosis, talcosis, and berylliosis. Pneumoconioses are diffuse interstitial lung diseases caused by inorganic dusts, most often related to occupational exposures. Mining, sandblasting, gravestone engraving, and pottery are some occupations in which workers may be exposed to silica dust with resultant silicosis; as identified in the name, coal workers' pneumoconiosis is seen in coal miners. Berylliosis is an uncommon chronic pneumoconiosis that may be encountered in individuals who mine beryllium, who manufacture beryllium ceramics, or who previously manufactured beryllium lighting (these types of lights are no longer manufactured because of the high risk of acute and chronic berylliosis). Talcosis may occur as a result of the mining of talc or excessive inhalation of talcum powder and in intravenous drug abusers. Thyroid carcinoma is the prototypic tumor that produces thousands of tiny micronodular metastases and may appear as a nodular interstitial lung disease. Breast cancer may also produce this pattern of metastasis; other primary tumors rarely produce a micronodular pattern of lung metastasis.

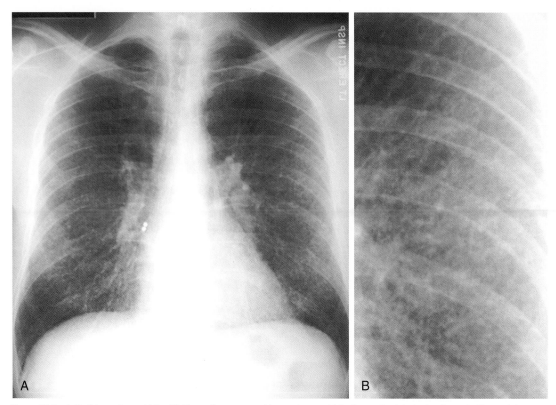

**Figure 19-3. A,** Nodular pattern of interstitial lung disease caused by cryptococcal infection on frontal chest radiograph. Note subtle, tiny nodular densities throughout lung fields bilaterally. **B,** Magnified view of chest radiograph. Note subtle, tiny nodular densities throughout lung.

10. **Discuss the smoking-related lung diseases that cause micronodular lung disease.**
    There are two smoking-related lung diseases that cause a micronodular lung disease: Langerhans cell histiocytosis and respiratory bronchiolitis interstitial lung disease. Langerhans cell histiocytosis may also produce a nodular pattern of interstitial lung disease. In most cases, pulmonary Langerhans cell histiocytosis is associated with a history of smoking and typically manifests as persistent cough or dyspnea or both in young and middle-aged adults. In the early stages of disease, the patient develops small nodular areas of interstitial fibrosis. As the disorder progresses, cystic lesions may develop in association with an obstructive lung disease. Respiratory bronchiolitis interstitial lung disease is a smoking-related disease that manifests as very fine nodules on chest CT. This micronodular disease cannot be seen on chest radiographs but can occasionally be a cause for chronic respiratory disability.

11. **What is the chest radiographic staging system for sarcoidosis, and what is the clinical significance?**
    Table 19-1 summarizes the staging system for sarcoidosis. The higher the stage of sarcoidosis, the greater the likelihood that the patient will experience chronic respiratory deficits.

12. **Give some examples of hypersensitivity pneumonitis (extrinsic allergic alveolitis).**
    Farmer's lung is the prototypic example of a hypersensitivity pneumonitis. There are a wide variety of other hypersensitivity pneumonitides; some of the many other causes are listed in Table 19-2. These disorders represent an allergic lung reaction to various organic dusts that can initially manifest as capillary leak pulmonary edema, but chronically result in granulomatous interstitial fibrosis. In most cases, the offending antigens are microorganisms that grow within decaying vegetable matter. Antigens from these organisms are delivered to the lung via inhalation of dust or aerosolized contaminated water. Notable exceptions to this general concept are bird-related hypersensitivity pneumonitides. In bird fancier's lung, hypersensitivity occurs against bird-related antigens, such as those found in bird feathers.

13. **Why do intravenous drug abusers get talcosis?**
    Not all intravenous drug abusers get talcosis. The process that can result in talcosis is the intravenous injection of oral medications. These medications are ground into a fine powder, suspended in fluid, and injected intravenously. Pills contain fillers, including talc and methylcellulose, which are inorganic substances that embolize to the lung microvasculature and result in a foreign body giant cell granulomatous reaction, which may appear as small nodules on chest radiography.

**Table 19-1.** Chest Radiographic Staging System for Sarcoidosis

| STAGE | RADIOGRAPHIC APPEARANCE |
|---|---|
| 0 | Chest radiograph appears normal |
| I | Chest radiographic evidence of hilar or mediastinal lymphadenopathy without evidence of interstitial lung disease |
| II | Chest radiographic evidence of hilar or mediastinal lymphadenopathy and evidence of interstitial lung disease |
| III | Chest radiographic evidence of interstitial lung disease without evidence of hilar or mediastinal lymphadenopathy |
| IV | Chest radiographic evidence of interstitial fibrosis with distortion of pulmonary structures, such as blood vessels, without evidence of hilar or mediastinal lymphadenopathy |

**Table 19-2.** Causes of Hypersensitivity Pneumonitis

| EXPOSURES | CAUSES |
|---|---|
| Occupational | Organic dust |
|   Farmer's lung | Hay |
|   Baker's lung | Flour |
|   Sugar cane worker's lung | Sugar cane dust |
|   Cotton worker's lung | Cotton dust |
|   Mushroom worker's lung | Mushrooms |
| Hobbies | |
|   Bird fancier's lung | Bird feathers |
| Other exposures | |
|   Down pillows and comforters | Bird feathers |
|   Hot tubs | Aerosolized water |
|   Humidifiers | Aerosolized water |

14. **What radiographic feature of nodular pneumoconioses is most strongly associated with respiratory deficits?**

Progressive massive fibrosis (PMF), also known as *conglomerate masses*, is the radiographic feature most strongly associated with respiratory deficits. In PMF, the small nodular areas of fibrosis associated with nodular pneumoconioses progressively coalesce into large (>3 cm) fibrotic masses. These masses are typically found in the upper lung zones and result in fibrotic distortion of the surrounding lung parenchyma. All of the nodular pneumoconioses can cause PMF, but it is most strongly associated with silicosis. Many patients with simple silicosis (nodular interstitial disease without PMF) are clinically asymptomatic. Nearly all patients with complicated silicosis (nodular interstitial disease with PMF) have dyspnea, however. The causes of the nodular interstitial pattern are reviewed in Table 19-3.

15. **What are the radiographic characteristics of the peripheral reticular pattern?**

The peripheral reticular pattern has two distinguishing features:
- Small size of the holes (typically <5 mm) seen within a network of fine crisscrossing linear opacities
- Peripheral and basilar distribution of the network

The network typically is seen filling the costophrenic angles on frontal and lateral chest radiographs (Figures 19-4 and 19-5).

16. **Which diseases cause the peripheral reticular pattern?**

Although various disorders may occasionally result in the peripheral reticular pattern, most cases are caused by idiopathic pulmonary fibrosis (IPF), a connective tissue disorder, or asbestosis.

17. **What demographic features can help distinguish the cause of the peripheral reticular pattern?**

Asbestosis and IPF are disorders of elderly patients, usually individuals older than 50, whereas connective tissue disorders tend to affect younger individuals, often in their 30s and 40s. Patients must have had an extensive exposure to asbestos dust to acquire asbestosis. Nearly all patients with asbestosis have an occupational exposure to asbestos, such as from mining, roofing, car brake shoe repair, shipyard work, or boiler making. Asbestosis is almost exclusively seen in men because few women have sufficient asbestos dust exposure to acquire the disease. Connective tissue

**Table 19-3.** Causes of Nodular Interstitial Lung Disease Pattern

| CATEGORY | DISEASES |
|---|---|
| Granulomatous diseases | Sarcoidosis<br>Miliary infections<br>Tuberculosis<br>Histoplasmosis<br>Coccidioidomycosis<br>Cryptococcosis<br>Blastomycosis<br>Hypersensitivity pneumonitis |
| Nodular pneumoconiosis | Silicosis<br>Coal workers' pneumoconiosis<br>Berylliosis<br>Talcosis |
| Metastasis | Thyroid carcinoma<br>Other malignancies |
| Smoking-related diseases | Langerhans cell histiocytosis<br>Respiratory bronchiolitis interstitial lung disease |

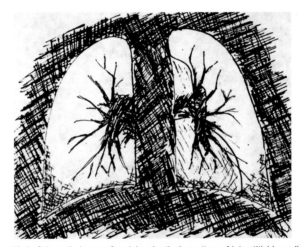

**Figure 19-4.** Schematic image of peripheral reticular pattern of interstitial lung disease.

disorders are more commonly encountered in women, and more patients with connective tissue–related interstitial lung disease are women.

18. **Which connective tissue disorders can result in interstitial disease?**
   *Scleroderma*, or *progressive systemic sclerosis*, has the highest incidence of interstitial fibrosis among all connective tissue disorders. *Rheumatoid arthritis* has the highest prevalence of interstitial disease because it is one of the most common connective tissue disorders and may occasionally cause interstitial fibrosis. *Dermatomyositis/polymyositis* may also result in interstitial fibrosis. By virtue of its potential to overlap with progressive systemic sclerosis, rheumatoid arthritis, or dermatomyositis/polymyositis, *mixed connective tissue disorder* may also cause interstitial fibrosis. *Systemic lupus erythematosus* is one of the most prevalent connective tissue disorders but only rarely produces clinically significant interstitial fibrosis. Although pathologic and radiologic studies may show mild abnormalities, it is quite rare for patients with systemic lupus erythematosus to have respiratory symptoms related to interstitial fibrosis. When these disorders cause interstitial fibrosis, they produce a peripheral reticular interstitial pattern on chest radiography.

19. **Are there any imaging features that can help distinguish the cause of the peripheral reticular pattern?**
   In most cases, there are no imaging features that help distinguish the different causes of the peripheral reticular pattern. Occasionally, extrapulmonary findings help, however, in the differential diagnosis of the peripheral reticular pattern. Approximately two thirds of patients with asbestosis also have asbestos-related pleural plaques. Patients with

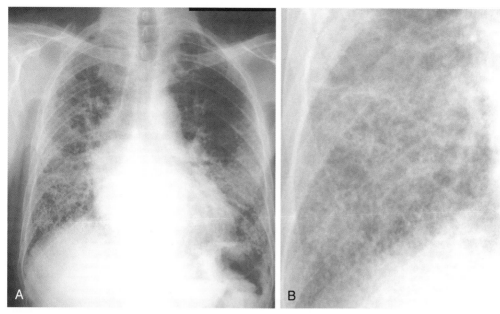

**Figure 19-5. A,** Peripheral reticular pattern of interstitial lung disease secondary to idiopathic pulmonary fibrosis on frontal chest radiograph. Note peripheral and basilar distribution. **B,** Magnified view of chest radiograph. Note network of fine crisscrossing linear opacities in peripheral and basilar distribution of lungs forming small holes between opacities.

---

**Box 19-1.** Causes of Peripheral Reticular Interstitial Lung Disease Pattern

Idiopathic pulmonary fibrosis (IPF)
Connective tissue disorders
    Scleroderma, or progressive systemic sclerosis
    Rheumatoid arthritis
    Polymyositis/dermatomyositis
    Mixed connective tissue disorder
    Systemic lupus erythematosus
Asbestosis

---

progressive systemic sclerosis may have a radiographically identifiable dilated esophagus as a result of CREST syndrome; *CREST* stands for *c*alcinosis cutis, *R*aynaud phenomenon, *e*sophageal dysfunction, *s*clerodactyly, and *t*elangiectasia. Patients with rheumatoid arthritis may have erosions of the distal clavicles as a result of acromioclavicular arthritis. Causes of the peripheral reticular pattern of interstitial lung disease are reviewed in Box 19-1.

20. **Describe the imaging characteristics of the linear pattern on chest radiography.**
The lines visible on a normal chest radiograph represent the branching pulmonary arteries and veins. These begin centrally and radiate from the hilum toward the periphery of the lung. The linear pattern appears as increased numbers of lines radiating from the central hila bilaterally. In addition, the linear pattern may produce Kerley B lines. These are thin horizontal lines 1 to 2 cm long, extending from the lateral chest wall toward the central lung (Figures 19-6 and 19-7). The most common cause of the linear pattern is congestive heart failure, and to the degree that an interstitial abnormality resembles congestive heart failure, it is more likely to represent the linear pattern of interstitial disease. Novice radiologists should take care not to overdiagnose the linear interstitial pattern. There is a wide variation in the normal appearance of chest radiographs. If one is unsure of whether there is an interstitial abnormality present on a chest radiograph, it is usually best to assume that the examination is normal.

21. **What disorders cause the linear pattern of interstitial disease?**
Causes of the linear interstitial pattern include:
- Interstitial pulmonary edema
- Lymphangitic carcinomatosis
- Sarcoidosis
    Congestive heart failure and other causes of *interstitial pulmonary edema* are the most common causes of the linear pattern. In nearly all cases, the presence of a linear interstitial pattern should be assumed to represent

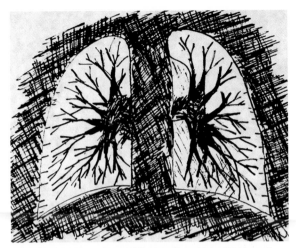

**Figure 19-6.** Schematic image of linear pattern of interstitial lung disease.

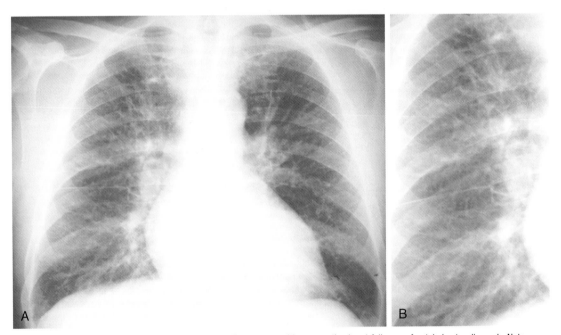

**Figure 19-7. A,** Central linear pattern of interstitial lung disease caused by congestive heart failure on frontal chest radiograph. Note symmetrically increased number of lines radiating from bilateral hila. **B,** Magnified view of chest radiograph. Note symmetrically increased number of lines radiating from the bilateral hila.

interstitial pulmonary edema. *Lymphangitic carcinomatosis* is the most common chronic cause for the linear pattern. This is a form of hematogenous metastasis that grows along the interstitial framework of the lung, rather than growing concentrically as nodules. Breast and lung cancers are the malignancies most likely to cause a pattern of lymphangitic metastasis. Gastric, pancreatic, and ovarian carcinomas are other causes of lymphangitic carcinomatosis. *Sarcoidosis* typically causes peribronchial granulomas, which may also result in interstitial lung disease with a pattern of lines radiating from the hilum of the lung, producing a linear pattern.

22. **Are there any imaging clues that may help to distinguish the cause of the linear interstitial pattern?**
    In most cases, no imaging clues help to distinguish the cause of the linear pattern of interstitial disease. One notable exception is the recognition of a markedly asymmetric linear pattern, in which one lung is considerably more affected than the other. This imaging finding is virtually always associated with lymphangitic carcinomatosis.

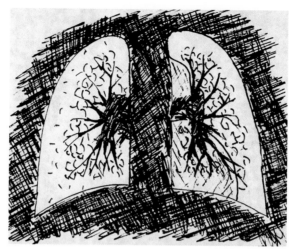

**Figure 19-8.** Schematic image of cystic pattern of interstitial lung disease.

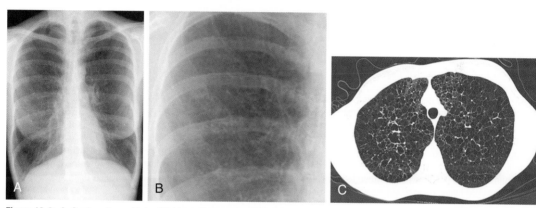

**Figure 19-9. A,** Cystic pattern of interstitial lung disease caused by Langerhans cell histiocytosis on frontal chest radiograph. Note network of fine ring shadows in more central lung and larger holes between opacities (compared with smaller holes in peripheral reticular pattern). **B,** Magnified view of chest radiograph. Note network of fine ring shadows in more central lung and larger holes between opacities (compared with smaller holes in peripheral reticular pattern). **C,** Cystic pattern of interstitial lung disease caused by Langerhans cell histiocytosis on CT. Note multiple cysts of variable size throughout lungs.

23. What are the imaging characteristics of the cystic pattern of interstitial lung disease?
    This pattern is characterized by a group of curved lines that produce a network of fine ring shadows in the more central lung. Although a reticular pattern, the cystic pattern is quite distinct from the peripheral reticular pattern. In the cystic pattern, the holes are, on average, approximately 10 mm in diameter, which are much larger than the holes seen in the peripheral reticular pattern. The rings of the cystic pattern are distributed in the more central lung, whereas the peripheral reticular pattern characteristically affects the subpleural and basilar lung (Figures 19-8 and 19-9).

24. What disorders produce the cystic interstitial pattern?
    The cystic interstitial pattern is the least common of the interstitial patterns on chest radiography, and the most common cause of the cystic pattern is not interstitial lung disease, but emphysema. *Emphysema* usually appears as a decrease in the number and conspicuity of the normal lines seen on chest radiography. It has been recognized for many years, however, that emphysema occasionally appears as an increase in the number and conspicuity of interstitial lines. When emphysema does this, it appears in the cystic interstitial pattern. *Diffuse bronchiectasis* may also appear as many ring shadows distributed throughout the lung parenchyma. Two rare disorders that may also cause this pattern are *Langerhans cell histiocytosis* (which was previously discussed along with the nodular pattern) and lymphangioleiomyomatosis. *Lymphangioleiomyomatosis* is a rare hormonally mediated disorder of young and middle-aged women. Proliferation of interstitial smooth muscle results in air trapping and production of small uniform cystic spaces in the lung. Box 19-2 lists the causes of the cystic interstitial lung disease pattern.

25. What disorders cause diffuse bronchiectasis?
    Although various disorders may result in bronchiectasis, only a few diseases cause widespread bronchiectasis that involves most of the lung parenchyma. The most common of these is cystic fibrosis. Other diseases include primary

**Box 19-2.** Causes of Cystic Interstitial Lung Disease Pattern

Emphysema
Cystic lung disease
    Langerhans cell histiocytosis (eosinophilic granuloma)
    Lymphangioleiomyomatosis
Diffuse bronchiectasis
    Cystic fibrosis
    Primary cilia dyskinesia
    Allergic bronchopulmonary aspergillosis
    Immunodeficiency states
      • Common variable immunodeficiency
      • Hyper-IgE syndrome

cilia dyskinesia; allergic bronchopulmonary aspergillosis; and various immunodeficiency states, such as common variable immunodeficiency syndrome, natural killer cell deficiency, and hyper-IgE syndrome.

26. **Are there any radiographic imaging features that help to distinguish the cause of the cystic pattern?**
In many cases, the disorders that cause the cystic pattern produce radiographically indistinguishable disease. One notable exception is diffuse bronchiectasis. The cystic spaces caused by bronchiectasis typically produce thick-walled, distinct ring shadows, whereas the other disorders often cause very faint rings (see Box 19-2 for causes of the cystic interstitial pattern). Also, primary cilia dyskinesia is associated with situs inversus, where the internal organs are left-right inverted.

27. **When is computed tomography (CT) scanning indicated for the evaluation of interstitial lung disease?**
CT is more sensitive and more specific than chest radiography for interstitial abnormalities. In advanced cases with obvious chest radiographic findings, chest radiographs may be diagnostic. However, in most cases, CT will provide increased information about the distribution and severity of disease. Patients with apparently normal or minimally abnormal chest radiographs in whom there is a clinical suspicion of interstitial lung disease should receive a thin-section chest CT scan to evaluate better for the presence of interstitial lung disease. Patients with chest radiographs that are nonspecific may benefit from a CT study, which in many cases allows the clinician to narrow the differential diagnosis. Lastly, CT provides improved characterization of the extent of disease. In cases in which therapeutic decisions are based on imaging evidence of progression, stability, or regression of disease, CT scanning is indicated.

28. **What type of CT scan is indicated for the evaluation of interstitial lung disease?**
CT scanning has inherently less spatial resolution than standard chest radiography. As interstitial lung diseases are typified by very fine spatial abnormalities, it is necessary to maximize the spatial resolution of CT images by minimizing the slice thickness, usually to 0.5 to 1.5 mm. Modern multislice helical CT scanners are typically set to generate thin-slice images in nearly all chest CT studies and generate so-called high-resolution CT (HRCT) chest CT scans because of the improved spatial resolution that is characteristic of the studies. Thin-section expiratory CT images are also often obtained to detect presence of pulmonary air trapping, which may occur in association with interstitial lung disease. Furthermore, prone CT images may be acquired if posterior peripheral interstitial lung disease is suspected in order to minimize obscuration and confounding by dependent atelectasis present in the supine position.

## KEY POINTS

- Interstitial pulmonary edema, usually caused by congestive heart failure, is the most common interstitial abnormality encountered in daily practice.
- The nodular pattern of interstitial lung disease appears as increased numbers of nodular opacities (<10 mm) that are randomly distributed throughout the lung parenchyma. The four broad groups of disorders that cause nodular interstitial disease are granulomatous lung diseases, nodular pneumoconioses, small metastases, and smoking-related lung diseases.
- The two distinguishing features of the peripheral reticular pattern of interstitial lung disease are the small size of the holes (typically <5 mm) seen within a network of fine crisscrossing linear opacities and a peripheral and basilar distribution of this network. Most cases are caused by IPF, a connective tissue disorder, or asbestosis.
- The linear pattern of interstitial lung disease appears as increased numbers of lines radiating from the hila centrally. This pattern also may produce peripheral Kerley B lines. The most common cause of this pattern is congestive heart failure, although lymphangitic carcinomatosis is the most common chronic cause of this pattern.
- The cystic pattern is characterized by a group of curved lines that produce a network of fine ring shadows in the more central lung with larger holes than are seen in the peripheral reticular pattern. The most common cause of this pattern is emphysema.

## BIBLIOGRAPHY

Webb WR, Muller NL, Naidich DP. *High-resolution CT of the lung*. 5th ed. Philadelphia: Wolters Kluwer Health; 2015.

Reed JC. *Chest radiology: plain film patterns and differential diagnoses*. 6th ed. Philadelphia: Elsevier; 2011.

Hansell DM, Lynch D, McAdams HP, et al. *Imaging of diseases of the chest*. 5th ed. Philadelphia: Elsevier; 2010.

Miller WT Jr. Radiographic evaluation of diffuse interstitial lung disease: review of a dying art. *Semin Ultrasound CT MR*. 2002;23(4):324-338.

# CHAPTER 20

# IMAGING OF MEDIASTINAL DISEASE

*Drew A. Torigian, MD, MA, FSAR, Charles T. Lau, MD, MBA, and Wallace T. Miller, Jr., MD*

1. Describe the anatomy of the mediastinum.

   The mediastinum is located centrally within the thorax between the pleural cavities laterally, the sternum anteriorly, the spine posteriorly, the thoracic inlet superiorly, and the diaphragm inferiorly. It is usually divided into anterior, middle, and posterior compartments to help categorize tumors and diseases by their site of origin and location. Processes that arise in these different compartments are generally related to the anatomic structures located within the compartments. Figure 20-1, *A*, shows the normal appearance of the mediastinum on frontal chest radiography.

2. What are the three compartments of the mediastinum?

   - The **anterior mediastinal compartment** is a space posterior to the sternum and anterior to the heart and trachea extending from the thoracic inlet to the diaphragm; it contains the thymus, thyroid gland, fat, and lymph nodes.
   - The **middle mediastinal compartment** is a space that contains the heart and pericardium, the ascending aorta and aortic arch, brachiocephalic vessels, venae cavae, main pulmonary arteries and veins, trachea and bronchi, fat, and lymph nodes.
   - The **posterior mediastinal compartment** is a space posterior to the middle mediastinal compartment that contains the descending thoracic aorta, esophagus, azygos and hemiazygos veins, autonomic ganglia and nerves, thoracic duct, fat, and lymph nodes.

     Figure 20-1*B*, delineates the three compartments of the mediastinum on lateral chest radiography.

3. List the differential diagnosis of major anterior mediastinal lesions.

   In the following list, an asterisk (*) indicates the most common causes:

   Thymic Masses
   - Lymphoma*
   - Thymoma*
   - Thymic carcinoma
   - Thymic carcinoid
   - Thymolipoma
   - Thymic cyst
   - Thymic hyperplasia

   Thyroid Masses
   - Thyroid goiter*
   - Thyroid cyst
   - Thyroid adenoma
   - Thyroid carcinoma

   Germ Cell Tumors
   - Teratoma and teratocarcinoma*
   - Seminoma
   - Mixed germ cell tumors

4. List the differential diagnosis of major middle mediastinal lesions.

   In the following list, an asterisk (*) indicates the most common causes:
   - Goiter
   - Lymphadenopathy
   - Metastatic disease* (lung cancer is the most common etiologic factor)
   - Lymphoma (non-Hodgkin lymphoma and Hodgkin lymphoma) or leukemia*
   - Granulomatous infection (fungus, tuberculosis, nontuberculous mycobacterium)
   - Sarcoidosis
   - Inhalational lung disease (silicosis, coal workers' pneumoconiosis, or berylliosis)
   - Castleman disease
   - Aortic abnormalities: aneurysm,* dissection,* traumatic aortic rupture
   - Bronchopulmonary foregut cysts
   - Tracheal tumor
   - Esophageal abnormalities: neoplasms (carcinoma, leiomyoma, leiomyosarcoma), achalasia
   - Hiatal hernia* (often contains air-fluid level) (Figure 20-2)
   - Cardiac tumor

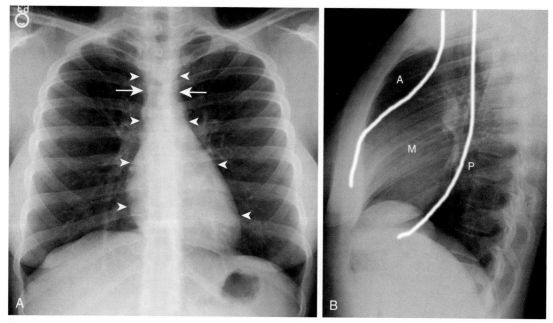

**Figure 20-1.** **A,** Normal frontal chest radiograph. Note normal width of mediastinum (*between arrows*) and sharp demarcation of mediastinal contours (*arrowheads*) against adjacent lungs. **B,** Normal lateral chest radiograph. Note lines separating anterior (*A*), middle (*M*), and posterior (*P*) compartments of mediastinum.

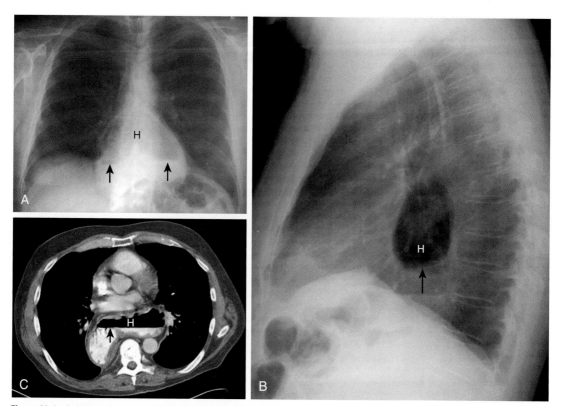

**Figure 20-2.** **A,** Hiatal hernia on frontal chest radiograph. Note gas-filled structure (*H*) with air-fluid level (*arrows*) overlying mediastinum. **B,** Hiatal hernia on lateral chest radiograph. Note gas-filled structure (*H*) with air-fluid level (*arrow*) posterior to heart in posterior mediastinum. **C,** Hiatal hernia on CT. Note structure (*H*) with gas-contrast level (*arrow*) lined by rugal folds posterior to heart in posterior mediastinum indicating stomach.

- Left ventricular or thoracic aortic aneurysm or pseudoaneurysm
- Pulmonary artery aneurysm
- Neurogenic tumor of the vagus nerve

5. **List the differential diagnosis of major posterior mediastinal lesions.**
In the following list, an asterisk (*) indicates the most common causes:
- Neurogenic tumors* (peripheral nerve, sympathetic ganglion, or parasympathetic involvement)
- Primary or metastatic bone tumor of the thoracic spine
- Osteomyelitis or paraspinal abscess of the thoracic spine
- Extramedullary hematopoiesis

6. **List the differential diagnosis of fat-containing mediastinal lesions.**
- Lipoma
- Mature teratoma
- Thymolipoma
- Well-differentiated liposarcoma
- Mediastinal lipomatosis
- Fat-containing hernia (hiatal, Bochdalek, or Morgagni hernia)
- Posterior mediastinal angiomyolipoma

7. **List the differential diagnosis of cystic mediastinal lesions.**
Cystic lesions with thin, smooth wall:
- Pericardial cyst
- Bronchogenic cyst
- Esophageal duplication cyst
- Thymic cyst
- Neurenteric cyst
- Mediastinal pancreatic pseudocyst
- Intrathoracic meningocele
Cyst lesions with thick wall, mural nodularity, or internal septations:
- Thymic teratoma
- Any mediastinal tumor with necrosis or cystic change
- Mediastinal abscess

8. **Name different collections that may occur within the mediastinum.**
- Fluid: mediastinal edema or pericardial effusion
- Blood: mediastinal hematoma or hemopericardium
- Pus: mediastinal abscess, pericardial abscess, or acute mediastinitis
- Air: pneumomediastinum and pneumopericardium
- Fat: mediastinal lipomatosis
- Fibrosis: fibrosing mediastinitis
- Cells: mediastinal tumor

9. **What clinical symptoms and signs can be associated with mediastinal lesions?**
Compression or invasion of the trachea or bronchi, recurrent laryngeal nerve, or esophagus may produce cough, dyspnea, chest pain, respiratory infection, hoarseness, or dysphagia. Compression or invasion of the adjacent cardiovascular structures may produce superior vena cava syndrome; cardiac dysrhythmias; constrictive pathophysiology; cardiac tamponade; or, rarely, sudden death. About 75% of mediastinal tumors in asymptomatic patients are benign, whereas about 66% of those in symptomatic patients are malignant.

10. **What is a thymoma?**
A thymoma is an uncommon thymic epithelial tumor that is the most common primary tumor of the thymus and of the anterior mediastinum. It occurs in men and women equally and most often occurs after age 40. It is an epithelial neoplasm composed of a mixture of epithelial cells and mature lymphocytes. About 33% are invasive, and the remainder are encapsulated. Complete surgical resection is the major treatment for a thymoma. Radiation therapy or chemotherapy may be used for an invasive thymoma, an incompletely resected thymoma, or a disseminated thymoma. Most patients with an encapsulated thymoma are cured with surgical resection, and many with microscopically invasive thymoma are cured with surgery and adjunctive radiation therapy. Patients with macroscopic invasion often have a prolonged course with slowly growing metastatic disease. The Masaoka-Koga staging system is used in patients with thymoma (Box 20-1).

11. **Describe the clinical presentation of a thymoma.**
Most patients are asymptomatic, although 33% may be symptomatic because of compression or invasion of adjacent structures. Of patients, 50% may have a paraneoplastic syndrome, such as myasthenia gravis, hypogammaglobulinemia, or pure red blood cell aplasia. About 30% to 50% of patients with a thymoma may develop myasthenia gravis, whereas 15% of patients with myasthenia gravis have a thymoma. Ten percent of patients with a

**Box 20-1.** Masaoka-Koga Staging System of Thymic Epithelial Tumors

I—Macroscopically, completely encapsulated; microscopically, no capsular invasion
II—Macroscopic invasion into surrounding fatty tissue or mediastinal pleura; or microscopic invasion into capsule
III—Macroscopic invasion into neighboring organs (pericardium, lung, or great vessels)
IVA—Pleural or pericardial dissemination
IVB—Lymphogenous or hematogenous metastases

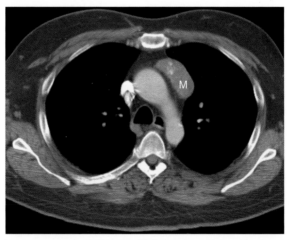

**Figure 20-3.** Anterior mediastinal mass secondary to thymoma on CT. Note ovoid, partially calcified mass (*M*) anterior to aortic arch within anterior mediastinum.

thymoma may develop hypogammaglobulinemia, whereas 5% of patients with hypogammaglobulinemia have a thymoma. Five percent of patients with a thymoma may develop red blood cell aplasia, whereas 50% of patients with red blood cell aplasia have a thymoma.

12. Describe the imaging findings of a thymoma.
    One typically sees a well-defined, rounded, or lobulated anterosuperior mediastinal soft tissue mass arising from one of the thymic lobes with asymmetric growth toward one side of the midline, occasionally with necrotic, cystic, hemorrhagic, or calcific changes (Figure 20-3). About 33% of thymomas invade through the capsule and involve adjacent tissues or structures such as the mediastinal fat, pleura, pericardium, great vessels, heart, or lung and may extend through the diaphragm into the peritoneal cavity or retroperitoneum. Metastatic disease is most commonly to the pleura, often mimicking malignant pleural mesothelioma with unilateral pleural thickening, masses, or diffuse nodular circumferential pleural thickening encasing the ipsilateral lung. Pleural effusions, lymphadenopathy, or distant hematogenous metastases are present less commonly.

13. What is thymic carcinoma?
    Thymic carcinoma is an aggressive epithelial malignancy that often includes early local invasion, lymphadenopathy, and distant metastatic disease. Squamous cell carcinoma and lymphoepithelioma-like carcinoma are the most common cell types and most often occur in middle-aged men. On imaging, thymic carcinomas are commonly large, poorly defined, infiltrative anterior mediastinal masses that may have cystic or necrotic changes, often with pleural and pericardial effusions (Figure 20-4). Treatment and prognosis depend on the stage and histologic grade of the tumor. Avid uptake of fluorodeoxyglucose (FDG) on positron emission tomography (PET) imaging is typically seen, generally to a greater degree than in thymomas.

14. What is thymic carcinoid?
    Thymic carcinoid is a rare neuroendocrine tumor that typically affects men in the fourth to fifth decades of life. About 50% of patients have endocrine abnormalities, most commonly Cushing syndrome resulting from ectopic adrenocorticotropic hormone (ACTH) production or multiple endocrine neoplasia syndrome. Classic carcinoid syndrome caused by serotonin secretion is rarely associated with thymic carcinoid. Symptoms and signs secondary to local mass effect and invasion may also occur. A large lobulated and usually invasive anterior mediastinal mass is seen that may be associated with cystic, necrotic, hemorrhagic, or calcific change. Lymphadenopathy and distant metastases may be seen in 75% of cases. Complete surgical excision is the treatment of choice, and radiotherapy and chemotherapy may be used for more advanced disease.

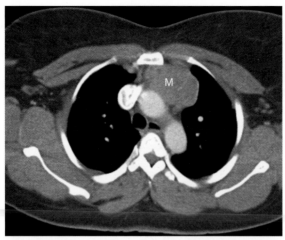

**Figure 20-4.** Anterior mediastinal mass secondary to thymic carcinoma on CT. Note ovoid soft tissue attenuation mass (*M*) anterior to ascending aorta within anterior mediastinum.

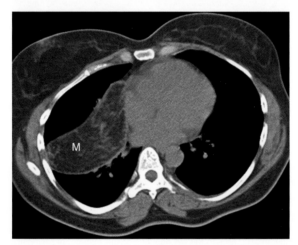

**Figure 20-5.** Anterior mediastinal mass secondary to thymolipoma on CT. Note predominantly fat attenuation mass (*M*) anterior and to right of heart within anterior mediastinum.

15. What is thymolipoma?

Thymolipoma is a rare, benign, slow-growing thymic neoplasm that may occur in any age group, although young adults are most commonly affected. It is a large, soft, encapsulated mass composed of mature adipose cells and thymic tissue. About 50% of patients are asymptomatic. On imaging, a thymolipoma often presents as a large anterior mediastinal mass that droops into the anteroinferior mediastinum, may occupy one or both hemithoraces, and is characterized by its ability to conform to adjacent structures and to change in shape after changes in patient positioning. Predominant fat attenuation on computed tomography (CT) (Figure 20-5) or fat signal intensity on magnetic resonance imaging (MRI) with intermixed soft tissue components is seen. Complete surgical resection is curative.

16. What is a mediastinal germ cell tumor?

Mediastinal germ cell tumors are a heterogeneous group of benign and malignant neoplasms that originate from primitive germ cells that remain in the mediastinum after early embryogenesis. The anterior mediastinum is the most common extragonadal primary site of germ cell tumors. Mediastinal germ cell tumors usually occur in young adults. Although mature teratomas occur equally in men and women, most malignant germ cell tumors occur in men. $\alpha$-fetoprotein and $\beta$-human chorionic gonadotropin serum levels may be abnormally elevated in patients with malignant mediastinal germ cell tumors. Primary testicular or ovarian germ cell tumors need to be excluded when a mediastinal germ cell tumor is discovered because the mediastinum may be a site of metastasis from gonadal germ cell tumors.

17. What is a mediastinal teratoma?

Teratomas are the most common mediastinal germ cell tumor, composed of tissues from more than one of the three primitive germ cell layers (teeth, skin, and hair from ectoderm; cartilage and bone from mesoderm; and bronchial, intestinal, or pancreatic tissue from endoderm). Most teratomas are well-differentiated and benign (mature). However, on rare occasions teratomas may contain fetal tissue and either recur or metastasize (when immature). Mediastinal teratomas occur most commonly in children and young adults. Although usually asymptomatic, large tumors may cause symptoms because of local mass effect. On imaging, mature teratoma appears as a lobulated, well-defined heterogeneous anterior mediastinal mass usually located to one side of the midline with fat attenuation or signal intensity foci, along with multilocular cysts, and very high attenuation/very low signal intensity teeth, calcifications, or bone. The presence of fat, fluid, and soft tissue elements within an anterior mediastinal mass is virtually diagnostic of a mediastinal teratoma. Surgical excision is curative.

18. Name a rare but highly specific clinical presentation of mediastinal teratoma.
Expectoration of hair (trichoptysis) or sebum is a rare but pathognomonic sign of ruptured mediastinal teratoma. This presentation is due to secretion of digestive enzymes by intestinal mucosa or pancreatic tissue in the tumor, precipitating rupture into the bronchi.

19. What is mediastinal thyroid goiter?
Mediastinal thyroid goiter is an encapsulated, lobulated heterogeneous enlargement of part or all of the thyroid gland, most commonly in asymptomatic women with a palpable cervical goiter. Occasionally, local compressive symptoms are present; 20% of lesions extend inferiorly into the thorax, usually into the left anterosuperior mediastinum, and less commonly into the middle or posterior mediastinal compartment. On imaging, a well-defined, lobulated heterogeneous lesion, often in the anterosuperior mediastinum, with areas of cystic, hemorrhagic, or calcific change is seen, often with tracheal displacement in the neck. Tracheal displacement on a chest radiograph indicates a mass of thyroid origin or a goiter. On CT and MRI, identification of contiguity of the mass with the thyroid gland establishes a thyroid origin (Figure 20-6). Surgical resection is the treatment of choice for symptomatic lesions, although most patients with a goiter are asymptomatic and require no therapy other than iodine or hormonal replacement.

20. Define mediastinal lipoma and mediastinal lipomatosis.
Mediastinal lipoma is a benign, well-circumscribed mesenchymal tumor that originates from adipose tissue, predominantly occurring in the anterior mediastinum, often without clinical symptoms or signs. On imaging, it is generally a well-circumscribed, oval or round homogeneous fat attenuation or signal intensity lesion.

Mediastinal lipomatosis is due to excessive unencapsulated fat deposition within the mediastinum. It is commonly associated with obesity and chronic exogenous corticosteroid administration and appears as widening of the mediastinum on radiography and as an increase in mediastinal fat on CT or MRI.

21. What is Hodgkin lymphoma (HL)?
HL accounts for about 25% to 30% of lymphomas. Of patients with mediastinal involvement by lymphoma, 85% may have Hodgkin lymphoma. Hodgkin lymphoma occurs with a bimodal age distribution, with peaks during adolescence and early adulthood and after the fifth decade of life, most often occurring above the diaphragm. The diagnosis is established on pathologic study by identification of Reed-Sternberg cells, generally in a background of inflammation and fibrosis. On imaging, one generally observes enlarged lymph nodes or conglomerate masses, sometimes with hemorrhagic, necrotic, cystic, or calcific change, and almost always involving the anterior mediastinum, often involving contiguous nodal groups. Avid uptake of FDG on PET imaging is often seen. The Ann Arbor staging system is used in patients with lymphoma (Box 20-2).

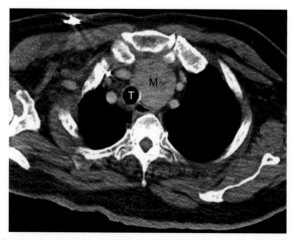

**Figure 20-6.** Middle mediastinal mass secondary to thyroid goiter on CT. Note soft tissue mass (*M*) within middle mediastinum to left of trachea (*T*). This was seen to be contiguous with inferior aspect of thyroid gland (not shown) confirming thyroid origin.

**Box 20-2.** Ann Arbor Staging System of Lymphoma (HL and NHL)

I—Involvement of a single lymphatic site (nodal region, Waldeyer's ring, thymus, or spleen)
  IE—Localized involvement of a single extralymphatic site
II—Involvement of ≥2 lymph node regions on the same side of the diaphragm
  IIE—Localized involvement of a single extralymphatic site associated with regional lymph node involvement without or with involvement of other lymph node regions on the same side of the diaphragm
III—Involvement of lymph node regions on both sides of the diaphragm
  IIIE—Involvement of lymph node regions on both sides of the diaphragm accompanied by extralymphatic extension
  IIIS—Involvement of lymph node regions on both sides of the diaphragm accompanied by involvement of the spleen
  IIIES—Involvement of lymph node regions on both sides of the diaphragm accompanied by extralymphatic extension and involvement of the spleen
IV—Diffuse or disseminated involvement of ≥1 extralymphatic organ without or with lymph node involvement, or isolated extralymphatic organ involvement in absence of adjacent regional lymph node involvement but with disease in distant site(s); this includes any involvement of the liver, bone marrow, lungs (other than by direct extension from another site), or cerebrospinal fluid

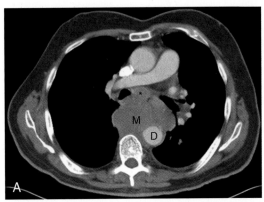 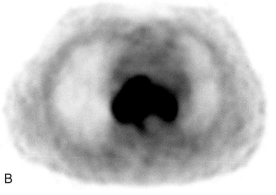

**Figure 20-7. A,** Middle and posterior mediastinal mass secondary to lymphoma on CT. Note large homogeneous soft tissue attenuation mass (*M*) in subcarinal station of middle mediastinum (*) and in posterior mediastinum surrounding descending thoracic aorta (*D*).
**B,** Middle and posterior mediastinal mass secondary to lymphoma on FDG PET. Note avid FDG uptake in location of mediastinal mass.

22. What is non-Hodgkin lymphoma (NHL)?
    NHL may occur in all age groups, although older patients tend to be affected most commonly. Most patients present with advanced disease. On pathologic specimens, one observes a predominance of malignant lymphocytes that are generally homogeneous and uniformly cellular. On imaging, one may see enlarged lymph nodes anywhere within the thorax, but extranodal disease is common, generally appearing as homogeneous soft tissue masses that may involve nearly any organ in the body. Cystic, necrotic, or calcific changes are uncommon but may occasionally be seen. Avid uptake of FDG on PET imaging is often present (Figure 20-7).

23. What are the most common causes of mediastinal lymphadenopathy?
    The four most common causes of radiographically detectable mediastinal lymphadenopathy are sarcoidosis, lymphoma, metastatic tumor, and granulomatous infections. In younger patients with bilateral hilar and mediastinal lymphadenopathy, sarcoidosis should be the diagnosis of exclusion because it is the most common cause. In older individuals, lymphoma and metastatic tumor are the most common causes of mediastinal lymphadenopathy. It would seem logical that any pulmonary infection could lead to mediastinal lymphadenopathy; however, only granulomatous infections commonly cause mediastinal or hilar lymphadenopathy. These include primary tuberculosis, histoplasmosis, cryptococcosis, and coccidioidomycosis.

24. Which vascular disorders can appear as mediastinal masses?
    Aortic aneurysm, aortic pseudoaneurysm, aortic dissection, and traumatic aortic rupture can appear as a mediastinal mass, most often projecting from the left side of the mediastinum on chest radiography. Cross-sectional imaging shows enlargement of the aorta in the setting of aortic aneurysm and sometimes in the setting of the latter two conditions. Also, mediastinal hematoma may be seen if aortic rupture has occurred (Figure 20-8).

25. Describe the congenital foregut cysts.
    Bronchogenic cysts represent 50% to 60% of all mediastinal cysts, esophageal duplication cysts represent 5% to 10%, and neurenteric cysts represent 2% to 5%. About 85% of bronchogenic cysts are located close to the trachea, mainstem bronchi, or carina, and 15% may occur in the lungs. Esophageal duplication cysts are almost always found

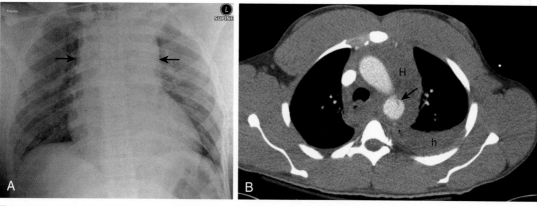

**Figure 20-8. A,** Mediastinal hematoma secondary to traumatic aortic transection on supine frontal chest radiograph. Note widening of mediastinum (*between arrows*). **B,** Mediastinal hematoma secondary to traumatic aortic transection on CT. Note high attenuation mediastinal hemorrhage (*H*) and left hemothorax (*h*) along with abnormal contour of transected descending thoracic aorta (*arrow*).

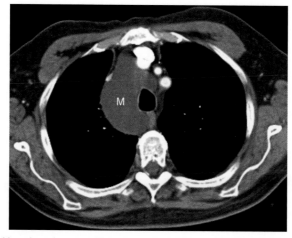

**Figure 20-9.** Mediastinal bronchogenic cyst on CT. Note fluid attenuation mass (*M*) with lobulated contours in mediastinum.

within the esophageal wall or adherent to the esophagus. Neurenteric cysts may occur in isolation within the mediastinum or may be connected by a fibrous tract to the spine. On imaging, cysts are generally round, smooth, thin-walled lesions that contain simple fluid or sometimes complex fluid (Figure 20-9). Symptoms may occur from compression of mediastinal structures or superinfection.

26. What is a mediastinal pancreatic pseudocyst?

    A mediastinal pancreatic pseudocyst is an encapsulated collection of pancreatic secretions that does not have an epithelial lining and is almost always located in the inferoposterior mediastinum. A mediastinal pancreatic pseudocyst is due to extension of fluid through the esophageal or aortic hiatus of the diaphragm in the setting of pancreatitis.

27. What is pneumomediastinum?

    Pneumomediastinum is gas within the mediastinum. On imaging, one sees streaky linear or curvilinear lucent, very low attenuation, or very low signal intensity gas in the mediastinum that outlines mediastinal structures (Figure 20-10). Although pneumopericardium (gas within the pericardial space) is confined to the distribution of the pericardial reflection, pneumomediastinum may occur anywhere within the mediastinum. The causes of pneumomediastinum include:

    - Air trapping from obstructive lung disease such as emphysema or asthma.
    - Straining against a closed glottis from vomiting, parturition, weightlifting, or marijuana use.
    - Blunt/penetrating trauma or iatrogenic injury to the trachea, bronchi, or esophagus.
    - Barotrauma from mechanical ventilation, sudden decrease in atmospheric pressure, or coughing.
    - Erosion of the trachea or esophagus by tumor.
    - Esophageal rupture from Boerhaave syndrome, alcoholism, or diabetic ketoacidosis.
    - Extension of gas from pneumothorax, pneumoperitoneum, or pneumoretroperitoneum.
    - Recent thoracic surgery.

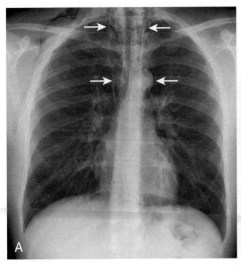

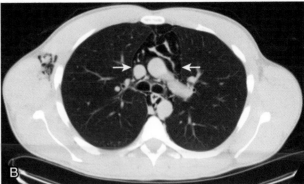

**Figure 20-10. A,** Pneumomediastinum on frontal chest radiograph. Note streaky linear lucent gas (*arrows*) in mediastinum that outlines mediastinal structures. **B,** Pneumomediastinum on CT. Note very low attenuation gas (*between arrows*) in mediastinum that outlines mediastinal structures.

28. What is acute mediastinitis?

Acute mediastinitis is an uncommon but potentially life-threatening infectious condition that requires early diagnosis and treatment. In 90% of cases, it is secondary to esophageal rupture. Other causes include tumor necrosis, spread of infection from contiguous areas such as the neck, retroperitoneum, pleura, and lungs, or infection after thoracic surgery. Patients tend to be very ill with fever, chills, chest pain, and tachycardia, although some patients present with symptoms and signs that mimic other disease conditions. Therefore, a high index of suspicion is required in order to arrive at the correct diagnosis in a timely fashion.

29. Describe the imaging features of acute mediastinitis.

Imaging features may include mediastinal widening; pneumomediastinum; infiltration of the mediastinal fat due to edema, inflammation, or infection; mediastinal fluid; or a mediastinal abscess. Associated findings of esophageal rupture, infection in adjacent tissues, or recent thoracic surgery may also be seen.

30. What is a mediastinal abscess?

A mediastinal abscess is a loculated collection of pus. Major causes of mediastinal abscess include surgery, esophageal perforation, tracheobronchial perforation, spread of infection from a contiguous location, or penetrating trauma. On imaging, one may see a loculated fluid collection that tends to have a thick, enhancing wall and that may contain gas. Acute infection of the mediastinum is often fulminant and life-threatening, and is treated urgently.

31. What is fibrosing mediastinitis?

Fibrosing mediastinitis is an uncommon benign disorder characterized by proliferation of dense mediastinal fibrous tissue. It typically occurs in young patients who present with symptoms and signs owing to obstruction of vital mediastinal structures. Fibrosing mediastinitis is sometimes related to histoplasmosis infection but is often idiopathic in etiology. On imaging, one often sees nonspecific mediastinal widening, sometimes with hilar involvement, by focal or diffuse confluent soft tissue that is commonly calcified. Encasement, narrowing, or occlusion of the mediastinal airway or vascular structures is also often seen.

32. What are neurogenic tumors?

Neurogenic tumors are the most common cause of posterior mediastinal masses. Schwannomas and neurofibromas arise from peripheral nerves and are more common in adults. Ganglioneuromas, ganglioneuroblastomas, and neuroblastomas arise from sympathetic ganglia and are more common in children. Paragangliomas arise from paraganglia and are less common.

Schwannomas and neurofibromas are the most common mediastinal neurogenic tumors and are benign. Schwannomas are encapsulated tumors composed of Schwann cells and loose reticular tissue; arise from the nerve sheath; and are often heterogeneous with hemorrhagic, cystic, necrotic, calcific, or fatty change. Neurofibromas are usually homogeneous nonencapsulated tumors composed of Schwann cells, nerve fibers, and fibroblasts.

33. Describe the imaging appearance of neurogenic tumors.

On imaging, peripheral nerve neurogenic tumors may appear as lobulated spherical or fusiform masses in the paraspinal region of the thorax, sometimes with a dumbbell configuration if there is extension into a neural foramen. A plexiform neurofibroma, pathognomonic for neurofibromatosis type 1 (NF1), usually involves an entire nerve trunk or

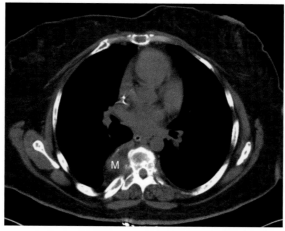

**Figure 20-11.** Posterior mediastinal mass secondary to ganglioneuroma on CT. Note well-circumscribed mixed soft tissue and fat attenuation mass (*M*) within posterior mediastinum to right of thoracic spine.

plexus. Associated smooth pressure erosions of the adjacent inferior rib surfaces and vertebrae or enlargement of the neural foramina may also be seen. Neurogenic tumors that arise from the sympathetic ganglia tend to appear as vertically oriented, elongated paraspinal masses with tapered borders. On CT and MRI, fluid attenuation or signal intensity components owing to cystic change or necrosis, soft tissue attenuation or signal intensity components, fat attenuation or signal intensity components secondary to fatty degeneration, and very high attenuation or very low signal intensity calcification may be visualized (Figure 20-11).

34. What is an intrathoracic meningocele?

An intrathoracic meningocele is an anomalous herniation of leptomeninges through an intervertebral foramen or a defect in the vertebral body, commonly associated with NF-I. On imaging, one sees a well-circumscribed, smooth, lobulated or round paraspinal cystic lesion with enlargement of the intervertebral foramen or associated vertebral and rib anomalies or scoliosis. Diagnosis is confirmed by filling of the lesion with intraspinal contrast material on CT or fluoroscopy.

35. How do osseous tumors and infection within the posterior mediastinum differ on imaging?

Tumors of the thoracic spine generally are centered on the vertebrae without narrowing of the intervening disc spaces, whereas infections tend to be centered on the intervertebral disc spaces with disc space narrowing and involvement of the adjacent vertebral end plates.

36. What is extramedullary hematopoiesis?

Extramedullary hematopoiesis is caused by a proliferation of blood-forming elements in patients with thalassemia or other anemias and occurs most commonly in the liver and spleen and sometimes in the chest. On imaging, multiple lobulated masses along the thoracic spine or ribs may be seen with pressure erosions, often with associated osseous abnormalities and sometimes with associated splenomegaly. Fat attenuation or signal intensity components that are chronic may be visualized.

## KEY POINTS

- Processes that originate in the different compartments of the mediastinum are generally related to the anatomic structures located within the compartments.
- Most patients with asymptomatic mediastinal tumors have benign tumors, whereas most patients with symptomatic mediastinal tumors have malignant tumors.
- Thymoma is the most common primary tumor of the anterior mediastinum and of the thymus.
- Primary testicular or ovarian germ cell tumor should be excluded when a mediastinal germ cell tumor is discovered.
- Neurogenic tumor is the most common mass of the posterior mediastinum.

**BIBLIOGRAPHY**

Shahrzad M, Le TS, Silva M, et al. Anterior mediastinal masses. *AJR Am J Roentgenol.* 2014;203(2):W128-W138.
Vilstrup MH, Torigian DA. FDG PET in thoracic malignancies. *PET Clin.* 2014;9(4):391-420.
Kwee TC, Torigian DA, Alavi A. Oncological applications of positron emission tomography for evaluation of the thorax. *J Thorac Imaging.* 2013;28(1):11-24.
Marom EM. Advances in thymoma imaging. *J Thorac Imaging.* 2013;28(2):69-80, quiz 1-3.

McNeeley MF, Chung JH, Bhalla S, et al. Imaging of granulomatous fibrosing mediastinitis. *AJR Am J Roentgenol.* 2012;199(2):319-327.

Peterson CM, Buckley C, Holley S, et al. Teratomas: a multimodality review. *Curr Probl Diagn Radiol.* 2012;41(6):210-219.

Detterbeck FC, Nicholson AG, Kondo K, et al. The Masaoka-Koga stage classification for thymic malignancies: clarification and definition of terms. *J Thorac Oncol.* 2011;6(7 suppl 3):S1710-S1716.

Edge SB, Byrd DR, Compton CC, et al. Hodgkin and non-Hodgkin lymphomas. In: *AJCC cancer staging manual.* New York: Springer; 2010:607-612.

Masaoka A. Staging system of thymoma. *J Thorac Oncol.* 2010;5(10 suppl 4):S304-S312.

Bae YA, Lee KS. Cross-sectional evaluation of thoracic lymphoma. *Radiol Clin North Am.* 2008;46(2):253-264, viii.

Loevner LA, Kaplan SL, Cunnane ME, et al. Cross-sectional imaging of the thyroid gland. *Neuroimaging Clin N Am.* 2008;18(3):445-461, vii.

Gaerte SC, Meyer CA, Winer-Muram HT, et al. Fat-containing lesions of the chest. *Radiographics.* 2002;22:Spec No:S61-78.

Jeung MY, Gasser B, Gangi A, et al. Imaging of cystic masses of the mediastinum. *Radiographics.* 2002;22:Spec No:S79-93.

Rossi SE, McAdams HP, Rosado-de-Christenson ML, et al. Fibrosing mediastinitis. *Radiographics.* 2001;21(3):737-757.

Dunnick NR. Image interpretation session: 1999. Extramedullary hematopoiesis in a patient with beta thalassemia. *Radiographics.* 2000;20(1):266-268.

Zylak CM, Standen JR, Barnes GR, et al. Pneumomediastinum revisited. *Radiographics.* 2000;20(4):1043-1057.

Strollo DC, Rosado de Christenson ML, Jett JR. Primary mediastinal tumors. Part 1: Tumors of the anterior mediastinum. *Chest.* 1997;112(2):511-522.

Strollo DC, Rosado-de-Christenson ML, Jett JR. Primary mediastinal tumors: Part II. Tumors of the middle and posterior mediastinum. *Chest.* 1997;112(5):1344-1357.

# CHAPTER 21

# IMAGING OF PLEURAL DISEASE

*Drew A. Torigian, MD, MA, FSAR, Charles T. Lau, MD, MBA, and Wallace T. Miller, Jr., MD*

1. Describe the normal pleural anatomy and physiologic features.

   The pleural space is a potential space that contains 2 to 10 mL of pleural fluid between the visceral and parietal pleural layers that essentially represents interstitial fluid from the parietal pleura (an ultrafiltrate of plasma). The pleural space is contiguous with the interlobar fissures of the lungs. The pleura is a thin, serous layer that covers the lungs (visceral pleura) and is reflected onto the chest wall and pericardium (parietal pleura). The visceral pleura is supplied by the pulmonary arterial system and drains into the pulmonary venous system, whereas the parietal pleura is supplied by the systemic arterial system and drains into the systemic venous system. Figure 21-1 shows the normal appearance of the pleura on chest radiography.

2. List the major tumors that may affect the pleura.
   - Pleural metastasis
   - Solitary fibrous tumor of the pleura
   - Malignant pleural mesothelioma
   - Pleural lipoma
   - Pleural lymphoma

3. What are the major substances that may collect within the pleural space?
   - Fluid: pleural effusion (plasma ultrafiltrate, chyle, bile, urine, gastrointestinal contents, or ascites)
   - Blood: hemothorax
   - Gas: pneumothorax
   - Pus: empyema
   - Cells: pleural tumor
   - Fibrosis: fibrothorax

4. What is the differential diagnosis of major causes of pleural effusion?
   For the answer, see Box 21-1.

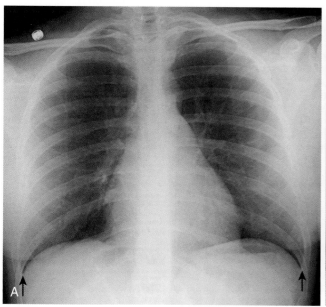
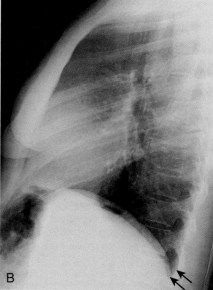

**Figure 21-1. A,** Normal frontal chest radiograph. Note sharp lateral costophrenic angles (arrows) bilaterally and clear demarcation of hemidiaphragms. **B,** Normal lateral chest radiograph. Note sharp posterior costophrenic angles (arrows) bilaterally and clear demarcation of hemidiaphragms.

---

**Box 21-1.** Differential Diagnosis of Pleural Effusion

**Transudative**

Congestive heart failure*
Cirrhosis*
Renal failure
Hypoalbuminemia

**Exudative**

Malignancy
  Metastases*
  Malignant pleural mesothelioma
  Lymphoma
Inflammatory disease
  Infection (bacterial, mycobacterial, viral, fungal, parasitic)
    • Empyema

Parapneumonic effusion*
Collagen vascular disease: systemic lupus erythematosus,
  rheumatoid arthritis, systemic sclerosis
Trauma
Thoracic or abdominal surgery*
Acute pulmonary embolism*
Abdominopelvic pathologic conditions*
  Ascites
  Pancreatitis
  Peritonitis
  Other disease conditions of the abdomen or pelvis
Chylothorax
Hemothorax

*Indicates most common causes.

---

5. List the major mechanisms of pleural effusion formation.
   • Increased hydrostatic pressure in the microvascular circulation (e.g., congestive heart failure).
   • Decreased oncotic pressure in the microvascular circulation (e.g., hypoalbuminemia).
   • Decreased pressure in the pleural space (e.g., with pulmonary atelectasis or restrictive lung disease).
   • Increased permeability of the microvascular circulation (e.g., from pleural inflammation or neoplasm).
   • Impaired lymphatic drainage from the pleural space caused by blockage in the lymphatic system.
   • Transit of fluid from the peritoneal cavity through the diaphragm to the pleural space.

6. What are the two major types of pleural effusions?
   Transudative pleural effusions are usually caused by increased systemic or pulmonary capillary pressure and decreased oncotic pressure, resulting in increased filtration and decreased absorption of pleural fluid. Major causes include cirrhosis, congestive heart failure, renal failure, and hypoalbuminemia. Protein levels are less than 3 g/dL.

   Exudative pleural effusions occur when the pleural surface is damaged with associated capillary leak and increased permeability to protein or when there is decreased lymphatic drainage or decreased pleural pressure. Major causes include infection, noninfectious inflammatory disease, malignancy, recent surgery, and acute pulmonary embolism. Protein levels are greater than 3 g/dL, the pleural protein-to-serum protein ratio is greater than 0.5, and the pleural lactate dehydrogenase-to-serum lactate dehydrogenase ratio is greater than 0.6.

7. What are the major imaging findings of simple nonloculated pleural effusions on upright chest radiography?
   The most common imaging finding of a pleural effusion is blunting of the lateral costophrenic sulcus on upright frontal chest radiography or blunting of the posterior costophrenic sulcus on upright lateral chest radiography. A pleural effusion usually has a sharply marginated, concave–upward curved border between the lung and pleural space, which is known as the "meniscus" sign. Because the posterior costophrenic angle is more dependent than the lateral costophrenic angle, smaller pleural effusions are more apparent on the lateral view (with >75 mL of fluid) than on the frontal view (with >200 mL of fluid). Moderate to large pleural effusions usually obscure the ipsilateral hemidiaphragm (Figure 21-2, *A*). Less common manifestations of pleural effusions include apparent elevation and medial flattening of the hemidiaphragm with lateral displacement of the diaphragmatic apex and an increase in distance (>2 cm) between the inferior surface of the lung and the gastric bubble on the left. The lateral decubitus view is the most sensitive radiographic view for detection of a pleural effusion and can detect 5 mL of pleural fluid.

8. Describe the major imaging findings related to simple nonloculated pleural effusions on portable supine and semi-upright chest radiography, computed tomography (CT), and magnetic resonance imaging (MRI).
   A little-understood fact is that blunting of the costophrenic angles is a rare manifestation of pleural effusions on portable supine and semi-upright chest radiographs. On these views, pleural effusions most often appear as increased opacity of the hemithorax without obscuration of vascular markings or of the ipsilateral hemithorax because fluid layers in the posterior pleural space dependently behind the more anterior nondependent lung. If the patient is supine, this layering appears as a uniform haze of the ipsilateral hemithorax. On semi-upright radiographs, the density produced by the pleural effusion increases from superior to inferior because free-flowing pleural fluid falls dependently into the more inferior portions of the pleural space. Rarely, if the patient is imaged in the Trendelenburg position, the pleural fluid collects as a crescentic opacity over the lung apex, which is known as an apical cap. On CT, fluid attenuation is seen within the dependent aspect of the pleural space, often with a meniscus along its non-dependent aspect (Figure 21-2, *B*). On MRI, low signal intensity fluid on T1-weighted images and very high signal intensity fluid on T2-weighted images relative to skeletal muscle without enhancement are observed.

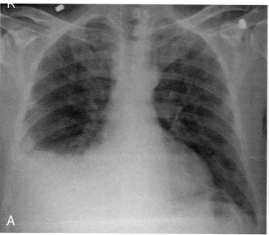
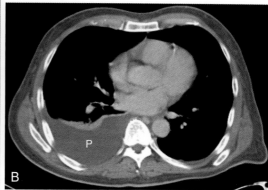

**Figure 21-2. A,** Simple pleural effusion on frontal upright chest radiograph. Note blunting of right lateral costophrenic angle with meniscus sign and obscuration of right hemidiaphragm. **B,** Simple pleural effusion on CT. Note fluid attenuation pleural effusion (*P*) in dependent right hemithorax. Note higher attenuation mild passive right lower lobe atelectasis of lung anterior to pleural effusion.

9. **What are the major imaging findings associated with complex loculated pleural effusions?**
Complex pleural effusions (often seen with exudative effusions) are often located in nondependent portions of the pleural space and do not shift freely in the pleural space on lateral decubitus chest radiography because of adhesions between the visceral and parietal pleurae. CT and MRI scans may also sometimes show associated pleural thickening and enhancement, internal septations, attenuation greater than that of water (i.e., >20 HU), increased signal intensity on T1-weighted images, or decreased signal intensity on T2-weighted images. Occasionally, loculated pleural fluid in the interlobar fissure may mimic a pseudomass on chest radiography, often appearing as a poorly marginated opacity on frontal chest radiography and as an elliptical opacity in the location of a major or minor interlobar fissure on lateral chest radiography.

10. **List the differential diagnosis of major causes of hemothorax.**
   • Trauma (blunt or penetrating or iatrogenic) (most common cause)
   • Bleeding diathesis (e.g., anticoagulation, protein S or C deficiency)
   • Malignancy
   • Infection
   • Acute pulmonary embolism
   • Thoracic aortic rupture (from aneurysm, pseudoaneurysm, dissection, penetrating aortic ulcer, or transection)

11. **What is pneumothorax?**
Pneumothorax is gas within the pleural space; this occurs either through a communication between the outside world and the pleural space via a defect in the chest wall or through a communication between the gas-containing bronchi or alveoli and the pleural space via a defect in the visceral pleura. Free intrapleural gas preferentially moves to the nondependent aspects of the pleural spaces (apicolateral location on upright chest radiography and basilar or anteromedial location on supine chest radiography).

12. **What are the radiographic imaging findings of pneumothorax?**
The pathognomonic finding is a thin, sharply defined, visceral pleural "white" line between radiolucent lung (with vascular markings) and radiolucent "black" free gas in the peripheral pleural space (without vascular markings). On supine chest radiography, one may see sharp visualization of the right cardiac border, superior and inferior vena cavae, left subclavian artery, and anterior junction line; a deep lucent cardiophrenic sulcus ("deep sulcus" sign); hyperlucency at the lung bases; and associated atelectasis of the adjacent lung.

13. **How much gas in a pneumothorax is required for radiographic visualization?**
On upright chest radiographs, small amounts of gas (about 50 mL) are generally visible at the lung apex, whereas on supine radiographs, about 500 mL of gas is needed to be visible.

14. **What radiographic maneuvers can be performed to show a subtle pneumothorax?**
Expiratory chest radiography or contralateral decubitus chest radiography (i.e., left side down if looking for a right pneumothorax and vice versa) can often help reveal a small pneumothorax that may not be seen on standard inspiratory frontal chest radiography. Alternatively, cross-table lateral chest radiography with the patient in the supine position can also show a subtle pneumothorax.

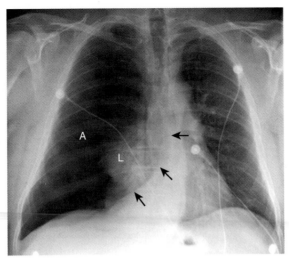

**Figure 21-3.** Tension pneumothorax on frontal chest radiograph. Note thin, sharply defined visceral pleural "white" line between radiolucent lung (*L*) and radiolucent "black" free gas (*A*) in right peripheral pleural space, in addition to leftward mediastinal shift (*arrows*) and inferior right hemidiaphragmatic shift caused by gas under tension.

15. What is a tension pneumothorax?

    Uncommonly, gas in the pleural space can develop positive pressure, most often as a result of mechanical ventilation, and can compress the mediastinum with resultant decreased venous return to the heart. This can be a medical emergency because rapid cardiopulmonary compromise and death may ensue if the patient is not immediately treated. The radiographic clues to a tension pneumothorax are the presence of a pneumothorax in association with contralateral mediastinal shift and inferior displacement of the ipsilateral hemidiaphragm (Figure 21-3). These findings are not diagnostic of a tension pneumothorax, however, which can occur without these findings. The diagnosis is based on radiographic recognition of a pneumothorax and clinical findings of hypotension and tachycardia. Immediate decompression by thoracentesis through the second rib interspace in the midclavicular line or with chest thoracostomy is typically performed for emergent treatment of a tension pneumothorax.

16. What is the differential diagnosis of major causes of pneumothorax?

    In the following list, an asterisk (*) indicates the most common causes:
    - Idiopathic*: most often because of rupture of an apical bleb
    - Trauma*: blunt or penetrating injury, iatrogenic injury (e.g., central venous line placement), barotrauma (mechanical ventilation)
    - Obstructive lung disease (e.g., chronic obstructive pulmonary disease, asthma)
    - Cystic lung disease (e.g., Langerhans cell histiocytosis, lymphangiomyomatosis, tuberous sclerosis)
    - Bronchiectasis or cavitary lung disease (e.g., cystic fibrosis, tuberculosis, *Pneumocystis carinii* (*jiroveci*) pneumonia)
    - Advanced interstitial lung disease with honeycombing (e.g., usual interstitial pneumonia, sarcoidosis, chronic hypersensitivity pneumonitis)
    - Adult respiratory distress syndrome (ARDS)
    - Endometriosis (e.g., catamenial pneumothorax)
    - Bronchopulmonary fistula (e.g., after lung surgery or transplantation)

17. When should treatment of a patient with a pneumothorax be considered?

    Many pneumothoraces resolve spontaneously, and only patients at risk for complications of the pneumothorax require intervention. Generally, treatment with thoracostomy is necessary if the patient has respiratory compromise as a result of the pneumothorax. Findings such as shortness of breath, dyspnea, hypoxemia, or hypotension indicate the need for drainage of the pneumothorax. If the pneumothorax increases in size on serial chest radiographs, treatment also may become necessary. If clinical and radiographic findings indicate a tension pneumothorax, decompression and drainage of the pneumothorax are necessary. Finally, most patients receiving positive-pressure ventilation require chest tube drainage because of the increased risk of developing a tension pneumothorax.

18. How is the diagnosis of an empyema obtained?

    Diagnosis is made when pleural fluid is grossly purulent, when pleural fluid has a positive Gram stain or culture, or when the white blood cell count is greater than $5 \times 10^9$ cells per liter. Anaerobic bacteria, usually streptococci or gram-negative rods, are responsible in about 75% of cases. Chest radiographic findings of empyema are similar to findings of other loculated pleural fluid collections. CT findings may include increased attenuation of the fluid caused by protein, cells, or hemorrhage; septations and loculation; foci of very low attenuation gas; thickened enhancing pleural surfaces (the "split-pleura" sign); or increased attenuation of the extrapleural fat (Figure 21-4). MRI findings

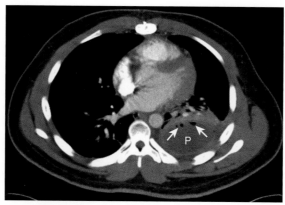

**Figure 21-4.** Empyema on CT. Note ovoid loculated pleural effusion (*P*) in left hemithorax surrounded by thickened enhancing visceral and parietal pleural surfaces ("split pleura" sign) and containing nondependent very low attenuation foci of gas (*arrows*). Note higher attenuation mild passive left lower lobe atelectasis of lung anterior to empyema.

may include increased signal intensity of the fluid on T1-weighted images, decreased signal intensity of the fluid on T2-weighted images, very low signal intensity foci of gas, internal septations, and thickened enhancing pleural surfaces.

19. When is empyema usually treated?
Empyemas with pH <7 or a glucose level <40 mg/dL may require thoracostomy. If simple drainage fails or if a fibrinous peel forms on the lung, decortication is usually curative.

20. What is empyema necessitatis?
Empyema necessitatis is an uncommon complication of an empyema in which the inflammatory process within the pleural space decompresses and extends into the soft tissues of the chest wall, forming a subcutaneous abscess, which may or may not communicate directly with the skin surface. The most common etiologic factor is tuberculosis, and the most common clinical presentation is a palpable mass in the chest wall, sometimes with a cutaneous fistula. This extension into the chest wall usually is not evident on chest radiographs but may be detected with CT or MRI of the thorax.

21. List causes of pleural calcification.
• Chronic infection/inflammation (tuberculosis, empyema)
• Chronic hemothorax
• Asbestos exposure

22. What are pleural plaques?
Pleural plaques are collections of hyalinized collagen in the parietal pleura, and are a common benign finding of prior asbestos exposure. These are virtually pathognomonic for confirming prior asbestos exposure, and typically appear more than 20 years after such exposure. When noncalcified, they appear as small plateau-shaped areas of pleural thickening when seen in profile and may mimic pulmonary nodules when seen en face. They often calcify, however. When visualized tangentially on a chest radiograph, a linear or curvilinear calcification along the pleural surface is seen, whereas when seen en face, irregular linear, stippled, or geographic calcification overlying the hemithorax is seen (Figure 21-5).

23. What is malignant pleural mesothelioma?
Malignant pleural mesothelioma is an uncommon neoplasm that arises from the parietal pleura or, rarely, from the pericardium or peritoneum. Histologic subtypes include epithelioid, sarcomatoid (fibrous), and mixed (biphasic), with epithelioid being the most common. About 2000 to 3000 new cases are diagnosed in the United States each year. This is the most common primary pleural malignancy, and its incidence has been increasing over the past 30 years.

24. What are risk factors for the development of malignant pleural mesothelioma?
Exposure to asbestos is the most important risk factor (amphibole fibers, including crocidolite and amosite, are the most potent causes). Other asbestos-related minerals and simian virus 40 (SV40) are also risk factors. About 80% of cases occur in patients with a history of asbestos exposure, with a lifetime risk of 10%. The latency period after exposure is an average of 40 years, with a range of approximately 15 to 65 years.

25. Describe symptoms and signs of malignant pleural mesothelioma.
Nonspecific dull chest or shoulder pain, shortness of breath, dyspnea, dry cough, fatigue, weight loss, digital clubbing, hypertrophic osteoarthropathy, superior vena cava syndrome, lymphadenopathy, chest wall masses, dysrhythmias, pleural effusion, pericardial effusion, ascites, or bowel obstruction due to spread to the peritoneal cavity may be seen.

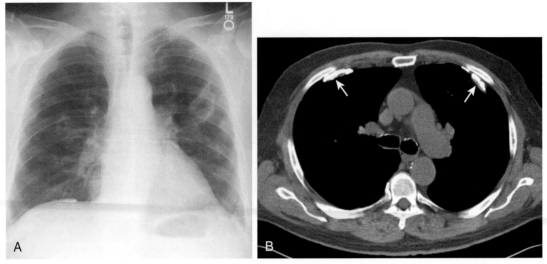

**Figure 21-5. A,** Calcified asbestos-related pleural plaques on frontal chest radiograph. Note linear or curvilinear dense calcifications along inferior aspects of hemithoraces (seen tangentially) and irregular geographic calcifications overlying hemithoraces (seen en face). **B,** Calcified asbestos-related pleural plaques on CT. Note curvilinear dense calcifications (*arrows*) along anterior pleural surfaces.

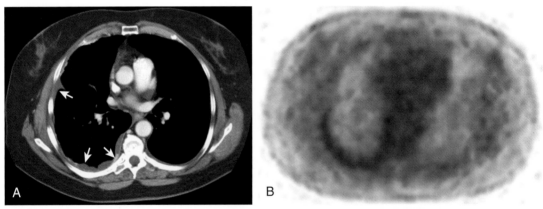

**Figure 21-6. A,** Malignant pleural mesothelioma on CT. Note small right loculated pleural effusion (*arrows*) with several areas of nodular pleural thickening. **B,** Malignant pleural mesothelioma on FDG PET. Note avid FDG uptake in peripheral right hemithorax corresponding to abnormalities on CT.

Chest wall pain is an important sign of chest wall involvement by tumor. Malignant pleural mesothelioma should be considered in any patient with either pleural effusion or pleural thickening, especially if chest pain is present.

26. What are the imaging findings of malignant pleural mesothelioma?
    The most common chest radiographic finding of malignant pleural mesothelioma is a loculated pleural effusion. Unilateral pleural masses and plaquelike or nodular, irregular pleural thickening with encasement of the entire lung are also common findings that are highly suggestive of mesothelioma. Extension into the interlobar fissures, lung, mediastinum, chest wall, diaphragm, and biopsy tracts may occur. As a result of constriction of the lung by adherent pleural tumor, ipsilateral volume loss of the hemithorax with ipsilateral mediastinal shift, narrowing of the intercostal spaces, and elevation of the ipsilateral hemidiaphragm are commonly present. Pleural calcification resulting from prior asbestos exposure is seen in two thirds of cases, and intrathoracic lymphadenopathy, extension to the peritoneum or retroperitoneum, and hematogenous metastases anywhere in body may be seen on CT or MRI in later stages. Increased FDG uptake is commonly observed on $^{18}$F-fluorodeoxyglucose positron emission tomography (FDG PET) (Figure 21-6).

27. What diagnostic tests may be used in the diagnosis or staging of malignant pleural mesothelioma?
    Chest radiography, CT, MRI, FDG PET, ultrasonography (US), thoracentesis, and biopsy are used in the diagnosis or staging of malignant pleural mesothelioma. Chest radiographs may sometimes appear normal, and negative pleural

biopsy and cytology results do not exclude mesothelioma. US, CT, and FDG PET scanning may be used to guide biopsy, however, and increase diagnostic yield. CT and MRI are nearly equivalent in staging accuracy, although MRI is superior to CT for detection of diaphragmatic, endothoracic fascial, or focal chest wall invasion and is often used as a problem-solving tool after CT. FDG PET is also very useful for staging and preoperative evaluation and has increased accuracy for detecting malignant lymphadenopathy or occult extrathoracic metastases. Tumor metabolic activity on FDG PET and patient survival are inversely proportional.

28. **What is the prognosis for malignant pleural mesothelioma?**
Prognosis is generally poor, with a median survival of 8 to 18 months because the tumor is generally progressive. Favorable prognostic factors include limited extent of disease and an epithelioid histologic subtype. Unfavorable prognostic factors include sarcomatoid or mixed histologic subtypes; more advanced stages of disease, such as with intrathoracic lymphadenopathy; extensive pleural involvement; distant metastatic disease; and older age.

29. **Describe the general treatment approach to malignant pleural mesothelioma.**
Radical surgery (either radical pleurectomy-decortication or extrapleural pneumonectomy with removal of the pleura, mediastinal lymph nodes, ipsilateral pericardium, and diaphragm) is considered when there is tumor without lymphadenopathy. Radiotherapy, chemotherapy, and photodynamic therapy may also be used with surgery as adjuvant treatments. Talc pleurodesis or video-assisted thoracoscopic pleurectomy may also be used to control pleural effusions and are less invasive than open pleurectomy and decortication. Radiotherapy may be used palliatively to relieve pain in about 50% of cases or can be used prophylactically at biopsy sites to prevent seeding by tumor. Pain medications are used as needed.

30. **What is solitary fibrous tumor of the pleura?**
Solitary fibrous tumor of the pleura is a rare mesenchymal neoplasm that most commonly affects the pleura, uncommonly affects the lungs and mediastinum, and rarely involves extrathoracic sites. It is unrelated to asbestos exposure and may be either benign (about 90%) or malignant (about 10%). Most patients present in the fifth through eighth decades of life and have a much better prognosis than patients with malignant pleural mesothelioma. Of these neoplasms, 80% arise from the visceral pleura, and 20% arise from the parietal pleura, although a few are intrapulmonary in location. Of neoplasms, 20% to 50% are pedunculated, and they are composed of spindle-shaped, fibroblast-like cells with a variable amount of collagenous stroma, vascularity, and myxoid or cystic degeneration.

31. **Name clinical presentations of solitary fibrous tumor of the pleura.**
Of solitary fibrous tumors of the pleura, 50% may be asymptomatic. Symptoms and signs, when present, may include cough, dyspnea, hemoptysis, chest pain, and sensation of a mass. Paraneoplastic syndromes, such as hypoglycemia, digital clubbing, and hypertrophic osteoarthropathy, are uncommon but may be associated with an intrathoracic mass.

32. **What are the imaging features of solitary fibrous tumor of the pleura?**
Typically, a well-defined, usually sharply marginated, lobulated, and solitary mass is identified within the thorax adjacent to the chest wall or diaphragm (Figure 21-7). It may be very small or very large. When large, a solitary fibrous tumor of the pleura can fill the inferior aspect of the hemithorax and mimic an elevated hemidiaphragm on a chest radiograph. The tumor is typically connected to the chest wall by a thin pedicle or stalk. Changes in patient positioning, such as with decubitus radiographs, may result in changes in position of the mass within the thorax. On CT or MRI, intense enhancement, myxoid or cystic degeneration, hemorrhage, or calcification may be seen, and no

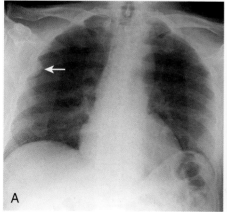
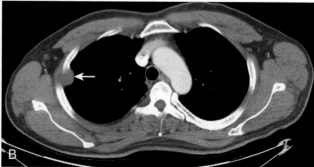

**Figure 21-7. A,** Solitary fibrous tumor of pleura on frontal chest radiograph. Note small, well-defined, sharply marginated solitary lesion (*arrow*) within right hemithorax forming obtuse angle margins with adjacent chest wall. **B,** Solitary fibrous tumor of pleura on CT. Note small, well-defined, sharply marginated soft tissue attenuation lesion (*arrow*) within right hemithorax forming obtuse angle margins with adjacent chest wall.

imaging findings other than presence of metastatic disease can help differentiate between benignancy and malignancy of the lesion.

33. What is the treatment for solitary fibrous tumor of the pleura?

Treatment involves surgical resection, which is often curative, although some patients have local recurrence, malignant transformation, or distant metastatic disease. Complete surgical excision is overall the best prognostic indicator.

## KEY POINTS

- If a pneumothorax is seen on chest radiography that is associated with contralateral mediastinal shift and inferior displacement of the ipsilateral hemidiaphragm, the physician caring for the patient must be notified immediately because a tension pneumothorax may be present, requiring emergent treatment to prevent rapid death.
- Malignant pleural mesothelioma is the most common primary malignancy of the pleura and is most often related to prior asbestos exposure.
- Malignant pleural mesothelioma should be considered in any patient with either pleural effusion or pleural thickening, especially if chest pain is present.
- Normal chest radiography and negative pleural biopsy and cytology results do not exclude malignant pleural mesothelioma.
- Paraneoplastic syndromes—such as hypoglycemia, digital clubbing, and hypertrophic osteoarthropathy—may suggest the diagnosis of solitary fibrous tumor of the pleura when associated with an intrathoracic mass.

**BIBLIOGRAPHY**

Nickell LT Jr, Lichtenberger JP 3rd, Khorashadi L, et al. Multimodality imaging for characterization, classification, and staging of malignant pleural mesothelioma. *Radiographics.* 2014;34(6):1692-1706.

Vilstrup MH, Torigian DA. FDG PET in thoracic malignancies. *PET Clin.* 2014;9(4):391-420.

Armato SG 3rd, Labby ZE, Coolen J, et al. Imaging in pleural mesothelioma: a review of the 11th International Conference of the International Mesothelioma Interest Group. *Lung Cancer.* 2013;82(2):190-196.

Kwee TC, Torigian DA, Alavi A. Oncological applications of positron emission tomography for evaluation of the thorax. *J Thorac Imaging.* 2013;28(1):11-24.

Truong MT, Viswanathan C, Godoy MB, et al. Malignant pleural mesothelioma: role of CT, MRI, and PET/CT in staging evaluation and treatment considerations. *Semin Roentgenol.* 2013;48(4):323-334.

Hussein-Jelen T, Bankier AA, Eisenberg RL. Solid pleural lesions. *AJR Am J Roentgenol.* 2012;198(6):W512-W520.

Makis W, Ciarallo A, Hickeson M, et al. Spectrum of malignant pleural and pericardial disease on FDG PET/CT. *AJR Am J Roentgenol.* 2012;198(3):678-685.

Myers R. Asbestos-related pleural disease. *Curr Opin Pulm Med.* 2012;18(4):377-381.

Weldon E, Williams J. Pleural disease in the emergency department. *Emerg Med Clin North Am.* 2012;30(2):475-499, ix-x.

Ginat DT, Bokhari A, Bhatt S, et al. Imaging features of solitary fibrous tumors. *AJR Am J Roentgenol.* 2011;196(3):487-495.

Light RW. Pleural effusions. *Med Clin North Am.* 2011;95(6):1055-1070.

Ayres J, Gleeson F. Imaging of the pleura. *Semin Respir Crit Care Med.* 2010;31(6):674-688.

Jeong YJ, Kim S, Kwak SW, et al. Neoplastic and nonneoplastic conditions of serosal membrane origin: CT findings. *Radiographics.* 2008;28(3):801-817, discussion 817-18; quiz 912.

Qureshi NR, Gleeson FV. Imaging of pleural disease. *Clin Chest Med.* 2006;27(2):193-213.

Rosado-de-Christenson ML, Abbott GF, McAdams HP, et al. From the archives of the AFIP: localized fibrous tumor of the pleura. *Radiographics.* 2003;23(3):759-783.

Sahn SA, Heffner JE. Spontaneous pneumothorax. *N Engl J Med.* 2000;342(12):868-874.

# TUBES, LINES, CATHETERS, AND OTHER DEVICES

Drew A. Torigian, MD, MA, FSAR, and Charles T. Lau, MD, MBA

1. **What is the radiographic appearance of an endotracheal tube (ETT), and where is it optimally placed?**

   An ETT usually appears as a faintly radiopaque tube with a thin, densely radiopaque line along its length, and its position should be determined relative to the carina, which if not seen on a chest radiograph can be approximated by following the course of the mainstem bronchi medially at the T5-T7 level. In adults, the tip of an ETT should be below the thoracic inlet and approximately 5 to 7 cm above the carina when the patient's head is in neutral position, as flexion or extension of the neck can cause the tube to move either 2 cm higher or lower, respectively. The optimal width of the tube should be one half to two thirds of the tracheal width (generally <3 cm), and the inflated cuff should not distend the trachea because tracheal injury may occur.

2. **Describe how an ETT may be malpositioned; list other potential complications of ETT placement.**

   If an ETT is inserted beyond the carina (i.e., with unilateral bronchial intubation), preferential hyperaeration and potential barotrauma of the intubated lung (more commonly the right) and hypoaeration and atelectasis of the contralateral lung may occur (Figure 22-1). If the tube is not advanced far enough, inadvertent extubation or possible vocal cord damage caused by the inflated cuff may occur. Esophageal intubation is another potential complication, which can be detected clinically by gurgling sounds and distention of the stomach as air is insufflated and radiographically by lateral extension of the tube margins beyond the tracheal margins, visualization of the tracheal air column to the side of the tube, gastric distention, and lung hypoinflation. Other complications of ETT placement include:
   - Pharyngeal, laryngeal, or tracheobronchial injury (particularly if placed too high or if the cuff is overinflated).
   - Aspiration.
   - Sinusitis.
   - Dislodgment of teeth or dental appliances.

3. **What is the optimal positioning of a tracheostomy tube?**

   A tracheostomy tube tip is optimally located one half to two thirds of the distance from the stoma to the carina. The tube itself should overlie the trachea, and the width of the tube should be about two thirds of the tracheal width.

4. **Name potential complications after tracheostomy tube placement.**
   - Injury of the recurrent laryngeal nerve with resultant vocal cord paralysis.
   - Injury of the lung apex with development of pneumothorax or pneumomediastinum.
   - Injury of the trachea with development of tracheomalacia or stricture.
   - Soft tissue infection, leading to tracheal ulceration and perforation with tracheal–innominate artery fistula, tracheoesophageal fistula, or cervical abscess formation.

5. **What is the radiographic appearance and ideal positioning of a nasogastric tube (NGT) or orogastric tube (OGT)?**

   An NGT or OGT usually appears as a faintly radiopaque tube with a thin, densely radiopaque line along the entire length of the tube (Figure 22-2). Unlike an ETT, the thin, densely radiopaque line is interrupted near the distal tip of the NGT/OGT, representing a distal side hole. The tube should course inferiorly along the midline of the chest, with its tip located at least 10 cm within the stomach so that the distal side hole is situated in the stomach rather than in the esophagus.

6. **Describe the radiographic appearance and optimal location of an enteral feeding tube.**

   An enteral feeding tube usually appears as a faintly radiopaque tube, though without a thin, densely radiopaque line along its length (seen with ETTs, NGTs, and OGTs). Compared to NGT/OGTs, enteral feeding tubes are more narrow in caliber. Some, but not all, enteral feeding tubes have a radiopaque marker at their tip. The optimal location of an enteral feeding tube tip is beyond the gastric pylorus within the duodenum, optimally at the duodenojejunal junction (ligament of Treitz). On a frontal radiograph, the tube generally curves to follow the C-shaped loop of the duodenum, and on a lateral radiograph, the tube curves posteriorly from the gastric antrum and first portion of the duodenum as it enters the retroperitoneal second portion of the duodenum (Figure 22-3).

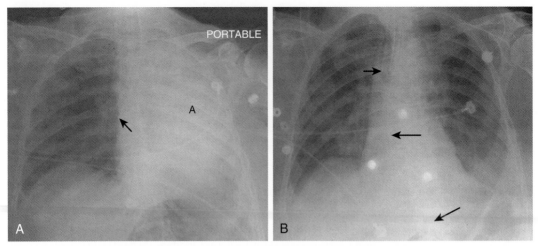

**Figure 22-1.** **A,** Malpositioned ETT on frontal chest radiograph. Note tip of ETT within proximal right mainstem bronchus (*arrow*) with complete atelectasis (*A*) of left lung. **B,** Repositioning of ETT on frontal chest radiograph. Note tip of ETT (*arrow*) now appropriately positioned within distal trachea with resolution of previously noted left lung atelectasis. Also note the normal course of newly placed NGT (*long arrows*), which follows expected course of esophagus before entering abdomen.

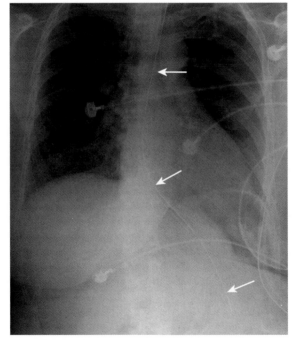

**Figure 22-2.** Appropriately positioned NGT on frontal radiograph. Note thin radiopaque curvilinear strip along entire length of NGT (*arrows*), which extends inferiorly along midline of chest in expected location of esophagus with tip overlying expected location of stomach.

7. Discuss ways in which an NGT, OGT, or feeding tube may be malpositioned, including other potential complications.

Coiling within the pharynx or esophagus may occur even if the tip of the tube is in the appropriate position; this may sometimes induce vomiting and subsequent aspiration (Figure 22-4). Vomiting and aspiration may also occur if the tip is situated above the gastroesophageal junction. With tracheobronchial placement, a tube follows the course of the trachea and bronchi; lung perforation and entry into the pleural space can occasionally occur, leading to intrabronchial or intrapleural infusion of feedings, pneumonia, lung abscess, empyema, hydropneumothorax, or pneumothorax (Figure 22-5). Esophageal perforation is a rare but serious complication. However, extraesophageal tube placement is difficult to detect on a frontal radiograph unless other views or water-soluble contrast agent injection are performed, which may show a tube that does not follow the expected course of the esophagus, a widened mediastinum,

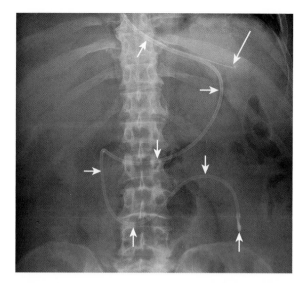

**Figure 22-3.** Appropriately positioned feeding tube on frontal abdominal radiograph. Note feeding tube (*short arrows*) that curves to follow C-shaped loop of duodenum with radiopaque marker at tip overlying expected located of duodenojejunal junction (ligament of Treitz). Also note appropriately positioned tip of NGT (*long arrow*) overlying expected location of stomach in left upper quadrant of abdomen with thin radiopaque curvilinear strip along its visualized portion.

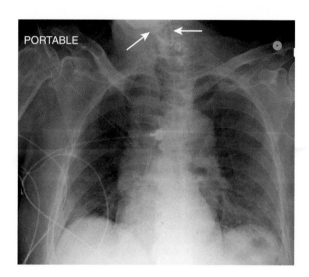

**Figure 22-4.** Malpositioned feeding tube on frontal chest radiograph. Note portion of feeding tube (*arrows*) curled within pharynx and upper thoracic esophagus.

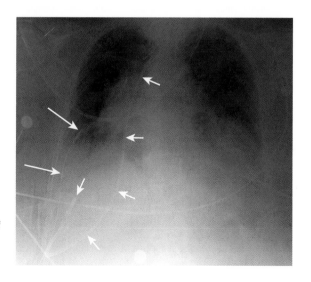

**Figure 22-5.** Malpositioned feeding tube on frontal chest radiograph. Note feeding tube (*short arrows*) following course of right bronchi and terminating in inferior right hemithorax within pleural space. Also note right thoracostomy tube (*long arrows*) within right pleural space to drain complex pleural fluid.

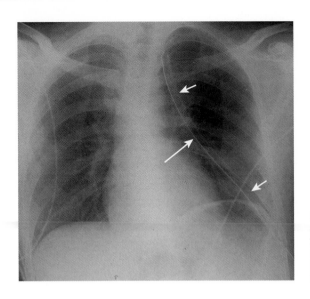

**Figure 22-6.** Appropriately positioned thoracostomy tube for pneumothorax on frontal chest radiograph. Note gentle curve of thoracostomy tube (*short arrows*) with curvilinear radiopaque stripe and short-segment interruption because of side hole (*long arrow*) with tip located near lung apex directed anterosuperiorly.

pneumomediastinum, a unilateral pleural effusion, or contrast agent leak from the esophagus into other thoracic compartments.

8. If an NGT, OGT, or feeding tube is misplaced within the tracheobronchial tree, what should one do before removing the tube?
One should have a thoracostomy tube set ready at the patient's bedside before removing the tube, in case the tube has entered the pleural space and a pneumothorax suddenly develops when the tube is removed.

9. When is a thoracostomy tube generally used?
A thoracostomy tube is usually placed for drainage of air (pneumothorax), particularly when persistent (i.e., with a bronchopleural fistula), large, increasing, or symptomatic (i.e., under tension). Thoracostomy tubes are also placed for drainage of fluid (pleural effusion), blood (hemothorax), chylous fluid (chylothorax), or pus (empyema) from the pleural space. They are also sometimes placed for drainage of a lung abscess.

10. What is the radiographic appearance of a thoracostomy tube, and where should its tip be located?
A thoracostomy tube usually appears as a faintly radiopaque tube with a thin, densely radiopaque line along the entire length of the tube. Similar to an NGT/OGT, the thin, densely radiopaque line is interrupted near the tip of the thoracostomy, representing the site of a side hole. Thoracostomy tubes should curve gently within the thorax (Figure 22-6), because kinks may prevent appropriate drainage. For drainage of a pneumothorax, the tube should be positioned near the lung apex at the anterior axillary line and directed anterosuperiorly, whereas for drainage of a pleural effusion, the tube may be positioned at the midaxillary line and directed posteroinferiorly through the sixth through eighth intercostal spaces. In either case, the side hole should always be located medial to the ribs within the pleural space and not within the chest wall. Computed tomography (CT) is indicated when a thoracostomy tube does not drain air or fluid properly, and the chest radiograph is noncontributory.

11. Discuss potential complications of thoracostomy tube placement.
Persistent pneumothorax and extensive subcutaneous emphysema may occur if side holes are located external to the rib cage and pleural space (Figure 22-7). Lung laceration (Figure 22-8) with bronchopleural fistula may also occur with a persistent pneumothorax, pneumomediastinum, or extensive subcutaneous emphysema and is more commonly seen with preexisting lung disease or pleural adhesions. Laceration or injury of an intercostal artery, phrenic nerve, thoracic duct, diaphragm, liver, spleen, stomach, mediastinum, heart, breast, or pectoralis muscle may also occur. Placement within an interlobar fissure is common, which may cause poor tube function, and is best seen on CT. Soft tissue or pleural infection may occur adjacent to the tube insertion site. Unilateral reexpansion pulmonary edema may be seen with rapid pleural decompression, and rapid development of an infiltrate at the tip or side holes may be due to pulmonary infarction from suction of lung tissue. High insertion in the posterior chest wall may lead to Horner syndrome, and recurrence of a pleural collection, pleurocutaneous fistula, or retention of a tube fragment are potential complications after tube removal.

12. How can I decrease the chance of injury to an intercostal artery or vein during thoracostomy tube placement?
Place the tube just superior to a rib to avoid the neurovascular bundle that is located near the inferior aspect of each rib.

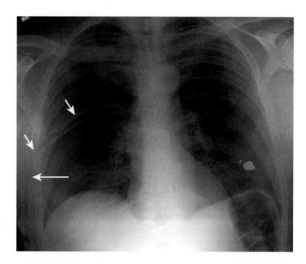

**Figure 22-7.** Malpositioned thoracostomy tube on frontal chest radiograph. Note thoracostomy tube (*short arrow*) with side hole (*long arrow*) located external to rib cage.

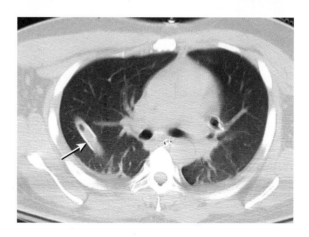

**Figure 22-8.** Malpositioned thoracostomy tube on CT. Note thoracostomy tube (*arrow*) located within right lung parenchyma instead of pleural space.

13. Describe the basic normal venous anatomy of the chest.

The deeply situated brachial veins and the superficially situated basilic and cephalic veins of the upper extremities converge centrally to form the axillary veins. The axillary veins become the subclavian veins at the lateral aspects of the first ribs. The superficially situated external jugular veins drain from the neck into the subclavian veins. More centrally, the subclavian veins and the internal jugular veins from the neck converge to form the brachiocephalic veins (longer on the left than on the right), which then join to form the superior vena cava (SVC), finally leading to the right atrium. The vertical segment of the azygos vein is located to the right of the thoracic spine and drains superiorly toward its horizontal segment, which enters the posterior SVC above the right mainstem bronchus. The hemiazygos venous system is located toward the left of the thoracic spine and has variable communication with the azygos system.

14. What is the radiographic appearance and optimal location of a central venous line (CVL) and a peripherally inserted central catheter (PICC)?

A CVL appears as a thin, moderately radiopaque linear or curvilinear tube that usually extends centrally from a subclavian or internal jugular vein when in the chest (Figure 22-9), whereas a PICC appears as a thin radiopaque curvilinear tube that extends from the upper extremity (because it is placed peripherally within the lower arm or upper forearm usually via the basilic vein) centrally into the chest. The optimal location of the tip of a CVL and PICC is within the lower third of the SVC or at the junction of the SVC and right atrium.

15. What are potential complications of CVL or PICC placement?

An early complication of CVL insertion is pneumothorax, which is more commonly encountered in subclavian approaches. Early complications of CVL or PICC placement include malpositioning within a vein or artery or in the heart; arterial injury with pseudoaneurysm formation or thromboembolism; venous injury; perforation through a vein with extravascular malpositioning in the pleural space, mediastinum, or soft tissue; cardiac injury with risk of myocardial perforation and cardiac tamponade; hemorrhage or hematoma; air embolism; and catheter knotting, fracture, and embolism. Late complications include catheter occlusion, migration, knotting, fracture, and embolism;

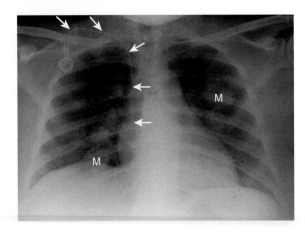

**Figure 22-9.** Appropriately positioned chemoport CVL for history of uterine sarcoma on frontal chest radiograph. Note thin, moderately radiopaque curvilinear tube (*arrows*) that overlies right internal jugular vein with tip overlying caval-atrial junction. Also note multiple pulmonary nodules and masses (*M*) in lungs due to metastases.

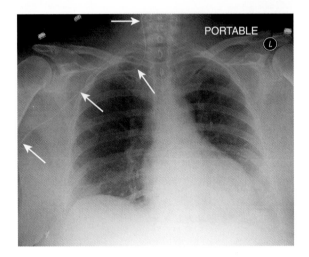

**Figure 22-10.** Malpositioned PICC on frontal chest radiograph. Note right PICC (*arrows*) seen as thin radiopaque curvilinear tube extending from right upper extremity into right neck overlying expected location of right internal jugular vein.

venous thrombosis; central venous stenosis; soft tissue infection; bacteremia/septicemia; and cardiac dysrhythmias, which usually occur with low right atrial placement.

16. List locations where a CVL or PICC may be malpositioned when inserted through a vein.
    For a PICC or subclavian vein CVL, malpositioning may occur in the ipsilateral internal jugular vein (Figure 22-10); contralateral brachiocephalic vein; contralateral subclavian vein; internal jugular vein; right atrium; right ventricle; pulmonary artery; inferior vena cava; hepatic vein; azygos vein; or central venous collaterals, including the external jugular vein, inferior thyroidal vein, superior intercostal vein, internal thoracic vein, or pericardiacophrenic vein.
    For an internal jugular vein CVL, malpositioning within the ipsilateral subclavian vein may also occur. Intracardiac malpositioning of a CVL inserted via the subclavian vein approach is more common when inserted on the right (30%) than on the left (12%).

17. Name some clues of inadvertent arterial puncture with a CVL, PICC, or Swan-Ganz catheter (SGC).
    At the time of catheter placement, bright red and pulsatile backflow of blood may be seen, although in patients with hypoxia or hypotension, the blood may be nonpulsatile and dark, mimicking venous blood. On a chest radiograph, arterial location of a catheter should be suspected when the course of the catheter follows the expected course of an artery rather than a vein or when the tip is located in a midsternal or left paravertebral location. Confirmation of an arterial puncture may be performed by analysis of blood gas levels of blood samples drawn through the catheter.

18. What should one consider in the differential diagnosis for rapid development of an ipsilateral pleural effusion or mediastinal widening after CVL, PICC, or SGC placement?
    Rapid development of an ipsilateral pleural effusion or mediastinal widening after venous catheter placement should make one consider (1) perforation of a vein by the catheter, with the tip located in the pleural space or mediastinum after catheter infusion, or (2) vessel injury by the catheter with associated hemothorax or mediastinal hematoma. Associated pneumothorax may occur with vessel injury in this setting.

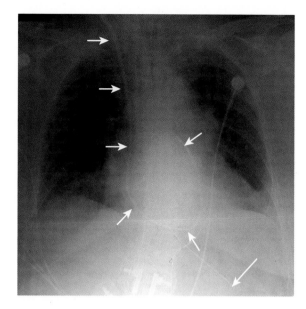

**Figure 22-11.** Appropriately positioned SGC on frontal chest radiograph. Note thin, moderately radiopaque curvilinear tube (*short arrows*) that overlies right internal jugular vein in neck and successively follows course of right brachiocephalic vein, SVC, right atrium, right ventricle, and pulmonary outflow tract, with tip located over main pulmonary artery. Also note appropriately positioned tip of NGT overlying stomach in left upper quadrant of abdomen (*long arrow*).

19. If air embolism is suspected during catheter placement, what should one do to treat the patient?

    When air embolism is suspected (usually when a sucking sound during patient inspiration is heard through a catheter at the time of placement or if inadvertent injection of air through a catheter occurs), the patient should immediately be placed in the left lateral decubitus position (i.e., left side down) to keep the air trapped in the right heart chambers, supplemental oxygen should be administered, and vital signs should be monitored.

20. How do I prevent air embolism during catheter placement in the first place?

    Air embolism during line placement can be reduced by keeping a finger over the open end of the catheter until the catheter is flushed with saline and capped.

21. Describe the radiographic appearance of an SGC and its optimal location.

    SGC (or pulmonary arterial catheter) appears as a thin, moderately radiopaque curvilinear tube that originates centrally from a subclavian or internal jugular vein and passes successively through the brachiocephalic vein, SVC, right atrium, right ventricle, and pulmonary outflow tract, with its tip optimally located in the main, right, or left pulmonary artery or within a proximal lobar pulmonary arterial branch (Figure 22-11). SGCs are occasionally inserted via a femoral vein approach, entering the right atrium via the inferior vena cava (IVC). When the balloon at the catheter tip is inflated for pulmonary capillary wedge pressure measurement, a 1-cm round radiolucency at the catheter tip may be seen radiographically. A thin, short linear tubular radiopacity is also generally seen at the skin entry site, which is the vascular sheath that surrounds the SGC. The SGC can be removed while the sheath still remains in place.

22. What are potential complications of SGC placement?

    Potential complications of SGC placement include the complications listed previously for CVL or PICC placement and malpositioning within the right atrium, right ventricle, pulmonary outflow tract, or peripheral pulmonary arterial branch; coiling within cardiac chambers (Figure 22-12) with associated cardiac injury, thrombus formation, or atrial or ventricular cardiac dysrhythmias; tricuspid or pulmonic valve injury; pulmonary arterial injury/rupture, occasionally with formation of either a pseudoaneurysm or a pulmonary artery to bronchial fistula; pulmonary thromboembolism; and pulmonary infarction.

23. Why can pulmonary infarction occur as a complication of SGC placement?

    Pulmonary infarction with SGC placement results from obstruction of pulmonary blood flow because of tip placement too peripherally within a pulmonary arterial branch or persistent inflation of the balloon at the catheter tip. Generally, the extent of pulmonary infarction is directly related to the caliber of the occluded vessel and to the portions of lung supplied by it. In general, if the tip of the SGC is situated more than 2 cm lateral to the pulmonary hilum on a frontal chest radiograph, it may be too peripheral in location and should be pulled back. The balloon should be inflated only during the measurement of wedge pressures.

24. How does an intraaortic counterpulsation balloon (IACB) work?

    An IACB is inserted percutaneously via the common femoral artery and subsequently passes through the external iliac artery, common iliac artery, and abdominal aorta to reach the descending thoracic aorta. A long, inflatable balloon is situated around the distal catheter segment and cyclically inflated during early diastole and deflated during early

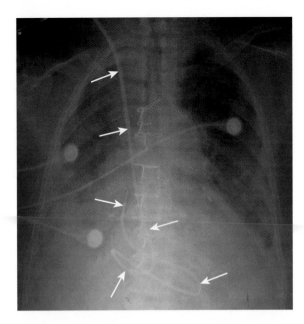

**Figure 22-12.** Malpositioned SGC on frontal chest radiograph. Note SGC (*arrows*) curled over right heart with tip overlying superior aspect of right atrium.

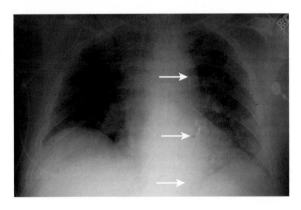

**Figure 22-13.** Appropriately positioned IACB on frontal chest radiograph. Note linear radiopaque IACB (*arrows*) overlying descending thoracic aorta to left of midline with small radiopaque rectangle at tip overlying proximal descending thoracic aorta inferior to aortic knob.

systole of each cardiac cycle. This helps to increase myocardial oxygenation and decrease myocardial oxygenation demand, mainly through improved coronary and peripheral arterial blood flow and decreased cardiac afterload.

25. **What are the major indications and contraindications for placement of IACB?**
    An IACB is often used in critically ill patients with left ventricular failure, unstable angina, acute myocardial ischemia/infarction associated with percutaneous transluminal angioplasty, or severe mitral regurgitation. Major contraindications to IACB placement include severe aortic insufficiency, aortic dissection, severe peripheral vascular disease, or contraindication to systemic anticoagulation.

26. **Describe the radiographic appearance of an IACB and its optimal position.**
    An IACB usually appears as a thin tube coursing vertically, just left of midline, along the expected course of the descending thoracic aorta. A small, radiopaque rectangle is usually visible at the tip of an IACB on a frontal chest radiograph and should be located just distal to the left subclavian artery within the proximal descending thoracic aorta below the level of the aortic knob (Figure 22-13).

27. **What are the potential complications of IACB?**
    Potential complications include arterial injury and hemorrhage; aortic dissection; arterial thromboembolism with associated limb, visceral, or cerebral ischemia; malpositioning within the aorta proximal to the left subclavian artery or far distal to the aortic arch; venous malpositioning; balloon rupture with potential air embolism if helium gas is used for balloon inflation; thrombocytopenia; soft tissue infection or hematoma formation at the percutaneous site of insertion; or bacteremia/septicemia. If the balloon is situated upstream from the left subclavian artery origin, potential occlusion of the arterial branch vessels of the aortic arch (i.e., innominate, left common carotid, and left subclavian arteries) is possible. When the balloon is located too far downstream from the aortic arch, counterpulsation is less effective, and potential occlusion of the visceral branch vessels is also possible.

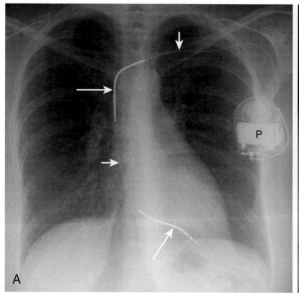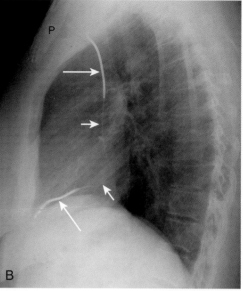

**Figure 22-14. A,** Appropriately positioned AICD on frontal chest radiograph. Note power/generator pack (*P*) over left pectoral area as radiopaque ovoid structure connected to thin curvilinear metallic lead (*short arrow*) with tip overlying right ventricular apex to left of midline. Also note thicker, short segments of spring defibrillation coils (*long arrows*). **B,** Appropriately positioned AICD on lateral chest radiograph. Note power/generator pack (*P*) over anterior chest wall connected to thin curvilinear metallic lead (*short arrows*) with tip overlying right ventricular apex anteriorly and inferiorly. Also note thicker, short segments of spring defibrillation coils (*long arrows*).

28. What is the radiographic appearance of a transvenous pacemaker or automatic implantable cardioverter defibrillator (AICD)?

The power/generator pack for a transvenous pacemaker or AICD is located subcutaneously in the pectoral area of the anterior chest wall and appears as a radiopaque, round, ovoid, or rectangular structure that is approximately 5 cm in diameter on a frontal chest radiograph. The metallic lead or leads appear as dense, thin curvilinear radiopacities (with associated thicker short segments of spring defibrillation coils in the case of an AICD) that usually course through the subclavian or internal jugular vein from the generator pack to pass through the brachiocephalic vein and SVC, subsequently terminating in the right atrium, right ventricle, or coronary sinus (Figures 22-14 and 22-15, *A*).

29. Where should the leads of a transvenous pacemaker or AICD be located?

A right atrial lead (usually in the right atrial appendage) curves around the right side of the heart just below the SVC on a frontal chest radiograph. A right ventricular lead should project slightly to the left of midline, overlapping the ventricular apex on a frontal chest radiograph, and should project anteriorly and inferiorly near the ventricular apex on a lateral chest radiograph. A lead within the coronary sinus projects superiorly and to the left over the heart on a frontal chest radiograph and is situated posteriorly along the course of the atrioventricular groove on a lateral chest radiograph.

30. What are potential complications of transvenous pacemaker/AICD placement?

Potential complications of transvenous pacemaker/AICD placement include all of the complications of SGC, CVL, and PICC placement previously listed as well as hematoma or abscess formation around the generator pack; lead malpositioning, redundancy, tautness, dislodgment (Figure 22-15, *B*), migration, or fracture with or without embolism (Figure 22-16); twiddler's syndrome; cardiac perforation; loss of pacing or cardioversion/defibrillation function; and induction of cardiac dysrhythmias. Cardiac perforation by a lead should be suspected on a chest radiograph (particularly on the lateral view) if the lead extends beyond the margin of the cardiac silhouette.

31. What is twiddler's syndrome?

Twiddler's syndrome is an uncommon disorder that occurs when a patient causes malfunction of a transvenous pacemaker, AICD, or chest port by manipulating, or "twiddling," the subcutaneously placed pacing generator pack or port. This may be facilitated when the generator pack or chest port is situated in a large subcutaneous pocket or loose subcutaneous tissue, leading to dislodgment of the pacing leads or chest port catheter. A chest radiograph is the key to diagnosis and typically shows twisting or coiling of the lead around the axis of the pacemaker and possible lead fracture, displacement, or migration.

32. Name two retained foreign bodies that may be encountered in the postoperative setting.

Two retained foreign bodies that may be encountered in the postoperative setting are laparotomy pads (surgical sponges) and suture needles. Laparotomy pads are not radiopaque but usually have a thin ribbon-like radiopaque strip

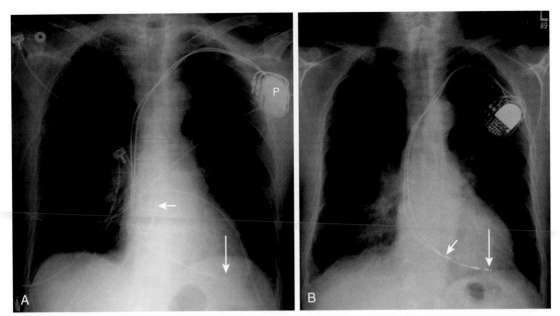

**Figure 22-15. A,** Appropriately positioned transvenous pacemaker on frontal chest radiograph. Note power/generator pack (*P*) over left pectoral area as a radiopaque ovoid structure connected to leads with tip in right atrium (*short arrow*) overlying right side of heart and tip in right ventricle (*long arrow*) overlying ventricular apex. **B,** Subsequent dislodgment of right atrial lead of transvenous pacemaker with migration to right ventricle on frontal chest radiograph. Note new position of right atrial lead (*short arrow*) compared with **A,** similar to right ventricular lead (*long arrow*).

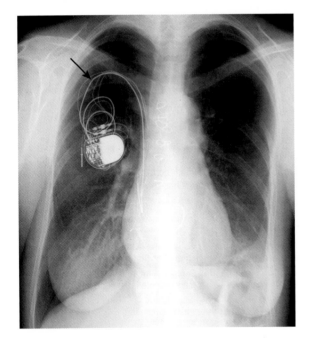

**Figure 22-16.** Fracture of pacemaker lead on frontal chest radiograph. Note discontinuity (*arrow*) of one pacemaker lead.

embedded within them so that they may be visualized on a radiograph (Figure 22-17). Suture needles usually appear as thin small curvilinear radiopacities (Figure 22-18) and can sometimes mimic the appearance of a surgical clip on a radiograph when viewed "edge-on"; therefore, two orthogonal radiographs are preferable when searching for a retained foreign body.

33. What are some procedure types and risk factors that may increase the risk of retention of a surgical foreign body?
    Abdominal surgical procedures are most commonly associated with retention of a foreign body, followed by gynecologic procedures, urologic and vascular procedures, and orthopedic and spinal procedures. In addition, complex

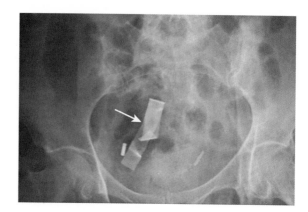

**Figure 22-17.** Retained surgical sponge on frontal pelvic radiograph. Note thin ribbon-like radiopaque strip (*arrow*) in pelvis representing embedded marker.

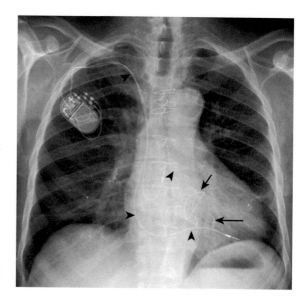

**Figure 22-18.** Retained suture needle on frontal chest radiograph. Note thin small curvilinear radiopacity (*long arrow*) representing retained surgical needle. Also note right subclavian dual-chambered pacemaker with leads in right atrium and right ventricle (*arrowheads*), mitral annuloplasty ring (*short arrow*), and median sternotomy wires.

surgical procedures (e.g., involving more than one surgical team, a large number of instruments/instrument sets, or surgery upon more than one body cavity), damage control procedures, emergency surgical procedures, and prolonged surgical procedures increase the risk of a retained foreign body. The risk also increases with increasing body mass index of the patient.

34. What are the potential complications of retained foreign bodies?
    Potential complications associated with retained foreign bodies may vary but include infection (leading to events such as abscess formation or sepsis), erosion or perforation of adjacent vessels or organs, fistulization to other organs or skin, bleeding, inflammation/fibrosis, and pain. Sometimes, retained foreign bodies may be asymptomatic.

**KEY POINTS**

- If an NGT, OGT, or feeding tube is seen to extend into a distal bronchus, lung, or pleural space, the clinical staff should be notified immediately, and the radiologist should suggest that tube removal be performed only after a thoracostomy tube set is at the bedside in case a significant pneumothorax develops.
- Rapid development of an ipsilateral pleural effusion or mediastinal widening after venous catheter placement should lead one to consider venous perforation, with the tip located in the pleural space or mediastinum after catheter infusion, or vessel injury with associated hemithorax or mediastinal hematoma.
- When air embolism is suspected during line placement or use, the patient should immediately be placed in the left lateral position to keep the air trapped in the right heart chambers, supplemental oxygen should be administered, and vital signs should be monitored.

## BIBLIOGRAPHY

Nayeemuddin M, Pherwani AD, Asquith JR. Imaging and management of complications of central venous catheters. *Clin Radiol.* 2013;68(5):529-544.

Ananthakrishnan G, McDonald R, Moss J, et al. Central venous access port devices—a pictorial review of common complications from the interventional radiology perspective. *J Vasc Access.* 2012;13(1):9-15.

Costelloe CM, Murphy WA Jr, Gladish GW, et al. Radiography of pacemakers and implantable cardioverter defibrillators. *AJR Am J Roentgenol.* 2012;199(6):1252-1258.

Godoy MC, Leitman BS, de Groot PM, et al. Chest radiography in the ICU: Part 1, Evaluation of airway, enteric, and pleural tubes. *AJR Am J Roentgenol.* 2012;198(3):563-571.

Godoy MC, Leitman BS, de Groot PM, et al. Chest radiography in the ICU: Part 2, Evaluation of cardiovascular lines and other devices. *AJR Am J Roentgenol.* 2012;198(3):572-581.

Aguilera AL, Volokhina YV, Fisher KL. Radiography of cardiac conduction devices: a comprehensive review. *Radiographics.* 2011;31(6):1669-1682.

Amerasekera SS, Jones CM, Patel R, et al. Imaging of the complications of peripherally inserted central venous catheters. *Clin Radiol.* 2009;64(8):832-840.

Stawicki SP, Evans DC, Cipolla J, et al. Retained surgical foreign bodies: a comprehensive review of risks and preventive strategies. *Scand J Surg.* 2009;98(1):8-17.

Taljanovic MS, Hunter TB, Freundlich IM, et al. Misplaced devices in the chest, abdomen, and pelvis: Part I. *Semin Ultrasound CT MR.* 2006;27(2):78-97.

Taljanovic MS, Hunter TB, Freundlich IM, et al. Misplaced devices in the chest, abdomen, and pelvis: Part II. *Semin Ultrasound CT MR.* 2006;27(2):98-110.

Hunter TB, Taljanovic MS, Tsau PH, et al. Medical devices of the chest. *Radiographics.* 2004;24(6):1725-1746.

Stone GW, Ohman EM, Miller MF, et al. Contemporary utilization and outcomes of intra-aortic balloon counterpulsation in acute myocardial infarction: the benchmark registry. *J Am Coll Cardiol.* 2003;41(11):1940-1945.

Gayer G, Rozenman J, Hoffmann C, et al. CT diagnosis of malpositioned chest tubes. *Br J Radiol.* 2000;73(871):786-790.

Cardall TY, Brady WJ, Chan TC, et al. Permanent cardiac pacemakers: issues relevant to the emergency physician, part II. *J Emerg Med.* 1999;17(4):697-709.

Levy H. Nasogastric and nasoenteric feeding tubes. *Gastrointest Endosc Clin N Am.* 1998;8(3):529-549.

Peterson JC, Cook DJ. Intra-aortic balloon counterpulsation pump therapy: a critical appraisal of the evidence for patients with acute myocardial infarction. *Crit Care.* 1998;2(1):3-8.

Henschke CI, Yankelevitz DF, Wand A, et al. Chest radiography in the ICU. *Clin Imaging.* 1997;21(2):90-103.

Zarshenas Z, Sparschu RA. Catheter placement and misplacement. *Crit Care Clin.* 1994;10(2):417-436.

Gilbert TB, McGrath BJ, Soberman M. Chest tubes: indications, placement, management, and complications. *J Intensive Care Med.* 1993;8(2):73-86.

Steiner RM, Tegtmeyer CJ, Morse D, et al. The radiology of cardiac pacemakers. *Radiographics.* 1986;6(3):373-399.

Dunbar RD. Radiologic appearance of compromised thoracic catheters, tubes, and wires. *Radiol Clin North Am.* 1984;22(3):699-722.

# V

# GASTROINTESTINAL IMAGING

# CHAPTER 23

# ABDOMINAL RADIOGRAPHY

*Stephen E. Rubesin, MD*

1. **What is a "flat plate" of the abdomen?**

   Flat plate is a historical term that refers to a past method of radiography when radiographs were recorded on flat plates of glass coated with an emulsion sensitive to x-rays. This examination also has been termed a plain abdominal radiograph, plain film of the abdomen, abdominal plain film, and KUB. KUB refers to the kidney, ureters, and bladder; this term is not preferred because the ureters are not visible on the plain radiograph, and other organs are visible. The term plain film of the abdomen is not accurate if the image is recorded either on a phosphor plate or directly by electronic means, stored electronically, and displayed on a monitor or plasma screen. No "film" is involved. The preferred terms are **plain radiograph of the abdomen** or **plain abdominal radiograph**.

2. **What structures are visible on a plain abdominal radiograph?**

   Structures are visible on a plain radiograph as a result of differential attenuation of the x-ray beam by air, fat, soft tissue, calcium, and various metals. The edge of an organ composed of soft tissue is visible only where it interfaces with fat of the retroperitoneum or mesenteries, gas within the lumen of the adjacent bowel, or gas within the intraperitoneal or retroperitoneal spaces (Figure 23-1). Interfaces are best shown when the x-ray beam is tangential to the interface. Calcium density is detected in bones or abnormal calcifications, such as gallstones or kidney stones, or within vessel lumens or vascular walls.

   The inferior edge of the liver may be visible. The soft tissue of the spleen may be outlined by air in the stomach and gas in the splenic flexure of the colon. The kidneys and lateral border of the psoas muscles are outlined by retroperitoneal fat. A moderately distended urinary bladder may be outlined by pelvic fat. Portions of the uterus may also be outlined by pelvic fat.

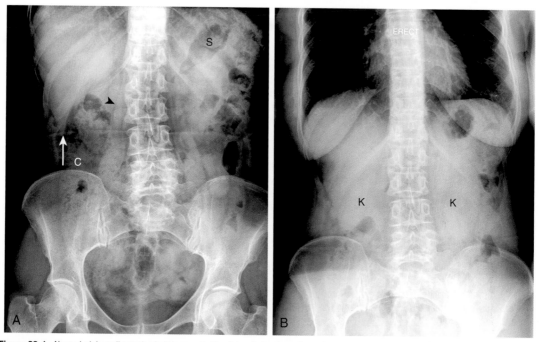

**Figure 23-1.** Normal plain radiograph of abdomen. **A,** Frontal radiograph performed with patient in supine position. Lower ribs, lumbar spine, pelvis, and femoral heads have bone density. Stomach (*S*), seen under left hemidiaphragm, has air density. Right psoas margin (*arrowhead*) is seen because of interface of retroperitoneal fat and muscle soft tissue density. Tip of liver (*arrow*) is demonstrated because gas in hepatic flexure abuts soft tissue density of liver tip, creating interface. Feces in colon (*C*) has mottled density of soft tissue and gas. **B,** Frontal radiograph performed with patient in upright position. No air-fluid levels are seen, as there is no fluid in stomach or right colon. Kidneys (*K*) are outlined by interface of retroperitoneal fat and soft tissue of kidneys.

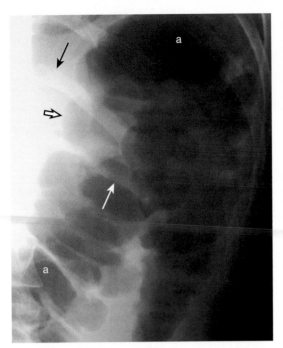

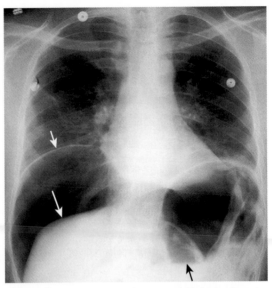

**Figure 23-3.** Free intraperitoneal gas on upright chest radiograph. Large amount of air density free intraperitoneal gas separates right hemidiaphragm (*small white arrow*) from superior edge of liver (*large white arrow*). Air-fluid level (*black arrow*) in small bowel loop reveals that this chest radiograph was obtained with patient in upright position.

**Figure 23-2.** Coned-down plain abdominal radiograph of left upper quadrant obtained with patient standing. Air density (*a*) varies from black to gray. Bone density is shown in lower left ribs (*black arrow* on left eleventh rib). The colon is identified by its air-filled haustral sacculations (*hollow black arrow*), interfaced with adjacent soft tissue density. Interhaustral folds of splenic flexure of colon are thick (*white arrow*) in this patient diagnosed with fulminant colitis ("toxic megacolon"). The interhaustral fold density is representative of soft tissue density.

The stomach is defined by its rugal folds. Air and fluid in a nondistended stomach is a normal finding. The duodenal bulb may be shown by air. Small bowel is identified by its thin, transverse folds (valvulae conniventes). The large bowel is defined by its haustral sacculations (Figure 23-2). A small amount of gas may be present in nondistended small bowel. Gas may outline the nondependent portions of the large bowel, in particular, the transverse colon. Although the lung bases and posterior costophrenic angles are usually underexposed during chest radiography, they are well shown on plain abdominal radiographs.

3. What is an anteroposterior radiograph?

The standard plain abdominal radiograph is obtained with the patient in a recumbent position, lying on his or her back, and is termed a **supine radiograph** (see Figure 23-1, *A*). The x-ray tube is anterior (superior) to the patient, and the radiographic image capture device is posterior (inferior) to the patient. The x-ray beam travels from anterior to the patient to be captured posterior to the patient. By convention, this is termed an **anteroposterior radiograph**.

4. What is a lateral decubitus radiograph?

The term **decubitus** means lying down. Without qualification, the term decubitus radiograph is meaningless. A "decub" is obtained with the patient lying with his or her left or right side down. A right lateral decubitus radiograph is an image obtained with the patient lying with his or her right side down, the x-ray tube oriented in a horizontal position on one side of the patient, and the image capture device (usually a "cassette") oriented perpendicular (upright) to the tube on the other side of the patient. To prevent any confusion, the best terms are **right-side-down decubitus** and **left-side-down decubitus** views, referring to the position of the patient.

5. What is the purpose of an image obtained with the patient in a lateral decubitus or erect position?

Images obtained with the patient in an erect position (chest or abdominal image) or images obtained with the patient in a lateral decubitus position are used to show air-fluid levels in the gastrointestinal (GI) tract or free intraperitoneal gas (Figure 23-3). These views are important in patients with suspected perforation or bowel obstruction. An erect view is used in patients who can stand; lateral decubitus views are performed in patients who are unable to stand.

6. List indications for obtaining a plain radiograph of the abdomen.
   - Acute or subacute abdominal pain.
   - Suspected calculus in any viscus.
   - Suspected bowel obstruction or adynamic ileus.
   - Suspected perforation of a viscus.
   - Abdominal trauma.
   - Abdominal distention.
   - Determination of presence and location of a tube, catheter, intravascular device, or potential radiopaque foreign body.

7. What are the advantages and disadvantages of a plain abdominal radiograph versus a computed tomography (CT) scan?
   A plain abdominal radiograph is a low-cost procedure that is easy to perform with inexpensive radiographic equipment. A radiograph requires little cooperation from the patient. The radiation dose is small. A CT scan is a high-cost procedure that also requires little cooperation from the patient. CT equipment is expensive and delivers a higher radiation dose to the patient. Given the rapid speed of new CT scanners, the time that a patient is lying on the scanner tabletop is nearly equal for a plain radiograph of the abdomen and a CT scan. A plain abdominal radiograph requires no patient preparation. There is about a 1-hour preparation time for a CT scan that uses intravenous (IV) and oral contrast agents.

   CT has far greater contrast resolution than a plain abdominal radiograph and is far superior in showing abnormal calcifications or fluid/gas patterns in the viscera or peritoneal space. CT is tremendously superior for assessment of the solid organs. A plain radiograph has better spatial resolution than CT, in particular, the overview scout image of a CT scan (variously termed **scanogram** or **topogram**). A plain abdominal radiograph provides an overall "big picture" for bowel obstruction superior to a CT scan. This advantage is greatly surpassed, however, by the ability of CT to demonstrate individual bowel loops, fluid-filled bowel loops, bowel wall thickness, and intravenous contrast enhancement patterns.

8. In the era of fast CT scanners, what is the role of a plain radiograph?
   Plain abdominal radiographs are helpful when patients require serial studies, such as patients undergoing decompression for small bowel obstruction or follow-up for resolution of postoperative adynamic ileus. Plain radiographs are also helpful in determining positions of various tubes placed in the abdomen. If there is any question, however, that a tube tip is not within its expected location, a contrast study is performed.

   Plain radiographs may be valuable in patients in the intensive care unit (ICU) who are too seriously ill to move. The physicians have to balance the risk of patient transport from the ICU to the CT scanner to obtain greater information obtained by a CT scan with the mediocre diagnostic capability but high safety level of a plain abdominal radiograph obtained with portable radiographic equipment. In situations that require extreme speed, a CT scan without the use of either oral or intravenous contrast material still provides much more information than a plain abdominal radiograph.

9. Why is the term *free air* a misnomer?
   Gas in the stomach is initially similar in composition to atmospheric air swallowed by the patient. When various digestive processes occur, the gas in the small or large bowel no longer has the same composition as atmospheric air. Carbon dioxide is generated when acid secreted by the stomach combines with bicarbonate secreted by the pancreas. Oxygen and carbon dioxide are resorbed in the small bowel. Nitrogen is not absorbed. Colonic gas is also composed of gases such as methane and hydrogen sulfide, produced by bacterial fermentation.

   Gas in the peritoneal cavity ascends to a nondependent position under the anterior abdominal wall with the patient in a supine position and underneath the diaphragm with the patient in an erect position. Intraperitoneal gas is also trapped in various crevices of the organs and mesenteries. A patient should generally be positioned in an erect or lateral decubitus position for about 5 minutes before a radiograph is obtained to look for "free intraperitoneal gas."

10. What are the best patient positions to detect free intraperitoneal gas on a plain radiograph?
    Free intraperitoneal gas is best shown on an erect chest x-ray centered over the diaphragm (see Figure 23-3); 1 mL of gas may be detected under the curve of a hemidiaphragm. A left-side-down lateral decubitus view to show gas above or under the liver edge is the second best choice.

11. What percentage of supine radiographs shows free intraperitoneal gas?
    In some patients, an erect chest, erect abdominal, or lateral decubitus radiograph is impossible, and an image can be obtained only with the patient in a supine position. A supine abdominal radiograph shows free intraperitoneal gas in about 60% of patients with free intraperitoneal gas.

12. What is the "Rigler" sign?
    "Rigler" sign is named after the radiologist Leo Rigler, MD, who described a sign of pneumoperitoneum in 1941. Normally, gas outlines only the luminal side of a bowel loop. The soft tissue side of the bowel is not visible as a sharp edge because there is no difference in density between the soft tissue of the bowel wall and the remainder of the abdomen. When free intraperitoneal gas abuts a gas-filled loop of bowel, gas surrounds both sides of the bowel wall.

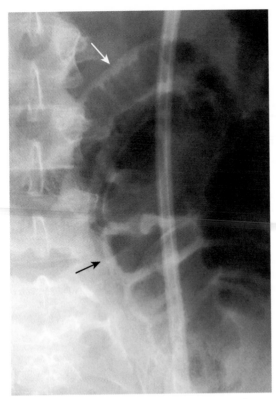

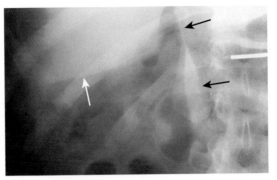

**Figure 23-5.** "Falciform ligament" sign of free intraperitoneal gas on plain abdominal radiograph. Falciform ligament (*black arrows*) and inferior edge of liver (*white arrow*) are outlined by radiolucent free intraperitoneal gas.

**Figure 23-4.** "Rigler" sign of free intraperitoneal gas on supine plain abdominal radiograph. Outer walls of small and large bowel are normally invisible. Radiolucent free intraperitoneal gas outlines outer wall of loop of small bowel (*white arrow*) and proximal sigmoid colon (*black arrow*). Colon is identified by its sacculated outer contour structure, whereas small bowel is identified by smooth outer contour.

If the interfaces of gas and bowel wall are perpendicular to the x-ray beam, the bowel wall is visible and appears as a thin stripe of soft tissue (Figure 23-4).

13. In what abdominal quadrant is free intraperitoneal gas best detected?
    Signs of free intraperitoneal gas are most commonly seen in the right upper quadrant, as lucency over the liver; curvilinear, triangular, or linear streaks of gas outlining the edge of liver near the porta hepatis; or gas outlining the falciform ligament (Figure 23-5). Other signs of free intraperitoneal gas include a curved lucency under the mid-diaphragm resembling a "cupola," gas trapped in the interhaustral folds (the "triangle" sign), and gas in the pelvis outlining the lateral umbilical folds (Figure 23-6).

14. A coned-down image of the abdominal right upper quadrant is presented in Figure 23-7. What structure is outlined by gas, and where is the gas located?
    The right kidney is outlined by retroperitoneal gas in this example. Gas in the retroperitoneal space usually results from iatrogenic causes or gas-forming infections. Retroperitoneal gas originates from the following retroperitoneal structures: the second through fourth portions of the duodenum; pancreas and distal common bile duct; ascending colon, descending colon, and rectum; kidneys, ureters, and urinary bladder; and abdominal aorta and its branches. Gas rarely arises from the retroperitoneal adrenal glands.

15. What is the most common non-iatrogenic cause of pneumobilia?
    Gas in the biliary tree, or pneumobilia, usually results from communication of bowel with the biliary tree, not a gas-forming infection. The most common cause of pneumobilia is probably endoscopically or surgically performed sphincterotomy or a choledochoenteric anastomosis. In patients who have not undergone iatrogenic interventions, the most common cause of pneumobilia is a penetrating duodenal ulcer. Other etiologic factors include choledochoduodenal or cholecystoduodenal fistula owing to gallstones eroding into the duodenum.

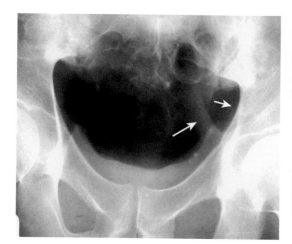

**Figure 23-6.** Free intraperitoneal gas in pelvis on coned-down supine pelvic radiograph. Radiolucent free intraperitoneal gas outlines lateral umbilical folds (*left fold identified by long arrow*) and inferior left (*short arrow*) and right paracolic gutters.

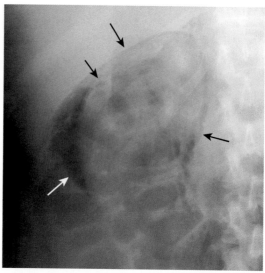

**Figure 23-7.** Retroperitoneal gas on coned-down plain abdominal radiograph of right upper quadrant. Ovoid lucency outlines right kidney (*long arrows*). Lobules of perirenal fat appear as 0.5- to 1-cm lucencies surrounded by rings of soft tissue (*short arrow*). This retroperitoneal gas was secondary to rectal perforation at endoscopy.

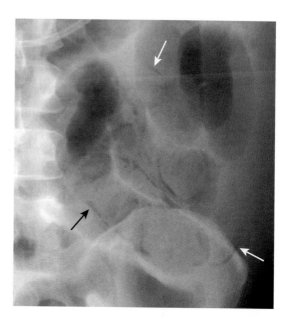

**Figure 23-8.** Linear form of pneumatosis on coned-down supine plain abdominal radiograph. Note linear streaks of radiolucent gas (*arrows*) within smooth-surfaced walls of small bowel. Soft tissue within lumen of bowel represents fluid and debris composed of blood and sloughed cells (the "small bowel feces" sign). This patient was hypotensive, and bowel ischemia with transmural necrosis was found at surgery.

16. What is the Rigler triad?

The combination of gas in the biliary tree; small bowel dilation; and a calcified, ectopic gallstone is a triad of findings described by Rigler. It also has been termed **gallstone ileus**. This triad is seen in less than half of patients in whom a gallstone erodes into the bowel and causes an obstruction in the distal ileum or the sigmoid colon, the narrowest areas of the small and large bowel, respectively. The triad is uncommon in patients in whom a gallstone erodes into bowel because only a few gallstones are calcified; bowel obstruction is not always present; and the fistula may close, resulting in a lack of biliary gas.

17. What does the linear form of pneumatosis imply?

Pneumatosis is gas in the bowel wall. Linear streaks of gas within the small or large bowel wall (Figures 23-8 and 23-9) suggest bowel ischemia but not irreversible necrosis. In patients with bowel ischemia, bowel does not contract normally and dilates. Ischemia is one of the most common causes of severe small bowel dilation. Edema, blood, or

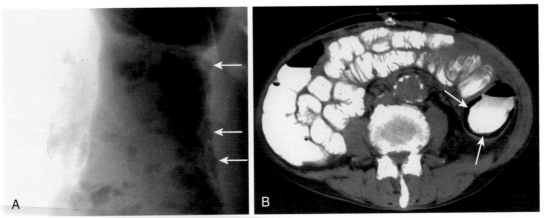

**Figure 23-9.** Pneumatosis coli on abdominal radiograph and CT. **A,** Coned-down supine plain abdominal radiograph shows small (1 to 2 mm) irregularly shaped bubbles of radiolucent gas overlying descending colon. Where colonic wall is shown in profile, bubbles of gas (*arrows*) are shown to be located in colonic wall. This hypotensive patient had infarction in portion of colon that is at transition (watershed) zone of arterial supply between superior mesenteric artery and inferior mesenteric artery. **B,** Axial CT image through abdomen shows curvilinear air attenuation (*arrows*) between contrast-filled lumen of descending colon and soft tissue of colonic wall.

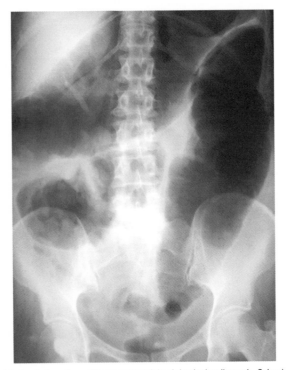

**Figure 23-10.** Thumbprinting in fulminant ulcerative colitis on supine plain abdominal radiograph. Colon is moderately and diffusely distended by gas. Ovoid and polygonally shaped soft tissue nodules seen in cecum have been described as "thumbprints" by imaginative radiologists. This finding implies mucosal necrosis or submucosal edema or hemorrhage associated with ischemia. Combination of diffusely dilated colon with thumbprinting in various forms of colitis (ulcerative colitis, Crohn's disease, *C. difficile* colitis, etc.) has been termed "toxic megacolon." Colon need not be dilated to be necrotic in this entity, and therefore, appropriate term is "fulminant colitis."

necrotic tissue in the mucosa or submucosa of the bowel wall associated with bowel ischemia may appear as nodular soft tissue densities resembling "thumbprints" (Figure 23-10).

Rounded air collections in bowel wall may be due to benign causes of rents in the mucosa, termed **pneumatosis cystoides intestinalis** or **benign pneumatosis coli**. The gas-filled blebs are most commonly detected in the colon and are associated with various clinical conditions, such as scleroderma, corticosteroid use, and celiac disease.

18. In what portions of the GI tract is normal gas located when the patient is radiographed in supine and prone positions?

Gas collects in nondependent portions of the GI tract. When the patient is lying in a supine position, the gastric antrum and transverse colon are the most anterior (nondependent) portions of the GI tract. An air-filled transverse colon less than 5 to 7 cm in diameter is a normal finding on a supine radiograph. When the patient lies in a prone position, the gastric fundus, ascending and descending colon, and midrectum are the most posterior (nondependent) portions of the GI tract.

19. What does the term *ileus* mean?

Ileus is from the Greek *eilein*, meaning "to roll." The term initially was used to describe patients "doubled-over" with abdominal pain. The term later was used to describe bowel dilation. The term ileus, meaning dilation, needs a qualifier to imply either atony or obstruction. **Mechanical ileus** means bowel obstruction. The terms **adynamic ileus, paralytic ileus,** or **functional ileus** describe diminished bowel contraction or peristalsis, not obstruction, with accumulation of gas and fluid in the intestinal lumen.

20. Which study is superior in diagnosing small bowel obstruction: plain radiograph or CT?

Before the advent of CT, plain abdominal radiographs (Figure 23-11) and barium studies were used to diagnose small bowel obstruction. CT has become the imaging modality of choice, however, in patients with suspected small bowel obstruction. CT is superior in diagnosing the presence, location, and etiologic factors of small bowel obstruction. The value of plain radiographs is in follow-up of the resolution or progression of small bowel obstruction in patients who do not undergo surgery.

21. What are the pitfalls of plain radiographic diagnosis of small bowel obstruction?

A small bowel loop is identified on plain abdominal radiography by intraluminal gas outlining valvulae conniventes. If a small bowel loop is completely filled with fluid, it cannot be identified on a plain abdominal radiograph. Plain abdominal radiography misses fluid-filled loops, underdiagnoses small bowel obstruction, and is unable to estimate the level of obstruction accurately. In contrast, CT can identify fluid-filled bowel loops just proximal to the site of obstruction that plain radiography cannot identify.

The clue to an obstruction is a transition between dilated small bowel proximal to an obstructing lesion and collapsed small bowel distal to the site of obstruction (Figure 23-11). False-negative diagnosis may be made with CT and plain abdominal radiography when bowel is not dilated owing to vomiting or nasogastric tube/long tube decompression or when an examination is performed before fluid can accumulate proximal to the obstruction. False-positive diagnosis of obstruction is frequent with CT and plain abdominal radiography and may be made in patients with an adynamic ileus predominantly involving the small bowel (Figure 23-12). Plain abdominal radiography detects about 80% of small bowel obstructions.

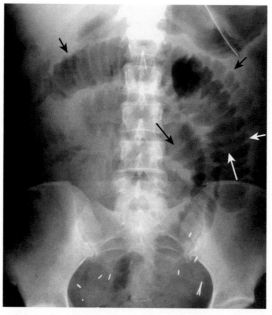

**Figure 23-11.** Closed-loop small bowel obstruction with ischemia on supine plain abdominal radiograph. Mid–small bowel is disproportionately dilated. Small bowel loops are "radially arranged" (*short arrows*) with their mesenteric origin in right lower quadrant. Whereas normal valvulae conniventes are 1 to 2 mm thick, small bowel folds appear markedly thickened, about 4 to 5 mm (*long arrows*), in this patient.

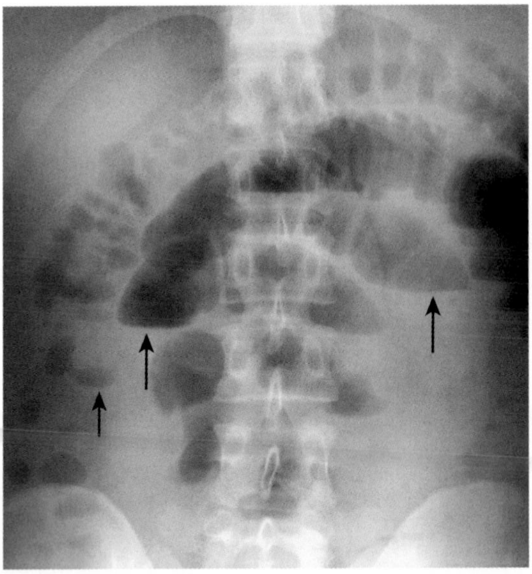

**Figure 23-12.** Adynamic ileus mimicking small bowel obstruction on upright plain abdominal radiograph. Mid–small bowel is disproportionately dilated, and air-fluid levels (*long arrows*) are seen in small bowel lumen. Nondistended colon is identified by its haustral sacculations. Air-fluid levels are also present in colon (*short arrow*) and are suggestive that this patient had (bacterial) enteritis with hypersecretory state.

22. What imaging modality is able to diagnose a bowel obstruction complicated by ischemia?
    Ischemia may occur when the mesentery is twisted during a closed loop obstruction in a hernia or under an adhesion, compromising venous return and arterial inflow. Ischemia may also occur during any obstruction in which luminal dilation results in decreased or absent blood flow to the mucosa. CT is the best radiologic modality to identify bowel ischemia. CT diagnosis depends on identification of thick-walled bowel that either does not enhance or has a mural stratification pattern because of marked submucosal edema (Figure 23-13). In some patients, there is increased attenuation of the bowel wall on unenhanced scans because of intramural hemorrhage. Enlargement of veins in the mesentery may be present in patients with venous obstruction. The mesentery may have increased attenuation because of edema.

23. Can CT show adhesions?
    CT diagnosis of small bowel obstruction relies on identification of the transition zone between dilated and nondilated portions of bowel. CT can identify causes of bowel obstruction that have bulk, such as a primary carcinoma or a metastasis, and CT can show an external hernia. CT identifies extrinsic inflammatory processes, such as appendicitis or diverticulitis, that may secondarily obstruct small bowel. CT diagnosis of adhesions as a cause of bowel obstruction is a presumptive diagnosis only, however, made when no identifiable cause of obstruction is seen at the transition zone.

24. In what situations are barium studies most helpful for the diagnosis of small bowel obstruction?
    Barium studies are superior to CT in diagnosing low-grade or intermittent small bowel obstructions. The site of obstruction is identified more reliably by a barium study than with CT. Barium studies are superior in determining whether a stricture in a patient with Crohn's disease is functionally obstructive. Barium studies also are superior to CT in showing intraluminal tumors as a cause of intussusception/obstruction.

25. What is the most common form of colonic volvulus?
    Sigmoid volvulus accounts for about three fourths of cases of colonic volvulus (Figure 23-14). Radiographically, an inverted U-shaped loop of dilated colon extends far out of the pelvis into the upper abdomen. If the inner walls of the ascending and descending portions of the sigmoid loop are apposed to each other, a thick soft tissue stripe is seen radiating toward the pelvis. This has been described as resembling a coffee bean. The colon and even the small bowel proximal to the twist also are dilated.

26. What patient groups have a greater incidence of sigmoid volvulus?
    Patients with elongated, dilated sigmoid colons are predisposed to sigmoid volvulus. Sigmoid volvulus is common in parts of the world (e.g., Africa) where people have high-fiber diets, bulky stools, and large colons. In the United States, sigmoid volvulus is common in patients who are either bedridden or taking medications that cause colonic hypomotility; patients in nursing homes and mental institutions are at the most risk for sigmoid volvulus.

27. What is wrong with the term *cecal volvulus*?
    The ascending colon is fused to the retroperitoneum in most people. In patients in whom the right colon has incompletely fused to the retroperitoneum, the ascending colon can twist on its mesentery and become obstructed.

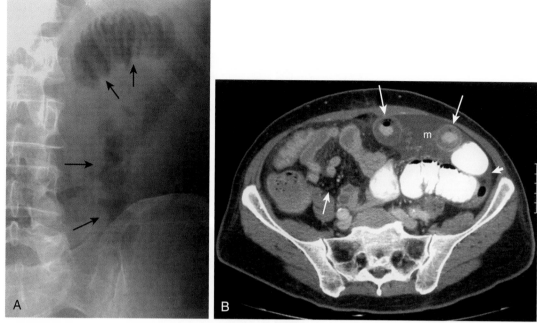

**Figure 23-13.** Small bowel ischemia shown by comparison on plain abdominal radiograph and CT. **A,** Coned-down supine plain abdominal radiograph of left upper quadrant shows mildly dilated loop of small bowel with thick valvulae conniventes (*short arrows*). Smooth 1-cm nodules (*long arrows*) seen on mesenteric border of second left upper quadrant loop are examples of "thumbprinting" owing to severe submucosal edema (in this case) or hemorrhage. **B,** Axial CT image through abdomen at level of upper sacrum shows two loops of ileum with mural stratification pattern ("target" sign) (*long arrows*). High-attenuation oral contrast material and air attenuation bubbles of gas are seen within ileal lumen surrounded by thick annular band of fluid attenuation in submucosa surrounded by thin annular soft tissue attenuation in muscularis propria. Ascites is present in paracolic gutters (*left paracolic gutter identified by short thick arrow*). Mesentery supplying these abnormal loops is engorged and of fluid attenuation (*m*) compared with normal fat attenuation of normal small bowel mesentery (*short thin arrow*) of nonischemic loops.

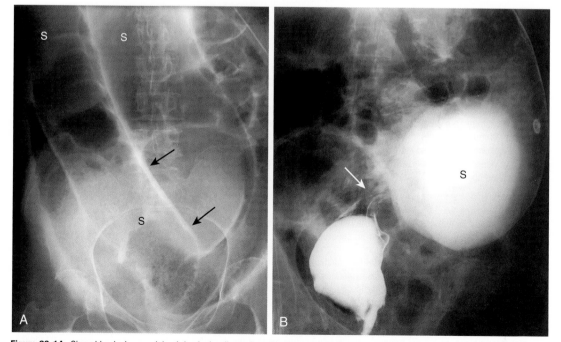

**Figure 23-14.** Sigmoid volvulus on plain abdominal radiograph and barium enema. **A,** Plain radiograph of abdomen shows markedly dilated sigmoid colon (*S*). Thick soft tissue stripe (*arrows*) is seen between adjacent limbs of dilated sigmoid colon representing walls of two adjacent loops coapted together. This overall appearance is said to resemble a coffee bean (radiologists are very imaginative individuals). **B,** Overhead image from subsequent single contrast barium enema shows smooth narrowing (*arrow*) distal to massively dilated sigmoid colon (*S*). When obstruction has been shown, radiologist does not fill colon proximal to an obstruction with much barium because barium can form concretions in colon behind obstruction. (Barium would not form concretions in obstructed small bowel.)

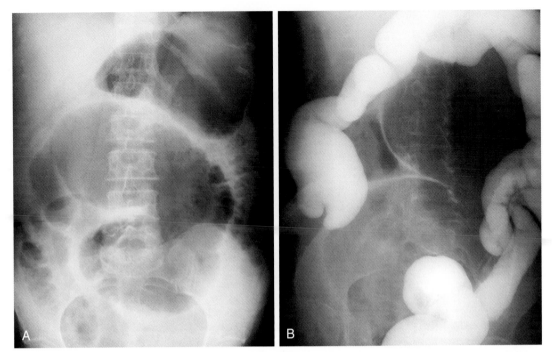

**Figure 23-15.** Cecal volvulus on plain abdominal radiograph and barium enema. **A,** Plain supine radiograph of abdomen demonstrates large reverse C-shaped viscus in midabdomen. This viscus is identified as colon by its haustral sacculations and as cecum and ascending colon by its lack of connection to rectum. **B,** Single contrast barium enema demonstrates abrupt cut-off of flow of barium in ascending colon. Dilated air-filled structure does not fill with barium and therefore cannot be sigmoid colon. Air-filled dilated colon on plain radiograph is confirmed by barium enema to be dilated cecum and proximal ascending colon.

The colon proximal to the twist, in particular the cecum, becomes dilated and is located in the mid-left abdomen or in the left upper quadrant. This condition is poorly termed a cecal volvulus, when, in reality, it is a volvulus of the mesentery of the ascending colon (Figure 23-15).

28. What percentage of gallstones is calcified?

About 15% of gallstones are radiopaque on plain abdominal radiography (Figure 23-16). Calcification is detected in about 30% to 40% of gallstones on CT. CT detects about 80% of calcified or noncalcified gallstones (Figure 23-17). Cholesterol gallstones appear as low-attenuation filling defects, often floating in bile, although often similar in attenuation to surrounding bile. Ultrasonography (US) detects about 95% of gallstones.

Gallstones are an example of concretions formed in the abdomen. The calcification in such concretions usually occurs around a central nidus of organic or inorganic foreign matter, thrombus, focal pus, or cellular debris. Such calcifications occur within the lumina of tubular structures, such as blood vessels, bile ducts, or ureters, or within hollow viscera such as the gallbladder or urinary bladder. Concretions may have a round, ovoid, branched, or spiculated shape.

29. A plain radiograph of the abdomen is obtained in a patient who has a palpable abdominal mass (Figure 23-18). What is the diagnosis?

There is a curvilinear calcification in the left midabdomen centered at the L2 vertebral body level, in keeping with a diagnosis of a calcified abdominal aortic aneurysm.

Linear or curvilinear calcifications are seen in tubular or cystic structures. In the walls of tubular structures, such as blood vessels and vasa deferentia, the calcifications are usually discontinuous and of varying thickness. If a tubular structure is seen en face, a thick, discontinuous ring of calcification may be detected. This type of calcification is typical of arterial calcifications, in particular, atherosclerotic calcification.

Calcifications in the walls of cystic structures appear as a curvilinear rim of calcification. This rim is often incomplete. Various lesions give this appearance, including renal cysts and renal cell carcinoma, aneurysms of the aorta and other major vessels, echinococcal cysts in the liver or spleen, pancreatic pseudocysts, adrenal cysts, mesenteric cysts, mucinous tumors of the appendix, and cystic tumors of the ovaries. Calcification of the gallbladder wall in chronic cholecystitis (porcelain gallbladder) has a similar appearance (Figure 23-19). The location of an abnormality is a clue to the location of a calcification in the abdomen detected on plain abdominal radiography. CT shows the organ of origin and the underlying cause of a calcified lesion in most cases.

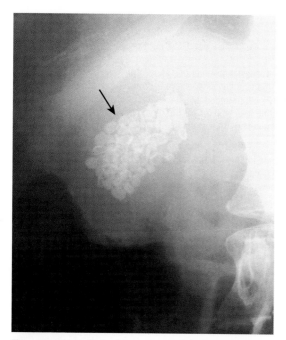

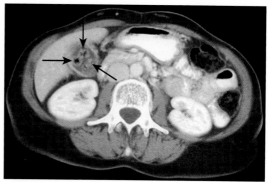

**Figure 23-17.** Noncalcified gallstones on CT. Note three noncalcified gallstones (*arrows*) within gallbladder. Periphery of stones has higher attenuation than that of surrounding bile. Tiny bubbles of air attenuation are seen in two stones, representing trapped nitrogen gas.

**Figure 23-16.** Calcified gallstones on coned-down supine plain abdominal radiograph. Note numerous 2- to 3-mm polygonal calcified faceted gallstones (*arrow*).

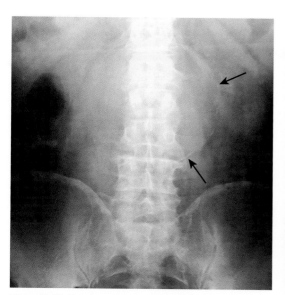

**Figure 23-18.** Vascular calcification on plain abdominal radiograph. Note discontinuous ring of curvilinear calcification (*arrows*) surrounding soft tissue mass (11 cm in diameter) in midabdomen. This was due to saccular abdominal aortic aneurysm with vascular calcification caused by atherosclerosis.

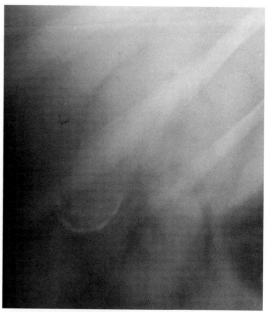

**Figure 23-19.** Porcelain gallbladder on coned-down plain abdominal radiograph of right upper quadrant. Note curvilinear calcification associated with oval-shaped soft tissue density. Punctate calcifications superior to curvilinear calcification are also present. Curvilinear calcification is lateral and separate from soft tissue density of right kidney. Therefore, calcified renal mass is unlikely. This calcification in wall of chronically inflamed gallbladder wall has been termed "porcelain" gallbladder. Gallbladder cancer is found to present in about 22% of patients with porcelain gallbladder diagnosed with plain abdominal radiography.

30. A coned-down view of the upper abdomen (Figure 23-20) is obtained in a man with chronic abdominal pain. What is the diagnosis?

Dense, sharply angulated clumps of calcium are confined to a 4-cm area just to the right of the L2 vertebral body, in keeping with a diagnosis of chronic calcific pancreatitis.

Calcifications in abdominal masses and inflammatory processes have various shapes and sizes. Calcifications in mucin-producing tumors appear amorphous or punctate. Intraductal calcifications in patients with alcoholic pancreatitis appear as small clumps overlying the pancreas (see Figure 23-20). Mottled, slightly irregular, ovoid masses of calcification are typically seen in calcified lymph nodes. Uterine leiomyomas are the most common pelvic tumor to calcify. These benign tumors may have peripheral rim, central whorled, or clumplike calcification (Figure 23-21).

31. A patient has a palpable abdominal mass (Figure 23-22). What organ is enlarged?

The spleen is enlarged in this patient. CT, magnetic resonance imaging (MRI), and US are now the imaging modalities of choice in the workup of a palpable abdominal mass. If gynecologic disease is suspected, US or MRI of the pelvis is the preferred examination. For upper abdominal masses, abdominal CT or MRI is indicated.

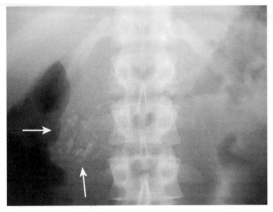

**Figure 23-20.** Chronic calcific pancreatitis on coned-down plain abdominal radiograph of upper abdomen. Note radiodense clumps of calcification (*arrows*) to right of L2 vertebral body. These calcifications are not in pancreatic parenchyma but are within dilated pancreatic ducts. This patient had a history of chronic alcohol abuse.

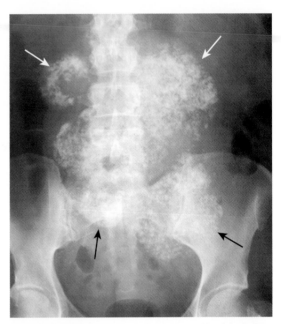

**Figure 23-21.** Calcified uterine leiomyomas on plain abdominal radiograph. Note four round calcified masses confluent in midline (*arrows*) in lower abdomen and upper pelvis. These calcifications are dense and punctate, but some are said to resemble "popcorn." This type of calcification is typically seen in uterine leiomyomas.

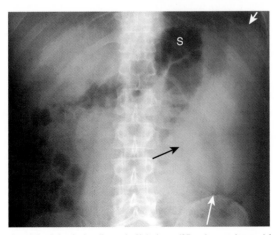

**Figure 23-22.** Splenomegaly on supine plain abdominal radiograph. Note large (25 cm) mass (*arrows*) in left upper quadrant that displaces splenic flexure of colon (*S*) medially. This "mass" represents enlarged spleen in patient with leukemia.

32. A 45-year-old man has recently received a liver transplant. Identify the type and location of the two tubular structures below the diaphragm in Figure 23-23, *A*. What has the radiologist done in Figures 23-23, *B* and *C*?

Answers are provided in the associated figure legend. A wide variety of manmade devices are placed in the abdomen at surgery or through various orifices. Clinically placed foreign objects are better seen on plain radiographs when a radiodense substance has been incorporated into the device by the manufacturer. Injection of various tubes with water-soluble contrast material can confirm the location of the tubes (see Figure 23-19, *C*). Radiopaque wires and tubes outside of the patient make radiographic interpretation more difficult, unless the radiologist knows exactly what is supposed to lie inside or outside of the patient. The location of a tube in the GI tract is suggested by its configuration.

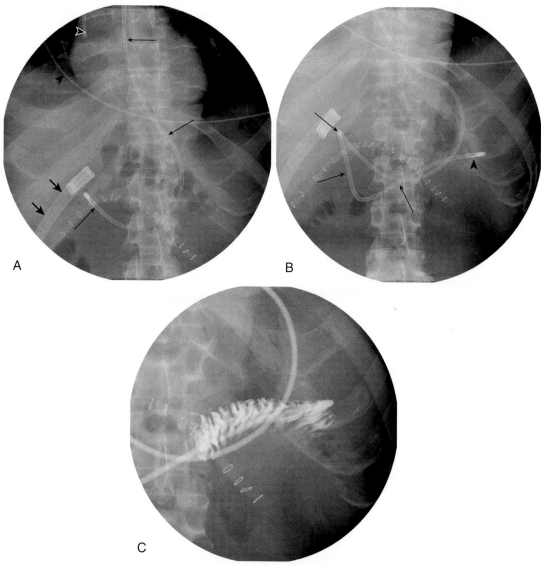

**Figure 23-23.** Tube and device assessment on spot radiographs of upper abdomen obtained during fluoroscopy. **A,** Note thin (5 mm) radiopaque tubular structure (*long arrows*) coursing parallel to lower thoracic spine, entering mid-upper abdomen, then curving gently to right, coursing along greater curvature of stomach, with its tip overlying distal gastric antrum, representing feeding tube. Second tube (*short arrows*) is folded over itself in right upper quadrant. This tube has four lumina and multiple small holes and represents Jackson-Pratt drainage tube that was placed in subhepatic space. Tip of right venous catheter (*white/black arrowhead*) overlies caval-atrial junction. Metallic wire representing electrocardiogram lead (*black arrowheads*) crosses lower chest and is outside of patient because it does not conform to any anatomic structure. Multiple metallic skin staples are present in curvilinear configuration in upper abdomen. **B,** Under fluoroscopic guidance, radiologist has advanced feeding tube tip (*arrowhead*) from gastric antrum to duodenal-jejunal junction. Configuration of feeding tube (*arrows*) mimics "C" shape of duodenum. **C,** Injection of feeding tube with water-soluble contrast material confirms that tip of feeding tube is at duodenal-jejunal junction.

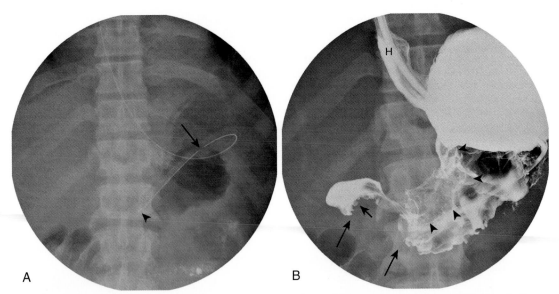

**Figure 23-24.** Tube assessment on spot radiographs of upper abdomen obtained during fluoroscopy. **A,** Note radiopaque tube of caliber much wider than feeding tube shown in Figure 23-19, *A.* Tube is looped in gastric fundus, and its tip (*arrowhead*) overlies distal gastric body. Side hole of tube (*arrow*) is identified. This represents nasogastric tube, typically used to decompress stomach or small bowel. Stomach is not dilated. **B,** Spot radiograph obtained 30 minutes after nasogastric tube was injected with high-density barium. Complete gastric outlet obstruction is shown because no barium has left stomach. There is 4-cm-long annular constriction of proximal gastric antrum (between long arrows) with nodular mucosa (*short arrow*). Plaquelike flattening and mucosal nodularity extend up lesser curvature (*arrowheads*). Thick rugal folds are seen along distal greater curvature. Also note reflux of barium into small hiatal hernia (*H*) and distal esophagus. This gastric mass was due to adenocarcinoma of stomach infiltrating lower gastric body and proximal gastric antrum causing complete gastric outlet obstruction. These images show how plain radiography only provides limited information in some cases. Nasogastric decompression has removed fluid and made stomach of normal size on plain radiograph, without any indication of complete gastric outlet obstruction. Vomiting can also decompress obstructed stomach.

33. A 38-year-old man complains of nausea and vomiting (Figure 23-24). What type of tube has been placed in Figure 23-24, *A*?

Tubes used for decompression are typically of larger caliber than tubes used for feeding. The nasogastric tube used for decompression seen in Figure 23-24, *A*, is wider than the enteral feeding tube seen in Figure 23-23, *A*.

## KEY POINTS

- Plain radiographs of the abdomen have largely been replaced by CT, US, and MRI in patients with acute clinical problems.
- Plain radiographs are helpful to show the location of various tubes and to evaluate ICU patients or patients who require serial studies.
- The first examination one generally obtains for a patient with suspected small bowel obstruction is a CT scan.
- Free intraperitoneal gas is detected on a supine plain radiograph in 60% of patients with bowel perforation.
- Linear pneumatosis is highly suggestive of bowel ischemia.

**BIBLIOGRAPHY**

Baker SR. Abdominal calcifications. In: Gore RM, Levine MS, eds. *Textbook of gastrointestinal radiology.* 4th ed. Philadelphia: Elsevier Saunders; 2015:197-204.

Messmer JM, Levine MS. Gas and soft tissue abnormalities. In: Gore RM, Levine MS, eds. *Textbook of gastrointestinal radiology.* 4th ed. Philadelphia: Elsevier Saunders; 2015:178-196.

Thompson WM. Abdomen: normal anatomy and examination techniques. In: Gore RM, Levine MS, eds. *Textbook of gastrointestinal radiology.* 4th ed. Philadelphia: Elsevier Saunders; 2015:165-177.

Baker SR, Cho KC. *The abdominal plain film with correlative imaging.* 2nd ed. Stamford, CT: Appleton & Lange; 1999.

Miller RE, Nelson SW. The roentgenologic demonstration of tiny amounts of free intraperitoneal gas: experimental and clinical studies. *Am J Roentgenol Radium Ther Nucl Med.* 1971;112(3):574-585.

# CHAPTER 24

# FLUOROSCOPY OF THE UPPER GASTROINTESTINAL TRACT

Stephen E. Rubesin, MD

1. **What organs are studied during an upper gastrointestinal (GI) series?**

   The esophagus, stomach, and duodenum are studied. The radiologist evaluates the morphology and motility of these organs.

2. **What organs are studied during a pharyngoesophagogram?**

   The radiologist evaluates the motility of the oral cavity, pharynx, and esophagus, and the morphology of the pharynx, esophagus, and gastric cardia. The radiologist records the fluoroscopic images of oral, pharyngeal, and esophageal motility directly into the picture archiving and communication system (PACS), into a proprietary computer system, onto a videocassette recorder (VCR), via a digital video disc (DVD) recorder, or on film ("cine"). Film has been almost completely replaced as the recording medium for motility because of increased radiation exposure, cost, and difficulty of film processing. The term "cine-esophagram" is outdated.

3. **What organ is shown in Figure 24-1?**

   Figure 24-1 shows a normal lower thoracic esophagus. The esophagus is a muscular tube within the mediastinum. The esophagus is usually collapsed unless distended by liquid or solid food; swallowed air; or, in this image, swallowed air and barium. In this patient, swallowed high-density barium coats the mucosa. The swallowed carbon dioxide (effervescent agent) and swallowed air distend the lumen of the esophagus. The mucosa of the esophageal tube seen in profile appears as a white line (arrows). The mucosal surface of the normal esophagus seen en face is smooth and varies from white to gray (representative mucosa identified by $S$). Normal structures in the mediastinum push on the distended esophagus, manifested as alterations of the normal straight tubular contour of the esophagus. These indentations are identified as the bottom of the aortic arch ($a$), the left mainstem bronchus ($b$), and the left atrium ($l$).

4. **What organs are shown in Figure 24-2? Identify the numbered parts of the organs as labeled, along with the curvatures labeled by arrows.**

   For the answer, see the figure legend.

5. **Why does the gastric fundus appear white in Figure 24-2, whereas the gastric antrum appears gray?**

   Barium sulfate absorbs and scatters x-rays, but air does not. X-rays passing through barium are blocked and do not reach the x-ray detector. X-rays easily pass through gastrointestinal (GI) structures filled with air and reach the x-ray detector. The relatively exposed areas of the x-ray detector appear as shades of black; the relatively unexposed areas of the x-ray detector appear as shades of white. The heavy barium falls to the lowest or most "dependent" portion of the stomach. This image was obtained with the patient recumbent, with the back against the fluoroscopic tabletop (i.e., a supine radiograph). The gastric fundus is posterior to the gastric antrum; barium falls into the gastric fundus when the patient lies in a supine position. Because barium absorbs more x-rays than air, the gastric fundus appears "white." In this radiograph, the anteriorly located gastric antrum is filled with air and is also "etched in white" by a thin layer of barium. Most of the x-rays, but not all, pass through the antrum, partially exposing the x-ray detector. The gastric antrum appears gray, not black as a purely air-filled structure would appear.

   Today, most radiographs are not obtained using real film as the recording medium but instead use some type of image capture device. The relative exposures on the image capture device are digitized and are assigned gray-scale values, from white to black. The images are displayed on a monitor or flat panel. Depending on the radiologist, large exposures are assigned either "white" or "black" values. In the United States, barium is usually assigned a "white" value, air a "black value"; in Japan, barium often is assigned a "black" value and air a "white" value.

6. **Two images of the esophagus are presented in Figure 24-3. What is your diagnosis?**

   This is a semiannular carcinoma of the esophagus. The tumor originated on the side of contour irregularity and has begun to spread circumferentially. The wall opposite the tumor is smooth and uninvolved by the tumor but has been pulled inward by the desmoplastic tumor. The barium pool in Figure 24-3, *A*, shows the contour of a luminal organ but obscures mucosal detail. The air contrast image in Figure 24-3, *B*, reveals the luminal contour in profile, as does the barium pool. The air contrast image also reveals the mucosal surface en face. In this case, the air contrast image shows the surface and the edge of the semiannular cancer.

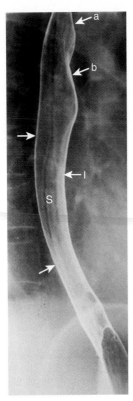

**Figure 24-1.** Normal esophagus on double-contrast upper GI examination (see text above for description).

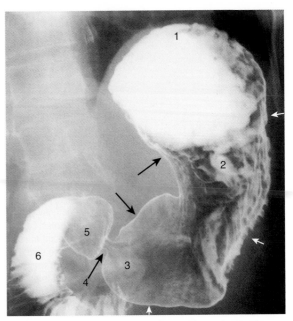

**Figure 24-2.** Normal stomach and proximal duodenum on double-contrast upper GI examination. 1 = gastric fundus, 2 = gastric body, 3 = gastric antrum, 4 = pylorus (pyloric channel), 5 = duodenal bulb, and 6 = second portion of duodenum. Black arrows indicate lesser curvature of stomach. White arrows indicate greater curvature of stomach.

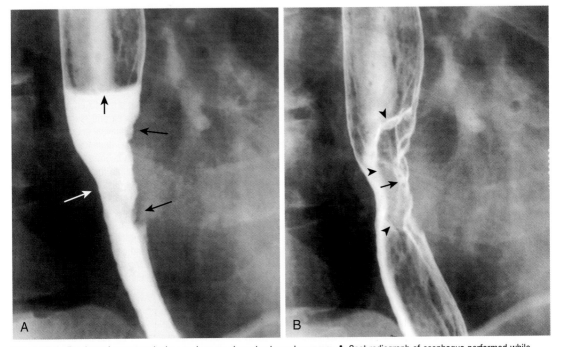

**Figure 24-3.** Esophageal cancer on barium pool versus air contrast esophagogram. **A,** Spot radiograph of esophagus performed while patient stands and drinks high-density barium shows column of barium (with air-barium level, *short black arrow*) in midesophagus. Focal circumferential narrowing of esophagus, 3 cm in length, is present, which appears smooth on one wall (*white arrow*) and has irregular contour on opposite wall (*black arrows*). **B,** Spot radiograph performed seconds later after barium column has passed through esophagus shows same circumferential narrowing with smooth contour on one side and irregular contour on other. Mucosal surface is now seen en face as well, however, revealing focal mucosal nodularity (*short black arrow*) and barium-coated lines (*arrowheads*) that disrupt the normal smooth surface of esophagus and outline outer margin of mass.

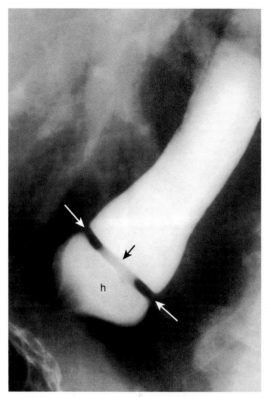

**Figure 24-4.** Schatzki ring on single-contrast esophagogram (see question regarding single-contrast for description).

7. What does "single contrast" mean?

A single-contrast study of a GI structure means that one contrast agent is used, such as a suspension of barium sulfate, an ionic water-soluble contrast agent such as diatrizoate meglumine (Gastroview/Gastrografin), or a nonionic water-soluble contrast agent such as iohexol (Omnipaque). Figure 24-4 is an example of a single-contrast image obtained with the patient swallowing barium while lying in a prone position. A column of "thin" barium fills the distal esophageal lumen. The radiologist examines the luminal contour in profile for abnormalities that either protrude into the lumen or protrude outside of the expected luminal contour of the organ. The radiologist also looks for abnormalities en face. Large protrusions into the lumen displace the barium column, allow x-rays to pass through the esophagus, and appear as radiolucent "filling defects" in the barium column. Large protrusions outside the luminal contour fill with barium and, when seen en face, appear as a "double density" of barium.

In this patient, there is a small hiatal hernia (*h*). At the esophagogastric junction, a thin, smooth, symmetric ringlike narrowing, 3 mm in height, is seen in profile as a shelflike indentation of the luminal contour (*white arrows*). En face, the ring is manifested as a thin radiolucent filling defect in the barium column (*black arrow*). This is a Schatzki ring, a narrowing that commonly causes dysphagia with solids.

8. What does "double contrast" mean?

In a double-contrast study, the radiologist uses two contrast agents to examine the organs in question. A double-contrast upper GI series uses an effervescent agent that creates carbon dioxide to distend the luminal organs and high-density barium to "scrub and paint" the mucosa. This study is also known as an *air contrast upper GI series* or a *biphasic upper GI series*. Figure 24-5 is a double-contrast image of the distal stomach. Rugal folds are seen as radiolucent filling defects in the barium pool (white arrow) and as parallel barium etched lines (*black arrows*). Rugal folds are composed of mucosa and submucosa and are most prominent along the greater curvature of the stomach. The normal gastric antrum (*A*) has few, if any, rugal folds in most patients.

9. What are clinical indications for performing an upper GI study?

Clinical indications for performing an upper GI study include heartburn, dysphagia, or odynophagia referred to a substernal location; upper abdominal pain or discomfort; upper GI bleeding; and vomiting.

10. What are clinical indications for performing a video/DVD pharyngoesophagogram?

Clinical indications for performing a video/DVD pharyngoesophagogram include dysphagia or odynophagia referred to the head, neck, and suprasternal regions; history of globus sensation; chronic cough; aspiration pneumonia or cerebrovascular accident; dribbling from the mouth; abnormal tongue motions; and history of surgery or radiation of the tongue, palate, pharynx, or larynx.

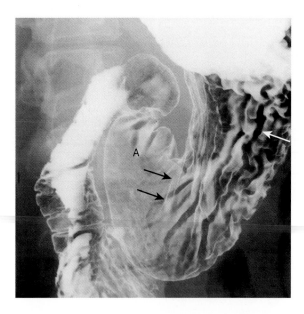

**Figure 24-5.** Normal distal stomach on double-contrast upper GI examination (see question regarding double-contrast for description).

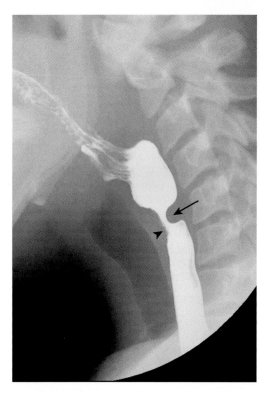

**Figure 24-6.** Incomplete opening (relaxation) of cricopharyngeal muscle on pharyngoesophagogram. Image was obtained while patient drank barium and stood in lateral position. Note smooth-surfaced hemispheric soft tissue indentation (*arrow*) on posterior wall of pharyngoesophageal segment due to incomplete opening (relaxation) of cricopharyngeus, representing compensatory response to protect pharynx and larynx from gastroesophageal reflux. Pharyngoesophageal segment is identified by redundant, undulating mucosa in its anterior wall (*arrowhead*), as this region abuts cricoid cartilage.

11. A 23-year-old woman complains of a lump in her throat at all times of the day (a globus sensation). An image of the lower pharynx and upper cervical esophagus is obtained (Figure 24-6). What is your diagnosis?

Figure 24-6 shows incomplete opening of the cricopharyngeal muscle, depicted as a smooth, hemispheric radiolucent extrinsic impression on the posterior wall of the pharyngoesophageal segment.

A globus sensation is usually related to delayed opening, incomplete opening, or early closure of the cricopharyngeal muscle. Abnormal cricopharyngeal opening is usually a vagal-mediated reflex response to gastroesophageal reflux. When a patient refluxes, the normally tonically contracted upper esophageal sphincter

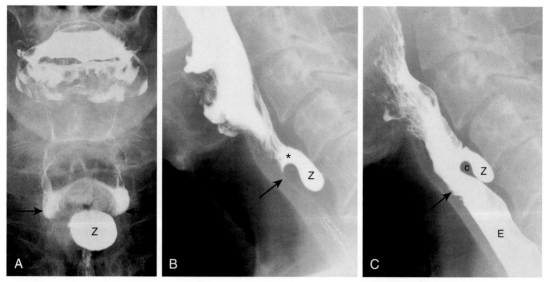

**Figure 24-7.** Zenker's diverticulum on pharyngoesophagogram. **A,** Image obtained while patient stands in frontal position. Note 2 × 3 cm smooth-surfaced, ovoid sacculation (Z) in midline below tips of piriform sinuses (*arrows*). **B** and **C,** Images obtained while patient drinks barium and stands in lateral position. In **B**, barium contrast bolus has just arrived in distal hypopharynx. Barium goes through opening of diverticulum (*) and fills sac (Z). Pharyngoesophageal segment (*arrow*) has not yet opened. In **C**, barium contrast bolus has now nearly completely passed through pharynx into cervical esophagus (E). Pharyngoesophageal segment (*arrow*) is now open. Zenker's diverticulum (Z) is seen posterior to cricopharyngeal muscle (c) and uppermost portion of posterior wall of cervical esophagus.

(comprised mainly of the cricopharyngeal muscle) remains tight to prevent reflux of esophageal contents into the pharynx and hence to prevent aspiration.

This is an example of the interrelationship of esophageal and pharyngeal function. Abnormalities in the esophagus often result in symptoms in the neck. For example, when food is stuck in the distal esophagus, the patient often complains of food being stuck in the throat. This is also an example of why a pharyngoesophagram on an outpatient should include images of the oral, pharyngeal, and esophageal phases of swallowing. This is also an example of why, if an upper GI series is ordered for gastroesophageal reflux rather than a pharyngoesophagram, the radiologist should look for complications of gastroesophageal reflux in the pharynx, especially abnormal epiglottic tilt with resulting laryngeal penetration and abnormal cricopharyngeal opening.

12. A 74-year-old man complains of a lump in his throat and regurgitation of food into his mouth. Images of the lower pharynx and upper cervical esophagus are obtained (Figure 24-7). What is your diagnosis?

Figure 24-7 shows a Zenker's diverticulum. Zenker's diverticulum is an acquired herniation of mucosa and tunica propria through Killian's dehiscence, an area of congenital weakness between the thyropharyngeal muscles and the cricopharyngeal muscle on the posterior wall of the pharyngoesophageal segment. Although the pathogenesis is uncertain, there is a strong association between the development of a Zenker's diverticulum and the presence of a hiatal hernia and gastroesophageal reflux disease. It is postulated that the presence of gastroesophageal reflux leads to incomplete opening of the cricopharyngeal muscle, such that a pulsion-type diverticulum (the Zenker's diverticulum) forms in the area of muscle weakness above the cricopharyngeal muscle. Zenker's diverticulum is another example of the interrelationship between the esophagus and the pharynx and the reason that the radiologist should evaluate both regions given the appropriate clinical history and fluoroscopic findings.

13. Describe the preparation for an upper GI study or pharyngoesophagogram.

Each hospital or outpatient facility has its own preparation routines for these studies. These preparations should be available from the radiologists in hard copy form or in an institutional document online. At our institution, a handout describing the examination and explaining the preparation (see the following) is available to all referring physicians:

1. Patients should have nothing by mouth after 9 PM.
2. Insulin-dependent diabetics should eliminate or decrease the dose of insulin the morning of the examination.
3. Patients should not take antacids or bismuth subsalicylate (Pepto-Bismol) on the morning of the examination.
4. Patients should wear dentures or other swallowing appliances.
5. If patients have solid food dysphagia, they should bring a type of food that causes dysphagia.
6. After the examination, patients are encouraged to drink liquids and may take a laxative if additional radiologic tests are scheduled or if there is a history of colonic hypomotility.

14. What are contraindications to a barium study of the upper GI tract?
Contraindications include:
- Known or suspected gastrointestinal tract perforation.
- Inability to swallow.
- In the case of inability to swallow, an examination of the stomach and small bowel may be performed by sending the patient to fluoroscopy with a nasogastric tube placed in the stomach.

15. What type of contrast agent should be requested first in patients with suspected upper GI perforation?
In patients with known or suspected perforations of the pharynx, esophagus, or duodenum, an ionic water-soluble contrast agent such as diatrizoate meglumine (Gastroview or Gastrografin) should be used initially. This type of agent is readily absorbed from the soft tissues of the neck, mediastinum, and peritoneal cavity. This type of agent, if aspirated, has the theoretical potential to cause pulmonary edema because it is hyperosmolar and draws fluid into the lungs. If aspiration is a likely possibility, the radiologist may start with a nonionic water-soluble contrast agent that is either only mildly hyperosmolar (iohexol [Omnipaque for Oral Use]) or iso-osmolar. Other radiologists start with barium if a perforation of the pharynx or esophagus is suspected, and there is a high risk of aspiration because barium in the soft tissues of the neck or mediastinum is relatively harmless. Barium entering the peritoneal cavity from a gastric or duodenal perforation can potentially cause mild barium peritonitis. This situation is not as serious, however, as barium entering the peritoneal space from a colonic perforation. The combination of barium and feces entering the peritoneal space during a barium enema has a much greater likelihood of causing peritonitis and has a high mortality rate.

16. When is a single-contrast upper GI series performed?
Double-contrast examinations focus on showing mucosal detail. Single-contrast examinations focus only on the big picture to detect obstruction, perforation, abnormal motility, or fistulas. A single-contrast examination is performed to detect a complication along a staple/suture line, at an anastomosis, or near a wound; to evaluate an organ as it passes through a surgically created tunnel; or to identify a rent in a mesentery. A single-contrast examination may also be performed to evaluate emptying of surgically created pouches after surgery for morbid obesity and in conjunction with a small bowel follow-through examination.

17. What portion of the GI tract is shown in Figure 24-8?
For the answer, see the figure legend.

18. What portion of the GI tract is shown in Figure 24-9?
For the answer, see the figure legend.

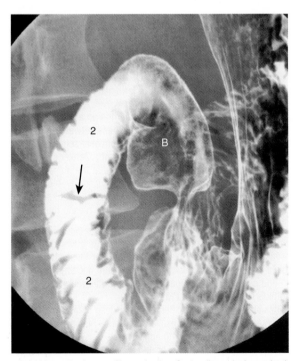

**Figure 24-8.** Proximal duodenum on double-contrast upper GI examination. Spot radiograph shows duodenal bulb (*B*) and second portion of duodenum (*2*). Duodenal folds (folds of Kerckring) (*arrow*) cross duodenum except at level of papilla of Vater.

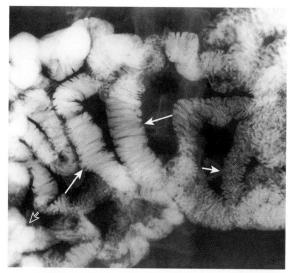

**Figure 24-9.** Small bowel on small bowel follow-through examination. Many loops of small bowel are visible. Two loops are well distended (*long arrows*) and show that valvulae conniventes lie perpendicular to longitudinal axis of small bowel. Some loops are partially collapsed, and valvulae conniventes overlap each other, giving folds "feathery" (*short arrow*) appearance. Some loops overlap and no morphologic detail is visible (*open arrow*).

19. What are the indications for a small bowel follow-through?

A small bowel follow-through may be performed whenever small bowel disease is suspected. The patient drinks a large volume (750 to 1000 mL) of thin barium, and a single-contrast examination of the esophagus, stomach, and small bowel is performed. Barium filling of the small bowel is limited by gastric emptying at the pylorus. The radiologist is unable to distend all the loops of small bowel either quickly or at the same time. A small bowel follow-through is also limited by the normal 30- to 120-minute transit time from the pylorus to the ileocecal valve. The radiologist cannot stand in the fluoroscopic suite for 1 to 2 hours and watch the barium flow down the small bowel. The radiologist examines the patient at 15- to 30-minute intervals, palpating loops of small bowel when they are optimally distended with barium. A small bowel follow-through relies on fluoroscopically obtained spot radiographs, not overhead images.

A water-soluble contrast agent is used if bowel perforation is strongly suspected. A water-soluble contrast study of the small bowel is often suboptimal, however, because the hyperosmolar water-soluble contrast agent draws fluid into the lumen and prevents fluid resorption. The water-soluble contrast agent is diluted, and the images are very difficult to interpret. If a gastric or proximal small bowel leak is suspected, a water-soluble contrast upper GI study and proximal small bowel follow-through usually suffice. If a mid- to distal small bowel leak is suspected, a computed tomography (CT) scan may be the better initial test. If a very distal small bowel leak or anastomotic leak is suspected in a patient with an ileocolic anastomosis, a water-soluble contrast enema is probably the best examination.

20. Figure 24-10 is an overhead image obtained from what type of study? What organ is being imaged?

For the answer, see the figure legend.

21. What layers of the bowel wall comprise the valvulae conniventes?

Valvulae conniventes (plicae circulares, folds of Kerckring) are composed of mucosa and submucosa. These folds increase the surface area of the small bowel. The villi of the small intestine are about 1 mm in cross-section and are just at the radiographic limits of resolution.

22. What are the indications for enteroclysis (small bowel enema)?

Small bowel enemas are difficult to perform and often are uncomfortable for the patient. They are superior, however, to small bowel follow-through examination for showing short lesions and the valvulae conniventes. Indications include the following:

- Unexplained anemia or GI bleeding; a patient should have a normal upper or lower endoscopy or normal double-contrast upper GI study and barium enema before enteroclysis.
- Malabsorption.
- Demonstration of skip lesions in a patient with known Crohn's disease.
- Suspected tumor of any kind.

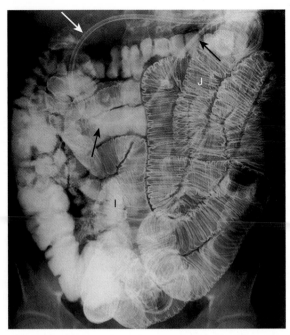

**Figure 24-10.** Small bowel on overhead radiograph from enteroclysis, or small bowel enema. During this examination, tube is passed through patient's mouth or nose, down throat, through esophagus, around stomach, through duodenum, and past duodenal-jejunal junction. Passage of tube (*arrows*) eliminates pylorus as rate-limiting factor of barium passage into small bowel. In this particular case, radiologist has injected medium-density barium to coat mucosa and methylcellulose to distend lumen. Double-contrast (but not air contrast) image is obtained. Jejunum (*J*) is in left upper quadrant, and ileum (*I*) is in right lower quadrant. Enteroclysis may be performed as single-contrast study with low-density barium or as double-contrast study using barium to coat mucosa and either air or methylcellulose to distend lumen.

23. What is the preparation for enteroclysis?
    Residual fluid and feces should be removed from the small bowel and right colon. The patient should not eat after 9 PM. Bisacodyl tablets are given with water at 10 PM the night before the examination to stimulate the right colon to contract. The patient does not drink fluids after midnight. Insulin-dependent diabetic patients do not take their morning dose of insulin. Other hospitals request that a full barium enema preparation be administered.

24. Figure 24-11 is a spot radiograph of the terminal ileum in a young man with chronic diarrhea. What disease does this patient have?
    Figure 24-11 is an image obtained during a per-oral pneumocolon in this patient with Crohn's disease. This is a specialized air contrast examination of the distal ileum, terminal ileum, cecum, and ascending colon. The patient undergoes a barium enema preparation the day before the examination to empty the terminal ileum and colon of feces. The patient then undergoes a routine small bowel follow-through examination. At the end of that examination, the per-oral pneumocolon study is performed. The patient receives 1 mg of glucagon intravenously to relax the colon, ileocecal valve, and small bowel. Air is insufflated into the rectum via a small soft catheter (e.g., a Foley catheter). The radiologist distends the colon with air and attempts to reflux air into the terminal ileum. Air refluxes into the terminal ileum in most patients (85%), enabling double-contrast images of the terminal ileum that are superior to the images obtained during small bowel follow-through examination alone. A per-oral pneumocolon study may be valuable to show subtle mucosal changes of Crohn's disease and to evaluate the right colon and ileocecal valve if these areas were not seen at either endoscopy or barium enema.

25. Figure 24-12 is from a double-contrast esophagogram performed in an immunocompromised patient with acute odynophagia. What is your diagnosis?
    For the answer, see the figure legend.

26. Figure 24-13 is an image performed during an esophagogram while the patient lies prone and rapidly drinks thin barium. This patient had long-standing dysphagia for solids and chronic heartburn. What is your diagnosis?
    Endoscopy and barium studies diagnose reflux esophagitis in about 40% of patients with biopsy-proven reflux esophagitis. Endoscopy has the ability to obtain biopsy specimens, whereas an upper GI series is more accurate in the diagnosis of gastroesophageal reflux itself because only a small percentage of patients (10%) who have gastroesophageal reflux have reflux esophagitis. An upper GI study detects gastroesophageal reflux in about 50% to

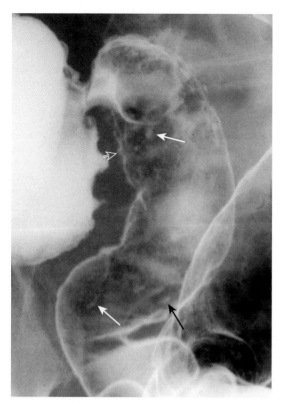

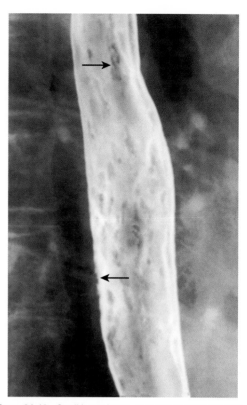

**Figure 24-11.** Crohn's disease on per-oral pneumocolon. Spot radiograph of terminal ileum shows numerous aphthoid ulcers en face as 2- to 5-mm punctate or slightly elongated collections of barium surrounded by radiolucent halos (*arrows*). In profile, aphthoid ulcers appear as 2- to 4-mm punctate barium collections (*open arrow*) protruding outside expected luminal contour. In patients with chronic diarrhea, aphthoid ulcers in terminal ileum strongly suggest diagnosis of Crohn's disease. *(From Rubesin SE, Bronner M. Radiologic-pathologic concepts in Crohn's disease. Gastrointest Radiol. 1991;1:27-55.)*

**Figure 24-12.** *Candida* esophagitis on double-contrast upper GI examination. Note numerous 1- to 4-mm elongated radiolucent filling defects aligned longitudinally (*top arrow*). Intervening mucosa is smooth and normal. In profile, filling defects are shown to be mildly elevated plaques (*bottom arrow*). These small, elevated plaques are almost pathognomonic for *Candida* esophagitis. Double-contrast esophagography has 90% to 95% sensitivity for detecting *Candida* esophagitis in immunocompromised patients.

70% of patients who have pH probe–proven gastroesophageal reflux. Barium studies are superior to endoscopy in the diagnosis of reflux-induced strictures because subtle tapered strictures are easily missed at endoscopy.

27. Figure 24-14 is an image performed during an esophagram in another patient with long-standing dysphagia. What is your diagnosis?

    In most patients with fully developed achalasia, primary peristalsis of the esophagus is absent and there is abnormal opening of the lower esophageal sphincter. These findings are seen during fluoroscopy. The radiographic findings include a variably dilated esophagus and a smooth, short, "beak-like" narrowing of the distal esophagus whose tip is just above the esophagogastric junction. Early primary achalasia may have less obvious abnormal peristalsis and less esophageal dilation.

    Secondary achalasia can be the result of tumor invasion of the myenteric plexus at the esophagogastric junction or the result of a paraneoplastic syndrome to circulating antigens. Gastric cancer directly invading the esophagus or metastasis to the esophagogastric junction may result in secondary achalasia. In Chagas disease, the bite of a triatomine bug transmits the protozoan *Trypanosoma cruzi*, and its amastigotes destroy the intramural autonomic neurons of the esophagus. In secondary achalasia, the "beak-like" narrowing is typically longer. If gastric cancer invading the esophagus causes secondary achalasia, the mucosa near the esophagogastric junction is nodular.

28. Figure 24-15 shows two images of the lesser curvature of the stomach from a double-contrast upper GI series performed in a young patient with 1 week of abdominal pain. What is your diagnosis?

    A double-contrast upper GI series can be used to diagnose an ulcer confidently as a benign gastric ulcer in two thirds of patients with ulcers. In the remaining one third of patients, ulcers are either equivocally benign, requiring endoscopic biopsy, or are frankly malignant.

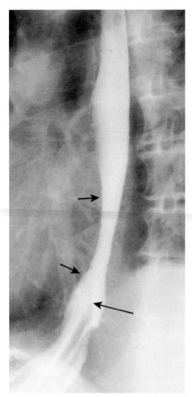

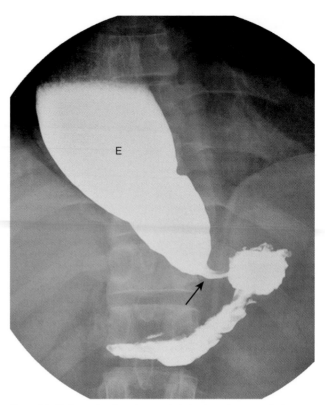

**Figure 24-13.** Reflux-induced esophageal stricture on single-contrast esophagogram. Note long (4 cm), tapered narrowing of distal esophagus (*short arrows*) with 8-mm luminal diameter. Small hiatal hernia is also present (*long arrow* identifies top of gastric fold, and esophagogastric junction is above diaphragm). Given radiographic appearance of benign distal esophageal stricture, chance of Barrett's esophagus is about 10% to 20%.

**Figure 24-14.** Long-standing primary achalasia of esophagus on single-contrast esophagogram. Spot radiograph of lower esophagus shows markedly dilated esophagus (*E*) with short, smooth, beak-like narrowing (*arrow*) near esophagogastric junction. No peristalsis was seen at fluoroscopy. Area of narrowing intermittently opened by small amount.

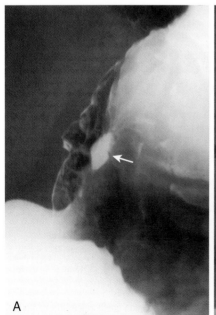

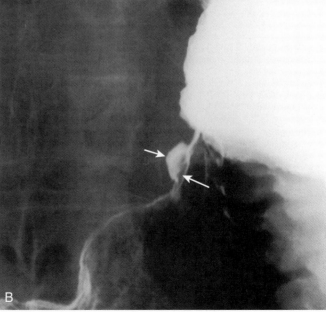

A          B

**Figure 24-15.** Benign gastric ulcer on double-contrast upper GI examination. **A,** 6-mm focal barium collection (*arrow*) is seen en face. No mass effect is seen. **B,** Ulcer niche (crater) filled with barium (*short arrow*) is seen in profile and protrudes beyond expected contour of stomach. No mass or mucosal nodularity is seen to indicate presence of tumor. As ulcer extends into soft submucosal fat, it spreads laterally, burrowing under mucosa. This undermined mucosa is seen as lucency (*long arrow*) crossing edge of ulcer, termed *Hampton line*. These are typical findings of benign gastric ulcer.

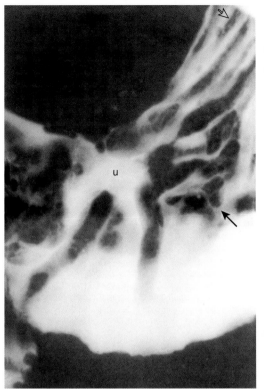

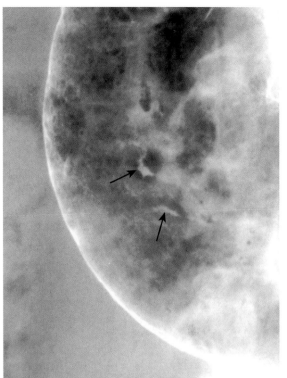

**Figure 24-16.** Malignant gastric ulcer on double-contrast upper GI examination. Coarsely lobulated, nodular folds radiate toward central barium collection (*u*). Compare normal-sized fold (*open arrow*) with enlarged, lobulated fold (*black arrow*). These radiographic findings are that of malignant tumor, proved at surgery to be due to adenocarcinoma.

**Figure 24-17.** Erosive gastritis on double-contrast upper GI examination. In gastric antrum, there are two thin, serpentine barium collections (*arrows*) surrounded by radiolucent halos. These are radiographic findings of erosive gastritis. Erosions are most commonly caused by nonsteroidal anti-inflammatory drugs (NSAIDs) but also may be caused by alcohol, viral infection, hypotension, or iatrogenic trauma (electrocautery). Linear erosions, as depicted in this figure, are usually related to NSAID use. This patient with rheumatoid arthritis was taking aspirin.

29. Figure 24-16 is an image of the gastric antrum from a double-contrast upper GI series performed in a 52-year-old woman with anemia. What is your diagnosis?
For the answer, see the figure legend.

30. Figure 24-17 is a close-up of the distal greater curvature of the stomach obtained during a double-contrast upper GI series performed in a patient with abdominal pain and rheumatoid arthritis. What is your diagnosis?
For the answer, see the figure legend.

31. A coned-down image of the gastric fundus obtained during a double-contrast upper GI series is shown in Figure 24-18. What is your diagnosis?
For the answer, see the figure legend.

32. A coned-down image of the gastric fundus obtained during a double-contrast upper GI series is shown in Figure 24-19. What is your diagnosis?
Figure 24-19 shows the typical appearance of a submucosal mass. A smooth-surfaced tumor protrudes into the lumen. The tumor has an abrupt interface with the normal adjacent contour manifested, in profile, as sharp angulation with the lumen and, en face, as a ring shadow or sharp-edged barium pool. Central ulceration is shown in about 50% of submucosal masses. The most common submucosal mass in the stomach is a gastrointestinal stromal tumor (GIST). Lymphoma, granular cell tumor, and metastases are other common submucosal masses.

33. Figure 24-20 is an image of the gastric antrum from a double-contrast upper GI series performed in a 43-year-old man with anemia. What is your diagnosis?
For the answer, see the figure legend.

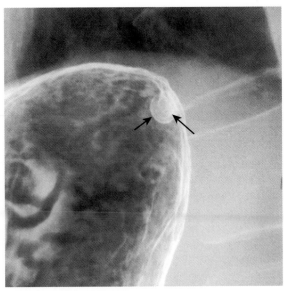

**Figure 24-18.** Hyperplastic gastric polyp on double-contrast upper GI examination. Small (6 mm) area of increased density is coated by barium (*short arrow*). Subtle ring shadow (*long arrow*) is seen centrally. These are radiographic findings of pedunculated polyp seen en face. Head of polyp (*short arrow*) is manifested as outer barium-etched ring. Pedicle of polyp (*long arrow*) is etched in white and is seen toward center of polyp. Biopsy specimen demonstrated hyperplastic polyp.

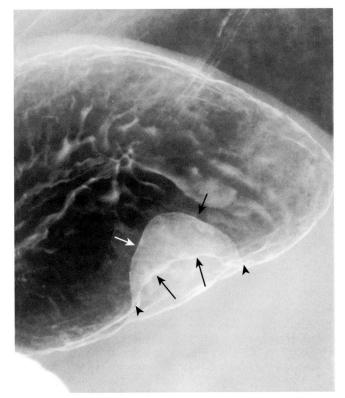

**Figure 24-19.** Gastrointestinal stromal tumor (GIST) of stomach on double-contrast upper GI examination. Note 4-cm, smooth-surfaced mass (*short arrows*) protruding into stomach, which has sharp angles to luminal contour (*arrowheads*). There is sharp line between obliquely oriented tumor and mucosal surface (*long arrows*). These are classic findings of mass arising in submucosa or muscularis propria, variably termed *submucosal* or *extramucosal mass*. This proved to be due to GIST in this patient.

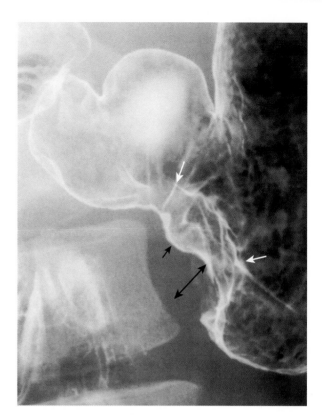

**Figure 24-20.** Gastric adenocarcinoma on double-contrast upper GI examination. Note mass shown in profile as focal loss of mucosal contour of greater curvature of gastric antrum with area of soft tissue density (*double arrow*) protruding into lumen. En face, mass appears as numerous lobulated, barium-coated lines (*white arrows*) disrupting mucosal surface. This mass has central ulceration (*black arrow*) that is not filled with barium, because mass is located on anterior wall of stomach and barium has fallen into dependent portion of stomach (gastric fundus). These radiographic findings are typical of mass of mucosal origin—in this case, gastric adenocarcinoma. Compare nodular surface of this mucosal tumor with smooth surface of submucosal tumor in Figure 24-19.

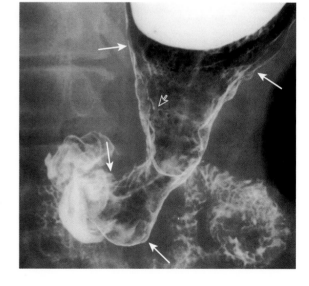

**Figure 24-21.** Linitis plastica due to gastric adenocarcinoma on double-contrast upper GI examination. Note long, circumferential, tapered narrowing of distal gastric body and proximal gastric antrum (between arrows on greater and lesser curvatures). Mucosal surface is only focally nodular (*open arrow*). These are radiographic findings of linitis plastica, proved in this case to be due to signet-ring cell adenocarcinoma of stomach broadly infiltrating submucosa. Carcinomas of stomach may spread longitudinally in submucosal tissue. If desmoplastic (scirrhous) response occurs, large portions of stomach may be narrowed. Most common causes of long gastric narrowing include adenocarcinoma, metastatic breast cancer, and corrosive ingestion.

34. An elderly man complains of early satiety. A spot radiograph of the stomach from a double-contrast upper GI series is provided (Figure 24-21). What is your diagnosis?
    For the answer, see the figure legend.

35. Figure 24-22 is a spot radiograph of the lower stomach obtained from a double-contrast upper GI series in a man who has had 4 months of abdominal discomfort. What is your differential diagnosis?
    For the answer, see the figure legend.

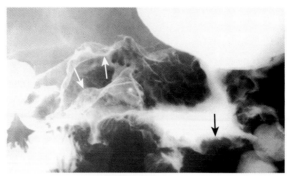

**Figure 24-22.** Gastric lymphoma on double-contrast upper GI examination. Rugal folds are composed of mucosa and submucosa. Rugal fold enlargement indicates pathology in mucosa and submucosa. Radiographically, normal rugal folds are smooth, about 5 mm in size, and slightly more undulating along greater curvature. Normal rugal folds also diminish in size from gastric fundus to antrum. Well-distended gastric antrum usually does not have rugal folds. In this image, folds of gastric antrum and body are markedly enlarged, lobulated, sometimes smooth (*white arrows*), and sometimes nodular (*black arrow*). Differential diagnosis includes tumor of mucosa (adenocarcinoma) or submucosa (lymphoma), and hyperplasia of component of mucosa (Ménétrier's disease [i.e., hyperplasia of the surface foveolar cells]). This appearance cannot represent parietal cell hyperplasia seen in Zollinger-Ellison syndrome because parietal cells are not located in gastric antrum, and folds are larger than folds typically seen in Zollinger-Ellison syndrome. This patient had lymphoma of stomach.

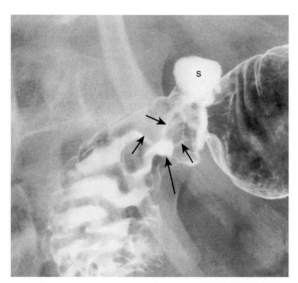

**Figure 24-23.** Acute benign duodenal ulcer on double-contrast upper GI examination. Note 6-mm barium collection (*long arrow*) in duodenal bulb. Smooth folds (*short arrows*) radiate to margin of collection. These are typical radiographic findings of acute, benign ulcer of posterior wall of duodenal bulb. Sacculation of superior fornix of duodenal bulb (*s*) reflects scarring process radiating to ulcer.

36. A young man complains of acute right upper quadrant pain. Figure 24-23 is a spot radiograph from a double-contrast upper GI series. What is your diagnosis?
Ulcers in the duodenal bulb are invariably benign. Barium examinations are very effective (95%) at detecting acute duodenal bulb ulcers in patients who do not have scarring and sacculations related to chronic scarring. In about 20% of patients with recurrent ulcer disease, however, small ulcers may be missed in scarred or sacculated duodenal bulbs.

37. Figure 24-24, *A*, is a coned-down image of the mid–small bowel obtained in a man with unexplained heme-positive stool. Figure 24-24, *B*, is an axial image from a CT scan that was performed several days later. What is your differential diagnosis?
For the answer, see the figure legend.

38. What is the best radiologic test to show small bowel tumors?
Enteroclysis (small bowel enema) is the best radiologic test to show most small bowel tumors. Enteroclysis is poor at showing arteriovenous malformations, however. In patients with known metastatic melanoma, enteroclysis can be performed if there is a clinical question of small bowel metastases (Figure 24-25).

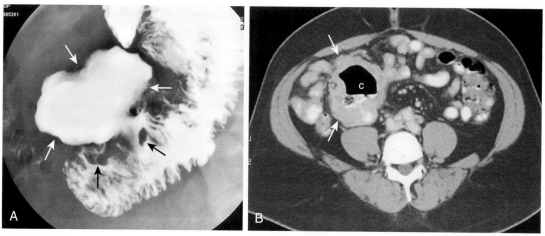

**Figure 24-24.** Malignant GIST of small bowel on small bowel follow-through. **A,** Note large (6 cm) barium-filled cavity (*white arrows*) protruding from mesenteric border of small bowel. Lobulated folds are seen on mesenteric border of bowel (*black arrows*). **B,** Soft tissue mass (*arrows*) is seen in right midabdomen. Central cavity (*c*) is filled with oral contrast material, debris, and gas. These are radiographic findings of cavitary tumor originating in small bowel. Highly cellular tumors, such as lymphoma or metastatic melanoma, or highly vascular tumors, such as GIST, are most common cavitary masses in small bowel. This patient had malignant GIST.

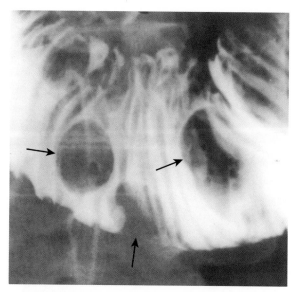

**Figure 24-25.** Metastatic melanoma to small bowel on enteroclysis. Spot radiograph of mid–small bowel obtained during single-contrast phase of enteroclysis shows at least five smooth-surfaced round/ovoid radiolucent filling defects (*arrows*) in barium column. These findings are typical of submucosal masses. Most common cause of multiple submucosal masses in small bowel is metastatic melanoma. Disseminated lymphoma, other hematogenous metastases, or Kaposi sarcoma may have similar appearance.

39. A young man complains of increasing abdominal distention and subacute right lower quadrant pain. Two images from a computed tomography (CT) scan are presented (Figure 24-26). Although a specific diagnosis is not possible, describe what is happening.

    CT is an excellent first examination in patients with vomiting and abdominal distention and a suspected clinical diagnosis of small bowel obstruction. CT is a rapidly performed procedure compared with a small bowel follow-through in a patient with an obstruction. The radiologist looks for a transition zone between dilated, fluid-filled bowel and collapsed bowel. CT can detect strictures related to Crohn's disease, primary or metastatic tumors, internal or external hernias, and polypoid tumors causing intussusception. CT cannot directly show adhesions, the most common cause of small bowel obstruction in patients who previously have undergone surgery. The CT diagnosis of adhesion is a diagnosis of exclusion; if an abnormality is not seen at the transition zone, a diagnosis of adhesion is made.

40. A young man complains of diarrhea for 4 weeks. Figure 24-27 is a spot image of the terminal ileum from a small bowel follow-through. What is your diagnosis?

    For the answer, see the figure legend.

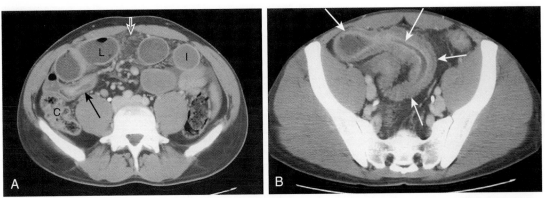

**Figure 24-26.** Crohn's disease on CT. **A,** Axial image at level of iliac crests shows moderately dilated loops of ileum. Some ileal loops are completely filled with fluid (*l*) and are not visible on radiograph; other loops (*L*) have small amount of intraluminal gas. Collapsed loop of ileum has mildly thickened wall (*arrow*). Portion of small bowel mesentery is hazy (*open arrow*) because of inflammatory stranding of mesenteric fat. Cecum (*c*) is identified. **B,** Axial image more caudally located reveals markedly thick-walled distal small bowel (*short arrows*). Mucosal surface (*long arrow*) is enhancing more than skeletal muscle, and submucosa is of low attenuation, in keeping with mural stratification pattern indicating nonneoplastic disease. Diagnosis of partial small bowel obstruction can be made, manifested as disproportionate dilation of proximal small bowel, but specific diagnosis of cause of bowel wall thickening cannot be made. Bowel obstruction was shown on separate small bowel follow-through examination to be caused by Crohn's disease.

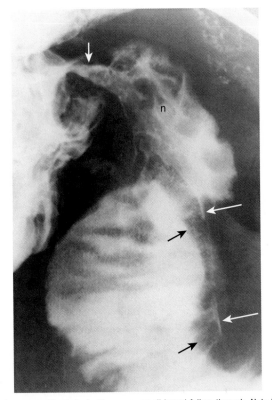

**Figure 24-27.** Mesenteric border ulcer caused by Crohn's disease on small bowel follow-through. Note long, thin barium collection (*long white arrows*) on mesenteric border of terminal ileum, paralleled by radiolucent mound of edema (*black arrows*). These are radiographic findings of mesenteric border ulcer, which is almost pathognomonic of Crohn's disease. Also present are thick, slightly nodular folds in terminal ileum (*n*) and mild stricture of ileocecal valve (*short white arrow*). *(From Rubesin SE, Bronner M. Radiologic-pathologic concepts in Crohn's disease. Gastrointest Radiol. 1991;1:27-55.)*

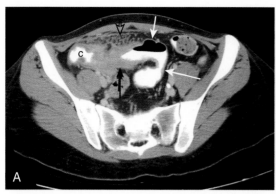 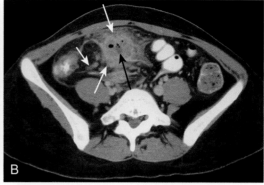

**Figure 24-28.** Detection of complications of Crohn's disease on CT. **A,** Axial image through pelvis shows varying degrees of bowel wall thickening in this patient with known Crohn's disease. Thickness of wall of terminal ileum varies from normal (*short white arrow*) to mildly thickened (*long white arrow*) to markedly thickened (*black arrow*). Wall of cecum (*C*) is mildly thickened and has mural stratification pattern. Omental fat (*open black arrow*) anterior to ileum has numerous linear soft tissue strands (so-called dirty or hazy fat). **B,** Axial image more cephalad in pelvis shows unsuspected abscess (*long white arrows*). 5-cm inhomogeneous mass in right lower quadrant has areas of soft tissue, fluid (*black arrow*), and air attenuation. Surrounding fat has soft tissue stranding. There is also regional lymphadenopathy (*short white arrow*). These images demonstrate ability of CT to show serious complications in patients with known Crohn's disease. *(From Rubesin SE, Bartram CI, Laufer I. Inflammatory bowel disease. In: Levine MS, Rubesin SE, Laufer I, eds. Double contrast gastrointestinal radiology. Philadelphia: Saunders; 2000. p. 417-470.)*

41. A patient with known Crohn's disease comes to the emergency department with abdominal pain (Figure 24-28). What radiologic test should be performed first?
    A CT scan shows an unsuspected complication in about 25% of symptomatic patients with Crohn's disease. Figures 24-26 to 24-28 are representative examples of imaging in Crohn's disease. In patients with a known diagnosis of moderate to severe Crohn's disease and acute symptoms, CT is the first examination of choice, as it demonstrates the severe complications of Crohn's disease. However, a barium examination of the small bowel or colon will demonstrate pathognomonic findings of Crohn's disease (aphthoid ulcers, mesenteric border ulcers, and cobblestoning) that are not visible on a CT study. A barium study is more specific than CT because it directly looks at the mucosal surface. Therefore, in a patient with mild or chronic symptoms, if the clinical question is (1) Does this patient have Crohn's disease? or (2) Does this patient have recurrent Crohn's disease?, a barium study is superior to CT in the demonstration of mild Crohn's disease and is more specific in the diagnosis of Crohn's disease.

42. A middle-aged woman has peripheral lymphadenopathy and heme-positive stool. Figure 24-29 is an image of the terminal ileum and ileocecal valve from the single-contrast phase of a small bowel enema. What are the diagnostic possibilities?
    For the answer, see the figure legend.

43. A middle-aged woman has foul-smelling yellow stools. Figure 24-30 is a spot image of the proximal jejunum obtained during enteroclysis. The double arrows represent 1 inch. What is your diagnosis?
    Diseases that cause malabsorption usually involve the mucosa, submucosa, and lymphatics and mesenteric lymph nodes. Enteroclysis is superior to small bowel follow-through in the workup of malabsorption because enteroclysis shows the mucosal surface and valvulae conniventes better than a small bowel follow-through. For the answer, see the figure legend.

44. A 35-year-old woman has right lower quadrant pain and diarrhea. The results of the CT scan were normal. Figure 24-31 is a spot radiograph of the distal ileum from a small bowel follow-through. What is your diagnosis?
    Although CT is excellent at showing disease outside of the small bowel and markedly thickened bowel wall, CT cannot show the mucosal surface or subtle wall abnormalities, and it cannot be used to make specific diagnoses in most cases. For the answer, see the figure legend.

45. A 44-year-old man had surgery for a persistent duodenal ulcer (Figure 24-32). What operation was performed?
    For the answer, see the figure legend. Surgical treatment for peptic ulcer disease is reserved for complications such as perforation, severe hemorrhage, and obstruction. Vagotomy, in its various forms, denervates the body-type mucosa, reducing acid production. Acid secretion can be reduced further by resecting the gastric antrum, eliminating gastrin-secreting G cells. The remaining upper stomach is connected to the duodenum (termed **gastroduodenostomy/Billroth I reconstruction**) or to the jejunum (**gastrojejunostomy/Billroth II reconstruction**). If an antrectomy is not performed, a pyloroplasty is done because vagotomy alters pyloric sphincter function, reducing gastric emptying.

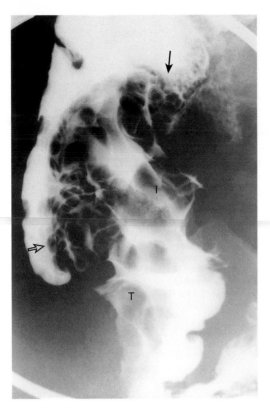

**Figure 24-29.** Ileocecal lymphoma on enteroclysis. Folds of terminal ileum (*T*), ileocecal valve (*I*), medial wall of cecum (*open arrow*), and proximal ascending colon (*arrow*) are markedly thickened and slightly lobulated but smooth-surfaced. There are no pathognomonic findings of Crohn's disease (e.g., aphthoid ulcers, mesenteric border ulcers, cobblestoning, fissures, fistulas). Folds are much larger than would be seen in Crohn's disease. Two most likely possibilities are lymphoma or carcinoma of ileocecal valve invading terminal ileum. This proved to be mantle cell lymphoma of ileocecal region. This case shows that not all fold thickening in terminal ileum during barium studies or wall thickening on CT is due to Crohn's disease. Acute or semi-acute infections (e.g., *Yersinia* enterocolitis), tuberculosis in patients from endemic areas or in patients with acquired immunodeficiency syndrome, and lymphoma can cause thick ileal folds. Unless aforementioned pathognomonic findings of Crohn's disease are present, biopsy, stool culture, or follow-up imaging is indicated.

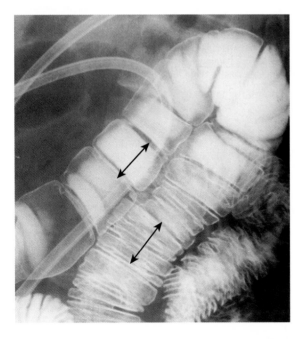

**Figure 24-30.** Gluten-sensitive enteropathy on enteroclysis. Note diminished number of valvulae conniventes per inch in more superior loop of jejunum than in inferior loop. Only two folds per inch are seen superiorly, whereas about five to six folds per inch are seen inferiorly (double arrows). Loss of valvulae conniventes indicates that there is loss of mucosal surface area. These radiographic findings are macroscopic correlates of villous atrophy seen in gluten-sensitive enteropathy (celiac disease, nontropical sprue). Celiac disease is underdiagnosed in adult patients. Currently, antibodies are found in 70% to 90% of patients with gluten-sensitive enteropathy and in about 1 in 200 adults. Diagnosis of celiac disease requires biopsy-shown improvement of villous atrophy after trial of gluten-free diet. Role of enteroclysis in symptomatic patients with celiac disease is to exclude development of complications such as ulcerative jejunoileitis or tumors including adenocarcinoma or lymphoma of small bowel.

46. **What are the physiologic sequelae of gastric operations?**
    Truncal vagotomy accelerates liquid emptying from the stomach but diminishes solid emptying. Truncal vagotomy diminishes pancreatic exocrine secretion and biliary secretion after a meal. **A dumping syndrome** may occur immediately or several hours after a meal. Dumping syndrome includes GI symptoms such as nausea or epigastric discomfort and systemic symptoms such as palpitations, dizziness, or syncope. **Alkaline reflux gastritis** is the term for gastritis induced by reflux of pancreaticobiliary secretions into the remaining stomach. This causes nausea, pain, or vomiting.

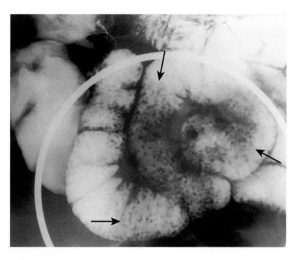

**Figure 24-31.** Lymphoid hyperplasia of ileum on small bowel follow-through. Multiple uniformly round, radiolucent filling defects (1 to 2 mm in size) (*arrows*) are in barium column of distal-most three loops of ileum. Normal smooth mucosa separates these nodules. These findings are characteristic of extensive lymphoid hyperplasia. Causes of extensive lymphoid hyperplasia in ileum include recent enteric infection and immunodeficiency states, such as common variable immunodeficiency and IgA deficiency. After barium study, diagnosis of common variable immunodeficiency was made in this patient.

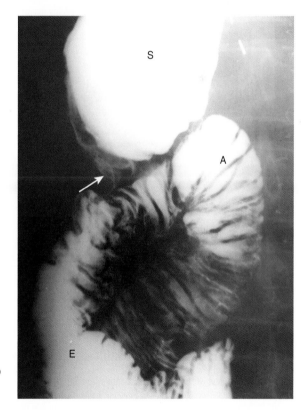

**Figure 24-32.** Antrectomy with gastrojejunostomy (Billroth II procedure) on double-contrast upper GI examination. Spot radiograph shows remaining upper stomach (*S*) filled with barium. Gastrojejunal anastomosis (*arrow*), efferent limb (*E*), and afferent limb (*A*) are identified. In this patient, afferent limb is on left side of anastomosis, but loop curves back to right to join duodenum.

47. A 62-year-old man complains of abdominal pain 20 years after an antrectomy with gastroduodenostomy was performed for intractable duodenal ulcer disease (Figure 24-33). What is your differential diagnosis?
    Chronic reflux of pancreaticobiliary secretions (bile reflux) results in progression from chronic inflammation to development of mucosal hyperplasia, gastric metaplasia, and dysplasia, with the possible development of adenocarcinoma. Lack of eradication of *Helicobacter pylori* in the postoperative stomach can result in a similar cascade. If large, lobulated folds and nodular mucosa are seen long after gastric surgery, the differential diagnosis includes severe *H. pylori* gastritis or bile reflux gastritis complicated by hyperplasia, dysplasia, or adenocarcinoma. An adenocarcinoma was found in this patient.

48. A 45-year-old woman complains of vomiting. She had surgery for morbid obesity 2 years previously (Figure 24-34). What operation did this patient have? Why is she vomiting?
    For the answer, see the figure legend.

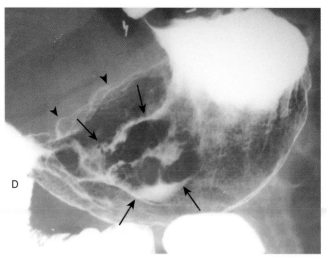

**Figure 24-33.** Gastric cancer arising after gastroduodenostomy (Billroth I procedure) on double-contrast upper GI examination. Spot radiograph of stomach shows large, lobulated folds (*arrows*) in distal gastric body. Contour of lesser curvature is undulating (*arrowheads*). Gastroduodenostomy is seen in overlap, and proximal duodenum (*D*) is identified.

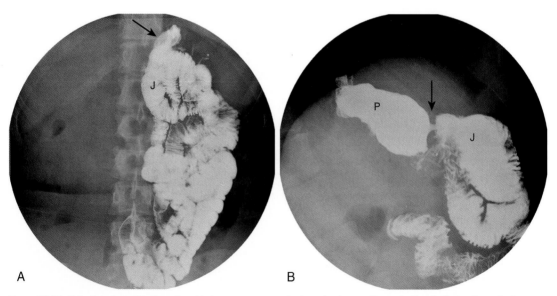

**Figure 24-34.** Detection of complications of gastric bypass surgery on single-contrast upper GI examination. **A,** Spot radiograph of abdomen obtained at low magnification shows small portion of stomach, i.e., gastric pouch (*arrow*). Remainder of stomach, pylorus, and duodenum is not filled with barium. Barium enters jejunum (*J*). **B,** Spot radiograph of left upper quadrant obtained with patient in left-side down lateral position shows gastric pouch (*P*), gastrojejunal anastomosis (*arrow*), and proximal jejunum (*J*), in keeping with prior gastric bypass surgery. Almost all of stomach, all of duodenum, and first 50 to 150 cm of jejunum have been "bypassed." In normal postoperative patients, gastric pouch is small, holding about 15 to 60 mL of volume. In this patient, gastric pouch is dilated because of chronic obstruction at gastrojejunal anastomosis, resulting in vomiting. Gastrojejunal anastomosis (*arrow*) measures 5 mm in luminal diameter but normally measures about 9 to 10 mm at our institution. Bypassed stomach, duodenum, and proximal jejunum are connected to jejunum by jejunojejunostomy. This author prefers term "alimentary limb" for portion of jejunum between pouch and jejunojejunostomy and "pancreaticobiliary limb" for bypassed stomach, duodenum, and jejunum proximal to jejunojejunostomy.

49. A 42-year-old woman has undergone surgery for morbid obesity (Figure 24-35). What operation was performed?

 For the answer, see the figure legend. Gastric bypass results in better weight loss than vertical banded gastroplasty. As a result, gastric bypass improves type 2 diabetes to a better degree than vertical banded gastroplasty. Gastric bypass has a greater incidence of immediate postoperative leaks. In the remote postoperative period, gastric bypass has a greater incidence of pouch ulceration, pouch outlet stenosis, vitamin $B_{12}$ deficiency, and iron-deficiency anemia.

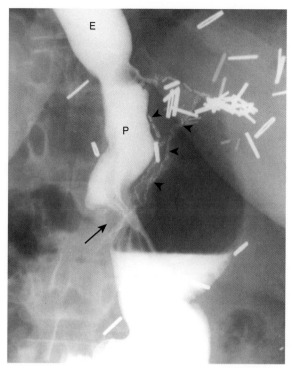

**Figure 24-35.** Vertical banded gastroplasty on single-contrast upper GI examination. Spot radiograph of stomach is performed with patient standing. Distal esophagus (*E*) is identified. Elongated gastric pouch (*P*) is present along lesser curvature, separated from upper stomach by staple line (*arrowheads*). Pouch outlet (*arrow*) communicates with gastric body. Gastric fundus is filled with air with patient in upright position. In vertical banded gastroplasty, hole is made by staple gun about 5 cm inferior to gastric cardia. Gastric pouch is constructed by firing stapling device between hole and angle of His, creating band of tissue between cardia and greater curvature (hence the term *vertical band*). Outlet of pouch is formed by mesh wrapped around stomach, from hole to lesser curvature. Vertical banded gastroplasties have been replaced by newer procedures. However, they are permanent surgery, and therefore the clinician must note difference between this outdated surgery and other procedures for morbid obesity, as many patients with this procedure are still living.

50. A 41-year-old woman had undergone surgery for morbid obesity (Figure 24-36). What operation was performed?
    For the answer, see the figure legend.

51. A 27-year-old woman underwent surgery for morbid obesity and now presents with left upper quadrant pain and regurgitation. Figure 24-37, *A*, is a spot radiograph from a study performed 14 months before the image shown in Figure 24-37, *B*. What has happened?
    For the answer, see the figure legend. Complications of laparoscopic band surgery include port infections and inadequate weight loss. The stomach may form ulcers where the band compresses the upper gastric body, or the band may fully erode into the stomach. Slippage of the stomach through the band may result in obstruction.

52. A 29-year-old woman had a sleeve gastrectomy 6 weeks ago and now complains of vomiting after small meals. Figure 24-38 is from an upper GI series. What is your diagnosis?
    For the answer, see the figure legend. During a sleeve gastrectomy, the surgeon removes a large portion of the proximal greater curvature of the stomach. This resection removes gastric body–type mucosa and a large portion of the oxyntic cells that secrete grehlin, a peptide hormone that stimulates appetite. Grehlin acts on hypothalamic cells to increase hunger, stimulate gastric secretion, and increase gastric motility. Thus, a sleeve gastrectomy is in part restrictive, with a small gastric pouch, and also physiologic, as it causes the patient to eat less.

---

**KEY POINTS**

- Single-contrast GI examinations use "thin barium" or water-soluble contrast material (no gas used) and are easier to perform in sick patients who cannot turn to detect bowel obstruction, perforation, or fistulas.
- Double-contrast GI examinations use high-density barium and air/carbon dioxide, require patients to turn, and are more sensitive than single-contrast examinations for detecting mucosal abnormalities.

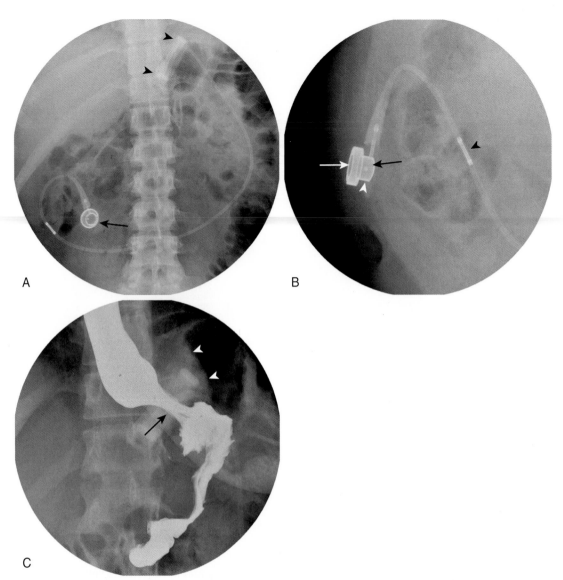

**Figure 24-36.** Laparoscopic band procedure on single-contrast upper GI examination. **A,** Spot radiograph of upper abdomen obtained at low magnification shows "band" of radiopaque material (*arrowheads*) just to left of T10 and T11 vertebral bodies. Radiopaque tube connects band to port (*arrow*). This band has been placed just below gastric cardia and contains balloon that can be filled with variable amounts of fluid via port/tubing. **B,** Spot radiograph with patient in lateral position shows structure of port. Opening of port appears as thin metallic ring (*white arrow*) and is covered by membrane. Reservoir of port (*white arrowhead*) holds variable amount of fluid, depending on band/manufacturer, usually 4 to 14 mL. Small metal ball (*black arrow*) falls to most dependent portion of port. This pellet helps guide needle entry into port. Connector (*black arrowhead*) connects port complex to band. **C,** Spot radiograph obtained while patient stands and drinks barium. Mild constriction of stomach by band is identified (*arrow*). This narrowing is not distal esophagus, as tiny pouch of stomach lies above band. Compression by band on fundus is manifested as soft tissue indentation into air-filled fundus (*arrowheads*). Band is angled normally, with outer margin superior to inner margin, between 30 and 60 degrees from horizontal.

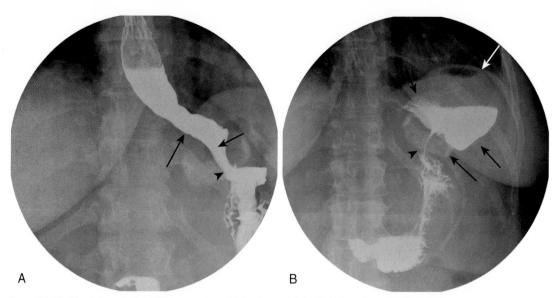

**Figure 24-37.** Slip of stomach through laparoscopic gastric band associated with high-grade gastric obstruction on upper GI examination. **A,** Baseline spot radiograph performed while patient was asymptomatic shows small pouch (*short arrow*) above band. Esophagogastric junction is seen as thin indentation (*long arrow*). Note width of lumen of stomach as it passes through band (*arrowhead*) and normal angle of band. **B,** Spot radiograph performed 14 months later shows large "pouch," including gastric fundus and upper gastric body (*short arrows*) superior to band. Lumen of stomach is markedly narrowed (to about 1 mm) as it goes through band (*arrowhead*). Band is now angled inferiorly (*long arrow*). Residual fluid in gastric fundus (note air-fluid and fluid-barium levels) is also indicative of obstruction.

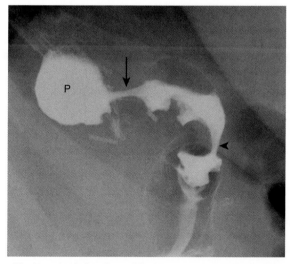

**Figure 24-38.** Stricture in mid–gastric sleeve developing after gastric sleeve procedure on double-contrast upper GI examination. Spot radiograph performed with patient in upright position shows focal 2-cm smooth narrowing of proximal gastric sleeve (*arrow*) and round dilation of unoperated fundus of stomach (*P*) proximal to narrowing. Gastric sleeve outlet is also narrow (*arrowhead*). Normal gastric sleeve should have a more tubular configuration.

## BIBLIOGRAPHY

Gore RM, Levine MS. *Textbook of gastrointestinal radiology*. 4th ed. Philadelphia: Elsevier Saunders; 2015.

Meyers MA, Charnsangavej C, Oliphant M. *Meyers' dynamic radiology of the abdomen: normal and pathologic anatomy*. 6th ed. New York, NY: Springer; 2011.

Lee JKT, Sagel SS, Stanley RJ, et al. *Computed body tomography with MRI correlation*. 4th ed. Philadelphia: Lippincott Williams & Wilkins; 2003.

Levine MS, Rubesin SE, Laufer I. *Double contrast gastrointestinal radiology*. 3rd ed. Philadelphia: Saunders; 2000.

Herlinger H, Maglinte D, Birnbaum BA. *Clinical radiology of the small intestine*. 2nd ed. New York: Springer-Verlag; 1999.

# CHAPTER 25

# CT AND MRI OF THE UPPER GASTROINTESTINAL TRACT

*Drew A. Torigian, MD, MA, FSAR*

1. **What are the general indications for routine computed tomography (CT) and magnetic resonance imaging (MRI) of the upper gastrointestinal (GI) tract?**

   General indications for routine abdominopelvic CT or MRI evaluation of the upper GI tract include:
   - Assessment of patients with clinical symptoms or signs potentially related to GI tract pathology for detection and characterization of the underlying etiologies.
   - Staging, pretreatment planning, response assessment, and restaging of patients with known GI tract malignancy.
   - Assessment of patients with suspected or known infectious, inflammatory, or ischemic bowel disease.
   - Assessment of patients with traumatic injury to the abdomen or pelvis for detection of bowel injury.
   - Evaluation of patients with known bowel obstruction to elucidate the underlying etiology.

   Routine CT is typically performed using axial 5-mm sections during the venous phase of intravenous contrast enhancement following the administration of barium- or iodine-based positive oral contrast material. Positive oral contrast material increases the attenuation of the bowel lumen relative to the bowel wall while simultaneously distending the bowel lumen. Therefore, this type of oral contrast material is most often used to improve the detection of intraluminal bowel pathology and to detect and localize bowel leaks, particularly after prior bowel surgery.

   Routine MRI is typically performed using multiplanar T1-weighted, T2-weighted, and diffusion-weighted image acquisitions, followed by dynamic contrast-enhanced T1-weighted imaging. However, oral contrast material is generally not administered.

2. **How are computed tomographic enterography (CTE) and magnetic resonance enterography (MRE) different from routine CT or MRI scans of the abdomen and pelvis?**

   CTE and MRE are tailored specifically for detailed evaluation of the small bowel. They are both obtained through the abdomen and pelvis after the administration of large volumes (>1 L) of neutral oral contrast material. Neutral oral contrast material has fluid attenuation on CT and fluid signal intensity on MRI (i.e., low T1-weighted and high T2-weighted signal intensity). This improves the distinction between the bowel wall and the bowel lumen while simultaneously distending the bowel lumen, allowing for improved detection of abnormal bowel wall pathology. Multiplanar thin section images are then typically obtained during one or more phases of intravenous contrast enhancement. MRE has superior soft tissue contrast compared to CTE, improving the detection of mural edema and mural hyperenhancement, and involves no radiation exposure but is more expensive and takes longer to perform than CTE.

3. **What are the major clinical indications for CTE and MRE?**

   CTE and MRE are most often performed for:
   - Assessment of patients with suspected or known Crohn's disease to determine disease activity, disease extent, presence of disease complications, and disease response to therapeutic intervention.
   - Assessment of patients with obscure GI bleeding to detect the presence, site, and etiology of GI hemorrhage.

4. **What is the normal CT and MRI appearance of the upper GI tract?**

   The normal bowel wall is generally ≤3 mm in thickness when well distended. However, the gastric antrum and pylorus may normally measure up to 11 mm, and underdistended portions of normal bowel may also appear to be thicker than 3 mm but without asymmetric thickening or abnormal enhancement (Figure 25-1). On unenhanced CT and MR images, the wall of the bowel attenuation and signal intensity are similar to those of skeletal muscle. On contrast-enhanced CT and MR images, the bowel wall normally has uniform homogeneous enhancement that is typically less than or similar to that of the liver. However, the normal gastric wall may sometimes have a stratified enhancement pattern, where the mucosal layer (and sometimes the serosal layer) has greater enhancement than the submucosal layer.

   The esophagus typically appears underdistended, and the stomach may be variably distended on cross-sectional imaging. The small bowel is generally ≤3 cm in caliber, and the jejunum typically has thicker, taller, and more numerous (4 to 7 per inch) valvulae conniventes (also called folds of Kerckring or plicae circulares) than the ileum (2 to 4 per inch).

5. **What is the hallmark of GI tract pathology on cross-sectional imaging?**

   Wall (mural) thickening is the hallmark of GI tract pathology seen on cross-sectional imaging. In general, the greater the degree of mural thickening, the more likely that malignancy is the underlying etiology. Bowel wall thickness

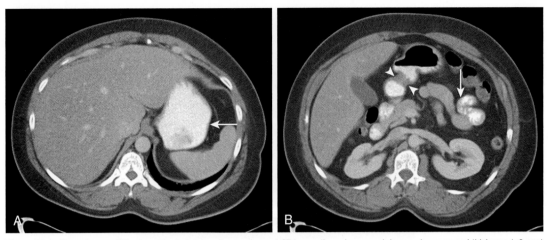

**Figure 25-1.** Normal upper GI tract on CT. **A,** Axial contrast-enhanced CT image through upper abdomen shows normal thickness (≤3 mm) of gastric body wall (*arrow*). Note moderate distention of stomach by positive oral contrast material. **B,** Axial contrast-enhanced CT image more inferiorly through abdomen shows normal thicker wall of gastric pylorus (*arrowheads*) as well as normal (≤3 mm in thickness) wall of well-distended loop of jejunum (*arrow*).

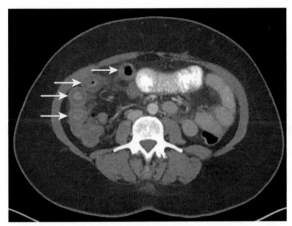

**Figure 25-2.** "Target" sign of small bowel on CT. Note moderate wall thickening of multiple loops of small bowel (*arrows*) in right abdomen and mild perienteric fat stranding. Also note associated bright soft tissue attenuation inner layer, dark low-attenuation middle layer (secondary to submucosal edema), and bright soft tissue attenuation outer layer representing "target" sign. In small bowel, presence of "target" sign is highly specific for nonneoplastic disease. This patient presented with acute abdominal pain caused by small bowel angioedema secondary to angiotensin converting enzyme (ACE) inhibitor drug therapy.

<1.5 cm is generally nonneoplastic in etiology, whereas bowel wall thickness >1.5 cm is usually due to malignancy. Asymmetric wall thickening and focal wall thickening are also generally suggestive features of malignancy, although nonneoplastic diseases of the bowel may sometimes also be asymmetric or focal. Surrounding fat stranding greater than the degree of wall thickening favors an inflammatory etiology.

6. What is the "target" sign?
   On CT, the "target" sign, also known as mural stratification, refers to visualization of a bright soft tissue attenuation inner layer (representing mucosa, lamina propria, and hypertrophied muscularis mucosae, sometimes with hyperemia), a dark low-attenuation middle layer (representing edematous submucosa), and sometimes a bright soft tissue attenuation outer layer (representing muscularis propria and serosa); the alternating layers correspond to the rings of a target (Figure 25-2). On MRI, a similar bright-dark-bright pattern is seen on contrast-enhanced fat-suppressed T1-weighted images, whereas a dark-bright-dark pattern is seen on T2-weighted images, because fluid and edema are high in signal intensity on T2-weighted images.

   This sign is not specific for a particular disease condition but is highly specific for the diagnosis of nonneoplastic disease (edema, infection, inflammation, ischemia) when encountered in the small bowel. However, this specificity for nonneoplastic disease does not hold when it is encountered in the stomach, as scirrhous carcinoma may also have a "target" sign.

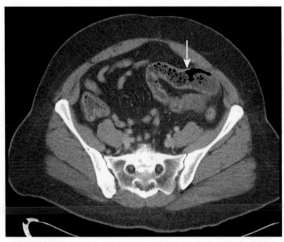

**Figure 25-3.** "Small bowel feces" sign of small bowel on CT. Note particulate debris and gas bubbles with mildly dilated loop of small bowel (*arrow*) mimicking appearance of fecal material in large bowel related to low-grade partial small bowel obstruction secondary to nonvisualized adhesions.

7. What is the "fat halo" sign?

The "fat halo" sign indicates the sequelae of prior inflammatory disease and is characterized by fat attenuation in the submucosa with relative hyperattenuation of the mucosa and muscularis propria or serosa on CT. On MRI, fat signal intensity is seen in the submucosa. This finding is nonspecific and can also be seen in normal bowel.

8. What is the "comb" sign?

The "comb" sign is due to engorgement of the perienteric or pericolic vessels which, when viewed en face, mimic the tines of a comb radiating away from the bowel. This is usually encountered with infectious or inflammatory disease of the bowel, most often with Crohn's disease.

9. What is the "small bowel feces" sign?

The "small bowel feces" sign is due to the mixture of particulate debris and gas bubbles within the small bowel lumen, mimicking the appearance of fecal material that is normally encountered in the large bowel. It is due to incompletely digested food, bacterial overgrowth, and/or increased water absorption secondary to stasis. This finding generally indicates presence of a small bowel obstruction and is typically encountered just proximal to the site of obstruction (Figure 25-3).

10. What does active GI bleeding look like on CTE or MRE images?

Active GI bleeding typically appears as a focus of high attenuation or high signal intensity contrast material within the lumen of a portion of the bowel during the arterial phase of enhancement, which then progressively enlarges over time during the venous or delayed phases of enhancement.

11. What are some cross-sectional imaging features that suggest presence of bowel malrotation?

- Malposition of the duodenojejunal junction (ligament of Treitz) from its normal location to the left of the spine at the level of the duodenal bulb
- A predominance of small bowel loops in the right abdomen and of large bowel loops in the left abdomen (Figure 25-4)
- Inversion of the normal relationship of the superior mesenteric vein (SMV) and superior mesenteric artery (SMA). The proximal SMV is normally seen anterior to and to the right of the proximal SMA, but in the setting of bowel malrotation, the proximal SMV may instead be located anterior to and to the left of the proximal SMA

12. What are some causes of esophagitis?

For the answer, see Box 25-1. Gastroesophageal reflux (GER) and infectious esophagitis (typically in immunocompromised patients) are the most common causes of esophagitis, and *Candida albicans* is the most common cause of infectious esophagitis. Caustic ingestion is most often due to the ingestion of lye (sodium hydroxide), either accidentally in children or during suicide attempts in adults.

13. What are the typical imaging features of esophagitis on CT and MRI?

Segmental or diffuse smooth circumferential wall thickening of the esophagus is seen (Figure 25-5). Sometimes, increased mural enhancement, increased mural T2-weighted signal intensity relative to skeletal muscle, a "target" sign, luminal narrowing, surrounding fat stranding, intramural tract or abscess formation, or fistula formation between the esophagus and other structures such as the tracheobronchial tree or stomach may also be seen.

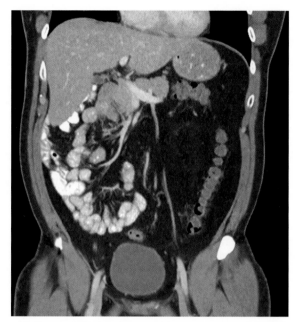

**Figure 25-4.** Bowel malrotation on CT. Note predominance of small bowel loops in right abdomen and of large bowel loops in left abdomen.

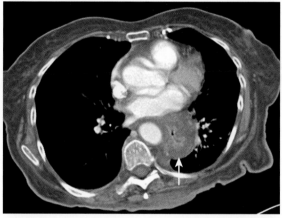

**Figure 25-5.** Esophagitis on CT. Note marked smooth circumferential wall thickening of esophagus (*arrow*) along with "target" sign and luminal narrowing.

**Box 25-1.** Some Causes of Esophagitis

- GER
- Infection
  - *Candida albicans*
  - Herpes simplex virus (HSV) type 1
  - Cytomegalovirus (CMV)
  - Human immunodeficiency virus (HIV)
  - Mycobacterial infection
- Oral medications
  - NSAIDs
  - Tetracycline or doxycycline
  - Potassium chloride
- Radiation therapy
- Caustic ingestion
- Crohn's disease

14. What is achalasia?

Achalasia is an uncommon esophageal dysmotility disorder in which there is absent esophageal peristalsis and impaired or absent relaxation of the lower esophageal sphincter during deglutition. The two major forms are primary achalasia and secondary achalasia.

Primary, or idiopathic, achalasia is caused by degeneration of myenteric plexi in the esophageal wall, whereas secondary achalasia (or pseudo-achalasia) is a less common form caused by other conditions (especially malignant tumors) that lead to an achalasia-like motility disorder. Differentiation of these two forms is important because primary achalasia is generally treated with botulinum toxin injection, pneumatic dilation, or laparoscopic myotomy, whereas secondary achalasia usually requires diagnostic workup and treatment of the underlying malignancy.

15. How can one distinguish between primary achalasia and secondary achalasia based on clinical and cross-sectional imaging features?

Primary achalasia typically presents clinically with long-standing slowly progressive dysphagia usually in adult patients <50 to 60 years of age. On cross-sectional imaging, smooth tapered narrowing of the distal esophagus is seen, sometimes with mild smooth wall thickening, in association with upstream esophageal dilation, which can be massive and associated with retained ingested debris. No soft tissue mass at the gastroesophageal junction, regional lymphadenopathy, or distant metastases are seen (Figure 25-6).

Secondary achalasia typically presents clinically with a more acute onset and a more rapid progression of symptoms (usually within 6 months) in older patients (usually >60 years of age). On cross-sectional imaging, upstream esophageal dilation is again seen, but additional suggestive imaging features may be present including distal esophageal wall thickening that is nodular, lobulated, or asymmetric; a soft tissue mass at the gastroesophageal junction; regional lymphadenopathy or distant metastatic disease. Adenocarcinoma of the gastric cardia, gastric fundus, or distal esophagus is the most frequent tumor that causes secondary achalasia.

16. What are esophageal varices, and what is their appearance on CT and MRI?

Esophageal varices are dilated venous collaterals in or around the esophageal wall. On CT and MRI, they appear as tubular or serpentine structures in or around the esophageal wall that enhance to a degree similar to that of other systemic veins, resulting in a thickened lobulated appearance of the esophageal wall (Figure 25-7).

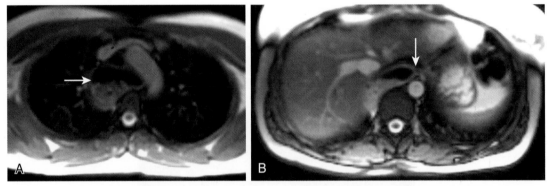

**Figure 25-6.** Primary achalasia on MRI. **A,** Axial bright-blood MR image through upper chest shows marked dilation of upper esophagus (*arrow*) with layering retained ingested debris. **B,** Axial bright-blood MR image through lower chest demonstrates smooth tapered narrowing of distal esophagus (*arrow*). Note absence of associated soft tissue mass.

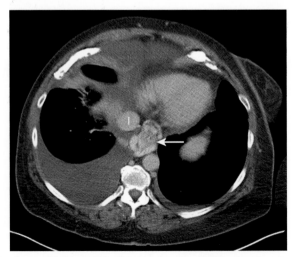

**Figure 25-7.** Uphill esophageal varices on CT. Note multiple dilated tubular serpentine structures in and around wall of distal esophagus that enhance to similar degree as inferior vena cava (*I*) representing varices. This patient has portal hypertension secondary to cirrhosis.

17. **What is the difference between uphill and downhill varices of the esophagus?**

Uphill varices of the esophagus are secondary to portal hypertension and are typically seen in the lower third of the esophagus (see Figure 25-7). Downhill varices of the esophagus are secondary to superior vena cava (SVC) occlusion and are typically seen in the upper and middle thirds of the esophagus (if the site of obstruction is superior to the junction of the azygos vein and SVC) or in the esophagus diffusely (if the site of obstruction is inferior to the junction of the azygos vein and SVC).

18. **What types of esophageal diverticula are there?**

A pulsion diverticulum, the most common type, occurs due to increased intraluminal pressure related to esophageal dysmotility, is usually encountered in the middle to lower thirds of the esophagus, and often occurs with multiple other pulsion diverticula. It typically appears as an ovoid or round outpouching of the esophagus with a wide neck.

An epiphrenic diverticulum, a subtype of pulsion diverticulum, is located in the distal esophagus and is usually solitary.

A traction diverticulum occurs due to fibrosis in adjacent tissues, is usually seen in the middle third of the esophagus, and is usually solitary. It typically has a tented or triangular shape due to tethering by the adjacent scar tissue.

19. **Can diverticula occur in the remainder of the upper GI tract?**

Yes. Gastric diverticula almost always occur in the posterior aspect of the gastric fundus. Duodenal diverticula are most often seen along the medial aspect of the second portion of the duodenum and to a lesser extent in the third and fourth portions of the duodenum. Jejunal and ileal diverticula can also occur but are uncommon. Meckel's diverticulum, a congenital true diverticulum, typically arises from the antimesenteric border of the distal ileum within 100 cm of the ileocecal valve.

On CT and MRI, diverticula of the upper GI tract may be filled with gas, fluid, and/or oral contrast material. When completely fluid-filled, they may sometimes mimic the appearance of cystic lesions arising from adjacent organs. When large in size, they may exert mass effect upon adjacent structures.

20. **What is the most common benign tumor of the esophagus?**

Leiomyoma is the most common benign tumor of the esophagus. It typically appears as a small smooth homogeneous soft tissue mass in the wall of the distal esophagus.

21. **What is an esophageal fibrovascular polyp?**

An esophageal fibrovascular polyp is a rare benign lesion that arises from the cervical esophagus that usually occurs in older men. It appears as a smoothly marginated pedunculated intraluminal esophageal mass with fat, soft tissue, and/or vascular components on CT and MRI. Associated esophageal luminal distention may also be seen when large in size. It is usually surgically removed because there is a risk for polyp regurgitation and potentially lethal acute laryngeal occlusion.

22. **What are the two major types of esophageal cancers?**

Squamous cell carcinoma of the esophagus is associated with tobacco use and alcohol use and usually arises within the upper or middle thirds of the esophagus. Adenocarcinoma of the esophagus is associated with Barrett's esophagus (replacement of normal esophageal squamous epithelium by metaplastic columnar epithelium) and usually arises within the lower or middle thirds of the esophagus or at the gastroesophageal junction.

23. **What are the cross-sectional imaging features of esophageal malignancy?**

Esophageal malignancy typically appears as either focal or segmental esophageal wall thickening or as a focal homogeneous or heterogeneous soft tissue enhancing mass of the esophagus, often with associated luminal narrowing (Figure 25-8). Direct spread of tumor into the surrounding mediastinal structures (e.g., mediastinal fat,

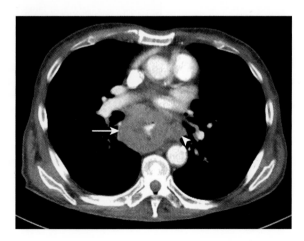

**Figure 25-8.** Esophageal cancer on CT. Note marked and asymmetric wall thickening of esophageal wall (*arrow*). Also note enlarged periesophageal lymph node (*arrowhead*) secondary to metastatic disease spread to regional lymph node.

tracheobronchial tree, lungs, thoracic aorta, thyroid gland, or diaphragm) may occur, as manifested by a loss of intervening fat planes; by displacement, indentation, or encasement of adjacent structures by soft tissue tumor; or by fistula formation. In more advanced stages of disease, regional lymphadenopathy, distant metastatic disease (most commonly involving the lungs, liver, osseous structures, and adrenal glands), or direct spread to the peritoneal cavity may be encountered.

24. What is a hiatal hernia, and what types are there?

A hiatal hernia is a herniation of abdominal organs (most often a portion of the stomach and less often portions of the mesenteric fat or of other organs) through the esophageal hiatus of the diaphragm. There are two types of hiatal hernias.

An axial hiatal hernia is the most common type (98%), where the gastroesophageal junction is located above the esophageal hiatus (Figure 25-9). This type is often seen in the setting of gastroesophageal reflux (GER) and may either occur as a sliding subtype (which is only seen when the patient is recumbent) or as a fixed subtype.

A paraesophageal hiatal hernia is an uncommon type (2%), where the gastroesophageal junction remains below the esophageal hiatus but a portion of the stomach (most commonly the gastric fundus) herniates through the esophageal hiatus alongside the distal esophagus. This type is not associated with GER but is associated with an increased risk of gastric incarceration, strangulation, and perforation.

25. What are some causes of gastric wall thickening?

For the answer, see Box 25-2. Gastritis and gastric malignancy are the most common causes of gastric wall thickening. Gastritis can be acute or chronic and is caused by various etiologies including aspirin and other nonsteroidal anti-inflammatory drugs (NSAIDs), alcohol, tobacco, stress, trauma, burn injury, Crohn's disease, or infection. Of the various infectious etiologies, *Helicobacter pylori* is the most common cause of chronic gastritis. Ménétrier's disease is a rare idiopathic cause of gastric wall thickening and usually involves the gastric fundus and body. Zollinger-Ellison syndrome (ZES) is related to increased gastric acid secretion and associated severe peptic ulcer disease caused by the increased secretion of the hormone gastrin by a gastrinoma or carcinoid tumor.

26. What are the typical imaging features of gastritis on CT and MRI?

Segmental or diffuse smooth wall thickening of the stomach is typically seen. Sometimes, increased mural enhancement, increased mural T2-weighted signal intensity relative to skeletal muscle, a "target" sign, luminal narrowing, ulceration, or perigastric fat stranding may also be seen in the setting of acute gastritis (Figure 25-10).

27. What is the major differential diagnosis for gas seen in the wall of the stomach?

Emphysematous gastritis is a rare type of infectious gastritis caused by gas-forming organisms following gastric ischemia or infarction secondary to severe injury from various causes including caustic ingestion, surgery, or gastric

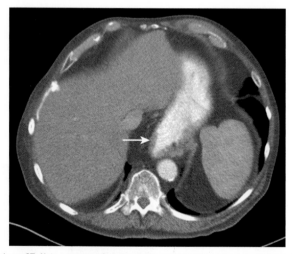

**Figure 25-9.** Axial hiatal hernia on CT. Note presence of gastroesophageal junction and proximal stomach (*arrow*) within inferior chest.

**Box 25-2.** Some Causes of Gastric Wall Thickening

- Gastritis
- Malignancy (adenocarcinoma, lymphoma, metastatic disease)
- Ménétrier's disease
- Zollinger-Ellison syndrome (ZES)
- Caustic ingestion
- Radiation therapy
- Gastric varices
- Acute pancreatitis

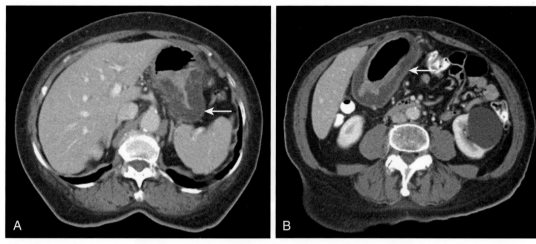

**Figure 25-10.** Acute gastritis on CT. **A,** Axial contrast-enhanced CT image through upper abdomen shows marked diffuse smooth wall thickening of gastric body (*arrow*) and associated decreased attenuation of gastric wall due to submucosal edema. **B,** Axial contrast-enhanced CT image through lower abdomen shows marked diffuse smooth wall thickening of gastric antrum (*arrow*) with associated "target" sign.

---

**Box 25-3.** Major Types of GI Tract Malignancies

- Adenocarcinoma
- Lymphoma
- GIST
- Carcinoid tumor
- Metastatic disease

---

volvulus. Patients with this condition are typically acutely ill, and there is an associated high mortality rate. On cross-sectional imaging, multiple gas bubbles are seen in the gastric wall, which may be thickened.

Gastric emphysema is secondary to a mucosal rent that allows gas to extend into the gastric wall. This condition may occur secondary to gastric outlet obstruction or gastric iatrogenic injury during endoscopy or other instrumentation. Patients with this condition are typically asymptomatic. On cross-sectional imaging, long linear foci of gas are typically seen circumferentially in the gastric wall.

Gastric pneumatosis is a very rare form of pneumatosis intestinalis in which multiple gas-filled cysts or blebs are present in the gastric wall. Patients with this condition are typically asymptomatic. On cross-sectional imaging, multiple gas bubbles are seen in the gastric wall.

28. What are the major types of GI tract malignancies?
For the answer, see Box 25-3. Adenocarcinoma is the most common gastric malignancy, carcinoid tumor is the most common small bowel malignancy, and gastrointestinal stromal tumor (GIST) is the most common mesenchymal tumor of the GI tract. Gastric adenocarcinoma is overall the second most common cause of cancer death worldwide (where lung cancer is the most common cause).

29. What is linitis plastica?
Linitis plastica is a descriptive term referring to a particular imaging appearance of the stomach comprised of gastric wall thickening, luminal narrowing, and luminal nondistensibility, which may partially or diffusely involve the stomach (Figure 25-11). Scirrhous adenocarcinoma, metastatic breast cancer, and lymphoma are the malignancies that most commonly lead to linitis plastica, caused by intramural tumor infiltration and/or an associated desmoplastic response. Causes of severe gastric inflammation or injury, such as caustic ingestion or radiation therapy, may also lead to this appearance.

30. What are the cross-sectional imaging features of GI tract adenocarcinoma?
In the stomach, focal or diffuse wall thickening, often irregular in contour and with associated luminal narrowing, or a soft tissue enhancing mass with an intraluminal polypoid or plaquelike component is seen, sometimes with areas of ulceration, necrosis, or calcification. Direct spread of tumor into the perigastric fat or into other surrounding organs (e.g., distal esophagus, duodenum, transverse colon, liver, spleen, or pancreas) may also occur. In more advanced stages of disease, regional lymphadenopathy, distant metastatic disease (most commonly involving the lungs, liver, osseous structures, and adrenal glands), or direct spread to the peritoneal cavity may be encountered (Figure 25-12).

In the small bowel, adenocarcinoma is uncommon but most commonly occurs in the duodenum or proximal jejunum and occurs with increased frequency in the distal ileum in the setting of Crohn's disease. Focal small bowel wall thickening (often asymmetric or lobulated in contour) or an annular mass with luminal narrowing is typically seen,

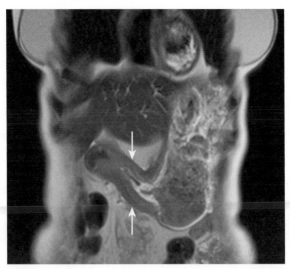

**Figure 25-11.** Linitis plastica on MRI. Coronal heavily T2-weighted image through abdomen shows wall thickening of gastric antrum and distal gastric body (*arrows*) with associated luminal narrowing and upstream retained ingested debris. This was due to metastatic breast cancer to gastric wall.

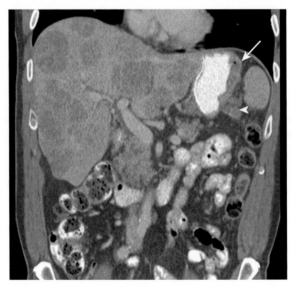

**Figure 25-12.** Gastric adenocarcinoma on CT. Note focal plaquelike wall thickening (*arrow*) of gastric body representing primary tumor. Also note regional gastric lymphadenopathy (*arrowhead*) along with multiple hypoattenuating hepatic metastases.

often with associated bowel obstruction. Direct spread into the peritoneal cavity, regional lymphadenopathy, and distant metastatic disease may also be present.

31. What are the cross-sectional imaging features of GI tract lymphoma?

GI tract lymphoma most commonly occurs in the stomach (70%) (most often in the gastric antrum and body), followed by small bowel (20%) (most often in the ileum) and ileocecal region (10%). It is most commonly due to non-Hodgkin's lymphoma of B cell origin.

Bowel wall thickening or focal soft tissue enhancing mass, which is typically homogeneous, may be seen. In the stomach, the wall thickening may be focal, segmental, or diffuse, and luminal narrowing may be present. In the small bowel, focal or segmental involvement may occur along with aneurysmal dilation of the affected bowel loops due to tumor infiltration of the myenteric plexus, although bowel obstruction is uncommonly seen. Intraluminal and/or exophytic soft tissue tumor components are commonly present, and direct spread of tumor to adjacent organs or to the peritoneal space may be encountered. Lymphadenopathy is commonly present, and involvement of distant sites may also be seen (Figure 25-13).

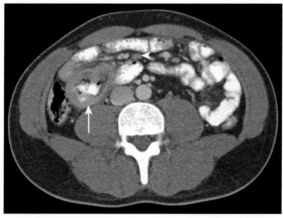

**Figure 25-13.** Small bowel lymphoma on CT. Note homogeneous segmental wall thickening of loop of small bowel (*arrow*) in right lower quadrant of abdomen with associated mild aneurysmal dilation. Also note enlarged mesenteric lymph node (*arrowhead*) representing mesenteric lymphadenopathy involved by lymphoma.

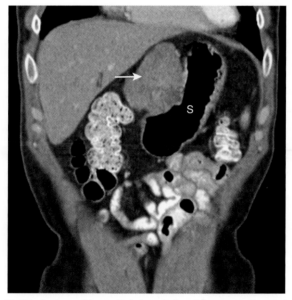

**Figure 25-14.** Gastric GIST on CT. Note focal smoothly marginated exophytic soft tissue mass (*arrow*) along right aspect of stomach (*S*).

32. What are the cross-sectional imaging features of gastrointestinal stromal tumor (GIST)?

GIST arises from the interstitial cells of Cajal, uniquely expresses CD117, and may have benign or malignant biologic behavior. It most commonly occurs in the stomach (60%) (most often in the gastric fundus and body), followed by small bowel (25%) (usually in the jejunum), and anorectum (10%).

A focal soft tissue enhancing mass is typically seen, often with intraluminal and/or exophytic soft tissue tumor components. Small (<5 cm) lesions tend to be homogeneous, whereas large (>5 cm) lesions tend to be heterogeneous secondary to presence of hemorrhage, calcification, cystic change, and/or necrotic change. Unlike other GI tract malignancies, lymphadenopathy is very uncommon, although distant metastases (most commonly to the liver) and extension to the peritoneal cavity may be encountered (Figure 25-14).

33. What are the cross-sectional imaging features of GI tract carcinoid tumor?

Carcinoid tumor is a well-differentiated neuroendocrine neoplasm with malignant potential that most commonly occurs in the small bowel (40%) (most often in the distal ileum), followed by rectum (27%), appendix (24%), and stomach (9%). The biologic behavior of carcinoid tumor varies with the site of origin. For example, small bowel carcinoid tumors often have an aggressive biologic behavior whereas appendiceal and rectal carcinoids tend to have a more indolent biologic behavior.

One or more smooth small (<2 cm) soft tissue hyperenhancing polypoid or intramural masses or areas of bowel wall thickening are typically seen in the bowel wall, although in many cases the primary tumor is not visualized. An irregular mesenteric soft tissue mass secondary to mesenteric tumor spread and associated desmoplastic response may be visualized, frequently with calcification and associated tethering, angulation, and/or thickening of adjacent small bowel loops. Distant metastases, which are characteristically hyperenhancing during the arterial phase of enhancement and most often seen in the liver, may also be encountered (Figure 25-15).

34. What is carcinoid syndrome, and how often does it occur in patients with carcinoid tumor?
Carcinoid syndrome is a syndrome that clinically presents with cutaneous flushing, sweating, bronchospasm, colicky abdominal pain, diarrhea, and right-sided cardiac valvular fibrosis and occurs in less than 10% of patients with carcinoid tumor. The syndrome is due to the secretion of vasoactive substances (e.g., serotonin) by the tumor and most commonly occurs in patients with hepatic metastases, as the secreted substances are then able to enter the systemic circulation without undergoing hepatic degradation.

35. What types of malignancies most often metastasize hematogenously to the GI tract?
Hematogenous metastatic spread of tumor to the bowel is usually seen in patients with widespread metastatic disease and is most commonly due to melanoma, lung cancer, and breast cancer. On cross-sectional imaging, multiple submucosal masses of the bowel wall are typically visualized, sometimes with areas of necrosis or ulceration (Figure 25-16). In the setting of metastatic breast cancer involving the stomach, a linitis plastica appearance of the stomach may be seen due to cellular infiltration of the gastric wall (see Figure 25-11).

36. What are the main causes of small bowel wall thickening based on the spatial extent of bowel involvement?
For the answer, see Box 25-4.

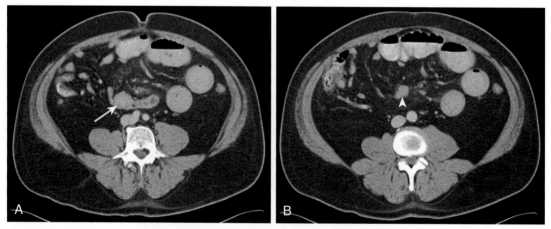

**Figure 25-15.** Small bowel carcinoid tumor on CT. **A,** Axial contrast-enhanced CT image through lower abdomen shows small enhancing intramural soft tissue mass (*arrow*) of distal ileum. **B,** Axial contrast-enhanced CT image more superior shows adjacent mesenteric soft tissue mass (*arrowhead*) representing mesenteric lymphadenopathy involved by metastatic carcinoid tumor.

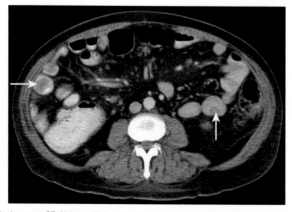

**Figure 25-16.** Small bowel metastases on CT. Note multiple polypoid masses (*arrows*) involving several loops of small bowel. This patient has a history of metastatic melanoma of skin.

**Box 25-4.** Major Causes of Small Bowel Wall Thickening Based on the Spatial Extent of Bowel Involvement

Diffuse involvement
- Edema (cirrhosis, hypoproteinemia)
- Infection

Segmental involvement
- Infection
- Inflammation (Crohn's disease, vasculitis, radiation therapy)

- Ischemia
- Intramural hemorrhage
- Lymphoma

Focal involvement
- Malignancy
- Crohn's disease

37. **What is Crohn's disease?**

Crohn's disease is an idiopathic inflammatory disease condition that can affect any part of the GI tract. The peak age of patients affected is 15 to 25 years of age. The small bowel is most commonly affected (most often involving the terminal ileum), followed by the large bowel, stomach (most often involving the gastric antrum and body) and duodenum, and the esophagus. When the stomach, duodenum, or esophagus is involved, there is almost always involvement of either the jejunum/ileum or large bowel as well. Skip lesions, where abnormal segments of bowel are separated by intervening normal segments of bowel, are characteristically seen. Patients have an increased risk of GI tract adenocarcinoma and lymphoma as well.

Differentiation of active inflammatory Crohn's disease from fibrostenotic Crohn's disease is important because the former is typically treated medically whereas the latter is typically treated with stricturoplasty or surgical resection. However, mixed fibrostenotic and active inflammatory Crohn's disease may occur.

38. **What are the cross-sectional imaging features of Crohn's disease in the GI tract?**

Findings of active inflammatory Crohn's disease include a "target" sign or increased mural T2-weighted signal intensity relative to skeletal muscle due to submucosal edema, mural restricted diffusion due to inflammatory cell infiltration, increased mural enhancement (either homogeneously in the wall or with mural stratification to predominantly involve the mucosal layer ± serosal layer), mural ulcerations, and inflammatory pseudopolyps (seen as polypoid intraluminal filling defects secondary to islands of residual bowel mucosa surrounded by areas of ulceration). Ancillary findings include surrounding fat stranding, a "comb" sign, and enlarged or hyperenhancing reactive lymph nodes.

Findings of inactive or quiescent Crohn's disease include lack of a "target" sign, presence of low to intermediate mural T2-weighted signal intensity relative to skeletal muscle, lack of mural restricted diffusion, presence of a "fat halo" sign, normal mural enhancement, and lack of the ancillary findings of active inflammatory disease listed above.

Fibrostenotic Crohn's disease is present when there is a bowel stricture (seen as an area of bowel wall thickening that is associated with fixed luminal narrowing and upstream bowel dilation). This may occur either with mixed fibrostenotic and active inflammatory Crohn's disease or in the setting of inactive Crohn's disease.

Penetrating Crohn's disease (which may occur in the setting of active inflammatory Crohn's disease or mixed fibrostenotic and active inflammatory Crohn's disease) is present when there is fistula formation (seen as linear or curvilinear enhancing soft tissue tracts that connect two epithelial surfaces, such as enterocutaneous, enteroenteric, enterocolic, enterovesical, and enterovaginal fistulae), sinus tract formation (seen as linear or curvilinear enhancing soft tissue tracts that extend from mural defects but blindly end in the surrounding fat without connection to adjacent epithelial surfaces), abscess formation, or uncommonly, bowel perforation.

Wall thickening (focal or segmental, circumferential or asymmetric) and fibrofatty proliferation (seen as increased fat adjacent to abnormal segments of bowel) may be seen with active inflammatory, inactive, or fibrostenotic Crohn's disease. Luminal narrowing may be seen with active inflammatory or fibrostenotic Crohn's disease (Figure 25-17).

39. **What are the cross-sectional imaging features of Crohn's disease outside of the GI tract?**
- Primary sclerosing cholangitis.
- Cholelithiasis.
- Nephrolithiasis (particularly calcium oxalate calculi).
- Sacroiliitis.
- Avascular necrosis (AVN) (usually of the femoral heads).
- Venous thrombosis (superior mesenteric vein, portal vein).

40. **What is an enteric duplication cyst?**

An enteric duplication cyst is a rare congenital abnormality of the GI tract that contains all the layers of bowel. On cross-sectional imaging, it typically appears as a solitary round or elongated unilocular cystic lesion with a thick enhancing wall that is located adjacent to a loop of bowel, most commonly the duodenum or distal ileum.

41. **What is the difference between an external hernia and an internal hernia?**

An external hernia involves passage of visceral tissue through a defect in the body wall and is common. An internal hernia involves passage of visceral tissue through a defect in the peritoneum, omentum, mesentery, or mesocolon within the confines of the body wall and is rare.

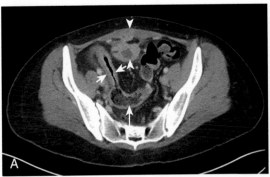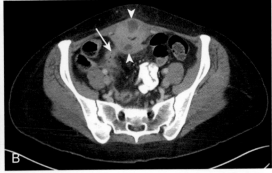

**Figure 25-17.** Mixed fibrostenotic and active inflammatory Crohn's disease of small bowel on CT. **A,** Axial contrast-enhanced CT image through upper pelvis shows moderate segmental wall thickening and mucosal hyperenhancement of distal ileum (*short arrows*) with associated luminal narrowing, upstream small bowel dilation (*long arrow*), and "small bowel feces" sign indicating presence of small bowel stricture. Loculated fluid collection with surrounding soft tissue (*arrows*) in anterior pelvic mesentery and anterior pelvic body wall is also seen due to abscess. **B,** Axial contrast-enhanced CT image more superiorly through pelvis reveals linear soft tissue attenuation gas-filled structure (*arrow*) extending from distal ileum to abscess (*arrowheads*) representing sinus tract. Presence of sinus tract and abscess indicate penetrating Crohn's disease.

42. **What is the role of CT and MRI in the evaluation of patients with a hernia?**
    These techniques provide superior anatomic detail for hernia detection, hernia classification, determination of hernia size and contents, detection of hernia-related complications, and detection of posthernia repair complications.
    Prone or lateral decubitus positioning along with acquisition of images during a Valsalva maneuver may be useful to improve the conspicuity of hernias (in up to 50%) and to reveal otherwise occult subtle or reducible hernias (in up to 10%).

43. **What is the most common type of external hernia?**
    Indirect inguinal hernia is the most common type of external hernia. It is also the most common type of pediatric hernia.

44. **What are the boundaries of Hesselbach's triangle?**
    The inguinal ligament is located inferiorly, the inferior epigastric vessels are located superiorly and laterally, and the rectus abdominis muscle is located medially.

45. **How can one distinguish direct inguinal hernias from indirect inguinal hernias on cross-sectional imaging?**
    All inguinal hernias are superiorly located to the inguinal ligament (which extends from the anterior superior iliac spine of the iliac bone to the pubic tubercle of the ipsilateral pubic bone) and are more commonly seen in men than in women.
    Direct inguinal hernias occur through Hesselbach's triangle secondary to acquired weakness of the transversalis fascia and are therefore located inferior and medial to the inferior epigastric vessels in the groin region.
    Indirect inguinal hernias occur lateral to Hesselbach's triangle through the inguinal canal secondary to a patent processus vaginalis or acquired weakness and dilation of the deep inguinal ring and are therefore located lateral to the inferior epigastric vessels in the groin region (Figure 25-18).

46. **What is a femoral hernia?**
    A femoral hernia is another type of external hernia that occurs in the groin region and is much more commonly seen in women than in men. This type of hernia is also more commonly associated with bowel strangulation due to its narrow neck. The hernia passes through the femoral ring into the femoral canal, just medial to the common femoral vein, and is inferiorly located to the inguinal ligament. Associated mass effect upon the common femoral vein is therefore typically seen, whereas this finding is not typically seen in inguinal hernias unless large in size.

47. **What is a Richter hernia?**
    A Richter hernia is an external hernia that involves only the antimesenteric aspect of a loop of bowel. It occurs most commonly in femoral hernias and at laparoscopy port sites and is also more prone to strangulation.

48. **What are the boundaries of the superior lumbar triangle?**
    The twelfth rib is located superiorly, the internal oblique muscle is located anteriorly, and the erector spinae muscle is located posteriorly.

49. **What are the boundaries of the inferior lumbar triangle?**
    The iliac crest is located inferiorly, the external oblique muscle is located anteriorly, and the latissimus dorsi muscle is located posteriorly.

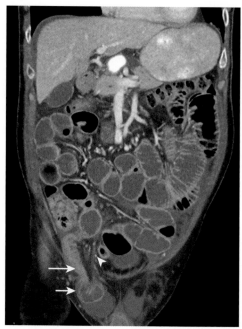

**Figure 25-18.** Incarcerated indirect inguinal hernia with small bowel obstruction on CT. Note entrapped dilated loop of small bowel (*short arrow*) in right inguinal region external to body wall representing incarcerated inguinal hernia. Note that contiguous small bowel loop (*long arrow*) is located lateral to right inferior epigastric artery (*arrowhead*) indicating indirect type of inguinal hernia. Multiple upstream dilated loops of small bowel are also seen in keeping with small bowel obstruction.

50. What is a lumbar hernia?

    A lumbar hernia is an uncommon type of external hernia that occurs through either the superior or inferior lumbar triangle. Superior lumbar triangle hernias (also called Grynfeltt-Lesshaft hernias) are more common than inferior lumbar triangle hernias (also called Petit hernias).

51. What are the major potential complications of a hernia?
    - Bowel incarceration (i.e., presence of an irreducible hernia sac) (see Figure 25-18).
    - Closed loop bowel obstruction (i.e., obstruction along two separate locations along the course of the bowel).
    - Bowel strangulation (i.e., bowel ischemia/infarction).
    - Bowel perforation.

## KEY POINTS

- On cross-sectional imaging, the normal bowel wall is generally ≤3 mm in thickness when well distended, although the gastric antrum and pylorus may normally measure up to 11 mm in thickness.
- Wall (mural) thickening is the hallmark of GI tract pathology. In general, the greater the degree of mural thickening, the more likely that malignancy is the underlying etiology. Asymmetric wall thickening and focal wall thickening are also generally suggestive features of malignancy.
- The "target" sign, also known as mural stratification, is highly specific for the diagnosis of nonneoplastic disease when encountered in the small bowel. However, this specificity for nonneoplastic disease does not hold when it is encountered in the stomach.
- CTE and MRE are most often performed to assess patients with either suspected or known Crohn's disease or with obscure GI bleeding.
- Bowel incarceration, obstruction, strangulation, and perforation are the major potential complications of a hernia.

**BIBLIOGRAPHY**

Baker ME, Hara AK, Platt JF, et al. CT enterography for Crohn's disease: optimal technique and imaging issues. *Abdom Imaging.* 2015;40(5):938-952.

Allen BC, Leyendecker JR. MR enterography for assessment and management of small bowel Crohn disease. *Radiol Clin North Am.* 2014;52(4):799-810.

Fernandes T, Oliveira MI, Castro R, et al. Bowel wall thickening at CT: simplifying the diagnosis. *Insights Imaging.* 2014;5(2):195-208.

Lewis RB, Mehrotra AK, Rodriguez P, et al. From the radiologic pathology archives: Gastrointestinal lymphoma: radiologic and pathologic findings. *Radiographics.* 2014;34(7):1934-1953.

Licurse MY, Levine MS, Torigian DA, et al. Utility of chest CT for differentiating primary and secondary achalasia. *Clin Radiol.* 2014;69(10): 1019-1026.

Murphy KP, O'Connor OJ, Maher MM. Adult abdominal hernias. *AJR Am J Roentgenol.* 2014;202(6):W506-W511.

Qiu Y, Mao R, Chen BL, et al. Systematic review with meta-analysis: magnetic resonance enterography vs. computed tomography enterography for evaluating disease activity in small bowel Crohn's disease. *Aliment Pharmacol Ther.* 2014;40(2):134-146.

Grand DJ, Beland M, Harris A. Magnetic resonance enterography. *Radiol Clin North Am.* 2013;51(1):99-112.

Hallinan JT, Venkatesh SK. Gastric carcinoma: imaging diagnosis, staging and assessment of treatment response. *Cancer Imaging.* 2013;13:212-227.

Lewis RB, Mehrotra AK, Rodriguez P, et al. From the radiologic pathology archives: Esophageal neoplasms: radiologic-pathologic correlation. *Radiographics.* 2013;33(4):1083-1108.

Trainer V, Leung C, Owen RE, et al. External anterior abdominal wall and pelvic hernias with emphasis on the key diagnostic features on MDCT. *Clin Radiol.* 2013;68(4):388-396.

Burkhardt JH, Arshanskiy Y, Munson JL, et al. Diagnosis of inguinal region hernias with axial CT: the lateral crescent sign and other key findings. *Radiographics.* 2011;31(2):E1-E12.

Cronin CG, Delappe E, Lohan DG, et al. Normal small bowel wall characteristics on MR enterography. *Eur J Radiol.* 2010;75(2):207-211.

Ba-Ssalamah A, Zacherl J, Noebauer-Huhmann IM, et al. Dedicated multi-detector CT of the esophagus: spectrum of diseases. *Abdom Imaging.* 2009;34(1):3-18.

Levy AD, Sobin LH. From the archives of the AFIP: Gastrointestinal carcinoids: imaging features with clinicopathologic comparison. *Radiographics.* 2007;27(1):237-257.

Macari M, Megibow AJ, Balthazar EJ. A pattern approach to the abnormal small bowel: observations at MDCT and CT enterography. *AJR Am J Roentgenol.* 2007;188(5):1344-1355.

Martin LC, Merkle EM, Thompson WM. Review of internal hernias: radiographic and clinical findings. *AJR Am J Roentgenol.* 2006;186(3):703-717.

Takeyama N, Gokan T, Ohgiya Y, et al. CT of internal hernias. *Radiographics.* 2005;25(4):997-1015.

Levy AD, Remotti HE, Thompson WM, et al. From the archives of the AFIP: Gastrointestinal stromal tumors: radiologic features with pathologic correlation. *Radiographics.* 2003;23(2):283-304.

Pickhardt PJ, Asher DB. Wall thickening of the gastric antrum as a normal finding: multidetector CT with cadaveric comparison. *AJR Am J Roentgenol.* 2003;181(4):973-979.

Wittenberg J, Harisinghani MG, Jhaveri K, et al. Algorithmic approach to CT diagnosis of the abnormal bowel wall. *Radiographics.* 2002;22(5):1093-1107, discussion 107-109.

# CHAPTER 26

# FLUOROSCOPY OF THE LOWER GASTROINTESTINAL TRACT

*Stephen E. Rubesin, MD*

1. Identify the parts of the colon (numbers 1 through 8) labeled in Figure 26-1.
   For the answer, see the figure legend.

2. What are haustra?

   The longitudinal muscle layer of the colon is divided into three thick bands, termed the **taeniae coli**. There is a paucity of longitudinal muscle between the three tenial bands. Haustra are sacculations of colon protruding between the three rows of taeniae coli (Figures 26-2 and 26-3). At the edges of the haustral sacculations, folds, termed **interhaustral folds**, radiate toward the taeniae coli. The colon is identified by its haustral sacculations and interhaustral folds on any radiologic study—whether plain abdominal radiograph, computed tomography (CT), magnetic resonance imaging (MRI), or barium enema. Rounded, air-filled pockets are seen in a nondependent (anterior) position. Fluid-filled or contrast-filled rounded sacculations are seen on the dependent (inferior) surface.

   Haustra are relatively fixed structures in the right and transverse colon. Haustra are intermittently seen structures in the descending and proximal sigmoid colon, depending on the stage of colonic contraction. The left colon may intermittently appear "ahaustral," depending on the degree of colonic contraction. Although the edge of the colon has a sacculated appearance, the edge of the small bowel is relatively straight, altered only by its thin valvulae conniventes. Valvulae conniventes are thinner than interhaustral folds and cross the entire lumen of the bowel, whereas interhaustral folds cross about one third of the colonic diameter when seen in profile. Seen en face, the interhaustral folds may falsely appear to cross the entire lumen of the colon.

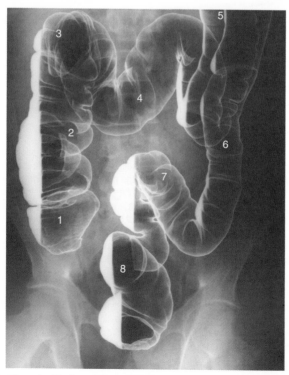

**Figure 26-1.** Normal colon on double-contrast barium enema examination. *1* = cecum, *2* = ascending colon, *3* = hepatic flexure, *4* = mid-transverse colon, *5* = splenic flexure (partially imaged), *6* = descending colon, *7* = sigmoid colon, and *8* = rectum.

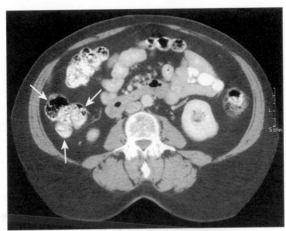

**Figure 26-2.** Colonic haustra on CT. Axial image through lower abdomen shows three rows of haustral sacculations (*arrows*) in ascending colon. Feces in ascending colon have mottled appearance of black air; soft tissue appears gray; oral contrast material appears white. Feces are not seen in mid–small bowel loops.

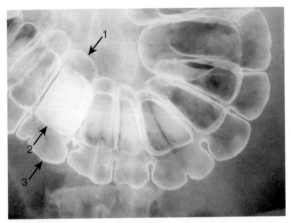

**Figure 26-3.** Colonic haustra on double-contrast barium enema examination. Spot radiograph of transverse colon shows three rows of haustral sacculations (edges of three haustral rows are identified by black arrows and numbered). Most dependent haustral row is partially filled with barium.

3. Figure 26-4 is from what type of examination?
A double-contrast (or air-contrast) barium enema examination uses two contrast agents to image the colon. A medium-density, medium-viscosity barium suspension is instilled into the colon via a rectal tube. This barium scrubs residual feces and fluid into the suspension and then coats the mucosal surface with barium. Air (or carbon dioxide) is insufflated via the rectal tube to distend the colon and render it "translucent." The end result is that the mucosal surface is "etched" in white by barium, and the colonic walls are widely separated. Spot radiographs and overhead images are then obtained. A colonic hypotonic agent (1 mg of intravenous glucagon) is routinely administered at our hospital. Other hospitals use glucagon only if there is colonic spasm, excessive patient discomfort, or inability to retain the contrast agent. In other countries, an anticholinergic agent (e.g., hyoscine butylbromide [Buscopan]) may be used to induce colonic hypotonia.

4. In what position is the patient lying on the tabletop of the fluoroscope in Figure 26-1?
Air-barium levels are the clue to the patient's position. Barium is heavier than air; barium identifies the "down" side of the patient. The air-barium levels show that the patient is lying with his or her right side down. The x-ray tube is positioned in a **cross-table position**, with the x-ray tube at one side of the tabletop, so the x-ray beam parallels the tabletop. A cassette is placed in an upright position, perpendicular to the tabletop, in front or in back of the patient. This image is termed a **right-side-down decubitus view**.

5. What type of patient is capable of undergoing a double-contrast barium enema examination?
A patient has to be able to hold the barium and air in his or her colon; anal sphincter tone must be normal. The patient must be able to roll upon the tabletop of the fluoroscope; he or she must be strong enough to roll over in bed. The

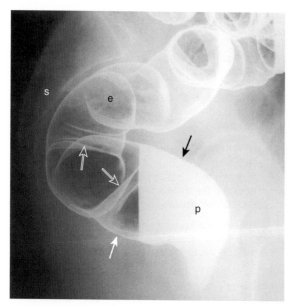

**Figure 26-4.** Normal rectum on double-contrast barium enema examination. Spot radiograph of rectum where patient lies in prone position and x-ray beam is "shot" across patient; this is termed *cross-table image.* Mucosal detail is seen en face in air contrast (*e*), but obscured by barium pool (*p*). Radiologist looks at contour of colon in barium pool (*black arrow*) and in air (*white arrow*). Two valves of Houston are identified (*open arrows*). Proximal and midrectum parallel the sacrum (*s*).

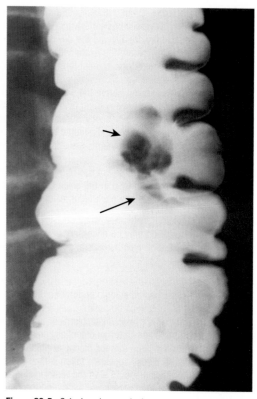

**Figure 26-5.** Colonic polyp on single-contrast barium enema examination. Spot radiograph of ascending colon. Radiologist evaluates contour and barium column. In this patient, luminal contour has normal sacculations. There is a 1.5-cm lobulated radiolucent filling defect (*short arrow*) connected to smooth tubular filling defect (*long arrow*), typical of pedunculated polyp. Barium in interstices of lesion indicates its villous or tubulovillous nature. Polyp proved to be tubulovillous adenoma. *(From Rubesin SE, Stuzin N, Laufer I. Tumors of the colon. Semin Colon Rect Surg. 1993;4:94-111.)*

radiologist must be able to communicate with the patient. If the patient does not speak the same language as the radiologist, a translator must be provided. The patient must have enough mental acuity to be able to understand and respond to the following commands: "Don't breathe/breathe," "Turn left/turn right," and "Hold the barium in your rectum."

6. Figure 26-5 is an image from what type of examination?
   This is a spot radiograph from a single-contrast barium enema examination. This type of examination uses one contrast agent: low-density barium. Under fluoroscopic control, the colon is filled with barium. Spot radiographs and overhead images of the entire colon are obtained. Postevacuation spot radiographs or overhead images are also obtained.

7. What are the indications for a double-contrast barium enema examination?
   Indications for double-contrast barium enema examination include rectal bleeding, diarrhea, abdominal pain, screening for colorectal neoplasia, or involvement of the colon by extracolonic inflammatory or neoplastic masses.

8. What are the indications for a single-contrast barium enema examination?
   A single-contrast barium enema examination may be performed in patients with suspected fistula, high-grade colonic obstruction, or Hirschsprung's disease. If a distal small bowel obstruction is suspected, a single-contrast barium enema examination with reflux of barium into the distal ileum to the point of obstruction may be performed as a complementary study to CT.

9. What is your hospital's preparation for a barium enema?
   Each hospital has its own preparation for a barium enema that should be available from the department of radiology. Preparations generally include (1) a period during which solid food is limited in an effort to reduce undigested material

reaching the colon, (2) an oral laxative, and (3) a medication that induces colonic contraction. The preparation at the Hospital of the University of Pennsylvania includes the following:

- Clear liquids only are allowed the day before the examination.
- At 5 PM the day before the examination, 10 to 16 oz of magnesium citrate is given.
- The patient should drink at least three to four 8 oz glasses of water throughout the day of the examination to maintain hydration.
- At 10 PM the evening before the examination, four 5 mg bisacodyl tablets are taken with 8 oz of water.
- The patient should have nothing by mouth after midnight the night before until after the examination.
- The patient is given a bisacodyl suppository the morning of the examination.
- Insulin dose is reduced or eliminated the morning of the examination.
- After the examination, patients are encouraged to drink water and take laxatives if they have colonic hypomotility.

At our hospital, we do not use large-volume colonic lavage agents that are used for colonoscopy because they leave large amounts of fluid in the colon that degrade barium coating of the mucosa. Cleansing enemas are discouraged because they push fecal residue into the right colon and leave residual fluid in the colon.

10. **Which types of patients may require more than the standard barium enema preparation?**
A 2-day preparation may be necessary in immobile or bedridden patients, patients with hypomotility disorders such as diabetes mellitus or hypothyroidism, postoperative patients, or patients taking opiates or drugs with anticholinergic side effects.

11. **List the contraindications for a barium enema examination.**
- Known or suspected colonic perforation. If a perforation is suspected, CT or an enema using a water-soluble contrast agent should be used.
- Fulminant colitis ("toxic megacolon") or any severe colitis.
- A recent procedure that has potentially created a hole in the colonic mucosa. A barium enema should be postponed for 1 week if a large forceps biopsy at rigid sigmoidoscopy, a snare polypectomy, or a hot biopsy has been performed. A biopsy specimen taken with small forceps via a flexible endoscope is not a contraindication.
- Also, the clinician should alert the radiologist if a patient has a latex allergy, so all products containing latex can be removed from the fluoroscopic suite, and the room can be cleaned before a procedure.

12. **What are the contraindications for the use of intravenous glucagon?**
Patients with known or suspected insulinoma or pheochromocytoma should not receive intravenous glucagon.

13. **Which types of patients should be scheduled early in the day?**
Patients with latex allergy should be scheduled first in the day, after the room has been cleaned. Insulin-dependent diabetic patients, patients with hypoglycemia, and other patients who require breakfast should be scheduled as early in the day as possible.

14. **What are the complications of a barium enema examination?**
- The examination may fail to image the entire colon if the patient has colonic spasm or poor sphincter tone and is unable to retain barium or air.
- Distention of the colon may cause the patient to complain of cramps, but it rarely produces syncope.
- Colonic perforation occurs in about 1 in 40,000 examinations. Perforation is usually retroperitoneal and related to distention of a rectal balloon. If a free intraperitoneal perforation occurs, it is usually in a patient who has severe colitis or ischemia. In contrast to the rarity of barium enema perforation, perforation occurs in about 1 in 1000 colonoscopies.
- Rarely, barium impaction occurs in patients who have colonic hypomotility, such as bedridden patients, patients taking narcotics or other drugs that cause hypomotility, and diabetic patients. Barium impaction can be prevented, in part, by having patients take oral laxatives after the procedure.
- Allergic reactions to the barium, glucagon, or colonic preparation are rare but have been reported. Although allergic reactions to latex in barium enema balloons have occurred, the manufacturers have removed the latex from the balloons attached to the enema tips.
- Rarely, patients develop myocardial ischemia during a barium enema examination.

15. **Is antibiotic prophylaxis needed before administration of a barium enema?**
There is conflicting evidence regarding bacteremia during barium enema examination. Routine antibiotic prophylaxis is probably unnecessary except in susceptible patients with cardiac lesions who have a history of endocarditis or a prosthetic valve.

16. **What is the most important radiographic predictor of malignancy arising in a polyp?**
Size is the most important predictor of malignancy present in a polyp; the larger the polyp, the greater the chance of malignancy. The amount of villous change is a much less important factor. About 1% of tubular adenomas smaller than 1 cm are malignant (Figure 26-6); 10% of tubular adenomas 1 to 2 cm are malignant, and 35% of tubular adenomas larger than 2 cm are malignant. About 10% of villous adenomas less than 2 cm are malignant, and about 50% of villous adenomas larger than 2 cm are malignant. The presence of a pedicle longer than 1 cm means that a

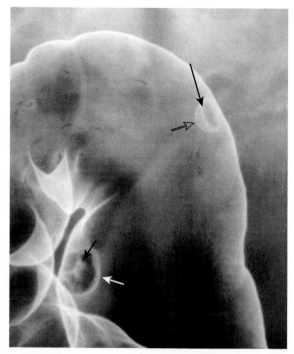

**Figure 26-6.** Colonic polyps on double-contrast barium enema examination. Spot radiograph of splenic flexure shows two polyps. Small polyp resembles hat, where top of hat (*open arrow*) represents top of polyp, and brim of hat (*long black arrow*) represents barium trapped between mucosa and polyp as it is retracted by its stalk. This polyp was due to tubular adenoma. Second polyp has more worrisome morphology—that of an umbilicated, sessile polyp. Small barium collection (*short black arrow*) fills central umbilication or ulceration. Edge of polyp is coated by barium (or "etched in white") (*white arrow*). This polyp was due to tubulovillous adenoma.

pedunculated polyp has a greater than 95% chance of benign behavior, regardless of the histology in the head of the polyp.

17. What does fine lobulation of the surface of a polyp mean?
    Barium enters the interstices between fronds of a polyp (see Figure 26-5), and the greater the number of lobules, the greater the amount of villous change in a polyp. A polyp with more than several lobules is in the spectrum of tubulovillous to villous adenoma (Figure 26-7) and has a slightly greater risk of malignancy. A villous tumor 6 to 10 mm in size has a 10% chance of malignancy. Therefore, if a 6 to 10 mm in size finely lobulated polyp is seen at barium enema, it should be removed.

18. What percentage of colonic cancers is out of reach of the flexible sigmoidoscope?
    Over the past 4 decades, the distribution of colon cancers has shifted toward the right colon (Figure 26-8). About 40% to 50% of colonic cancers are out of reach of the flexible sigmoidoscope. This is why screening for colonic carcinoma requires a total colonic examination, either by colonoscopy or by double-contrast barium enema examination.

19. Which of the following morphologic shapes is the most common form of symptomatic colonic carcinoma: polypoid, carpet, plaquelike, or annular?
    About 50% of advanced cancers in symptomatic patients are annular cancers. Obstructive symptoms result when annular lesions narrow the lumen. When an annular cancer is seen radiographically (Figure 26-9), there is a 98% chance of serosal invasion, a 50% chance of lymph node metastasis, and about a 15% chance of liver metastasis.
    Polypoid cancers are most commonly found in the rectum or cecum. Polypoid cancers may cause colonic bleeding but do not usually result in obstructive symptoms unless intussusception occurs. Polypoid cancers have a better prognosis: 55% of patients have serosal invasion, and 25% have lymph node metastasis.

20. What is the most common cause of colonic intussusception in adults?
    Colonic cancers are the most common cause of colonic intussusception in adults. Less likely causes include adenomas and lipomas.

21. Hyperplastic polyps are found most commonly in what part of the colon?
    Hyperplastic polyps are small (<5 mm), smooth-surfaced polyps most commonly found in the rectum on the crest of folds. In contrast to adenomatous polyps, hyperplastic polyps are not premalignant.

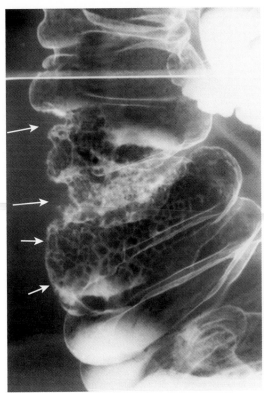

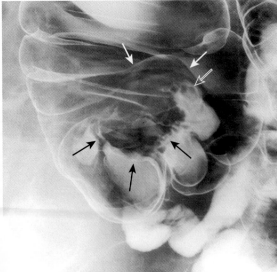

**Figure 26-8.** Polypoid carcinoma of ileocecal valve on double-contrast barium enema examination. Spot radiograph of cecum shows 3-cm, finely lobulated mass (*black arrows*) expanding contour of inferior lip of ileocecal valve. Normal-sized and smooth superior lip of ileocecal valve is labeled (*white arrows*) for comparison. Lumen of ileocecal valve (*open white arrow*) is nodular, indicating tumor spread into ileum.

**Figure 26-7.** Adenocarcinoma arising in villous adenoma of ascending colon on double-contrast barium enema examination. Spot radiograph shows 4-cm area of polygonal nodules with barium filling interstices between tumor lobules. Flat nature of tumor is evident in profile where luminal contour is neither pushed in nor excavated out (*short arrows*). Adenocarcinoma is present where lesion disrupts luminal contour (*long arrows*). This flat lesion has been called "carpet lesion" by some authors. (*From Rubesin SE, Laufer I. Pictorial glossary. In: Gore RM, Levine MS. Textbook of gastrointestinal radiology. 2nd ed. Philadelphia: Saunders; 2000.*)

22. What is the most common tumor arising in the submucosa of the colon?
    Lipomas are the most common submucosal tumors arising in the colon. Internal hemorrhoids are the most common lesions arising in the submucosa. Lipomas are most commonly found in the right colon as sessile or broadly pedunculated, smooth-surfaced polyps or masses (Figure 26-10). These tumors change size and shape with palpation and varying degrees of colonic distention.

23. What tumors commonly spread to the intraperitoneal space?
    Ovarian cancer is the most common type of tumor that spreads to the peritoneal space in women. In men, cancers of the colon, pancreas, and stomach are the primary tumors that most frequently spread to the intraperitoneal space. Hepatocellular carcinomas spread to the peritoneal space, but they are less common in the United States compared with Asia or Africa.

24. What are the differences in distribution between ulcerative colitis and Crohn's disease?
    Ulcerative colitis (Table 26-1) is left-sided colonic disease, beginning at the anorectal junction and extending continuously and retrogradely a variable distance (proctosigmoiditis, left-sided colitis, pancolitis) (Figure 26-11). Ulcerative colitis symmetrically involves a bowel segment (Figure 26-12). Crohn's disease involves the colon and terminal ileum in 55% of patients. Terminal ileal involvement alone is seen in 14% of patients. Terminal ileal and distal small bowel involvement alone is seen in 13% of patients. Pure colonic involvement is seen in about 15% of patients. Crohn's disease is discontinuous, having patchy involvement locally and between loops, called skip areas. Crohn's disease is asymmetric, first involving the mesenteric side of bowel.

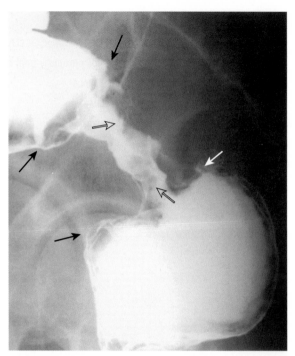

**Figure 26-9.** Annular adenocarcinoma of rectum on single-contrast barium enema examination. Spot radiograph shows 5-cm-long, circumferential narrowing of proximal rectum. This lesion has abrupt shelf-like margins (*black and white arrows*) and irregular surface (*open arrows*). This has been called an "apple core" lesion, but this is a misnomer because tumor represents the part of the apple that has been eaten away, and lumen would be the "apple core."

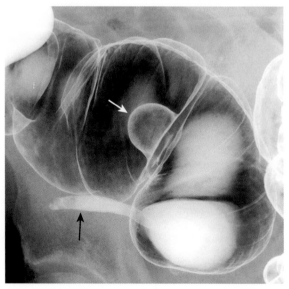

**Figure 26-10.** Colonic lipoma on double-contrast barium enema examination. Spot radiograph of cecum shows smooth-surfaced, 2-cm polypoid lesion (*white arrow*) arising from superior lip of ileocecal valve. This smooth appearance is typical of colonic lipoma on barium enema examination. Appendix is identified (*black arrow*).

25. Aphthoid ulcers are characteristic of which chronic inflammatory bowel disease?

In an American with long-standing symptoms, aphthoid ulcers are almost pathognomonic for Crohn's disease (Figure 26-13). They are also seen in patients with acute diarrheal states, such as yersiniosis, amebiasis, and viral (cytomegalovirus/herpes virus) infection. An aphthoid ulcer results from breakdown of the mucosa above an inflamed lymph aggregate in the lamina propria or submucosa. Other characteristic radiographic findings in Crohn's disease

**Table 26-1.** Comparison of Crohn's Disease and Ulcerative Colitis

| CROHN'S DISEASE | ULCERATIVE COLITIS |
| --- | --- |
| Right-sided | Extends proximally from rectum |
| Discontinuous | Continuous |
| Asymmetric | Symmetric |
| Terminal ileal changes in 85% | Backwash ileitis in 10% |
| Aphthoid ulcers | Mucosal granularity |
| Ulcers on background of normal mucosa | Ulcers on background of mucosal granularity |
| Severe perianal disease | Colon cancer in larger percentage of patients |
| Sinus tracks and fistulas | Sclerosing cholangitis in larger percentage of patients |
| Abscess formation | |

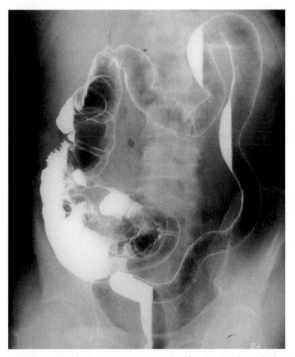

**Figure 26-11.** Ulcerative colitis on double-contrast barium enema examination. Overhead radiograph shows that transverse, descending, and sigmoid colon and rectum have tubular configuration. Colon is narrowed, and haustral sacculations have disappeared. Rectum is narrowed, and valves of Houston are gone. In this patient, ascending colon appears normal. *(From Rubesin SE, Bartram CI, Laufer I. Inflammatory bowel disease. In: Levine MS, Rubesin SE, Laufer I, eds. Double contrast gastrointestinal radiology. Philadelphia: Saunders; 2000:417-470.)*

include mesenteric border ulcers and crisscrossing knifelike clefts resulting in cobblestoning (see Table 26-1). Strictures, fissures, and fistulas are seen with transmural disease. Pathologically, granulomas are detected in 25% to 70% of patients. The characteristic radiographic findings in ulcerative colitis are granular mucosa (see Figure 26-12), ulcers on a background of inflammatory granularity, shortening of the colon, and loss of haustration.

26. **What is the first radiographic study that is performed in symptomatic patients with previously diagnosed Crohn's disease?**
CT is performed first, primarily to exclude an intra-abdominal abscess and to show the cause of separated bowel loops—whether abscess, inflammation, or fibrofatty proliferation. Fat does not creep or proliferate, so "fibrofatty proliferation" is a misnomer. Prominent fat may be related to retraction of fat secondary to inflammation spreading along lymphatic and venous channels.

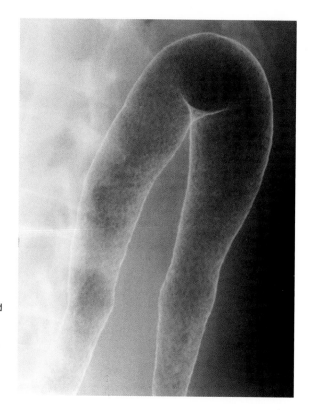

**Figure 26-12.** Ulcerative colitis on double-contrast barium enema examination. Spot radiograph of splenic flexure shows innumerable diminutive radiolucencies surrounded by linear and punctate barium collections. This very fine mucosal nodularity has been described as granular mucosa. It involves entire surface of bowel. Colon is tubular in shape without haustration. *(From Rubesin SE, Bartram CI, Laufer I. Inflammatory bowel disease. In: Levine MS, Rubesin SE, Laufer I, eds.* Double contrast gastrointestinal radiology. *Philadelphia: Saunders; 2000:417-470.)*

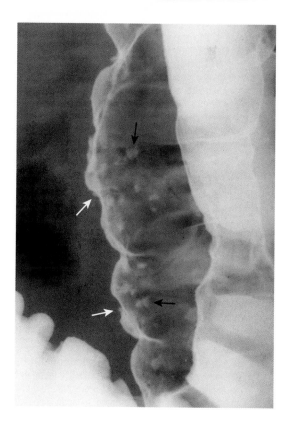

**Figure 26-13.** Aphthoid ulcers of colon in Crohn's disease on double-contrast barium enema examination. Spot radiograph of splenic flexure of colon shows numerous 2- to 3-mm punctate and stellate barium collections surrounded by radiolucent halos. Several aphthoid ulcers are identified in profile (*white arrows*) and en face (*black arrows*). Large portion of mucosa is smooth and normal. *(From Rubesin SE, Bartram CI, Laufer I. Inflammatory bowel disease. In: Levine MS, Rubesin SE, Laufer I, eds.* Double contrast gastrointestinal radiology. *Philadelphia: Saunders; 2000:417-470.)*

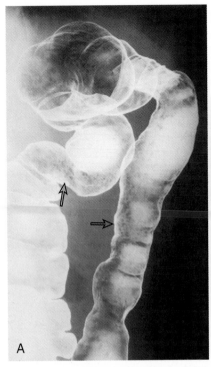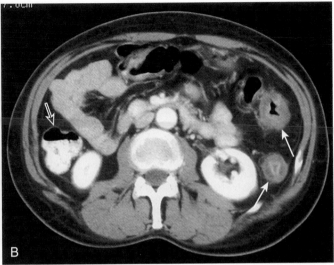

**Figure 26-14.** Ischemic colitis on double-contrast barium enema examination and CT. **A,** Spot radiograph of splenic flexure shows diffuse narrowing of lumen, loss of normal haustral pattern, and fine nodularity of mucosa (*open arrows*). (*From Rubesin SE, Bartram CI, Laufer I. Inflammatory bowel disease. In: Levine MS, Rubesin SE, Laufer I, eds.* Double contrast gastrointestinal radiology. *Philadelphia: Saunders; 2000:417-470.*) **B,** Axial CT image through upper descending colon shows mural stratification pattern in splenic flexure and descending colon (*arrows*). Low attenuation of submucosa represents submucosal edema related to ischemia. Compare thickness and attenuation of wall in areas of ischemia with wall of normal ascending colon (*open arrow*).

27. What is the most common form of colitis in an outpatient older than 50 years?
    The most common form of colitis in an outpatient older than 50 years is ischemic colitis. The most common causes of ischemic colitis are low-flow states, such as congestive heart failure, shock, or dysrhythmia. Occlusion of large vessels owing to atherosclerosis or embolism infrequently causes colonic ischemia because large collateral arterial arcs (arc of Riolan, marginal artery of Drummond) can compensate for central vascular occlusion.

    Ischemia may occur in any part of the colon; however, it commonly involves the distal transverse colon and descending colon (Figure 26-14) because these regions are the sites of transition between the blood supply from the superior mesenteric and inferior mesenteric arteries. The splenic flexure region is known as the "watershed" area of the colonic arterial supply.

28. A woman with a history of cervical cancer now has rectal bleeding (Figure 26-15). What is the most likely diagnosis?
    Radiation-induced stricture is the most likely diagnosis (see Figure 26-15 legend for discussion). Radiation acutely causes necrosis in the bowel walls. With time, blood vessels and lymphatics are obliterated, resulting in chronic ischemia with mucosal atrophy, fibrosis, and occasional stricture formation. Radiation-induced changes in the rectum, sigmoid colon, and pelvic ileum are common causes of gastrointestinal bleeding or obstruction. Radiation-induced colitis and enteritis are most commonly encountered in patients who have been irradiated for cervical or prostatic carcinoma.

29. What are colonic diverticula?
    Colonic diverticula are protrusions of mucosa and submucosa through areas of colonic wall weakness (Figure 26-16), primarily where the end arteries perforate the colonic wall (on the mesenteric side of the antimesenteric taeniae). The diverticula protrude into the pericolic fat, separated from the pericolonic fat by a thin layer of longitudinal muscle. **Diverticulum** is the singular form; **diverticula** is the plural form. "Diverticuli" and "diverticulae" are incorrect plural forms.

30. Describe the distribution of colonic diverticula.
    In patients with diverticulosis, diverticula are found in the sigmoid colon in 90% of patients, in the descending colon in 30%, and throughout the colon in 26%. Isolated right-sided diverticula, although uncommon in the United States (about 4% of patients), are common in Japan. Appendiceal diverticula are found in 0.2% to 2% of patients.

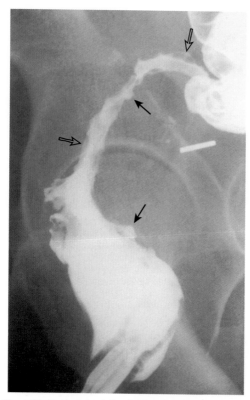

**Figure 26-15.** Radiation-induced stricture of colon on single-contrast barium enema examination. Spot radiograph of rectum shows 10-cm-long, focal narrowing of distal sigmoid colon and proximal rectum with tapered margins. Contour is irregular, mucosa is nodular (*open arrows*), and focal ulceration (*black arrows*) is present. Clips present in pelvis indicate prior surgery. In conjunction with clinical history provided, diagnosis of radiation-induced stricture can be made. If no clinical history was available, stricture resulting from Crohn's disease, lymphogranuloma venereum, or rare infiltrating carcinoma could give similar radiographic appearance.

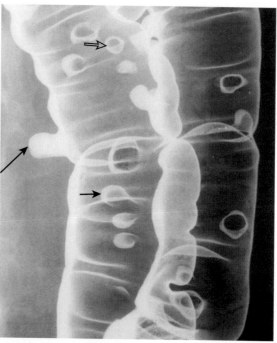

**Figure 26-16.** Diverticulosis of colon on double-contrast barium enema examination. Coned-down overhead image of splenic flexure with patient in right-side-down decubitus position reveals numerous diverticula. Some barium-filled diverticula are seen in profile (*long black arrow*). Most diverticula seen en face have a small pool of barium on their dependent surface resembling meniscus (*short black arrow*). Other diverticula are devoid of barium meniscus and are depicted only as barium-coated ring shadows (*open arrow*). Normal haustral sacculations and interhaustral folds are preserved.

31. What is the primary muscle abnormality in diverticular disease?

The longitudinal muscle layer of the colon is primarily divided into three bands, termed the **taeniae coli**. In diverticular disease, elastin deposits between normal muscle fibers in the taeniae coli. Macroscopically, the taeniae coli are shortened and thickened, resulting in overall shortening and straightening of the colon and redundancy of the circular muscle fibers and mucosa. The circular muscle forms thick, 180-degree bands of muscle that cross the colon. This "bunching" together of the circular muscle layer and the mucosa of the colon occurs particularly in the sigmoid colon. The muscle abnormality is termed **myochosis**. The longitudinal muscle abnormality has also been termed **circular muscle thickening**, **hypertrophy**, or **bunching**. The term **diverticular disease** implies circular muscle bunching (Figure 26-17). The term **diverticulosis** implies presence of diverticula with or without circular muscle bunching.

32. An elderly patient presents with acute left lower abdominal pain. The clinical concern is acute diverticulitis. What examination is performed first?

CT of the abdomen is the first study performed in most adults with acute left lower abdominal pain. Ultrasonography (US) is the first examination performed, particularly in women of childbearing age, if the clinician suspects disease originating in the adnexa or uterus.

33. Figure 26-18 is an image from a CT scan in a patient with acute left lower quadrant abdominal pain. What is your diagnosis?

An abscess is seen to abut the sigmoid colon, a finding suggestive of acute diverticulitis. CT is superior to barium enema examination in the diagnosis of diverticulitis. CT shows the presence and size of pericolic abscesses, and it is superior in diagnosing other complications of diverticulitis (e.g., liver abscess, venous thrombosis, small bowel obstruction). CT is also slightly safer than contrast enema examination. Although most patients with diverticulitis have walled-off pericolonic inflammation or abscess formation, a small percentage (<1%) of patients with diverticulitis have

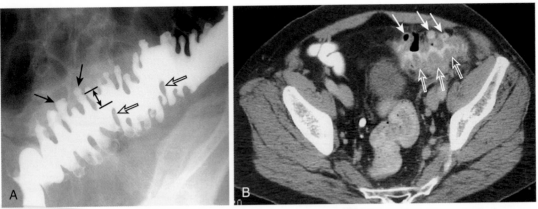

**Figure 26-17.** Diverticular disease of sigmoid colon on single-contrast barium enema examination and CT. **A,** Spot radiograph shows circular muscle thickening and diverticulosis of sigmoid colon. Lumen has zigzag, accordion-like, or concertina-like appearance created by thick folds of circular muscle and redundant mucosa protruding into lumen. Diverticula (*black arrows*) are small, barium-filled saccular protrusions outside of expected luminal contour. Representative circular muscle folds are identified (*open arrows*). The height of one thick, circular muscle fold is identified by double arrow. **B,** Axial CT image of different patient with diverticular disease shows thick, undulating wall (*open arrows*) in sigmoid colon, corresponding to circular muscle "bunching." Contrast-filled and air-filled diverticula are present (*white arrows*).

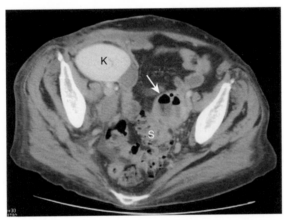

**Figure 26-18.** Pericolic abscess related to sigmoid diverticulitis on CT. Axial CT image through pelvis reveals 4-cm heterogeneous lesion (*arrow*) adjacent to sigmoid colon (*S*). Fluid attenuation and air bubbles are seen centrally in pericolic lesion. Thick rind of soft tissue is seen in its periphery. These findings are in keeping with pericolic abscess in this patient with diverticulitis. No colonic wall thickening or intrinsic colonic mass is present to suggest perforated colonic carcinoma. Right pelvic renal transplant (*K*) is also present.

free perforation into the peritoneal space. Barium enema examination would be potentially dangerous in this tiny subset of patients with free perforation.

CT and contrast enema examination are superior to endoscopy in the diagnosis of left lower quadrant pain. CT is inferior to barium studies in diagnosing a perforated colon cancer as the cause of a pericolic abscess. If CT shows focal colonic wall thickening, a mass, or pericolic lymphadenopathy, endoscopy or barium enema may be indicated to exclude a perforated carcinoma, after the acute inflammatory process heals. Some patients with subacute abdominal pain undergo barium enema examination. The findings of diverticulitis (Figure 26-19) are the demonstration of air or contrast material outside of the expected luminal contour, and the extrinsic inflammatory effect of a pericolic abscess upon the colon.

34. A young woman complains of left lower quadrant pain (Figure 26-20). What is your diagnosis?
The diagnosis is endometriosis involving the sigmoid colon. Disease in the peritoneal space descends to the rectovesical space in men and to the rectouterine space (pouch of Douglas) in women. This is most commonly seen with intraperitoneal metastases from the colon, pancreas, or stomach in men or ovarian cancer in women. Pelvic diseases can directly invade the rectosigmoid colon—primary tumors from the ovary, cervix, or prostate gland, or abscesses related to the ovaries, appendix, or colon. Barium studies and CT are superior to endoscopy in diagnosing extrinsic disease involving the colon.

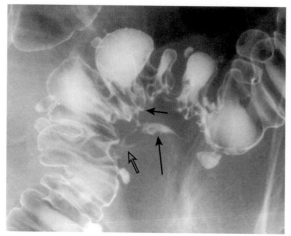

**Figure 26-19.** Colonic diverticulitis on double-contrast barium enema examination. Spot radiograph of sigmoid colon shows several small barium-filled tracks (*open arrow*) forming flame-shaped collection (*long arrow*) in pericolic space. Wall of adjacent sigmoid colon has spiculated contour (*short arrow*). There is extrinsic mass impression on inferior wall of sigmoid colon. Compare asymmetric inflammatory changes with normal contour of opposite colonic wall. *(From Rubesin SE, Laufer I. Diverticular disease. In: Levine MS, Rubesin SE, Laufer I, eds. Double contrast gastrointestinal radiology. Philadelphia: Saunders; 2000:471-494.)*

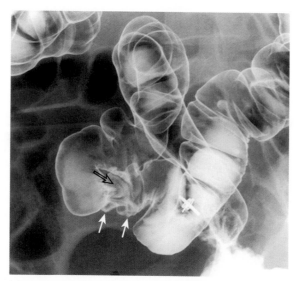

**Figure 26-20.** Endometriosis involving colon on double-contrast barium enema examination. Spot radiograph shows spiculation of inferior border of sigmoid colon (*white arrows*). Colon is tethered, manifested as smooth thin folds (*open arrow*), pulled toward inferior contour. These are findings of disease extrinsic to colon. This young woman has known endometriosis.

35. What is defecography?

Defecography is an examination that records a patient defecating a thick, stool-like barium paste. This is a dynamic examination recorded on videotape or digital video disc (DVD) recorder. Defecography is also known as **voiding proctography** and is often performed in conjunction with cystography.

36. What types of symptoms are indications for defecography?

Patients complaining of incontinence, painful defecation, incomplete defecation, or constipation may benefit from defecography.

37. What happens to a patient during defecography?

The patient, if a woman, ingests a moderate volume of barium (500 mL) to opacify the small intestine. If the patient is a woman, a small amount (3-5 mL) of thick barium is instilled into the vagina to opacify the vagina. A tiny lead marker (e.g., a metallic nipple marker used in chest radiography) is placed on the perineal body. Thick barium paste that mimics soft, formed stool is instilled into the rectum. The patient then sits on a commode and defecates. The radiologist takes images before, during, and after defecation. The images show the relationships between the small bowel, vagina, and rectum during defecation.

38. What abnormalities are detected during defecography that are not identified during endoscopy or barium enema?

Defecography can show rectocele, enterocele (Figure 26-21), abnormal anal sphincter opening, abnormal "relaxation" of the puborectalis muscle of the pelvic floor, abnormal rectal contraction, and varying degrees of prolapse of the rectal or anal tissue either through the anal canal or through the vagina (Figure 26-22).

39. What are the indications for a water-soluble contrast enema?

Water-soluble contrast agents use iodine as the x-ray absorber rather than barium. A water-soluble enema is used if there is concern for a colonic perforation because water-soluble contrast material is safer in the peritoneal space than barium. Water-soluble contrast agents are rapidly resorbed from the peritoneal cavity, and the iodine is excreted by the kidneys. In comparison, if barium and feces spill into the peritoneal cavity, a severe, potentially life-threatening granulomatous peritonitis may ensue.

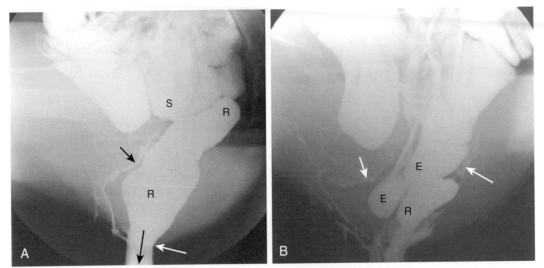

**Figure 26-21.** Development of enterocele during defecation on defecography. **A,** Lateral image of pelvis at beginning of defecation shows barium in small bowel (*S*), rectum (*R*), and vagina (*short black arrow*). Anal sphincter (*white arrow*) is opening normally while patient defecates paste (*long black arrow*). **B,** Lateral image of pelvis at end of defecation shows residual barium stasis in small rectocele (*R*). Several barium-filled loops of small bowel (E) have dipped deep into pelvis between vagina (*short arrow*) and collapsed rectum (*long arrow*). This represents enterocele. Enteroceles typically appear at end of defecation or during straining after defecation.

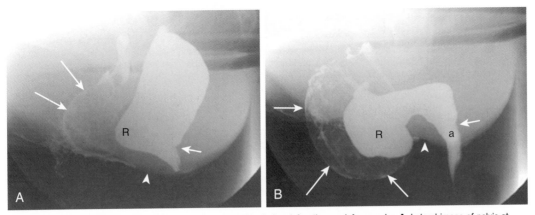

**Figure 26-22.** Development of rectocele prolapsing through vagina during defecation on defecography. **A,** Lateral image of pelvis at beginning of defecation shows mild bulging of anterior wall of rectum (*R*), representing beginning of rectocele formation. Anal canal has not completely opened, and impression of puborectalis muscle (*short arrow*) is still present. Vagina (*long arrows*) bulges slightly forward. Arrowhead identifies metallic marker placed on perineal body. **B,** Lateral image of pelvis at end of defecation. Puborectalis impression has normally disappeared (*short arrow*). Anal canal (*a*) remains open. Vagina (*long arrows*) and large rectocele (*R*) now prolapse out of vaginal introitus. Arrowhead identifies metallic marker placed on perineal body.

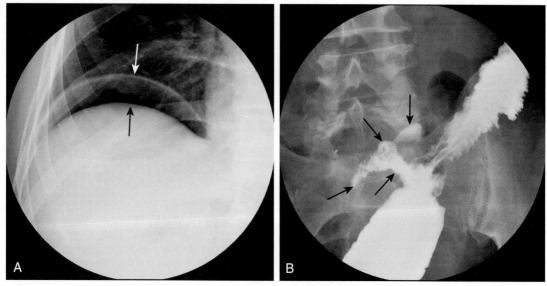

**Figure 26-23.** Leak at end-to-end colorectal anastomosis 11 days after partial colectomy for adenocarcinoma of descending colon on plain radiograph and water-soluble contrast enema examination. **A,** Coned-down view of right hemidiaphragm shows persistence of free peritoneal gas in greater amount than would be expected 11 days after surgery. Radiolucent space separates right hemidiaphragm (*white arrow*) from superior edge of liver (*black arrow*). **B,** Spot radiograph from water-soluble contrast enema shows 3-cm-long collection (*arrows*) arising from right lateral wall of known end-to-end colorectal anastomosis. This has irregular contour inferiorly and lobulated contour superiorly. This collection should not be mistaken for colonic stump of side-to-end colorectal anastomosis.

Some surgeons prefer that water-soluble contrast agents are used in patients with suspected colonic obstruction because the presence of residual barium in the colon would make spillage of colonic contrast agent at surgery more problematic. Water-soluble contrast agents may also be used in patients who may have a difficult time expelling barium from the colon before it forms concretions. These patients include debilitated, bedridden patients; patients on narcotic medications or medications with anticholinergic side effects; or patients in whom an oral preparation is contraindicated, such as patients with small bowel obstruction.

40. A water-soluble contrast enema is performed in a patient with a hand-sewn end-to-end colorectal anastomosis, after resection of a colonic adenocarcinoma. What is the diagnosis in Figure 26-23?
    For the answer, see the figure legend.

## KEY POINTS

- Know or have access to your institution's preparation instructions for barium enema.
- Contraindications for barium enema include suspected bowel perforation, fulminant colitis (toxic megacolon), recent polypectomy/deep biopsy, and latex or barium allergy.
- A patient with latex allergy should be the first patient scheduled in the morning, after the fluoroscopic room has been cleaned; diabetic patients should be scheduled early in the day.
- Know the difference between a double-contrast and single-contrast barium enema, and know what types of patients are capable of undergoing a double-contrast barium enema.
- A CT scan is the examination of choice in patients with suspected colonic diverticulitis.

## BIBLIOGRAPHY

Cunnane ME, Rubesin SE, Furth EE, et al. Small flat umbilicated tumors of the colon: radiographic and pathologic findings. *AJR Am J Roentgenol.* 2000;175(3):747-749.

Rubesin SE, Bartram CI, Laufer I. Inflammatory bowel disease. In: Levine MS, Rubesin SE, Laufer I, eds. *Double contrast gastrointestinal radiology.* Philadelphia: Saunders; 2000:417-470.

Rubesin SE, Laufer I. Diverticular disease. In: Levine MS, Rubesin SE, Laufer I, eds. *Double contrast gastrointestinal radiology.* Philadelphia: Saunders; 2000:471-494.

Rubesin SE, Laufer I. Tumors of the colon. In: Levine MS, Rubesin SE, Laufer I, eds. *Double contrast gastrointestinal radiology.* Philadelphia: Saunders; 2000:357-416.

McCarthy PA, Rubesin SE, Levine MS, et al. Colon cancer: morphology detected with barium enema examination versus histopathologic stage. *Radiology.* 1995;197(3):683-687.

# CHAPTER 27

# CT AND MRI OF THE LOWER GASTROINTESTINAL TRACT

*Hanna Zafar, MD, MHS*

1. **What is shown in Figure 27-1?**
   A topogram from a computed tomographic colonography (CTC), an examination tailored to evaluate for colorectal polyps and masses.

2. **What is the adenoma-carcinoma sequence?**
   The adenoma-carcinoma sequence refers to a series of genetic mutations whereby small adenomatous colon polyps (<5 mm) transform into large adenomatous polyps (>1 cm), noninvasive carcinomas, and then invasive carcinomas. This entire process takes, on average, 10 years, which serves as the basis for colorectal cancer screening. Up to 90% of colorectal carcinomas, predominantly adenocarcinomas, develop through the adenoma-carcinoma sequence, rendering colorectal cancer a virtually preventable disease through regular screening.

3. **What is the risk of malignancy in a colonic adenomatous polyp measuring <1 cm?**
   1%.

4. **What is the risk of malignancy in a colonic adenomatous polyp measuring 1 cm?**
   10%.

5. **What is the diagnostic performance of CTC compared to traditional or optical colonoscopy (OC) for adenomatous polyps?**
   The diagnostic performance of CTC improves with increased polyp size. For the answer, see Table 27-1.

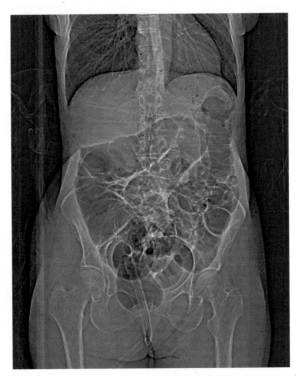

**Figure 27-1.** Topogram on CTC. Note presence of gas throughout colon from level of rectum to cecum and visualization of rectal tube within rectum.

**Table 27-1.** Diagnostic Performance of CTC Versus OC Based on Polyp Size

| POLYP SIZE | CTC | OC |
|---|---|---|
| 6 mm | Sensitivity 78-89%<br>Specificity 80-88% | Sensitivity 92% |
| ≥10 mm | Sensitivity 90-94%<br>Specificity 86-96% | Sensitivity 88% |

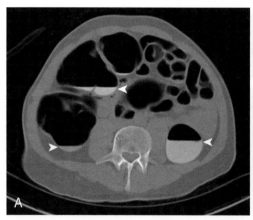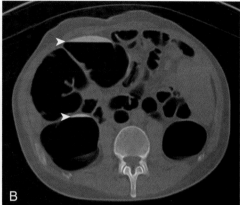

**Figure 27-2.** Primary 2D images on CTC. **A,** Axial supine images through upper abdomen using polyp window reveal homogenously tagged fluid in hepatic flexure, ascending colon, and descending colon (*arrowheads*). **B,** Axial prone images using polyp window reveal fluid shift either to opposite colonic wall (*arrowheads*) or out-of-field of view, ensuring that these segments are adequately visualized between both positions. Adequate colonic distension ensures that polyps can be visualized against gas-filled colonic lumen.

6. What is the protocol for CTC?
   The typical preparation for CTC involves a combination of a low residue diet, cathartic bowel preparation, and fecal tagging (i.e., labeling of fecal residue) using both barium sulfate (Tagitol) and water-soluble iodinated contrast material (Gastroview). When CTC is performed on the same day as an incomplete OC, Gastroview is administered after sedation has worn off and 2 to 3 hours prior to scanning.

7. Can CTC be performed without a cathartic bowel preparation?
   Yes. The preparation for laxative free CTC is accomplished using a combination of fecal tagging and low residue diet. However, the absence of a cathartic bowel preparation affects the diagnostic performance of this test and does not permit same day polypectomy. Specifically, the sensitivity and specificity of laxative free CTC is 91% and 86%, respectively, for polyps ≥10 mm, but is 59% and 88%, respectively, for polyps ≥6 mm. As such, laxative free CTC is generally reserved for patients unwilling to undergo a cathartic bowel preparation for either CTC or OC.

8. What are the three factors that should be optimized on CTC?
   • **Colonic cleansing/fecal tagging** to ensure that adherent or retained stool can be distinguished from potential polyps to avoid false-positive results.
   • **Colonic distension** so that polyps can be visualized against an air-filled lumen.
   • **Patient positioning** using at least two positions to assess for lesion mobility, to shift fluid to increase exposed colonic lumen, and to shift gas to distend colonic segments. If patients are unable to lie prone, decubitus images may be performed as an alternative (Figure 27-2).

9. What are the differences between a primary "2D" and a primary "3D" read on CTC?
   For the answer, see Table 27-2.

10. What is the "polyp" window?
    The "polyp" window is used for primary 2D review, where the contrast and brightness settings of display of the images are set between those used for lung and bone windows. This window optimizes the contrast between the gas-filled colonic lumen and intraluminal polyps or masses (see Figure 27-2).

11. What is the differential diagnosis for a focal mass projecting into the colon lumen on 3D images (prior to correlation with the 2D images)?
    The differential diagnosis for a focal mass identified on 3D images includes tagged stool, impacted fecalith, bulbous fold, lipoma, and polyp (Figure 27-3). This differential diagnosis underscores the importance of correlating all focal abnormalities detected on 3D images with the 2D images.

**Table 27-2.** Differences Between Primary 2D and 3D Interpretation of CTC

|  | PRIMARY 2D | PRIMARY 3D |
|---|---|---|
| Image visualization | Thin-section cross-sectional images. | Endoluminal volume-rendered (VR) images. |
| Technique | Visualization of the colon from rectum to cecum focusing on short segments in order to trace from the "floor" to the "ceiling." In other words, every wall of the colon must be visualized for a given segment. | Fly-through visualization of the colon from rectum to cecum BOTH antegrade and retrograde. Retrograde views are necessary to view lesions on the back of a colonic fold. |
| Lesion characterization | Soft tissue windows on 2D images. | Soft tissue windows on 2D images. |
| Limitations | Usually takes a longer amount of time to perform than primary 3D review. | Nonvisualization of colonic walls submerged in fluid. Suboptimal visualization of poorly distended segments. |

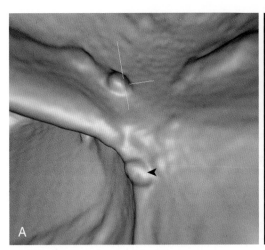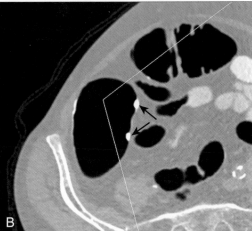

**Figure 27-3.** Primary 3D image on CTC. **A,** Endoluminal image in cecum depicts polypoid lesion located along fold (*crosshairs*). Similar polypoid lesion is visualized immediately below this lesion (*arrowhead*). **B,** Correlation with 2D image demonstrates that both lesions correspond to foci of tagged high attenuation fecal material (*arrows*). This example demonstrates need to correlate all 3D image findings with those of 2D images.

12. What is the major differential diagnosis for a focal polypoid soft tissue attenuation colonic lesion on CTC?
    Colon cancer, adenomatous polyp, hyperplastic polyp, and pseudolesion (untagged stool or mucosal fold) (Figure 27-4).

13. How is a colonic diverticulum diagnosed on CTC?
    The presence of a ring shadow or dark curvilinear focus surrounding the orifice of the lesion indicates a colonic diverticulum (Figure 27-5). Recognition of these findings allows the reader to confidently ignore them on a primary 3D review.

14. How do diverticula of the gastrointestinal tract form?
    Bowel diverticula are the result of one of three processes: (1) pulsion diverticula due to increased intraluminal pressure, (2) traction diverticula due to traction on the wall of the bowel by scarring, and (3) congenital diverticula due to abnormal development. The most common type of diverticula are pulsion diverticula, which are seen predominantly in the colon.

15. What are the three methods utilized to distinguish stool from polyps on CTC?
    For the answer, see Table 27-3.

16. What is the definition of a "clinically significant polyp" on CTC?
    The size threshold for a clinically significant polyp on CTC is 6 mm or greater. This cutoff is based on large patient series which demonstrate that lesions less than 6 mm on CTC often represent hyperplastic polyps or normal mucosal skin tags. Hyperplastic polyps almost never undergo malignant degeneration and so there is minimal to no risk of cancer developing in these lesions. The majority of polyps less than 5 mm are adenomas that will not undergo the adenoma-carcinoma sequence.

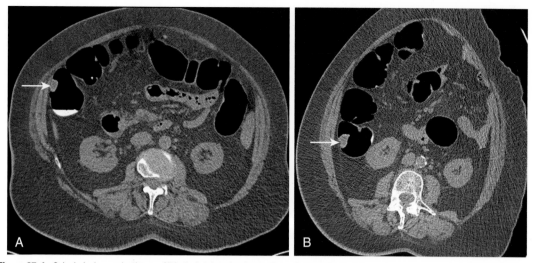

**Figure 27-4.** Colonic lesion evaluation on CTC. **A,** Axial supine image through ascending colon using soft tissue window depicts 2-cm soft tissue attenuation polypoid lesion arising from lateral wall of colon (*arrow*). **B,** Axial left lateral decubitus image through ascending colon using soft tissue window demonstrates that lesion does not move with changes in patient positioning. On basis of soft tissue attenuation, lack of mobility, and size, this patient must be referred to endoscopy for tissue sampling.

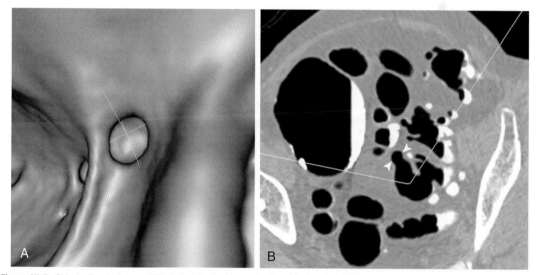

**Figure 27-5.** Colonic diverticulum on CTC. **A,** Endoluminal image in sigmoid colon depicts ring shadow (*crosshairs*). **B,** Axial left lateral decubitus image shows that this corresponds to colonic diverticulum (*arrowheads*). Presence of ring shadow on primary 3D review does not require correlation with 2D images.

17. How frequently should CTC be performed?
   There is little long-term data on the optimal frequency at which CTC should be performed. However, according to joint guidelines from the American Cancer Society (ACS), the US Multi-Society Task Force on Colorectal Cancer, and the American College of Radiology (ACR), CTC should be performed every 5 years, similar to double-contrast barium enema. This is compared to every 10 years for OC among patients with no polyps.

18. What are the most commonly observed indications for CTC?
   The most common indication for CTC is incomplete OC, which can be performed the same day as OC, as well as a history of prior difficult OC. Less frequently encountered indications include sedation risk, chronic anticoagulation, evaluation of the colon proximal to an obstructing mass or stricture that precludes passage of an endoscope, and characterization of an indeterminate colorectal lesion on OC. Of note, CTC can be performed safely in patients with colonic anastomoses.
   Coverage for screening CTC remains controversial due to concerns over cost-effectiveness, the ability of CTC to reach the previously unscreened population, extracolonic findings (findings outside of the colonic lumen visible on CTC

**Table 27-3.** Three Methods to Distinguish Fecal Material from Polyps on CTC

| | |
|---|---|
| Attenuation | Fecal material should be immediately characterized on an adequately tagged examination by the presence of high attenuation barium infused within the lesion. Polyps can be identified as soft tissue attenuation masses which may be coated, but not infused, with high attenuation contrast. *Pearl:* When fecal tagging is suboptimal, the presence of gas within a lesion is diagnostic of fecal material. |
| Mobility | Fecal material will shift with patient positioning, whereas polyps will remain fixed to the colon wall. *Pearl:* Polyps within intraperitoneal colonic segments located on a mesentery (i.e., sigmoid colon, transverse colon, and cecum) may appear to shift. Careful inspection of multiplanar 2D images should help one to make this distinction. |
| Morphology | Fecal material generally demonstrates angular geographic borders in contrast to polyps which demonstrate smooth borders. *Pearl:* All lesions detected on 3D images, even those with smooth borders, must be correlated with 2D images. Tagged stool, fecaliths, and submucosal masses such as lipomas may demonstrate smooth walls. |

but not OC), and radiation risk. In some regions of the country, CTC is reimbursed as a method of colorectal cancer screening, although most insurers including the Centers for Medicaid and Medicare (CMS) do not currently cover this modality for screening.

19. **When is CTC not recommended?**
CTC is not advised for surveillance of patients at high risk for cancer including patients with hereditary syndromes (e.g., Lynch syndrome, hereditary polyposis, or nonpolyposis syndrome). This examination is not advised on the same day as OC where a deep biopsy or polypectomy is performed. CTC is also not appropriate for patients with acute colitis, recent surgery, symptomatic colon-containing abdominal wall hernia, known or suspected bowel perforation, and high-grade small bowel obstruction.

20. **What is the role of routine computed tomography (CT) and magnetic resonance imaging (MRI) in colon cancer screening?**
None.

21. **What are the complications of CTC?**
The main risk of CTC is perforation, which is seen in 0 to 7 out of 1,000 elderly patients (compared to 12 out of 1,000 elderly patients who receive OC).

22. **What is the radiation dose for CTC?**
Both supine and prone position imaging can be performed at a dose of less than 12 mSv, using an effective tube current of 50 mAs or modulated dose protocols. This radiation dose is similar to or lower than that from a double-contrast barium enema and ≤50% the diagnostic reference level for routine abdominopelvic CT.

23. **Why do patients prefer CTC to OC?**
75% of patients prefer CTC to OC for the following reasons: noninvasiveness, lack of sedation, improved comfort, and avoidance of OC risks (i.e., perforation).

24. **What is the normal cross-sectional imaging appearance of the colon?**
The normal wall thickness of the colon is paper thin (i.e., <3 mm) when well distended. The diameter of the colon varies greatly, where the cecum generally has the greatest diameter and is usually <9 cm, the transverse colon is usually <6 cm, and the descending colon and sigmoid colon are slightly smaller in caliber. Gas, fecal material, and fluid are normally present in the colon.

25. **What are the major nonneoplastic causes of colonic wall thickening?**
For the answer, see Box 27-1.

26. **What is the "target" sign, and what is its significance?**
On CT, the "target" sign (Figure 27-6), also known as mural stratification, refers to visualization of a bright soft tissue attenuation inner layer (representing mucosa, lamina propria, and hypertrophied muscularis mucosae, sometimes with hyperemia), a dark low attenuation middle layer (representing edematous submucosa), and sometimes a bright soft tissue attenuation outer layer (representing muscularis propria and serosa); the alternating layers correspond to the rings of a target. On MRI, a similar bright-dark-bright pattern is seen on contrast-enhanced fat-suppressed T1-weighted images, whereas a dark-bright-dark pattern is seen on T2-weighted images, since fluid and edema are high in signal intensity on T2-weighted images. This sign is not specific for a particular disease condition, as it can be seen in a variety of inflammatory processes including pseudomembranous colitis, ischemic colitis, and inflammatory bowel disease, but is highly specific for diagnosis of nonneoplastic disease when encountered in the colon.

**Box 27-1.** Major Nonneoplastic Causes of Colonic Wall Thickening

**A. Infection**

1. *Clostridium difficile* (pseudomembranous colitis)
2. Neutropenic colitis (typhlitis)
3. *Salmonella*
4. *Shigella*
5. *Yersinia*
6. Amoeba
7. Cytomegalovirus

**B. Ischemia**

**C. Inflammatory bowel disease**

1. Crohn's disease
2. Ulcerative colitis

**D. Hypoproteinemia**

1. Cirrhosis
2. Other

(Adapted from Zafar HM, Miller Jr. WT. Imaging of the bowel. In: Diagnostic abdominal imaging. New York: McGraw Hill; 2013:15-160.)

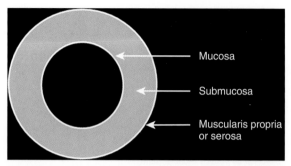

**Figure 27-6.** "Target" sign of bowel on CT. This appearance, also known as mural stratification, is due to soft tissue attenuation of mucosa (*bright inner ring*), low attenuation edema of submucosa (*dark middle ring*), and soft tissue attenuation of muscularis propria or serosa (*bright outer ring*). Although nonspecific, this finding indicates nonneoplastic disease when seen in colon.

27. What are the CT and MR imaging features of infectious colitis?

Segmental or diffuse colonic wall thickening is seen, typically with homogeneous enhancement, and often with pericolic inflammatory fat stranding. A "target" sign may also be seen, and pericolic fluid or ascites may also be present.

28. What is the etiology of pseudomembranous colitis?

Pseudomembranous colitis results from toxins produced by an overgrowth of the bacteria *Clostridium difficile* resulting in watery diarrhea, abdominal pain, and fever. This diagnosis is most commonly seen as a complication of antibiotic therapy but has also been associated with hypotensive episodes, chemotherapeutic agents, and abdominal surgery.

29. How is pseudomembranous colitis diagnosed?

Pseudomembranous colitis is typically diagnosed through stool assays or visualization of characteristic adherent yellow plaques on endoscopy. Yet, in some cases, the diagnosis is not clinically suspected and is first suggested based on imaging. When left untreated, pseudomembranous colitis can result in significant mortality and morbidity. Therefore, recognition of the characteristic imaging findings of this disease is important.

30. What are the cross-sectional imaging features that are helpful to distinguish pseudomembranous colitis from other forms of colitis?

For the answer, see Table 27-4. Also see Figure 27-7.

31. What is the treatment for pseudomembranous colitis?

Metronidazole and vancomycin are usually effective for the treatment of pseudomembranous colitis. Less than 1% of patients will not respond to medical therapy and require colectomy or other surgical procedures.

32. What is the role of CT in the management of pseudomembranous colitis?

CT is helpful to evaluate disease extent, severity, and presence of complications (e.g., perforation). However, CT findings alone do not predict which patients will require surgical intervention.

33. What is typhlitis?

Typhlitis, also called neutropenic enterocolitis, occurs in patients undergoing treatment for malignancy such as acute leukemia, aplastic anemia, lymphoma, acquired immunodeficiency syndrome (AIDS), and solid organ transplantation. The exact etiology is unknown but is thought to be mucosal injury initiated by a combination of ischemia, infection, hemorrhage, and neoplastic infiltration of the bowel wall.

34. How is typhlitis diagnosed?

CT is the examination of choice for the diagnosis of typhlitis given the increased risk of bowel perforation through endoscopy or contrast enema examination. This diagnosis should be suggested when a neutropenic patient presents

**Table 27-4.** Cross-sectional Imaging Features Suggestive of Pseudomembranous Colitis

| | |
|---|---|
| Wall thickening | Generally greater in degree than any other inflammatory or infectious disease of the colon, save Crohn's disease. Of note, wall thickening in pseudomembranous colitis is asymmetric and irregular compared to that of Crohn's disease, which is generally symmetric and homogeneous. When severe, trapping of barium within thickened haustral folds produces the "accordion" sign (see Figure 27-7). |
| Distribution | Classically seen as a pancolitis from rectum to cecum, although it can also present with a segmental distribution. |
| Bowel enhancement pattern | "Target" sign may be present, although this may also be seen with other colitides. |
| Luminal dilation | Thought to reflect transmural inflammation. |
| Pericolic fat stranding | Generally mild relative to the degree of wall thickening, but may also be seen with other colitides. |

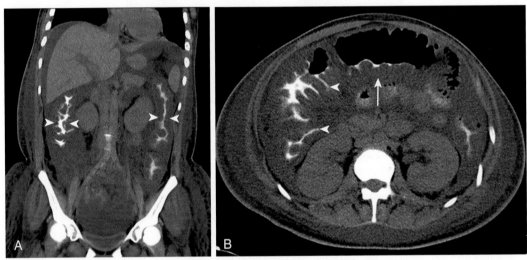

**Figure 27-7.** Pseudomembranous colitis on CT. **A,** Coronal image with oral but no intravenous contrast material of 18-year-old woman presenting with abdominal pain following antibiotic therapy demonstrates marked wall thickening (*arrowheads*) involving visualized ascending and descending colon. Low attenuation within colon wall corresponds to edema. **B,** Axial image demonstrates positive oral contrast material trapped between edematous haustral folds resulting in "accordion" sign (*arrowheads*). Note that wall thickening along dependent wall of transverse colon is irregular (*arrow*), and that there is dilation of that colonic segment. These imaging findings, in constellation with provided history of antibiotic use, are highly suggestive of pseudomembranous colitis. Moderate ascites is secondary to acute hepatic and renal failure from other causes.

with wall thickening involving the terminal ileum, cecum, and ascending colon. Submucosal edema may be present, seen as low attenuation in the bowel wall, and fat stranding of the adjacent mesenteric fat due to edema and/or inflammation is common. In addition to diagnosis, CT is further useful in evaluating treatment response and detecting complications requiring surgery such as pneumatosis, bowel perforation, and pericolic fluid collections (Figure 27-8).

35. What is the treatment of typhlitis?

Resolution of typhlitis corresponds to the adequate return of functioning neutrophils. Supportive treatment includes bowel rest, total parenteral nutrition, antibiotics, and aggressive fluid and electrolyte replacement. Surgery is reserved for patients with uncontrolled gastrointestinal bleeding or sepsis, bowel obstruction, abscess formation, transmural necrosis, or bowel perforation.

36. What are the causes of ischemic colitis?

For the answer, see Box 27-2.

37. What is the most common cause of ischemic colitis?

Hypoperfusion (nonocclusive ischemic disease).

38. What is the most common finding of ischemic colitis on CT?

Circumferential symmetric colonic wall thickening between 3 mm to 2 cm, with fold enlargement. In up to 25% of cases, the "target" sign may be present. This finding is best appreciated during the late arterial and venous phases of

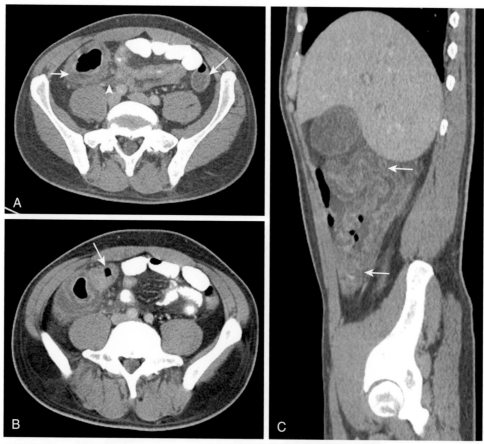

**Figure 27-8.** Typhlitis on CT. **A,** Axial image in 36-year-old man with acute myelogenous leukemia reveals wall thickening involving dilated cecum (*short arrow*) and adjacent fat stranding (*arrowhead*). Note normal wall thickness of fluid-filled descending colon (*long arrow*). **B,** Axial image located more superiorly demonstrates that wall thickening also involves terminal ileum (*arrow*). **C,** Sagittal image at level of ascending colon shows that wall thickening extends from cecum to hepatic flexure (*arrows*). This distribution of wall thickening in setting of neutropenia is highly suggestive of typhlitis.

---

**Box 27-2.** Causes of Ischemic Colitis

**Arterial Occlusive Disease**

1. Thromboembolism
   i. Atrial fibrillation
   ii. Endocarditis
   iii. Other
2. Arterial stenosis
   i. Atherosclerosis
   ii. Vasculitis
   iii. Fibromuscular dysplasia
   iv. Other
3. Hypercoagulable states
   i. Antiphospholipid antibody syndrome
   ii. Protein C deficiency
   iii. Protein S deficiency
4. Invasive malignancy

**Venous Occlusive Disease**

1. Hypercoagulable states
2. Invasive malignancy
3. Extrinsic venous compression
   i. Bowel obstruction
   ii. Invasive malignancy

**Hypoperfusion**

1. Heart failure
2. Hemorrhagic or septic shock
3. Medications affecting blood pressure

(Adapted from Zafar HM, Miller Jr. WT. Imaging of the bowel. In: *Diagnostic abdominal imaging.* New York: McGraw Hill; 2013:15-160.)

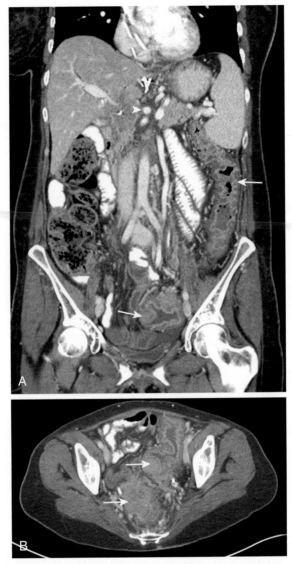

**Figure 27-9.** Ischemic colitis on CT. **A,** Coronal image in 45-year-old woman with metastatic ovarian cancer reveals segmental colonic wall thickening from descending colon to rectum (*arrows*) and normal wall thickness of more proximal colon. "Target" sign is also seen in descending colon and rectum. Note confluent soft tissue metastatic implant in porta hepatis that encases and occludes main portal vein (*arrowhead*). **B,** Axial image shows peritoneal implants in pelvis that invade sigmoid colon and proximal rectum (*arrows*). The distribution of colonic wall thickening in setting of portal vein encasement and metastatic disease favors ischemic colitis, thought to be secondary to inferior mesenteric vein congestion.

enhancement following administration of negative (water attenuation) oral contrast material as well as intravenous contrast material (Figure 27-9).

39. What causes colonic wall thickening in ischemic colitis?
   A combination of mural edema, congestion, hemorrhage, and/or superinfection of the ischemic bowel wall.

40. What generally causes more severe bowel wall thickening, arterial or venous occlusion?
   Venous occlusion.

41. Does the degree of bowel wall thickening correlate with the severity of ischemia?
   No.

42. What are other ancillary findings of ischemic bowel?
   Bowel dilation indicating disruption of normal peristalsis, and pneumatosis and portal venous gas indicating bowel wall necrosis.

43. What is the preferred imaging modality for evaluation of bowel ischemia?

CT with negative oral contrast material is the preferred imaging modality to evaluate the presence and distribution of bowel ischemia as well as potential underlying causes. Conventional angiography is useful in the diagnosis and treatment of occlusive vascular disease but is insensitive for the diagnosis of nonocclusive mesenteric ischemia.

44. What are the "watershed" regions of the colon?

The splenic flexure, which is at the junction of the superior and inferior mesenteric artery distributions, and the rectosigmoid colon, which is at the junction of the inferior mesenteric and sigmoid artery distributions. These areas are susceptible to hypoperfusion due to their location at the junctions of two vascular distributions.

45. What is the role of CT and MRI in the detection of early inflammatory bowel disease?

Early manifestations of Crohn's disease including enlarged lymphoid follicles, erosions, and aphthoid ulcers are only detectable on colonoscopy and conventional enteroclysis. CT and MRI can help identify and characterize abnormal bowel segments in advanced disease and identify extraluminal findings in order to guide treatment, including surgery when indicated (e.g., when there is bowel stenosis, perforation, or fistulas).

46. How are Crohn's disease and ulcerative colitis distinguished on cross-sectional imaging?

For the answer, see Table 27-5. Also see Figures 27-10, 27-11, and 27-12.

47. What percent of patients with Crohn's disease present with isolated colonic involvement?

20%.

48. What is the most common finding of inflammatory bowel disease on CT and MRI?

Bowel wall thickening, which is greater in Crohn's disease due to transmural involvement compared to ulcerative colitis, which is restricted to the mucosa.

49. What is the "comb" sign?

Engorgement of the pericolic or perienteric vessels which, when viewed en face, mimic the tines of a comb radiating away from the colon or small bowel (see Figures 27-11 and 27-12).

50. What are the MRI findings of active Crohn's disease?

Bowel wall thickening with increased T2-weighted signal intensity indicating acute edema (best appreciated on fat-suppressed images), ulcers characterized by linear, high signal intensity protrusions into the bowel wall (best appreciated on T2-weighted images), and mesenteric edema which is seen as increased T2-weighted signal intensity

**Table 27-5.** Comparison of Cross-sectional Imaging Features of Crohn's Disease and Ulcerative Colitis

| | CROHN'S DISEASE | ULCERATIVE COLITIS |
|---|---|---|
| Distribution | May involve any part of the gastrointestinal tract; most commonly affects small bowel, followed by colon, and less commonly esophagus, stomach, or duodenum | Involves colon starting at the rectum and moving proximally |
| Pattern of spread | Skip lesions | Continuous |
| Mean wall thickness | 12 mm | 8 mm |
| Wall morphology | Eccentric, segmental, sometimes with pseudosacculations | Diffuse, symmetric |
| Enhancement pattern | "Target" sign in active disease, "fat halo" sign in chronic disease | "Target" sign in active disease, "fat halo" sign in chronic disease |
| Terminal ileal involvement | 95% | 25% backwash ileitis in setting of pancolitis |
| Distribution of fibrofatty change | Mesenteric distribution | Perirectal distribution; associated with widening of the presacral space |
| Mesenteric lymphadenopathy | Yes | No |
| Complications | Fistulas, sinus tracts, and abscess formation (due to transmural extent of disease), stricture formation, colorectal cancer, lymphoma | Toxic megacolon, stricture formation, sclerosing cholangitis, colorectal cancer (higher risk than in Crohn's disease), lymphoma |

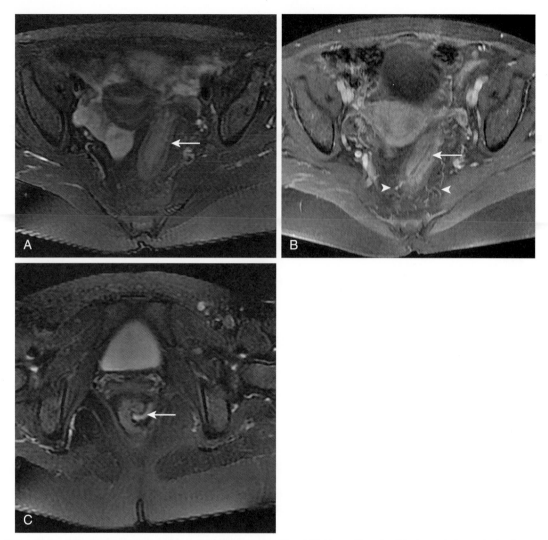

**Figure 27-10.** Active Crohn's disease on MRI. **A,** Axial fat-suppressed T2-weighted image through pelvis demonstrates marked wall thickening involving rectosigmoid colon (*arrow*) with increased signal intensity of mucosa and submucosa. **B,** Axial contrast-enhanced fat-suppressed T1-weighted image shows increased enhancement of mucosa and submucosa (*arrow*) in same colonic segment with mild fat stranding and engorgement of adjacent vessels (*arrowheads*). **C,** Axial fat-suppressed T2-weighted image through lower pelvis reveals high signal intensity anal fistula (*arrow*) arising from 3:00 position. Although involvement of distal colon may be seen in either Crohn's disease or UC, presence of perianal fistula is highly specific for Crohn's disease.

within the mesenteric fat. On diffusion-weighted images (DWI), restricted diffusion may be seen due to acute inflammatory cellular infiltration within the bowel wall. Additional findings in the bowel seen on both MRI and CT include mucosal fold thickening and hyperenhancement, the "target" sign, and the "comb" sign. The presence of fistulas, sinus tracts, and abscesses is helpful to suggest this diagnosis on either MRI or CT (see Figure 27-10). MRI is generally superior to CT for detection and delineation of perianal fistulas and sinus tracts, given its superior soft tissue contrast resolution.

51. What is the significance of the degree of bowel wall enhancement in inflammatory bowel disease?

Mural hyperenhancement is the most sensitive finding of active inflammatory bowel disease, best depicted following administration of negative oral contrast material along with intravenous contrast material on CT enterography (CTE) or magnetic resonance enterography (MRE). This results in accentuation of the "target" sign on contrast-enhanced images, as the inner ring of mucosa appears even more bright relative to the dark submucosal layer. Mild or no increased enhancement is present in the setting of chronic inflammatory bowel disease. For this reason, the degree of mural enhancement can be used to guide management.

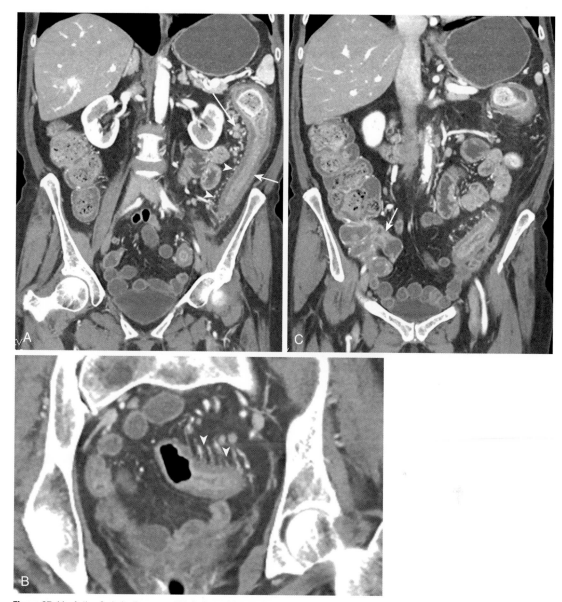

**Figure 27-11.** Active Crohn's disease on CT. **A,** Coronal image through abdomen and pelvis reveals segmental wall thickening of descending colon (*short arrow*) with "target" sign. There is associated engorgement of pericolic vessels (*arrowheads*) representing "comb" sign, as well as multiple adjacent enlarged mesenteric lymph nodes (*long arrow*). **B,** Small field-of-view coronal image at level of sigmoid colon better demonstrates "comb" sign whereby engorged pericolic vessels mimic tines of comb (*arrowheads*). **C,** Coronal image more anteriorly through abdomen and pelvis shows wall thickening of terminal ileum wall with luminal narrowing (*arrow*), in keeping with skip lesion. Note normal appearing adjacent ascending colon. These findings are highly suggestive of active Crohn's disease.

52. What is the significance of the "fat halo" sign?
    In the setting of known inflammatory bowel disease, the "fat halo" sign (Figure 27-13) indicates chronic disease characterized by fat deposition with the submucosa with relative hyperattenuation of the mucosa and muscularis propria or serosa on CT. On MRI, fat signal intensity is seen in the submucosa. This finding is present in up to 60% of patients with UC, but in only 8% of patients with Crohn's disease. Of note, this finding is nonspecific and can be seen in nondiseased individuals as well.

53. What is the best technique for the evaluation of colovesical fistula?
    CT imaging following the administration of oral contrast material without intravenous contrast material is the best way to evaluate for a colovesical fistula. This eliminates the possibility that positive contrast material seen in the bladder may be from urinary tract excretion of intravenous contrast material as opposed to oral contrast material from the

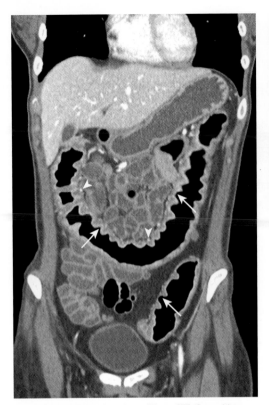

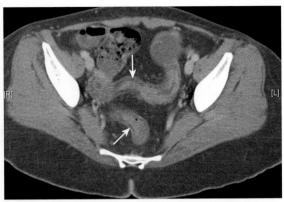

**Figure 27-13.** "Fat halo" sign on CT. Axial image through pelvis reveals fat attenuation within submucosa of thickened rectosigmoid colon indicating "fat halo" sign (*arrows*). There is also apparent increased amounts of visceral fat surrounding these bowel segments. These findings are suggestive of chronic inflammatory bowel disease, in this case chronic ulcerative colitis.

**Figure 27-12.** Active ulcerative colitis on CTE. Coronal image following administration of negative oral material and intravenous contrast material reveals continuous colonic wall thickening and associated "target" sign from rectum to transverse colon with irregularity of mucosa (*arrows*), outlined by nondependent gas. There is also dilation of subjacent pericolic vessels (*arrowheads*) indicating "comb" sign. Note normal wall thickness of small bowel loops.

bowel. The presence of gas in the bladder in the setting of active colonic inflammation and no history of recent instrumentation is highly specific for presence of a colovesical (or enterovesical) fistula.

54. Is colorectal cancer common?
    Colorectal cancer is the third most common cancer in the United States (after prostate cancer [in men], breast cancer [in women], and lung cancer). It is also the third leading cause of cancer death in the United States.

55. What proportion of patients with colorectal cancer have synchronous colonic cancers?
    5%.

56. What is the frequency of metastatic disease on initial presentation of colorectal cancer?
    Less than 15%.

57. What are the most common locations of metastases in colorectal cancer?
    The liver is the most common site because the portal vein receives the majority of colonic venous drainage. Other common sites include the lungs, adrenal glands, and osseous structures. The rectum has dual venous drainage into the portal venous system (via the superior hemorrhoidal vein) and into the systemic venous system (via the middle and inferior hemorrhoidal veins to the inferior vena cava). For this reason, rectal cancer has a predilection to lead to lung cancer metastases, sometimes without liver metastases.

58. What are the CT and MRI findings of colorectal cancer?
    Focal (<5 cm) colonic wall thickening or mass is seen, often moderate-marked in degree, irregular, and asymmetric, with soft tissue attenuation on CT images and increased T2-weighted signal intensity and restricted diffusion on MR images. There tends to be abrupt shouldering at the transition between normal and abnormal portions of colon. Minimal to no pericolic fat stranding or fluid is seen, which is more typically seen in colitis (Figure 27-14). In some patients, a polypoid intraluminal component may also be seen, and in other patients, extraluminal spread of soft tissue tumor into the surrounding fat or subjacent organs may be detected. Large bowel obstruction can occur when there is

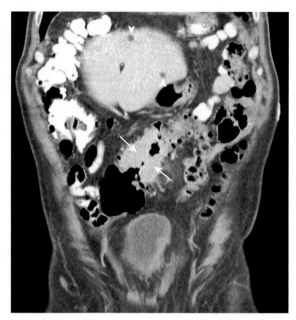

**Figure 27-14.** Colon adenocarcinoma on CT. Coronal image in 73-year-old man with weight loss and blood in stools reveals short segment of moderate-marked asymmetric wall thickening of sigmoid colon (*arrows*) with irregular walls and luminal narrowing. Note abrupt shouldering at transition site between involved and uninvolved colon with only minimal fat stranding of adjacent pericolic fat. These findings are pathognomonic for colon adenocarcinoma. Hypoattenuating lesions in liver (*arrowheads*) are due to cysts as characterized by subsequent MRI (*not shown*).

sufficient luminal narrowing. Adjacent pericolic lymph nodes may be present, which are assumed to represent regional nodal metastases until proven otherwise when they are ≥3 mm in size. Peritoneal spread of tumor as well as distant metastases may also be encountered.

59. What is the most sensitive imaging study to detect colorectal cancer in the setting of a negative routine CT study and rising carcinoembryonic antigen (CEA) levels?
$^{18}$F-fluorodeoxyglucose positron emission tomography/computed tomography (FDG PET/CT).

60. What is the frequency of primary colonic lymphoma?
0.4% of all colorectal malignancies.

61. What are the most common locations of colonic lymphoma?
The cecum and the rectum.

62. What are the cross-sectional imaging features that help to distinguish colorectal lymphoma from adenocarcinoma?
For the answer, see Table 27-6.

63. What is the most common site of extrapulmonary tuberculosis?
The abdomen.

64. What percentage of patients with gastrointestinal tuberculosis demonstrate no evidence of pulmonary tuberculosis?
Up to 25%.

65. What is the most common site of abdominal tuberculosis?
The ileocecal region, which is thought to reflect the higher proportion of lymphoid tissue in this location.

66. What are the findings of abdominal tuberculosis on CT and MRI?
Circumferential mural thickening of the cecum and terminal ileum are usually seen. Occasionally, there is asymmetric thickening of the medial wall of the cecum and ileocecal valve that extends into the adjacent tissues with resultant engulfment of the terminal ileum; a presentation that may mimic that of lymphoma. Abdominal lymphadenopathy, which is the most common manifestation of abdominal tuberculosis, is present in up to two thirds of patients. Typically, the abnormal lymph nodes demonstrate central hypoattenuation, central high T2-weighted signal intensity (relative to skeletal muscle), and central nonenhancement related to central necrosis, along with peripheral

**Table 27-6.** Comparison of Cross-sectional Imaging Features of Colorectal Lymphoma and Colorectal Adenocarcinoma

| | LYMPHOMA | ADENOCARCINOMA |
|---|---|---|
| Effect on adjacent soft tissues | General preservation of surrounding visceral fat | May be associated with invasion of adjacent visceral fat and other organs |
| Bowel obstruction | No | Yes |
| Bowel lumen | Aneurysmal dilation | Annular narrowing |
| Wall thickening | Mild, smooth, concentric | Severe, irregular, eccentric |
| Transition from normal to abnormal wall thickness | Gradual | Abrupt with shouldering |
| Length of affected segment | Segmental or focal | Focal (<5 cm) |
| Lymphadenopathy | Bulky mesenteric and/or retroperitoneal lymph nodes are common | Enlarged lymph nodes tend to be less bulky than in lymphoma, predominantly in pericolic or mesenteric locations |

hyperenhancement related to granulation tissue, inflammation, and hypervascularity. Despite their bulky appearance, these nodes seldom cause obstruction of the adjacent bowel or ureters. Peritoneal spread of infection may be encountered, as manifested by exudative ascites, peritoneal thickening, peritoneal enhancement, and omental/mesenteric soft tissue infiltration or caking. Nonspecific appearing lesions in abdominal solid organs may also be encountered.

67. What is familial adenomatous polyposis (FAP)?
    FAP is an autosomal dominant syndrome characterized by innumerable bowel polyps and other findings. Spontaneous genetic mutations occasionally result in this syndrome.

68. What is the most common location of the polyps in patients with FAP?
    Colon > stomach > duodenum > small bowel.

69. What are the major variants of FAP?
    Attenuated FAP, characterized by <100 adenomatous polyps in the colon and older age of diagnosis; familial polyposis coli, characterized by multiple enteric polyps; and Gardner's syndrome, characterized by a combination of enteric polyps, osteomas, soft tissue tumors (e.g., desmoid tumors, ampullary/duodenal tumors, and papillary thyroid cancers), and dental abnormalities.

70. What is the risk of colorectal cancer among patients with untreated FAP?
    Virtually 100% by approximately 35 years of age.

71. What is the treatment for FAP?
    Prophylactic total colectomy at about 20 years of age.

72. What is an appendiceal mucocele?
    Chronic cystic dilation of the appendiceal lumen by mucin accumulation.

73. What do appendiceal mucoceles correspond to on pathology?
    Focal or diffuse mucosal hyperplasia, mucinous cystadenoma, or mucinous cystadenocarcinoma.

74. What are the cross-sectional imaging findings of an appendiceal mucocele?
    On CT and MRI, appendiceal mucoceles present as well-defined cystic masses in the right lower quadrant with near water attenuation/signal intensity and curvilinear calcifications (seen only on CT) (Figure 27-15). The presence of thickened nodular walls, irregular serosal contours, or nodular enhancing components should raise suspicion for mucinous cystadenocarcinoma.

75. What is pseudomyxoma peritonei?
    Pseudomyxoma peritonei is a rare condition where mucinous ascites arises from rupture of a mucinous appendiceal adenoma. It has a strong association with synchronous or metachronous colorectal adenoma and carcinoma, such that surveillance of the entire large bowel is warranted.

76. What is the treatment for an appendiceal mucocele?
    Surgical resection.

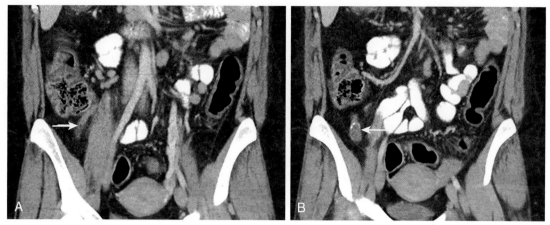

**Figure 27-15.** Appendiceal mucocele on CT. **A,** Coronal image through pelvis reveals normal caliber of proximal appendix (*arrow*). **B,** Coronal image more anteriorly through pelvis shows focal dilation of distal appendix (*arrow*) with luminal fluid attenuation and high attenuation mural calcification. These findings are highly suggestive of appendiceal mucocele.

## KEY POINTS

- CTC is comparable to OC in the detection of polyps ≥6 mm, the size cutoff for polyps reported on this imaging modality.
- CTC is not indicated for surveillance of patients at high risk for colorectal cancer, including patients with hereditary syndromes, and should not be performed the same day that a deep biopsy or polypectomy on OC is performed. CTC is also not appropriate among patients with acute colitis, recent surgery, symptomatic colon-containing abdominal wall hernia, and known or suspected bowel perforation or high-grade small bowel obstruction.
- All focal abnormalities detected on 3D evaluation of CTC must be correlated with 2D images using soft tissue windows.
- On CT, the "target" sign, also known as mural stratification, refers to visualization of a bright soft tissue attenuation inner layer (representing mucosa, lamina propria, and hypertrophied muscularis mucosae, sometimes with hyperemia), a dark low attenuation middle layer (representing edematous submucosa), and sometimes a bright soft tissue attenuation outer layer (representing muscularis propria and serosa); the alternating layers correspond to the rings of a target. This sign is not specific for a particular disease condition but is highly specific for diagnosis of nonneoplastic disease when encountered in the colon.
- The intensity of bowel wall enhancement in Crohn's disease relates to disease activity and can be used to guide patient management.

## BIBLIOGRAPHY

Yee J, Kim DH, Rosen MP, et al. ACR appropriateness criteria colorectal cancer screening. *J Am Coll Radiol.* 2014;11(6):543-551.

Zafar HM, Harhay MO, Yang J, et al. Adverse events following computed tomographic colonography compared to optical colonoscopy in the elderly. *Prev Med Rep.* 2014;1:3-8.

Zafar HM, Miller WT Jr. Imaging of the bowel. In: *Diagnostic abdominal imaging.* New York: McGraw Hill; 2013:15-160.

Zalis ME, Blake MA, Cai W, et al. Diagnostic accuracy of laxative-free computed tomographic colonography for detection of adenomatous polyps in asymptomatic adults: a prospective evaluation. *Ann Intern Med.* 2012;156(10):692-702.

Tolan DJ, Greenhalgh R, Zealley IA, et al. MR enterographic manifestations of small bowel Crohn disease. *Radiographics.* 2010;30(2): 367-384.

McFarland EG, Fletcher JG, Pickhardt P, et al. ACR Colon Cancer Committee white paper: status of CT colonography 2009. *J Am Coll Radiol.* 2009;6(11):756-772 e4.

Johnson CD, Chen MH, Toledano AY, et al. Accuracy of CT colonography for detection of large adenomas and cancers. *N Engl J Med.* 2008;359(12):1207-1217.

McFarland EG, Levin B, Lieberman DA, et al. Revised colorectal screening guidelines: joint effort of the American Cancer Society, U.S. Multisociety Task Force on Colorectal Cancer, and American College of Radiology. *Radiology.* 2008;248(3):717-720.

Ahualli J. The target sign: bowel wall. *Radiology.* 2005;234(2):549-550.

Pereira JM, Sirlin CB, Pinto PS, et al. Disproportionate fat stranding: a helpful CT sign in patients with acute abdominal pain. *Radiographics.* 2004;24(3):703-715.

Pickhardt PJ, Choi JR, Hwang I, et al. Computed tomographic virtual colonoscopy to screen for colorectal neoplasia in asymptomatic adults. *N Engl J Med.* 2003;349(23):2191-2200.

Pickhardt PJ, Levy AD, Rohrmann CA Jr, et al. Primary neoplasms of the appendix: radiologic spectrum of disease with pathologic correlation. *Radiographics.* 2003;23(3):645-662.

Horton KM, Corl FM, Fishman EK. CT evaluation of the colon: inflammatory disease. *Radiographics.* 2000;20(2):399-418.

# CHAPTER 28

# CT AND MRI OF THE LIVER, GALLBLADDER, AND BILIARY TRACT

*Anil Chauhan, MD, and Drew A. Torigian, MD, MA, FSAR*

1. **What are the common indications for computed tomography (CT) and magnetic resonance imaging (MRI) of the liver, gallbladder, and biliary tree?**
   The most common clinical indications include:
   - Characterization of indeterminate hepatic lesions detected on prior cross-sectional imaging.
   - Surveillance of cirrhotic patients for hepatocellular carcinoma (HCC).
   - Surveillance of patients with primary sclerosing cholangitis (PSC) for cholangiocarcinoma.
   - Staging and response assessment of patients with hepatobiliary malignancies.
   - Pretreatment and post-treatment evaluation of patients undergoing liver transplantation.
   - Evaluation of patients with abdominal symptoms or signs (e.g., right upper quadrant pain, abnormal liver function tests) that may be secondary to hepatobiliary disease.
   - Assessment for traumatic injury to liver, biliary tree, or gallbladder (mainly using CT).
   - Assessment for presence, location, and causes of biliary obstruction (mainly using MRI).
   - Diagnosis and response assessment in patients with primary (genetic) hemochromatosis (using MRI).
   - Providing guidance for percutaneous biopsy or intervention for hepatobiliary disease.

2. **What are the typical MRI sequences that are acquired for hepatobiliary imaging?**
   - Multiplanar heavily T2-weighted images (echo time [TE] 90 to 180 msec).
   - Axial in-phase and out-of-phase T1-weighted gradient recalled echo (GRE) images.
   - Axial fat-suppressed T2-weighted images.
   - Axial diffusion-weighted images (DWI) with apparent diffusion coefficient (ADC) parametric map images.
   - Coronal (and sometimes axial) very heavily T2-weighted magnetic resonance cholangiopancreatography (MRCP) images (TE >500 msec).
   - Axial pre- and postcontrast fat-suppressed T1-weighted images.

3. **What is magnetic resonance cholangiopancreatography (MRCP)?**
   MRCP is a noninvasive fluid-sensitive heavily T2-weighted sequence, which is primarily used to assess the biliary and pancreatic ductal systems. Fluid-containing structures (bile ducts, pancreatic duct, bowel, etc.) appear very high in signal intensity relative to a dark tissue background. MRCP can be displayed with a thin-section technique (2- to 5-mm thick slices) or a thick slab technique (projection images 20 to 60 mm in thickness shown in coronal and oblique coronal planes). Thick slab MRCP images are useful to quickly assess for the presence of biliary and pancreatic ductal dilation, whereas thin-section MRCP images are useful to assess for the presence and location of transition sites of ductal obstruction along with detection of abnormal internal contents within the ductal systems such as may be caused by calculi, debris, or tumors.

4. **What are hepatobiliary MRI contrast agents?**
   Hepatobiliary MRI contrast agents are in part taken up by functioning hepatocytes and excreted into the biliary system. Gadoxetate disodium (Eovist, Bayer HealthCare Pharmaceuticals Inc.) and gadobenate dimeglumine (Multihance, Bracco Diagnostics Inc.) are the two commonly used hepatobiliary MRI contrast agents used in clinical practice. Eovist has approximately 50% biliary excretion, while Multihance has 2% to 5% biliary excretion.
   The most common indications for use of hepatobiliary MRI contrast agents in clinical practice are to differentiate focal nodular hyperplasia (FNH) from hepatic adenoma, to characterize indeterminate hepatic lesions in patients with cirrhosis, and to assess for presence of bile leak.

5. **What is the normal appearance of the liver on CT and MRI?**
   The liver is the largest organ in the abdomen and has attenuation of 50 to 70 Hounsfield units (HU) on CT, which on average is about 10 HU greater than that of the spleen. On MRI, the liver has high T1-weighted signal intensity relative to spleen secondary to abundant intracellular protein and paramagnetic substances (Figure 28-1, *A*), whereas the liver has low T2-weighted signal intensity relative to spleen (Figure 28-1, *B*). The normal contour of the liver is smooth, and the liver parenchyma normally homogeneously enhances.
   Following the intravenous administration of contrast material, sequential phases of enhancement of the liver are seen as follows:
   - The early arterial (or hepatic arterial) phase of enhancement occurs ≈10 to 20 seconds after contrast administration, when arteries will enhance but portal and hepatic veins do not enhance. This phase is useful for delineation of arterial anatomy prior to therapeutic intervention.

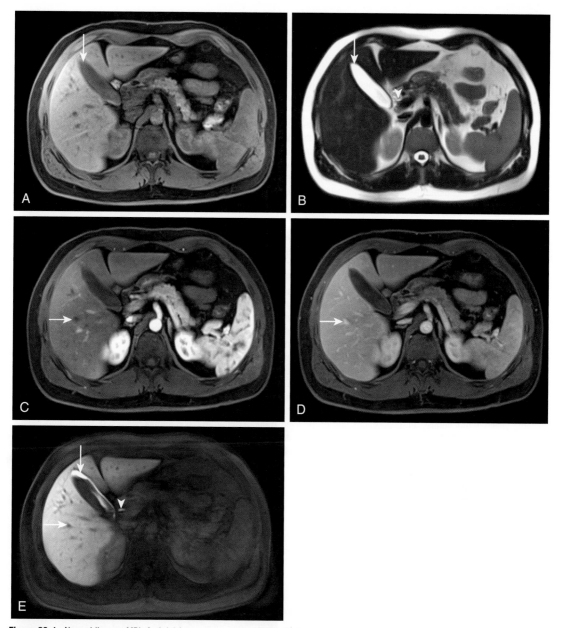

**Figure 28-1.** Normal liver on MRI. **A,** Axial fat-suppressed T1-weighted MR image through abdomen shows high signal intensity of liver relative to spleen. Note normal low signal intensity fluid within gallbladder (*arrow*). **B,** Axial heavily T2-weighted MR image through abdomen demonstrates low signal intensity of liver relative to spleen. Note normal very high signal intensity fluid within thin-walled gallbladder (*arrow*) and extrahepatic bile duct (*arrowhead*). **C,** Axial late arterial phase contrast-enhanced fat-suppressed T1-weighted MR image through abdomen shows enhancement of arteries and portal veins but lack of enhancement of hepatic veins (*arrow*). **D,** Axial venous phase contrast-enhanced fat-suppressed T1-weighted MR image through abdomen now demonstrates enhancement of liver parenchyma and portal veins as well as of hepatic veins (*arrow*). **E,** Axial hepatobiliary phase contrast-enhanced fat-suppressed T1-weighted MR image through abdomen shows persistent enhancement of liver parenchyma relative to skeletal muscle and excretion of contrast material into gallbladder (*long arrow*) and extrahepatic bile duct (*arrowhead*) but lack of enhancement of hepatic vessels including hepatic veins (*short arrow*).

- The late arterial (or portal inflow) phase of enhancement occurs ≈25 to 35 seconds after contrast administration, when arteries enhance and portal veins begin to enhance, but hepatic veins do not enhance. In this phase, the spleen has heterogeneous enhancement, the kidneys are usually in the corticomedullary phase of enhancement, and hypervascular lesions are seen to best effect (Figure 28-1, *C*).
- The hepatic venous (or portal venous or parenchymal) phase of enhancement occurs ≈50 to 90 seconds after contrast administration, when hepatic veins enhance. In this phase, the spleen has homogeneous enhancement, the kidneys may be in the corticomedullary or nephrographic phase of enhancement, the liver parenchyma

homogeneously enhances, hypovascular lesions are seen to best effect, and hypervascular lesions may have washout of enhancement relative to liver parenchyma (Figure 28-1, *D*).

- The delayed (or excretory or equilibrium) phase of enhancement occurs ≈>120 to 180 seconds after contrast administration, when liver parenchyma and vessels decrease in enhancement, while the renal collecting systems increasingly opacify with excreted intravenous contrast material. This phase is useful to more definitely characterize certain hepatic lesions, including hemangioma (which has persistent delayed phase enhancement), FNH (which has delayed phase central scar enhancement), and cholangiocarcinoma (which often has delayed phase enhancement of fibrous stroma).
- The hepatobiliary phase of enhancement is subsequently visualized on MRI if a hepatobiliary MRI contrast agent was intravenously administered, using T1-weighted MR images typically acquired >20 minutes after contrast administration. In this phase, the liver parenchyma homogeneously retains contrast material and appears hyperintense relative to skeletal muscle, the hepatic vessels appear hypointense relative to liver parenchyma, and the biliary tree, gallbladder, and renal collecting systems (given the ≈1:1 ratio of hepatobiliary:renal excretion of gadoxetate disodium) become opacified with excreted intravenous contrast material (Figure 28-1, *E*).

6. What is the normal segmental anatomy of the liver, and how are hepatic lobes and segments identified on cross-sectional imaging?

The liver is subdivided into right, left, and caudate lobes. The right hepatic lobe is further subdivided into anterior and posterior segments, and the left hepatic lobe is further subdivided into medial and lateral segments. Whereas the hepatic veins are located between segments of the liver (i.e., are intersegmental in location), the portal veins, hepatic arteries, and bile ducts are located within segments of the liver (i.e., are intrasegmental in location). Superiorly, the middle hepatic vein delineates the boundary between the left and right hepatic lobes, the right hepatic vein delineates the boundary between the anterior and posterior segments, and the left hepatic vein delineates the boundary between the medial and lateral segments. Inferiorly, the interlobar fissure, which is in the plane of the gallbladder fossa, delineates the boundary between the left and right hepatic lobes, and the fissure for the falciform ligament (or left intersegmental fissure) delineates the boundary between the medial and lateral segments.

The Bismuth-Couinaud system is often used to provide a segmental nomenclature for localizing focal hepatic lesions. In this system, vertically oriented planes along the right, middle, and left hepatic veins are maintained and further divided by a horizontal plane through the right and left portal veins to divide the liver into 9 "segments" comprised of the caudate lobe and 8 hepatic subsegments.

Segment I is the caudate lobe of the liver, which is located posterior to the fissure for the ligamentum venosum, and which is functionally an autonomous part of the liver. It has a separate blood supply, venous drainage, and biliary drainage. Segments II, IVa, VIII, and VII are the lateral, medial, anterior, and posterior segments of the liver, respectively, located above the plane of the portal vein. Segments III, IVb, V, and VI are the lateral, medial, anterior, and posterior segments of the liver, respectively, located below the plane of the portal vein (Figure 28-2).

7. What is the normal appearance of the biliary tree and gallbladder on cross-sectional imaging?

The intrahepatic bile ducts are normally ≤2 mm in caliber, and they coalesce to form segmental bile ducts. The segmental bile ducts then join to form the right and left hepatic ducts, which subsequently coalesce to form the extrahepatic bile duct.

The extrahepatic bile duct extends from the liver to the second portion of the duodenum within the hepatoduodenal ligament, anterior to the main portal vein and lateral to the hepatic artery. It is comprised of

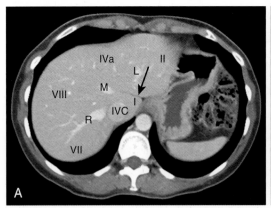
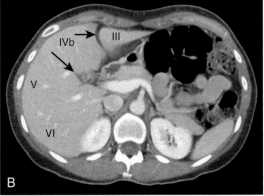

**Figure 28-2.** Normal segmental anatomy of liver on CT. **A,** Axial contrast-enhanced CT image through liver above plane of portal vein shows right (*R*), middle (*M*), and left (*L*) hepatic veins between hepatic segments that drain to inferior vena cava (*IVC*). Note fissure for ligamentum venosum (*arrow*) anterior to caudate lobe (*I*), as well as lateral (*II*), medial (*IVa*), anterior (*VIII*), and posterior (*VII*) segments. **B,** Axial contrast-enhanced CT image through liver below plane of portal vein shows left intersegmental fissure (*short arrow*) and interlobar fissure (*long arrow*), as well as lateral (*III*), medial (*IVb*), anterior (*V*), and posterior (*VI*) segments.

the more superiorly located common hepatic duct (CHD), which is normally ≤6 mm in caliber, and the more inferiorly located common bile duct (CBD), which is normally ≤8 mm in caliber (see Figure 28-1, *B*). The cystic duct, which communicates with the gallbladder, joins to the CHD to form the CBD. The CBD then joins inferiorly with the main pancreatic duct to form the ampulla of Vater, which then drains into the second portion of the duodenum via the major duodenal papilla.

Bile duct walls are normally thin and smooth, and no filling defects are normally seen in the biliary tree or gallbladder.

The gallbladder is ≈10 cm long and 3 to 5 cm in diameter and is located inferiorly to the liver along the interlobar fissure in the gallbladder fossa. The normal gallbladder wall thickness is ≤3 mm, and the surrounding visceral fat is normally homogeneous and similar in attenuation and signal intensity to fat elsewhere in the body (see Figure 28-1, *B*).

8. What are the common MR imaging features to determine if a focal hepatic lesion is hepatocellular or extrahepatocellular in origin?

Determination of the origin of a focal hepatic lesion as hepatocellular or extrahepatocellular is useful to establish a definitive diagnosis for the lesion. Commonly encountered lesions of hepatocellular origin include FNH, hepatic adenoma, focal hepatic steatosis, regenerative nodule, and HCC.

In general, lesions that are isointense to hyperintense in signal intensity relative to liver parenchyma on in-phase T1-weighted images are hepatocellular in origin, whereas lesions that are low in signal intensity relative to liver parenchyma are generally extrahepatocellular in origin. Presence of intralesional lipid content, as manifested by a loss of signal intensity within a hepatocellular origin hepatic lesion on out-of-phase T1-weighted images relative to in-phase T1-weighted images, is often seen in all of the hepatocellular origin hepatic lesions listed above except for FNH but is not seen in most extrahepatocellular origin hepatic lesions with the exception of lipid-containing hepatic metastases from clear cell renal cell carcinoma or adrenocortical carcinoma. Retention of hepatobiliary MRI contrast material within a lesion during the hepatobiliary phase of enhancement generally indicates presence of either focal hepatic steatosis, regenerative nodule, or FNH, whereas all other hepatic lesions appear hypointense relative to surrounding liver parenchyma during this phase of enhancement. Lesions with high T2-weighted signal intensity relative to liver but intermediate signal intensity relative to spleen tend to be due to a malignant neoplasm, whereas lesions with high T2-weighted signal intensity relative to both liver and spleen parenchyma are most often due to cysts or hemangiomas.

See Tables 28-1 and 28-2 below for summaries of the MRI features of hepatic lesions of hepatocellular and extrahepatocellular origin.

**Table 28-1.** MRI Features of Hepatic Lesions of Hepatocellular Origin

| LESION | T1-W | T2-W | HEAVILY T2-W | POSTCONTRAST T1-W | OTHER |
|---|---|---|---|---|---|
| Focal steatosis | = | = to ↑ | = | = on all phases | Often geographic in shape and in particular distribution, no mass effect upon vessels |
| FNH | =; ↓ of central scar | =; ↑ of central scar | = | ↑↑↑ on A phase; = on V, D, and HB phases; ↑ of central scar on D phase | Homogeneous enhancement, central scar, no lipid content |
| Hepatic adenoma | = to ↑; ↑↑ if hemorrhagic | = to ↑ | = | ↑↑ on A phase; = to ↓ on V and D phases; ↓ on HB phase | More heterogeneous, a/w oral contraceptive use |
| Regenerative nodule | = to ↑; ↓ if siderotic | = to ↓ | = | = on all phases | Small, multiple, in cirrhotic liver |
| HCC | = to ↓ | = to ↑ | = | ↑↑ on A phase; = to ↓ on V and D phases; ↓ on HB phase | More heterogeneous, often in cirrhotic liver, ± vascular invasion, ± metastatic disease |

Table legend: *T1-W* means T1-weighted; *T2-W* means T2-weighted; = means approximately isointense to liver parenchyma; ↑ means increased signal intensity relative to liver parenchyma; ↓ means decreased signal intensity relative to liver parenchyma; *A* means arterial; *V* means venous; *D* means delayed; *HB* means hepatobiliary; *a/w* means associated with.

**Table 28-2.** MRI Features of Hepatic Lesions of Extrahepatocellular Origin

| LESION | T1-W | T2-W | HEAVILY T2-W | POSTCONTRAST T1-W | OTHER |
|---|---|---|---|---|---|
| Cyst | ↓↓↓; ↓↓ to ↑↑ if proteinaceous or hemorrhagic | ↑↑↑; ↓↓ to ↑↑ if proteinaceous or hemorrhagic | ↑↑↑; ↓↓ to ↑↑ if proteinaceous or hemorrhagic | No or minimal thin rim enhancement | |
| Hemangioma | ↓ | ↑↑ | ↑↑ | Peripheral nodular discontinuous enhancement on A phase; centripetal fill-in on V phase; persistent enhancement on D phase | Sometimes flash-filling in A phase when small in size; often central cleftlike area of cystic degeneration or liquefaction when large in size |
| Hepatic metastasis | ↓ | ↑ | = to ↑ | Variable, may have continuous rim enhancement, ± "peripheral washout" sign in V or D phase | History of primary tumor often known, often heterogeneous, usually multiple, ± extrahepatic metastatic disease, no cirrhosis present |
| Abscess | ↓↓; ↓↓↓ if contains foci of gas | ↑↑↑; ↓↓↓ if contains foci of gas | ↑; ↓↓↓ if contains foci of gas | Rim and septal enhancement in A or V phase that persists in D phase, regional hyperenhancement | Often clustered, may be surrounded by edema |
| Intrahepatic cholangiocarcinoma | ↓ | ↑ | = to ↑ | Heterogeneous peripheral enhancement in A and V phases with gradual centripetal fill-in on D phase | Heterogeneous, ± biliary obstruction, ± capsular retraction, ± extrahepatic metastatic disease |
| Hepatic lymphoma | ↓ | ↑ | = to ↑ | Hypoenhancing on all phases | Homogeneous, usually multiple, often associated with lymphadenopathy |

Table legend: *T1-W* means T1-weighted; *T2-W* means T2-weighted; = means approximately isointense to liver parenchyma; ↑ means increased signal intensity relative to liver parenchyma; ↓ means decreased signal intensity relative to liver parenchyma; *A* means arterial; *V* means venous; *D* means delayed.

9. **What is the role of CT and MRI in hepatic transplantation?**

   CT and MRI play an important role in preoperative evaluation of liver transplant donors, as well as in pre- and postoperative evaluation of recipients of liver transplants.

   In potential liver donors, preoperative evaluation can be performed with three-phase dynamic contrast-enhanced CT or MRI (depending on particular institution) to delineate the hepatic arterial, portal venous, hepatic venous, and biliary anatomy (because anatomic variations are common) and to measure hepatic lobar volumes. This imaging evaluation is also performed to identify any incidental lesions in the abdomen of the donors, which may or may not need attention prior to surgery.

   In potential liver transplant recipients, preoperative evaluation is helpful to delineate the underlying hepatobiliary and vascular anatomy, to evaluate for preexisting hepatobiliary disease, and to stage underlying hepatic malignancy.

   Post-transplant evaluation in liver transplant recipients is primarily focused on vascular or biliary complications. Although ultrasonography (US) is often the initial imaging modality to evaluate these patients, CT and MRI are often used for problem-solving. Commonly encountered vascular complications following liver transplantation include thrombosis or stenosis of arteries or veins and arterial pseudo-aneurysm formation. Commonly encountered biliary complications following liver transplantation include biliary stenosis (most commonly at the anastomosis), bile duct strictures, biliary leak, biloma formation, choledocholithiasis, and bile duct necrosis. Other important complications include abdominal abscess, hematoma, recurrence of preexisting malignancy, recurrence of cirrhosis, transplant rejection, and post-transplant lymphoproliferative disorder (PTLD).

10. **What is FNH, and what are its CT and MR imaging features?**

    FNH is the most commonly encountered benign hepatic lesion of hepatocellular origin, and is more frequently seen in women. FNH, usually identified as an incidental lesion on CT and MRI, is a focal regenerative response of hepatocytes to an underlying hepatic vascular malformation, which also contains Kupffer cells.

    On MRI, FNH is typically isointense on T1-weighted images and T2-weighted images relative to liver parenchyma. On dynamic contrast-enhanced images, FNH shows intense homogeneous arterial phase enhancement, which becomes isointense to liver parenchyma on venous and delayed phase images. A central scar is often present, which has low T1-weighted and high T2-weighted signal intensity relative to liver parenchyma and does not enhance on arterial phase images, although delayed phase enhancement is typically seen. On hepatobiliary phase T1-weighted images, FNH retains hepatobiliary contrast material such that portions of the lesion will appear isointense or hyperintense to liver parenchyma (Figure 28-3).

    FNH is usually not identifiable on unenhanced CT images, and it has no associated calcifications. The enhancement pattern of FNH on CT is similar to that on MRI.

11. **What is hepatic adenoma, and what are its CT and MR imaging features?**

    Hepatic adenoma is the second most common benign lesion of hepatocellular origin, and it is most commonly encountered in young women, especially in those who are taking oral contraceptives. It may also be associated with anabolic corticosteroid use as well as type I glycogen storage (von Gierke's) disease. Hepatic adenoma, although a benign neoplasm, is often treated with surgical resection given the risk of hemorrhage, especially for lesions that are ≥3 to 4 cm and/or located in the subcapsular region of the liver. Hepatic adenomatosis is a specific rarer condition, which is defined by presence of more than 10 hepatic adenomas in the liver and which is associated with a small but increased risk of malignant transformation into HCC.

    On MRI, hepatic adenoma is isointense to hyperintense relative to liver parenchyma on T1-weighted images (Figure 28-4, *A*), often contains intralesional lipid (seen by loss of signal intensity on out-of-phase T1-weighted images relative to in-phase T1-weighted images), and is isointense to slightly hyperintense relative to liver parenchyma on T2-weighted images. When subacute hemorrhage is present, foci of very high T1-weighted signal intensity will be visualized. Following contrast administration, variably heterogeneous mild to moderate arterial phase enhancement is usually present (Figure 28-4, *B*), along with isointensity or hypointensity relative to liver parenchyma on venous and delayed phases of enhancement (Figure 28-4, *C*). On hepatobiliary phase T1-weighted images, hepatic adenoma will appear hypointense relative to liver parenchyma because it does not retain hepatobiliary contrast material (Figure 28-4, *D*).

    On CT, hepatic adenoma may have variable attenuation relative to liver parenchyma depending on lipid content and presence of hemorrhage, and it has similar enhancement characteristics to those described on MRI (Figure 28-4, *E*).

12. **How does one differentiate FNH from hepatic adenoma on cross-sectional imaging?**

    For the answer, see Table 28-3.

13. **How does one differentiate FNH from fibrolamellar hepatocellular carcinoma (HCC) on cross-sectional imaging?**

    Fibrolamellar HCC is a rare form of HCC that typically affects young adults and can mimic the imaging appearance of FNH. However, some cross-sectional imaging features that may be useful to help differentiate between them are as follows:

    - FNH is typically small in size (<5 cm) and homogeneous, whereas fibrolamellar HCC is typically large in size and heterogenous.
    - The central scar of FNH is hyperintense on T2-weighted images and noncalcified, whereas the central scar of fibrolamellar HCC is hypointense on T2-weighted images and sometimes calcified.

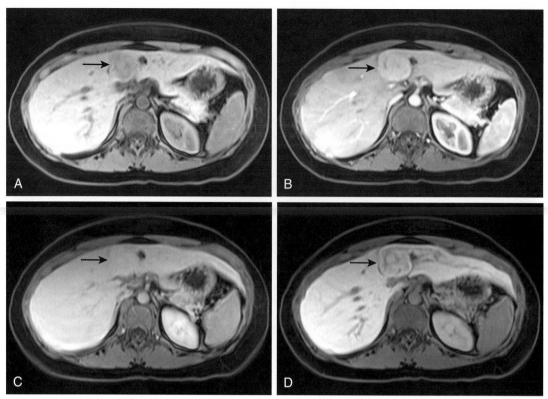

**Figure 28-3.** FNH on MRI. **A,** Axial fat-suppressed T1-weighted MR image through liver shows hepatic lesion (*arrow*) that is slightly hypointense-isointense in signal intensity relative to liver parenchyma. **B,** Axial arterial phase, **C,** Axial venous phase, and **D,** Axial hepatobiliary phase contrast-enhanced MR images through liver show that hepatic lesion (*arrow*) has intense homogeneous arterial phase enhancement, venous phase enhancement similar to liver parenchyma, and hepatobiliary phase retained enhancement similar to liver parenchyma.

**Table 28-3.** Imaging Features to Differentiate FNH and Hepatic Adenoma

| IMAGING FEATURE | FNH | HEPATIC ADENOMA |
|---|---|---|
| Associated with oral contraceptive use | – | +++ |
| Intralesional lipid content | – | +++ |
| Intralesional hemorrhage | – | +++ |
| Multifocality | + | +++ |
| Marked arterial phase enhancement | +++ | + |
| Presence of central scar | +++ | + |
| Retention of hepatobiliary contrast material | +++ | – |

14. **What are the two most commonly encountered benign hepatic lesions?**
    Hepatic cysts and hemangiomas are the two most common benign hepatic lesions, occurring in up to 20% of adults, more commonly in women.

15. **What are the CT and MR imaging features of a hepatic cyst?**
    A hepatic cyst is round or oval in shape and composed of simple fluid. Therefore, on CT, it will have fluid attenuation, and on MRI, it will have low signal intensity on T1-weighted images, very high signal intensity on T2-weighted images, and very high signal intensity on heavily T2-weighted images relative to liver parenchyma. It either has no enhancement or has minimal thin rim enhancement (Figure 28-5).

16. **What are the CT and MR imaging features of a hepatic hemangioma?**
    Hepatic hemangioma is the most common benign hepatic neoplasm, and it is composed of vascular channels and fibrous stroma. On CT, hepatic hemangioma appears as a well-defined lobulated low attenuation lesion. On MRI, it is

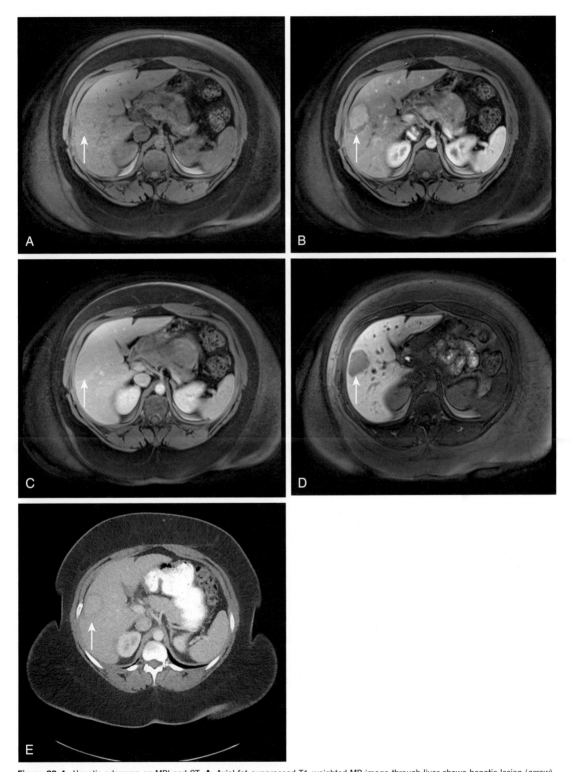

**Figure 28-4.** Hepatic adenoma on MRI and CT. **A,** Axial fat-suppressed T1-weighted MR image through liver shows hepatic lesion (*arrow*) that is slightly hypointense-isointense in signal intensity relative to liver parenchyma. **B,** Axial arterial phase, **C,** Axial venous phase, and **D,** Axial hepatobiliary phase contrast-enhanced MR images through liver show that hepatic lesion (*arrow*) has moderate heterogeneous arterial phase enhancement, mild venous phase washout relative to liver parenchyma, and hepatobiliary phase hypointense signal intensity relative to liver parenchyma. **E,** Axial arterial phase contrast-enhanced CT image through liver again reveals that hepatic lesion (*arrow*) has moderate heterogeneous arterial phase enhancement.

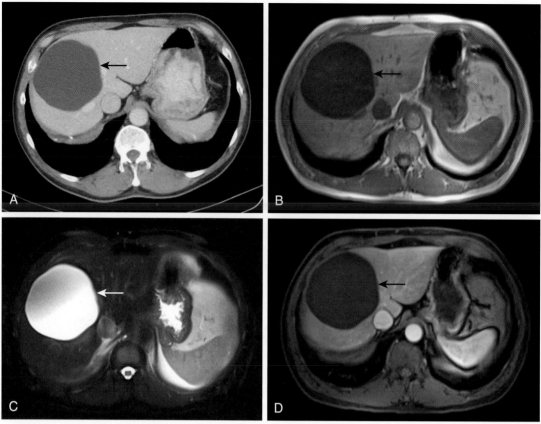

**Figure 28-5.** Hepatic cyst on CT and MRI. **A,** Axial venous phase contrast-enhanced CT image through liver shows hepatic lesion (*arrow*) with round shape, fluid attenuation, and no enhancement. **B,** Axial T1-weighted and **C,** Axial fat-suppressed T2-weighted MR images through liver demonstrate hepatic lesion (*arrow*) with low T1-weighted and very high T2-weighted signal intensity relative to liver parenchyma. **D,** Axial venous phase contrast-enhanced fat-suppressed T1-weighted MR image through liver again reveals that hepatic lesion (*arrow*) has no enhancement.

hypointense on T1-weighted images (Figure 28-6, *A*) and hyperintense on T2-weighted images relative to liver parenchyma. On heavily T2-weighted images, it remains hyperintense relative to liver parenchyma and spleen, although with signal intensity less than simple fluid (Figure 28-6, *B*).

Peripheral nodular discontinuous enhancement (following the enhancement of the aorta) with subsequent centripetal fill-in and persistent delayed phase enhancement is the characteristic enhancement pattern of hepatic hemangioma, and it is pathognomonic of this diagnosis (Figures 28-6, *C*, through 28-6, *E*). Small hemangiomas (<1.5 cm) may sometimes demonstrate homogeneous arterial phase ("flash filling") enhancement, potentially mimicking hypervascular hepatic malignancies. However, hemangiomas will have persistent hyperenhancement in the venous and delayed phases of enhancement relative to liver parenchyma, whereas malignant lesions will tend to become isoenhancing or hypoenhancing relative to liver parenchyma in the venous or delayed phases of enhancement. Large hemangiomas (>4 to 5 cm) almost always have a central cleft-like area of cystic degeneration or liquefaction that has low attenuation, low T1-weighted signal intensity, and very high T2-weighted signal intensity, without enhancement.

17. What is nonalcoholic fatty liver disease (NAFLD), and what is nonalcoholic steatohepatitis (NASH)?

NAFLD is secondary to excessive lipid accumulation in the hepatocytes (i.e., steatosis), where other etiologies including alcoholism have been excluded. NAFLD is rising in incidence at an alarming rate in the United States and is currently thought to affect 20% to 30% of patients in the general population and 85% to 90% of patients undergoing evaluation for weight-reduction surgeries. It is the most common cause of chronic liver disease in the United States. Obesity, diabetes mellitus, and hyperlipidemia are known risk factors. NAFLD has been long considered the hepatic manifestation of metabolic syndrome. Patients with uncomplicated NAFLD are usually asymptomatic, although some patients may have right upper quadrant pain or abnormal liver function tests.

NAFLD can progress to NASH in approximately 10% of patients, which is a histologic diagnosis based on steatosis and inflammation along with variable amounts of fibrosis. NASH, which can be reversible in early stages by

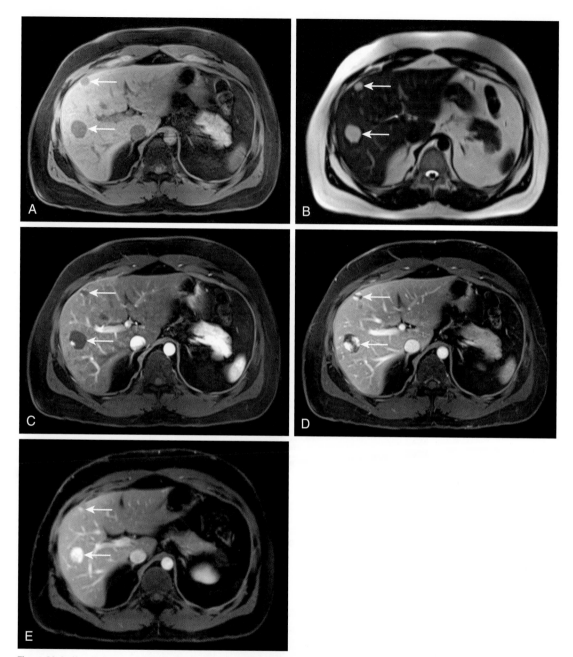

**Figure 28-6.** Hepatic hemangiomas on MRI. **A,** Axial fat-suppressed T1-weighted and **B,** Axial heavily T2-weighted MR images through liver demonstrate hepatic lesions (*arrows*) with low T1-weighted and very high T2-weighted signal intensity relative to liver parenchyma. **C,** Axial arterial phase, **D,** Axial venous phase, and **E,** Axial delayed phase contrast-enhanced MR images through liver show that hepatic lesions (*arrows*) have peripheral nodular discontinuous enhancement with subsequent centripetal fill-in and persistent delayed phase enhancement.

dietary modification, exercise, and/or weight-reduction surgeries, is the leading cause of cryptogenic cirrhosis (occurring in up to one third of patients).

18. What are the CT and MR imaging features of hepatic steatosis?

Hepatic steatosis is most commonly diffuse but may alternatively be focal, multifocal, subcapsular, or perivascular in distribution. When focal or multifocal, geographic shapes with linear, angulated, or interdigitated margins are typically encountered, characteristically without mass effect upon hepatic vessels.

On CT, areas of hepatic steatosis have decreased attenuation in the liver relative to the spleen by at least 10 HU on unenhanced CT images or by at least 25 HU on contrast-enhanced CT images (Figure 28-7). Hepatic attenuation of <40 HU is also suggestive. However, CT is less sensitive than MRI for detection of hepatic steatosis.

On MRI, hepatic steatosis is confirmed when there is loss of signal intensity on out-of-phase T1-weighted images relative to in-phase T1-weighted images.

19. **What does hepatic iron deposition look like on CT and MRI, and what are its major causes?**
Iron deposition leads to diffusely increased hepatic attenuation >75 HU on CT and decreased T1-weighted and T2-weighted signal intensity of the liver on MRI, which is particularly accentuated on in-phase T1-weighted MR images.

In primary (genetic) hemochromatosis, an autosomal recessive condition, there is increased iron overload related to abnormally increased iron absorption through the duodenum and jejunum. As a result, iron is primarily deposited in the liver parenchyma, and to a lesser extent in the pancreas, myocardium, joints, endocrine glands, and skin, leading to organ damage (Figure 28-8). Iron deposition in the spleen and bone marrow is not seen. Cirrhosis occurs in one third of patients, and patients have an approximately 200-fold increased risk of HCC.

In secondary hemosiderosis, there is iron accumulation in the reticuloendothelial system, namely the liver, spleen, and bone marrow, secondary to either high dietary iron intake or chronic anemia with repeated blood transfusions (Figure 28-9). However, organ function is usually preserved.

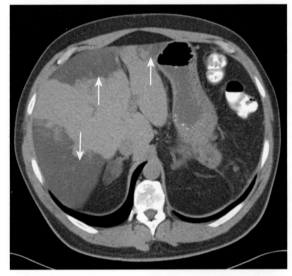

**Figure 28-7.** Multifocal hepatic steatosis on CT. Note multiple geographic regions of low attenuation in liver with linear, angulated, or interdigitated margins (*arrows*).

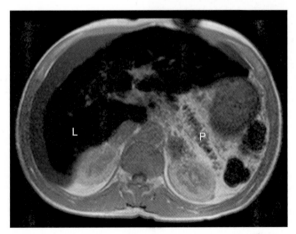

**Figure 28-8.** Primary (genetic) hemochromatosis on MRI. Note diffusely decreased signal intensity of liver (*L*) along with diffusely decreased signal intensity of pancreas (*P*). These findings are secondary to parenchymal iron deposition.

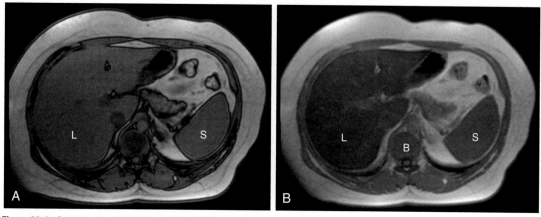

**Figure 28-9.** Secondary hemosiderosis on MRI. **A,** Axial out-of-phase and **B,** Axial in-phase T1-weighted MR images through liver demonstrate diffuse loss of signal intensity of liver (*L*) and spleen (*S*) on in-phase images relative to out-of-phase images. Also note diffusely low signal intensity of bone marrow (*B*) on in-phase images. These findings are secondary to iron deposition in reticuloendothelial system.

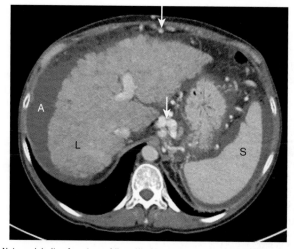

**Figure 28-10.** Cirrhosis on CT. Note nodularity of contour of liver (*L*). Also note enlargement of spleen (*S*), varices (*arrows*), and ascites (*A*) indicating portal hypertension.

20. What are the hepatic and extrahepatic imaging features of cirrhosis?

Cirrhosis is histologically defined by presence of disorganized liver parenchymal architecture with areas of fibrosis and regenerative nodules. It is a major cause of death in the United States, where it is most often related to viral hepatitis (secondary to Hepatitis C virus [HCV] more commonly than Hepatitis B virus [HBV]), alcohol abuse, and cryptogenic causes (commonly related to NAFLD).

On CT and MRI, the morphologic changes of cirrhosis include enlargement or diminution of hepatic size, hepatic surface nodularity, hypertrophy of the lateral segment and caudate lobe, atrophy of the medial segment and right hepatic lobe (sometimes leading to enlargement of the pericholecystic space, also called the "expanded gallbladder fossa" sign), prominence of the hepatic fissures, and the "right posterior hepatic notch" sign, which manifests as a sharp indentation or notch along the right posterior hepatic contour (Figure 28-10). Hepatic steatosis, regenerative nodules, and hepatic fibrosis can also be seen.

Regenerative nodules generally appear similar to normal hepatic parenchyma, and on MRI, they typically appear isointense to hyperintense relative to liver parenchyma on T1-weighted images, often contain intralesional lipid, and are isointense to hypointense relative to liver parenchyma on T2-weighted images. Regenerative nodules can sometimes contain iron, called siderotic regenerative nodules, and instead have low signal intensity on in-phase T1-weighted images. No arterial phase enhancement is seen, but mild venous and delayed enhancement is usually present.

Hepatic fibrosis generally occurs in a diffuse lacelike pattern in the liver between regenerative nodules, is hypointense on T1-weighted images and mildly hyperintense relative to liver parenchyma on T2-weighted images, and demonstrates delayed phase enhancement. Sometimes, more geographic conglomerate regions of confluent hepatic fibrosis may also be encountered with similar signal intensity and enhancement characteristics, sometimes adjacent to areas of capsular retraction.

Extrahepatic findings of cirrhosis pertain to the presence and severity of portal hypertension and include ascites, splenomegaly, portosystemic varices, gallbladder wall thickening with submucosal edema, bowel wall thickening with submucosal edema, and subcutaneous or visceral fat edema. Reactively enlarged periportal and portacaval lymph nodes may also be seen.

21. What is HCC, and what are its CT and MR imaging features?

HCC is the most common primary malignant tumor of the liver, is more commonly seen in men than in women, usually in patients who are >50 years of age in the Western hemisphere, and typically occurs in the setting of chronic liver damage, most often related to chronic hepatitis or cirrhosis. It is solitary in 50%, multifocal in 40%, and diffuse in 10% of cases and may sometimes be associated with direct extrahepatic extension, regional lymphadenopathy, or distant metastatic disease.

Regenerative changes in the liver in response to liver damage lead to formation of regenerative nodules. With time, a regenerative nodule can progress to a dysplastic nodule, and then potentially to HCC. HCC predominantly receives hepatic arterial blood supply, whereas a regenerative nodule predominantly receives portal venous blood supply, accounting for differences in their enhancement patterns observed on cross-sectional imaging.

The classic enhancement pattern of HCC on both CT and MRI often includes heterogeneous arterial phase enhancement, venous phase washout (i.e., low attenuation or low signal intensity relative to liver parenchyma), presence of an enhancing pseudocapsule (representing a peripheral rim of compressed hepatic parenchyma) on delayed phase images, and hypointense signal intensity relative to liver parenchyma on hepatobiliary phase images given the lack of retention of hepatobiliary contrast material. On MRI, high T2-weighted signal intensity relative to liver parenchyma (but similar to spleen) and restricted diffusion are additional highly suggestive findings for presence of HCC, especially when encountered within a cirrhotic liver (Figure 28-11).

Note that although similar imaging features may be seen with metastases to the liver, metastatic disease to a cirrhotic liver is extremely rare. Therefore, when lesions with suspicious imaging features are seen in a cirrhotic liver, they are assumed to be caused by HCC until proven otherwise, even in patients with known extrahepatic cancer.

Small arterial phase enhancing foci in a cirrhotic liver may sometimes be secondary to arterioportal venous shunts and/or altered hepatic blood flow dynamics. However, these changes are not visualized during other phases of contrast enhancement or on precontrast images. On follow-up cross-sectional imaging, these will generally resolve, decrease in size, or remain stable, whereas HCC tends to grow over time.

Tumor thrombus within the portal or hepatic veins is an additional imaging manifestation of HCC. Compared to bland thrombus, tumor thrombus can be suggested by the presence of high T2-weighted signal intensity and restricted diffusion, enhancement, venous luminal expansion, or presence of contiguous adjacent HCC.

22. What are the Milan criteria?

The Milan criteria are used in patients with HCC to determine which patients may receive a liver transplant and have a good clinical outcome. The criteria are as follows:
- Solitary HCC ≤5 cm in size.
- ≤3 HCCs, each ≤3 cm in size.
- No hepatic vascular invasion by tumor.
- No presence of metastatic disease.

23. What are the CT and MR imaging features of hepatic metastatic disease?

Hepatic metastasis is the most common malignant tumor of the liver and is about 20 times more common than HCC. It is more commonly seen in men than in women, usually in those who are >50 years of age.

Metastatic disease is suspected when an enhancing hepatic lesion is seen in a patient with a history of primary malignancy (unless cirrhosis is present, in which case HCC is more likely). In general, the liver is the second most common site of metastatic disease in the body (lymph nodes are the most common site). A hepatic metastasis can be hypervascular or hypovascular, depending on the nature of the primary tumor. The suspicion for metastatic disease is greater when lesions are multifocal, are heterogeneous but with similar enhancement patterns, have ill-defined margins, invade vascular structures, obstruct the biliary tree, grow over time, or are associated with direct perihepatic extension, regional lymphadenopathy, or extrahepatic metastatic disease.

On CT, hepatic metastases will vary in their attenuation and enhancement properties depending on their tissue composition and are often heterogeneous in appearance. Low attenuation components relative to liver parenchyma may be present secondary to presence of mucinous, myxoid, cystic, or necrotic tissue components (generally best visualized on venous phase images). Higher attenuation components relative to liver parenchyma may also be present secondary to hyperenhancing soft tissue components (generally best visualized on arterial phase images), calcification, hemorrhage, or increased tissue cellularity.

On MRI, hepatic metastases will similarly vary in signal intensity and enhancement properties depending on their tissue composition, and again are often heterogeneous. However, isointense T2-weighted signal intensity relative to spleen and restricted diffusion are additional highly suggestive findings that add specificity for the presence of metastatic disease.

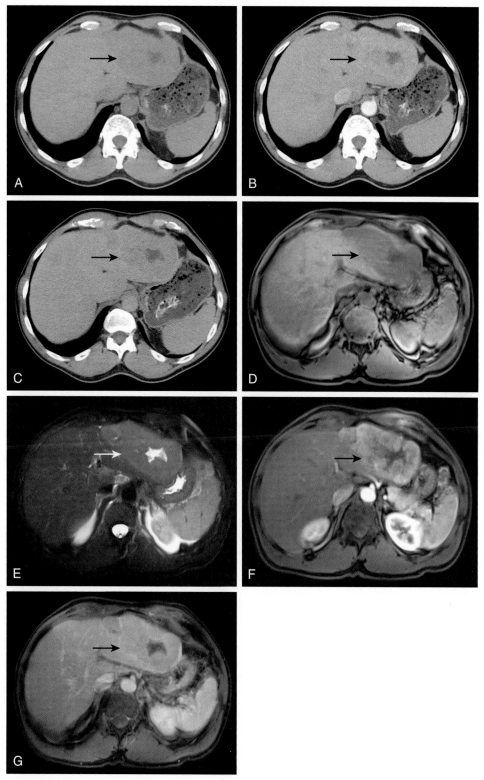

**Figure 28-11.** HCC on CT and MRI. **A,** Axial unenhanced, **B,** Axial arterial phase contrast-enhanced, and **C,** Axial venous phase contrast-enhanced CT images through liver show heterogeneous attenuation mass (*arrow*) in left hepatic lobe that has heterogeneous arterial phase enhancement and venous phase washout relative to liver parenchyma. **D,** Axial fat-suppressed T1-weighted and **E,** Axial fat-suppressed T2-weighted MR images through liver demonstrate that hepatic mass (*arrow*) has heterogeneously low-intermediate T1-weighted and heterogeneously high T2-weighted signal intensity relative to liver parenchyma (but with T2-weighted signal intensity predominantly similar to spleen). **F,** Axial arterial phase and **G,** Axial delayed phase postcontrast fat-suppressed T1-weighted MR images through liver again reveal that hepatic mass (*arrow*) has heterogeneous arterial phase enhancement and delayed phase washout relative to liver parenchyma. Also note delayed phase peripheral rim of enhancement representing pseudocapsule (composed of compressed hepatic parenchyma).

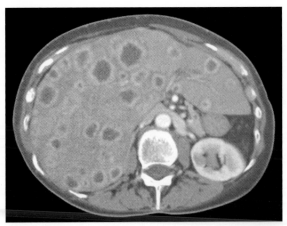

**Figure 28-12.** Hepatic metastases secondary to breast cancer on CT. Note multiple masses throughout liver with peripheral continuous rim enhancement, many of which have central low attenuation secondary to cystic or necrotic change.

Peripheral continuous rim enhancement is classically seen in hepatic metastases (Figure 28-12) and should not be confused with the peripheral nodular discontinuous enhancement pattern of hepatic hemangiomas. However, the enhancement pattern of hepatic metastases can be variable, ranging from minimal to marked, as well as from homogeneous to heterogeneous. A "peripheral washout" sign may sometimes be seen on delayed phase images. It manifests as a peripheral rim of decreased enhancement relative to the lesion center and is more commonly present in hypervascular metastases. Hypointense signal intensity relative to liver parenchyma is also typically encountered on hepatobiliary phase images given the lack of retention of hepatobiliary contrast material.

24. List the types of malignant tumors that most commonly lead to hyperenhancing hepatic lesions on arterial phase postcontrast CT or MR images.
    - HCC.
    - Renal cell carcinoma (RCC).
    - Thyroid cancer.
    - Breast cancer.
    - Neuroendocrine tumors (carcinoid tumor, pheochromocytoma, paraganglioma, islet cell tumor).
    - Choriocarcinoma.
    - Melanoma.

25. What are the CT and MR imaging features of a hepatic pyogenic abscess?
    A hepatic pyogenic abscess may arise from biliary tree infection, from direct spread of infection in adjacent organs, from hematogenous infection, following traumatic injury, or with superinfection of a preexisting hepatic hematoma or necrotic tumor. It is most often caused by gram negative bacilli, most commonly *Escherichia coli* in adults.
    On CT and MRI, a heterogeneous multiloculated cystic lesion is seen, more frequently in the right than left hepatic lobe, commonly with thick rim enhancement and internal septal enhancement, perilesional edema, and perilesional enhancement, and occasionally with internal foci of very low attenuation or very low signal intensity gas that are highly specific for this diagnosis. A "cluster" sign is a characteristic finding, where multiple lesions are clustered in the same region of the liver (Figure 28-13).

26. What CT imaging findings may be encountered in hepatic trauma?
    The liver is the most commonly injured solid organ in penetrating trauma, and the second most commonly injured solid organ in blunt trauma (following the spleen). The right hepatic lobe is more commonly involved by traumatic injury than the left hepatic lobe. CT is the mainstay of imaging evaluation of patients for potential hepatic trauma. Currently, the most widely used CT grading system for hepatic injury is based on the American Association for the Surgery of Trauma (AAST) scale. The spectrum of hepatic injuries includes contusion, hematoma, laceration, avulsion, infarction, active hemorrhage, and vascular injuries including hepatic arterial pseudoaneurysm and juxtahepatic (hepatic vein, portal vein, or inferior vena cava) venous injuries. Patients with higher grade injuries (IV to VI) are more likely to be unstable and in need of surgical or percutaneous vascular intervention.
    Hepatic hematomas appear as foci of nonenhancing high attenuation (30 to 70 HU) hemorrhagic fluid on CT, either subcapsular or intraparenchymal in location. When active hemorrhage is present, one sees focal areas of increased attenuation on contrast-enhanced images similar to that of enhancing vessels that do not conform to known vascular structures and that persist or increase in size on more delayed phase acquisitions (Figure 28-14). Hepatic arterial pseudoaneurysms also appear as well-circumscribed foci of contrast enhancement with attenuation similar to adjacent contrast-enhanced arteries but decrease in attenuation on more delayed phase acquisitions.

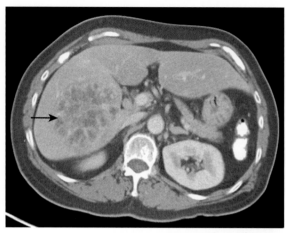

**Figure 28-13.** Hepatic pyogenic abscess on CT. Note heterogeneous multiloculated cystic lesion (*arrow*) in right hepatic lobe with "cluster" sign (caused by clustering of multiple lesions in same region of liver), thick rim enhancement, and internal septal enhancement.

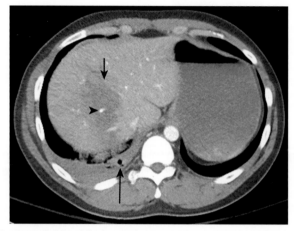

**Figure 28-14.** Hepatic penetrating traumatic injury following gunshot wound injury on CT. Note linear irregular nonenhancing low attenuation region in right hepatic dome (*short arrow*) representing hepatic laceration filled with high attenuation hemorrhagic fluid. Also note focal area of increased attenuation (*arrowhead*) within laceration similar to attenuation of enhancing vessels which does not conform to known vascular structures indicating active hemorrhage. Small right hemopneumothorax (*long arrow*) is also seen. Patient was subsequently treated with percutaneous coil embolization of bleeding hepatic arterial pseudoaneurysm (*not shown*).

Hepatic contusions appear as focal or more diffuse areas of hypoattenuation within the liver, although they may sometimes be isoattenuating relative to surrounding liver parenchyma or hyperattenuating when there is associated hemorrhage.

Hepatic lacerations appear as linear, irregular, or branching nonenhancing low attenuation parenchymal defects in the liver, often paralleling intrahepatic venous structures, and often with adjacent areas of high attenuation hemorrhage (see Figure 28-14). When severe, portions of hepatic parenchyma may even avulse from the remainder of the liver.

Hepatic infarcts appear as peripheral, often wedge-shaped, areas of nonenhancement in the hepatic parenchyma.

27. What is cholelithiasis, and what is choledocholithiasis?

Cholelithiasis is the presence of calculi in the gallbladder and is common, occurring in up to 15% of men and in up to 40% of women >60 years of age. It is secondary to cholesterol calculi in 70% and bile pigment calculi in 30%.

Choledocholithiasis is the presence of calculi in the biliary tree and is the most common cause of bile duct obstruction. It is seen in ≈15% of patients with cholelithiasis, although calculi can also form de novo within the biliary system.

28. What are the CT and MR imaging features of gallbladder and biliary tree calculi?

Calculi appear as nonenhancing round, oval, or polygonal filling defects in the gallbladder or biliary tree and are usually mobile and seen to be layering along the dependent luminal surface.

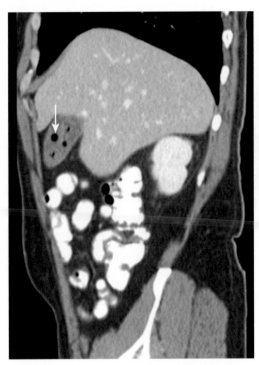

**Figure 28-15.** Cholelithiasis on CT. Sagittal contrast-enhanced CT image through abdomen shows multiple very low attenuation foci (*arrow*) within gallbladder representing nitrogen gas–containing gallstones.

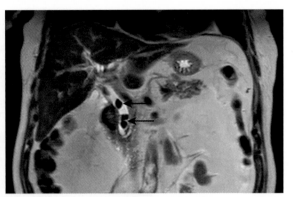

**Figure 28-16.** Choledocholithiasis on MRI. Coronal heavily T2-weighted image through abdomen shows multiple polygonal low signal intensity filling defects (*arrows*) within extrahepatic bile duct secondary to calculi.

On CT, calculi may sometimes have attenuation similar to bile, in which case they are not visible. This accounts for the suboptimal sensitivity of CT (≈75% to 80%) for the detection of calculi in the gallbladder and biliary tree. In other cases, they may either have low attenuation (related to cholesterol content) or high attenuation (related to calcium content) components relative to bile and are then visible. Occasionally, very low attenuation stellate foci of nitrogen gas may be seen within central fissures of the calculi, leading to the "Mercedes Benz" sign (Figure 28-15).

On MRI, calculi have low signal intensity on T2-weighted images relative to surrounding high signal intensity bile and may either have low T1-weighted signal intensity relative to bile when composed of cholesterol or high T1-weighted signal intensity relative to bile when composed of biliary pigments (Figure 28-16). The sensitivity of MRI for detection of calculi in the gallbladder and biliary tree is >95%. Associated upstream bile duct dilation may be visualized when there is biliary obstruction.

Please note that complications of calculi including acute cholecystitis, acute cholangitis, and acute pancreatitis will be discussed in chapter 32 on the acute abdomen and pelvis.

29. **What is primary sclerosing cholangitis (PSC), and what are its CT and MR imaging features?**
    PSC is a chronic idiopathic fibroinflammatory biliary disease that is typically seen in young adults, more commonly in men than in women, and is associated with ulcerative colitis in up to 70% of patients. It can lead to cirrhosis and is associated with an increased risk of cholangiocarcinoma.
    On CT and MRI, multifocal segmental areas of bile duct dilation and stenosis are typically seen, leading to a beaded appearance of the biliary tree (Figure 28-17). Pruning of the peripheral intrahepatic bile ducts and intraductal calculi may also be encountered. Bile duct wall thickening and increased enhancement are often seen, sometimes with surrounding edema or patchy increased enhancement in the surrounding liver parenchyma. Cirrhosis, characteristically with atrophy of the lateral and posterior segments, and reactively enlarged periportal and portacaval lymph nodes can also be visualized.

30. **Describe the classification and cross-sectional imaging features of choledochal cysts.**
    Choledochal cysts are congenital cystic dilations of the bile ducts, with the vast majority presenting in childhood, more commonly seen in women than in men. These are divided into 5 subtypes as per the Todani Classification. Table 28-4 details the classification and imaging findings. It is important to recognize, and potentially surgically resect, choledochal cysts, given the increased risk of recurrent ascending cholangitis, calculus formation, and cholangiocarcinoma. In types I through V, focal or multifocal dilation of the bile ducts is seen, sometimes with presence of intraductal calculi. In type V, the "central dot" sign may also be encountered, which appears within the liver as an enhancing portal venous radicle surrounded by dilated bile duct radicles.

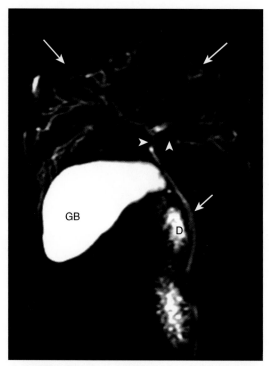

**Figure 28-17.** PSC on MRI. Oblique coronal MRCP image through abdomen demonstrates multifocal segmental areas of perihilar bile duct stenosis (*arrowheads*) leading to beaded appearance of biliary tree, with associated peripheral upstream intrahepatic bile duct dilation (*long arrows*). Note normal CBD (*short arrow*), gallbladder (*GB*), and second portion of duodenum (*D*).

**Table 28-4.** Todani Classification of Choledochal Cysts

| TYPE | DESCRIPTION | OTHER |
|---|---|---|
| I(a-c) | Diffuse or segmental fusiform dilation of extrahepatic bile duct | Most common type (80% to 90%) |
| II | Saccular bile duct diverticulum | Rare type (2%) |
| III | Focal dilation of intramural segment of distal CBD in 2nd portion of duodenum | Also known as a choledochocele, uncommon type (5%) |
| IVa | Multifocal dilation of intrahepatic and extrahepatic bile ducts | Second most common type (10%) |
| IVb | Multifocal dilation of extrahepatic bile ducts | |
| V | Multifocal dilation of intrahepatic bile ducts | Also known as Caroli's disease, rare type; may be associated with congenital hepatic fibrosis, medullary sponge kidney, and cystic renal disease |

31. What is the cross-sectional imaging appearance and clinical significance of a gallbladder polyp?

    A gallbladder polyp is usually an incidental finding on imaging and is usually benign in nature. On CT and MRI, a gallbladder polyp appears as an intraluminal enhancing lesion that is attached to the gallbladder wall. It is generally considered as benign if less than 5 mm in size, and it can be followed up with US, CT, or MRI when 5 to 10 mm. Surgical consultation can be obtained when a polyp exceeds 10 mm in size, increases in size over time, or is symptomatic, because there is increased likelihood of developing malignancy in such scenarios. Extra caution is taken in patients with a history of primary malignancy (especially in patients with melanoma or breast cancer), as metastatic disease to the gallbladder is also possible.

32. What is gallbladder carcinoma, and what are its CT and MR imaging features?

    Gallbladder carcinoma, most often due to adenocarcinoma, is the most common primary malignancy of the biliary system, is more common in women than in men, and usually occurs in patients who are >50 years of age. It is associated with a poor clinical prognosis because it often presents in an advanced stage of disease.

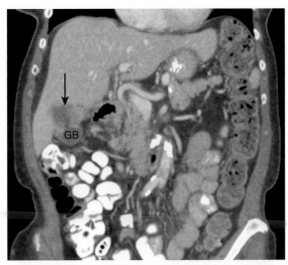

**Figure 28-18.** Gallbladder carcinoma on CT. Coronal contrast-enhanced CT image through abdomen shows heterogeneously enhancing poorly defined exophytic mass (*arrow*) centered in gallbladder fossa arising from superior gallbladder (*GB*) with invasion of subjacent liver parenchyma.

On CT or MRI, it typically presents as a heterogeneously enhancing mass centered in the gallbladder fossa with or without invasion of surrounding organs. Additional imaging appearances may include focal or diffuse gallbladder wall thickening (often poorly defined) with enhancement, or a polypoid enhancing intraluminal gallbladder mass lesion. Presence of direct extension into surrounding organs, regional lymphadenopathy, or distant metastatic disease helps to differentiate gallbladder cancer, particularly when perforated, from acute cholecystitis (Figure 28-18).

33. What is cholangiocarcinoma, and what are its CT and MR imaging features?
Cholangiocarcinoma is the second most common primary hepatic malignancy, is more common in women than in men, usually occurs in patients who are >50 years of age, and is most often due to adenocarcinoma. It can be intrahepatic (10%), hilar (60%), or extrahepatic (30%) in location.

Intrahepatic cholangiocarcinoma presents as a masslike infiltrative hepatic lesion on CT and MRI that typically demonstrates heterogeneous mild to moderate arterial phase enhancement, peripheral venous or delayed phase washout, delayed phase central enhancement (secondary to extensive intratumoral fibrosis), and hypointense signal intensity relative to liver parenchyma on hepatobiliary phase images. Compared with HCC, vascular invasion is less commonly seen. However, segmental or lobar intrahepatic bile duct dilation and associated hepatic parenchymal atrophy are more commonly seen in the setting of cholangiocarcinoma.

Hilar cholangiocarcinoma, also known as Klatskin tumor, tends to present with biliary strictures involving the right hepatic duct, the left hepatic duct, or bifurcation of the CHD, secondary to periductal tumor infiltration and extensive fibrosis associated with this tumor. The tumor is often difficult to visualize owing to its superficial spread but may appear either as a focal enhancing bile duct mass (when exophytic or polypoid intraluminal in configuration) or as a focal enhancing region of bile duct wall thickening with associated luminal narrowing. Associated upstream bile duct dilation may be present. Heterogeneous perfusional changes or atrophy involving a segment or lobe of the liver may also be seen. Regional lymphadenopathy or distant metastatic disease may also be encountered.

Extrahepatic cholangiocarcinoma involves the CHD or CBD and demonstrates similar imaging features to those of hilar cholangiocarcinoma described above (Figure 28-19).

**KEY POINTS**

- Most hepatic lesions are hypointense relative to liver parenchyma on T1-weighted images. Lesion isointensity relative to liver on T1-weighted images suggests that it is of hepatocellular origin.
- Out-of-phase T1-weighted images are useful to detect hepatic steatosis and lipid content in certain hepatic neoplasms.
- On T2-weighted images, malignant hepatic lesions tends to have similar signal intensity as the spleen, whereas hepatic cysts and hemangiomas are hyperintense relative to the spleen and remain hyperintense on heavily T2-weighted images.
- Metastatic disease to a cirrhotic liver is extremely rare. A focal hepatic lesion in a cirrhotic liver that either demonstrates arterial phase enhancement or isointensity to spleen on T2-weighted images is considered as HCC until proven otherwise.
- MRI has higher sensitivity than CT for the detection and localization of calculi within the gallbladder and biliary tree.

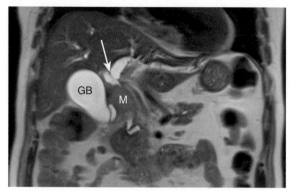

**Figure 28-19.** Extrahepatic cholangiocarcinoma on MRI. Coronal heavily T2-weighted image through abdomen reveals focal mass (*M*) arising from extrahepatic bile duct with associated upstream dilation of biliary tree (*arrow*) and gallbladder (*GB*).

## BIBLIOGRAPHY

Hope TA, Ohliger MA, Qayyum A. MR imaging of diffuse liver disease: from technique to diagnosis. *Radiol Clin North Am.* 2014;52(4): 709-724.

Siegelman ES, Chauhan A. MR characterization of focal liver lesions: pearls and pitfalls. *Magn Reson Imaging Clin N Am.* 2014;22(3): 295-313.

Wells SA. Quantification of hepatic fat and iron with magnetic resonance imaging. *Magn Reson Imaging Clin N Am.* 2014;22(3):397-416.

Yam BL, Siegelman ES. MR imaging of the biliary system. *Radiol Clin North Am.* 2014;52(4):725-755.

Tan CH, Lim KS. MRI of gallbladder cancer. *Diagn Interv Radiol.* 2013;19(4):312-319.

Torigian DA, Kitazono MT. *Netter's correlative imaging: abdominal and pelvic anatomy.* 1st ed. Philadephia: Elsevier; 2013:1-499.

Goodwin MD, Dobson JE, Sirlin CB, et al. Diagnostic challenges and pitfalls in MR imaging with hepatocyte-specific contrast agents. *Radiographics.* 2011;31(6):1547-1568.

Singh AK, Cronin CG, Verma HA, et al. Imaging of preoperative liver transplantation in adults: what radiologists should know. *Radiographics.* 2011;31(4):1017-1030.

van Aalten SM, Thomeer MG, Terkivatan T, et al. Hepatocellular adenomas: correlation of MR imaging findings with pathologic subtype classification. *Radiology.* 2011;261(1):172-181.

Musso G, Gambino R, Cassader M. Non-alcoholic fatty liver disease from pathogenesis to management: an update. *Obes Rev.* 2010;11(6):430-445.

Anderson SW, Kruskal JB, Kane RA. Benign hepatic tumors and iatrogenic pseudotumors. *Radiographics.* 2009;29(1):211-229.

Jang HJ, Yu H, Kim TK. Imaging of focal liver lesions. *Semin Roentgenol.* 2009;44(4):266-282.

Queiroz-Andrade M, Blasbalg R, Ortega CD, et al. MR imaging findings of iron overload. *Radiographics.* 2009;29(6):1575-1589.

Seale MK, Catalano OA, Saini S, et al. Hepatobiliary-specific MR contrast agents: role in imaging the liver and biliary tree. *Radiographics.* 2009;29(6):1725-1748.

Catalano OA, Sahani DV, Kalva SP, et al. MR imaging of the gallbladder: a pictorial essay. *Radiographics.* 2008;28(1):135-155, quiz 324.

Hanna RF, Aguirre DA, Kased N, et al. Cirrhosis-associated hepatocellular nodules: correlation of histopathologic and MR imaging features. *Radiographics.* 2008;28(3):747-769.

Menias CO, Surabhi VR, Prasad SR, et al. Mimics of cholangiocarcinoma: spectrum of disease. *Radiographics.* 2008;28(4):1115-1129.

Sainani NI, Catalano OA, Holalkere NS, et al. Cholangiocarcinoma: current and novel imaging techniques. *Radiographics.* 2008;28(5):1263-1287.

Willatt JM, Hussain HK, Adusumilli S, et al. MR Imaging of hepatocellular carcinoma in the cirrhotic liver: challenges and controversies. *Radiology.* 2008;247(2):311-330.

Brancatelli G, Federle MP, Ambrosini R, et al. Cirrhosis: CT and MR imaging evaluation. *Eur J Radiol.* 2007;61(1):57-69.

Mortele KJ, Rocha TC, Streeter JL, et al. Multimodality imaging of pancreatic and biliary congenital anomalies. *Radiographics.* 2006;26(3):715-731.

Hussain SM, Terkivatan T, Zondervan PE, et al. Focal nodular hyperplasia: findings at state-of-the-art MR imaging, US, CT, and pathologic analysis. *Radiographics.* 2004;24(1):3-17, discussion 8-9.

Mortele KJ, Segatto E, Ros PR. The infected liver: radiologic-pathologic correlation. *Radiographics.* 2004;24(4):937-955.

Moore EE, Cogbill TH, Jurkovich GJ, et al. Organ injury scaling: spleen and liver (1994 revision). *J Trauma.* 1995;38(3):323-324.

# CHAPTER 29

# CT AND MRI OF THE SPLEEN

*Drew A. Torigian, MD, MA, FSAR*

1. What is the normal CT and MRI appearance of the spleen?

   The normal spleen has homogeneous soft tissue attenuation on unenhanced CT, usually 5 to 10 HU less than liver, and appears slightly hypointense on T1-weighted images and hyperintense on T2-weighted images relative to liver (Figure 29-1). It is typically less than 13 cm in craniocaudal dimension and has an average volume of ≈225 ml in adults. Splenic clefts are commonly seen, which are smooth curvilinear infoldings of the splenic surface without surrounding fluid (Figure 29-1, *A*).

2. What is the normal enhancement pattern of the spleen?

   During the arterial phase of enhancement (≈20 to 35 seconds after intravenous [IV] contrast administration), the spleen typically appears to have alternating bands of low and high CT attenuation or T1-weighted MRI signal intensity known as the arciform enhancement pattern (Figure 29-2, *A*). Variation from this pattern suggests presence of diffuse splenic disease. During the venous phase of enhancement (≈50 to 75 seconds after IV contrast administration), contrast material equilibrates in the spleen such that homogeneous intense enhancement is observed (Figure 29-2, *B*).

3. What is the difference between white pulp and red pulp?

   The spleen is composed of white pulp and red pulp, which are indistinguishable on CT or MR images. The white pulp is comprised of lymphatic tissue, whereas the red pulp is composed of venous sinuses and cellular splenic cords.

4. What is an accessory spleen?

   An accessory spleen (also known as a splenule) is a discrete focus of normal splenic tissue that is separate from the spleen, usually 1 to 2 cm in size, and may be single or multiple. CT attenuation and MRI signal intensity properties of an accessory spleen are identical to those of the normal spleen (Figure 29-3). This is encountered in ≈10% to 30% of patients, usually within the splenic hilum or near/within the pancreatic tail, and is important to recognize prior to planned splenectomy for treatment of patients with hematologic or autoimmune disorders.

5. What is an upside-down spleen?

   This is a normal variant due to abnormal splenic rotation, where the hilum is superiorly located and the convex border is medial and adjacent to the left kidney.

6. What is splenosis?

   Splenosis is the spread of splenic tissue anywhere within the torso, most commonly in the peritoneal cavity, due to prior trauma or splenectomy. This is a potential mimic of peritoneal spread of tumor, although the attenuation, signal intensity, and enhancement properties are similar to those of normal splenic tissue. Uptake of [99m]Tc sulfur colloid or [99m]Tc heat damaged red blood cells on scintigraphy is diagnostic.

7. What is the major differential diagnosis of splenomegaly?

   Major causes of splenomegaly include congestion (e.g., portal hypertension, splenic vein occlusion), malignancy (e.g., lymphoma, leukemia), hematologic disorders (e.g., thalassemia), myeloproliferative disorders (e.g., polycythemia vera, myelofibrosis), infectious and inflammatory disorders (e.g., Epstein-Barr virus infection, sarcoidosis, Felty's syndrome), and storage disorders (e.g., Gaucher's disease, amyloidosis).

8. What is the most common cause of a small spleen?

   Sickle cell disease resulting in splenic autoinfarction is the most common cause of a small spleen. The spleen will typically have diffusely very high attenuation due to calcification, as well as diffusely very low signal intensity due to iron deposition from chronic blood transfusions.

9. What are some causes of splenic calcification?

   Major causes include fungal infection (most commonly histoplasmosis), mycobacterial infection, *Pneumocystis jiroveci* infection, prior splenic infarction, systemic lupus erythematosus, and pseudocyst formation related to prior infection or hemorrhage.

10. What does splenic iron deposition look like on MRI, and what are some major causes of iron deposition in the spleen?

    Iron deposition leads to decreased T1-weighted and T2-weighted signal intensity of the spleen relative to normal splenic tissue, which is particularly accentuated on in-phase T1-weighted gradient recalled echo MR images. Punctate foci of iron deposition, known as Gamna Gandy bodies, result from intraparenchymal hemorrhages in the setting of portal hypertension. Focal iron deposition may also occur with prior splenic infarction. Diffuse iron deposition in the

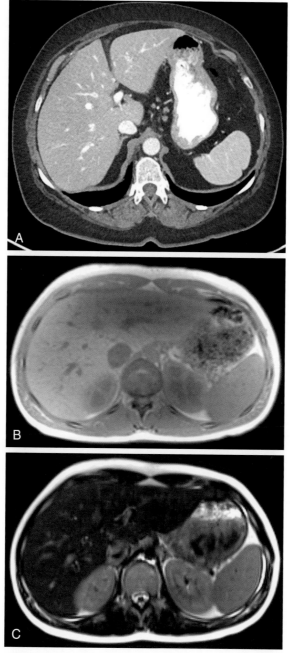

**Figure 29-1. A,** Normal spleen on CT. Note homogeneous attenuation of spleen along with smooth curvilinear infolding of lateral splenic surface without surrounding fluid due to splenic cleft. **B,** Normal spleen on T1-weighted MRI. Note slight hypointense signal intensity of spleen relative to liver. **C,** Normal spleen on T2-weighted MRI. Note hyperintense signal intensity of spleen relative to liver.

spleen is most commonly due to secondary hemosiderosis related to repeated blood transfusions, where iron is taken up by reticuloendothelial cells. Diffuse iron deposition in the liver and bone marrow is also commonly seen. In contrast, genetic (primary) hemochromatosis, an inherited condition leading to excess iron absorption from the bowel, leads to diffuse iron deposition in the liver, pancreas, and myocardium, with sparing of the spleen.

11. What are the CT and MRI findings of splenic infarction?
    A splenic infarct is typically seen on contrast-enhanced CT or MR images as a wedge-shaped peripheral region of nonenhancement in the spleen (Figure 29-4). Major etiologies include bland and septic embolism, pancreatitis, coagulopathy, sickle cell disease, lymphoma, and leukemia.

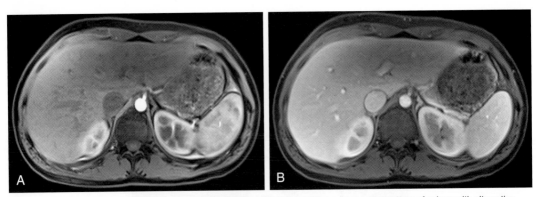

**Figure 29-2. A,** Normal arterial phase enhancement of spleen on MRI. Note arciform enhancement pattern of spleen with alternating bands of low and high signal intensity. **B,** Normal venous phase enhancement of spleen on MRI. Note homogeneous enhancement of spleen.

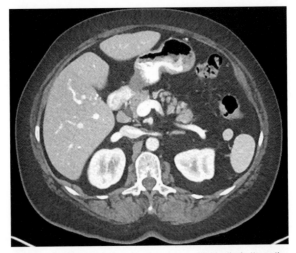

**Figure 29-3.** Splenule on CT. Note 2-cm discrete round focus of splenic tissue with identical attenuation as spleen located more laterally.

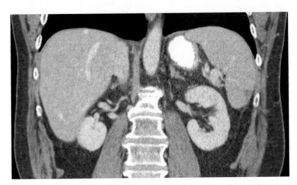

**Figure 29-4.** Splenic infarct on CT. Note small peripheral wedge-shaped region of nonenhancement in inferolateral spleen.

12. **What abdominal organ is most commonly injured due to blunt abdominal trauma?**
    The spleen is the most commonly injured organ in blunt abdominal trauma, accounting for up to 50% of visceral injuries, and CT is highly accurate in diagnosing splenic injury. Currently, the most widely used CT grading system for splenic injury is based on the American Association for the Surgery of Trauma (AAST) scale, although a more recent CT-based grading system has been shown to provide improved accuracy to predict the need for angiography or surgery. The spectrum of splenic injuries includes hematoma, laceration, infarction, active hemorrhage, and vascular injuries including pseudoaneurysm and arteriovenous fistula (AVF).

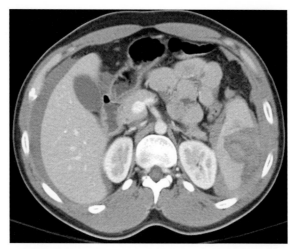

**Figure 29-5.** Splenic laceration on CT in setting of trauma. Note irregular linear focus of hypoattenuation within spleen containing high attenuation hemorrhage, along with high attenuation hemorrhage surrounding spleen.

Intraparenchymal hematomas appear as round, ovoid, or irregular foci of nonenhancing high attenuation (30 to 70 HU) hemorrhagic fluid within the spleen; subcapsular hematomas are crescentic and peripheral in location and exert mass effect upon the splenic contour; and perisplenic hematomas surround the spleen in the peritoneal space without deforming the splenic contour. On MRI, subacute hemorrhage has high T1-weighted signal intensity.

Splenic lacerations appear as irregular, linear, branching, or stellate nonenhancing low attenuation parenchymal defects in the spleen, often with adjacent areas of high attenuation hemorrhage (Figure 29-5). When active hemorrhage is present, one sees focal areas of increased attenuation on contrast-enhanced images similar to that of enhancing vessels which do not conform to known vascular structures and which persist or increase in size on more delayed phase acquisitions. Splenic pseudoaneurysms and AVF also appear as well-circumscribed foci of contrast enhancement with attenuation similar to adjacent contrast-enhanced arteries but decrease in attenuation on more delayed phase acquisitions. Presence of active hemorrhage or of vascular injuries on CT are generally predictive of the need for splenic angiography and transcatheter embolization or splenic surgery.

13. What are some benign cystic lesions that may involve the spleen?

Cyst, pseudocyst, lymphangioma, pyogenic abscess, hydatid cyst, fungal microabscess, and mycobacterial microabscess.

Cysts (lined by epithelium), pseudocysts (lined by fibrotic tissue), and lymphangiomas typically have fluid attenuation (0 to 20 HU), low T1-weighted and very high T2-weighted signal intensity, thin walls, and no solid enhancement. Peripheral calcifications are sometimes seen in pseudocysts, and thin internal septations are often seen in lymphangiomas.

Pyogenic abscesses have low attenuation, low T1-weighted and high T2-weighted signal intensity, internal septations, and thick rim enhancement, sometimes with very low attenuation and very low signal intensity foci of gas (Figure 29-6).

Hydatid cyst due to *Echinococcus granulosus* parasitic infection typically contains multiple daughter cysts creating a multilocular appearance along with a low signal intensity rim, which may be calcified, usually without enhancement. Some loculations may have increased attenuation or T1-weighted signal intensity. The presence of internal collapsed membranes (the "water lily" sign) is considered to be pathognomonic.

Microabscesses due to fungal or mycobacterial infection tend to be multiple, <1 cm in size, and have low attenuation, low T1-weighted and high T2-weighted signal intensity relative to spleen, and rim enhancement. These are most often due to candidiasis in immunocompromised patients and are commonly seen to also involve the liver.

14. What are some benign solid lesions that may involve the spleen?

Hemangioma, hamartoma, and sarcoidosis.

Hemangioma is the most common benign vascular neoplasm of the spleen, is typically <2 cm in size, and has low attenuation, low-intermediate T1-weighted and high T2-weighted signal intensity, peripheral enhancement, and centripetal fill-in of enhancement on delayed phase postcontrast images (Figure 29-7).

Hamartoma is an uncommon nonneoplastic benign lesion which is typically solitary and round in shape, has intermediate attenuation, intermediate T1-weighted and high T2-weighted signal intensity relative to spleen, and diffuse early enhancement which becomes isointense to spleen on delayed phase images.

Sarcoidosis, due to idiopathic formation of noncaseating granulomas, may demonstrate low attenuation, low signal intensity, and hypoenhancing lesions in the spleen along with splenomegaly (the most common finding), hepatomegaly, hepatic lesions, and lymphadenopathy.

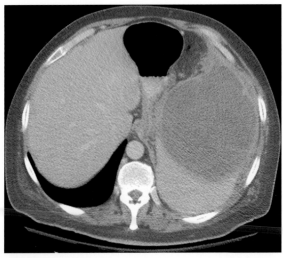

**Figure 29-6.** Splenic pyogenic abscess on CT. Note large round heterogeneous low attenuation lesion in anterior spleen with thick rim enhancement and surrounding inflammatory fat stranding.

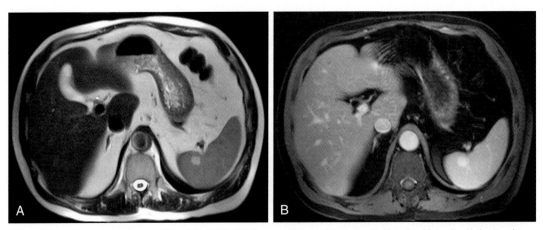

**Figure 29-7. A,** Splenic hemangioma on T2-weighted MRI. Note 2-cm ovoid lesion in spleen with high signal intensity relative to spleen and lower signal intensity than cerebrospinal fluid. **B,** Splenic hemangioma on delayed phase postcontrast MRI. Note homogeneous delayed phase hyperenhancement of lesion relative to spleen.

15. What are some malignant lesions that may involve the spleen?

Lymphoma, leukemia, metastatic disease, and angiosarcoma.

Lymphoma is the most common splenic malignancy and is most commonly due to secondary involvement by non-Hodgkin's lymphoma in up to 40% of patients. The most common appearance of lymphoma is splenomegaly. In some patients, one or more focal hypoenhancing splenic lesions are seen, which are typically homogeneous in appearance, have low attenuation and intermediate T1-weighted and low-intermediate T2-weighted signal intensity relative to spleen, and have hypoenhancement, often along with areas of lymphadenopathy (Figure 29-8).

Leukemia in the spleen also most commonly appears as splenomegaly, sometimes with multiple small hypoenhancing splenic lesions.

Metastatic disease uncommonly affects the spleen in up to 7% of patients with malignancy, most often due to melanoma and breast cancer and less often from cancers of the lung, colon, stomach, ovary, endometrium, and prostate gland. These are often poorly marginated, heterogeneous, and multiple, and have low attenuation and low-intermediate T1-weighted and intermediate-high T2-weighted signal intensity relative to spleen, along with heterogeneous enhancement, usually with peripheral rim enhancement. When present, cystic/necrotic areas have fluid attenuation, low T1-weighted and very high T2-weighted signal intensity, hemorrhagic components have soft tissue attenuation and high T1-weighted signal intensity, and calcifications have very high attenuation and are difficult to visualize on MR images.

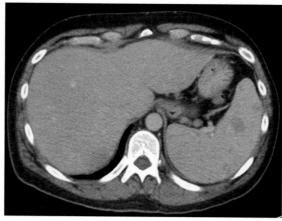

**Figure 29-8.** Splenic lymphoma on CT. Note multiple homogeneous low attenuation lesions within spleen along with mild splenomegaly. A subtle low attenuation lesion is also present within liver.

Angiosarcoma is the most common primary malignant nonlymphoid tumor of the spleen and is highly aggressive with a poor prognosis, but it is exceedingly rare. Typically, a nodular heterogeneous ill-defined splenic mass with solid enhancing and cystic components is encountered, often in association with splenomegaly and metastatic disease.

16. How are incidentally detected splenic lesions generally managed?

In patients without a history of cancer, indeterminate splenic lesions are followed over time with imaging if no suspicious features are present, whereas lesions with suspicious features are further evaluated with MRI, [18]F-fluorodeoxyglucose positron emission tomography (FDG PET), or tissue sampling. Suspicious imaging features include heterogeneous attenuation or signal intensity, solid areas of enhancement, irregular margins, presence of necrotic areas, splenic parenchymal or vascular invasion, large size, and growth over time. In patients with a history of cancer, subcentimeter splenic lesions are followed over time with imaging, whereas lesions ≥1 cm are further evaluated with MRI, FDG PET, or tissue sampling given the greater likelihood of metastatic disease.

17. What is polysplenia?

Polysplenia is defined as presence of multiple small spleens in place of a single spleen. This is associated with bilateral left-sidedness in patients with organ heterotaxy, the abnormal arrangement of organs and vessels in the body. Polysplenia is associated with cardiac septal defects (acyanotic), interruption of the inferior vena cava with azygos continuation, bilateral bilobed lungs, bilateral hyparterial bronchi (with mainstem bronchi inferior to pulmonary arteries), a midline liver, and a hypoplastic pancreatic body and tail.

18. What is asplenia?

Asplenia is defined as congenital absence of the spleen and is associated with bilateral right-sidedness in patients with organ heterotaxy. Asplenia is associated with more severe, cyanotic cardiac defects than is polysplenia, a left-sided inferior vena cava, bilateral trilobed lungs, bilateral eparterial bronchi (with mainstem bronchi superior to pulmonary arteries), and a midline liver.

## KEY POINTS

- The normal spleen demonstrates alternating bands of low and high attenuation or signal intensity during the arterial phase of enhancement and appears homogeneous in the venous phase of enhancement.
- A splenic laceration is associated with a history of trauma, is irregular or branching in configuration, and is associated with adjacent areas of fluid, whereas a developmental splenic cleft is smooth without presence of surrounding fluid.
- CT and MRI are less specific in the characterization of splenic lesions than they are for characterization of hepatic, adrenal, or renal lesions.

**BIBLIOGRAPHY**

Heller MT, Harisinghani M, Neitlich JD, et al. Managing incidental findings on abdominal and pelvic CT and MRI, part 3: white paper of the ACR Incidental Findings Committee II on Splenic and Nodal Findings. *J Am Coll Radiol*. 2013;10(11):833-839.

Boscak A, Shanmuganathan K. Splenic trauma: what is new? *Radiol Clin North Am*. 2012;50(1):105-122.

Kaza RK, Azar S, Al-Hawary MM, et al. Primary and secondary neoplasms of the spleen. *Cancer Imaging*. 2010;10:173-182.

Marmery H, Shanmuganathan K, Alexander MT, et al. Optimization of selection for nonoperative management of blunt splenic injury: comparison of MDCT grading systems. *AJR Am J Roentgenol*. 2007;189(6):1421-1427.

Meier JM, Alavi A, Iruvuri S, et al. Assessment of age-related changes in abdominal organ structure and function with computed tomography and positron emission tomography. *Semin Nucl Med.* 2007;37(3):154-172.

Gayer G, Hertz M, Strauss S, et al. Congenital anomalies of the spleen. *Semin Ultrasound CT MR.* 2006;27(5):358-369.

Elsayes KM, Narra VR, Mukundan G, et al. MR imaging of the spleen: spectrum of abnormalities. *Radiographics.* 2005;25(4):967-982.

Abbott RM, Levy AD, Aguilera NS, et al. From the archives of the AFIP: primary vascular neoplasms of the spleen: radiologic-pathologic correlation. *Radiographics.* 2004;24(4):1137-1163.

Paterson A, Frush DP, Donnelly LF, et al. A pattern-oriented approach to splenic imaging in infants and children. *Radiographics.* 1999;19(6):1465-1485.

Moore EE, Cogbill TH, Jurkovich GJ, et al. Organ injury scaling: spleen and liver (1994 revision). *J Trauma.* 1995;38(3):323-324.

# CT AND MRI OF THE PANCREAS

*Drew A. Torigian, MD, MA, FSAR*

# CHAPTER 30

1. **What are the general indications for computed tomography (CT) and magnetic resonance imaging (MRI) of the pancreas?**

   CT and MRI are commonly used to assess the extent and severity of disease in patients suspected of having pancreatitis, to evaluate for associated complications of pancreatitis, and to provide guidance for percutaneous drainage of peripancreatic fluid collections or percutaneous biopsy of pancreatic lesions. They are also useful to detect and characterize pancreatic lesions in patients at increased risk for pancreatic neoplasms, with symptoms or signs suggestive of pancreatic pathology, or with previously detected incidental pancreatic lesions on other imaging studies. In particular, MRI is often used as a problem-solving tool when an indeterminate pancreatic lesion is detected on other imaging studies, when the patient cannot receive iodinated contrast material for CT examination, or when the patient is pregnant. CT and MRI are also useful for the staging and pretreatment planning of patients with pancreatic malignancy (e.g., to determine the resectability of pancreatic malignancy), for response assessment of tumor following therapy, and for restaging assessment to detect recurrent tumor.

   Given its superior soft tissue resolution, MRI is particularly useful for detection of cholelithiasis and choledocholithiasis, assessment of pancreatic duct disruption, identification of pancreaticobiliary developmental abnormalities (e.g., annular pancreas and pancreas divisum), improved assessment of pancreatic and peripancreatic fluid collections, improved detection and characterization of focal cystic or solid pancreatic lesions, particularly when small (<2 cm) in size, and assessment of iron deposition within the pancreas and other organs in the setting of primary (genetic) hemochromatosis.

2. **What is magnetic resonance cholangiopancreatography (MRCP), and how does it compare with endoscopic retrograde cholangiopancreatography (ERCP)?**

   MRCP is a noninvasive MR imaging technique that is performed through acquisition of very heavily T2-weighted images such that only fluid-filled structures, in particular the pancreaticobiliary tree, have very high signal intensity, whereas other background tissues and organs have very low signal intensity (Figure 30-1). It is typically performed as part of a complete abdominal MRI examination, so that information about the surrounding soft tissues is also provided.

   ERCP is an invasive technique that is performed by gastroenterologists during patient sedation by passage of an endoscope into the stomach and duodenum. It allows for direct visualization of the mucosa of the stomach and

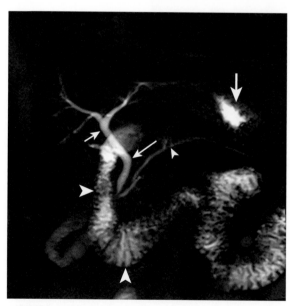

**Figure 30-1.** Normal MRCP. Coronal MRCP image shows normal caliber main pancreatic duct (*small arrowhead*), common bile duct (*long thin arrow*), and common hepatic duct (*short thin arrow*). Also note fluid-filled stomach (*thick arrow*) and duodenum (*large arrowheads*).

duodenum, direct visualization of the ampulla, and biopsy of lesions encountered. Contrast material is injected into the common bile duct and pancreatic duct, and then x-ray fluoroscopic images are acquired to create images of these ductal systems. Since the advent of MRCP, ERCP is performed less often for diagnostic purposes unless a therapeutic procedure is also planned such as removal of calculi, dilation of a sphincter, dilation of a stricture, or stent placement.

3. What is the normal CT and MRI appearance of the pancreas?

The pancreas is approximately 15 cm in length and 2 to 3 cm in width and is located within the anterior pararenal space of the retroperitoneum. It can be subdivided into the pancreatic uncinate process, head, neck, body, and tail. The pancreatic head is located to the left of the second portion of the duodenum, and the pancreatic body and tail are located posteriorly to the gastric body and antrum. In general, the pancreatic body and tail are slightly more superiorly located than the pancreatic head and uncinate process. Pancreatic size tends to decrease with increasing age. In younger people, the pancreas typically has a smooth contour and homogeneous attenuation, signal intensity, and enhancement (Figure 30-2), whereas in older people, the pancreas typically becomes more lobulated and more inhomogeneous due to fatty change (which may be diffuse or focal). On MRI, the pancreas typically has the highest T1-weighted signal intensity among all abdominal organs (excluding abdominal fat).

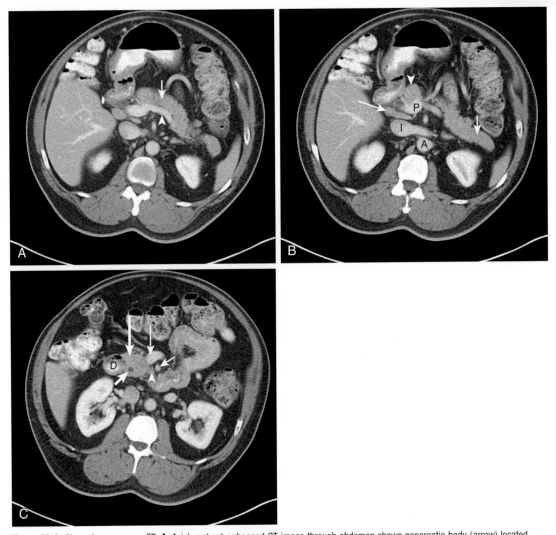

**Figure 30-2.** Normal pancreas on CT. **A,** Axial contrast-enhanced CT image through abdomen shows pancreatic body (*arrow*) located anterior to splenic vein (*arrowhead*). **B,** Axial contrast-enhanced CT image more inferiorly demonstrates pancreatic neck (*arrowhead*) located anterior to portal vein confluence (*P*) along with pancreatic tail (*short arrow*). Note normal size portacaval lymph node (*long arrow*) in portacaval space between portal vein confluence (*P*) and inferior vena cava (*I*). Abdominal aorta (*A*) is also visualized. **C,** Axial contrast-enhanced CT image even more inferiorly reveals pancreatic head (*long thick arrow*) located medial to 2nd portion of duodenum (*D*) and uncinate process (*arrowhead*) which is posteriorly located to proximal SMV (*long thin arrow*) and SMA (*short thin arrow*). Note common bile duct (*short thick arrow*) passing through right posterolateral aspect of pancreatic head.

The main pancreatic duct is normally ≤2 to 3 mm in caliber but may measure up to 5 mm in caliber in elderly patients. The main pancreatic duct (of Wirsung) typically joins the common bile duct to form the ampulla of Vater and then drains into the second portion of the duodenum through the major duodenal papilla (of Vater). An accessory pancreatic duct (of Santorini) may occasionally be present more superiorly, which drains more superiorly and anteriorly into the second portion of the duodenum through the minor duodenal papilla. The common bile duct is typically located in the right posterolateral aspect of the pancreatic head (see Figure 30-2, *C*). Approximately 20 to 35 short pancreatic ductal side branches join perpendicularly to the main pancreatic duct.

4. **What blood vessels are found near the pancreas?**
The splenic vein and artery are located posteriorly to the body and tail of the pancreas (see Figure 30-2, *A*), where the former is larger in caliber, is less tortuous, and is more inferiorly located than the latter. The splenic vein is a reliable landmark to help identify the location of the pancreatic body and tail. The portal vein confluence (where the superior mesenteric [SMV] and splenic veins join), proximal SMV, and proximal superior mesenteric artery (SMA) pass posteriorly to the pancreatic neck and anteriorly to the uncinate process, where the proximal SMA is normally located posteriorly and to the left of the proximal SMV (see Figure 30-2, *C*). The gastroduodenal artery (GDA) arises from the common hepatic artery and extends inferiorly along the anterolateral aspect of the pancreatic head.

5. **What structures may be seen in the portacaval space?**
The portacaval space is located between the main portal vein and inferior vena cava. Portacaval lymph nodes (see Figure 30-2, *B*), the uncinate process of the pancreas, and an accessory or replaced right hepatic artery arising from the SMA may be seen in this location.

6. **What is pancreas divisum?**
Pancreas divisum is the most common congenital anomaly of the pancreas, occurring in up to 15% of patients. It results from failure of the dorsal and ventral pancreatic anlagen of the ductal systems to fully fuse during development. The duct in the pancreatic body and tail (derived from the dorsal pancreatic anlage) drains into the duodenum through the accessory duct (of Santorini) and minor duodenal papilla, whereas the separate, more posteriorly and inferiorly located duct in the pancreatic head and uncinate process (derived from the ventral pancreatic anlage) joins the distal common bile duct and drains into the duodenum through the major duodenal papilla (of Vater). Some investigators believe that this anomaly may be associated with an increased incidence of recurrent idiopathic pancreatitis, although others believe that the association is incidental.

7. **What is an annular pancreas?**
An annular pancreas is a rare congenital anomaly of the pancreas, where pancreatic tissue partially or completely surrounds the second portion of the duodenum. On cross-sectional imaging, pancreatic parenchyma will be seen to encircle the duodenum, sometimes with associated duodenal luminal narrowing (Figure 30-3). Sometimes, there may be associated duodenal obstruction.

8. **What is an intrapancreatic splenule?**
An intrapancreatic splenule is a congenital anomaly where an accessory spleen is located in the pancreatic tail. On CT and MRI, a 1- to 3-cm well-circumscribed structure is seen in the pancreatic tail that has similar attenuation, signal intensity, and enhancement properties as normal splenic parenchyma. It is asymptomatic and of no clinical significance, but awareness of this anomaly is of critical importance to prevent unnecessary surgical resection for a mistakenly suspected pancreatic neoplasm. A technetium-99m ($^{99m}$Tc) heat-denatured red blood cell (RBC) scan or a

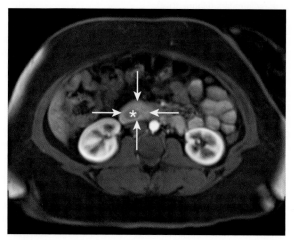

**Figure 30-3.** Annular pancreas on MRI. Axial contrast-enhanced T1-weighted MR image through abdomen shows high signal intensity pancreatic parenchyma (*arrows*) completely surrounding 2nd portion of duodenum (*).

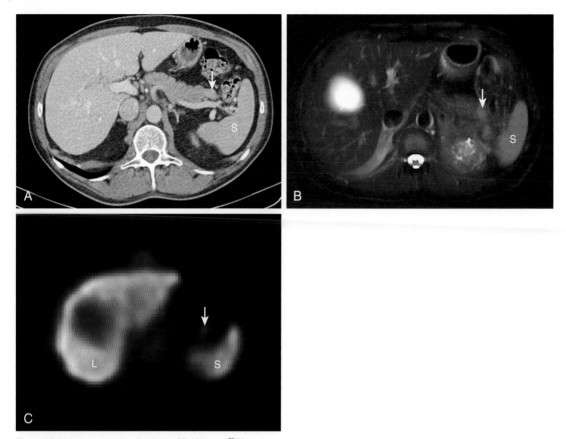

**Figure 30-4.** Intrapancreatic splenule on CT, MRI, and $^{99m}$Tc sulfur colloid single photon emission computed tomography (SPECT). **A,** Axial contrast-enhanced CT image through abdomen shows ovoid well-circumscribed enhancing structure in pancreatic tail (*arrow*) with similar attenuation as spleen (*S*). **B,** Axial fat-suppressed T2-weighted image similarly shows that pancreatic tail structure (*arrow*) has similar signal intensity as spleen (*S*). **C,** Axial $^{99m}$Tc sulfur colloid SPECT image reveals radiotracer uptake in structure (*arrow*) confirming presence of reticuloendothelial tissue composition and therefore of diagnosis of intrapancreatic splenule. Note normal radiotracer uptake in liver (*L*) and spleen (*S*) and round photopenic area in liver due to cyst.

$^{99m}$Tc sulfur colloid scan may be performed as needed to confirm this diagnosis, because splenic tissue will demonstrate uptake of these radiotracers (Figure 30-4).

9. What are some causes of pancreatic fatty replacement?

Fatty replacement, either diffuse or focal, can be seen with older age, cystic fibrosis (Figure 30-5), diabetes mellitus, obesity, corticosteroid use, chronic obstruction of the pancreatic duct (such as by tumor or calculus), and prior pancreatitis. When focal, it can sometimes mimic a hypoattenuating pancreatic mass on CT. However, focal fatty replacement typically occurs in the anterior pancreatic head with a smooth well-demarcated border from a platelike or triangular higher attenuation area of fatty sparing in the posterior pancreatic head and uncinate process and generally remains stable over time (Figure 30-6). Furthermore, there is preservation of the normal pancreatic contour and lobular appearance of the parenchyma, and no additional features of malignancy such as ductal obstruction, vascular encasement, lymphadenopathy, or metastatic disease are seen. On MRI, regions of focal fatty replacement have intermediate-high signal intensity on in-phase T1-weighted images with loss of signal intensity seen on out-of-phase T1-weighted images.

10. What does pancreatic iron deposition look like on MRI, and what is the major cause?

On MRI, iron deposition leads to low signal intensity of the pancreatic parenchyma on in-phase T1-weighted images compared to out-of-phase T1-weighted images. The major cause of pancreatic iron deposition is primary (genetic) hemochromatosis, which is an autosomal recessive disorder in which abnormal iron metabolism results in iron deposition in the liver and sometimes in the pancreas or myocardium. There is absence of iron deposition in the spleen or bone marrow, which instead would be seen in the setting of secondary hemosiderosis related to multiple blood transfusions, chronic hemodialysis, or hemolytic anemias.

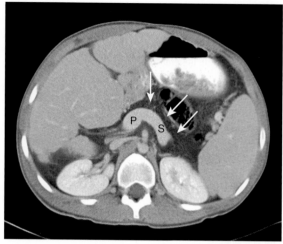

**Figure 30-5.** Diffuse pancreatic fatty replacement secondary to cystic fibrosis on CT. Note fat attenuation of pancreatic body and tail (*arrows*) located anterior to splenic vein (*S*), which connects to portal vein confluence (*P*).

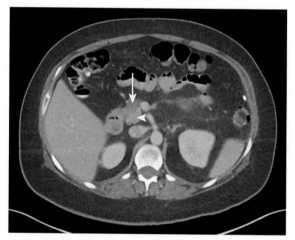

**Figure 30-6.** Focal fatty replacement on CT. Note geographic low attenuation area in anterior pancreatic head (*arrow*) with well-defined demarcation from triangular area of fatty sparing in posterior pancreatic head (*arrowhead*).

11. What is the role of CT and MRI in the assessment of patients with acute pancreatitis?

CT is the mainstay of imaging evaluation of patients with acute pancreatitis, whereas MRI is more commonly used as a problem-solving tool. When performed, CT is typically obtained after 3 days from the onset of symptoms or when clinical findings worsen. Major indications for CT and MRI in this clinical setting are:
- To confirm the clinical diagnosis of acute pancreatitis (if the diagnosis is uncertain) while simultaneously excluding other potential causes of acute abdominal symptoms and signs.
- To assess the severity of acute pancreatitis involving the pancreas and peripancreatic tissues including the presence of complications.
- To determine the underlying etiology of acute pancreatitis.
- To guide treatment (e.g., percutaneous drainage of collections) and to monitor treatment response.

12. What are the most common causes of acute pancreatitis?

Alcoholism and gallstones are the most common causes of acute pancreatitis, accounting for 90% of cases in the United States. Less common causes include certain medications, chemicals, or toxins, abdominal trauma, ERCP, pancreatic tumors, hypertriglyceridemia, hypercalcemia, viral or parasitic infection, autoimmune disease, hereditary pancreatitis, and idiopathic pancreatitis.

13. What are the two major types of acute pancreatitis, and how do they appear on cross-sectional imaging?

Interstitial edematous pancreatitis and necrotizing pancreatitis.

In interstitial edematous pancreatitis, diffuse or localized enlargement of the pancreas is seen, with normal homogeneous enhancement or slightly heterogeneous enhancement of the pancreatic parenchyma due to edema and inflammation. Sometimes, peripancreatic fat stranding, peripancreatic fluid, retroperitoneal fascial plane thickening, or reactive bowel wall thickening may also be seen (Figure 30-7). Note that visualization of a normal appearing pancreas on cross-sectional imaging does not exclude the presence of acute pancreatitis.

In necrotizing pancreatitis, areas of nonenhancement are seen in the pancreas and/or surrounding peripancreatic tissues due to tissue necrosis, which may be sterile or superinfected (Figure 30-8). Presence of necrosis and larger amounts of necrosis (particularly when >30% of the pancreas) are associated with increased patient morbidity and mortality.

14. Describe the four types of pancreatic and peripancreatic collections that may occur in the setting of acute pancreatitis.
    1. Acute peripancreatic fluid collections (APFC) occur in the peripancreatic tissues within ≤4 weeks of symptom onset and have homogeneous fluid attenuation and signal intensity but have no discernible walls (see Figure 30-7).
    2. Pseudocysts occur in the peripancreatic tissues usually after >4 weeks of symptom onset and are well-circumscribed round or oval collections with homogeneous fluid attenuation and signal intensity, with discernible enhancing nonepithelialized walls made of fibrous or granulation tissue. The majority of pseudocysts spontaneously resolve, whereas ones that are >4 to 6 cm in size, are increasing in size, are associated with symptoms, or are superinfected may require drainage.
    3. Acute necrotic collections (ANC) may occur in the pancreas or peripancreatic tissues within ≤4 weeks of symptom onset, have heterogeneous attenuation and signal intensity with nonliquefied necrotic material and are variably loculated but have no discernible walls.

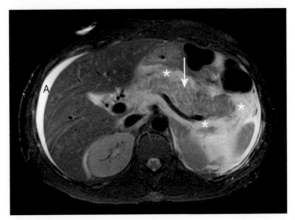

**Figure 30-7.** Interstitial edematous pancreatitis on MRI. Axial fat-suppressed T2-weighted image through abdomen shows diffuse enlargement of pancreatic body and tail (*arrow*) with increased parenchymal signal intensity due to edema/inflammation. Also note high signal intensity peripancreatic APFCs (*) and small ascites (*A*).

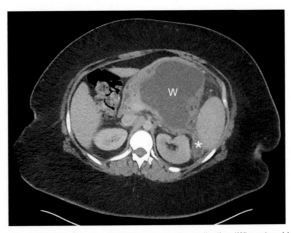

**Figure 30-8.** Necrotizing pancreatitis on CT. Note large loculated low attenuation collection (*W*) centered in pancreatic body and tail with discernible enhancing walls representing WON. Also note smaller focus of extrapancreatic WON (*) in left retroperitoneum.

4. Walled-off necrosis (WON) may occur in the pancreas or peripancreatic tissues after >4 weeks of symptom onset, have heterogeneous attenuation and signal intensity with nonliquefied necrotic material, are variably loculated, and have discernible enhancing walls (see Figure 30-8).

Superinfection of any of these collections may occur and is suspected when foci of very low attenuation and very low signal intensity gas are seen in a collection. However, presence of gas may alternatively be caused by fistulization of a collection with the gastrointestinal tract or by prior intervention. When infection is present, percutaneous, endoscopic, or surgical intervention is usually required.

15. **What are some other local complications of acute pancreatitis?**
    - Hemorrhage.
    - Venous thrombosis (splenic vein, portal vein, SMV).
    - Arterial pseudoaneurysm formation (splenic artery, GDA).
    - Extrahepatic bile duct obstruction.
    - Ascites.

16. **What are the CT and MR imaging features of chronic pancreatitis?**
    Chronic pancreatitis is secondary to prolonged inflammation with associated fibrotic change and is most often encountered in the setting of alcoholism. On CT and MRI, pancreatic parenchymal atrophy with fatty change and focal calcifications are characteristically seen. Irregular or beaded dilation of the main pancreatic duct and side branches, often with focal strictures or intraductal calculi, is also seen (Figure 30-9). Sometimes, focal pancreatic enlargement mimicking a pancreatic neoplasm may occur, which may require tissue sampling for definitive diagnosis. However, the "penetrating duct" sign may also sometimes be present, where a normal or minimally narrowed pancreatic duct passes through the region of focal pancreatic enlargement, which is more suggestive of a nonneoplastic etiology. Additional findings such as pseudocyst formation or splenic vein thrombosis may also be present.

17. **What is groove pancreatitis?**
    Groove pancreatitis is a form of segmental pancreatitis where fluid, inflammation, and/or fibrosis extend into the groove between the pancreatic head and the duodenum, and it is typically seen in men with a history of alcoholism. On cross-sectional imaging, fluid, fat stranding, and/or fibrous tissue are seen predominantly between the pancreatic head and the duodenum. Associated duodenal wall thickening or pseudocyst formation may also be present (Figure 30-10).

18. **Are there any CT or MR imaging features that may indicate the presence of autoimmune pancreatitis?**
    Diffuse pancreatic enlargement with a sausage-like appearance is typically seen in autoimmune pancreatitis. A characteristic peripancreatic fibroinflammatory soft tissue rim may also be present, which has low attenuation, low signal intensity, and delayed phase enhancement relative to pancreatic parenchyma. Presence of extrapancreatic disease, such as sclerosing cholangitis, renal lesions, pulmonary nodules or opacities, sclerosing mesenteritis, retroperitoneal fibrosis, orbital pseudotumor, and salivary and lacrimal gland enlargement, may also suggest the diagnosis. Corticosteroids are the mainstay for initial treatment, with high rates of remission. Immunomodulatory drugs are administered as needed in patients with relapse or corticosteroid-resistant disease.

19. **What cross-sectional imaging findings may be encountered in pancreatic trauma?**
    Pancreatic injuries are uncommon but most commonly occur from penetrating trauma and less commonly occur from blunt trauma when there is severe compression of the pancreas against the spine during seat belt, deceleration, or

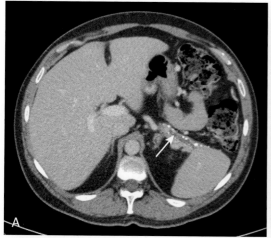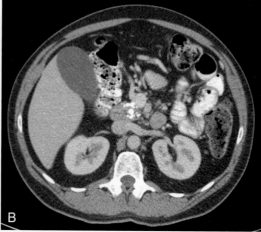

**Figure 30-9.** Chronic pancreatitis on CT. **A,** Note diffuse parenchymal atrophy of pancreatic body and tail along with dilation of main pancreatic duct (*arrow*) and very high attenuation calcifications. **B,** Note very high attenuation calcifications in pancreatic head as well.

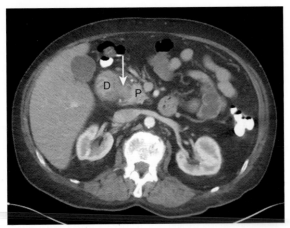

**Figure 30-10.** Groove pancreatitis on CT. Note amorphous soft tissue and fat stranding (*arrow*) in between pancreatic head (*P*) and 2nd portion of duodenum (*D*). Associated thickening of medial wall of duodenum is also present.

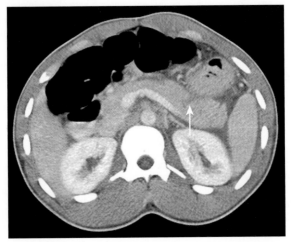

**Figure 30-11.** Pancreatic trauma on CT. Note linear nonenhancing low attenuation focus (*arrow*) in pancreatic tail representing pancreatic laceration. Also note mild diffuse enlargement of pancreatic tail and mild surrounding fat stranding secondary to pancreatic contusion and/ or mild pancreatitis.

handlebar compression injury. The pancreatic body is most commonly injured in the setting of blunt abdominal trauma, and overall, pancreatic injury has a mortality rate of up to 20%.

Currently, the most widely used CT grading system for pancreatic injury is based on the American Association for the Surgery of Trauma (AAST) scale. The spectrum of pancreatic injuries includes contusion, hematoma, laceration without or with ductal injury, and complete organ disruption. The most important factor that determines clinical outcome (and whether or not surgical intervention will be required) is the integrity or the pancreatic duct. Assessment of the pancreatic duct is difficult to perform on CT but is facilitated through use of MRCP or ERCP.

The pancreas, when injured, may sometimes appear normal on cross-sectional imaging.

Pancreatic hematomas appear as foci of nonenhancing high attenuation (30 to 70 HU) hemorrhagic fluid on CT. When active hemorrhage is present, one sees focal areas of increased attenuation on contrast-enhanced images similar to that of enhancing vessels that do not conform to known vascular structures and that persist or increase in size on more delayed phase acquisitions.

Pancreatic contusions appear as focal or more diffuse areas of hypoattenuation within the pancreas, although they may sometimes be isoattenuating relative to surrounding pancreatic parenchyma or hyperattenuating when there is associated hemorrhage. Associated pancreatic enlargement as well as peripancreatic fluid, hemorrhage, or fat stranding may also be seen.

Pancreatic lacerations appear as linear nonenhancing low attenuation parenchymal defects in the pancreas, often with adjacent areas of high attenuation hemorrhage (Figure 30-11).

Associated findings of pancreatitis (including any of the local complications of pancreatitis listed above) or of fistula formation to adjacent organs may also be visualized.

**Box 30-1.** Major Differential Diagnosis of Focal Pancreatic Lesions

True epithelial cyst
Lymphangioma
Focal pancreatitis (acute or chronic)
Pseudocyst/WON
Cystic pancreatic neoplasms
• Serous cystadenoma
• Mucinous cystadenoma/cystadenocarcinoma
• IPMN
  • Side branch type
  • Main duct type
• SPN

• Adenocarcinoma (with cystic change or necrosis)
• Neuroendocrine tumor (with cystic change or necrosis)
• Metastasis (with cystic change or necrosis)
Solid pancreatic neoplasms
• Adenocarcinoma
• Neuroendocrine tumor
• SPN
• Metastasis
• Lymphoma
• Acinar cell carcinoma

20. What cross-sectional imaging findings suggest presence of a pancreatic ductal injury?
    • Presence of a deep (>50%) laceration of the pancreas.
    • Presence of a collection that is seen to communicate with the pancreatic duct.
    • Visualization of discontinuity of the pancreatic duct.

21. What is the major differential diagnosis for focal pancreatic lesions?
    For the answer, see Box 30-1.

22. What lesion can mimic a pancreatic cystic lesion on cross-sectional imaging?
    A duodenal diverticulum can occasionally mimic a cystic lesion of the pancreas when it is completely fluid-filled. Contiguity with the duodenal lumen and presence of internal gas or oral contrast material are specific diagnostic features for this specific diagnosis on cross-sectional imaging.

23. How are incidentally detected pancreatic cystic lesions generally managed?
    Pancreatic cystic lesions that are >3 cm in size, have mural nodules or solid enhancing components, or are associated with main pancreatic duct dilation are more likely malignant in nature and therefore are generally managed with tissue sampling (fluid aspiration) followed by surgical resection (when appropriate). Pancreatic cystic lesions that are ≤3 cm in size, have no mural nodules or solid enhancing components, are not associated with main pancreatic duct dilation, and are asymptomatic are more likely benign in nature and therefore are generally managed more conservatively with CT or MR imaging follow-up.

24. What conditions are associated with pancreatic epithelial cyst formation?
    • von Hippel-Lindau (vHL) syndrome.
    • Autosomal dominant polycystic kidney disease (ADPKD).
    • Cystic fibrosis (CF).

25. What pancreatic lesions are associated with vHL syndrome?
    Pancreatic serous cystadenomas, pancreatic epithelial cysts, and pancreatic neuroendocrine tumors are associated with vHL syndrome. Retinal or central nervous system hemangioblastomas, hepatic and renal cysts, renal cell carcinoma (RCC), pheochromocytomas/paragangliomas, endolymphatic sac tumors, and epididymal papillary cystadenomas are extrapancreatic lesions that are associated with vHL syndrome.

26. What is a pancreatic serous cystadenoma?
    A pancreatic serous cystadenoma is a benign glycogen-rich serous epithelial pancreatic neoplasm that can occur anywhere in the pancreas and is typically encountered in elderly women. The microcystic type occurs in about two thirds of cases, where multiple (>6) small (<2 cm) clustered cystic foci separated by thin septations are typically seen in the lesion on cross-sectional imaging (Figure 30-12). A characteristic enhancing, sometimes calcified, stellate central scar may also be visualized. The macrocystic or oligocystic type occurs in the remaining one third of cases, where one or a few cystic foci are seen in the lesion without a central scar, which may not be distinguishable from other pancreatic cystic neoplasms based on cross-sectional imaging features alone. No communication between the lesion and the pancreatic ductal system is seen. Because this lesion is benign, management is generally conservative unless the lesion is symptomatic or ≥4 cm in size.

27. What are the different types of pancreatic mucinous cystic neoplasms?
    Pancreatic mucinous cystadenoma (and cystadenocarcinoma) is a rare mucinous epithelial pancreatic neoplasm which may range from premalignant to frankly malignant. This tumor most commonly occurs in the pancreatic body or tail and is typically encountered in middle-aged women. On cross-sectional imaging, a unilocular or multilocular cystic lesion in the pancreas is seen, typically containing <6 clustered cystic foci that are >2 cm in size, sometimes with variably increased attenuation, increased T1-weighted signal intensity, or decreased T2-weighted signal intensity of the internal fluid contents (Figure 30-13). Wall thickening, septal thickening, mural nodules, solid enhancing components, or peripheral calcifications may sometimes be present. However, no communication between the lesion

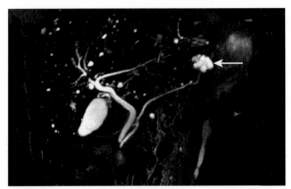

**Figure 30-12.** Pancreatic serous cystadenoma in elderly woman on MRI. Coronal MRCP image shows well-circumscribed cystic lesion (*arrow*) in pancreatic tail composed of multiple (>6) small (<2 cm) clustered cystic foci separated by thin septations.

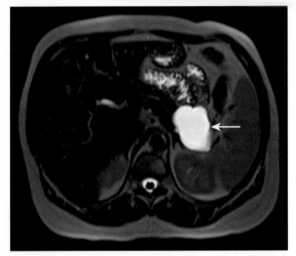

**Figure 30-13.** Pancreatic mucinous cystadenoma in middle-aged woman on MRI. Axial heavily T2-weighted image through abdomen demonstrates large minimally septated cystic lesion (*arrow*) in pancreatic tail.

and the pancreatic ductal system is seen. Mesenteric vascular encasement, regional lymphadenopathy, or distant metastatic disease may be encountered in some patients as well.

Intraductal papillary mucinous neoplasm (IPMN) is an uncommon mucinous epithelial pancreatic neoplasm which may range from premalignant to frankly malignant. This tumor most commonly occurs in the pancreatic head and uncinate process and is often encountered in elderly men. There are two subtypes of IPMN: the main pancreatic duct subtype (which may also involve the side branches) and the side branch subtype; the former is more likely to be malignant than the latter. On cross-sectional imaging, the main pancreatic duct subtype typically appears as segmental or diffuse main pancreatic duct dilation (typically out of proportion to the degree of pancreatic parenchymal atrophy), sometimes with side branch dilation or bulging of the duodenal papilla (Figure 30-14). The side branch subtype typically appears as a unilocular or multilocular cystic lesion in the pancreatic head or uncinate process that communicates with the pancreatic ductal system. Wall thickening, septal thickening, mural nodules, and solid enhancing components may sometimes be present, although calcifications are not generally seen. Patients with pancreatic IPMN also have an increased risk (5% to 10%) of developing a metachronous pancreatic adenocarcinoma in the future.

28. What is pancreatic adenocarcinoma, and what are its CT and MR imaging features?
Pancreatic adenocarcinoma is the most common pancreatic malignancy, the most common cause of a solid pancreatic mass, and the fourth leading cause of cancer death in the United States. It occurs more commonly in men than in women, predominantly occurs in older adults, usually presents with advanced unresectable disease, and is associated with a poor prognosis.

A pancreatic mass with poorly defined borders is seen, sometimes in association with a focal contour abnormality, typically with soft tissue attenuation, low-intermediate signal intensity on T1-weighted images, and intermediate-slightly high signal intensity on T2-weighted images, as well as hypoenhancement on arterial phase contrast-enhanced images (secondary to presence of desmoplastic stroma). Sometimes, cystic or necrotic change

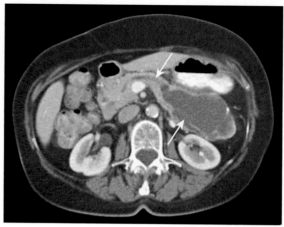

**Figure 30-14.** Pancreatic main duct subtype IPMN on CT. Note dilation of main pancreatic duct (*arrows*), most marked in pancreatic tail, along with some internal septations.

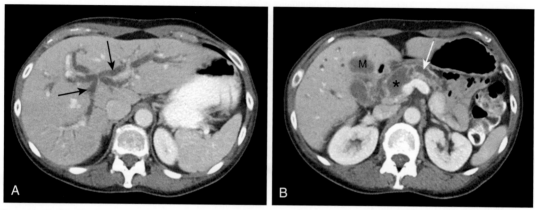

**Figure 30-15.** "Double duct" sign secondary to pancreatic adenocarcinoma on CT. **A,** Note marked dilation of intrahepatic bile ducts (*arrows*). Extrahepatic bile duct dilation was also present (*not shown*). **B,** Note heterogeneous low attenuation mass (*) in pancreatic head secondary to pancreatic adenocarcinoma, associated upstream pancreatic parenchymal atrophy, upstream pancreatic ductal dilation (*arrow*), and heterogeneous hypoattenuating hepatic metastasis (*M*). Simultaneous upstream dilation of biliary tree and main pancreatic duct comprise "double duct" sign.

within the mass may be present, which appears as nonenhancing components with attenuation and signal intensity characteristics similar to fluid. About 70% arise in the pancreatic head, with the remainder occurring in other regions of the pancreas. Associated features such as biliary ductal dilation, upstream pancreatic ductal dilation often with abrupt transition (the "interrupted duct" sign), upstream pancreatic parenchymal atrophy, local invasion of surrounding organs and tissues, regional lymphadenopathy, and distant metastatic disease may sometimes be encountered as well (Figure 30-15).

29. What CT and MR imaging findings indicate unresectability of pancreatic adenocarcinoma?
    - Tumor encasement of the arterial mesenteric vasculature (celiac artery, SMA, common hepatic artery). This is seen as obliteration of the normal fat around an artery, >180° of contact of tumor with an artery, or arterial luminal narrowing on cross-sectional imaging. If there is ≤180° of contact of tumor with an artery or short segment encasement of the common hepatic artery >1 cm from its origin, then the tumor may still be resectable.
    - Tumor encasement of the venous mesenteric vasculature (SMV, portal vein). This is seen as obliteration of the normal fat around a vein, >180° of contact of tumor with a vein, venous luminal narrowing, or a teardrop configuration of the vein on cross-sectional imaging. Dilation of adjacent venous collaterals is also suggestive of unresectable tumor. If there is limited short segment nonocclusive involvement of the vein, then the tumor may still be resectable.
    - Presence of direct tumor invasion of organs (other than the duodenum).
    - Presence of distant metastatic disease (most often encountered in the liver, peritoneum, and nonregional lymph nodes, and less often seen in the lungs and bone marrow) (see Figure 30-15, *B*).

30. What is the "double duct" sign?

The "double duct" sign refers to simultaneous upstream dilation of the biliary tree and main pancreatic duct (see Figure 30-15). This sign is highly suggestive of presence of pancreatic head adenocarcinoma, although other less common etiologies such as an ampulla of Vater carcinoma, cholangiocarcinoma of the distal common bile duct, focal chronic pancreatitis in the pancreatic head, or ampullary stenosis may also lead to this imaging appearance.

31. What are pancreatic neuroendocrine tumors?

Pancreatic neuroendocrine tumors comprise a heterogeneous group of neoplasms that arise from cells of the neuroendocrine system. They all have malignant potential, but may be benign or malignant in their biologic behavior, and are typically associated with a better prognosis than pancreatic adenocarcinomas. Eighty-five percent are symptomatic due to the effects of secreted hormones and are typically detected when small in size, whereas 15% are symptomatic related to mass effect on adjacent abdominal structures and are typically detected when large in size.

On cross-sectional imaging, a pancreatic mass is seen, sometimes in association with a focal contour abnormality, typically with soft tissue attenuation, low-intermediate signal intensity on T1-weighted images, intermediate-slightly high signal intensity on T2-weighted images, as well as hyperenhancement on arterial phase contrast-enhanced images (Figure 30-16). Cystic or necrotic change may sometimes be present, which appears as nonenhancing components with attenuation and signal intensity characteristics similar to fluid. Very high attenuation calcification may sometimes also be seen on CT. In general, small lesions tend to be homogeneous whereas large lesions tend to be heterogeneous in appearance. Associated biliary ductal dilation, upstream pancreatic ductal dilation, upstream pancreatic parenchymal atrophy, local invasion of surrounding organs and tissues, regional lymphadenopathy, and distant metastatic disease may occur, but less commonly than with pancreatic adenocarcinoma. Presence of regional lymphadenopathy or distant metastatic disease indicates that the pancreatic neuroendocrine tumor is malignant in behavior.

32. What are the two most common types of pancreatic neuroendocrine tumor?

Insulinoma is the most common type, which is most often <2 cm in size, solitary, and benign in biologic behavior.

Gastrinoma is the second most common type, which is usually malignant in biologic behavior and most often located in the "gastrinoma triangle" (located between the junction of the pancreatic neck and body medially, the junction of the cystic and common bile ducts superiorly, and the junction of the second and third portions of the duodenum inferiorly).

33. What characteristic clinical presentations are associated with specific types of functional pancreatic neuroendocrine tumors?

For the answer, see Table 30-1.

34. What genetic syndromes may be associated with pancreatic neuroendocrine tumors?

- Multiple endocrine neoplasia (MEN) type I.
- vHL.
- Neurofibromatosis type 1 (NF-1).
- Tuberous sclerosis (TS).

35. What is a pancreatic solid pseudopapillary neoplasm (SPN)?

A pancreatic SPN is a rare neoplasm of low-grade malignant potential, which is typically encountered in young (20- to 30-year-old) women. Eighty-five percent have an indolent biologic behavior, whereas 15% are associated with

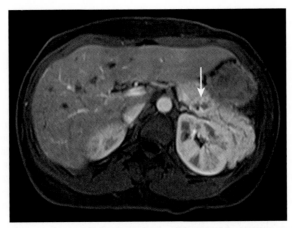

**Figure 30-16.** Pancreatic neuroendocrine tumor on MRI. Axial fat-suppressed arterial phase contrast-enhanced T1-weighted image through abdomen shows mass (*arrow*) in pancreatic tail with hyperenhancement relative to surrounding normal pancreatic parenchyma. Nonenhancing hypointense foci seen in mass represent areas of cystic or necrotic change, leading to its heterogeneous appearance.

**Table 30-1.** Characteristic Clinical Presentations Associated with Specific Types of Functional Pancreatic Neuroendocrine Tumors

| TUMOR TYPE | CLINICAL PRESENTATION |
|---|---|
| Insulinoma | Whipple's triad (fasting hypoglycemia, symptoms of hypoglycemia, and symptomatic relief with intravenous glucose administration) |
| Gastrinoma | Zollinger-Ellison syndrome (severe gastroesophageal reflux disease [GERD], severe peptic ulcer disease [PUD], diarrhea) |
| Glucagonoma | 4D syndrome (<u>d</u>iabetes mellitus, <u>d</u>ermatitis, <u>d</u>eep venous thrombosis [DVT], <u>d</u>epression) |
| VIPoma | WDHA syndrome (<u>w</u>atery <u>d</u>iarrhea, <u>h</u>ypokalemia, <u>a</u>chlorhydria) (where VIP stands for vasoactive intestinal peptide) |
| Somatostatinoma | Inhibitory syndrome (diabetes mellitus or glucose intolerance, cholelithiasis, weight loss, diarrhea ± steatorrhea, hypochlorhydria/achlorhydria) |

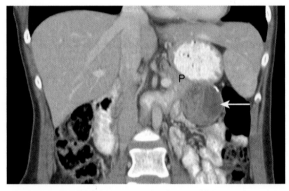

**Figure 30-17.** Pancreatic SPN in young woman on CT. Coronal contrast-enhanced CT image shows heterogeneous well-circumscribed mass (*arrow*) with soft tissue attenuation and fluid attenuation components that arises exophytically from pancreatic tail (*P*). Note very high attenuation peripheral calcification as well.

presence of distant metastatic disease. On cross-sectional imaging, a large round encapsulated mass with cystic and solid enhancing components is typically seen, most often in the pancreatic tail. Very high attenuation calcification may be present in 30% (Figure 30-17). Complete surgical resection is generally performed for treatment.

36. **What are the most common primary tumors that metastasize hematogenously to the pancreas?**
RCC and lung cancer (and less commonly breast cancer and melanoma) are the most common primary tumors that metastasize hematogenously to the pancreas. Metastatic disease involving the pancreas is usually encountered in patients with an advanced stage of malignancy.

## KEY POINTS

- The presence of necrosis and larger amounts of necrosis (particularly when >30% of the pancreas) in the setting of acute pancreatitis are associated with increased patient morbidity and mortality.
- In the setting of pancreatic trauma, the most important factor that determines clinical outcome (and whether or not surgical intervention will be required) is the integrity of the pancreatic duct.
- Pancreatic adenocarcinomas typically hypoenhance during the arterial phase of enhancement relative to the pancreas, whereas pancreatic neuroendocrine tumors typically hyperenhance.
- Pancreatic adenocarcinoma is generally unresectable when there is encasement of the mesenteric vasculature, invasion of organs other than the duodenum, or presence of distant metastatic disease.
- The "double duct" sign is highly suggestive of presence of pancreatic head adenocarcinoma, although other less common etiologies such as an ampulla of Vater carcinoma or focal chronic pancreatitis of the pancreatic head may also be associated with this imaging finding.

**BIBLIOGRAPHY**

Hungerford JP, Neill Magarik MA, Hardie AD. The breadth of imaging findings of groove pancreatitis. *Clin Imaging.* 2015;39(3):363-366.
Al-Hawary MM, Francis IR, Chari ST, et al. Pancreatic ductal adenocarcinoma radiology reporting template: consensus statement of the Society of Abdominal Radiology and the American Pancreatic Association. *Radiology.* 2014;270(1):248-260.

Khandelwal A, Shanbhogue AK, Takahashi N, et al. Recent advances in the diagnosis and management of autoimmune pancreatitis. *AJR Am J Roentgenol.* 2014;202(5):1007-1021.

Borghei P, Sokhandon F, Shirkhoda A, et al. Anomalies, anatomic variants, and sources of diagnostic pitfalls in pancreatic imaging. *Radiology.* 2013;266(1):28-36.

Sahani DV, Bonaffini PA, Fernandez-Del Castillo C, et al. Gastroenteropancreatic neuroendocrine tumors: role of imaging in diagnosis and management. *Radiology.* 2013;266(1):38-61.

Coakley FV, Hanley-Knutson K, Mongan J, et al. Pancreatic imaging mimics: part 1, imaging mimics of pancreatic adenocarcinoma. *AJR Am J Roentgenol.* 2012;199(2):301-308.

Perez-Johnston R, Sainani NI, Sahani DV. Imaging of chronic pancreatitis (including groove and autoimmune pancreatitis). *Radiol Clin North Am.* 2012;50(3):447-466.

Raman SP, Hruban RH, Cameron JL, et al. Pancreatic imaging mimics: part 2, pancreatic neuroendocrine tumors and their mimics. *AJR Am J Roentgenol.* 2012;199(2):309-318.

Tanaka M, Fernandez-del Castillo C, Adsay V, et al. International consensus guidelines 2012 for the management of IPMN and MCN of the pancreas. *Pancreatology.* 2012;12(3):183-197.

Thoeni RF. The revised Atlanta classification of acute pancreatitis: its importance for the radiologist and its effect on treatment. *Radiology.* 2012;262(3):751-764.

Khan A, Khosa F, Eisenberg RL. Cystic lesions of the pancreas. *AJR Am J Roentgenol.* 2011;196(6):W668-W677.

Low G, Panu A, Millo N, et al. Multimodality imaging of neoplastic and nonneoplastic solid lesions of the pancreas. *Radiographics.* 2011;31(4):993-1015.

Berland LL, Silverman SG, Gore RM, et al. Managing incidental findings on abdominal CT: white paper of the ACR incidental findings committee. *J Am Coll Radiol.* 2010;7(10):754-773.

Lewis RB, Lattin GE Jr, Paal E. Pancreatic endocrine tumors: radiologic-clinicopathologic correlation. *Radiographics.* 2010;30(6):1445-1464.

Sandrasegaran K, Patel A, Fogel EL, et al. Annular pancreas in adults. *AJR Am J Roentgenol.* 2009;193(2):455-460.

Leung RS, Biswas SV, Duncan M, et al. Imaging features of von Hippel-Lindau disease. *Radiographics.* 2008;28(1):65-79, quiz 323.

Linsenmaier U, Wirth S, Reiser M, et al. Diagnosis and classification of pancreatic and duodenal injuries in emergency radiology. *Radiographics.* 2008;28(6):1591-1602.

Ahualli J. The double duct sign. *Radiology.* 2007;244(1):314-315.

Cooper JA. Solid pseudopapillary tumor of the pancreas. *Radiographics.* 2006;26(4):1210.

Yu J, Turner MA, Fulcher AS, et al. Congenital anomalies and normal variants of the pancreaticobiliary tract and the pancreas in adults: part 2, pancreatic duct and pancreas. *AJR Am J Roentgenol.* 2006;187(6):1544-1553.

Macari M, Lazarus D, Israel G, et al. Duodenal diverticula mimicking cystic neoplasms of the pancreas: CT and MR imaging findings in seven patients. *AJR Am J Roentgenol.* 2003;180(1):195-199.

Moore EE, Cogbill TH, Malangoni MA, et al. Organ injury scaling, II: pancreas, duodenum, small bowel, colon, and rectum. *J Trauma.* 1990;30(11):1427-1429.

# CHAPTER 31

# CT AND MRI OF THE PERITONEUM, OMENTUM, AND MESENTERY

*Drew A. Torigian, MD, MA, FSAR*

1. ### What is the peritoneum?

   The peritoneum is the largest and most complexly arranged serous membrane in the body. It is closed in men and open to the ends of the fallopian tubes in women. The parietal layer lines the abdominal wall, whereas the visceral layer lines the visceral organs. It contains a potential space, the peritoneal space, which normally contains a small amount of fluid. Its major function is to provide for unimpeded activity and mobility of contained viscera, although it also has absorptive and immune functions.

2. ### What are peritoneal ligaments, small bowel mesentery, mesocolon, and omentum?

   The various "ligaments" of the peritoneum are actually peritoneal reflections that may contain fat, blood vessels, nerves, lymphatics, and lymph nodes.

   The small bowel mesentery is a double-layered fold of visceral peritoneum that contains subperitoneal fat, mesenteric blood vessels, nerves, lymphatics, and lymph nodes and connects the small bowel to the posterior body wall, extending from the left upper quadrant at the ligament of Treitz to the right lower quadrant at the ileocecal valve.

   The mesocolon is similarly a double-layered fold of visceral peritoneum that connects intraperitoneal portions of the large bowel (i.e., the transverse colon and sigmoid colon) to the posterior body wall.

   The lesser omentum is a double-layered peritoneal fold comprised of the gastrohepatic and hepatoduodenal ligaments that extends from the lesser curvature of the stomach and first portion of the duodenum to the liver.

   The greater omentum is a large peritoneal fold comprised of the gastrosplenic and gastrocolic ligaments. It hangs from the greater curvature of the stomach in the anterior abdomen, folds upon itself, and then heads superiorly and posteriorly to attach to the posterior abdominal wall just superior to the attachment of the transverse mesocolon. Its redundant portion in the anterior abdomen fuses to itself during development inferior to the level of the transverse colon and is therefore comprised of 4 layers of visceral peritoneum. A portion of the greater omentum also extends between the stomach and spleen.

   The peritoneal ligaments, small bowel mesentery, mesocolon, and omentum are often involved by disease processes and may serve as either barriers to or conduits of disease spread.

3. ### What is the anatomy of the abdominal peritoneal cavity?

   The abdominal peritoneal cavity can be divided into supramesocolic and inframesocolic compartments, where the former is located superior to the transverse mesocolon and the latter is located inferior to the transverse mesocolon. The supramesocolic component is further subdivided into the subphrenic space (located inferior to the diaphragm), the subhepatic space (located inferior to the liver), and the lesser sac (located anterior to the pancreas and posterior to the stomach). The lesser sac communicates with the greater sac (which includes the subphrenic, subhepatic, infracolic, and paracolic spaces) via the foramen of Winslow (also called the epiploic foramen), which is located posterior to the hepatoduodenal ligament and anterior to the inferior vena cava. The inframesocolic component is further subdivided into the infracolic spaces (located medial to the ascending and descending portions of the large bowel and lateral to the small bowel mesentery) and the paracolic spaces (located lateral to the ascending and descending portions of the large bowel).

4. ### What is the anatomy of the pelvic peritoneal cavity?

   The pelvic peritoneal cavity can be divided into paravesical and rectovesical spaces. The paravesical space is further subdivided into the supravesical space (located superior to the bladder and medial to the medial umbilical folds), the medial inguinal fossae (located lateral to the medial umbilical folds and medial to the lateral umbilical folds), and the lateral inguinal fossae (located lateral to the lateral umbilical folds). The median umbilical fold of parietal peritoneum is located anteriorly in the midline adjacent to the obliterated urachus (also called the median umbilical ligament), whereas the paired medial umbilical folds of parietal peritoneum are adjacent to the obliterated umbilical arteries (also called the medial umbilical ligaments) and the paired lateral umbilical folds of parietal peritoneum are adjacent to the inferior epigastric vessels.

   In men, the rectovesical space is located between the rectum and the bladder. In women, the rectovesical space is further subdivided into the vesicouterine space (located between the uterus and bladder) and the rectouterine pouch of Douglas (located between the uterus and rectum).

**Table 31-1.** Nonparenchymal Cystic Lesions of the Abdomen and Pelvis

| | |
|---|---|
| Lymphatic origin | Urogenital cysts |
|    Simple lymphatic cyst | Other developmental lesions |
|    Lymphangioma |    Epidermoid cyst |
| Mesothelial origin |    Dermoid cyst |
|    Simple mesothelial cyst |    Mature cystic teratoma |
|    Benign cystic mesothelioma |    Lymphangioleiomyomatosis |
| Enteric origin |    Neurogenous choristoma |
|    Enteric duplication cyst | Pseudocysts and other loculated fluid collections |
|    Enteric cyst | Cystic or necrotic lymphadenopathy |
| Foregut origin | Cystic or necrotic neoplasms |
|    Bronchogenic cyst | Retained surgical sponge |
|    Extralobar pulmonary sequestration | |
| Hindgut origin | |
|    Tailgut cyst | |

5. What is the differential diagnosis for nonparenchymal cystic lesions in the abdomen and pelvis?

Nonparenchymal cystic lesions may infrequently be encountered in the omentum, mesentery, mesocolon, or retroperitoneum and are most often incidentally detected. For answers, see Table 31-1.

6. List some potential complications that may occur with nonparenchymal cystic lesions.

Potential complications include growth, hemorrhage, superinfection, torsion, rupture, and bowel obstruction. Whereas imaging surveillance may suffice for stable small asymptomatic nonaggressive-appearing cystic lesions, surgical resection may be performed to prevent potential complications, particularly for large or symptomatic lesions.

7. Are there any distinctive CT and MR imaging features of specific types of nonparenchymal cystic lesions?

Some imaging features listed below are useful to suggest specific types of nonparenchymal cystic lesions. Otherwise, there is much overlap in the CT and MR imaging appearance of nonparenchymal cystic lesions.

Lymphangiomas, benign cystic mesotheliomas, and tailgut cysts are typically multilocular, whereas simple lymphatic, simple mesothelial, enteric duplication, enteric, bronchogenic, epidermoid, and dermoid cysts are typically unilocular. Enteric duplication cysts have diffusely thickened walls because they contain all of the normal bowel wall layers, whereas enteric cysts have thin walls because they are lined only by enteric mucosa.

Enteric duplication cysts and enteric cysts are typically located adjacent to bowel loops, extrathoracic bronchogenic cysts and extralobar pulmonary sequestration are typically located in the subdiaphragmatic retroperitoneum, and tailgut cysts are typically retrorectal in location.

Mature cystic teratoma may contain fat attenuation or fat signal intensity components, whereas cystic or necrotic lymphadenopathy and cystic or necrotic neoplasms typically have residual soft tissue enhancing components.

Hemorrhagic fluid collections typically have nonenhancing high attenuation and high T1-weighted signal intensity fluid, sometimes with a hematocrit effect due to layering of cellular components of blood. Uriniferous fluid collections will characteristically be associated with leakage of excreted intravenous contrast material from the urothelium during the delayed phase of enhancement. Enteric and infectious fluid collections sometimes contain foci of very low attenuation and very low signal intensity gas.

8. What are the major causes of transudative ascites?

Hepatic failure, cirrhosis, renal failure, heart failure, and hypoproteinemia are the major causes of transudative ascites.

9. What are the major causes of exudative ascites?

Peritoneal malignancy, bowel perforation, infection, and noninfectious inflammatory disease conditions such as pancreatitis or peritonitis are the major causes of exudative ascites.

10. Are there CT and MR imaging features that can distinguish between transudative and exudative ascites?

Transudative ascites generally has water attenuation, low signal intensity on T1-weighted images, and very high signal intensity on T2-weighted images similar to fluid elsewhere in the body, is nonloculated, and tends to accumulate to a greater degree in the greater sac than in the lesser sac (Figure 31-1).

Exudative ascites has variably increased attenuation relative to fluid elsewhere in the body, variably increased signal intensity on T1-weighted images, and variably decreased signal intensity on T2-weighted images. Loculations, peritoneal thickening, and peritoneal enhancement are commonly seen as well. Fluid accumulation to a similar degree in both the greater and larger sacs favors a malignant etiology of ascites, whereas fluid accumulation to a greater degree in the lesser sac than in the greater sac favors inflammatory ascites related to pancreatitis.

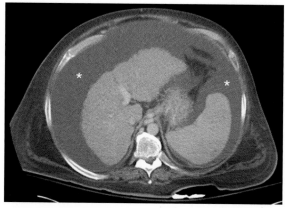

**Figure 31-1.** Transudative ascites on CT. Note large amount of water attenuation fluid (*) within greater sac of peritoneal cavity without loculations, peritoneal thickening, or peritoneal enhancement. Also note nodular contour of liver in keeping with cirrhosis.

| **Table 31-2.** Specific Types of Fluid Collection | |
| --- | --- |
| Simple | Enteric |
| Proteinaceous | Infectious |
| Hemorrhagic | Inflammatory noninfectious |
| Chylous | Malignant |
| Uriniferous | |

11. What specific types of fluid collection may occur?
    For the answer, see Table 31-2.

12. What are the major causes of pneumoperitoneum?
    Pneumoperitoneum (i.e., gas in the peritoneal cavity) is most often due to bowel perforation involving the intraperitoneal portions of bowel (i.e., the stomach, first portion of the duodenum, jejunum, ileum, cecum, transverse colon, sigmoid colon, and upper rectum) and recent abdominopelvic surgery. It is less commonly due to peritoneal infection, peritoneal dialysis, gastrostomy tube placement, rupture of pneumatosis cystoides intestinalis, rapid decompression after diving, extension of gas from the thorax (such as during mechanical ventilation), and extension of gas through the female genital tract (such as during pelvic physical examination). Very low attenuation and very low signal intensity gas within the peritoneal cavity is seen on CT and MR images, respectively (Figure 31-2).

13. What is pseudomyxoma peritonei, and what are its CT and MR imaging features?
    Pseudomyxoma peritonei is a rare condition where mucinous ascites arises from rupture of a mucinous appendiceal adenoma. It has a strong association with synchronous or metachronous colorectal adenoma and carcinoma, such that surveillance of the entire large bowel is warranted. Loculated ascites is typically seen with low attenuation, low-intermediate signal intensity on T1-weighted images, and high signal intensity on T2-weighted images relative to skeletal muscle. Thickened walls, internal septations, and scalloping of parenchymal organs such as the liver and spleen are often seen, sometimes with very high attenuation calcifications. However, lymphadenopathy and distant metastatic disease are absent.

14. What is peritoneal carcinomatosis, and what are its CT and MR imaging features?
    Peritoneal carcinomatosis is a more common condition due to the peritoneal spread of carcinoma. Common sites of origin include the ovary, stomach, large bowel, and pancreas, although any carcinoma can potentially spread to the peritoneal space. Complex ascites with variable attenuation and signal intensity properties may be seen, often in association with peritoneal, mesenteric, or omental masses or infiltrative soft tissue, as well as diffuse peritoneal thickening and enhancement (Figure 31-3). Very high attenuation calcifications may also sometimes be present. A primary tumor, along with lymphadenopathy or distant metastatic disease, may also be seen.

15. What is malignant peritoneal mesothelioma, and what are its CT and MR imaging features?
    Malignant peritoneal mesothelioma is a rare mesothelial neoplasm arising from the peritoneum. It is two to five times less common than malignant pleural mesothelioma and is more weakly associated with prior asbestos exposure. Nonspecific peritoneal, mesenteric, or omental thickening, nodularity, or mass formation is seen, indistinguishable from other peritoneal malignancies. Complex ascites may also be seen. Patients with small tumor nodules preferentially involving the greater omentum, free ascites, or minimal to absent small bowel/mesenteric involvement have a more favorable prognosis compared to those with larger soft tissue dissemination along the peritoneum or with entrapment/clumping of the small bowel.

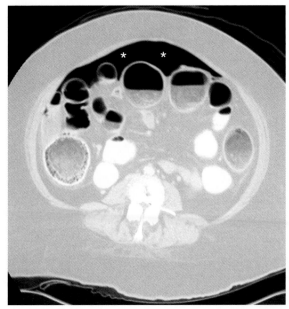

**Figure 31-2.** Pneumoperitoneum on CT. Note very low attenuation gas (*) within nondependent portion of abdominal peritoneal cavity that partially surrounds loops of bowel. This was due to cecal perforation secondary to large bowel obstruction caused by sigmoid colon cancer (*not shown*).

16. What is primary peritoneal carcinoma (PPC), and how can one distinguish this from peritoneal spread of ovarian cancer on CT and MR imaging?

    PPC is an uncommon malignancy that arises from the peritoneum, occurs in up to 7% of patients with suspected epithelial ovarian cancer, and predominantly affects postmenopausal women. Although the CT and MR imaging features of peritoneal involvement are identical to those that may be encountered with peritoneal spread of other cancers including ovarian cancer, PPC is more likely than ovarian cancer when no ovarian mass or enlargement is visualized.

17. What is intraabdominal desmoplastic small round cell tumor (DSRCT), and what are its CT and MR imaging features?

    Intraabdominal DSRCT is a rare highly aggressive malignant neoplasm, which predominantly affects adolescent and young adult males. Multiple nonspecific infiltrative soft tissue masses involving the peritoneum, omentum, or mesentery are seen, sometimes with ascites.

18. What is sclerosing mesenteritis?

    Sclerosing mesenteritis is a rare idiopathic fibroinflammatory disorder that affects the small bowel mesentery. Variable amounts of mesenteric inflammation, fat necrosis, and fibrosis are present, and treatment is generally conservative, most often with watchful waiting.

19. What are the CT and MR imaging features of sclerosing mesenteritis?

    Subtle infiltration of the mesenteric fat is typically seen, along with slightly low signal intensity on T1-weighted images, slightly high signal intensity on T2-weighted images, and mild delayed phase enhancement relative to other fat in the body. It is located predominantly in the left abdomen in the majority of cases, and preservation of the fat about the mesenteric vessels (i.e., the "fat ring" sign) is seen in 75% of cases. Mildly prominent mesenteric lymph nodes are also seen, sometimes with preservation of the surrounding fat, and a thin enhancing peripheral pseudocapsule may also be visualized (Figure 31-4). In some cases, a nonspecific well-circumscribed or infiltrative soft tissue mesenteric mass is present, which may be calcified and may tether or have mass effect upon adjacent small bowel loops.

20. What is pelvic lipomatosis?

    Pelvic lipomatosis is a rare idiopathic disorder characterized by benign hyperplastic overgrowth of pelvic extraperitoneal fatty tissue. It most often occurs in African American men and is associated with compression of the lower urinary tract and rectosigmoid colon. Patients have an increased risk of proliferative cystitis and bladder adenocarcinoma, and ≈40% require urinary diversion to prevent renal failure from obstructive uropathy.

21. What are the CT and MR imaging features of pelvic lipomatosis?

    Increased homogeneous nonencapsulated perivesical and perirectal pelvic visceral fat is seen, which surrounds the pelvic organs symmetrically. Superior displacement, a pear shape, or an inverted teardrop shape of the bladder,

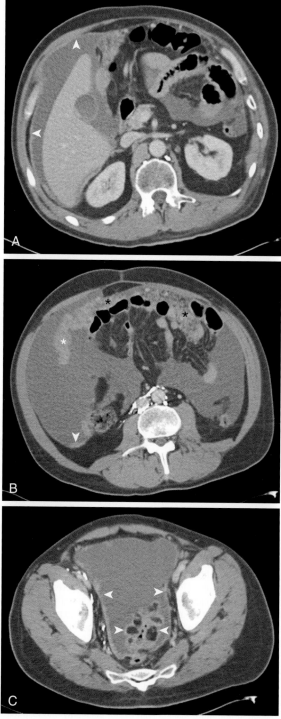

**Figure 31-3.** Peritoneal carcinomatosis on CT. **A-C,** Note areas of nodular peritoneal thickening and enhancement (*arrowheads*) in abdomen and pelvis, as well as soft tissue infiltration of omentum (i.e., omental caking) (*) and moderate exudative ascites due to peritoneal spread of lung cancer.

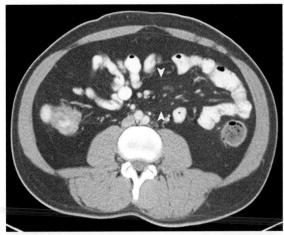

**Figure 31-4.** Sclerosing mesenteritis on CT. Note subtle infiltration of mesenteric fat compared to surrounding fat in left abdomen (*between arrowheads*). Mildly prominent mesenteric lymph nodes are also present.

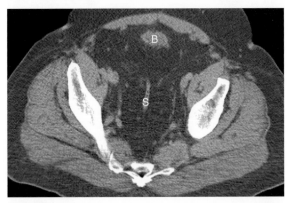

**Figure 31-5.** Pelvic lipomatosis on CT. Note increased amount of pelvic visceral fat with anterior displacement of urinary bladder (*B*) and smooth extrinsic narrowing of sigmoid colon (*S*).

superior displacement of the prostate gland, and smooth narrowing of the rectosigmoid colon are also characteristically seen. Unilateral or bilateral hydroureteronephrosis may also occur (Figure 31-5).

22. What is a desmoid tumor?

A desmoid tumor is an uncommon bland fibrous neoplasm that may arise sporadically or in association with familial adenomatous polyposis (FAP). Patients with FAP are at a thousand-fold increased risk of developing intraabdominal desmoid tumors, and patients who have had prior abdominal surgery are at increased risk for abdominal wall desmoid tumors. Sporadic intraabdominal desmoid tumors are more common in women, are solitary in >90% of cases, tend to be larger in size, and predominantly affect the pelvis and retroperitoneum. FAP-associated intraabdominal desmoid tumors are equally common in men and women, are multiple in 40% of cases, tend to be smaller in size, and predominantly affect the small bowel mesentery.

23. What are the CT and MR imaging features of desmoid tumors?

One or more well-circumscribed or infiltrative enhancing masses with soft tissue attenuation and low-intermediate signal intensity on T1-weighted and T2-weighted images are seen (Figure 31-6). High signal intensity on T2-weighted images may sometimes be seen in immature lesions with higher cellularity and less mature fibrosis. Associated findings of bowel or ureteral obstruction may be present as well. Occasionally, mesenteric desmoid tumors form a fistula with a bowel loop, where gas, fluid, or oral contrast material may be seen within the mass centrally.

24. What are the major types of peritonitis?

Infectious peritonitis is the most common type, and it is usually bacterial and less commonly mycobacterial or fungal in nature. Chemical (sterile) peritonitis is caused by irritant materials such as hemorrhage, bile, enteric fluid contents, contrast material, or other substances without peritoneal infection. Intraperitoneal rupture of a mature teratoma, familial Mediterranean fever (recurrent polyserositis), rheumatoid arthritis, and systemic lupus erythematosus are other sterile causes of peritonitis.

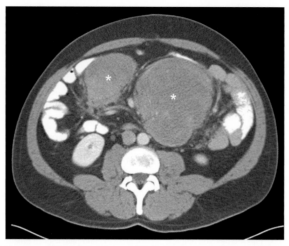

**Figure 31-6.** Mesenteric desmoid tumors on CT. Note two large mildly heterogeneous soft tissue attenuation mesenteric masses (*). Also note absence of colon in this patient with history of FAP.

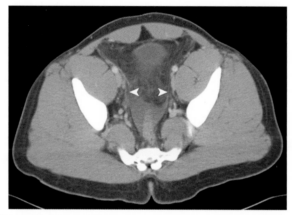

**Figure 31-7.** Peritonitis on CT. Note pelvic peritoneal thickening and enhancement (*arrowheads*) along with small ascites and subtle infiltration of pelvic visceral fat in this patient with acute appendicitis (*not shown*).

25. What are some differences between primary and secondary bacterial peritonitis?

Primary bacterial peritonitis (also known as spontaneous bacterial peritonitis) occurs without a known source of infection, particularly in patients with decompensated cirrhosis, and is usually monobacterial in nature. Secondary bacterial peritonitis is due to loss of integrity of the gastrointestinal or genitourinary tract with associated infection of the peritoneal space and is usually polymicrobial in etiology.

26. What are the CT and MR imaging features of peritonitis?

Peritoneal thickening and peritoneal enhancement are typically seen, often with presence of associated ascites (Figure 31-7). Findings of cirrhosis or portal hypertension may be seen in patients with primary bacterial peritonitis, whereas findings of other abdominopelvic pathology involving the gastrointestinal or genitourinary tract may be seen in patients with secondary bacterial peritonitis.

27. What is sclerosing encapsulating peritonitis, and what are its CT and MR imaging features?

Sclerosing encapsulating peritonitis is a rare but severe condition characterized by progressive peritoneal fibrosis, inflammation, calcification, and vascular alterations, with partial or total encasement of the small bowel. It is multifactorial in etiology but is most commonly associated with chronic ambulatory peritoneal dialysis. Often, one portion of the abdomen is more affected than others, forming a mass or "abdominal cocoon" usually containing small bowel loops and ascites. This condition generally has a poor prognosis due to bowel obstruction, malnutrition, septicemia, or postoperative complications.

Very high attenuation and very low signal intensity visceral and parietal peritoneal surfaces are seen due to peritoneal calcification or ossification. Diffuse smooth peritoneal thickening, peritoneal enhancement, loculated ascites, and adherent dilated loops of small bowel, sometimes with gas-fluid levels and wall thickening, may also be seen.

## KEY POINTS

- The most common cause of peritoneal malignancy is peritoneal spread of tumor. Other less common causes include pseudomyxoma peritonei, malignant peritoneal mesothelioma, primary peritoneal carcinoma, and intraabdominal desmoplastic small round cell tumor.
- Visualization of peritoneal thickening and enhancement in a patient with cirrhosis is suggestive of primary (spontaneous) bacterial peritonitis until proven otherwise.
- Pneumoperitoneum is most often due to bowel perforation involving the intraperitoneal portions of bowel and recent abdominopelvic surgery.

**BIBLIOGRAPHY**

Torigian DA, Kitazono MT. *Netter's correlative imaging: abdominal and pelvic anatomy.* 1st ed. Philadephia: Elsevier; 2013:1-499.

Torigian DA, Ramchandani P. CT and MRI of the retroperitoneum. In: Haaga JR, Lanzieri CF, Gilkeson RC, eds. *CT and MRI of the whole body.* 5th ed. Philadelphia: Elsevier; 2009:1953-2040.

Torigian DA, Siegelman ES. MRI of the retroperitoneum and peritoneum. In: Siegelman ES, ed. *Body MRI.* 1st ed. Philadelphia: WB Saunders; 2005:207-268.

Healy JC, Reznek RH. The peritoneum, mesenteries and omenta: normal anatomy and pathological processes. *Eur Radiol.* 1998;8(6):886-900.

Auh YH, Rubenstein WA, Markisz JA, et al. Intraperitoneal paravesical spaces: CT delineation with US correlation. *Radiology.* 1986;159(2):311-317.

# CHAPTER 32

# CT AND MRI OF THE ACUTE ABDOMEN AND PELVIS

*Drew A. Torigian, MD, MA, FSAR*

1. **Why is computed tomography (CT) commonly used initially for diagnostic purposes in patients with an acute abdomen or pelvis?**

   Accurate and timely diagnosis of life-threatening disease involving the abdomen and pelvis is essential to decrease potential morbidity and mortality. Clinical evaluation is sometimes difficult, and laboratory analysis and radiographic findings are not always useful in diagnosing the condition at hand. CT imaging of the abdomen and pelvis is a reliable, highly accurate, and fast imaging diagnostic modality for the evaluation of symptomatic patients. It is most useful in patients with a clinical presentation that is unrevealing or confusing. CT allows for direct visualization of anatomic structures in the abdomen and pelvis, along with detection and characterization of the nature and extent of disease, when present.

2. **When is magnetic resonance imaging (MRI) used for diagnostic purposes in patients with an acute abdomen or pelvis?**

   MRI is typically used as a problem-solving diagnostic modality following initial CT or ultrasonography (US) evaluation of patients with acute symptoms or signs of abdominopelvic disease, given its longer image acquisition times and greater expense. However, it is often utilized following nondiagnostic US for the evaluation of pregnant women who present with an acute abdomen or pelvis, given its lack of ionizing radiation. Furthermore, it is being utilized more and more often as the initial diagnostic test in many nonpregnant patients who present with an acute abdomen or pelvis, given its superior soft tissue contrast resolution (even when intravenous contrast material is not administered) and lack of ionizing radiation relative to CT.

3. **When are oral and intravenous contrast materials for CT and MRI administered to patients with an acute abdomen or pelvis?**

   Oral contrast material distends and opacifies the bowel, allowing for better characterization of bowel pathologic conditions and separation of bowel structures from nonbowel structures. Intravenous contrast material aids in the characterization of pathologic lesions and allows for opacification and evaluation of vascular and urothelial structures. Both types of contrast material are generally administered in patients with an acute abdomen or pelvis prior to CT scanning whenever possible. In patients with a history of intravenous contrast allergy or renal insufficiency, intravenous contrast material is generally not administered, unless the patient has received a corticosteroid preparation or is scheduled to undergo dialysis after the CT examination. In patients with suspected urolithiasis, unenhanced CT without oral or intravenous contrast material is generally performed because unenhanced images are often sufficient for making a diagnosis. In patients undergoing CT angiography evaluation of the arterial vasculature, oral contrast material is generally not administered because it can obscure normal vessels and vascular pathologic conditions during multiplanar image reconstruction.

   Oral contrast material is not routinely administered to patients undergoing MRI examination in the acute setting because the improved soft tissue contrast resolution allows for good visualization of the bowel wall and lumen. Intravenous gadolinium-based contrast material is routinely administered to patients undergoing MRI examination of the abdomen or pelvis in the acute setting. However, if there is a history of intravenous contrast allergy, renal insufficiency, or pregnancy, it is not administered.

4. **What is the major differential diagnosis for acute abdominopelvic conditions that can be diagnosed on CT and MRI?**

   This is a broad but important differential diagnosis, with representative etiologies as follows.
   - Inflammatory/infectious causes include acute hepatitis; acute cholecystitis; acute cholangitis; acute pancreatitis; acute pyelonephritis; peptic ulcer disease; acute infectious or inflammatory gastritis, enteritis, or colitis; acute diverticulitis; acute appendicitis; mesenteric lymphadenitis; peritonitis; epiploic appendagitis; segmental omental infarction; pelvic inflammatory disease (PID); abdominal or pelvic abscess; and Fournier gangrene.
   - Vascular causes include solid organ or neoplasm infarction; bowel (mesenteric) ischemia/infarction; hemorrhage (whether spontaneous or into a cyst or neoplasm); abdominal aortic aneurysm (AAA) rupture; abdominal aortic dissection or penetrating aortic ulcer; acute vascular occlusion; and adnexal torsion.
   - Traumatic causes include solid organ injury; hollow organ injury; and vascular injury.
   - Other causes include hollow organ (bowel, biliary tree, urothelial system) obstruction; bowel perforation; solid organ rupture; cyst or neoplasm rupture; abdominal compartment syndrome (ACS); and ectopic pregnancy.

5. What is an abscess, and what are its CT and MR imaging features?

An abscess is a loculated collection of pus.

On CT and MRI, an abscess appears as a complex loculated fluid collection that may contain debris, complex fluid, or hemorrhage with increased attenuation and T1-weighted signal intensity, sometimes with internal septations or very low attenuation/signal intensity gas bubbles. An abscess often has a thick enhancing rim of fibrous tissue peripherally (Figure 32-1). When an abscess arises within a parenchymal organ, multiple small adjacent abscesses (i.e., "satellite lesions") are also commonly encountered.

6. What is acute appendicitis?

Acute appendicitis is inflammation of the appendix that occurs after luminal obstruction, and it is one of the most common causes of acute abdominopelvic pain. Patients commonly present with right lower quadrant pain and tenderness, nausea, vomiting, fever, and leukocytosis. Early and accurate diagnosis with CT or MRI helps to minimize morbidity and mortality owing to appendiceal perforation and prevents unnecessary surgery for nonsurgical conditions that may mimic the clinical presentation of appendicitis. MRI is most often utilized when acute appendicitis is suspected in the setting of pregnancy.

7. Describe the CT and MR imaging features of acute appendicitis.

The most specific imaging finding is an abnormal appendix that is typically dilated to ≥6 mm and fluid-filled (Figures 32-2 and 32-3). Visualization of a calcified appendicolith (best seen on CT) with associated periappendiceal inflammatory fat stranding or edema is also highly specific. Other imaging findings may include:

- Hyperenhancement of the appendiceal wall.
- Thickening of the appendiceal wall (≥3 mm), sometimes with low attenuation/high T2-weighted signal intensity submucosal edema in the wall (leading to mural stratification or a "target" sign).

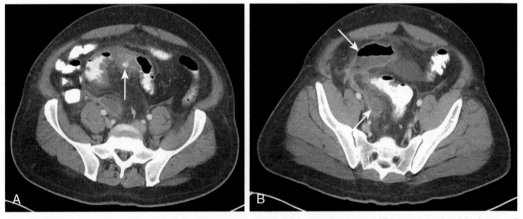

**Figure 32-1.** Acute sigmoid diverticulitis with abscess formation on CT. **A,** Axial contrast-enhanced CT image through pelvis shows wall thickening and enhancement of sigmoid diverticulum (*arrow*), segmental wall thickening of adjacent sigmoid colon, and pericolic fat stranding. **B,** Axial contrast-enhanced CT image more inferiorly through pelvis demonstrates two loculated fluid collections (*arrows*) with thick enhancing rims in right pelvis, one of which contains gas, in keeping with abscesses.

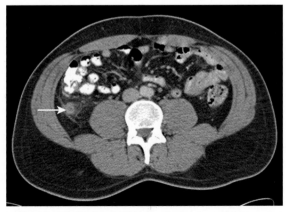

**Figure 32-2.** Acute appendicitis on CT. Axial contrast-enhanced CT image through lower abdomen reveals wall thickening and dilation of appendix (*arrow*) with periappendiceal inflammatory fat stranding.

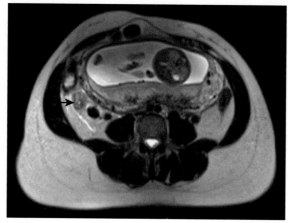

**Figure 32-3.** Acute appendicitis in setting of pregnancy on MRI. Axial T2-weighted MR image through lower abdomen shows wall thickening of appendix (*arrow*) with periappendiceal edema. Note intrauterine gestation as well.

- Reactive thickening of adjacent cecum or small bowel.
- Arrowhead-shaped funneling of the cecal apex toward the occluded appendiceal lumen ("arrowhead" sign).
- A curved soft tissue structure between the cecal lumen and an appendicolith, which is representative of an inflamed cecal or appendiceal wall ("cecal bar" sign).
- Periappendiceal fluid.
- Thickening and enhancement of the adjacent parietal peritoneum representing focal peritonitis.

Complications include appendiceal perforation with abscess formation, small bowel obstruction, and mesenteric venous thrombosis.

8. What is tip appendicitis?
In some patients, only the distal aspect of the appendix is inflamed, which is known as tip appendicitis. Therefore, the entirety of the appendix must be imaged and assessed on CT or MRI in patients with acute abdominopelvic symptoms to avoid missing this often subtle diagnosis.

9. What is acute large bowel diverticulitis, and what are its CT and MR imaging features?
Acute diverticulitis involving the large bowel is inflammation/infection in the setting of large bowel diverticulosis (i.e., the presence of multiple outpouchings of the wall of the large bowel). This condition most commonly occurs in elderly adults, most commonly (95%) in the distal descending and sigmoid colon, and much less commonly (5%) in the ascending colon and cecum. Patients present with fever, abdominal pain (often in the left lower quadrant), and leukocytosis.

CT and MRI findings include pericolic inflammatory fat stranding, thickening and enhancement of an inflamed diverticulum, inflammatory segmental wall thickening of the large bowel, pericolic gas bubbles owing to bowel microperforation, and pericolic fluid. Potential complications include abdominal or pelvic abscess formation, mesenteric or portal vein thrombosis or gas, bowel obstruction, and fistula formation between the affected large bowel segment and the bladder, vagina, small bowel, other portion of large bowel, or skin (see Figure 32-1).

10. Describe acute mesenteric lymphadenitis and its associated CT and MR imaging features.
Acute mesenteric lymphadenitis is a self-limited condition resulting from inflammation of ileal mesenteric lymph nodes, sometimes with associated terminal ileal and cecal inflammation. It often manifests with right lower quadrant pain and diarrhea and most often occurs in children and young adults. The most common causative agents include the bacteria *Campylobacter jejuni* and *Yersinia* species, although viruses may also be causative.

Characteristic CT and MRI findings include a cluster of three or more enlarged (≥5 mm) right lower quadrant mesenteric lymph nodes, sometimes with associated thickening of the cecum or terminal ileum, and a normal-appearing appendix.

11. Describe primary epiploic appendagitis (PEA) and segmental omental infarction and their associated CT and MR imaging features.
PEA and segmental omental infarction are self-limited conditions that often manifest with focal severe acute abdominal pain and tenderness and are treated with conservative therapy (e.g., analgesics). PEA is related to torsion, inflammation, and ischemia of an epiploic appendage, and segmental omental infarction is related to spontaneous infarction of a portion of the omentum.

CT and MRI findings of PEA include a small (1 to 5 cm) round or oval pedunculated fat attenuation/signal intensity structure with a soft tissue enhancing rim located adjacent to the serosal surface of the large bowel (in the expected location of an epiploic appendage), commonly with a high attenuation/low signal intensity central dot or line from thrombosis of a central vein or fibrosis. Associated inflammatory fat stranding and reactive bowel wall or peritoneal thickening may also be seen (Figure 32-4). PEA occurs most commonly adjacent to the sigmoid colon.

CT and MRI findings of segmental omental infarction include a large (5 to 10 cm) well-circumscribed focus of fat attenuation/signal intensity with associated inflammatory fat stranding. Typically, the infarction is located in the right anterolateral aspect of the abdomen between the colon and parietal peritoneum at or above the umbilical level (in the expected location of the greater omentum).

12. What is acute cholecystitis?

Acute cholecystitis is inflammation of the gallbladder wall owing to obstruction of the cystic duct or gallbladder neck. This is most often caused by gallstones (calculous cholecystitis), although in 5% to 10% of cases, gallstones are not present (acalculous cholecystitis). Acalculous cholecystitis tends to occur in the setting of prolonged illness, such as with prior traumatic or burn injury or with a prolonged intensive care unit stay. Most patients present with right upper quadrant pain and tenderness (Murphy sign), although in the setting of severe advanced inflammation, diabetes mellitus, or elderly age, these clinical findings may be less severe or absent. Treatment generally involves cholecystectomy (or percutaneous cholecystostomy for patients at high surgical risk) along with antimicrobial therapy.

13. List the CT and MR imaging findings of acute cholecystitis.

CT and MRI findings include smooth or irregular gallbladder wall thickening, generally ≥4 mm in thickness (sometimes with decreased attenuation/high T2-weighted signal intensity because of edema); gallbladder distention (>5 cm in width); pericholecystic inflammatory fat stranding or fluid; gallstones or gallbladder sludge; increased gallbladder wall enhancement; and transiently increased late arterial phase enhancement of the adjacent liver parenchyma owing to the inflammatory process (Figure 32-5). Both CT and MRI have high sensitivity and specificity for the diagnosis of acute cholecystitis. Note that only ≈75% of gallstones are detected on CT, whereas >95% are visualized on MRI.

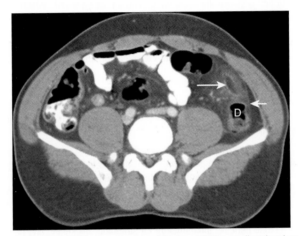

**Figure 32-4.** PEA on CT. Axial contrast-enhanced CT image through pelvis demonstrates small oval pedunculated fat attenuation structure with soft tissue enhancing rim (*long arrow*) and surrounding inflammatory fat stranding adjacent to descending colon (*D*). Also note thickening of adjacent parietal peritoneum (*short arrow*) secondary to reactive peritonitis.

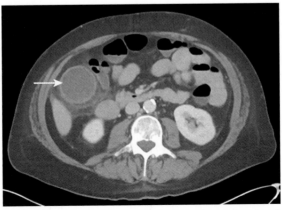

**Figure 32-5.** Acute cholecystitis on CT. Axial contrast-enhanced CT image through abdomen reveals wall thickening and distention of gallbladder (*arrow*) along with pericholecystic inflammatory fat stranding.

14. **What is gangrenous cholecystitis, and what are its CT and MR imaging features?**
    Gangrenous cholecystitis is a severe, advanced form of acute cholecystitis with ischemic necrosis of the gallbladder wall, which is associated with a higher rate of gallbladder perforation. This cholecystitis occurs more commonly in elderly men and in individuals with preexisting cardiovascular disease.
    CT and MRI findings include marked gallbladder wall thickening and distention; intraluminal membranes; intraluminal hemorrhage; irregularity or absence of the gallbladder wall; and lack of gallbladder wall enhancement. Gas may also sometimes be seen within the gallbladder wall or lumen, and a pericholecystic abscess may be seen with gallbladder perforation.

15. **Describe emphysematous cholecystitis and its CT and MR imaging features.**
    Emphysematous cholecystitis is a rare, rapidly progressive variant of acute cholecystitis, which is related to gas-forming infection (most often by *Clostridium welchii* and *Escherichia coli*) in the setting of gallbladder vascular insufficiency. 75% of cases occur in men, commonly in patients with diabetes mellitus, and are associated with a higher rate of gallbladder perforation.
    CT and MRI findings include gas within the gallbladder lumen or wall (sometimes with involvement of the pericholecystic tissues), along with other findings of acute cholecystitis described above.

16. **What is the major complication of acute, gangrenous, and emphysematous cholecystitis?**
    The major complication is gallbladder perforation, which most commonly occurs through the gallbladder fundus.
    On CT and MRI, a focal gallbladder wall defect, gallbladder contour irregularity, extraluminal gallstones, or a pericholecystic abscess may be seen. Other imaging findings may include bile peritonitis, pneumoperitoneum, fistula formation to an adjacent bowel loop, small bowel obstruction, and abdominal abscess formation.

17. **What is ascending cholangitis, and what are its CT and MR imaging features?**
    Ascending cholangitis is a biliary bacterial infection that occurs in the setting of bile duct obstruction, most often secondary to common bile duct calculi. Charcot's triad of right upper quadrant abdominal pain, fever, and jaundice is characteristic but not seen in all patients. Treatment generally involves biliary decompression along with antimicrobial therapy.
    CT and MRI findings include bile duct dilation; an underlying obstructive biliary lesion; bile duct wall thickening and hyperenhancement; periductal edema or transient late arterial phase hyperenhancement; pneumobilia; portal vein thrombosis; hepatic biloma or abscess formation; and bile peritonitis (Figure 32-6).

18. **What is acute pancreatitis?**
    Acute pancreatitis is pancreatic inflammation resulting from autodigestion by activated pancreatic enzymes, most commonly a result of alcohol abuse and gallstones. Patients often present with nausea, vomiting, and midepigastric pain and have a variable prognosis that is predominantly based on the severity of pancreatitis and the presence of complications.

19. **Describe the CT and MR imaging features of acute pancreatitis.**
    On CT and MRI, the pancreas can appear normal in the setting of mild pancreatitis. Imaging findings with increasing severity of pancreatitis include pancreatic enlargement (diffuse or focal); loss of the normal acinar pattern; decreased attenuation/T1-weighted signal intensity and increased T2-weighted signal intensity of the pancreas related to edema; haziness of the peripancreatic fat related to inflammation, edema, or peripancreatic fat necrosis; peripancreatic

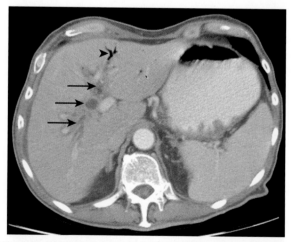

**Figure 32-6.** Ascending cholangitis on CT. Axial contrast-enhanced CT image through abdomen shows dilated bile ducts (*arrows*) with wall thickening and hyperenhancement, along with pneumobilia (*arrowhead*). Indwelling extrahepatic bile duct stent had become obstructed by tumor in-growth from pancreatic head adenocarcinoma (*not shown*).

collections (acute peripancreatic fluid collections [APFC] or acute necrotizing collections [ANC] [when ≤4 weeks of symptom onset] or pseudocysts or walled-off necrosis [WON] [when >4 weeks of symptom onset]), sometimes with presence of gas owing to fistula formation to adjacent bowel or superinfection; and pancreatic necrosis (seen as focal or diffuse lack of enhancement of pancreatic parenchyma), sometimes with sterile or infected ANC or WON. Collections are often present in the anterior pararenal space of the retroperitoneum but may also commonly involve the lesser sac of the peritoneal cavity and the transverse mesocolon.

Complications of acute pancreatitis may include formation of pancreatic or peripancreatic collections, superinfection of collections, hemorrhage, venous thrombosis (most commonly involving the splenic vein and superior mesenteric vein), and arterial pseudoaneurysm formation (often involving the splenic, gastroduodenal, pancreaticoduodenal, hepatic, and left gastric arteries) with the potential for subsequent rupture.

20. What is acute pyelonephritis, and what are its CT and MR imaging features?

Acute pyelonephritis is an infection of the kidney and renal pelvis. Patients often present with fever, chills, and flank pain and tenderness. It is most often due to ascending retrograde infection via the bladder, ureter, and collecting system with subsequent infection of the renal parenchyma.

CT and MRI findings may include normal-appearing kidneys; focal striated or wedge-shaped areas in the kidneys with increased T2-weighted signal intensity, restricted diffusion, or hypoattenuation/hypointensity on nephrographic phase contrast-enhanced images, resulting in a heterogeneous "striated nephrogram" pattern; a reversal of the striated nephrogram pattern on delayed phase contrast-enhanced images related to stasis of contrast material within edematous tubules; enlargement of the kidneys; perinephric inflammatory fat stranding; renal fascial thickening; and renal pelvic and ureteral thickening with hyperenhancement (Figure 32-7). Sometimes, associated hydroureteronephrosis (dilation of the collecting system and ureter), renal infarction, or renal or perinephric abscess formation may be seen.

21. What is emphysematous pyelonephritis, and what are its CT and MR imaging features?

Emphysematous pyelonephritis is a severe, life-threatening infection of the renal parenchyma by gas-forming bacteria. This condition most often occurs in diabetic patients and is often seen when there is obstruction of the collecting system. Rapid progression to septic shock may occur, and the overall mortality rate is as high as 50%.

On CT and MRI, the major imaging finding is very low attenuation/signal intensity gas within the renal parenchyma, often with a radial orientation within the renal pyramids, sometimes extending into the perinephric space, perinephric fascial planes, or collecting system. Associated findings of acute pyelonephritis, as previously described, are also commonly present. Treatment is typically with nephrectomy and antimicrobial therapy.

22. Describe the CT and MR imaging features of urolithiasis along with its associated complications.

Urinary tract calculi (i.e., "liths" or stones) may vary in size from less than 1 mm to many centimeters ("staghorn" calculi) and are typically seen as round, oval, or polygonal foci of very high attenuation on CT within the renal parenchyma, collecting system, ureter, or bladder. Occasionally, matrix calculi and concretions of protease inhibitors (used to treat patients with human immunodeficiency virus [HIV] infection) may be difficult to visualize on CT. MRI is less sensitive than CT for the detection of urinary tract calculi, especially when small in size. However, larger calculi

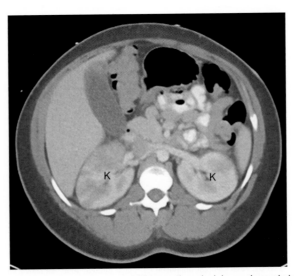

**Figure 32-7.** Acute pyelonephritis on CT. Axial contrast-enhanced CT image through abdomen demonstrates heterogeneous "striated nephrogram" pattern of kidneys (*K*).

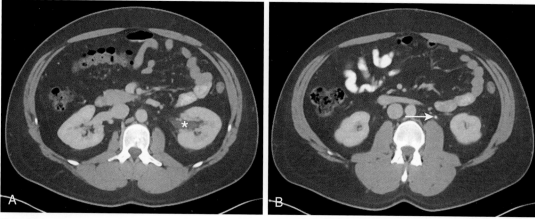

**Figure 32-8.** Obstructive urolithiasis on CT. **A,** Axial unenhanced CT image through abdomen reveals asymmetric dilation of left renal pelvis (*). **B,** Axial unenhanced CT image more inferiorly through abdomen shows 3 mm very high attenuation calculus (*arrow*) completely surrounded by thickened segment of left ureter ("soft tissue rim" sign).

may sometimes be visualized as very low signal intensity foci, often surrounded by very high T2-weighted signal intensity urine within the urothelial system.

When there is obstruction of the ureter by a calculus, which most often occurs at the ureteropelvic and ureterovesical junctions, CT and MRI findings may include dilation of the upstream ureter and collecting system; a thickened edematous segment of ureter completely surrounding the calculus ("soft tissue rim" sign); delayed enhancement of the ipsilateral kidney ("delayed nephrogram"); perinephric or periureteral stranding; renal enlargement; and perinephric fluid or urinoma formation (owing to rupture of a calyceal fornix with urine leak) that shows enhancement on excretory phase images (Figure 32-8).

Scanning of patients in the prone position is useful to differentiate between a recently passed calculus within the urinary bladder and a calculus that is impacted within the ureterovesical junction. The former will drop to the dependent bladder surface, whereas the latter will remain trapped within the ureterovesical junction.

23. What is pyonephrosis, and what are its CT and MR imaging features?

Pyonephrosis is the presence of pus within an obstructed collecting system and is considered to be a urologic emergency. It requires early diagnosis and early treatment with decompression/drainage and antimicrobial therapy to prevent rapid development of urosepsis and its associated complications.

On CT and MRI, hydronephrosis or hydroureteronephrosis upstream to an obstructive urothelial lesion is seen, sometimes containing complex-appearing fluid, layering debris, or foci of intraluminal gas. Inflammatory thickening of the renal pelvic wall or ureter may also be seen, and associated findings of acute pyelonephritis as previously described are also commonly present.

24. What is pelvic inflammatory disease (PID), and what are its CT and MR imaging features?

PID is common and covers a spectrum of infectious diseases involving the reproductive tract of women, including endometritis, cervicitis, salpingitis, and oophoritis, along with some more advanced manifestations of disease. Patients typically present with vaginal discharge, pelvic pain, fever, and leukocytosis. It is the most common cause for emergency room visits in the U.S.

CT and MRI findings include subtle mesenteric, omental, or pelvic visceral inflammatory fat stranding (the earliest imaging feature of PID); thickening of the uterosacral ligaments; pelvic peritoneal or endometrial fluid or gas; hyperenhancement or enlargement of the endometrium, cervix, fallopian tubes, or ovaries; thickening of the fallopian tubes (the most specific imaging feature of PID), sometimes with dilation by fluid or pus (i.e., hydrosalpinx or pyosalpinx), and often with ovarian involvement (tubo-ovarian abscess [TOA]); abdominopelvic abscess formation; and perihepatic inflammatory fat stranding or fluid, sometimes with peritoneal thickening and enhancement (Fitz-Hugh–Curtis syndrome) (Figure 32-9). When an intrauterine device is present, infection by *Actinomyces israelii* is more likely and should be considered in the differential diagnosis.

25. List the major causes of bowel obstruction.

The most common cause of small bowel obstruction is adhesions secondary to prior surgery. Small bowel obstruction secondary to hernia is the second most common cause. Some other causes of small bowel obstruction include primary and secondary small bowel tumors, Crohn's disease, volvulus, bowel malrotation, annular pancreas, endometriosis, foreign body, gallstone, bezoar, intussusception, and intramural hematoma.

Major causes of large bowel obstruction include adhesions, hernia, primary and secondary colorectal tumors, inflammatory bowel disease, sigmoid or cecal volvulus, diverticulitis, intussusception, large bowel stricture, and fecal impaction.

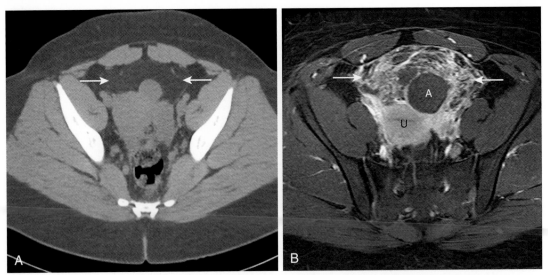

**Figure 32-9.** PID on CT and MRI. **A,** Axial unenhanced CT image through pelvis demonstrates subtle pelvic visceral inflammatory fat stranding (*between arrows*). **B,** Axial fat-suppressed contrast-enhanced T1-weighted image through pelvis obtained 8 months later reveals interval worsening of enhancing pelvic visceral inflammatory fat stranding (*between arrows*) and new pelvic abscess (*A*) formation. Uterus (*U*) is located more posteriorly in pelvis.

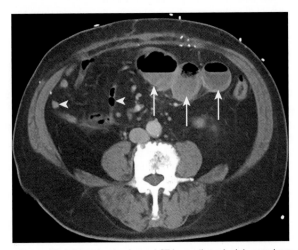

**Figure 32-10.** Small bowel obstruction on CT. Axial contrast-enhanced CT image through abdomen shows dilated loops of proximal small bowel (*arrows*) containing air-fluid levels in left abdomen along with collapsed loops of distal small bowel (*arrowheads*) in right abdomen. The underlying etiology was nonvisualized adhesions following prior abdominal surgery.

26. Describe the CT and MR imaging features of bowel obstruction.

The major imaging finding is upstream dilation and downstream collapse of bowel with respect to the site of obstruction (i.e., the transition zone) (Figure 32-10). Other findings may include focal bowel wall thickening; mass; luminal filling defect; luminal narrowing or angulation, tethering, or beaking of bowel at the transition zone; a mixture of particulate material and fluid within upstream dilated small bowel, mimicking the appearance of feces ("small bowel feces" sign); air-fluid levels within upstream dilated small bowel; and gradual dilution of oral contrast material when passing from proximal to distal in dilated bowel upstream to the site of obstruction. Associated findings of bowel ischemia/infarction described below may also be present.

27. What is a closed loop bowel obstruction, and what are its CT and MR imaging features?

A closed loop bowel obstruction is a surgical emergency and is secondary to obstruction of bowel at two separate locations along its course. This condition generally arises in the setting of volvulus, hernia, or adhesion formation, and it can rapidly progress to bowel ischemia, bowel infarction, bowel perforation, sepsis, and death.

CT and MRI findings include C-shaped or U-shaped loops of dilated bowel, often with a radial configuration and convergence of mesenteric vessels toward a central focus; mesenteric haziness and fluid related to edema; prominent

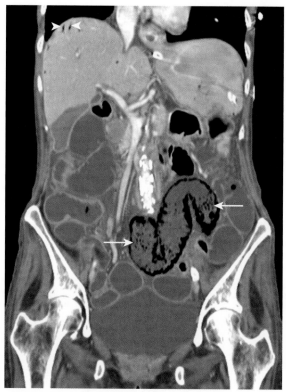

**Figure 32-11.** Acute small bowel infarction on CT. Coronal contrast-enhanced CT image through abdomen and pelvis demonstrates dilation of multiple small bowel loops along with very low attenuation gas bubbles within loop of small bowel (*arrows*) representing pneumatosis. Also note peripherally located foci of portal venous gas (*arrowheads*) within liver.

engorged mesenteric vessels; a swirling appearance of the mesentery and vessels adjacent to the transition zone ("whirl" sign); and beaking and tapering of bowel loops at the sites of obstruction ("beak" sign), often spatially located in close proximity to each other.

28. Describe the CT and MR imaging features of bowel ischemia/infarction.
On CT and MRI, one may see bowel wall thickening; mural hypoattenuation related to submucosal edema (sometimes with a "target" sign); mural hyperattenuation related to intramural hemorrhage; bowel dilation; perienteric or pericolic inflammatory fat stranding, fluid, or hemorrhage; ascites; absent, decreased, or increased mural enhancement; pneumatosis (gas bubbles in the bowel wall), mesenteric or portal venous gas, or pneumoperitoneum; and mesenteric arterial or venous occlusion (Figure 32-11).

If bowel ischemia/infarction is suspected, one should assess the patency of the celiac artery, superior mesenteric artery, inferior mesenteric artery, portal vein, superior mesenteric vein, and inferior mesenteric vein. When the central superior mesenteric vessels are affected, the entire small bowel, along with the large bowel proximal to the distal third of the transverse colon, tends to be affected. When the central inferior mesenteric vessels are affected, the distal third of the transverse colon, the descending colon, and the sigmoid colon are generally involved.

29. List some causes of bowel ischemia/infarction.
• Arterial causes include embolic disease, arterial thrombosis, vasculitis, aortic dissection extending into a mesenteric artery, tumor encasement of a mesenteric artery, and trauma.
• Venous causes include thrombosis, tumor encasement of a mesenteric vein, and trauma.
• Vessel hypoperfusion, systemic shock, radiation injury, bowel obstruction, infectious or inflammatory bowel disease, and some medications are other causes of bowel ischemia/infarction.

30. What is toxic megacolon, and what are its CT and MR imaging features?
Toxic megacolon, or fulminant colitis, is characterized by nonobstructive large bowel dilation and systemic toxicity. It is the most severe life-threatening complication of inflammatory bowel disease (most commonly ulcerative colitis [UC]), but it may also be seen in patients with pseudomembranous colitis or other colitides.

Characteristic CT and MRI features include segmental or diffuse marked large bowel dilation (>6 cm in caliber); loss of normal large bowel haustration; mural thickening; mural edema; decreased mural enhancement; nodular pseudopolyps; and intraluminal air-fluid levels (Figure 32-12). Pneumatosis, pericolic inflammatory fat stranding or

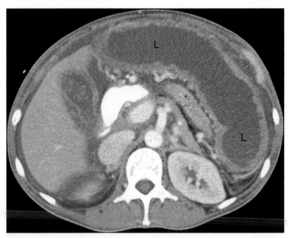

**Figure 32-12.** Toxic megacolon on CT. Axial contrast-enhanced CT image through abdomen reveals marked dilation of fluid-filled large bowel (*L*) with mural thickening and loss of normal haustration, along with small ascites.

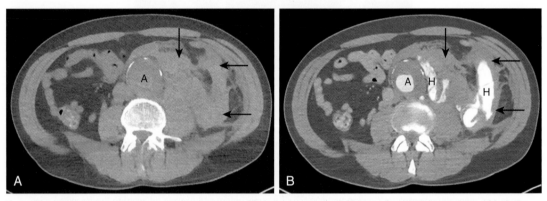

**Figure 32-13.** AAA rupture with active arterial hemorrhage on CT. **A,** Axial unenhanced CT image through abdomen shows AAA (*A*) along with periaortic and left retroperitoneal high attenuation acute hemorrhage (*arrows*) representing "sentinel clot" sign. **B,** Axial contrast-enhanced CT image through abdomen similarly demonstrates AAA (*A*) and nonenhancing high attenuation periaortic and left retroperitoneal acute hemorrhage (*arrows*). However, new foci of very high attenuation (*H*) are now visualized in left retroperitoneum with attenuation similar to that of contrast material within aortic lumen and which do not conform to known vascular structures, indicating active arterial hemorrhage.

edema, ascites, and peritonitis may additionally be present, and imaging findings of bowel perforation, as described below, may also be visualized.

31. List the major causes of bowel perforation.

Major causes of bowel perforation include bowel infarction, bowel obstruction (particularly closed loop obstruction), severe inflammatory bowel disease, peptic ulcer disease, bowel diverticular disease, foreign body perforation, traumatic or iatrogenic injury, and involvement of bowel by tumor.

32. What are the CT and MR imaging features of bowel perforation?

CT and MRI findings include direct visualization of a site of focal disruption in the wall of the bowel; pneumoperitoneum (when there is rupture of an intraperitoneal portion of bowel); pneumoretroperitoneum (when there is rupture of a retroperitoneal portion of bowel); gas bubbles, focal fluid, or inflammatory changes adjacent to the site of perforation; and leakage of fluid (bowel contents) or oral contrast material into the peritoneum or retroperitoneum. If associated peritonitis is present, thickening and enhancement of the peritoneum may be seen.

33. Describe the CT imaging features of acute hemorrhage and active arterial hemorrhage.

Hemorrhage may occur in any portion of the abdomen and pelvis, and generally appears on CT as nonenhancing high attenuation fluid, sometimes with a "hematocrit effect" as manifested by a dependent high attenuation layer and a low attenuation nondependent layer related to settling of red blood cells. Nonclotted acute hemorrhage generally has lower attenuation (30 to 45 HU) compared to clotted acute hemorrhage (45 to 70 HU). The presence of focal high attenuation clotted blood in the abdomen or pelvis may serve as an indicator of the source of hemorrhage ("sentinel clot" sign) (Figure 32-13). In patients with anemia, however, acute hemorrhage may have similar attenuation to that of simple fluid.

Active arterial hemorrhage appears as a round or linear focus of extraluminal intravenous contrast material with very high attenuation similar to that of contrast material within arterial vessels, which does not conform to a known vascular structure. It persists or increases in size on more delayed phase image acquisitions and is often surrounded by high attenuation acute hemorrhage (see Figure 32-13).

34. **Describe the CT imaging features of AAA rupture and impending rupture.**

    AAA rupture most commonly occurs along the posterolateral aspect of the abdominal aorta and is 2 to 4 times more common in women than in men. CT findings of AAA rupture include periaortic and retroperitoneal hemorrhage, sometimes with hemoperitoneum, and active arterial hemorrhage, as described above. Other imaging findings of rupture or impending rupture include high attenuation hemorrhage within the thrombus or wall of an AAA ("crescent" sign); interruption or outward displacement of atherosclerotic calcification, irregular contour, or defect of the aortic wall at the site of rupture; abnormal shape of an AAA; poor visualization of the posterior wall of an AAA that follows the vertebral contour of the spine ("draped aorta" sign); large size (up to 20% of AAA >5 cm rupture within 5 years); and rapid increase in the size of an AAA (see Figure 32-13).

35. **What are the CT and MR imaging features associated with shock, and what should one do upon seeing these findings?**

    CT and MRI findings of shock (also known as the hypoperfusion complex) include decreased caliber of the aorta and renal arteries (related to hypovolemia and compensatory vasoconstriction); flattening of the inferior vena cava ("flat cava" sign or "slit" sign); edema surrounding the inferior vena cava ("halo" sign); decreased or absent enhancement of the spleen; heterogeneous enhancement of the liver; persistent enhancement of the kidneys ("delayed nephrogram"); decreased or absent enhancement of the kidneys ("black kidney" sign); hyperenhancement of the adrenal glands; decreased or increased pancreatic enhancement with peripancreatic edema ("shock pancreas"); and diffuse thickening of the small bowel with dilation and patchy enhancement ("shock bowel"). Other imaging findings may include hemorrhage, sometimes with active bleeding, or ascites. When one sees findings of shock on CT or MRI, one should immediately check on the patient's condition and call for assistance from other clinical staff as needed.

36. **List the major CT imaging features associated with solid organ traumatic injury.**

    Contusions, lacerations, infarction, arterial pseudoaneurysm formation, and acute hemorrhage/hematomas with or without active bleeding are findings that may be encountered on CT in the setting of solid organ injury. Contusions usually appear as focal regions of hypoattenuation. Lacerations appear as irregular linear, curvilinear, or branching foci of hypoattenuation within the parenchyma of a solid organ, sometimes containing gas or high attenuation hemorrhage. When lacerations are severe, portions of organ parenchyma may even avulse from the remainder of the organ. Parenchymal infarctions typically appear as focal or diffuse areas of hypoattenuation owing to lack of enhancement, often peripheral in location and wedge-shaped when focal, and commonly with a preserved peripheral rim of enhancement resulting from capsular collateral vascular supply. Arterial pseudoaneurysms generally appear as focal, round, or oval well-circumscribed structures that enhance in the arterial phase and then wash out in the venous or delayed phase to a degree similar to that of other arterial vessels. Presence of active hemorrhage or of vascular injuries on CT are generally predictive of the need for angiography and transcatheter embolization or surgery.

37. **Describe the major CT imaging features related to hollow organ traumatic injury.**

    With hollow organ injury, CT may show contusion; ischemia or infarction; hemorrhage, sometimes with active bleeding; and perforation. Contusion of a hollow organ generally appears as wall thickening with patchy enhancement, sometimes with increased attenuation because of intramural hemorrhage. Adjacent mesenteric or retroperitoneal stranding, fluid, or hemorrhage may be visualized.

    With bowel injury, associated imaging features of bowel perforation, as previously described, may also be present.

    With bladder rupture, fluid attenuation urine may be seen in the extraperitoneal space (with extraperitoneal bladder rupture) or less commonly in the peritoneal space (with intraperitoneal bladder rupture) that opacifies with renally excreted intravenous contrast material during the excretory phase of enhancement. With rupture of the collecting system or ureter, similar findings of extraluminal fluid attenuation urine with contrast opacification during the excretory phase of enhancement may be seen in the retroperitoneum.

38. **What are the major CT and MR imaging features associated with vascular traumatic injury?**

    CT and MRI findings of vascular injury include an abrupt caliber change of a vessel (indicative of contained rupture or pseudoaneurysm formation); an intimal flap within an arterial vessel; lack of luminal enhancement and enlargement of vessel caliber owing to acute thrombosis; active extravasation of intravenous contrast material owing to active bleeding; high attenuation/intermediate-high T1-weighted signal intensity hemorrhage within the wall of a vessel (intramural hematoma) or surrounding a vessel; wall thickening, sometimes with an irregular contour; and secondary signs of solid organ infarction or bowel ischemia/infarction, as previously described.

39. **What is Fournier gangrene, and what are its CT and MR imaging features?**

    Fournier gangrene is an uncommon rapidly progressive necrotizing fasciitis of the perineal and genital regions, which has a potentially high mortality rate and is considered to be a urologic emergency. It occurs most often in immunocompromised men and is secondary to gas-forming infection, most notably by *Clostridium* species. Treatment

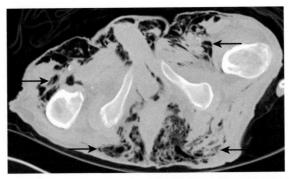

**Figure 32-14.** Fournier gangrene on CT. Axial unenhanced CT image through inferior pelvis reveals extensive very low attenuation gas (*arrows*) within fascial planes and subcutaneous fat of perineal and genital regions.

is with aggressive fluid resuscitation, broad-spectrum antimicrobial therapy, and early surgical debridement to prevent septic shock and death. Adjuvant hyperbaric oxygen therapy may be used in some patients as well.

CT and MRI findings include gas, fluid, or thickening of fascial planes in the perineal and genital regions, sometimes with extension to the thighs, pelvis, or abdomen along the fascial planes, subcutaneous fat, muscles, or deeper body wall layers; skin thickening or ulceration; and abscess formation (Figure 32-14).

40. **What is abdominal compartment syndrome (ACS), and what are its CT and MR imaging features?**
ACS is a life-threatening condition characterized by increased intraabdominal pressure (>20 mm Hg) with dysfunction of at least one thoracoabdominal organ. (Normal intraabdominal pressure is ≈5 mm Hg.) Potential etiologies of ACS include trauma, abdominal surgery, pancreatitis, sepsis, massive fluid resuscitation, and abdominal malignancy. Treatment is generally with decompressive laparotomy along with supportive therapy.

On CT and MRI, a rounded configuration of the abdomen is typically seen, with an anteroposterior : transverse abdominal diameter ratio of >0.8 ("round belly" sign). Other imaging findings may include ascites or hemoperitoneum; presence of retroperitoneal disease; flattening of the inferior vena cava or renal veins; bowel wall thickening and hyperenhancement; heterogeneous hepatic enhancement; and elevation of the diaphragm.

41. **What is ectopic pregnancy, and what are its CT and MR imaging features?**
An ectopic pregnancy refers to a pregnancy located anywhere outside of the endometrial cavity. It is most commonly encountered in the isthmic or ampullary portions of the fallopian tube.

CT and MRI findings include an ectopic gestational sac; a complex hemorrhagic adnexal mass; a hematosalpinx; hemoperitoneum, and lack of visualization of an intrauterine gestation in a patient with an elevated serum beta human chorionic gonadotropin (β-hCG) level.

42. **What is adnexal torsion, and what are its CT and MR imaging features?**
Adnexal torsion occurs when the adnexa and its vascular pedicle twist, resulting in ischemic injury to the ovary and/or fallopian tube. In the majority of cases, a predisposing functional cyst or neoplasm (most commonly a mature teratoma) is present. Treatment with urgent adnexal detorsion and oophoropexy is performed to prevent adnexal infarction when possible, along with removal of predisposing adnexal lesions when present. Otherwise, oophorectomy or salpingo-oophorectomy may be necessary.

On CT and MRI, an adnexal mass, ovarian enlargement, and simple or hemorrhagic pelvic fluid are commonly visualized. Other imaging findings include decreased or absent ovarian enhancement; ovarian stromal edema with peripheral follicles; visualization of a twisted vascular pedicle; fallopian tube wall thickening; ipsilateral uterine deviation; atypical location of the adnexa to the contralateral pelvis or midline; adnexal fat stranding; or hemorrhage within the ovary or fallopian tube.

## KEY POINTS

- Whenever you see visceral pelvic fat stranding on CT or MRI in a woman with an acute abdomen or pelvis, always consider the diagnosis of early PID and notify the clinical team. This will allow them to definitively establish or exclude the diagnosis of PID and to implement therapy as needed to prevent future complications of PID.
- Whenever you see findings of bowel obstruction on CT or MRI, always evaluate the etiology at the transition zone and exclude the presence of a closed loop obstruction because this constitutes a true surgical emergency.
- If you visualize imaging findings of active arterial extravasation of contrast material, shock, or AAA rupture on CT or MRI, immediately check on the status of the patient, start resuscitative measures if needed, and get help from your clinical colleagues right away.

**KEY POINTS** *(Continued)*

- If traumatic injury to the kidneys, ureters, or bladder is suspected clinically or on the basis of CT or MRI findings, obtain additional images through these areas during the excretory phase of enhancement to detect urothelial perforation as manifested by leakage of contrast-opacified urine.
- If you see a rounded configuration of the abdomen on CT or MRI, consider the diagnosis of ACS and notify the clinical team, because this is a life-threatening condition.

## Bibliography

Dreizin D, Munera F. Multidetector CT for penetrating torso trauma: state of the art. *Radiology.* 2015;277(2):338-355.

Uyeda JW, Gans BS, Sodickson A. Imaging of acute and emergent genitourinary conditions: what the radiologist needs to know. *AJR Am J Roentgenol.* 2015;204(6):W631-W639.

Ditkofsky NG, Singh A, Avery L, et al. The role of emergency MRI in the setting of acute abdominal pain. *Emerg Radiol.* 2014;21(6):615-624.

Furey EA, Bailey AA, Pedrosa I. Magnetic resonance imaging of acute abdominal and pelvic pain in pregnancy. *Top Magn Reson Imaging.* 2014;23(4):225-242.

Kao LY, Scheinfeld MH, Chernyak V, et al. Beyond ultrasound: CT and MRI of ectopic pregnancy. *AJR Am J Roentgenol.* 2014;202(4):904-911.

Lourenco AP, Swenson D, Tubbs RJ, et al. Ovarian and tubal torsion: imaging findings on US, CT, and MRI. *Emerg Radiol.* 2014;21(2):179-187.

Lozano JD, Munera F, Anderson SW, et al. Penetrating wounds to the torso: evaluation with triple-contrast multidetector CT. *Radiographics.* 2013;33(2):341-359.

Masselli G, Derchi L, McHugo J, et al. Acute abdominal and pelvic pain in pregnancy: ESUR recommendations. *Eur Radiol.* 2013;23(12):3485-3500.

Patel NB, Oto A, Thomas S. Multidetector CT of emergent biliary pathologic conditions. *Radiographics.* 2013;33(7):1867-1888.

Dreizin D, Munera F. Blunt polytrauma: evaluation with 64-section whole-body CT angiography. *Radiographics.* 2012;32(3):609-631.

Eun HW, Kim JH, Hong SS, et al. Assessment of acute cholangitis by MR imaging. *Eur J Radiol.* 2012;81(10):2476-2480.

Mullan CP, Siewert B, Eisenberg RL. Small bowel obstruction. *AJR Am J Roentgenol.* 2012;198(2):W105-W117.

Soto JA, Anderson SW. Multidetector CT of blunt abdominal trauma. *Radiology.* 2012;265(3):678-693.

Thoeni RF. The revised Atlanta classification of acute pancreatitis: its importance for the radiologist and its effect on treatment. *Radiology.* 2012;262(3):751-764.

Moulin V, Dellon P, Laurent O, et al. Toxic megacolon in patients with severe acute colitis: computed tomographic features. *Clin Imaging.* 2011;35(6):431-436.

Purysko AS, Remer EM, Filho HM, et al. Beyond appendicitis: common and uncommon gastrointestinal causes of right lower quadrant abdominal pain at multidetector CT. *Radiographics.* 2011;31(4):927-947.

Almeida AT, Melao L, Viamonte B, et al. Epiploic appendagitis: an entity frequently unknown to clinicians—diagnostic imaging, pitfalls, and look-alikes. *AJR Am J Roentgenol.* 2009;193(5):1243-1251.

Kaewlai R, Kurup D, Singh A. Imaging of abdomen and pelvis: uncommon acute pathologies. *Semin Roentgenol.* 2009;44(4):228-236.

Stoker J, van Randen A, Lameris W, et al. Imaging patients with acute abdominal pain. *Radiology.* 2009;253(1):31-46.

Vijayaraghavan G, Kurup D, Singh A. Imaging of acute abdomen and pelvis: common acute pathologies. *Semin Roentgenol.* 2009;44(4):221-227.

Levenson RB, Singh AK, Novelline RA. Fournier gangrene: role of imaging. *Radiographics.* 2008;28(2):519-528.

Patel A, Lall CG, Jennings SG, et al. Abdominal compartment syndrome. *AJR Am J Roentgenol.* 2007;189(5):1037-1043.

Schwartz SA, Taljanovic MS, Smyth S, et al. CT findings of rupture, impending rupture, and contained rupture of abdominal aortic aneurysms. *AJR Am J Roentgenol.* 2007;188(1):W57-W62.

Romano S, Lassandro F, Scaglione M, et al. Ischemia and infarction of the small bowel and colon: spectrum of imaging findings. *Abdom Imaging.* 2006;31(3):277-292.

Wiesner W, Khurana B, Ji H, et al. CT of acute bowel ischemia. *Radiology.* 2003;226(3):635-650.

Macari M, Hines J, Balthazar E, et al. Mesenteric adenitis: CT diagnosis of primary versus secondary causes, incidence, and clinical significance in pediatric and adult patients. *AJR Am J Roentgenol.* 2002;178(4):853-858.

Sam JW, Jacobs JE, Birnbaum BA. Spectrum of CT findings in acute pyogenic pelvic inflammatory disease. *Radiographics.* 2002;22(6):1327-1334.

Imbriaco M, Balthazar EJ. Toxic megacolon: role of CT in evaluation and detection of complications. *Clin Imaging.* 2001;25(5):349-354.

Birnbaum BA, Wilson SR. Appendicitis at the millennium. *Radiology.* 2000;215(2):337-348.

# VI

# GENITOURINARY IMAGING

# CHAPTER 33

# UROGRAPHY

*Parvati Ramchandani, MD, FACR, FSAR*

1. What is a urogram?

   A urogram is an imaging study that is used to evaluate both the anatomy and physiology of the urinary tract. The major indications for urography are to evaluate patients with gross or microscopic hematuria, history of urothelial carcinoma, urinary tract stones, and suspected post-surgical or post-traumatic ureteral leaks.

2. What are the different ways a urogram can be performed?

   There are three techniques for performing urography: intravenous urography (IVU), computed tomographic urography (CTU), and magnetic resonance urography (MRU). These are described in greater detail below.

3. What is IVU?

   IVU is a radiographic technique that provides anatomic and functional information about the urinary tract but has now largely been replaced by CTU for most indications. Radiographic contrast material is administered intravenously, and a series of images are obtained to show the kidneys, ureters, and urinary bladder (Figure 33-1). Other synonyms used for this study are **intravenous pyelography (IVP)** and **excretory urography**. Although IVP is probably the most commonly used term for this technique, it is inaccurate because pyelography literally means "a study of the renal pelvis." IVU provides far more information than just an anatomic depiction of the renal pelvis alone. The term **pyelography** is reserved for retrograde studies in which only the collecting system is visualized.

4. What is CTU?

   Thin-section multiplanar computed tomography (CT) is used to image the entire urinary tract in multiple phases. Initially, unenhanced images are obtained through the abdomen and pelvis to assess for calculi and calcifications. After a rapid infusion of intravenous contrast material, images through the kidneys are acquired in the nephrographic phase to assess for renal parenchymal abnormalities and renal masses, such as renal cell carcinoma (please refer to Chapter 35 for more details regarding the different phases of contrast enhancement in which the kidneys are examined). After a 10- to 12-minute delay from the start of contrast injection, coronal and sagittal reformatted images are created from image acquisition during the excretory phase, which provide "IVU-like images" of the collecting systems, ureters, and bladders (Figure 33-2). There are many techniques to perform CTU, with institutional variations, such as administration of a diuretic or saline infusion, to optimize distension and opacification of the collecting systems.

5. What is MRU?

   MRU uses magnetic resonance imaging (MRI) to evaluate the renal parenchyma and collecting systems for urothelial abnormalities. Intravenous administration of gadolinium-based contrast material as well as a diuretic are utilized to depict the collecting systems and ureters (Figure 33-3). MR images are acquired in axial, coronal, and sagittal planes.

6. What are the pros and cons of the three different imaging techniques available for urography?

   CT and MRI are comparable for evaluation of the renal parenchyma, and for assessment of renal masses. However, the ability of CTU to detect small urothelial lesions is much greater than that of MRU, making it the preferred technique for evaluating the collecting systems and ureters for urothelial neoplasms.

   IVU is much less sensitive than either CTU or MRU for detection of renal masses and evaluation of the parenchyma, making it less optimal than CTU or MRU in a patient undergoing evaluation for hematuria. In a patient undergoing evaluation for urothelial tumors, IVU has good sensitivity for depicting urothelial lesions. However, as detailed below, IVU requires a rigorous preprocedure preparation, making it uncomfortable for patients. For these reasons, IVU has ceded ground to CTU for most clinical indications in the evaluation of the urinary tract. It continues to be a valuable technique in evaluating patients postoperatively after urologic procedures, in order to exclude obstruction as a complication of the procedure.

   Due to the multiple phases of examination and the thin sections necessary for CTU, radiation exposure is a prime concern; it can range from 15 mSv to much higher. Evolving CT techniques are focused on reducing the radiation exposure for these examinations.

7. What preprocedure preparation is required for the different urographic techniques?

   Good-quality IVU requires preprocedural preparation, aimed at cleansing the colon so that overlying bowel contents do not obscure the upper urinary tract. Colon cleansing generally consists of laxatives taken the evening before the study. Patients are also asked to avoid solid food the day before the study and consume a clear liquid diet instead. In emergent situations, such as in the setting of a suspected ureteral leak, the study can be performed without preprocedural preparation, recognizing that the evaluation of the collecting systems for subtle abnormalities may be

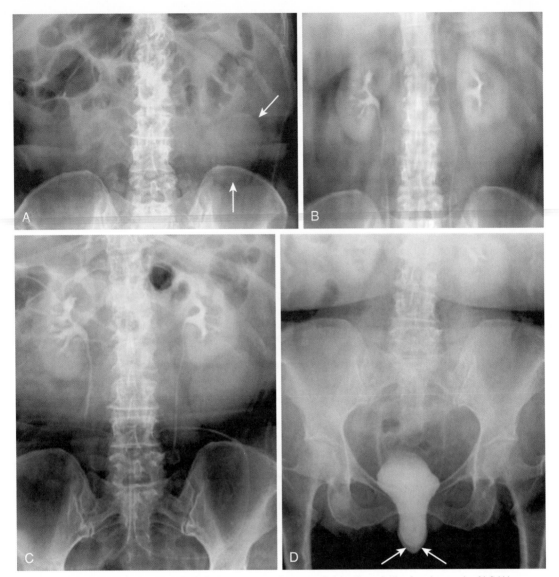

**Figure 33-1.** Renal cyst and cystocele on IVU. **A,** Preliminary image shows rounded density projecting from lower pole of left kidney (*arrows*), suggesting presence of left renal mass. **B,** Nephrotomogram demonstrates right kidney to be normal. Mass in left renal lower pole is seen well. US subsequently showed this to be due to simple renal cyst (*not shown*). **C,** Radiographic image at 12 minutes after intravenous contrast administration with abdominal compression reveals well-distended collecting systems and ureters, with ureteral contrast columns obstructed by compression balloons. Urothelial abnormalities are difficult to detect in underdistended collecting systems. **D,** Erect radiographic image shows near-complete drainage of contrast from collecting systems and ureters. Note abnormal descent of bladder below symphysis pubis (*arrows*) in this elderly woman representing cystocele caused by pelvic floor laxity (see Chapter 34 for more details regarding cystocele).

suboptimal without the bowel preparation. CTU requires neither a laxative preparation nor dietary modifications, making it the preferred technique for evaluation of the urinary tract.

For both CTU and MRU, normal renal function is a necessity. No special preprocedure preparation is required.

8. When is CTU or IVU contraindicated?
   - CTU and IVU require the administration of an intravenous contrast material and are not performed in patients who have a history of severe adverse reaction to iodinated contrast material (see Chapter 6 for more details).
   - Patients with renal insufficiency may have further deterioration in renal function after intravenous iodinated contrast administration. IVU and CTU are best avoided in such patients, and alternative imaging techniques are instead used to evaluate the urinary tract.
   - Pregnancy is a relative contraindication, with the primary concern being radiation exposure to the fetus, particularly in the first and second trimesters of pregnancy. All women of childbearing age are directly questioned to determine

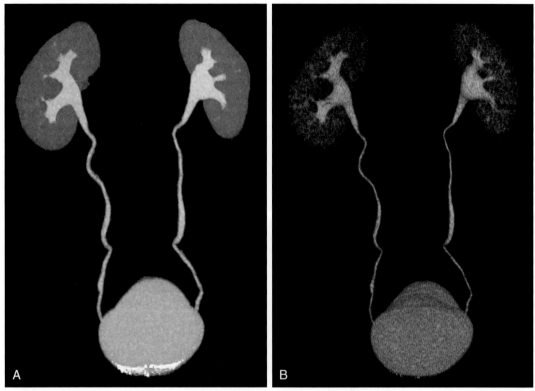

**Figure 33-2.** Normal CTU. **A,** Coronal maximum intensity projection (MIP) and **B,** Volume-rendered (VR) CT images through abdomen and pelvis acquired during excretory phase of enhancement demonstrate normal-appearing collecting systems, ureters, and urinary bladder. Thin-section CT images are also available for detailed evaluation of renal parenchyma and urothelium (*not shown*).

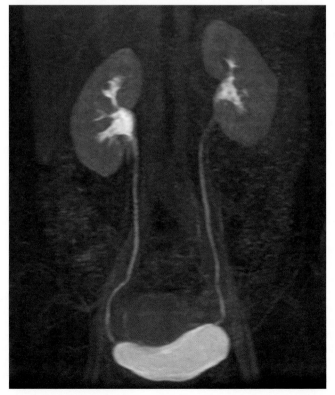

**Figure 33-3.** Normal MRU. Coronal maximum intensity projection (MIP) MR image through abdomen and pelvis acquired during excretory phase of enhancement reveals grossly normal-appearing collecting systems, ureters, and urinary bladder. Multiplanar T1-weighted and T2-weighted images are also available for detailed evaluation of the renal parenchyma and urothelium (*not shown*).

the date of the last menstrual period and to ascertain whether the patient could be pregnant. If there is concern, a pregnancy test is obtained before performing the study. If CTU or IVU is unavoidable in a pregnant patient, efforts are made to limit the radiation exposure using the ALARA principle (see Chapter 7 for more details).

- Patients taking oral hypoglycemic agents, such as metformin (Glucophage), should stop taking the medication at the time of CTU or IVU and not resume it until renal function has been confirmed as being normal to avoid the risk of lactic acidosis. Current guidelines do not require the patient to stop taking the medication before contrast administration.

9. When is MRU contraindicated?

MRU does not have the spatial resolution of CTU for detecting small urothelial lesions, thus making it inferior to CTU, IVU, and retrograde pyelography for evaluation of the collecting systems. MRU is a superb technique for delineating an obstructed urinary tract and for evaluating congenital anomalies. It is contraindicated in patients with a prior history of adverse reaction to gadolinium-based contrast material, in pregnant patients, and in patients with general contraindications to MRI, such as when certain metallic or electronic devices are present.

10. What is the sequence of images for an IVU?

The procedure (see Figure 33-1) begins with two radiographs, known as the **preliminary** or **scout** images, which are used to examine the soft tissues, bones, and bowel gas pattern. One radiograph is centered over the kidneys, and the second radiograph views the entire abdomen to the level of the pubic symphysis. Scout radiographs are particularly important for detecting radiopaque urinary tract stones because these stones have the same radiographic density as excreted contrast material and are often difficult to visualize when the collecting systems are opacified with contrast (Figure 33-4). In addition to calculi, the scout radiographs are also used to detect renal masses (see Figure 33-1, *A*).

The imaging sequence of IVU is aimed at evaluating the renal parenchyma for masses and the collecting systems for urothelial neoplasms and other abnormalities, such as papillary necrosis. Parenchymal evaluation is performed with a series of images called **nephrotomograms**, in which the x-ray tube moves over the patient in an arc with a fixed focal plane that is in sharp focus (see Figure 33-1, *B*). Structures anterior or posterior to the focal point are blurred.

Evaluation of the collecting systems for subtle abnormalities is aided by distention of the collecting systems. This requires compressing the abdomen with inflatable balloons so that the ureters are obstructed (see Figure 33-1, *C*). When the compression is released, contrast material floods the ureters, allowing for visualization of the entire length of the ureters. An image is also obtained in the upright position, which is very sensitive for showing low grades of obstruction (see Figure 33-1, *D*). An unobstructed collecting system should drain nearly completely on an upright image. Images of the urinary bladder are obtained with the bladder distended and then after the patient voids. The latter image allows for a rough estimate of bladder function and is sensitive for showing bladder masses.

11. How should a patient with hematuria be evaluated?

The upper and lower urinary tract of a patient with hematuria should be evaluated for stones, neoplasms, and other abnormalities that may cause hematuria. The upper urinary tract is usually evaluated with CTU for this purpose, as it is much more sensitive than IVU in diagnosing renal parenchymal abnormalities and in detecting small renal masses. The collecting systems are also satisfactorily evaluated with CTU. The urinary bladder is best evaluated with cystoscopy; all imaging studies are much less sensitive in showing pathologic conditions of the bladder compared to direct inspection by cystoscopy.

12. What should be done if IVU suggests the presence of a renal mass?

It is difficult to distinguish whether a renal mass seen on IVU represents a benign renal cyst (an extremely common occurrence in patients >50 years old) or a malignancy such as renal cell carcinoma. Any renal masses detected on IVU should be evaluated further with cross-sectional imaging techniques such as renal ultrasonography (US), renal CT, or renal MRI.

13. My patient presented with diffuse lung metastases and gross hematuria. What study would be best to look for a renal malignancy?

When looking for a primary renal tumor, CT and MRI are equivalent in detecting small masses and are usually performed with a "renal mass protocol" that involves obtaining images through the kidneys prior to the administration of contrast material as well as during the nephrographic phase following intravenous contrast administration to detect renal tumors. Evaluation of the urothelium is critical only in patients with a history of urothelial tumors, in which case a CTU is performed.

14. Why is urography necessary in patients with urothelial cancer of the urinary bladder?

Urothelial cancer (UC) is 50 times more common in the urinary bladder than in the upper urinary tract. UC is a multifocal process, however, and upper urinary tract involvement occurs in approximately 5% of patients with bladder cancer, either synchronously at the time of bladder cancer diagnosis, or in a metachronous fashion. The upper urinary tract of patients with bladder cancer must be kept under close surveillance, usually with periodic urograms. Patients with upper urinary tract UC have a 30% to 40% incidence of UC involving the opposite side. Treatment of upper tract UC is typically with nephroureterectomy, sometimes along with regional lymph node dissection, although segmental or endoscopic resection may be performed in selected cases. Chemotherapy is generally utilized when metastatic disease is present.

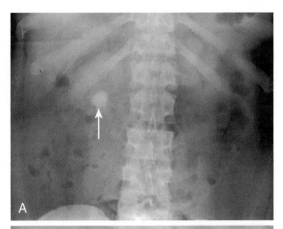
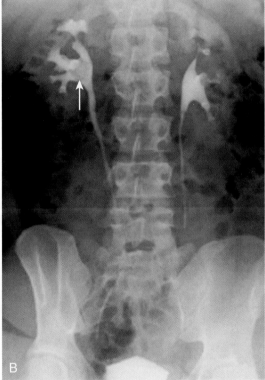

**Figure 33-4.** Renal calculus on IVU. **A,** Preliminary abdominal radiograph centered over kidneys shows radiopaque calculus in right kidney (*arrow*). **B,** Radiographic image acquired during excretory phase following intravenous contrast administration demonstrates filling defect due to calculus (*arrow*) in right renal pelvis partially obscured by high-density excreted contrast material.

15. What does upper tract UC look like on urography?

A persistent filling defect in the pyelocalyceal system or ureter is the most common imaging finding (Figure 33-5). With larger lesions, there may be obstruction of the ipsilateral collecting system by the tumor mass or blood clot. On CT and MRI, tumor masses will demonstrate enhancement, whereas blood clot will not.

16. What is bladder cancer?

Bladder cancer is the second most common genitourinary malignancy in the United States (where prostate cancer is the most common), most often arising in patients in the sixth to eighth decades of life, and occurring three times more commonly in men than in women. Ninety percent are due to urothelial (transitional cell) carcinoma, 5% are due to squamous cell carcinoma, 2% are due to adenocarcinoma, and 3% are due to other histologic subtypes. Tobacco use is the most common risk factor.

Seventy percent of bladder cancers are superficial to the detrusor muscle layer at presentation. Superficial bladder cancers are treated with transurethral resection of bladder tumor (TURBT) during cystoscopy as well as intravesical bacillus Calmette-Guérin (BCG) therapy. However, ≈70% of superficial bladder cancers recur, and up to

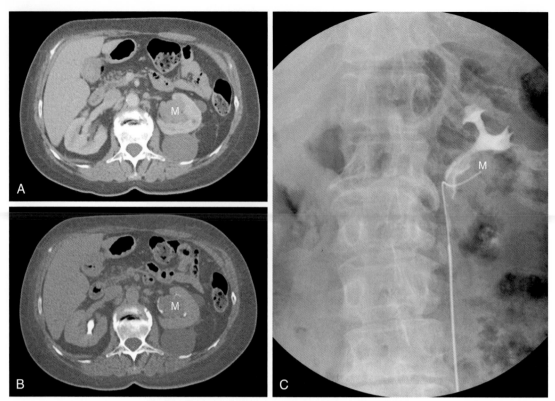

**Figure 33-5.** Upper tract urothelial cancer on CTU and retrograde pyelography. **A,** Axial nephrographic phase contrast-enhanced CT image through abdomen reveals large soft tissue attenuation mass (*M*) in left renal pelvis. Two exophytic left renal cysts are also visualized. **B,** Axial excretory phase contrast-enhanced CT image through abdomen shows mass (*M*) as filling defect within left renal pelvis surrounded by excreted high attenuation contrast material. **C,** Retrograde pyelogram image demonstrates irregular large filling defect corresponding to mass (*M*) in left renal pelvis. Note curvilinear radiodense structure with tip in region of mass representing brush biopsy device.

25% become muscle invasive. Thirty percent of bladder cancers are muscle invasive (i.e., involve the detrusor muscle) at presentation, and may sometimes extend beyond the bladder either locally or through lymphatic or hematogenous routes of metastatic spread. These more advanced stage tumors are treated with radical cystectomy or cystoprostatectomy, pelvic lymphadenectomy, radiation therapy, and/or chemotherapy depending on the spatial extent of disease.

17. What are the IVU, CT, and MR imaging features of bladder cancer?
    On IVU, an intraluminal filling defect in the bladder may be seen. This may be solitary or multifocal in spatial extent. On CT and MRI, an intraluminal enhancing bladder mass or focal asymmetric bladder wall thickening is seen, which may again be solitary or multifocal (Figure 33-6). Superficial calcification in the tumor may be seen in up to 5% of cases on CT. Restricted diffusion in tumor sites may also be visualized on diffusion-weighted images (DWI).

    Although CTU is superior to MRU for evaluation of the upper urothelial tract to detect urothelial cancer, MRI is superior to CT for the detection of detrusor muscle invasion by primary tumor, and hence is superior for the local staging and pretreatment planning of bladder cancer. The normal detrusor muscle appears as a low signal intensity layer in the bladder wall on T2-weighted images. If there is focal interruption of this low signal intensity layer by higher signal intensity tumor, particularly in association with restricted diffusion on DWI, then muscle-invasive tumor is likely present. Infiltration of the perivesical fat, invasion of adjacent organs including the body wall, presence of pelvic lymphadenopathy, and presence of distant metastatic disease are indicators of even more advanced stage bladder cancer and are detectable on CT and MRI.

18. What is the appearance of urinary tract stones on imaging studies?
    The terms **radiopaque** and **nonopaque**, when used to describe urinary stones, apply only to the ability to visualize stones on radiographs. All stones, regardless of their composition, are dense on CT and echogenic on US.

    Approximately 85% of urinary tract stones are composed of calcium oxalate and are radiopaque (and thus visible) on radiographs (see Figure 33-4, *A*). Ten percent of stones are composed of uric acid and are either nonopaque or very faintly opaque on radiographs, and they are therefore difficult to identify. Nonopaque stones are invisible on radiographs but are seen as filling defects in the contrast-opacified collecting system. Stones associated with chronic

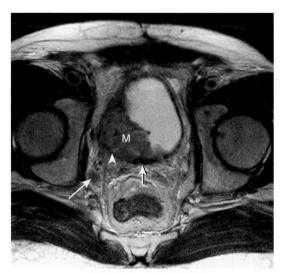

**Figure 33-6.** Bladder cancer on MRI. Axial T2-weighted MR image through pelvis reveals large mass (*M*) in right side of bladder that disrupts normal low signal intensity detrusor muscle (*arrowhead*), indicating muscle invasion. Note normal low signal intensity detrusor muscle posteriorly (*short arrow*) for comparison. Also note asymmetrically enlarged right obturator lymph node (*long arrow*) indicating metastatic nodal disease.

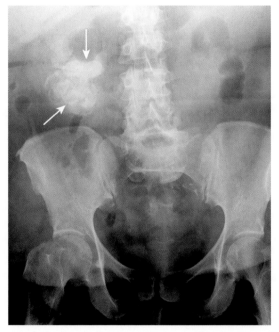

**Figure 33-7.** Staghorn calculus on abdominal radiograph. Note large radiopaque calculus (*arrows*) conforming to shape of right renal pyelocalyceal system. Such stones are usually related to chronic UTI and are composed of ammonium-magnesium-calcium phosphate.

or recurrent infection can grow to fill the entire collecting system (known as "staghorn calculi") (Figure 33-7). Other stone compositions, such as cystine and xanthine, are less common.

19. **Is a filling defect in the collecting system diagnostic of UC?**
No. Other pathologic conditions that can cause a filling defect are nonopaque stones, blood clots, fungus balls in patients with a fungal urinary tract infection (UTI), and subepithelial cysts associated with chronic infection or inflammation in a condition known as ureteritis cystica.

20. **How do I distinguish between these different pathologic conditions?**
If a filling defect is detected in the collecting system, a biopsy is the next step, so that cytopathologic analysis can be performed. The biopsy can be performed with fluoroscopic guidance by radiologists (as in Figure 33-5, *C*) or by

ureteroscopic guidance by a urologist. Nonopaque stones are mobile, whereas blood clots are always associated with gross hematuria. Fungus balls occur in immunocompromised patients with a fungal UTI. Ureteritis cystica usually occurs in patients with a history of UTI or stones, but if urine cytology is positive for UC in such a patient, then ureteroscopy is required to distinguish between a benign subepithelial cyst and a tumor, as definitive distinction cannot be made by imaging studies alone.

21. **What is the appearance of urinary tract obstruction on an IVU, CTU, and MRU?**
Obstruction of the urinary tract causes delay in the development of a nephrogram in the affected kidney, a delay in contrast excretion, and dilation of the upstream collecting system (Figure 33-8). Long-standing severe obstruction can cause atrophy of the renal parenchyma and is referred to as hydronephrotic atrophy. Obstruction can be related to intrinsic causes in the collecting system or ureter, such as stones or urothelial tumors, while extrinsic obstruction is due to compression by lesions adjacent to the collecting system or ureter, such as metastatic tumors or retroperitoneal fibrosis. The cause of urinary obstruction is best evaluated on cross-sectional imaging studies such as CT or MRI.

22. **What is the role of urography in a patient with suspected urinary tract obstruction?**
If the patient has renal insufficiency with elevation in the serum creatinine level, administration of a contrast material is contraindicated. Renal US is the best study to evaluate such a patient for a dilated collecting system, which would indicate obstruction. Renal scintigraphy may also be useful in this clinical scenario. Nondilated obstructive uropathy is rare. In patients with normal renal function and suspected obstruction, renal US and renal scintigraphy remain the mainstays for evaluation. In an occasional patient with equivocal results from other diagnostic tests, CTU or IVU may help. Prompt and symmetric nephrograms with bilateral contrast excretion and complete drainage of the collecting systems on an erect postvoid radiograph effectively exclude significant urinary tract obstruction. In postoperative patients in whom urinary diversion has been performed, a study in the first few months after surgery serves as a baseline to exclude strictures at the ureteral anastomotic sites.

23. **What is a stone-protocol CT?**
When a patient presents with suspected renal colic, the most common method used for evaluation is an abdominopelvic CT performed without oral or intravenous contrast material. This is referred to as a stone-protocol CT. The presence of a stone within the ureter, dilation of the upstream collecting system and ureter, and perinephric fluid and perinephric stranding are imaging findings that are highly suggestive of the presence of an obstructing stone. If a stone is impacted within the ureter, there may be surrounding soft tissue edema at the site, which is referred to as a "soft tissue rim" sign.

24. **My patient has severe flank pain. What study should I order to exclude renal colic as a cause of the flank pain?**
CT is the diagnostic modality of choice in evaluating patients who are suspected to have acute renal colic resulting from a stone. No intravenous or oral contrast administration is necessary. Nearly all stones larger than 2 to 3 mm are visible on CT.

25. **As a stone-protocol CT detects all renal stones, when is urography necessary in patients with urinary tract stones?**
IVU, CTU, and MRU are helpful to show the anatomy of the urinary tract in patients with recurrent stones, in patients in whom stone passage is arrested in the ureter, and in patients in whom surgical intervention is being considered to treat the stones. In such cases, urography helps identify congenital or acquired abnormalities that may be potentiating stone formation, collecting system damage related to chronic stone disease, and ureteral strictures that may prevent spontaneous passage of stones. Stones that are smaller than 5 to 6 mm almost always pass spontaneously, whereas larger stones may require surgical intervention.
    Urography may also show abnormalities, such as medullary nephrocalcinosis, that may be contributing to recurrent stone disease.

26. **What are calyceal diverticula?**
Calyceal diverticula are congenital outpouchings from the calyceal fornices, seen most frequently in the polar regions of the kidneys. They connect by a neck to the fornix they arise from, and the neck can be of variable width. If the neck is narrow, drainage from the diverticula may be impaired and result in complications such as stone formation or infection. A calyceal diverticulum can be confidently diagnosed on the excretory phase of contrast-enhanced CT or MRI, as the diverticulum will fill with excreted contrast material.

27. **What is medullary sponge kidney?**
This is also a congenital condition, in which the collecting ducts in the medullary pyramids are dilated and ectatic, giving the medullary pyramids a brush-like or sponge-like appearance. Stones form within these ducts, which can then erode into the collecting system. The findings are seen on the excretory phase of a CTU or on an IVU (Figure 33-9). Medullary renal cysts may also be encountered. The presence of clustered calcifications in the collecting ducts in the medullary pyramids is referred to as medullary nephrocalcinosis.
    The clinical importance of medullary nephrocalcinosis is that there is a very high incidence of stones passing from the renal parenchyma into the collecting systems; patients present with recurrent episodes of renal colic and stone-related complications.

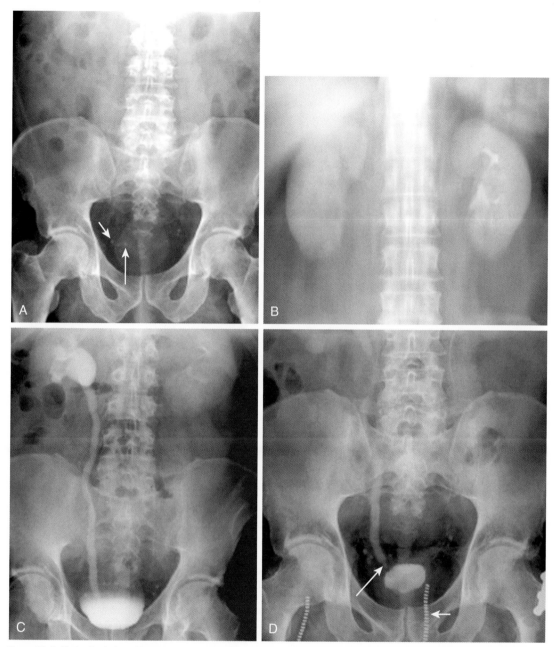

**Figure 33-8.** Ureteral calculus with partial urinary tract obstruction on IVU. **A,** Preliminary radiograph shows multiple calcific densities in pelvis in this patient with right flank pain. Long arrow marks irregular distal right ureteral stone. Other densities, including one marked by short arrow, represent smooth round calcified phleboliths. **B,** Nephrotomogram demonstrates delayed excretion of contrast material from right kidney. Left kidney is normal in appearance. **C,** Erect excretory phase radiographic image reveals column of excreted contrast material in dilated right collecting system and ureter to level of bladder. Stone seen on preliminary radiograph is obscured by contrast material on this image. Note near-complete drainage of contrast material from normal left collecting system and ureter. **D,** Post-void radiographic image shows continued right ureteral dilation to level of stone (*long arrow*). Other densities seen on preliminary image are outside of contrast-filled ureter, indicating that they are indeed phleboliths. Note zipper of trousers (*short arrow*) external to patient.

28. What is ureteropelvic junction (UPJ) obstruction?

   This is a congenital anomaly, in which the renal pelvis does not taper and funnel normally into the ureter, resulting in obstruction at the UPJ (Figure 33-10). The renal pelvis is located outside of the renal parenchyma (known as an extrarenal pelvis) and is usually large. The appearance of the ureter inserting into the large and dilated renal pelvis is referred to as a "balloon on a string" sign. Congenital UPJ, also known as congenital hydronephrosis, is a very

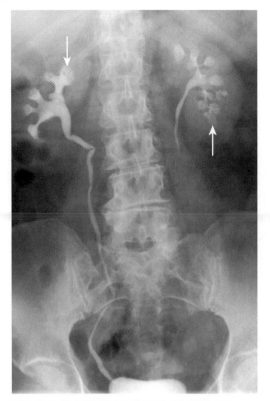

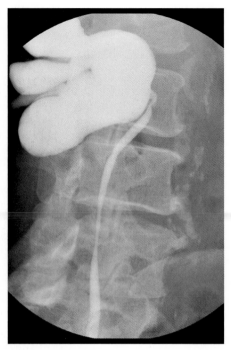

**Figure 33-10.** Congenital UPJ obstruction on retrograde pyelogram. Note dilated extrarenal pelvis of right kidney with poorly funneled ureteropelvic junction and normal caliber ureter, leading to "balloon on a string" sign.

**Figure 33-9.** Medullary sponge kidney on IVU. Radiographic image acquired during excretory phase following intravenous contrast administration demonstrates dilated collecting ducts in medullary pyramids (*arrows*) bilaterally leading to brush-like appearance. Subcentimeter radiopaque calculi are visible in several medullary pyramids on scout radiograph (*not shown*) but are obscured by excreted contrast material on this image.

common cause for an abdominal mass in a neonate. The treatment is surgical pyeloplasty and is usually performed laparoscopically.

29. What is an ectopic ureter?

The ureter normally inserts in the trigone of the urinary bladder. If the insertion is at any other site, it is referred to as ectopy. Caudal ectopy (i.e., insertion of the ureter below the trigone) is much more frequent than cranial ectopy (i.e., insertion of the ureter above the trigone). With caudal ectopy, the ureter can insert in the bladder neck, the urethra, or even the vagina in females. In most boys, ureteral ectopy is not associated with incontinence as the ureter almost always inserts above the striated sphincter, which is closed at rest and opens only during voiding. In girls, incontinence of variable severity often occurs with ureteral ectopy as the insertion may be in the vagina or the urethra distal to the sphincter, and necessitates a workup to determine where the ectopic ureter is inserting for appropriate surgical management.

30. What is meant by duplication of the collecting system, and what is its appearance on radiographic studies?

Duplication of the collecting system is a very common congenital anomaly and is a frequent finding on imaging studies. Embryologically, the ureter is derived from the mesonephric duct, and it ascends cephalad to meet with the primitive kidney, the metanephric blastema, to form the adult kidney and collecting system. If there are two buds developed from one mesonephric duct, there will be complete duplication of the collecting systems with two ureteral orifices in the bladder on the side of the duplication. In most completely duplicated systems, both ureters insert at the normal site in the bladder trigone, known as orthotopic insertion. However, there can be ectopic insertion of the ureters. The upper pole ureter usually inserts ectopically, below the bladder trigone, and is also obstructed, while the lower pole ureter inserts at the normal site in the bladder trigone but may have vesicoureteral reflux (VUR). This constellation of abnormalities is known as the Weigert-Meyer rule. The obstructed upper pole collecting system can cause mass effect on the lower pole ureter, and this appearance of the lower pole collecting system is referred to as a "drooping-lily" sign.

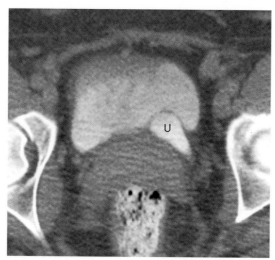

**Figure 33-11.** Orthotopic ureterocele on CTU. Axial excretory phase contrast-enhanced CT image through pelvis reveals dilated distal left ureter (*U*) with typical "cobra-head" appearance along with smooth and thin walls and no underlying lesion.

With partial or incomplete duplication, a single ureteral bud splits into two as it extends cephalad. It is important to determine where the two ureters join if urologic surgery is planned.

Duplication anomalies are well demonstrated on CTU, MRU, IVU, and retrograde pyelography. Awareness of these anomalies is important in patients undergoing urologic surgery, so that the surgeon can avoid inadvertent ureteral injury.

31. What is a ureterocele?

Ureterocele is literally dilation of the ureter. If the ureter is ectopic, it is referred to as an ectopic ureterocele, and it will be well demonstrated on a CTU or MRU.

Another type of ureterocele is referred to as an orthotopic ureterocele. Here, there is congenital narrowing of the ureteral orifice at the ureterovesical junction (UVJ). This causes dilation of the ureter in its course through the bladder wall, giving a "cobra-head" appearance to the dilated ureter (Figure 33-11). The walls of the ureterocele appear smooth and thin on imaging studies.

A pseudo-ureterocele is due to a stone or a tumor at the UVJ or adjacent bladder, which causes distal ureteral obstruction. There is irregularity of the UVJ due to the edema caused by these processes, so that the walls of the dilated ureter may appear irregular or thickened rather than smooth and thin as with an orthotopic ureterocele.

32. What is papillary necrosis?

The renal papilla is the portion of the medullary pyramid that projects into the cup of the renal calyx. In patients with sickle cell disease, diabetes mellitus, nonsteroidal anti-inflammatory drug (NSAID) abuse, and occasionally severe infections, the renal papillae can become ischemic and undergo necrosis. The calyces then become deformed and lose their normal cup shape. Contrast material from the calyces can extend into the necrotic papilla on the excretory phase of imaging studies; this appearance is known as a "lobster claw" or "ring" sign.

33. What is the imaging appearance of infections in the urinary tract?

Mild or initial episodes of acute pyelonephritis cause no permanent sequelae in the kidneys. Imaging is not indicated in clinically suspected acute pyelonephritis or in UTIs limited to the bladder. In patients with acute pyelonephritis who do not respond to appropriate antibiotic therapy, contrast-enhanced CT may be helpful to evaluate for complications such as a renal or perirenal abscess. CT is more sensitive than US in showing the presence and extent of complications. In patients who cannot receive iodinated contrast material, MRI may be performed as a good alternative.

With recurrent episodes of severe pyelonephritis, scarring may occur in the kidneys, and the calyces underlying the areas of scarring may be blunted or deformed. Urography may show a congenital abnormality or an obstructive lesion such as a stricture that may be contributory to the refractory UTI. In patients with VUR, the renal parenchymal scarring is most marked in the poles of the kidneys, with the upper pole of the kidney being the most severely affected.

Tuberculosis of the urinary tract usually is secondary to pulmonary tuberculosis and is seen commonly in areas of the world where this infection is prevalent. The process starts in the renal papilla, where cavitary changes may be seen. Presence of strictures in the infundibula of the collecting system and renal parenchymal calcifications clinch the diagnosis. The caseating tuberculous granulomas calcify, and if untreated, they eventually involve the entire kidney. An end-stage tuberculous kidney becomes calcified and atrophic and is referred to as a "putty" kidney. The process can descend to the ureters and urinary bladder causing strictures. Tuberculosis in the bladder results in a very small capacity, poorly distensible, and scarred bladder, known as a "thimble" bladder.

Schistosomiasis is an infection endemic in many parts of the world. The urinary tract is affected by *S. haematobium*, and heavy calcification is typically seen in the bladder. The bladder remains of normal capacity and distensible, unlike that involved by tuberculosis. The infection can ascend to involve the ureters, which can develop calcifications in the walls along with strictures. The calcifications in the urinary tract are best demonstrated on CT.

34. My patient is status post surgery for an abdominal tumor several days ago, and the surgical drains are putting out a lot of yellow fluid. What should I do?

Collecting system or ureteral injury can be iatrogenic or may be related to blunt or penetrating trauma. This patient can be evaluated either with IVU or contrast-enhanced CT including imaging during the excretory phase of enhancement. Both studies would show contrast leakage from the collecting system into the retroperitoneal tissues in the region of injury.

## KEY POINTS

- All urinary stones are dense on CT scans, including stones that are radiolucent (and undetectable) on radiographs.
- Patients with suspected acute renal colic are best evaluated with unenhanced CT. CT and MRI are comparable for evaluating renal masses.
- CTU is the imaging procedure of choice for evaluating the upper urinary tract in a patient with hematuria. Cystoscopy remains the procedure of choice to evaluate the urinary bladder for urothelial abnormalities.

**BIBLIOGRAPHY**

Potenta SE, D'Agostino R, Sternberg KM, et al. CT urography for evaluation of the ureter. *Radiographics*. 2015;35(3):709-726.

Surabhi VR, Menias CO, George V, et al. MDCT and MR urogram spectrum of congenital anomalies of the kidney and urinary tract diagnosed in adulthood. *AJR Am J Roentgenol*. 2015;205(3):W294-W304.

Ziemba J, Guzzo TJ, Ramchandani P. Evaluation of the patient with asymptomatic microscopic hematuria. *Acad Radiol*. 2015;22(8):1034-1037.

Koraishy FM, Ngo TT, Israel GM, et al. CT urography for the diagnosis of medullary sponge kidney. *Am J Nephrol*. 2014;39(2):165-170.

Wolin EA, Hartman DS, Olson JR. Nephrographic and pyelographic analysis of CT urography: differential diagnosis. *AJR Am J Roentgenol*. 2013;200(6):1197-1203.

Wolin EA, Hartman DS, Olson JR. Nephrographic and pyelographic analysis of CT urography: principles, patterns, and pathophysiology. *AJR Am J Roentgenol*. 2013;200(6):1210-1214.

Shebel HM, Elsayes KM, Abou El Atta HM, et al. Genitourinary schistosomiasis: life cycle and radiologic-pathologic findings. *Radiographics*. 2012;32(4):1031-1046.

Verma S, Rajesh A, Prasad SR, et al. Urinary bladder cancer: role of MR imaging. *Radiographics*. 2012;32(2):371-387.

O'Connor OJ, McLaughlin P, Maher MM. MR urography. *AJR Am J Roentgenol*. 2010;195(3):W201-W206.

Leyendecker JR, Gianini JW. Magnetic resonance urography. *Abdom Imaging*. 2009;34(4):527-540.

Silverman SG, Leyendecker JR, Amis ES Jr. What is the current role of CT urography and MR urography in the evaluation of the urinary tract? *Radiology*. 2009;250(2):309-323.

Vikram R, Sandler CM, Ng CS. Imaging and staging of transitional cell carcinoma: part 1, lower urinary tract. *AJR Am J Roentgenol*. 2009;192(6):1481-1487.

Vikram R, Sandler CM, Ng CS. Imaging and staging of transitional cell carcinoma: part 2, upper urinary tract. *AJR Am J Roentgenol*. 2009;192(6):1488-1493.

Leyendecker JR, Barnes CE, Zagoria RJ. MR urography: techniques and clinical applications. *Radiographics*. 2008;28(1):23-46, discussion 46-47.

Jindal G, Ramchandani P. Acute flank pain secondary to urolithiasis: radiologic evaluation and alternate diagnoses. *Radiol Clin North Am*. 2007;45(3):395-410, vii.

Dyer RB, Chen MY, Zagoria RJ. Intravenous urography: technique and interpretation. *Radiographics*. 2001;21(4):799-821, discussion 2-4.

# CHAPTER 34

# GENITOURINARY TRACT FLUOROSCOPY

*Parvati Ramchandani, MD, FACR, FSAR*

1. **What are genitourinary fluoroscopic examinations?**

   Genitourinary fluoroscopic examinations are studies that require "real-time" observation using fluoroscopy so that maximal information is obtained about the anatomy and function of the structure being studied. A radiographic iodinated contrast agent is injected into the various portions of the genitourinary tract for these examinations. Examples include retrograde pyelography to evaluate the upper urinary tract, cystography or voiding cystourethrography (VCUG) to evaluate the lower urinary tract, retrograde urethrography (RUG) to evaluate the urethra, and hysterosalpingography (HSG) to evaluate the uterus and fallopian tubes.

2. **What is a retrograde pyelogram, and how does it differ from a urogram?**

   As discussed in Chapter 33, a urogram (via intravenous urography [IVU] or computed tomographic urography [CTU]) requires intravenous administration of contrast material, after which imaging of the renal parenchyma is performed in the earlier nephrographic phase of enhancement and of the collecting system in the excretory phase of enhancement. A urogram provides physiologic information about the function of the kidneys, in addition to depicting the anatomy of the renal parenchyma and collecting systems. A retrograde pyelogram provides only anatomic information about the lumen of the collecting system and ureter, but the depiction of mucosal abnormalities is superior to that seen with urography. For performing a retrograde pyelogram, cystoscopy is initially performed by a surgeon, most commonly a urologist, and a catheter is placed through the ureterovesical junction into the renal pelvis under direct vision with a cystoscope. The patient is then transferred to the radiology department where contrast material is injected through this catheter under fluoroscopic guidance to evaluate the lumen of the pyelocalyceal system and ureter for mucosal abnormalities such as urothelial carcinoma. An alternative to placing a catheter into the collecting system is to inject contrast material directly into the ureterovesical junction through the cystoscope and obtain images in the operating room; this technique is useful if the ureter alone has to be evaluated for urothelial abnormalities but is unsuitable for complete evaluation of the collecting system (Figure 34-1, *A-B*).

3. **When is a retrograde pyelogram necessary?**

   A retrograde pyelogram is performed if the patient cannot receive an intravenous contrast material because of renal insufficiency or a history of severe adverse reaction to radiographic contrast agents. Retrograde examination can also be performed if a urogram fails to show the entire pyelocalyceal system or ureter, or to evaluate further an abnormality seen on a urogram (Figure 34-1, *C-E*).

4. **What is the difference between a cystogram and a voiding cystourethrogram?**

   A cystogram is tailored to evaluate the urinary bladder alone, whereas a voiding cystourethrogram includes evaluation of the bladder neck and urethra under fluoroscopic observation. Both studies require injection of radiographic contrast material into the urinary bladder through either an indwelling bladder drainage catheter or a catheter placed in the urinary bladder solely for the procedure. Cystography is limited to obtaining images of the bladder, whereas in voiding cystourethrography (VCUG), the catheter is removed after the bladder has been distended with contrast material, and the patient voids under fluoroscopic observation so that the bladder neck and urethra can also be evaluated.

5. **What are the indications for cystography and VCUG?**

   These studies are performed to evaluate the anatomy of the bladder and urethra in patients with voiding dysfunction or recurrent urinary tract infection (UTI) (Figure 34-2), to assess for a leak or fistula from the bladder after surgery or abdominal trauma (Figure 34-3), to evaluate for presence of vesicoureteral reflux (VUR) in patients with recurrent or refractory UTI, or to evaluate urinary incontinence.

6. **What is a retrograde urethrogram?**

   A retrograde urethrogram is a study used primarily to evaluate the anterior urethra in men (Figure 34-4). The male urethra is divided into two portions: the posterior urethra, consisting of the prostatic and membranous urethra, and the anterior urethra, consisting of the bulbar and pendulous urethra. The external urethral sphincter, located in the urogenital diaphragm, demarcates the posterior urethra from the anterior urethra. The posterior urethra has smooth muscle that relaxes when the detrusor muscle contracts during voiding and is best seen on VCUG. Although visualized on VCUG, the anterior urethra is better evaluated by retrograde urethrography (RUG), which is performed by placing a Foley catheter in the tip of the penis and injecting contrast material under fluoroscopic guidance. The urethra is usually opacified only to the level of the external sphincter on a retrograde urethrogram, because the sphincter is closed in the nonvoiding state, and contrast material cannot flow proximal to the closed sphincter.

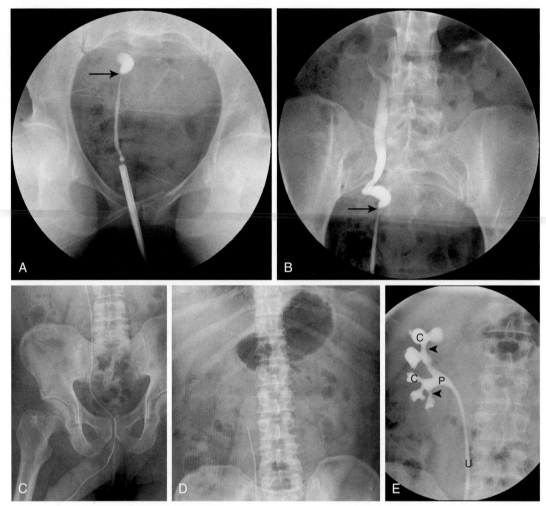

**Figure 34-1.** Retrograde pyelogram. **A** and **B,** Frontal fluoroscopic images through pelvis show cannula in right ureteral orifice placed through cystoscope through which contrast material is injected. Note excellent visualization of right ureter with tight narrowing in pelvic ureter (*arrow*) due to stricture along with upstream dilation of ureter. T-shaped radiodense structure in left pelvis represents indwelling intrauterine device (IUD) in this female patient. **C-D,** Frontal radiographs through pelvis and abdomen in different male patient demonstrate thin radiodense catheter placed through urethra and bladder into right lumbar ureter. **E,** Frontal fluoroscopic image through abdomen of same patient reveals opacification of normal-appearing right renal calyces (*C*), infundibula (*arrowheads*), renal pelvis (*P*), and ureter (*U*) by contrast material that was injected through ureteral catheter for retrograde pyelography. This allows better evaluation of collecting system than injection of contrast material through catheter at ureteral orifice as shown in **A** and **B**.

7. What are the indications for a retrograde urethrogram?
   The most common indication is to evaluate for a possible urethral stricture in a patient with a decreased force of urinary stream or a split stream; the procedure is also performed after repair of a urethral stricture to evaluate healing and to exclude a leak from the surgical site. Another indication is in a patient with trauma to the perineum, such as a straddle injury, or a pelvic fracture, which is usually sustained in a motor vehicle collision. Retrograde urethrograms are also useful in patients with suspected fistulae arising from the urethra, such as in a postoperative patient, in patients with inflammatory bowel disease, or after radiation therapy to the prostate gland.

8. How is the female urethra evaluated?
   The entire female urethra is well depicted on VCUG (see Figure 34-3). The short length of the female urethra makes RUG a difficult and unnecessary procedure in women.

9. What is a loopogram?
   In patients who have undergone cystectomy (usually performed for muscle-invasive bladder cancer), the ureters are connected to a loop of ileum known as an ileal conduit. The ileal conduit is excluded from the intestinal stream and is connected to the anterior abdominal wall through a stoma; a urinary drainage bag is applied to the stoma site to collect urine. A loopogram is performed to evaluate the conduit and the upper urinary tracts. A catheter is placed in

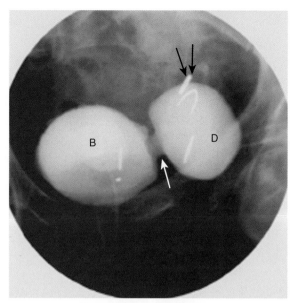

**Figure 34-2.** Bladder diverticulum on cystogram. Frontal fluoroscopic image through pelvis shows large contrast-opacified bladder diverticulum (*D*) arising from left side of urinary bladder (*B*) with wide neck (*white arrow*). Contrast material (and urine) fills diverticulum during voiding and then flows back into urinary bladder when voiding stops (*not shown*), accounting for patient's symptoms of incomplete emptying. Note surgical clip in pelvis (*black arrows*) from previous surgery.

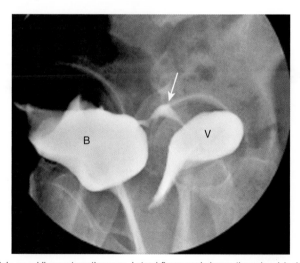

**Figure 34-3.** Vesicovaginal fistula on voiding cystourethrogram. Lateral fluoroscopic image through pelvis demonstrates contrast-opacified fistula (*arrow*) between posterior aspect of urinary bladder (*B*) and anterior aspect of vagina (*V*). Vesicovaginal fistulas can be complications of hysterectomy (as in this patient); difficult vaginal delivery, particularly if forceps are used; cesarean section; and gynecologic neoplasms, such as cervical cancer.

the ileal conduit, and contrast material is injected under fluoroscopic guidance until it refluxes in a retrograde fashion into the ureters and pyelocalyceal systems (Figure 34-5).

10. What is a pouchogram?

Urinary pouches are an alternative to an ileal conduit, for urine storage and drainage in patients who have undergone cystectomy; these pouches allow urine storage similar to the bladder, do not require a urinary drainage bag, are periodically emptied by either catheterization or voiding, and are therefore sometimes referred to as neo-bladders. They are of two main varieties: cutaneous and orthotopic. Many such pouches have been developed, and the names assigned to the pouches are assigned by the surgeon who developed them or the institution where they were developed. For instance, an "Indiana pouch," a form of cutaneous continent pouch, was developed at Indiana University in the United States, while a "Studer pouch," an orthotopic urinary pouch, was developed by Dr. Studer (Figure 34-6).

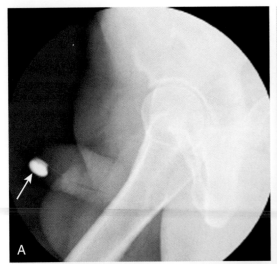

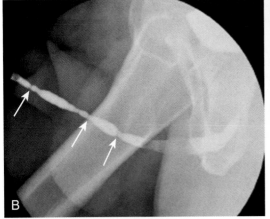

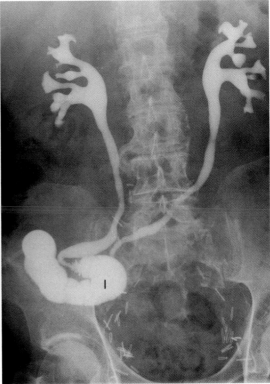

**Figure 34-5.** Normal loopogram. Frontal abdominopelvic radiograph following contrast injection into ileal conduit demonstrates normal-appearing collecting systems, ureters, and ileal conduit (*I*). Note surgical clips in pelvis related to prior cystectomy and lymph node resection in this patient with history of bladder cancer.

**Figure 34-4.** Urethral strictures on retrograde urethrogram. **A,** Lateral fluoroscopic image through pelvis reveals balloon of Foley catheter (*arrow*) in tip of penis distended and opacified with contrast material. Balloon is usually placed in fossa navicularis, an area of natural widening in glans penis. **B,** Lateral fluoroscopic image through pelvis shows anterior urethra opacified with contrast material. Multiple areas of urethral luminal narrowing (*arrows*) caused by strictures in penile urethra are typical of inflammatory disease. Bulbar urethra is located proximal to penile urethra, and wide caliber of proximal bulbar urethra as shown is normal. This male patient had history of gonorrheal STI.

It is not possible to detail the many continent pouches that are used in clinical practice currently. General principles are that the pouches are constructed of detubularized bowel and are made to have enough capacity to hold ≈500 ml or more of urine, and the ureters are anastomosed to the pouches. In a cutaneous pouch such as the Indiana pouch, the cecum and ascending colon are often used to form the pouch, and the patient catheterizes the pouch through a stoma made of a segment of the terminal ileum. In an orthotopic pouch, ileum is used to construct the pouch, which is anastomosed to the urethra so that the patient can void per urethra by straining and pushing on the pouch.

11. What is a hysterosalpingogram?
    A hysterosalpingogram is a study to evaluate the uterine cavity and fallopian tubes (Figure 34-7). After sterile cleansing of the vaginal canal and exocervix, a cannula is placed in the external cervical os, and contrast material is injected under fluoroscopic guidance. The procedure is performed in women with primary or secondary infertility as well as in women with recurrent miscarriages. It is the best study to demonstrate patency of the fallopian tubes, and to see abnormalities in nondilated fallopian tubes. The study is performed on days 7 to 12 after the first day of the last menstrual period and should not be performed in the phase after ovulation, to prevent inadvertent harm to an

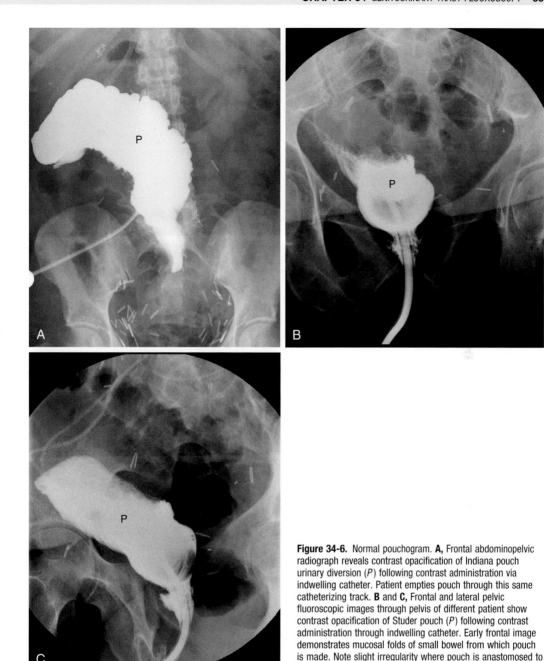

**Figure 34-6.** Normal pouchogram. **A,** Frontal abdominopelvic radiograph reveals contrast opacification of Indiana pouch urinary diversion (*P*) following contrast administration via indwelling catheter. Patient empties pouch through this same catheterizing track. **B** and **C,** Frontal and lateral pelvic fluoroscopic images through pelvis of different patient show contrast opacification of Studer pouch (*P*) following contrast administration through indwelling catheter. Early frontal image demonstrates mucosal folds of small bowel from which pouch is made. Note slight irregularity where pouch is anastomosed to urethra.

unexpected pregnancy. The study is contraindicated in patients with symptoms or signs suggestive of acute pelvic infection.

12. What is the normal appearance of the upper urinary tract on a retrograde pyelogram?
    There are 8 to 14 calyces in a normal collecting system, which drain through infundibulae into the renal pelvis (see Figure 34-1). The renal pelvis may sometimes protrude outside of the medial aspect of the renal parenchyma; this congenital variation is known as an extrarenal pelvis. An extrarenal pelvis may appear prominent because it is not compressed by the renal parenchyma, but it is important not to misconstrue this as hydronephrosis. The ureters insert on the posterior aspect of the bladder at the trigone.

13. What are some abnormalities that may be seen on a retrograde pyelogram?
    Urothelial tumors are seen as irregular filling defects in the collecting systems and ureters. Large lesions in the collecting system may cause obstruction of the calyces. There is often dilation of the ureter distal to the tumor on a

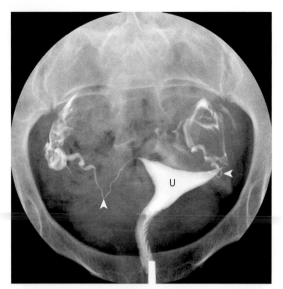

**Figure 34-7.** Normal hysterosalpingogram. Frontal fluoroscopic image through pelvis demonstrates metal cannula within external os at bottom of image. Uterine cavity (*U*) and both fallopian tubes (*arrowheads*) appear normal. There is contrast material spilling from both tubes into pelvic peritoneal cavity, which is normal. This young woman was undergoing evaluation for primary infertility.

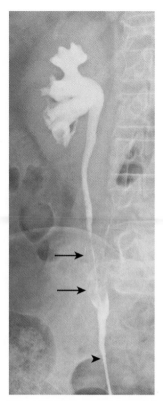

**Figure 34-8.** Ureteral urothelial cancer and pseudodiverticulosis on retrograde pyelogram. Frontal abdominopelvic radiograph following contrast injection through retrograde catheter demonstrates large filling defect in right ureter (*arrows*) caused by tumor. Note dilation of ureter just distal to filling defect indicating "goblet" sign. Also note tiny contrast-filled outpouchings of lumen of distal right ureter (*arrowhead*) representing ureteral pseudodiverticulosis.

retrograde pyelogram, which is referred to as a "goblet" sign (Figure 34-8). The ureter distal to a stone is usually small in caliber, and thus dilation of the ureter distal to a filling defect in the ureter is highly suggestive of a urothelial tumor.

Stones can be seen as filling defects in the collecting system, but they can be obscured by dense contrast material, as their radiodensity is similar to that of contrast material.

When a filling defect is seen in the collecting system or ureter, major differential diagnostic considerations include a urothelial tumor, a stone, a blood clot, and inflammatory processes such as ureteritis cystica. The latter process occurs in patients with long-standing presence of ureteral stents, stones, or infection, which can lead to reactive enlargement of submucosal glands in the ureter which then protrude into the lumen and appear as filling defects.

Another abnormality seen in the ureters is ureteral pseudodiverticulosis. Here, there are small erosions in the ureteral mucosa, so that contrast material collects into small protrusions from the lumen (see Figure 34-8). An association has been described between urothelial cancer of the bladder and the development of pseudodiverticulosis, although the etiology for this is not understood.

Ureteral strictures may be due to benign or malignant causes; when mild, they can be nonobstructing, and when more severe, they can cause partial or high-grade obstruction (see Figure 34-1, *A-B*). Chronic stone disease is one of the most common benign causes although endoscopic procedures such as ureteroscopic stone removal or other interventions can also lead to (iatrogenic) strictures. Ureteral narrowing due to malignancy can be caused by an intrinsic neoplasm of the ureter, such as a urothelial tumor, or by an extrinsic tumor that encases the ureter, which may be a primary tumor (e.g., cervical carcinoma that encases the pelvic ureter) or metastatic lymphadenopathy. A ureter encased by a malignant tumor is particularly likely to stricture after radiation therapy has been used to treat the tumor.

14. What are the causes of ureteral trauma, and how is it best evaluated?
    Iatrogenic injury is the most common cause for ureteral injuries, with gynecologic or other abdominal and pelvic surgeries being the common culprits.

Blunt abdominal trauma, such as by a motor vehicle collision, is an unusual cause for ureteral trauma, but penetrating trauma, such as by gunshot or stab wounds, can injure the ureter.

Computed tomography (CT) acquired in the excretory phase of enhancement is an effective way to assess the ureter for trauma; there is extravasation of contrast material from the injured segment, and there may also be some associated dilation of the affected ureter due to edema at the injury site causing slight obstruction. If ureteral injury is suspected intraoperatively, a retrograde pyelogram can be performed on the operating room table prior to completion of the surgery to assess the ureter for injury.

15. Why is vesicoureteral reflux (VUR) important, and how is it demonstrated?

VUR in children can cause recurrent UTIs and lead to permanent renal scarring, termed *reflux nephropathy*. This condition can cause complications such as hypertension and renal insufficiency; 10% to 30% of all cases of end-stage renal disease may be related to reflux nephropathy. In adults, VUR has less clinical significance, although it can be associated with recurrent or intractable UTIs, and rarely even flank pain. VUR is reliably shown by fluoroscopically monitored VCUG. However, if the bladder is not distended to the point of voiding, VUR may not be shown. In children, radionuclide cystography is an alternative study to minimize radiation exposure to the pelvic organs.

16. What is the normal appearance of the bladder on fluoroscopic studies?

The underdistended bladder may show slightly irregular contours and is wider in the left-right direction than in the craniocaudal direction. The fully distended bladder is usually smooth in outline, unless there is bladder wall thickening due to muscle hypertrophy to overcome bladder outlet obstruction; this is usually seen in older men with an enlarged prostate gland, and it is referred to as bladder trabeculation.

The bladder neck is the widest part of the outlet of the bladder. It is closed at rest and opens only during voiding.

17. What is a cystocele?

In perimenopausal and menopausal women, particularly those who have had vaginal childbirth, the support structures of the bladder and urethra become atrophic and lax. This leads to downward descent of the bladder and bladder neck, as well as protrusion of the bladder through the anterior wall of the vagina. Descent of the bladder neck below the level of the pubic symphysis is known as a cystocele.

Assessment for a cystocele is usually performed clinically. On fluoroscopy, descent of the bladder neck over 2 cm below the pubic symphysis with straining maneuvers such as a Valsalva maneuver is indicative of a cystocele.

18. What are some causes of incontinence?

There are many causes of incontinence, ranging from neurologic disorders to damage of the sphincters in the bladder neck or urethra by surgery or radiation therapy, to menopause resulting in stress incontinence. In a patient presenting with symptoms suggestive of incontinence, a thorough neurologic evaluation as well as a clinical evaluation with urodynamic studies is performed in a urologist's office. Imaging plays a relatively minor role in the evaluation of such patients. If there are symptoms of stress incontinence, leakage of contrast material into the urethra from the bladder may be seen during fluoroscopic observation if the patient is asked to perform straining maneuvers such as a Valsalva maneuver or is asked to cough.

19. Is a cystogram sensitive in excluding a leak from the bladder?

Leakage of urine from the bladder may be of clinical concern in a patient who has sustained trauma or has undergone pelvic or bladder surgery. To evaluate the bladder for a leak, the technique of the procedure is very important. The urinary bladder should be distended with a contrast agent until a detrusor contraction occurs, which indicates that the bladder capacity has been reached. Otherwise, small bladder leaks may not be shown. There is a great deal of variation in the amount of bladder filling required to produce a detrusor contraction, but most patients require 300 to 600 mL of contrast material to reach this point. A detrusor contraction is recognized by one of the following: (1) the patient voids, (2) there is resistance to injection of contrast material through a hand-held syringe so that the barrel of the syringe starts to move back out, or (3) flow through a contrast agent–filled bag suspended 35 to 40 cm above the fluoroscopy table stops or reverses.

20. A patient is brought to the emergency department with blunt abdominal trauma and pelvic fractures. Does this patient need both an abdominopelvic CT scan and a fluoroscopic cystogram?

No. The bladder can be distended with contrast material while the patient is on the CT scanner table to perform a CT cystogram to evaluate for a leak. CT cystography is as sensitive as a fluoroscopic cystography, if not more so, to exclude a leak from the urinary bladder. Before a catheter is placed in the urinary bladder in a patient with pelvic fractures, however, the urethra should be evaluated for injuries with RUG. A catheter is advanced through the urethra only if there is no urethral injury. Failure to follow this sequence could further traumatize an injured or partially disrupted urethra.

21. What kinds of injuries occur in the bladder?

Extraperitoneal bladder injuries are the most common injuries of the bladder and occur in patients with blunt trauma and associated pelvic fractures. These injuries are managed conservatively with Foley catheter drainage, and patients rarely require surgery to repair such injuries. If there is a forceful blow to the abdomen when the bladder is very full, tears occur at the dome of the bladder, which is covered by the peritoneum, such that the injury can also involve the peritoneum. The leakage of urine then occurs into the peritoneal cavity and results in urinary ascites. Such injuries usually require operative management, because they do not heal with Foley catheter drainage alone.

22. What are the imaging findings of cystitis?

In most patients, imaging is not indicated in the evaluation of cystitis. As mentioned above, in patients who have recurrent UTI, a voiding cystourethrogram may be performed to exclude VUR as the underlying etiology.

In patients with advanced genitourinary tuberculosis, the bladder becomes scarred and extremely small in capacity; this is referred to as a thimble bladder.

In diabetic patients with a severe gas-forming UTI, a special variant of cystitis called emphysematous cystitis may occur. Gas is seen within the bladder wall as well as in the lumen. The findings are best seen on CT images but may be discernible on abdominal radiographs in advanced cases. VCUG is not indicated in such patients, and the patients are managed with bladder drainage through a Foley catheter along with intravenous antibiotics until there is clinical defervescence.

23. What are the causes of bladder fistulae?

Colovesical fistulae, between the colon and bladder are related to colonic diverticulitis in >80% of cases. Colon carcinoma and inflammatory bowel disease, such as Crohn's disease, are less common causes.

Vesicovaginal fistulae, between the vaginal and bladder, are related to childbirth trauma in the majority of women, whether due to prolonged obstructed labor or traumatic forceps delivery (see Figure 34-3). Cesarean sections are a much less common cause of vesicovaginal fistulae. Tumors of the cervix can also erode into the bladder, resulting in fistulae, particularly after radiation therapy.

24. What is a bladder diverticulum?

Bladder diverticula most often occur in men with bladder outlet obstruction (see Figure 34-2). The diverticula are mucosal protrusions through the hypertrophied and thickened bladder wall. As diverticula have no muscle in their wall, they often empty poorly and may develop stones or tumors as a result. A congenital diverticulum called a "Hutch" diverticulum may be seen in the distal ureter near its insertion into the bladder and may cause ureteral compression or distort the ureterovesical junction (UVJ) enough to cause reflux.

25. What are some causes of urethral stricture?

Most strictures in the anterior urethra are related to sexually transmitted infection (STI) such as by gonorrhea or other nongonococcal pathogens (see Figure 34-4). Although uncommon in the developed world, granulomatous infections such as by tuberculosis can also cause strictures in the urethra. Both tuberculous and nontuberculous urethritis may cause fistulae to occur between the urethra and the adjacent soft tissues or perineal skin. When the fistulae are multiple, the process is referred to as a "watering can" perineum.

Chronic urethral strictures can cause difficulty in emptying the urinary bladder and result in complications such as bladder stone formation or recurrent infections. Chronic strictures are also a risk factor for the development of carcinoma at the stricture site. If a stricture has an irregular appearance on a urethrogram, endoscopic inspection of the urethra and biopsy as needed are performed.

Trauma to the anterior urethra, such as a straddle injury, can injure the bulbar urethra and result in a stricture. Pelvic fractures can injure the posterior urethra and result in strictures in the healing phase. Cystoscopy, particularly in young boys, can traumatize the urethra and result in strictures, most commonly at the urethral meatus, the penoscrotal junction, and the bulbomembranous junction; these sites are all areas of natural narrowing in the urethra, which makes them vulnerable to injury from prolonged endoscopic procedures. Chronic indwelling Foley catheters can also result in strictures at the same sites.

26. What is a urethral diverticulum?

A urethral diverticulum is often seen in women who present with a history of postvoid dribbling, dyspareunia, or a fluctuant mass on the anterior vaginal wall (Figure 34-9). The diverticulum results from infection in periurethral glands, which rupture into the periurethral soft tissues but continue to communicate with the urethra. Urethral diverticula can serve as a source of recurrent UTIs. Stones can form in urethral diverticula, and malignancy can also develop in the diverticula. Treatment is surgical resection; removal of the neck that connects the diverticulum to the urethra is important to prevent recurrence.

27. What kinds of traumatic injuries occur in the urethra?

Classification systems are available to categorize urethral injuries, but the most important assessment is to decide whether the injury is above the level of the external sphincter and membranous urethra or below the level of the external sphincter. Posterior urethral injuries, which are above the external sphincter, may lead to incontinence. Injuries below the external sphincter do not affect continence. As mentioned above, straddle injuries can cause injury to the bulbar urethra.

28. What is the normal appearance of the female genital tract on a hysterosalpingogram?

The uterine cavity has the shape of an inverted triangle. The fallopian tubes originate from the upper lateral aspects of the uterine fundus, and contrast material injected into the uterine cavity opacifies the tubes and then spills into the peritoneal cavity. The cornual portions of the tubes originate from the uterus and lead to the isthmic segments, which are thin and muscular portions of the tubes. The ampullary segments are wide portions of the tubes with

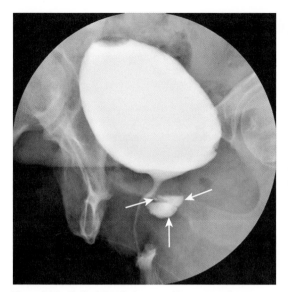

**Figure 34-9.** Urethral diverticulum on voiding cystourethrogram. Oblique frontal fluoroscopic image through pelvis reveals large pocket of contrast material along posterior aspect of urethra (*arrows*).

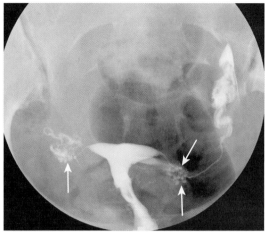

**Figure 34-10.** Salpingitis isthmica nodosa on hysterosalpingogram. Frontal fluoroscopic image through pelvis following contrast administration into uterine cavity shows contrast-opacified outpouchings (*arrows*) of proximal portions of fallopian tubes. This condition is the sequela of prior PID, is associated with tubal dysmotility and infertility, and is difficult to diagnose with any other imaging modality.

mucosal folds, while the fimbriated ends of the tubes overlie the ovaries but are not visualized distinctly on hysterosalpingography (HSG) (see Figure 34-7).

29. Does pelvic magnetic resonance imaging (MRI) or ultrasonography (US) provide the same information as HSG?
MRI and US are excellent for showing the anatomy of the uterus but are poor for showing the normal fallopian tubes, which are very small in size. Dilated fallopian tubes (hydrosalpinx) can be identified on MRI and US, but abnormality in nondilated tubes is best seen on a hysterosalpingogram. Tubal causes of infertility are the most common etiology of female infertility.

30. What are some abnormalities seen on a hysterosalpingogram?
Previous episodes of pelvic inflammatory disease (PID) or endometriosis can cause damage to the muscle of the fallopian tubes, the "myosalpinx," and result in tubal dilation known as hydrosalpinx. Such patients may have infertility or recurrent ectopic pregnancies in the abnormal tubes.

Salpingitis isthmica nodosa is another important cause of tubal infertility; it is seen in ≈25% of women with a previous history of PID. Outpouchings of contrast material are seen in the isthmic segments of the fallopian tubes on HSG. These outpouchings cause tubal dysmotility, leading to infertility or ectopic pregnancies (Figure 34-10).

Uterine abnormalities account for ≈10% of cases of infertility and early trimester pregnancy losses. Congenital anomalies may occur in the uterus but are usually associated with premature labor rather than miscarriages. Uterine leiomyomas are a common benign tumor in women but rarely cause infertility; they may be seen as filling defects in the endometrial cavity. Adenomyosis is a condition that occurs in women in their late 30s and early 40s and is associated with painful menstruation, pelvic pain, and infertility. MRI is the optimal method to evaluate for adenomyosis, but HSG may show outpouchings of contrast material from the endometrial cavity that suggest the diagnosis of adenomyosis.

Asherman's syndrome is a triad consisting of a history of D&C after a miscarriage or full-term pregnancy, followed by amenorrhea or scanty menstrual periods, and infertility. On HSG, the uterine cavity is irregular and small due to the presence of intrauterine synechiae.

31. If a female patient has a pelvic mass, what study would be helpful for further evaluation?
Either pelvic MRI or US would be useful to determine the organ of origin of the mass (e.g., gynecologic vs. nongynecologic, and uterine vs. ovarian) and to characterize it further. HSG has no role in this clinical situation.

32. Is a hysterosalpingogram useful for evaluation of the endometrium in a postmenopausal patient with vaginal bleeding?
Endometrial abnormalities, such as endometrial hyperplasia or endometrial cancer, can cause perimenopausal/postmenopausal bleeding and are best evaluated by transvaginal US or pelvic MRI. HSG has no role in this clinical situation.

## KEY POINTS

- The diagnosis of small leaks from the urinary bladder requires adequate bladder distention with contrast material until a detrusor contraction occurs, regardless of whether the evaluation is performed with CT or fluoroscopy.
- The anterior urethra in men is better evaluated on RUG. The posterior urethra in men is better evaluated on VCUG.
- In a man with pelvic trauma, the urethra should be evaluated with RUG before placement of a bladder drainage catheter.
- A retrograde pyelogram is an alternative study to a urogram (via IVU or CTU) to evaluate the urothelium in patients in whom intravenous contrast administration is contraindicated.
- A hysterosalpingogram is the most useful imaging study to evaluate the uterus and fallopian tubes in female patients with infertility.

## Bibliography

Dunnick R, Sandler C, Newhouse J. *Textbook of uroradiology.* 5th ed. Philadelphia, PA: Lippincott Williams & Wilkins; 2012.
Levine MS, Ramchandani P, Rubesin SE. *Practical fluoroscopy of the GI and GU tracts.* 1st ed. Cambridge, UK: Cambridge University Press; 2012.
Simpson WL Jr, Beitia LG, Mester J. Hysterosalpingography: a reemerging study. *Radiographics.* 2006;26(2):419-431.
Sandler CM, Goldman SM, Kawashima A. Lower urinary tract trauma. *World J Urol.* 1998;16(1):69-75.

# CHAPTER 35

# CT AND MRI OF THE KIDNEY

*Drew A. Torigian, MD, MA, FSAR, and Parvati Ramchandani, MD, FACR, FSAR*

1. **What are the common indications for computed tomography (CT) and magnetic resonance imaging (MRI) of the kidneys?**
   The most common clinical indications include:
   - Characterization of indeterminate renal lesions detected on prior cross-sectional imaging. This is done most frequently to distinguish a benign lesion such as a renal cyst from a malignant primary or metastatic neoplasm.
   - Surveillance of patients with genetic syndromes who are at increased risk for renal cell carcinoma (RCC).
   - Staging and response assessment of patients with renal malignancies.
   - Pretreatment and post-treatment evaluation of patients undergoing renal transplantation, as well as pretreatment evaluation of live renal donors.
   - Evaluation of patients with abdominal symptoms or signs (e.g., flank pain, hematuria) that are suspected to be secondary to renal disease.
   - Assessment for traumatic injury to the kidneys (mainly using contrast-enhanced CT).
   - Providing guidance for percutaneous biopsy or intervention for renal disease.

2. **What is the normal appearance of the kidneys on CT and MRI?**
   The kidneys have an attenuation of 30 to 50 Hounsfield units (HU) on unenhanced CT (Figure 35-1, *A*). On MRI, the renal cortices have low T1-weighted signal intensity relative to the medullary pyramids and low T2-weighted signal intensity relative to the medullary pyramids (Figure 35-2). The normal kidney is "bean shaped" and has a smooth contour. Persistent fetal lobation may sometimes be seen and can give the kidney a lobulated contour.

   Unenhanced CT images (but not MR images) are useful to detect renal calcifications that may be related to urinary stone disease, parenchymal calcifications due to varied causes such as hyperparathyroidism, or dystrophic calcifications in renal neoplasms. However, both CT and MR unenhanced images are useful to (1) detect presence of macroscopic fat within a renal mass to establish a specific diagnosis of renal angiomyolipoma (AML), a benign lesion, as well as to (2) serve as a reference of comparison for contrast-enhanced images to determine whether there are enhancing components within a renal lesion. In the vast majority of renal lesions, the presence of a soft tissue enhancing component is suspicious for a malignant lesion such as RCC.

   The kidneys receive ≈25% of the cardiac output and therefore enhance avidly and rapidly after contrast administration. Following the intravenous administration of contrast material, sequential phases of enhancement of the kidney are seen as follows:
   - The arterial phase of enhancement occurs 10 to 30 seconds after contrast administration, where the renal arteries predominantly enhance. This phase is useful for delineation of renal arterial anatomy and pathology, as in preoperative planning for renal donor evaluation or for a complex tumor resection.
   - The corticomedullary (or cortical) phase of enhancement occurs 25 to 70 seconds after contrast administration. Here, the renal cortices are enhanced but the medullary pyramids have not yet enhanced (Figure 35-1, *B*). In this phase, the intrarenal vasculature and hypervascular renal lesions are seen to best effect. However, some small renal lesions, particularly those located in the medullary pyramids, may be difficult to visualize during this phase of enhancement.
   - The nephrographic phase of enhancement occurs 60 to 180 seconds after contrast administration, where the renal cortices and medullary pyramids are homogeneously enhanced (Figure 35-1, *C*). In this phase, hypovascular renal lesions and the renal veins are seen to best effect; most renal lesions are seen as areas with less enhancement in the enhanced normal renal parenchyma. Hypervascular renal lesions may also have washout of enhancement relative to the enhanced normal renal parenchyma, and thus are easily identified.
   - The delayed (or excretory or equilibrium) phase of enhancement occurs starting >120 to 180 seconds after contrast administration, where renal parenchyma decreases in enhancement, and the renal collecting systems increasingly opacify with excreted intravenous contrast material (Figure 35-1, *D*). This phase is most useful to evaluate the collecting systems for urothelial tumors as in a CT urogram and to evaluate the integrity of the collecting systems in patients with severe renal trauma (blunt or penetrating).

3. **What is the role of CT and MRI in renal transplantation?**
   CT and MRI play an important role in the preoperative evaluation of renal transplant donors, as well as in the pre- and postoperative evaluation of recipients of renal transplants.

   In potential renal donors, preoperative evaluation can be performed with three-phase dynamic contrast-enhanced CT or MRI to delineate the renal arterial, venous, and urothelial anatomy, because anatomic variations are common.

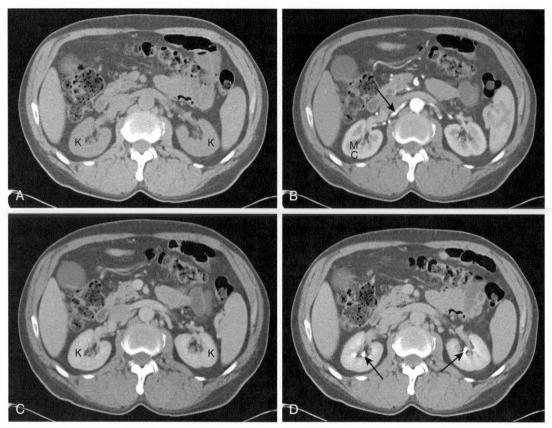

**Figure 35-1.** Normal kidneys and phases of renal enhancement on CT. **A,** Axial unenhanced CT image through abdomen shows normal kidneys (*K*) with homogeneous soft tissue attenuation and smooth external contours. **B,** Axial corticomedullary phase contrast-enhanced CT image through abdomen demonstrates enhancement of renal cortex (*C*) but lack of enhancement of medullary pyramids (*M*). Note avid enhancement of right renal artery (*arrow*) and other arteries including abdominal aorta. **C,** Axial nephrographic phase contrast-enhanced CT image through abdomen reveals homogeneous enhancement of kidneys (*K*) including cortices and medullary pyramids. **D,** Axial delayed phase contrast-enhanced CT image through abdomen shows decrease in enhancement of renal parenchyma and increased opacification of collecting systems (*arrows*) with excreted intravenous contrast material.

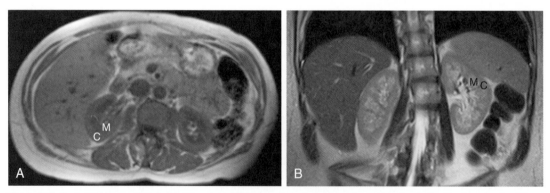

**Figure 35-2.** Normal kidneys on MRI. **A,** Axial T1-weighted MR image through abdomen shows high signal intensity of renal cortex (*C*) relative to medullary pyramids (*M*). **B,** Coronal heavily T2-weighted MR image through abdomen demonstrates low signal intensity of renal cortex (*C*) relative to medullary pyramids (*M*).

This imaging evaluation is also performed to identify any incidental lesions in the abdomen or pelvis of the donors, which may need attention prior to surgery.

In potential renal transplant recipients, preoperative evaluation is helpful to delineate the underlying anatomy and to evaluate for preexisting renal disease. Renal transplants are usually placed in the iliac fossa with vascular anastomosis to the external iliac vasculature and ureteral implantation into the bladder.

Post-transplant evaluation in renal transplant recipients is primarily focused on the detection of vascular, renal parenchymal, or urothelial complications. Although ultrasonography (US) is often the initial imaging modality to evaluate these patients, CT and MRI may be used for problem-solving. Commonly encountered vascular complications following renal transplantation include thrombosis or stenosis of the transplant renal arteries or veins, renal arteriovenous fistula (AVF), and renal arterial pseudoaneurysm formation (the latter two are often a complication of percutaneous biopsy of a renal transplant). Commonly encountered urothelial complications following renal transplantation include ureteral obstruction and leak at the site of ureteral anastomosis to the urinary bladder; such urologic complications account for 10% of postoperative complications in renal transplants and are an important cause of transplant failure. Other important complications seen in renal transplants include urolithiasis, peritransplant fluid collection (abscess, hematoma, lymphocele, or urinoma), renal infarct, acute tubular necrosis (ATN), transplant rejection, and post-transplant lymphoproliferative disorder (PTLD).

4. What is a horseshoe kidney?

A horseshoe kidney is the most common type of congenital renal fusion anomaly, occurring in 1 in 500 people, in which the lower poles of the kidneys are attached to each other across the midline, leading to a "horseshoe" configuration. The region of connection, called the isthmus, is composed of fibrous tissue or functioning renal parenchyma and is located just inferior to the inferior mesenteric artery (Figure 35-3).

Patients with a horseshoe kidney are generally asymptomatic but have an increased risk of a malformed ureteropelvic junction with resultant obstruction, vesicoureteral reflux (VUR), nephrolithiasis, renal traumatic injury to the isthmus in blunt abdominal trauma, urinary tract infections, and renal neoplasms including Wilms tumor and urothelial carcinoma.

5. What is the most common benign renal lesion?

A renal cyst is the most common benign renal lesion. It occurs with increasing frequency with increasing age and may be seen in up to one third of adults over the age of 60. It is round or oval in shape and is composed of simple fluid with a smooth thin wall. On CT, a simple renal cyst will have fluid attenuation (0 to 20 HU) on CT, and on MRI, it will have low signal intensity on T1-weighted images, very high signal intensity on T2-weighted images, and very high signal intensity on heavily T2-weighted images relative to renal parenchyma. Simple cysts do not demonstrate enhancement (Figure 35-4).

Sometimes, a cyst can become minimally complex secondary to hemorrhage or infection. When this occurs, on CT, the attenuation of the cyst contents will be higher than that in simple cysts. On MRI, the T1-weighted signal intensity of the cyst contents will be variably increased, and its T2-weighted signal intensity will be variably decreased relative to that of simple cysts. In addition, internal septations, fluid-debris levels, calcifications, or wall thickening may also be seen. However, no enhancing components will be present (Figure 35-5).

6. What is a cystic nephroma, and what are its CT and MR imaging features?

A cystic nephroma is a rare benign cystic renal neoplasm. In adults, it most commonly occurs in women in the fifth through seventh decades of life. It also occurs in young boys in the first decade of life. On CT and MRI, a well-circumscribed cystic renal lesion is typically seen, usually with multiple variably enhancing internal septations, and sometimes with herniation into the renal collecting system (Figure 35-6), which is a characteristic feature. Solid enhancing components, hemorrhage, venous extension, regional lymphadenopathy, and distant metastatic disease are generally not seen. However, surgical resection is generally performed because it is extremely difficult to distinguish a cystic nephroma from a cystic RCC.

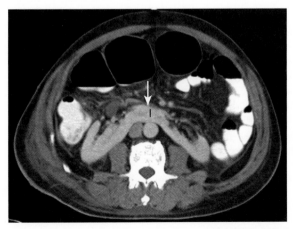

**Figure 35-3.** Horseshoe kidney on CT. Axial nephrographic phase contrast-enhanced CT image through abdomen reveals attachment of lower poles of kidneys across midline leading to "horseshoe" configuration. Note isthmus (*I*) located inferior and posterior to inferior mesenteric artery (*arrow*).

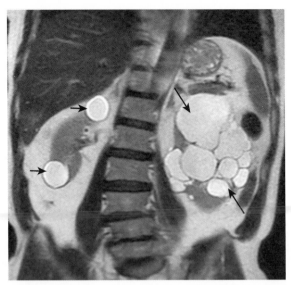

**Figure 35-4.** Simple renal cysts and localized cystic renal disease on MRI. Coronal heavily T2-weighted MR image through abdomen shows two round fluid signal intensity lesions in right kidney (*short arrows*) with smooth thin walls secondary to simple renal cysts (Bosniak I lesions). Also note cluster of tightly spaced variably sized simple cysts (Bosniak I lesions) and minimally septated cysts (Bosniak II lesions) within left kidney (*between longer arrows*) secondary to localized cystic renal disease.

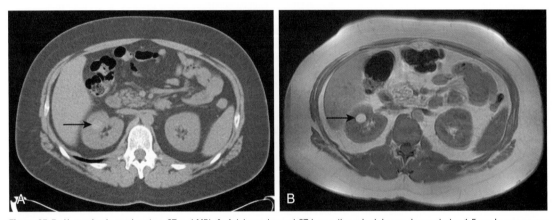

**Figure 35-5.** Hemorrhagic renal cyst on CT and MRI. **A,** Axial unenhanced CT image through abdomen demonstrates 1.5-cm homogeneous hyperattenuating fully intrarenal lesion in right kidney (*arrow*) which did not enhance on contrast-enhanced images (*not shown*) (Bosniak IIF lesion). **B,** Axial T1-weighted MR image through abdomen reveals homogeneous high signal intensity of lesion (*arrow*) secondary to hemorrhagic fluid contents. Lesion did not enhance on contrast-enhanced images (*not shown*) (Bosniak II lesion).

7. What is the Bosniak classification system for cystic renal lesions?
   The Bosniak classification system (Table 35-1) utilizes specific CT or MR imaging features to help classify cystic renal lesions into those that are likely benign (and do not require surgical resection) from those that are likely malignant (and thus require surgical resection).

8. What is the major differential diagnosis for polycystic kidney disease?
   The various conditions that lead to polycystic kidney disease may be subdivided into nonheritable causes and heritable causes.
      Non-heritable/idiopathic causes include the following conditions:
   - **Multiple incidental renal cysts**: When cysts involve the renal pelvis, they may either be secondary to (1) **peripelvic (renal sinus) cysts** that arise from the renal hilar lymphatics, which are usually small, multiple, and bilateral; or (2) **parapelvic cysts** that arise from the renal cortex and extend into the renal sinus fat, which are more commonly solitary and unilateral.
   - **Localized cystic renal disease**: This is a rare idiopathic benign condition in which a unilateral cluster of tightly spaced variably sized cysts are seen within a kidney. Presence of intervening normally enhancing renal parenchyma

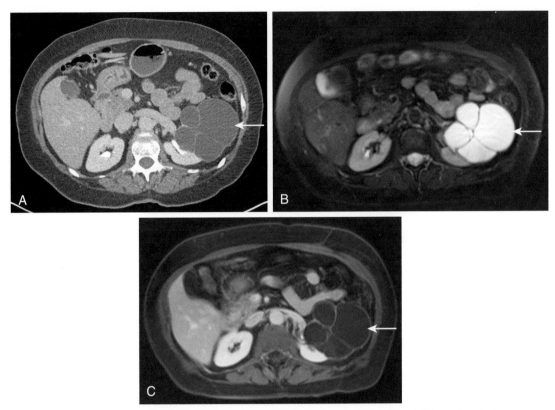

**Figure 35-6.** Cystic nephroma on CT and MRI. **A,** Axial nephrographic/delayed phase contrast-enhanced CT image through abdomen shows large well-circumscribed partially exophytic cystic lesion of left kidney (*arrow*) with multiple internal septations, some of which are thickened and enhancing (Bosniak III lesion). **B,** Axial fat-suppressed T2-weighted MR image through abdomen demonstrates fluid signal intensity within lesion (*arrow*) confirming cystic nature. **C,** Axial nephrographic phase contrast-enhanced MR image through abdomen again reveals multiple internal septations within lesion (*arrow*), some of which are thickened and enhancing.

**Table 35-1.** Bosniak Classification System for Cystic Renal Lesions

| CATEGORY | IMAGING FEATURES | MANAGEMENT |
|---|---|---|
| I: simple cyst | Fluid attenuation (CT)<br>Fluid signal intensity (MRI)<br>Thin smooth wall<br>No enhancement | 100% benign<br>No further follow-up |
| II: minimally complex cyst | Fine calcifications or a short segment of slightly thickened calcification (CT)<br>Few thin internal septations without enhancement<br>Homogeneously hyperattenuating (>20 HU) and nonenhancing but ≤3 cm and not fully intrarenal (CT)<br>Increased T1-weighted signal intensity or slightly decreased T2-weighted signal intensity relative to simple fluid but nonenhancing (MRI) | 100% benign<br>No further follow-up |
| IIF: probable minimally complex cyst | Small nodular calcifications (CT)<br>Multiple thin internal septations without enhancement<br>Minimal smooth thickening of wall or internal septations<br>Homogeneously hyperattenuating (>20 HU) and nonenhancing but either ≤3 cm and fully intrarenal or >3 cm (CT) | 95% benign<br>Follow-up imaging |
| III: probable cystic renal neoplasm | Thick or irregular walls or internal septations with enhancement | >50% malignant<br>Surgical resection |
| IV: cystic renal neoplasm | Solid nodular components with enhancement | >95% malignant<br>Surgical resection |

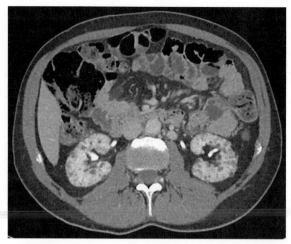

**Figure 35-7.** Lithium-induced nephrotoxicity on CT. Axial nephrographic/delayed phase contrast-enhanced CT image through abdomen shows multiple subcentimeter uniformly distributed cysts within normal-sized kidneys.

and the lack of a surrounding capsule are additional imaging features that are suggestive of this diagnosis (see Figure 35-4).

- **Multicystic dysplastic kidney (MCDK)**: This is a nonheritable developmental disorder that is often diagnosed in utero, where one kidney is partially or completely replaced by a cluster of nonfunctioning noncommunicating cysts, sometimes with atrophy of the ipsilateral ureter, renal collecting system, and renal vasculature. Compensatory hypertrophy of the contralateral kidney is often present as well.
- **Acquired cystic renal disease of dialysis (ACKD)**: Multiple renal cysts may occur in patients with end-stage renal disease and increase in frequency in proportion to the duration of dialysis. Multiple simple or complex cysts of varying size are typically seen throughout the small shrunken kidneys.
- **Lithium-induced nephrotoxicity**: This is secondary to long-term lithium therapy (usually in patients with depression or schizophrenia), where multiple subcentimeter (usually 1 to 2 mm) uniformly distributed cysts are seen throughout the normal-sized kidneys (Figure 35-7).
- **Glomerulocystic kidney disease (GCKD)**: This is a rare form of cystic renal disease that is most often seen in neonates and young children, where multiple small cysts are predominantly seen in the subcapsular cortices of the kidneys which may be normal or small in size.
  Heritable causes include the following conditions:
- **Autosomal dominant polycystic kidney disease (ADPKD)**: This is the most common heritable renal disorder. It typically presents in the third through fourth decades of life, where about 50% of patients develop end-stage renal disease, and is associated with an increased risk of cardiac valve abnormalities and intracranial aneurysms. Multiple cysts are typically seen bilaterally in the kidneys, which may be normal in size but can also be enormously enlarged. The cysts may be simple or minimally complex (Figure 35-8). Cysts are also commonly seen in the liver and less commonly seen in the pancreas, spleen, ovaries, and testes.
- **Autosomal recessive polycystic kidney disease (ARPKD)**: This is a rare heritable renal disorder, which may be diagnosed in utero, in neonates and infants, in children, or in adults but most often presents at the age of 2.5 years. Multiple uniform 1- to 2-mm tubular cysts are typically seen, predominantly in a medullary location, but sometimes larger 1- to 2-cm cysts are also encountered within the kidneys (which are typically large in size). Associated findings of congenital hepatic fibrosis, portal hypertension (including splenomegaly and ascites), and biliary cystic disease are typically present as well.
- **von Hippel Lindau (vHL) syndrome**: This is an autosomal dominant condition that is associated with development of renal cysts, RCC, pheochromocytomas, pancreatic cysts, pancreatic neoplasms including serous cystadenoma and neuroendocrine tumors, and central nervous system hemangioblastomas. In vHL syndrome, simple-appearing renal cysts often contain small foci of RCC.
- **Tuberous sclerosis (TS)**: This is the second most common phakomatosis (after neurofibromatosis type 1) and is an autosomal dominant condition that leads to hamartoma formation in the various organs of the body. Multiple bilateral renal AMLs are typically seen, which may enlarge and replace the kidneys, often in association with multiple renal cysts. Fat-containing hepatic AMLs and uniformly distributed cystic lung disease are additional suggestive imaging findings that may also be seen.
- **Medullary cystic renal disease**: This condition usually occurs in children and young adults. Multiple small 1- to 1.5-cm cysts are seen at the corticomedullary junctions in the kidneys (which are typically small in size).

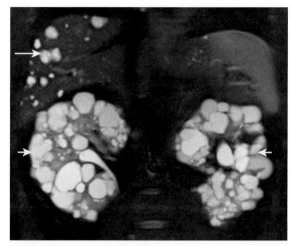

**Figure 35-8.** ADPKD on MRI. Coronal fat-suppressed heavily T2-weighted MR image through abdomen demonstrates multiple simple and minimally septated cysts (*short arrows*) within enlarged kidneys along with multiple hepatic cysts (*long arrow*).

---

**Box 35-1.** Major Differential Diagnosis for a Focal Renal Lesion

Cystic lesions
- Renal cyst
- Cystic nephroma
- Renal abscess
- Renal hematoma
- Cystic/necrotic renal malignancy (RCC, metastasis)

Solid lesions
- Renal contusion
- Renal infarct

- Focal pyelonephritis
- Renal AML
- Renal oncocytoma
- Solid renal malignancy (RCC, lymphoma, metastasis, urothelial cancer extending from collecting system)

---

9. **What is the major differential diagnosis for focal renal lesions?**
   For the answer, see Box 35-1.

10. **What is a renal AML, and what are its CT and MR imaging features?**
    A renal AML is the most common benign mesenchymal neoplasm of the kidney and is composed of variable amounts of fat, blood vessels, and smooth muscle. It may arise sporadically (in up to 70% of cases), 4 times more commonly in women, or may occur in the setting of TS with equal frequency in men and women. Renal AMLs have a >50% risk of spontaneous hemorrhage when >4 cm in size. Therefore, it is recommended that renal AMLs be treated prophylactically with catheter arterial embolization when they exceed 4 cm in size.

    On CT and MRI, visualization of the presence of macroscopic fat content within a renal mass is diagnostic of a renal AML. However, 5% of renal AMLs do not contain visible macroscopic fat and are known as lipid-poor AMLs. These may mimic other renal neoplasms such as RCC on cross-sectional imaging but tend to have homogeneous attenuation, homogeneous hypointense T2-weighted signal intensity relative to renal parenchyma, and homogeneous enhancement and often protrude from the renal parenchyma from a small parenchymal defect. Calcification is not typically seen (Figure 35-9). A small RCC may be very difficult to distinguish from a renal AML by imaging alone.

11. **What is a renal oncocytoma, and what are its CT and MR imaging features?**
    A renal oncocytoma is a benign renal neoplasm that occurs more commonly in men than in women, most commonly in the seventh decade of life. On CT and MRI, it appears as a solid enhancing well-circumscribed renal mass that is indistinguishable from RCC. A central stellate scar may be seen in ≈33% of cases with delayed phase enhancement, and hemorrhage is rare. Segmental enhancement inversion has been reported to be a fairly specific feature of renal oncocytomas, where one portion of a renal mass has avid enhancement during the corticomedullary phase and becomes less enhancing during the nephrographic phase, and another portion of a renal mass has low enhancement during the corticomedullary phase and becomes more enhancing during the nephrographic phase. No regional lymphadenopathy and no distant metastatic disease is seen with renal oncocytomas.

12. **What is acute pyelonephritis, and what are its CT and MR imaging features?**
    Acute pyelonephritis is inflammation of the renal parenchyma and renal pelvis and is most often due to an ascending urinary tract infection and less commonly a hematogenous infection. The diagnosis of acute pyelonephritis should be

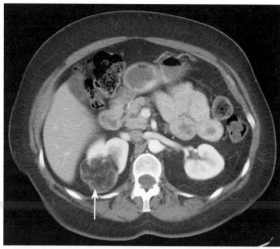

**Figure 35-9.** Renal AML on CT. Axial corticomedullary phase contrast-enhanced CT image through abdomen reveals large predominantly fat attenuation partially exophytic mass (*arrow*) of posterior upper pole of right kidney.

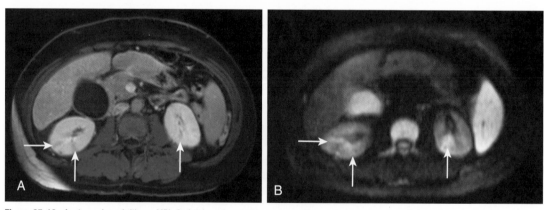

**Figure 35-10.** Acute pyelonephritis on MRI. **A,** Axial nephrographic phase contrast-enhanced MR image through abdomen shows alternating radially arranged linear and wedge-shaped areas of decreased enhancement (*arrows*) in kidneys with subjacent areas of normal enhancement representing "striated nephrogram" pattern. **B,** Axial DW MR image through abdomen demonstrates areas with high signal intensity restricted diffusion in kidneys (*arrows*) that correspond to areas of decreased enhancement.

made clinically, with imaging reserved for patients in whom there is no clinical improvement despite appropriate antibiotic therapy; imaging is then helpful in detecting the development of complications such as a renal abscess.

Heterogeneity of the renal parenchyma during the nephrographic phase of enhancement may be seen as linear or wedge-shaped areas of decreased enhancement alternating with areas of normal enhancement (known as the "striated nephrogram" pattern); this pattern is secondary to tubular obstruction caused by inflammatory debris, interstitial edema, and vasospasm. During the delayed phase of enhancement, a reversal of the striated nephrogram pattern may be seen, where contrast retention is seen in the linear or wedge-shaped areas that were hypoenhancing in the nephrographic phase. On MRI, areas of pyelonephritis appear hypointense on T1-weighted images, appear hyperintense on T2-weighted images, and restrict diffusion on diffusion-weighted images (DWI) relative to renal parenchyma (Figure 35-10). Other associated findings with acute pyelonephritis may include renal enlargement, inflammatory perinephric fat stranding, and thickening of the renal fascia. When pyelonephritis occurs focally, it may mimic the appearance of a renal mass.

13. **What are the CT and MR imaging features of a renal pyogenic abscess?**
   A renal abscess is most often secondary to Gram-negative bacilli and may complicate acute pyelonephritis or bacteremia. Seventy percent or more of renal abscesses occur in diabetic patients.

   On CT and MRI, an abscess is seen as a heterogeneous multiloculated cystic lesion, with thick rim enhancement and internal septal enhancement. The presence of gas in the lesion is highly specific for this diagnosis. Additional findings of coexistent acute pyelonephritis are also usually present.

14. **What is xanthogranulomatous pyelonephritis (XGP), and what are its CT and MR imaging features?**

XGP is an uncommon chronic granulomatous process that is secondary to bacterial infection and urolithiasis, in which there is replacement of the renal parenchyma by lipid-laden macrophages. This most often occurs in middle-aged patients and is twice as common in women than in men. Nephrolithiasis is almost always present, often with presence of a staghorn calculus.

On CT and MRI, unilateral renal enlargement is usually seen, which is diffuse in 90% of cases and focal in 10% of cases, along with decreased or absent excretion of contrast material. Multiple cystic-appearing areas secondary to inflammatory infiltrates replace the renal parenchyma, often in a configuration resembling the paw print of a bear, known as the "bear paw" sign. There is commonly extension of inflammatory tissue into the perinephric fat and even into the retroperitoneum or abdominal wall. Fistulae to adjacent structures are common, often to the skin or large bowel (Figure 35-11).

15. **What is the difference between nephrolithiasis and nephrocalcinosis?**

Nephrolithiasis is the presence of calculi (i.e., stones) in the kidneys, which can pass into the renal pelvis, ureter, or bladder. Patients may present acutely with flank pain or with complications related to obstruction of the collecting system or ureter.

Nephrocalcinosis is the deposition of calcification within the renal parenchyma, either within the renal cortex or within the renal medullary pyramids.

16. **What are the major causes of cortical nephrocalcinosis?**

Cortical nephrocalcinosis is secondary to deposition of calcification in the renal cortices (Figure 35-12). Major causes include chronic glomerulonephritis, acute cortical necrosis, and oxalosis.

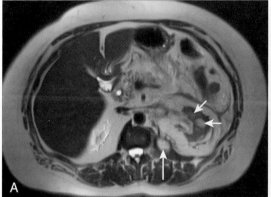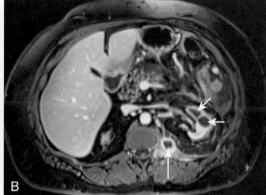

**Figure 35-11.** XGP with left psoas abscess on MRI. **A,** Axial heavily T2-weighted MR image through abdomen reveals several cystic-appearing foci within left kidney (*short arrows*) and left psoas muscle (*long arrow*). **B,** Axial nephrographic phase contrast-enhanced MR image through abdomen shows contracted left renal pelvis along with lack of enhancement of cystic foci within left kidney (*short arrows*). Also note thick rim enhancement of abscess in left psoas muscle (*long arrow*). Left staghorn calculus had previously been removed.

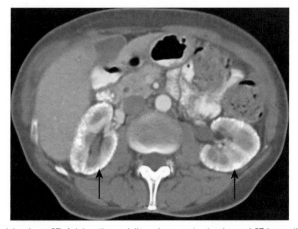

**Figure 35-12.** Cortical nephrocalcinosis on CT. Axial corticomedullary phase contrast-enhanced CT image through abdomen demonstrates diffuse calcification of renal cortices (*arrows*).

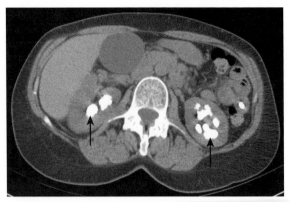

**Figure 35-13.** Medullary nephrocalcinosis secondary to type I RTA on CT. Axial unenhanced CT image through abdomen reveals heavy calcifications of medullary pyramids (*arrows*).

17. What are the major causes of medullary nephrocalcinosis?

Medullary nephrocalcinosis is secondary to deposition of calcification in the renal medulla and is more common than cortical nephrocalcinosis (Figure 35-13). Major causes include hyperparathyroidism, medullary sponge kidney, distal renal tubular acidosis (type 1 RTA), and oxalosis. The medullary calcifications can erode into the collecting system, causing patients to present with recurrent and intractable urinary stones.

18. What does renal iron deposition look like on MRI, and what are its major causes?

Renal cortical iron deposition is most commonly caused by intravascular hemolysis secondary to a malfunctioning prosthetic cardiac valve, paroxysmal nocturnal hemoglobinuria (PNH), or sickle cell disease. Renal medullary iron deposition, which is much less common, may be secondary to hemorrhagic fever with renal syndrome (HFRS) or renal vein thrombosis.

On MRI, iron deposition leads to decreased T1-weighted and T2-weighted signal intensity of the kidneys, which is particularly accentuated on in-phase T1-weighted MR images and most often involves the renal cortices.

19. What CT imaging findings may be encountered in renal trauma?

The kidney is injured in up to 10% of patients with blunt trauma and in up to 6% of patients with penetrating trauma. CT is the mainstay for imaging evaluation of patients with potential renal trauma. Currently, the most widely used CT grading system for renal injury is based on the American Association for the Surgery of Trauma (AAST) scale. The spectrum of renal injuries includes contusion, hematoma, laceration, avulsion, infarction, collecting system disruption, active hemorrhage, and vascular injuries including renal vascular pedicle injury, renal arterial pseudoaneurysm, and renal AVF. Patients with deep renal lacerations and vascular injuries are more likely to be unstable and in need of surgical or percutaneous intervention. However, the vast majority of patients with renal trauma respond well to conservative supportive treatment.

Renal contusions appear as focal areas of poorly defined hypoattenuation within the kidney, although they may sometimes be isoattenuating relative to surrounding renal parenchyma or hyperattenuating when there is associated hemorrhage. Perinephric fat stranding may also be seen.

Renal lacerations appear as linear, irregular, or branching nonenhancing low attenuation parenchymal defects in the kidney, often with adjacent areas of high attenuation hemorrhage (Figure 35-14, *A*). When severe, portions of renal parenchyma may even avulse from the remainder of the kidney.

Renal hematomas appear as foci of nonenhancing high attenuation (30 to 70 HU) hemorrhagic fluid on CT, either subcapsular or intraparenchymal in location. Subcapsular hematomas are well-circumscribed, are often crescentic in shape, and may distort the external renal contour. Because these hematomas are enclosed in a tight subcapsular space, they may cause ischemia of the underlying renal parenchyma due to mass effect, leading to hypertension; this is referred to as a "Page kidney." Perinephric hematomas within the retroperitoneum are generally more ill-defined and may displace the kidney but less often distort the external renal contour (Figure 35-14, *B*). When active hemorrhage is present, one sees focal areas of increased attenuation on contrast-enhanced images similar to that of enhancing vessels which do not conform to known vascular structures and which persist or increase in size on more delayed phase acquisitions.

Renal arterial pseudoaneurysms also appear as well-circumscribed round or oval foci of contrast enhancement with attenuation similar to adjacent contrast-enhanced arteries but decrease in attenuation on more delayed phase acquisitions. Renal AVF manifests as early enhancement of the renal vein during the arterial phase of enhancement. These may occur from spontaneous trauma or from iatrogenic trauma such as from percutaneous biopsy, percutaneous ablation, or percutaneous nephrostomy procedures. These are generally treated with catheter-directed embolotherapy or with surgical repair.

Renal vascular pedicle injury involves avulsion or thrombosis of the renal artery or vein. With renal artery injury, abrupt termination or complete nonenhancement of the renal artery is seen, along with nonenhancement of part or all

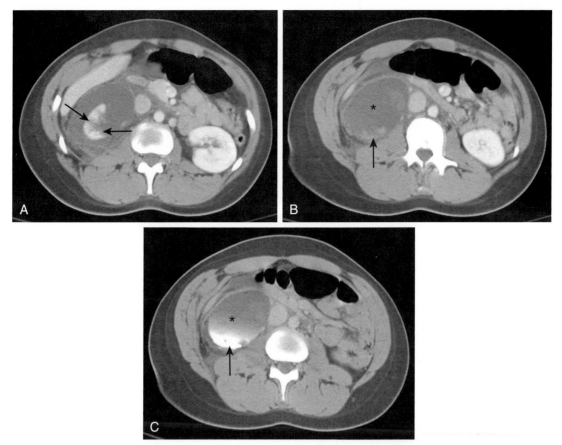

**Figure 35-14.** Renal trauma on CT. **A,** Axial nephrographic phase contrast-enhanced CT image through abdomen shows linear irregular nonenhancing low attenuation parenchymal defects in lower pole of left kidney (*arrows*) secondary to renal lacerations. **B,** Axial nephrographic phase contrast-enhanced CT image through abdomen more inferiorly demonstrates perinephric fluid collection (*) with dependent foci of high attenuation (*arrow*) representing perinephric hematoma. **C,** Axial delayed phase contrast-enhanced CT image through abdomen at same level reveals leakage of excreted intravenous contrast material (*arrow*) into perinephric fluid collection (*) indicating component of perinephric urinoma related to collecting system disruption.

of the renal parenchyma. With renal vein laceration, a medially or circumferentially located subcapsular or perinephric hematoma is seen, although the lacerated vein itself is generally difficult to visualize. With renal vein thrombosis, an intraluminal hypoattenuating filling defect secondary to thrombus is typically seen in an enlarged renal vein, in association with renal parenchymal enlargement and delayed enhancement.

Collecting system disruption appears as extraluminal fluid, representing urine, adjacent to the kidney, collecting system, or proximal ureter. In the excretory phase, excreted contrast accumulation is seen within the fluid collections (Figure 35-14, *C*). With deep lacerations of the renal parenchyma, the collecting system may also be involved.

20. What do renal infarcts look like on CT and MRI, and what are some causes of renal infarction?
    Renal infarcts appear as peripheral, often wedge-shaped, areas of nonenhancement in the renal parenchyma and are often multiple. A thin enhancing rim of cortical enhancement (i.e., the "cortical rim" sign) is typically seen in renal infarcts secondary to perfusion of the renal cortex by the renal capsular arteries (Figure 35-15).

    Some causes of renal infarction include traumatic renal injury, renal artery embolism, renal artery dissection, renal vein thrombosis, and vasculitis.

21. What are some risk factors for renal hemorrhage/hematoma?
    • Renal arterial aneurysm/pseudoaneurysm rupture.
    • Recent surgery.
    • Renal trauma.
    • Coagulopathy.
    • Renal malignancy.
    • Renal AML.

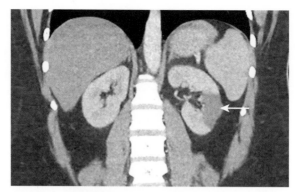

**Figure 35-15.** Renal infarct on CT. Coronal nephrographic phase contrast-enhanced CT image through abdomen shows peripheral wedge-shaped area of nonenhancement in left kidney (*arrow*).

22. **What is RCC, and what are its histologic subtypes?**

    RCC is the most common primary malignant tumor of the kidney, accounting for >90% of renal malignancies, most often arising in patients in the seventh through eighth decades of life, and occurring two to three times more commonly in men than in women. With the extensive use of cross-sectional imaging in clinical practice, 60% to 70% of renal neoplasms are discovered incidentally during imaging for other causes. The Fuhrman nuclear grading system is typically used to histopathologically grade RCC, where grade I carries the best prognosis and grade IV carries the worst prognosis. Treatment of RCC may involve total nephrectomy, partial nephrectomy, cryoablation, or radiofrequency ablation, and chemotherapy is administered when metastatic disease is present. Nephron sparing surgery is the treatment of choice, whenever feasible, with thermal ablation usually reserved for patients who are poor surgical candidates.

    Clear cell (conventional) RCC is the most common histologic subtype, accounting for 75% of cases, contains microscopic lipid, and is associated with the second worst prognosis.

    Papillary RCC accounts for 10% of cases and is generally associated with a good prognosis. Type I (basophilic) papillary RCC is more indolent, whereas type II (eosinophilic) papillary RCC is more aggressive.

    Chromophobe RCC accounts for 5% of cases and is associated with the best prognosis.

    Collecting duct RCC (including the renal medullary subtype) accounts for 1% of cases, is typically highly aggressive, and is associated with the worst prognosis. The renal medullary subtype is most commonly seen in young patients with sickle cell trait.

    The remaining 4% of RCC are unclassified.

23. **What are the CT and MR imaging features of RCC?**

    RCC is solitary in 95% of cases and may be intrarenal, exophytic, or both intrarenal and exophytic in configuration. A solid enhancing renal mass with soft tissue attenuation on CT or with low-intermediate T1-weighted signal intensity, variable T2-weighted signal intensity, and restricted diffusion relative to renal parenchyma on MRI is typically visualized. Presence of microscopic lipid content within the renal mass, as manifested by a loss of signal intensity on out-of-phase T1-weighted images relative to in-phase T1-weighted images, is a highly specific feature of the clear cell subtype of RCC, which may be seen in up to 60% of these tumors (Figure 35-16).

    RCC tends to be more homogeneous in appearance when small in size and more heterogeneous in appearance when large in size due to development of cystic or necrotic components, calcifications (seen in up to 30%), or hemorrhage. Fifteen percent of RCCs are cystic, most often the clear cell and papillary subtypes. The lesions have fluid attenuation or fluid signal intensity components in conjunction with thickened enhancing walls, thickened enhancing internal septations, and soft tissue nodular enhancing components (Figure 35-17). Soft tissue components tend to enhance more briskly and heterogeneously in the clear cell RCC but more mildly and homogeneously in the papillary and chromophobe RCCs. Washout of tumor enhancement relative to the renal parenchyma may be seen during the nephrographic or delayed phase of enhancement (see Figure 35-16).

    Peritumoral vascularity is sometimes seen, most often with the clear cell subtype. Associated direct extrarenal extension of tumor into surrounding tissues/organs, regional lymphadenopathy, or distant metastatic disease may sometimes also be present. Tumor extension into the renal vein or inferior vena cava (IVC) occurs in up to 20% of cases and appears as a high signal intensity filling defect on T1-weighted or T2-weighted images with restricted diffusion, enhancement, and occasional venous luminal expansion. The most common sites of distant metastatic disease include the lungs, bone marrow, liver, and lymph nodes. Metastases from RCC generally hyperenhance during the arterial phase of enhancement relative to surrounding tissues.

24. **What are some hereditary conditions and other risk factors associated with RCC?**

    - von Hippel Lindau (vHL) syndrome is associated with an increased risk of clear cell RCC (occurring in up to 40% of patients).

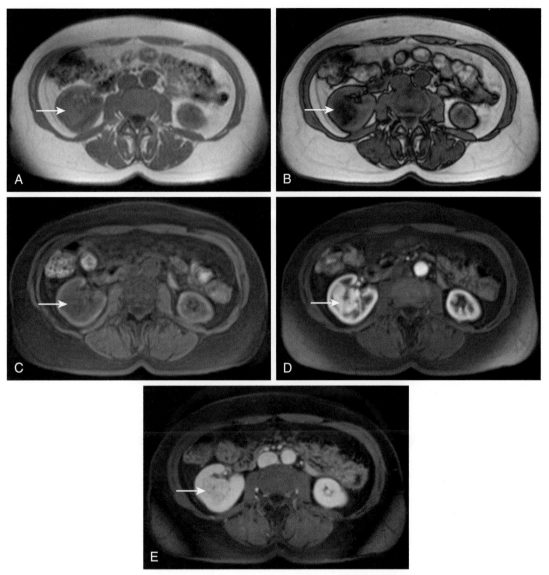

**Figure 35-16.** Clear cell RCC on MRI. **A,** Axial in-phase and **B,** Axial out-of-phase T1-weighted MR images through abdomen demonstrate large lesion in right kidney (*arrows*) with loss of signal intensity on out-of-phase images relative to in-phase images indicating presence of microscopic lipid content. **C,** Axial fat-suppressed T1-weighted unenhanced, **D,** Axial fat-suppressed T1-weighted corticomedullary phase contrast-enhanced, and **E,** Axial fat-suppressed T1-weighted nephrographic phase contrast-enhanced MR images through abdomen again reveal lesion in right kidney (*arrows*). Note avid heterogeneous corticomedullary phase enhancement and subsequent nephrographic phase washout of enhancement relative to renal parenchyma.

- Hereditary papillary renal carcinoma (HRPC) is an autosomal dominant condition that is associated with an increased risk of papillary RCC.
- Birt-Hogg-Dubé (BHD) syndrome is an autosomal dominant condition that is associated with various skin tumors and an increased risk of chromophobe RCC and renal oncocytomas. Cystic lung disease is also typically seen on CT.

  In the setting of these hereditary conditions, RCC is more frequently bilateral and multifocal, and it tends to present at a younger age.

  Other risk factors for RCC include tobacco use, obesity, exposure to various chemical compounds, and acquired cystic renal disease. Patients on long-term dialysis have a 3- to 6-fold increased risk of RCC compared to the general population.

25. Summarize the American Joint Committee on Cancer (AJCC) tumor node metastasis (TNM) staging system for renal cell carcinoma.
    For the answer, see Table 35-2.

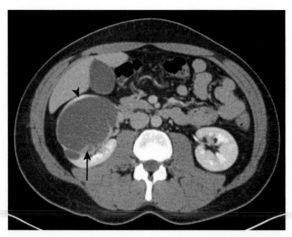

**Figure 35-17.** Cystic papillary RCC on CT. Axial nephrographic phase contrast-enhanced CT image through abdomen shows large complex cystic lesion of right kidney with multiple internal septations, thickened enhancing wall (*arrowhead*), and soft tissue nodular enhancing component (*arrow*) (Bosniak IV lesion).

**Table 35-2.** AJCC TNM Staging System of Renal Cell Carcinoma

| | |
|---|---|
| TX | Primary tumor cannot be assessed |
| T0 | No evidence of primary tumor |
| T1 | Tumor 7 cm or less in greatest dimension, limited to the kidney |
|   T1a | Tumor 4 cm or less in greatest dimension, limited to the kidney |
|   T1b | Tumor more than 4 cm but not more than 7 cm in greatest dimension, limited to the kidney |
| T2 | Tumor more than 7 cm in greatest dimension, limited to the kidney |
|   T2a | Tumor more than 7 cm but less than or equal to 10 cm in greatest dimension, limited to the kidney |
|   T2b | Tumor more than 10 cm in greatest dimension, limited to the kidney |
| T3 | Tumor extends into major veins or perinephric tissues but not into the ipsilateral adrenal gland and not beyond Gerota's fascia |
|   T3a | Tumor grossly extends into the renal vein or its segmental (muscle-containing) branches, or tumor invades perirenal and/or renal sinus fat but not beyond the Gerota fascia |
|   T3b | Tumor grossly extends into the vena cava below the diaphragm |
|   T3c | Tumor grossly extends into the vena cava above the diaphragm or invades the wall of the vena cava |
| T4 | Tumor invades beyond Gerota's fascia (including contiguous extension into the ipsilateral adrenal gland) |

**Regional lymph node (N)**

| | |
|---|---|
| NX | Regional lymph nodes cannot be assessed |
| N0 | No regional lymph node metastasis |
| N1 | Metastasis in regional lymph node(s) |

**Distant metastasis (M)**

| | |
|---|---|
| M0 | No distant metastasis |
| M1 | Distant metastasis |

**Anatomic stage/prognostic groups**

| Stage | T | N | M |
|---|---|---|---|
| I | T1 | N0 | M0 |
| II | T2 | N0 | M0 |
| III | T1-2 | N1 | M0 |
| | T3 | N0-1 | M0 |
| IV | T4 | Any N | M0 |
| | Any T | Any N | M1 |

*Note*: Any T3 or N1 lesion is at least stage III, and any T4 or M1 lesion is stage IV.
*(From Edge SB, Byrd DR, Compton CC, et al. AJCC Cancer Staging Manual. New York: Springer; 2010.)*

26. **What are the major indications for partial nephrectomy in patients with RCC?**
    Partial nephrectomy is used whenever possible to maximally preserve renal function. It is predominantly used when there is:
    - Tumor size <4 cm (although some surgeons will treat tumors up to 7 cm in size with nephron sparing techniques).
    - Peripheral tumor location.
    - Polar tumor location.
    - Lack of renal sinus fat or collecting system involvement by tumor.
    - Lack of venous extension of tumor.
    - Presence of contralateral renal disease.
    - Presence of a solitary functioning kidney.

27. **What are the CT and MR imaging features of renal lymphoma?**
    Renal lymphoma is uncommon, given the lack of lymphoid tissue in the kidneys, and is most often secondary to non-Hodgkin's lymphoma (occurring in 6% of patients at presentation). Treatment is with systemic therapy rather than with surgical resection.

    On CT and MRI, multiple renal masses are most commonly seen (in 50% to 60%), followed by direct contiguous spread from adjacent lymphadenopathy into the kidney (in 25% to 30%), diffuse renal infiltration (in 20%) which almost always occurs bilaterally, and a solitary renal mass (in <10%). Associated soft tissue extension into the perinephric tissues is sometimes also present. Lymphoma generally has soft tissue attenuation on CT, appears hypointense on T1-weighted images and isointense-slightly hyperintense on T2-weighted images relative to renal parenchyma, and restricts diffusion. Lymphomatous lesions are typically homogeneous, are hypoenhancing, and exert little mass effect upon subjacent structures. There is usually no venous extension or ureteral obstruction, but presence of abdominal lymphadenopathy is common (Figure 35-18).

28. **What are the CT and MR imaging features of metastatic disease to the kidneys?**
    Metastatic disease to the kidney is the most common malignant tumor of the kidney, is 4-fold more common than RCC in patients with a history of malignancy, and most often occurs in the setting of lung cancer, breast cancer, gastrointestinal malignancies, and melanoma.

    On CT and MRI, renal metastases will vary in their attenuation, signal intensity, and enhancement properties depending on their tissue composition, but they are often heterogeneous in appearance, usually restrict diffusion, and are usually hypoenhancing relative to renal parenchyma. The suspicion for metastatic disease is greater when the lesions are multifocal and bilateral, are heterogeneous but with similar enhancement patterns, have an infiltrative growth pattern, grow over time, or are seen in the presence of metastatic disease to other sites of the body. When necessary, percutaneous biopsy is performed to distinguish between renal metastatic disease and RCC.

29. **What are the CT and MR imaging features of urothelial cancers of the upper urinary tract?**
    Synchronous or metachronous urothelial malignancies occur in ≈5% of patients with a history of bladder cancer. The lesions are seen as filling defects or mucosal irregularities in the collecting system or ureter on a CT urogram, MR urogram, or intravenous urogram. Associated regional lymphadenopathy or distant metastatic disease may also be present. If the lesion invades the renal parenchyma, differentiation from a primary renal parenchymal neoplasm such as RCC is important, because the treatment of urothelial cancer of the kidney usually requires a complete nephroureterectomy.

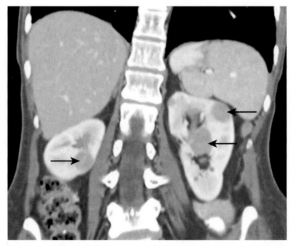

**Figure 35-18.** Renal lymphoma (diffuse large B cell subtype) on CT. Coronal corticomedullary phase contrast-enhanced CT image through abdomen demonstrates multiple bilateral homogeneous soft tissue attenuation hypoenhancing lesions within kidneys (*arrows*) with little mass effect upon adjacent structures.

## KEY POINTS

- An enhancing renal mass that does not contain macroscopic fat is considered to be secondary to RCC until proven otherwise.
- Cystic renal lesions that contain thick or irregular walls, thick or irregular internal septations, or solid nodular components with enhancement are considered as suspicious for cystic RCC until proven otherwise.
- Presence of macroscopic fat within a renal mass is diagnostic of a renal AML.
- Acquisition of delayed (or excretory) phase images is essential for detection of injury to the renal collecting systems or ureters in the setting of abdominal trauma.

### BIBLIOGRAPHY

Ramamurthy NK, Moosavi B, McInnes MD, et al. Multiparametric MRI of solid renal masses: pearls and pitfalls. *Clin Radiol.* 2015;70(3): 304-316.

Schieda N, Kielar AZ, Al Dandan O, et al. Ten uncommon and unusual variants of renal angiomyolipoma (AML): radiologic-pathologic correlation. *Clin Radiol.* 2015;70(2):206-220.

Wood CG 3rd, Stromberg LJ 3rd, Harmath CB, et al. CT and MR imaging for evaluation of cystic renal lesions and diseases. *Radiographics.* 2015;35(1):125-141.

Chung EM, Conran RM, Schroeder JW, et al. From the radiologic pathology archives: pediatric polycystic kidney disease and other ciliopathies: radiologic-pathologic correlation. *Radiographics.* 2014;34(1):155-178.

Heller MT, Schnor N. MDCT of renal trauma: correlation to AAST organ injury scale. *Clin Imaging.* 2014;38(4):410-417.

Weber TM, Lockhart ME. Renal transplant complications. *Abdom Imaging.* 2013;38(5):1144-1154.

Bosniak MA. The Bosniak renal cyst classification: 25 years later. *Radiology.* 2012;262(3):781-785.

Ifergan J, Pommier R, Brion MC, et al. Imaging in upper urinary tract infections. *Diag Interv Imag.* 2012;93(6):509-519.

Edge SB, Byrd DR, Compton CC, et al. Kidney. In: *AJCC cancer staging manual.* New York: Springer; 2010:479-490.

Katabathina VS, Kota G, Dasyam AK, et al. Adult renal cystic disease: a genetic, biological, and developmental primer. *Radiographics.* 2010;30(6):1509-1523.

Katabathina VS, Vikram R, Nagar AM, et al. Mesenchymal neoplasms of the kidney in adults: imaging spectrum with radiologic-pathologic correlation. *Radiographics.* 2010;30(6):1525-1540.

Alonso RC, Nacenta SB, Martinez PD, et al. Kidney in danger: CT findings of blunt and penetrating renal trauma. *Radiographics.* 2009;29(7):2033-2053.

Kim JI, Cho JY, Moon KC, et al. Segmental enhancement inversion at biphasic multidetector CT: characteristic finding of small renal oncocytoma. *Radiology.* 2009;252(2):441-448.

Craig WD, Wagner BJ, Travis MD. Pyelonephritis: radiologic-pathologic review. *Radiographics.* 2008;28(1):255-277, quiz 327-328.

Dyer R, DiSantis DJ, McClennan BL. Simplified imaging approach for evaluation of the solid renal mass in adults. *Radiology.* 2008;247(2):331-343.

Korkes F, Favoretto RL, Broglio M, et al. Xanthogranulomatous pyelonephritis: clinical experience with 41 cases. *Urology.* 2008;71(2): 178-180.

Ng CS, Wood CG, Silverman PM, et al. Renal cell carcinoma: diagnosis, staging, and surveillance. *AJR Am J Roentgenol.* 2008;191(4): 1220-1232.

Pedrosa I, Sun MR, Spencer M, et al. MR imaging of renal masses: correlation with findings at surgery and pathologic analysis. *Radiographics.* 2008;28(4):985-1003.

Demertzis J, Menias CO. State of the art: imaging of renal infections. *Emerg Radiol.* 2007;14(1):13-22.

Loffroy R, Guiu B, Watfa J, et al. Xanthogranulomatous pyelonephritis in adults: clinical and radiological findings in diffuse and focal forms. *Clin Radiol.* 2007;62(9):884-890.

Prasad SR, Humphrey PA, Catena JR, et al. Common and uncommon histologic subtypes of renal cell carcinoma: imaging spectrum with pathologic correlation. *Radiographics.* 2006;26(6):1795-1806, discussion 806-810.

Sheth S, Ali S, Fishman E. Imaging of renal lymphoma: patterns of disease with pathologic correlation. *Radiographics.* 2006;26(4): 1151-1168.

Jeong JY, Kim SH, Lee HJ, et al. Atypical low-signal-intensity renal parenchyma: causes and patterns. *Radiographics.* 2002;22(4):833-846.

Moore EE, Shackford SR, Pachter HL, et al. Organ injury scaling: spleen, liver, and kidney. *J Trauma.* 1989;29(12):1664-1666.

# CHAPTER 36

# CT AND MRI OF THE ADRENAL GLANDS

*Drew A. Torigian, MD, MA, FSAR, and Parvati Ramchandani, MD, FACR, FSAR*

1. **What are common indications for computed tomography (CT) and magnetic resonance imaging (MRI) of the adrenal glands?**

   The most common clinical indications include:
   - Characterization of indeterminate adrenal lesions incidentally detected on prior cross-sectional imaging. The main goal in this situation is to determine whether an adrenal lesion represents a benign lesion, such as an adenoma, or a malignant lesion.
   - Detection and characterization of culprit adrenal lesions in patients with symptoms or signs suggestive of an endocrine disorder such as hyperaldosteronism, hypercortisolism, or increased catecholamine secretion.
   - Staging and response assessment of patients with primary adrenal malignancies.
   - Staging and response assessment of patients with extraadrenal malignancies that may metastasize to the adrenal glands.
   - Providing guidance for percutaneous biopsy or intervention for an adrenal lesion.

2. **What is the normal appearance of the adrenal glands on CT and MRI?**

   The adrenal glands are anterosuperior to the upper poles of the kidneys and are located within the perinephric space of the retroperitoneum. The right adrenal gland is located anterior and lateral to the right diaphragmatic crus, posterior to the inferior vena cava, and medial to the right hepatic lobe. The left adrenal gland is located anterior and lateral to the left diaphragmatic crus, posterior to the splenic vessels at the level of the pancreas or stomach, and medial to the spleen.

   On CT, the adrenal glands have soft tissue attenuation, and on MRI, they have intermediate T1-weighted and slightly high T2-weighted signal intensity relative to skeletal muscle. Each adrenal gland is comprised of a body, a medial limb, and a lateral limb and often has an inverted letter "Y" or "V" configuration. Each adrenal gland limb is usually ≤6 mm in thickness (Figure 36-1). However, the left adrenal gland is generally thicker and more nodular than the right adrenal gland, and the adrenal glands often increase in thickness/volume and become more nodular with increasing age.

   The adrenal glands typically receive arterial blood supply from three separate arteries, although variations can occur: the superior adrenal arteries arise from the inferior phrenic arteries; the middle adrenal arteries arise from the lateral aspect of the abdominal aorta; and the inferior adrenal arteries arise from the superior aspect of the renal arteries. The right adrenal vein drains into the inferior vena cava, whereas the left adrenal vein joins with the left inferior phrenic vein before draining into the left renal vein, although variants are common.

   Unenhanced CT images (but not MR images) are useful to detect adrenal calcifications. Unenhanced images on both CT and MRI are useful to (1) detect presence of macroscopic fat within an adrenal nodule to establish a specific diagnosis of adrenal myelolipoma, (2) detect presence of microscopic lipid content within an adrenal nodule to establish a specific diagnosis of adrenal adenoma, and (3) serve as a reference of comparison for contrast-enhanced images for adrenal nodule characterization.

3. **What is a pancake adrenal gland?**

   A pancake adrenal gland is a congenital anomaly of the adrenal gland which may be seen when there is ipsilateral renal agenesis or renal ectopia. On cross-sectional imaging, the adrenal gland will appear to have a discoid or flattened configuration, and the ipsilateral kidney will not be visualized in its expected location (Figure 36-2).

4. **What is the significance of hyperenhancement of the adrenal glands?**

   Adrenal gland hyperenhancement (i.e., adrenal gland enhancement similar to that of adjacent vascular structures) is a finding that may indicate presence of shock or impending shock and tends to portend a poor clinical outcome. This may occur in the setting of trauma, pancreatitis, sepsis, or hemorrhage-induced hypotension.

5. **What are the major causes of adrenal gland calcification?**
   - Prior adrenal gland infection such as tuberculosis or histoplasmosis.
   - Prior adrenal gland hemorrhage.
   - Adrenal gland neoplasm such as adrenal myelolipoma or adrenal cortical carcinoma (ACC).

6. **How often are incidental adrenal lesions detected on cross-sectional imaging?**

   Adrenal incidentalomas are encountered in up to 7% of cross-sectional imaging studies and increase in prevalence with increasing age. Fifty percent to 80% of adrenal incidentalomas are secondary to nonhyperfunctioning adrenal adenomas (the most common cause), 5% to 10% are secondary to adrenal myelolipomas (the second most common

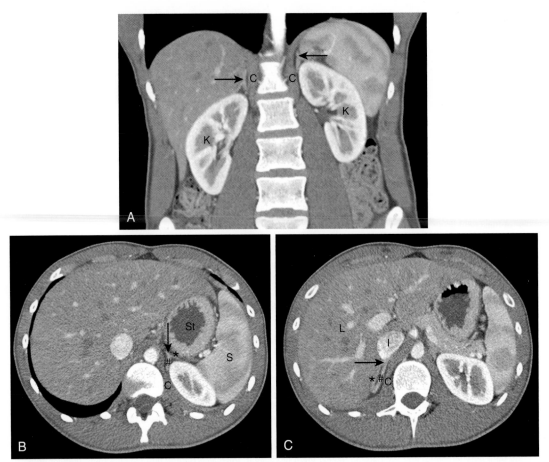

**Figure 36-1.** Normal adrenal glands on CT. **A,** Coronal contrast-enhanced CT image through abdomen shows normal adrenal glands (*arrows*) located superior to kidneys (*K*) and lateral to diaphragmatic crura (*C*). **B,** Axial contrast-enhanced CT image through abdomen demonstrates normal left adrenal gland located anterolateral to left diaphragmatic crus (*C*), posterior to stomach (*St*), and medial to spleen (*S*). Note left adrenal gland body (*arrow*), medial limb (*#*), and lateral limb (*\**). **C,** Axial contrast-enhanced CT through abdomen more inferiorly reveals normal right adrenal gland located anterolateral to right diaphragmatic crus (*C*), posterior to inferior vena cava (*I*), and medial to liver (*L*). Note right adrenal gland body (*arrow*), medial limb (*#*), and lateral limb (*\**).

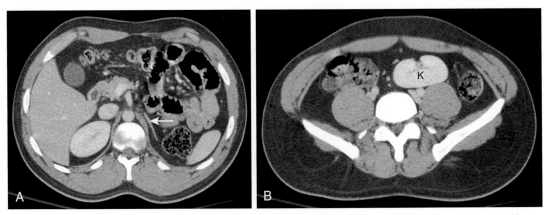

**Figure 36-2.** Pancake adrenal gland and renal ectopia on CT. **A,** Axial contrast-enhanced CT image through abdomen shows discoid or flattened configuration of left adrenal gland (*arrow*) and nonvisualization of ipsilateral left kidney. **B,** Axial image through pelvis demonstrates ectopic left kidney (*K*) in pelvis.

cause), and up to 5% are secondary to adrenal pheochromocytoma (the third most common cause). In patients without a history of cancer, adrenal incidentalomas are rarely malignant in etiology. However, in patients with a history of cancer, up to 50% of incidentally detected adrenal lesions are malignant in nature, most often secondary to metastatic disease.

7. What is the major differential diagnosis for a focal adrenal gland lesion?
For the answer, see Box 36-1.

8. What are the CT and MR imaging findings of adrenal hemorrhage/hematoma?
Adrenal hemorrhage/hematoma is rare. Eighty percent occurs unilaterally, more commonly on the right than on the left. It is often asymptomatic, but it may be associated with acute adrenal insufficiency (Addison's disease) when bilateral.

A masslike abnormality or diffuse thickening of the adrenal gland with maintenance of its normal inverted-Y or inverted-V configuration is seen, typically with high attenuation (30 to 70 HU) on CT (Figure 36-3). On MRI, low signal intensity on T1-weighted and T2-weighted images is seen in acute hemorrhage, whereas high signal intensity on T1-weighted images is seen in subacute hemorrhage. There is often associated infiltration of the surrounding fat and fascial planes by hemorrhagic fluid. Solid enhancing components or intralesional calcifications, when visualized, are suggestive of presence of an underlying adrenal neoplasm. Over time, adrenal hemorrhage/hematoma will decrease in size, decrease in attenuation, develop very low signal intensity components on T1-weighted and T2-weighted images secondary to hemosiderin or ferritin, and may either fully resolve, lead to adrenal pseudocyst formation, or lead to adrenal gland calcification.

9. What are some risk factors for adrenal hemorrhage/hematoma?
- Abdominal trauma (the most common risk factor); adrenal injuries are usually associated with other severe organ injury.
- Physiologic stress (such as from surgery, sepsis, burn injury, or hypotension).
- Coagulopathy or other hemorrhagic diathesis.
- Adrenal gland neoplasm.

---

**Box 36-1.** Major Differential Diagnosis for Focal Adrenal Gland Lesions

Nonneoplastic Lesions
- Cyst
- Hematoma
- Abscess

Neoplastic Lesions
- Adenoma (most common adrenal lesion)
- Myelolipoma

- Pheochromocytoma
- Metastasis (most common malignant adrenal lesion)
- ACC
- Lymphoma

---

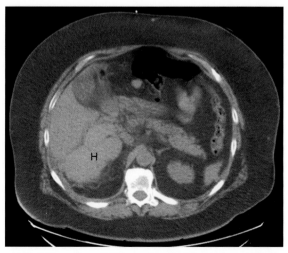

**Figure 36-3.** Adrenal hemorrhage on CT. Axial unenhanced CT image through abdomen shows high attenuation masslike hematoma of right adrenal gland (*H*). Note associated infiltration of surrounding retroperitoneal fat. No solid enhancing components were seen on contrast-enhanced images (*not shown*).

10. **What are the CT and MR imaging findings of adrenal cysts?**

    Adrenal cysts are rare and asymptomatic. They are most often secondary to endothelial cysts and pseudocysts (most often caused by prior adrenal hemorrhage) and less commonly secondary to epithelial or parasitic cysts. They are usually unilateral and appear as well-circumscribed round or oval fluid attenuation and fluid signal intensity cystic lesions of the adrenal gland with a smooth thin wall (Figure 36-4). Sometimes (most commonly with pseudocysts and parasitic cysts) the internal fluid may be proteinaceous or hemorrhagic with variably increased attenuation, increased T1-weighted signal intensity, or decreased T2-weighted signal intensity relative to simple fluid. Internal septations, fluid-debris levels, calcifications, or wall thickening may also be seen. However, no solid enhancing components will be visualized.

11. **What is adrenal hyperplasia, and what are its CT and MR imaging features?**

    Adrenal hyperplasia refers to nonmalignant proliferation of adrenal cortical cells. It may be symptomatic secondary to hormonal hyperfunction of the adrenal glands (such as in the setting of Conn's syndrome or adrenocorticotropic hormone [ACTH]-dependent Cushing's syndrome), or it may be asymptomatic.

    On CT and MRI, smooth diffuse adrenal gland thickening or adrenal gland multinodularity with maintenance of the normal inverted-Y or inverted-V configuration is typically seen, most often involving the adrenal glands bilaterally (Figure 36-5). However, the adrenal glands may sometimes have a normal appearance.

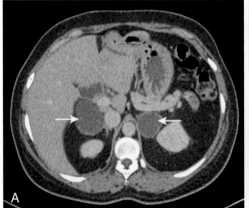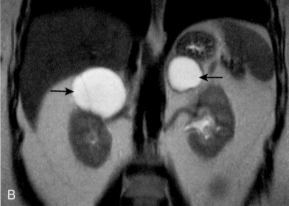

**Figure 36-4.** Adrenal pseudocysts on CT and MRI. **A,** Axial contrast-enhanced CT image through abdomen demonstrates bilateral oval fluid attenuation cystic lesions of adrenal glands (*arrows*) with smooth thin walls and without solid enhancing components. **B,** Coronal heavily T2-weighted MR image through abdomen reveals very high signal intensity of adrenal lesions (*arrows*) in keeping with cystic nature. Note thin internal septation in right adrenal gland lesion as well.

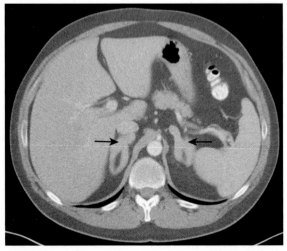

**Figure 36-5.** Adrenal hyperplasia on CT. Axial contrast-enhanced CT image through abdomen shows bilateral massive smooth diffuse enlargement of adrenal glands (*arrows*). Patient had ACTH-dependent Cushing's syndrome secondary to ACTH-producing well-differentiated neuroendocrine carcinoma in right pulmonary hilum (*not shown*).

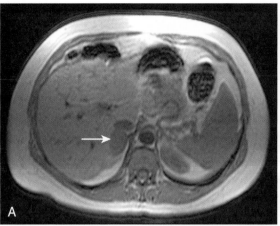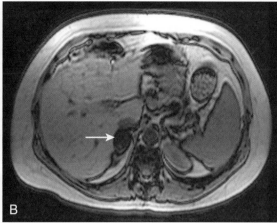

**Figure 36-6.** Adrenal adenoma on MRI. **A,** Axial in-phase and **B,** Axial out-of-phase T1-weighted MR images through abdomen demonstrate well-circumscribed right adrenal gland nodule (*arrows*) with uniform loss of signal intensity on out-of-phase images relative to in-phase images. This finding indicates presence of microscopic lipid and is characteristic of lipid-rich adrenal adenoma.

12. What is an adrenal adenoma, and what are its CT and MR imaging features?

Adrenal adenoma is the most common benign neoplasm of the adrenal gland and is often detected incidentally on cross-sectional imaging. Some may be hyperfunctional (i.e., hormonally active) and symptomatic, although they are more commonly nonhyperfunctional.

On CT and MRI, a well-circumscribed adrenal gland nodule or mass is visualized, often homogeneous and ≤3 to 4 cm in size. However, calcifications are rarely visualized. Stability of nodule size compared to imaging studies obtained >6 to 12 months prior to the current study is a very useful feature to indicate a benign etiology, which emphasizes the importance of comparison to prior studies whenever available. The majority of adrenal adenomas, ≈70% of cases, contain intracellular microscopic lipid.

Specific diagnostic features of a lipid-rich adrenal adenoma include (1) attenuation of <10 HU on unenhanced CT and (2) uniform loss of signal intensity on out-of-phase T1-weighted images relative to in-phase T1-weighted MR images (Figure 36-6), both secondary to presence of microscopic lipid.

13. Are CT and MRI able to distinguish between hyperfunctional and nonhyperfunctional adrenal adenomas?

CT and MRI are not generally able to distinguish between hyperfunctional and nonhyperfunctional adrenal adenomas. However, visualization of atrophy of the remainder of the adrenal gland tissue is suggestive of a hyperfunctional adrenal adenoma that is secreting increased levels of cortisol, because pituitary ACTH hormone secretion by the pituitary gland is suppressed in this scenario. Also, hyperfunctional adrenal adenomas tend to be smaller in size than nonhyperfunctional adrenal adenomas, because symptomatic patients tend to undergo abdominal imaging evaluation sooner than asymptomatic patients do.

14. What is an adrenal myelolipoma, and what are its CT and MR imaging features?

Adrenal myelolipoma is the second most common benign neoplasm of the adrenal gland and is composed of variable amounts of fat and hematopoietic tissue. It occurs with equal frequency in men and women, most often in the fifth through sixth decades of life, and is usually asymptomatic.

On CT and MRI, a well-circumscribed adrenal gland nodule or mass is visualized that contains macroscopic fat, which is the key diagnostic feature (Figure 36-7). Macroscopic fat has similar attenuation and signal intensity properties as subcutaneous and visceral fat within the torso. Non-fatty enhancing soft tissue components are also often present. Calcification may be seen in up to 20% of cases, and hemorrhagic components may be seen in up to 10% of cases.

15. What other types of adrenal gland nodules may contain microscopic lipid or macroscopic fat?

Adrenal gland metastases from clear cell renal cell carcinoma (RCC) or hepatocellular carcinoma (HCC) may rarely contain microscopic lipid, potentially mimicking adrenal adenomas. However, these usually occur in the setting of known malignancy and tend to grow over time. ACC may also contain microscopic lipid, but this is a rare tumor which tends to be large in size and heterogeneous in appearance, and thus easily distinguished from an adenoma.

Occasionally, small amounts of macroscopic fat may be seen within adrenal cortical neoplasms including degenerated adrenal adenomas and ACC secondary to myelolipomatous metaplasia, potentially mimicking adrenal myelolipomas. However, these tend to be more heterogeneous in appearance and are often large in size.

Finally, collision tumors of the adrenal gland may very rarely be encountered, where a malignant adrenal neoplasm such as by a metastasis or an ACC occurs in the setting of a preexisting adrenal adenoma or myelolipoma. In this setting, portions of the adrenal gland may contain microscopic lipid or macroscopic fat, whereas others do not.

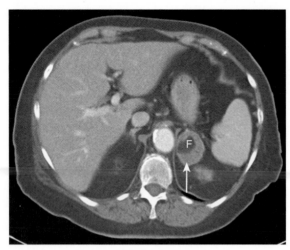

**Figure 36-7.** Adrenal myelolipoma on CT. Axial contrast-enhanced CT image through abdomen reveals well-circumscribed mass in left adrenal gland (*arrow*) that contains macroscopic fat (*F*) (similar in attenuation to subcutaneous and visceral fat elsewhere in abdomen) as well as nonfatty enhancing soft tissue.

Thus, if a lipid- or fat-containing adrenal gland nodule is large (>3 to 4 cm) in size, grows in size, or is heterogeneous in appearance, then a follow-up CT or MRI scan is generally warranted to exclude these other less common etiologies which may mimic the appearance of adrenal adenomas and myelolipomas.

16. If the CT or MR imaging features of an incidentally detected adrenal gland nodule are nondiagnostic, what are the next steps to determine its etiology?

If specific diagnostic features of a lipid-rich adrenal adenoma or other benign cause of an adrenal nodule (e.g., myelolipoma, hematoma, cyst) are not present, and no prior cross-sectional imaging studies are available to demonstrate long-term stability in size over time, then dedicated thin-section adrenal gland CT imaging with acquisition of unenhanced, venous phase contrast-enhanced, and 15-minute delayed phase contrast-enhanced images is performed. This is because adrenal adenomas are vascular lesions that enhance and wash out contrast on delayed phase images more than do malignant lesions. The washout of contrast from an adrenal nodule is calculated in one of two ways:

1. The absolute percentage washout (APW) = [venous phase attenuation (in HU) − 15-minute delayed phase attenuation (in HU)] / [venous phase attenuation (in HU) − unenhanced attenuation (in HU)] × 100%. An APW >60% is diagnostic of an adrenal adenoma (Figure 36-8).
2. The relative percentage washout (RPW) = [venous phase attenuation (in HU) − 15-minute delayed phase attenuation (in HU)] / [venous phase attenuation (in HU)] × 100%, which is used when unenhanced CT images were not obtained. An RPW >40% is also diagnostic of an adrenal adenoma.

Table 36-1 provides a summary of CT and MR imaging features that are useful to distinguish benign from malignant adrenal gland nodules. When these imaging features are not sufficient to determine whether or not an adrenal gland nodule is benign or malignant in nature, short-term follow-up CT or MR imaging may be performed to document size stability over time, which would favor a benign etiology. Fluorodeoxyglucose (FDG) positron emission tomography (PET) may also be performed, as benign adrenal nodules tend to have FDG uptake less than or equal to that of the liver. Otherwise, percutaneous biopsy or surgical removal is performed to obtain a definitive diagnosis.

17. What are the causes of Conn's syndrome?

Conn's syndrome, or primary hyperaldosteronism, is the most common cause of secondary hypertension, and is caused by a hyperfunctional adrenal adenoma in 65% of cases and by bilateral adrenal hyperplasia in 35% of cases. Hyperfunctional ACC and unilateral adrenal hyperplasia are rare causes of Conn's syndrome. Patients typically have an elevated serum aldosterone level, a low serum renin level, and a low serum potassium level. This is in contradistinction to patients who have secondary hyperaldosteronism (such as in the setting of renal artery stenosis) where there is instead physiologic activation of the renin-angiotensin-aldosterone axis.

In patients with Conn's syndrome, it is important to differentiate between unilateral versus bilateral adrenal pathologies as the underlying etiology. This is because an adrenal adenoma or unilateral adrenal hyperplasia may be treated with laparoscopic resection of the adrenal gland, whereas bilateral adrenal hyperplasia is usually managed medically. Adrenal vein sampling is also commonly performed to determine whether autonomous aldosterone production from the adrenal glands is unilateral or bilateral, as there is often discordance with cross-sectional imaging findings, particularly when the adrenal glands appear normal or when multiple bilateral adrenal gland nodules are present.

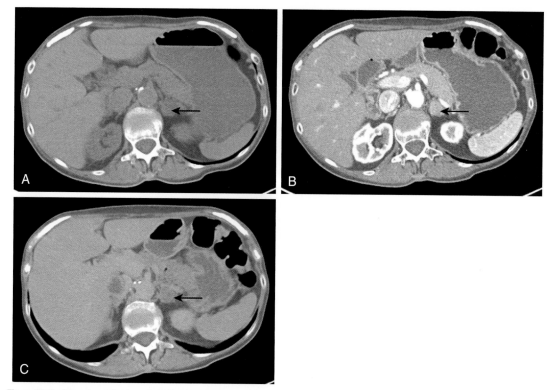

**Figure 36-8.** Adrenal nodule characterization based on percentage washout on CT. **A,** Axial unenhanced, **B,** Axial late arterial phase contrast-enhanced, and **C,** Axial 15-minute delayed phase contrast-enhanced CT images through abdomen show 1-cm well-circumscribed left adrenal gland nodule (*arrow*). Corresponding nodule attenuation measurements were 15 HU, 107 HU, and 37 HU, respectively, so that APW = 76% and RPW = 65%. Because APW is >60% and RPW is >40%, these findings are diagnostic of adrenal adenoma.

**Table 36-1.** CT and MR Imaging Features to Distinguish Benign from Malignant Adrenal Gland Nodules

| SUGGESTIVE BENIGN FEATURES | SUGGESTIVE MALIGNANT FEATURES |
| --- | --- |
| Small size (≤3-4 cm) | Large size (>4-5 cm) |
| Stability in size (over >6-12 months) | Growth in size (over >6-12 months) or new |
| Homogeneous attenuation or signal intensity | Heterogeneous attenuation or signal intensity |
| Smooth margins and no invasion of adjacent structures | Irregular margins or invasion of adjacent structures |
| Presence of macroscopic fat (myelolipoma) | |
| Presence of microscopic lipid (lipid-rich adenoma) | |
| APW >60%/RPW >40% (adenoma) | APW ≤60%/RPW ≤40% |
| Lack of enhancement (cyst, hematoma) | |

APW = absolute percentage washout; RPW = relative percentage washout

18. **What are the causes of Cushing's syndrome?**

    Cushing's syndrome (hypercortisolism) is ACTH dependent in 80% to 85% of cases, leading to excessive cortisol production by the adrenal glands and adrenal hyperplasia. Eighty percent to 85% of such cases are caused by a hyperfunctional pituitary adenoma (in which case the hypercortisolism is known as Cushing's disease), and 10% to 15% of such cases are caused by ectopic (nonpituitary) ACTH-secreting tumors (including small cell lung carcinoma, bronchial carcinoid tumor, thymoma, pancreatic neuroendocrine tumor, and medullary thyroid carcinoma).

    ACTH-independent Cushing's syndrome occurs in 15% to 20% of cases, and is most often secondary to a hyperfunctional adrenal adenoma, followed by a hyperfunctional ACC, and least commonly by adrenal hyperplasia. Exogenous administration of glucocorticoids is an additional cause of ACTH-independent Cushing's syndrome.

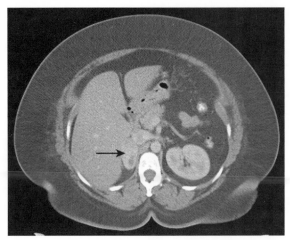

**Figure 36-9.** Adrenal pheochromocytoma on CT. Axial contrast-enhanced CT image through abdomen demonstrates well-circumscribed avidly enhancing right adrenal gland nodule (*arrow*) with low attenuation cystic component posteriorly.

19. What is an adrenal pheochromocytoma, and what are its CT and MR imaging features?

Adrenal pheochromocytoma is a relatively rare neuroendocrine tumor that is derived from the adrenal medulla, which may be benign or malignant in its biologic behavior. It affects women slightly more commonly than men, and it is most commonly seen in the third through fifth decades of life. Symptoms and signs, including headache, palpitations, diaphoresis, and hypertension, commonly occur secondary to catecholamine secretion, and detection of increased levels of catecholamines or metanephrines in the urine is essentially diagnostic. The "10% rule" is a useful mnemonic, because ≈10% of pheochromocytomas are malignant in their behavior, ≈10% occur bilaterally, ≈10% are extraadrenal in location (also known as paragangliomas), ≈10% are nonhyperfunctional, and ≈10% are associated with hereditary conditions.

On CT and MRI, an adrenal soft tissue nodule or mass is seen, which tends to be homogeneous in attenuation and signal intensity and avidly enhancing when small in size and heterogeneous when large in size secondary to hemorrhage, cystic change, and/or necrosis (Figure 36-9). Calcification is seen in ≈15% of cases. Occasionally, the lesion may be predominantly cystic in nature, potentially mimicking adrenal adenomas or cysts. Pheochromocytomas may also sometimes have an APW >60% or an RPW >40%, again potentially mimicking adrenal adenomas. A malignant behavior is suspected when invasion of adjacent organs, regional lymphadenopathy, or distant metastatic lesions are seen. Metastatic lesions from adrenal pheochromocytoma tend to avidly enhance during the arterial phase of enhancement.

20. What are some hereditary conditions associated with adrenal pheochromocytoma?
    - Multiple endocrine neoplasia (MEN) syndrome type II (including types IIA and IIB).
    - von Hippel Lindau (vHL) syndrome.
    - Neurofibromatosis type I (NF-1).
    - Hereditary paraganglioma-pheochromocytoma syndrome (HPPS) (related to genetic mutations in succinate dehydrogenase [SDH]).

21. What is adrenal cortical carcinoma (ACC), and what are its CT and MR imaging features?

ACC is the most common primary malignant tumor of the adrenal gland in adults; it arises from the adrenal cortex but is rare. It occurs slightly more commonly in women than in men and usually arises in infants and children <5 years old and in adults during the fourth to fifth decades of life. About 55% are hyperfunctional, most often leading to Cushing's syndrome, and are generally smaller in size than when nonhyperfunctional. Treatment generally involves surgical resection when feasible as well as chemotherapy and radiotherapy as needed.

On CT and MRI, a large (>5 cm) enhancing adrenal gland mass is typically seen, which is usually heterogeneous in attenuation and signal intensity. Microscopic lipid content may be visualized on out-of-phase T1-weighted images, and sometimes a small amount of macroscopic fat may be present. Additional findings that may be encountered include prominent peritumoral vascularity, calcification (in up to 30%), invasion of adjacent organs or tissues, venous extension, regional lymphadenopathy, and distant metastatic disease (most often to the liver, lungs, and bone marrow) (Figure 36-10).

22. What are the cross-sectional imaging features of metastatic disease to the adrenal glands?

Metastatic disease to the adrenal gland is the most common malignant tumor of the adrenal gland (occurring in up to 27% of patients with cancer at autopsy), and it most often occurs in the setting of lung cancer (most common), breast cancer, melanoma, gastrointestinal tract cancer, pancreatic cancer, and RCC. However, even in patients with known malignancy and an adrenal lesion, adrenal metastasis is less common than adrenal adenoma. CT, MRI, and FDG PET are commonly used for the detection and characterization of adrenal gland metastases in patients with known cancer.

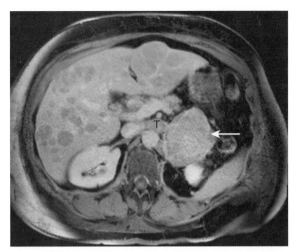

**Figure 36-10.** ACC on MRI. Axial contrast-enhanced T1-weighted MR image through abdomen reveals large, enhancing, heterogeneous, irregularly marginated left adrenal gland mass (*arrow*) with associated hypointense tumor thrombus (*T*) in left renal vein. Also note multiple heterogeneously enhancing hepatic lesions, in keeping with metastases.

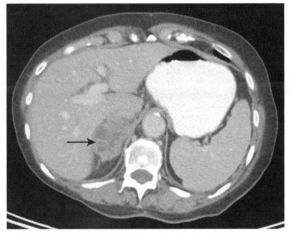

**Figure 36-11.** Adrenal metastasis on CT. Axial contrast-enhanced CT image through abdomen shows large, heterogeneous, irregularly marginated right adrenal gland mass (*arrow*). Patient had a history of melanoma.

On CT and MRI, the suspicion for adrenal metastatic disease is greater when the adrenal lesions are large (>4 to 5 cm in size), are multifocal and bilateral, are heterogeneous, have irregular margins, invade adjacent organs or tissues, grow over time or are new, or are seen in the presence of metastatic disease to other sites of the body (Figure 36-11). Specific diagnostic features of adrenal adenoma or other benign adrenal lesions will most often not be present on CT or MRI. On PET, adrenal nodule FDG uptake greater than that of liver is also suggestive of adrenal metastatic disease in a patient with known primary malignancy. When necessary, percutaneous biopsy is performed to distinguish between an adrenal metastatic disease and a benign adrenal lesion.

## KEY POINTS

- CT and MRI are useful to detect and characterize adrenal gland pathologies and to help distinguish benign and malignant etiologies of adrenal gland nodules.
- Most adrenal incidentalomas are benign in nature, and the most commonly detected incidental adrenal lesion is a nonhyperfunctional adrenal adenoma.
- Presence of microscopic lipid content within a small (≤3 cm in size) homogeneous adrenal gland nodule is essentially diagnostic of an adrenal adenoma.
- Presence of macroscopic fat within an adrenal gland nodule or mass is characteristic of an adrenal myelolipoma.
- Adrenal gland nodules/masses that have a large size (>4 to 5 cm), grow over time, are heterogeneous in appearance, or have irregular margins are more likely to be malignant in etiology.

## BIBLIOGRAPHY

Lacroix A, Feelders RA, Stratakis CA, et al. Cushing's syndrome. *Lancet.* 2015;386(9996):913-927.

Lattin GE Jr, Sturgill ED, Tujo CA, et al. From the radiologic pathology archives: adrenal tumors and tumor-like conditions in the adult: radiologic-pathologic correlation. *Radiographics.* 2014;34(3):805-829.

Song JH, Mayo-Smith WW. Current status of imaging for adrenal gland tumors. *Surg Oncol Clin N Am.* 2014;23(4):847-861.

Leung K, Stamm M, Raja A, et al. Pheochromocytoma: the range of appearances on ultrasound, CT, MRI, and functional imaging. *AJR Am J Roentgenol.* 2013;200(2):370-378.

Malayeri AA, Zaheer A, Fishman EK, et al. Adrenal masses: contemporary imaging characterization. *J Comput Assist Tomogr.* 2013;37(4): 528-542.

Raja A, Leung K, Stamm M, et al. Multimodality imaging findings of pheochromocytoma with associated clinical and biochemical features in 53 patients with histologically confirmed tumors. *AJR Am J Roentgenol.* 2013;201(4):825-833.

Jordan E, Poder L, Courtier J, et al. Imaging of nontraumatic adrenal hemorrhage. *AJR Am J Roentgenol.* 2012;199(1):W91-W98.

To'o KJ, Duddalwar VA. Imaging of traumatic adrenal injury. *Emerg Radiol.* 2012;19(6):499-503.

Bharwani N, Rockall AG, Sahdev A, et al. Adrenocortical carcinoma: the range of appearances on CT and MRI. *AJR Am J Roentgenol.* 2011;196(6):W706-W714.

Boland GW. Adrenal imaging: from Addison to algorithms. *Radiol Clin North Am.* 2011;49(3):511-528, vii.

Berland LL, Silverman SG, Gore RM, et al. Managing incidental findings on abdominal CT: white paper of the ACR incidental findings committee. *J Am Coll Radiol.* 2010;7(10):754-773.

Johnson PT, Horton KM, Fishman EK. Adrenal imaging with MDCT: nonneoplastic disease. *AJR Am J Roentgenol.* 2009;193(4):1128-1135.

Johnson PT, Horton KM, Fishman EK. Adrenal imaging with multidetector CT: evidence-based protocol optimization and interpretative practice. *Radiographics.* 2009;29(5):1319-1331.

Kempers MJ, Lenders JW, van Outheusden L, et al. Systematic review: diagnostic procedures to differentiate unilateral from bilateral adrenal abnormality in primary aldosteronism. *Ann Intern Med.* 2009;151(5):329-337.

Boland GW, Blake MA, Hahn PF, et al. Incidental adrenal lesions: principles, techniques, and algorithms for imaging characterization. *Radiology.* 2008;249(3):756-775.

Song JH, Chaudhry FS, Mayo-Smith WW. The incidental adrenal mass on CT: prevalence of adrenal disease in 1,049 consecutive adrenal masses in patients with no known malignancy. *AJR Am J Roentgenol.* 2008;190(5):1163-1168.

Ishibashi T, Satoh F, Yamada T, et al. Primary aldosteronism: a pictorial essay. *Abdom Imaging.* 2007;32(4):504-514.

Meier JM, Alavi A, Iruvuri S, et al. Assessment of age-related changes in abdominal organ structure and function with computed tomography and positron emission tomography. *Semin Nucl Med.* 2007;37(3):154-172.

Benitah N, Yeh BM, Qayyum A, et al. Minor morphologic abnormalities of adrenal glands at CT: prognostic importance in patients with lung cancer. *Radiology.* 2005;235(2):517-522.

Israel GM, Korobkin M, Wang C, et al. Comparison of unenhanced CT and chemical shift MRI in evaluating lipid-rich adrenal adenomas. *AJR Am J Roentgenol.* 2004;183(1):215-219.

Rockall AG, Babar SA, Sohaib SA, et al. CT and MR imaging of the adrenal glands in ACTH-independent cushing syndrome. *Radiographics.* 2004;24(2):435-452.

Caoili EM, Korobkin M, Francis IR, et al. Adrenal masses: characterization with combined unenhanced and delayed enhanced CT. *Radiology.* 2002;222(3):629-633.

Caoili EM, Korobkin M, Francis IR, et al. Delayed enhanced CT of lipid-poor adrenal adenomas. *AJR Am J Roentgenol.* 2000;175(5): 1411-1415.

Korobkin M, Brodeur FJ, Francis IR, et al. CT time-attenuation washout curves of adrenal adenomas and nonadenomas. *AJR Am J Roentgenol.* 1998;170(3):747-752.

# CHAPTER 37

# CT AND MRI OF THE RETROPERITONEUM

Drew A. Torigian, MD, MA, FSAR, and Parvati Ramchandani, MD, FACR, FSAR

1. What are the boundaries of the retroperitoneum?
The retroperitoneum is bounded anteriorly by the posterior parietal peritoneum and posteriorly by the transversalis fascia and extends from the diaphragm to the pelvic brim.

2. What are the compartments of the retroperitoneum and their contents?
The anterior pararenal space, perirenal space, and posterior pararenal space are the main retroperitoneal compartments, which are separated from each other by fascial planes (Figure 37-1). The anterior pararenal space, which contains the ascending colon, descending colon, second through fourth portions of the duodenum, and pancreas, is located anterior to the anterior renal fascia and medial to the lateroconal fascia and is contiguous across the midline. The bilateral perirenal (or perinephric) spaces contain the kidneys, renal pelves and proximal ureters, adrenal glands, and fat and are located between the anterior and posterior renal fascia. The posterior pararenal spaces contain fat are located posterior to the posterior renal fascia and external to the lateroconal fascia, and are contiguous with the properitoneal fat of the abdomen. The retroperitoneal fascial planes are not composed of single membranes but are laminated. As such, although they may serve as barriers to disease spread, these potentially expansile fascial planes may alternatively serve as conduits of disease spread to other compartments in the abdomen and pelvis.

3. What are the extraperitoneal spaces of the pelvis?
The prevesical space, also called the retropubic space or the space of Retzius, is an extraperitoneal space located anterior and lateral to the umbilicovesical fascia (UVF) and posterior to the pubic bones, extends posteriorly to communicate with the presacral space, and contains fat. It is a large potential space with multiple potential extensions and communications, allowing for bidirectional spread of fluid collections and other disease processes into the retroperitoneum and thighs. Prevesical fluid collections typically have a "molar tooth" configuration in the axial plane and can be large in size (Figure 37-2). The perivesical space is a small extraperitoneal space bounded by the UVF which contains the urinary bladder, urachus, obliterated umbilical arteries, and fat. Perivesical fluid collections are typically small in size. The perirectal space is surrounded by the perirectal fascia and contains the rectum, hemorrhoidal vessels, and fat.

4. Are the psoas muscles located within the retroperitoneum?
No. The psoas muscles are located within the retrofascial space posterior to the transversalis fascia (the posterior boundary of the retroperitoneum).

5. Which tumors most commonly occur in the retroperitoneum?
Most retroperitoneal tumors are malignant and are due to lymphoma, retroperitoneal sarcoma, or metastatic disease. Neurogenic tumors such as schwannoma, neurofibroma, and paraganglioma are less commonly encountered in the retroperitoneum.

6. What are the major types of retroperitoneal sarcoma?
Liposarcoma is the most common retroperitoneal sarcoma (40%), followed by leiomyosarcoma (30%) and malignant fibrous histiocytoma (MFH) (15%). Malignant peripheral nerve sheath tumor (MPNST) is more frequently encountered in patients with neurofibromatosis type 1 (NF-1).

7. How are computed tomography (CT) and magnetic resonance imaging (MRI) useful in patients with retroperitoneal sarcoma?
CT and MRI are useful to stage the extent of disease in patients with retroperitoneal sarcoma, to determine whether the tumor is fully resectable, and to detect presence of residual or recurrent tumor after treatment. The main pretreatment imaging features that indicate tumor unresectability include extensive vascular involvement by tumor, peritoneal spread of tumor, and presence of distant metastatic disease. Complete surgical resection is the key prognostic factor of clinical outcome in patients with retroperitoneal sarcoma.

8. What are the CT and MR imaging features of a retroperitoneal sarcoma?
Retroperitoneal sarcoma typically presents as a large retroperitoneal mass that may contain fat, soft tissue, myxoid tissue, cystic/necrotic change, hemorrhage, and/or calcification (Figure 37-3). Fatty components have attenuation and signal intensity properties similar to macroscopic fat located elsewhere in the body and when present indicate presence of a liposarcoma. Soft tissue components have soft tissue attenuation and in general low-intermediate T1-weighted and intermediate-high T2-weighted signal intensity relative to skeletal muscle with variable amounts of

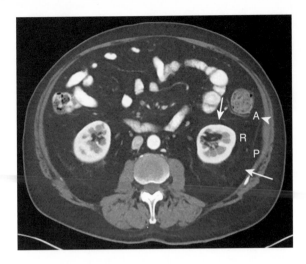

**Figure 37-1.** Normal retroperitoneal anatomy on CT. Note left aspect of anterior pararenal space (*A*) containing descending colon, left perirenal space (*R*) containing left kidney, and left posterior pararenal space (*P*) containing fat. Also note anterior renal fascia (*short arrow*), lateroconal fascia (*arrowhead*), and posterior renal fascia (*long arrow*).

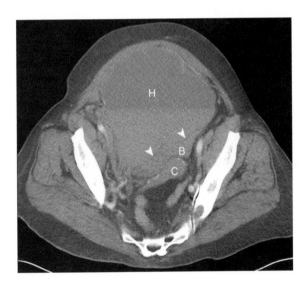

**Figure 37-2.** Prevesical space hematoma on CT. Note large high attenuation fluid collection (*H*) in anterior pelvis with typical "molar tooth" configuration and hematocrit effect as manifested by internal fluid-fluid level. Note intervening fat plane (*arrowheads*), located anterior to bladder (*B*) and posterior to nonvisualized umbilicovesical fascia (UVF), and posteriorly located cervix (*C*).

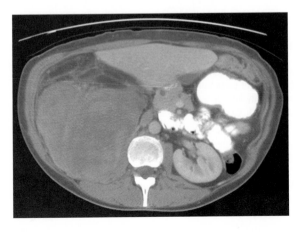

**Figure 37-3.** Retroperitoneal liposarcoma on CT. Note large right retroperitoneal mass that contains fat attenuation components anteriorly and heterogeneous soft tissue attenuation components posteriorly, with medial displacement of adjacent retroperitoneal structures such as the inferior vena cava and pancreas.

enhancement. Myxoid tissue and cystic/necrotic change both have fluid attenuation and very high T2-weighted signal intensity, although the former enhances, whereas the latter does not. Hemorrhagic areas typically show soft tissue attenuation (30 to 70 HU) and high T1-weighted signal intensity but do not enhance. Calcifications appear as very high attenuation foci on CT and are sometimes seen as very low signal intensity foci although they are much more difficult to visualize on MRI.

9. **What CT and MR imaging features favor a liposarcoma over a lipoma?**
Large size (>10 cm), thick septa (>2 mm), nodular and globular areas, nonadipose masslike areas, and decreased percentage of fat composition (<75% fat) favor liposarcoma.

10. **What clinical and imaging features favor presence of a retroperitoneal leiomyosarcoma?**
Retroperitoneal leiomyosarcoma occurs more commonly in women, whereas other retroperitoneal sarcomas occur more commonly in men or with similar frequencies in men and women. In addition, retroperitoneal leiomyosarcoma is often found in a location adjacent to or within the lumen of the inferior vena cava. Presence of these features may therefore favor this particular type of retroperitoneal sarcoma.

11. **What are some clinical, CT, and MR imaging features of schwannoma?**
Schwannomas account for 4% of retroperitoneal neoplasms, are benign peripheral nerve sheath tumors, and most commonly occur in the third to sixth decades of life. Most are asymptomatic, and malignant transformation is rare, but surgical resection may be performed when they are large in size or symptomatic.

A solitary well-circumscribed enhancing mass is usually seen, eccentric in location to the parent nerve when visualized, with similar or lower attenuation relative to skeletal muscle, low-intermediate signal intensity on T1-weighted images, and heterogeneous high signal intensity on T2-weighted images. Heterogeneity is more commonly seen than with neurofibroma due to the variable presence of fat, cystic, hemorrhagic, and calcific components, potentially mimicking retroperitoneal sarcoma in its imaging appearance on CT and MRI. Occasionally, a "target" sign may be encountered on T2-weighted images, which appears as central low signal intensity and peripheral high signal intensity, although this nonspecific finding may be seen with any type of neurogenic tumor.

12. **What are some clinical, CT, and MR imaging features of neurofibroma?**
Neurofibromas account for 5% of benign soft tissue neoplasms, are benign peripheral nerve sheath tumors, and most commonly occur in the third to fifth decades of life. The majority arise sporadically and are asymptomatic. However, 33% with a single neurofibroma have NF-1, and 99% with multiple or plexiform neurofibromas have NF-1. Surgical excision is usually performed when they are large in size, symptomatic, or suspicious for having undergone malignant transformation.

Solitary or multiple fusiform enhancing masses are usually seen in a retroperitoneal or paravertebral location, centered on parent nerves when visualized, often with a "bag of worms" configuration due to multiple diffusely thickened nerve branches as part of a plexiform neurofibroma. A dumbbell configuration may be seen when there is neural foraminal expansion by an involved spinal nerve. They usually have low soft tissue attenuation, low signal intensity on T1-weighted images, and high signal intensity on T2-weighted images relative to skeletal muscle, and they may be homogeneous or heterogeneous, sometimes with a "target" sign or else with a "whorled appearance" due to curvilinear low signal intensity foci on T2-weighted images (Figure 37-4).

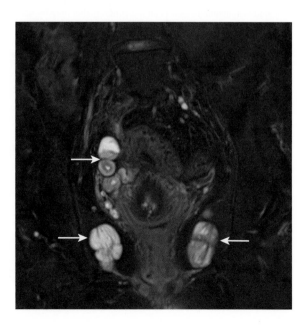

**Figure 37-4.** Neurofibromas in setting of NF-1 on T2-weighted MRI. Note multiple well-circumscribed high signal intensity extraperitoneal masses (*arrows*) in pelvis with "whorled appearance" due to curvilinear low signal intensity foci.

13. How often do patients with NF-1 develop neurofibromas?

Ten percent of patients with NF-1 develop one or more neurofibromas, which tend to be larger and located in deeper anatomic locations and occur at a younger age compared to those that arise sporadically.

14. When should one suspect malignant transformation of a neurofibroma into an MPNST?

Pain and rapid growth are the two main findings that raise suspicion for malignant transformation of a neurofibroma into an MPNST. Whereas malignant transformation of a neurofibroma into MPNST rarely occurs in sporadic cases, 2% to 5% of patients with NF-1 may develop an MPNST. MPNST arising in patients with NF-1 tends to have higher grade, larger size, and more aggressive behavior compared to that arising sporadically. A solitary, large, heterogeneous, enhancing retroperitoneal mass is typically seen with MPNST, although no specific CT or MR imaging features are available that can reliably differentiate MPNST from benign neurogenic tumors.

15. What are some clinical, CT, and MR imaging features of paraganglioma?

Paraganglioma, also known as an extraadrenal pheochromocytoma, is a rare neurogenic tumor that most commonly occurs in the fourth to fifth decades of life. In the abdomen, it most commonly arises in the retroperitoneum in the paired organs of Zuckerkandl that overlie the distal abdominal aorta. Ten percent of paragangliomas are multicentric, 40% are malignant (vs. 10% of adrenal pheochromocytomas), and 60% are functional (i.e., secrete catecholamines). Paragangliomas occurring in conjunction with gastrointestinal stromal tumors and pulmonary chondromas comprise Carney's triad and occur with increased incidence in multiple endocrine neoplasia (MEN) syndrome types IIA and IIB, NF-1, von Hippel Lindau syndrome, and hereditary paraganglioma- pheochromocytoma syndrome (HPPS) related to genetic mutations in succinate dehydrogenase (SDH). Detection of elevated urine catecholamine levels is suggestive of the diagnosis.

A retroperitoneal mass is typically visualized with soft tissue attenuation, low-intermediate signal intensity on T1-weighted images, and intermediate-high signal intensity on T2-weighted images relative to skeletal muscle, sometimes with areas of low T2-weighted signal intensity, and progressive enhancement. Heterogeneity due to cystic change, hemorrhage, or calcification is often seen. Functional tumors tends to be smaller in size than nonfunctional tumors, but otherwise the two cannot be distinguished from one another on CT or MR imaging. Similarly, the presence of metastatic disease is the only definitive imaging criterion of malignancy.

16. What are the CT and MR imaging features of retroperitoneal lymphoma?

Retroperitoneal lymphadenopathy or enhancing soft tissue masses, whether infiltrative or well-circumscribed, are seen, typically with homogeneous soft tissue attenuation, low-intermediate signal intensity on T1-weighted images, and high signal intensity relative to skeletal muscle (Figure 37-5). Central necrosis or calcification may be present, but most often after treatment, and low signal intensity on T2-weighted images after treatment may indicate nonviable tumor or fibrosis. When there is confluent lymphadenopathy sandwiching the mesenteric vessels, this is sometimes referred to as the "sandwich" sign. Whereas Hodgkin's lymphoma tends to spread to contiguous lymph node stations, non-Hodgkin's lymphoma is more likely to involve a variety of nodal groups and extranodal sites.

17. What CT and MR imaging findings can help distinguish benign from malignant lymph nodes?

Lymph nodes with a short axis diameter of <10 mm or with an oval shape are more likely to be benign in nature, whereas lymph nodes with a short axis diameter of ≥10 mm or with a spherical shape are more likely to be malignant in nature. However, these morphologic properties are nonspecific, as normal-sized lymph nodes may harbor malignancy and enlarged lymph nodes may be nonneoplastic in nature. Attenuation and signal intensity properties are also not accurate to differentiate between benign and malignant lymph nodes. Yet, malignant

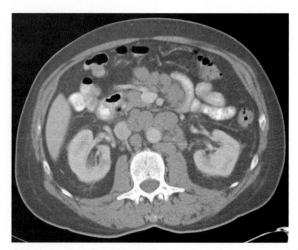

**Figure 37-5.** Retroperitoneal lymphadenopathy due to lymphoma on CT. Note enlarged homogeneous soft tissue attenuation retroperitoneal lymph nodes surrounding abdominal aorta and mesenteric vessels with associated anterior displacement of abdominal aorta from spine.

lymphadenopathy is more likely when there is associated anterior displacement of the abdominal aorta from the spine, lateral displacement of the ureters, or a history of known malignancy.

18. What is the differential diagnosis for abdominopelvic lymphadenopathy?

Lymphoma and metastatic disease are the most common causes of abdominopelvic lymphadenopathy. Less common causes include leukemia; mycobacterial, bacterial, viral, or fungal infection; and mesenteric lymphadenitis, sarcoidosis, amyloidosis, Castleman's disease, celiac sprue, inflammatory bowel disease, and other infectious or inflammatory disease conditions.

19. What are the major causes of necrotic lymph nodes?

Metastatic disease (especially from squamous cell carcinoma) and mycobacterial infection are the most common causes of necrotic lymph nodes. Bacterial infection, fungal infection, Whipple disease, and systemic lupus erythematosus are some less frequent causes.

20. What are the major causes of calcified lymph nodes?

Calcified lymph nodes are most commonly due to healed granulomatous disease (such as by fungal infection or sarcoidosis), metastatic disease, and lymphoma (most often after treatment), and they are less commonly due to amyloidosis and Castleman's disease.

21. What are the major causes of fatty lymph nodes?

Fatty lymph nodes may be seen with cavitary lymph node syndrome (associated with celiac disease and splenic atrophy), Whipple disease, multicentric angiomyolipoma, and metastatic germ cell tumor with a teratomatous component.

22. What are some imaging manifestations of retroperitoneal metastasis?

Retroperitoneal metastasis may appear as retroperitoneal lymphadenopathy via lymphatic spread (Figure 37-6), retroperitoneal nodules or masses via hematogenous spread, infiltrative soft tissue due to direct spread from a subjacent organ or tissue, or malignant retroperitoneal fibrosis (RPF) when there is an exuberant desmoplastic reaction to retroperitoneal metastatic foci.

23. Which malignant tumors most often spread to the retroperitoneum?

Any malignant tumor can spread to the retroperitoneum, but the most common types include lymphoma, melanoma, renal cell carcinoma, testicular cancer, prostate cancer, and cervical cancer.

24. What is RPF?

RPF is a rare fibroinflammatory retroperitoneal process that most commonly occurs in the fifth to sixth decades of life. Two thirds of cases are idiopathic in nature (in which case it is also known as Ormond's disease), and one third of cases develop in response to ergot derivatives and other medications or retroperitoneal metastatic disease (in which case it is called malignant RPF). Up to 15% of cases occur in association with other fibroinflammatory processes such as fibrosing mediastinitis, orbital pseudotumor, primary sclerosing cholangitis, and Reidel's thyroiditis. RPF typically arises in the inferior retroperitoneum at the lumbosacral level and may extend superiorly to the renal hila, sometimes encasing and obstructing one or both ureters.

25. What are the CT and MR imaging features of RPF?

Homogeneous soft tissue is typically seen in the retroperitoneum in a periaortic and pericaval distribution, sometimes with hydroureteronephrosis due to ureteral encasement. It has intermediate-slightly high attenuation, low-intermediate

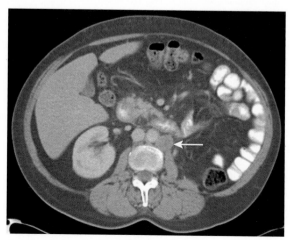

**Figure 37-6.** Retroperitoneal lymphadenopathy due to metastatic renal cell carcinoma on CT. Note enlarged heterogeneous soft tissue attenuation left para-aortic retroperitoneal lymph node.

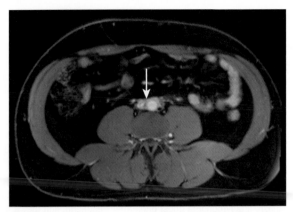

**Figure 37-7.** Retroperitoneal fibrosis (RPF) on postcontrast T1-weighted MRI. Note rim of confluent enhancing retroperitoneal soft tissue (*arrow*) surrounding abdominal aorta and inferior vena cava and lack of anterior displacement of abdominal aorta from spine.

signal intensity on T1-weighted images, either low signal intensity (when mature and benign) or high signal intensity (when immature or malignant) on T2-weighted images relative to skeletal muscle, and variable enhancement (Figure 37-7). Benign RPF typically does not cause anterior aortic displacement or lateral ureteral displacement. Malignant RPF is more likely to be present when lymphadenopathy or metastatic disease elsewhere in the body, an ill-defined heterogeneous mass, or adjacent osseous destruction is observed.

26. What are the major risk factors for retroperitoneal hemorrhage?

Retroperitoneal hemorrhage may be spontaneous or may be due to rupture of an abdominal aortic aneurysm, anticoagulation therapy, coagulopathy, trauma, surgery, arterial catheterization, or underlying parenchymal organ pathology with rupture.

27. What are the CT and MR imaging features of hemorrhage?

On CT, nonenhancing high attenuation (30 to 70 HU) hemorrhagic fluid is typically seen with acute hemorrhage, whereas acute hemorrhage in patients with anemia or more chronic hemorrhage may have lower attenuation (0 to 30 HU). A hematocrit effect manifesting as fluid-fluid levels due to layering of cellular components of blood also may be seen in acute hemorrhage (see Figure 37-2). Focal areas of extraluminal contrast material, when encountered, indicate the presence of active arterial hemorrhage. Over time, hematomas tend to decrease in size.

On MRI, acute hemorrhage has low signal intensity on T1-weighted and T2-weighted images due to deoxyhemoglobin, subacute hemorrhage has high T1-weighted and variable T2-weighted signal intensity due to methemoglobin, and chronic hemorrhage has very low signal intensity on T1-weighted and T2-weighted images due to hemosiderin and ferritin. The "concentric ring" sign, manifested by an inner rim of high signal intensity on T1-weighted images and an outer rim of very low signal intensity on T1-weighted and T2-weighted images, is specific for presence of a subacute hematoma.

28. What is a urinoma, and what are its major risk factors?

A urinoma is a fluid collection composed of urine caused by leakage of urine from the urothelial system, which most commonly occurs in the perirenal space of the retroperitoneum. Major risk factors include urinary obstruction, trauma, surgery, and instrumentation. Urinomas are generally managed conservatively when small in size but may be treated with percutaneous drainage along with repair of underlying sites of urothelial injury when large or superinfected.

29. What are the CT and MR imaging features of a urinoma?

A urinoma has fluid attenuation and low T1-weighted and very high T2-weighted signal intensity similar to fluid elsewhere in the body. Visualization of leakage of excreted intravenous contrast material from the urothelium into the fluid collection during the delayed phase of enhancement is diagnostic for a urinoma (Figure 37-8).

30. What are the major causes of pneumoretroperitoneum?

Pneumoretroperitoneum (i.e., gas in the retroperitoneum) is most often due to bowel perforation involving the retroperitoneal portions of bowel (i.e., the second through fourth portions of the duodenum, ascending colon, and descending colon). It is less commonly due to inferior extension of gas from the thorax, extracorporeal shock-wave lithotripsy, epidural anesthesia, percutaneous biopsy, abscess formation, necrotizing fasciitis, superinfected necrotizing pancreatitis, bowel infarction, and bowel pneumatosis. Very low attenuation and very low signal intensity gas surrounding retroperitoneal structures are seen on CT and MR images, respectively.

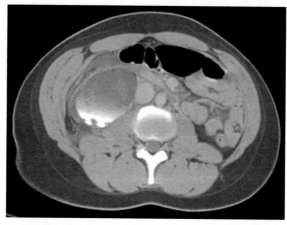

**Figure 37-8.** Retroperitoneal urinoma in setting of acute trauma on CT. Note right retroperitoneal fluid collection that demonstrates a dependent very high attenuation layer appearing only during the delayed phase of enhancement, indicating leakage of excreted intravenous contrast material from injured right urothelial system.

## KEY POINTS

- The anterior pararenal space, perirenal space, and posterior pararenal space are the main retroperitoneal compartments. The intervening retroperitoneal fascial planes are potentially expansile and may either serve as barriers to or conduits of disease spread to other compartments in the abdomen and pelvis.
- Most retroperitoneal tumors are malignant and are due to lymphoma, retroperitoneal sarcoma, or metastatic disease.
- Nonenhancing high attenuation fluid is suggestive of acute hemorrhage. When hemorrhage is seen, always assess for associated focal areas of extraluminal contrast material due to active arterial hemorrhage.
- Obtain delayed phase postcontrast images when a fluid collection is suspected to be due to a urinoma, such as in the setting of renal trauma, in order to make this specific diagnosis.
- Pneumoretroperitoneum is most often due to bowel perforation involving the retroperitoneal portions of bowel.

## BIBLIOGRAPHY

Torigian DA, Kitazono MT. *Netter's correlative imaging: abdominal and pelvic anatomy.* 1st ed. Philadephia: Elsevier; 2013:1-499.

Torigian DA, Ramchandani P. CT and MRI of the retroperitoneum. In: Haaga JR, Lanzieri CF, Gilkeson RC, eds. *CT and MRI of the whole body.* 5th ed. Philadelphia: Elsevier; 2009:1953-2040.

Torigian DA, Siegelman ES. MRI of the retroperitoneum and peritoneum. In: Siegelman ES, ed. *Body MRI.* 1st ed. Philadelphia: WB Saunders; 2005:207-268.

Rha SE, Byun JY, Jung SE, et al. Neurogenic tumors in the abdomen: tumor types and imaging characteristics. *Radiographics.* 2003;23(1):29-43.

Aizenstein RI, Owens C, Sabnis S, et al. The perinephric space and renal fascia: review of normal anatomy, pathology, and pathways of disease spread. *Crit Rev Diagn Imaging.* 1997;38(4):325-367.

Aizenstein RI, Wilbur AC, O'Neil HK. Interfascial and perinephric pathways in the spread of retroperitoneal disease: refined concepts based on CT observations. *AJR Am J Roentgenol.* 1997;168(3):639-643.

Korobkin M, Silverman PM, Quint LE, et al. CT of the extraperitoneal space: normal anatomy and fluid collections. *AJR Am J Roentgenol.* 1992;159(5):933-942.

Auh YH, Rubenstein WA, Schneider M, et al. Extraperitoneal paravesical spaces: CT delineation with US correlation. *Radiology.* 1986;159(2):319-328.

# CHAPTER 38

# IMAGING OF THE FEMALE PELVIS

*Ellie S. Kwak, MD, Sherelle L. Laifer-Narin, MD, and Elizabeth M. Hecht, MD*

1. **What is the first-line imaging modality of the female pelvis and why?**

   Common indications for pelvic imaging in a female patient include pelvic pain, pelvic masses, and abnormal bleeding. Ultrasonography (US) is the imaging modality of choice for evaluating the female pelvis because it offers excellent visualization of the pelvic organs. It is also fast, inexpensive, and portable and requires no intravenous or oral contrast material. If US results are inconclusive, magnetic resonance imaging (MRI) may be obtained for further evaluation. Computed tomography (CT) is generally reserved for emergent settings including trauma, hemodynamic instability, or acute lower abdominal or pelvic symptomatology when the differential diagnosis is broad, or for evaluation of patients with gynecologic malignancy. Positron emission tomography (PET) in combination with CT is most often performed for evaluation of suspected or known pelvic malignancy.

2. **How are US, CT, and MRI of the female pelvis performed?**

   US is performed using a transducer probe that sends and receives the ultrasound waves. Typically, images of the pelvis are initially obtained using a transabdominal approach (i.e., the transducer is placed over the abdomen and a conductive gel is applied) with a fluid-filled bladder. This is routinely followed by a transvaginal approach (i.e., a condom-covered sterilized transducer is placed in the vagina and covered in sterile conductive gel), preferably with an empty bladder. Transvaginal US typically demonstrates better delineation of the endometrium and adnexal regions, but these techniques are complementary. Images of the pelvic organs are obtained in the longitudinal and transverse planes. 2D and 3D imaging can be obtained, but 3D US requires specialized 3D transducers. Sonohysterography may be performed which combines hysterography with US. This is a slightly more invasive procedure because saline is infused into the endometrial canal. It is reserved for select patients with an abnormal endometrium. Transperineal and transrectal US are reserved for patients who are not candidates for transvaginal US and for assessment of pelvic organ prolapse. Although US is operator dependent and requires physical examination of the patient, it allows real-time imaging and is free of ionizing radiation. It takes at least 15 to 30 minutes to complete an examination, depending on its complexity.

   MRI utilizes strong magnetic fields to produce images, is similarly free of ionizing radiation, and is operator independent. For optimal image acquisition, a phased array coil is placed around the patient to optimize signal in the area of interest and to speed up image acquisition time. Patients must be screened prior to entering the MRI for any metallic devices. It can take up to 30 to 40 minutes to complete the examination, but with improvements in the technology, scan time continues to improve. 2D images may be acquired in any plane, and 3D imaging can also be performed. Multiple imaging sequences are obtained with different contrast weightings such as T1-weighted and T2-weighted images. Endovaginal and endorectal coils are occasionally used for urethral and perineal imaging. Gadolinium-based intravenous contrast material may be used if indicated. An antiperistalsis agent may sometimes be administered to decrease motion artifact from bowel peristalsis. Oral contrast material is sometimes administered for dedicated bowel imaging.

   CT is a technique that utilizes ionizing radiation. It is fast and nonoperator dependent. Scanning is performed in a single breath hold. Images are acquired in the transverse plane but can be reconstructed in coronal and sagittal planes, which are particularly helpful for evaluation of female pelvic anatomy and pathology. Iodinated intravenous contrast material and oral contrast material are often used for CT imaging.

3. **Which imaging modality best demonstrates the anatomy of the uterus?**

   MRI has superior soft tissue contrast compared to US or CT and best demonstrates uterine anatomy.

   The uterus consists of three zones with differential T2-weighted signal intensity on MRI: endometrium, inner myometrium (also called the junctional zone), and outer myometrium. The glandular endometrium has high T2-weighted signal intensity, the inner myometrium has low T2-weighted signal intensity due to presence of dense smooth muscle, and the outer myometrium has intermediate-slightly high T2-weighted signal intensity that contains more blood and less dense layers of smooth muscle (Figure 38-1). Sometimes, a very high T2-weighted signal intensity endometrial canal containing fluid is also seen.

   The cervix similarly demonstrates three distinct zones: a high T2-weighted signal intensity layer of endocervical glands (along with lower signal intensity longitudinal mucosal ridges [plicae palmitae]) that is contiguous with the endometrium, a low T2-weighted signal intensity inner cervical stroma that is contiguous with the junctional zone, and an intermediate-slightly high T2-weighted signal intensity outer cervical stroma that is contiguous with the outer myometrium. A very high T2-weighted signal intensity endocervical canal containing fluid may sometimes also be seen.

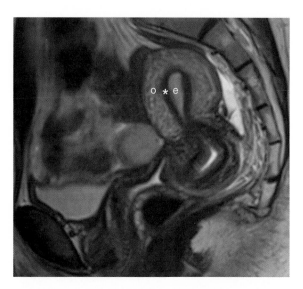

**Figure 38-1.** Normal uterine anatomy on MRI. Sagittal T2-weighted MR image in midline demonstrates zonal anatomy of uterus. Note intermediate-slightly high signal intensity outer myometrium (*o*), low signal intensity inner myometrium (*), and high signal intensity endometrium (*e*). Note similar zonal anatomy of cervix along with very high signal intensity endocervical fluid.

4. **What are the more common congenital uterine anomalies and their clinical significance?**

   Müllerian duct anomalies can cause abnormalities in uterine development that may be associated with infertility, miscarriage, and endometriosis. Accurate classification of müllerian duct anomalies is critical because treatment options vary depending on the type of underlying abnormality. MRI is the study of choice for delineation of uterine anomalies, while US and hysterosalpingography are often used for initial evaluation.

   The classification of anomalies relates to the embryology of uterine development. Two paired müllerian ducts develop into the anatomic structures of the female reproductive tract including the fallopian tubes, uterus, cervix, and upper two thirds of the vagina. The ovaries and lower third of the vagina are derived from different origins.

   There are three phases of development, and disruption of these processes can lead to anatomic variation and uterine anomalies. Failure of development during the organogenesis phase where one or both müllerian ducts do not fully develop can result in uterine agenesis, uterine hypoplasia, or a unicornuate uterus (Figure 38-2, *A-B*). The fusion phase refers to both lateral and vertical fusion of the paired müllerian ducts. Failure of lateral fusion can lead to bicornuate or didelphys uterus, and vertical fusion failure can result in incomplete development of the vagina. When the müllerian ducts fuse, a central septum is created which subsequently must then be resorbed to form a single uterine cavity. If not, this can lead to a septate uterus (Figure 38-2, *C-D*). Septate uterus is the most common type of congenital uterine anomaly and is associated with the highest risk of complications such as recurrent spontaneous abortions and premature delivery.

5. **What is the normal thickness of the endometrium in a premenopausal patient?**

   In premenopausal women, the appearance of the endometrium changes depending on the phase of the menstrual cycle. On US, during menstruation the endometrium is identified as a thin, echogenic line measuring 1 to 4 mm, sometimes with blood products or sloughed endometrial lining seen in the uterine cavity. During the proliferative phase, the endometrium is thicker, with a trilaminar appearance typically measuring 5 to 7 mm, composed of a thin echogenic central line, a hypoechoic functional layer, and a surrounding outer echogenic basal layer (Figure 38-3). During the secretory phase, the endometrium reaches its maximum thickness (up to about 16 mm) and is homogenously echogenic.

   On MRI, the endometrium is typically homogenous, is high in signal intensity on T2-weighted images and low in signal intensity on T1-weighted images, and can vary in thickness depending on the phase of the menstrual cycle. On CT, the measurement of endometrial thickness should be performed on sagittal reconstructed images and can be accurate and reproducible compared with that obtained from transvaginal US.

6. **What is the normal thickness of the endometrium in postmenopausal patients, and what is the significance of thickened endometrium in these patients?**

   The endometrium in postmenopausal women should appear as a thin, echogenic layer measuring less than 4 to 5 mm. Endometrial thickness greater than 5 mm with or without surface irregularity and endometrial heterogeneity in the setting of postmenopausal bleeding may be related to benign etiologies such as endometrial hyperplasia, submucosal leiomyomas (i.e., fibroids), or endometrial polyps. However, further workup should be pursued to exclude endometrial cancer, because US findings are often nonspecific.

7. **What are the most common causes of vaginal bleeding in a postmenopausal woman?**

   In postmenopausal women, atrophy of the endometrium is the most common etiology of vaginal bleeding. Other common causes include endometrial polyps, endometrial hyperplasia, and endometrial cancer. Less common etiologies include uterine leiomyomas, adenomyosis, hormone replacement therapy, and cervical cancer. Approximately 12% of

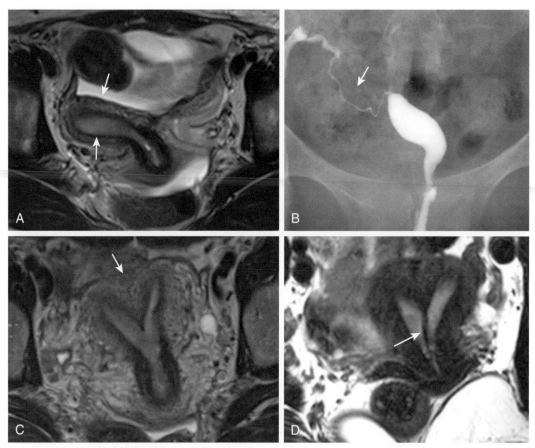

**Figure 38-2.** Müllerian duct anomalies of uterus on MRI and hysterosalpingography. **A,** Axial T2-weighted MR image shows unicornuate uterus (*arrows*) with small caliber "banana-shaped" uterine cavity in right pelvis. **B,** Hysterosalpingogram of same patient demonstrates contrast material in lumen of unicornuate uterus and right fallopian tube patency (*arrow*). **C,** Axial T2-weighted MR image in different patient shows partial septate uterus. Note flat outer fundal contour (*arrow*) which distinguishes septate uterus from bicornuate uterus. **D,** Axial T2-weighted MR image in another patient shows complete septate uterus (*arrow*).

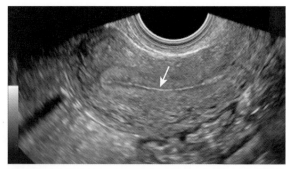

**Figure 38-3.** Normal uterus on transvaginal US. Sagittal image through uterus during proliferative phase of menstrual cycle reveals "trilaminar" appearance of endometrium with thin echogenic central line (*arrow*) representing interface between anterior and posterior endometrium. During secretory phase of menstrual cycle (*not shown*), endometrium becomes more uniformly echogenic.

women with postmenopausal bleeding have endometrial cancer. Endometrial cancer is one of the most common gynecologic malignancies, and the risk of development increases with age.

8. In a postmenopausal patient with vaginal bleeding, what is the role of imaging?
   Endometrial polyps, endometrial hyperplasia, submucosal fibroids, and endometrial cancer can all present with vaginal bleeding. Although vaginal bleeding is most often due to a benign etiology, imaging can be performed to exclude an underlying anatomic cause and potentially guide tissue sampling if needed. Transvaginal US is the first line of imaging

because it can visualize the endometrium and assess endometrial thickness. Endometrial thickness greater than 4 mm on US has a sensitivity of 98% for detection of endometrial cancer and requires further workup, whereas endometrial thickness of 4 mm or less has a negative predictive value of 99%. Sonohysterography and MRI may be performed for further evaluation as needed. Tissue sampling of the endometrium may be warranted using dilation and curettage (D&C) or hysteroscopy to enable visualization of the endometrium and directed biopsies. A diagnostic feature favoring endometrial cancer rather than endometrial hyperplasia or polyp is the presence of myometrial invasion or metastatic disease.

9. What is adenomyosis, and what are its imaging characteristics?

Adenomyosis is the presence of ectopic endometrial tissue that develops and grows within the muscular wall of the uterus (i.e., the myometrium). It typically affects women of reproductive age, and symptoms may include severe menstrual cramps, bloating, dysmenorrhea, and menorrhagia. Uterine adenomyosis can be focal, diffuse, or even masslike (i.e., an adenomyoma) and mimic leiomyomas. Transvaginal US is typically used as the first line of imaging. US features of adenomyosis include heterogeneous, most commonly hypoechoic, myometrium with striations and an ill-defined endomyometrial junction. The uterus may appear asymmetric with globular thickening of a wall in focal adenomyosis (Figure 38-4, *A-B*). MRI can be very helpful to confirm this diagnosis. On MRI, adenomyosis is identified as thickening of the junctional zone (≥12 mm), often with presence of subcentimeter foci of T2-weighted (and

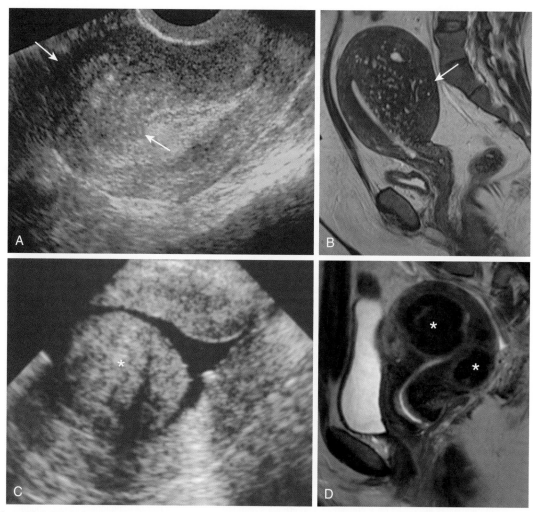

**Figure 38-4.** Focal adenomyosis and uterine leiomyomas on US and MRI. **A,** Sagittal transvaginal US image of uterus demonstrates focal thickening of myometrial wall with ill-defined endomyometrial junction (*arrows*) due to focal adenomyosis. **B,** Sagittal T2-weighted MR image in midline shows focal thickening of junctional zone along posterior myometrial wall with small high signal intensity cystic foci (*arrow*) due to segmental adenomyosis. Note lack of mass effect upon endometrium. **C,** Sagittal saline-infused sonohysterographic image demonstrates well-defined mass arising from posterior uterine wall and projecting into endometrial cavity representing intracavitary uterine leiomyoma (*). **D,** Sagittal T2-weighted MR image shows multiple well-circumscribed anterior and posterior intramural uterine leiomyomas (*). Note that anterior leiomyoma has submucosal component and exerts mass effect upon endometrium.

sometimes T1-weighted) hyperintensity representing ectopic endometrial glands. Focal adenomyosis typically has indistinct margins and does not exert much, if any, mass effect upon adjacent structures.

10. What is the most common neoplasm of the female genitourinary tract?

Leiomyoma, or fibroid, is the most common neoplasm of the female genitourinary tract, affecting up to 30% to 40% of women over the age of 35. Leiomyomas are benign smooth muscle tumors that are hormonally responsive, sometimes demonstrating dramatic growth during pregnancy, and are most often seen in the uterus, although they may also occur in other locations such as in the cervix or broad ligament. They may either be detected incidentally on imaging or may be associated with vaginal bleeding, pelvic pain, infertility, or a palpable abnormality. Leiomyomas may undergo various types of degeneration including hyaline (the most common), cystic, myxoid, red (hemorrhagic), or fatty degeneration (also called lipoleiomyoma).

On imaging, well-circumscribed myometrial masses are seen, which are more commonly multiple than solitary, may be homogeneous or heterogeneous in appearance, and typically exert mass effect upon adjacent structures such as the endometrium. On US, leiomyomas are usually hypoechoic but can be isoechoic or hyperechoic relative to the surrounding myometrium (see Figure 38-4, C). Anechoic or hypoechoic cystic components may be detected, and calcifications, when present, will appear as echogenic foci with posterior acoustic shadowing. On CT, leiomyomas have soft tissue attenuation with variable degrees of enhancement, and foci of very high attenuation calcification may also be present. On MRI, nondegenerated leiomyomas typically have homogeneous intermediate T1-weighted and low T2-weighted signal intensity relative to normal myometrium (see Figure 38-4, D). Cellular leiomyomas may have relatively increased T2-weighted signal intensity, whereas leiomyomas with hyaline degeneration have decreased T2-weighted signal intensity similar to nondegenerated leiomyomas. Areas of increased T1-weighted signal intensity may be seen with hemorrhagic or fatty degeneration, whereas loss of signal intensity will only occur with the latter on fat-suppressed T1-weighted images. Increased T2-weighted signal intensity components may be seen with cystic or myxoid degeneration, where the former does not enhance and the latter does enhance.

11. What is Asherman's syndrome, and what are its imaging characteristics?

Asherman's syndrome is due to the presence of intrauterine adhesions or synechiae and is the result of endometrial trauma, such as from prior D&C, surgery, abortion, or infection. This is associated with infertility and secondary amenorrhea or hypomenorrhea. On sonohysterography, hyperechoic bands may be seen within the endometrial canal. On MRI, low T2-weighted signal intensity bands are seen in the endometrial canal, sometimes with distortion or obliteration of the endometrial cavity.

12. What is the normal size of the ovaries in premenopausal versus postmenopausal women?

The ovaries in premenopausal women on average measure approximately 5 mL in volume, and multiple small <1 cm follicles are typically seen. Each month a dominant follicle develops and extrudes an egg during ovulation. In postmenopausal women, the ovaries on average measure approximately 2 mL in volume, are more homogenous and more frequently without the presence of follicles, and may be difficult to visualize on imaging. Ovarian volume is inversely proportional to patient age.

13. What are the most common benign lesions of the ovaries and their imaging characteristics?

The most common benign ovarian lesions include functional cysts and hemorrhagic cysts, which are typically diagnosed on transvaginal US. Functional cysts include follicular and corpus luteum cysts. A follicular cyst occurs when ovulation does not occur and the egg is not released due to lack of a luteinizing hormone (LH) surge. If ovulation occurs, a dominant follicle extrudes an egg and becomes a corpus luteum. If pregnancy occurs, the corpus luteum may fill with fluid or blood and becomes a corpus luteum cyst.

On US, a follicular cyst is identified as a unilocular anechoic ovoid or round lesion with posterior acoustic enhancement. A corpus luteum cyst is thick-walled and has increased vascularity with a classic "ring of fire" appearance on Doppler US (Figure 38-5, A-B). On MRI, functional ovarian cysts demonstrate homogenous hyperintense T2-weighted signal intensity similar to that of fluid and hypointense T1-weighted signal intensity with a thin wall.

Hemorrhagic cysts develop when there is hemorrhage within a functional cyst. US of a hemorrhagic cyst demonstrates mixed echogenicity and lacy interfaces due to the presence of blood products (Figure 38-5, C-D). On MRI, hemorrhagic cysts demonstrate varying imaging characteristics, with roughly two thirds appearing isointense or hypointense on T1-weighted images and one third appearing hyperintense. T2-weighted signal intensity is also variable.

14. What is the recommended management of an incidentally discovered asymptomatic simple ovarian cyst seen on US in premenopausal versus postmenopausal women?

Recommendations are based on a consensus conference statement from the Society of Radiologists in Ultrasound (SRU) that convened a panel of specialists from gynecology, radiology, and pathology in 2009. In premenopausal women, a simple cyst measuring less than 5 cm does not require follow-up. If the simple cyst measures greater than 5 cm, then yearly US is recommended to monitor changes in size although the lesion is considered most certainly benign. In postmenopausal women, a simple cyst measuring less than 1 cm does not require follow-up as it is most likely benign. For a simple cyst measuring greater than 1 cm, yearly US is recommended although it is likely benign. Both in pre- and postmenopausal women, any cyst measuring greater than 7 cm should undergo further workup with

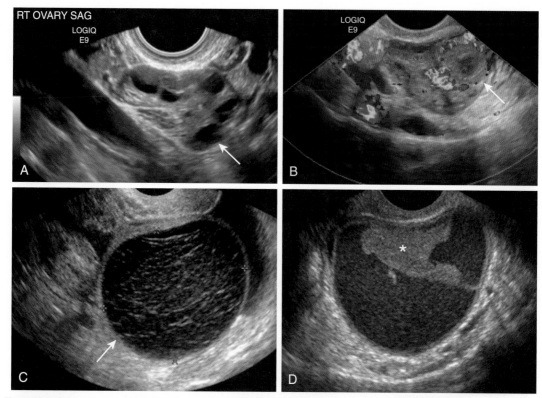

**Figure 38-5.** Normal ovary and benign ovarian cysts on transvaginal US. **A,** Sagittal image of normal right ovary in premenopausal patient with multiple anechoic follicles (*arrow*). **B,** Color Doppler image of right ovary demonstrates thick-walled corpus luteum with "ring of fire" appearance (*arrow*). **C** and **D,** Note ovarian hemorrhagic cysts with internal "lace-like" reticular echoes (*arrow*) and eccentric echogenic blood clot (*).

MRI or possibly surgical intervention because it may not be sufficiently assessed given the limitations of field of view with US.

15. **What are the imaging findings of endometriosis on US and MRI?**
    Endometriosis is defined as the presence of endometrial tissue outside the uterus, most commonly involving the ovaries, uterine ligaments, cul-de-sac, pelvic peritoneum, fallopian tubes, distal colon, and bladder. Endometriosis is commonly diffuse with scattered implants, but it can also be focal with a discrete endometrioma (also described as a "chocolate cyst" because of its appearance at pathology).

    On US, a typical endometrioma presents as a unilocular or multilocular cystic lesion with homogeneous low-level echoes (Figure 38-6, *A*) and no internal vascularity. In addition, the presence of ectogenic foci in the roll of a cystic mass that contains low level echoes would favor the diagnosis of endometrioma, and may be seen in one third of endometrioma. CT is not used commonly for evaluation of endometriosis, but it may visualize large endometriomas and complications such as rupture or bowel obstruction (Figure 38-6, *B*). On MRI, an endometrioma demonstrates T1-weighted hyperintensity that persists after fat suppression and T2-weighted hypointensity (also called "shading") (Figure 38-6, *C-D*). Another specific sign recently reported is the presence of more focal low T2-weighted signal intensity spots. Presence of multiple or bilateral high T1-weighted signal intensity ovarian lesions makes endometriomas more likely than hemorrhagic cysts. MRI also plays a role in revealing sites of deep fibrotic endometriosis involving structures such as the sigmoid colon, rectum, and cul-de-sac. Fibrotic endometriosis typically has low T2-weighted signal intensity and tethers adjacent structures.

16. **What are the major causes of hydrosalpinx and hematosalpinx, and what are their imaging features on US and MRI?**
    A hydrosalpinx is a dilated fluid-filled fallopian tube; it is most commonly due to prior pelvic inflammatory disease (PID) and less commonly due to endometriosis, prior pelvic surgery with adhesions, fallopian tube cancer, or ectopic pregnancy. On US, a tubular adnexal cystic lesion separate from the ovary is seen, sometimes with visualization of a characteristic "waist" sign due to indentation of the opposing walls or with a "cog-wheel" or "beads-on-a-string" appearance due to polypoid protrusions of the mucosa into the lumen. On MRI, low T1-weighted and very high T2-weighted signal intensity fluid contents are observed within a tubular adnexal cystic lesion, along with characteristic incomplete longitudinal folds representing mucosal plicae.

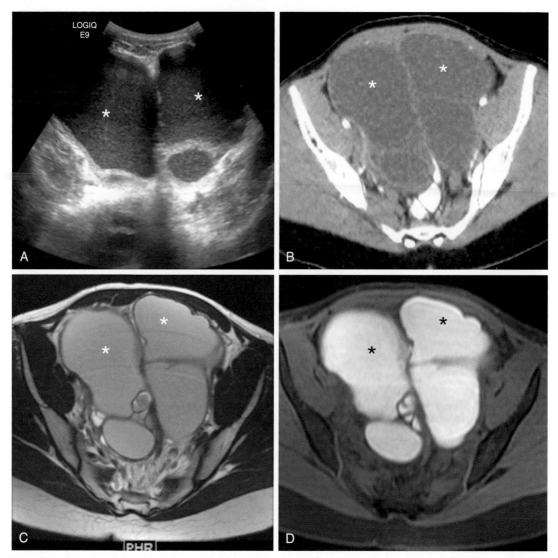

**Figure 38-6.** Bilateral ovarian endometriomas on US, CT, and MRI. **A,** US image shows adnexal cystic lesions (*) with low-level internal echoes representing endometriomas. **B,** Axial contrast-enhanced CT image demonstrates bilateral low attenuation adnexal lesions (*) with internal septations. **C,** Axial T2-weighted and **D,** Axial fat-suppressed T1-weighted MR images show bilateral cystic adnexal lesions (*) with slightly lower T2-weighted signal intensity than simple fluid and high T1-weighted signal intensity.

A hematosalpinx is a dilated hemorrhage-filled fallopian tube and is most commonly due to endometriosis in a nonpregnant female. Other causes include ectopic pregnancy, adnexal torsion, fallopian tube cancer, and retrograde menstruation in the setting of hematometrocolpos. On US, low-level echoes or laying echogenic material may be seen within the fallopian tube lumen. On MRI, high T1-weighted and variable T2-weighted signal intensity hemorrhagic fluid is observed.

17. What are the imaging features of a mature teratoma of the ovary?

A mature teratoma on US is identified as a cystic or echogenic mass with distinct features such as thin, echogenic lines representing hair, posterior acoustic shadowing from calcifications including bone and teeth, and fluid-fluid levels from sebum layering with serous fluid (Figure 38-7, *A*). On CT, fat attenuation with or without calcification is diagnostic for a mature teratoma (Figure 38-7, *B*). On MRI, high T1-weighted signal intensity may indicate the presence of fat or hemorrhage within a mass (Figure 38-7, *C-D*). Using fat suppression techniques on MRI, one can differentiate a mature teratoma from a hemorrhagic cyst or endometrioma, as the former will lose signal intensity on fat-suppressed T1-weighted images, whereas the latter will not. Mature teratoma can be associated with complications such as torsion (common), malignant degeneration (rare, <2%), or rupture (rare <1%), sometimes with associated chemical peritonitis.

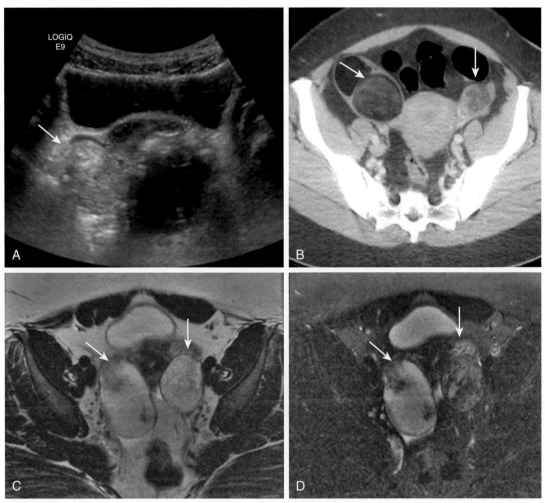

**Figure 38-7.** Bilateral ovarian teratomas on US, CT, and MRI. **A,** Transverse transabdominal US image of right adnexa demonstrates lobulated echogenic mass (*arrow*) with posterior acoustic shadowing consistent with calcification. **B,** Axial contrast-enhanced CT image through pelvis shows bilateral ovarian masses with fat attenuation components (*arrows*). **C,** Axial T2-weighted MR image in different patient reveals bilateral ovarian masses (*arrows*) with high signal intensity and lower signal intensity components. **D,** Axial fat-suppressed T2-weighted MR image shows loss of signal intensity in some areas of these lesions (*arrows*), left greater than right, confirming presence of macroscopic fat.

18. In a female patient with acute pelvic pain and suspected adnexal torsion, what is the study of choice, and what are the imaging findings of adnexal torsion?

    Adnexal torsion occurs when the adnexa and its vascular pedicle twist, resulting in ischemic injury to the ovary and/or fallopian tube. In the majority of cases, a predisposing ipsilateral functional cyst or neoplasm (most commonly mature teratoma) is present. When adnexal torsion is suspected, US is the initial study of choice. Common sonographic findings are an adnexal mass, an enlarged ovary, and pelvic fluid. The affected ovary may also demonstrate peripherally located follicles and may have an atypical location such as above the uterine fundus or adjacent to the contralateral ovary. Color Doppler US can demonstrate a "whirlpool" sign created by a twisted pedicle. Spectral Doppler US may demonstrate compromised blood flow depending on the extent of vascular obstruction (Figure 38-8A). On CT and MRI, an adnexal mass, an enlarged ovary, and simple or hemorrhagic pelvic fluid are commonly visualized (Figure 38-8B). Decreased or absent contrast enhancement of the ovary, visualization of a twisted vascular pedicle, fallopian tube wall thickening, deviation of the uterus toward the involved side, or atypical location of the adnexa to the contralateral pelvis or midline may also be seen. Hemorrhage within the ovary, fallopian tube, or pelvic peritoneal space when present has high attenuation on CT and high T1-weighted signal intensity on MRI.

19. How is polycystic ovarian syndrome (PCOS) diagnosed, and what is the role for imaging?

    A diagnosis of PCOS is established based on a combination of oligomenorrhea or anovulation, clinical or biochemical evidence of hyperandrogenism, and polycystic ovaries on US. Transvaginal US is the study of choice for evaluation of the ovaries. A diagnosis of polycystic ovaries is supported by imaging when there are 12 or more follicles measuring 2

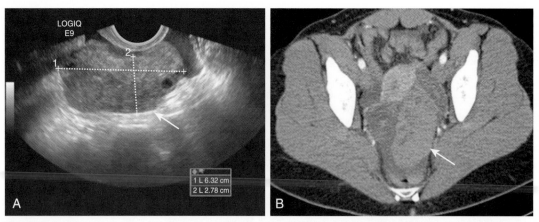

**Figure 38-8.** Right adnexal torsion on US and CT. **A,** Longitudinal transvaginal US image shows enlarged right ovary (*arrow*) in young woman with acute right lower quadrant pain. Color Doppler (*not shown*) demonstrates no arterial flow. **B,** Axial contrast-enhanced CT image through pelvis demonstrates right ovary enlargement (*arrow*) with atypical location in left side of pelvis and foci of high attenuation hemorrhage, along with hemorrhagic pelvic fluid. Surgery revealed necrotic right ovary and right fallopian tube with 360° torsion.

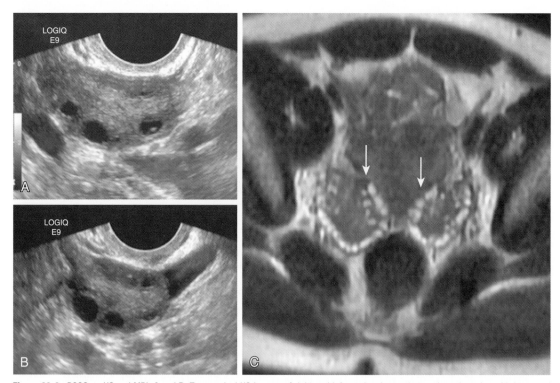

**Figure 38-9.** PCOS on US and MRI. **A** and **B,** Transvaginal US images of right and left ovaries demonstrate enlarged ovaries with increased central stroma and multiple peripherally located follicles. **C,** Axial T2-weighted MR image of different patient shows enlargement of both ovaries with numerous peripherally located follicles (*arrows*) and prominent central stroma.

to 9 mm in diameter, which are often peripherally located, or when the ovarian volume measures greater than 10 mL for at least one of the ovaries (Figure 38-9, *A-B*). Prominent central ovarian stroma may also be seen. MRI is reserved for cases where US is inconclusive (Figure 38-9, *C*).

20. **What are the most common malignancies of the female reproductive system?**
The most common malignancies of the female reproductive system worldwide are cervical cancer, endometrial cancer, and ovarian cancer in decreasing order of frequency. In the United States, endometrial cancer is the most common malignancy, followed by ovarian cancer and cervical cancer in decreasing order of frequency.

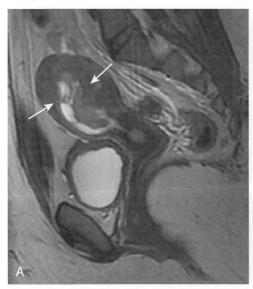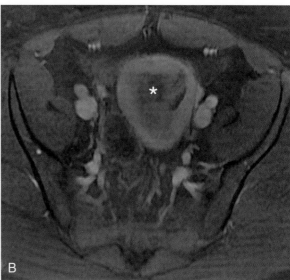

**Figure 38-10.** Endometrial cancer on MRI. **A,** Sagittal T2-weighted MR image through uterus demonstrates thickened and heterogeneous signal intensity endometrium (*arrows*). **B,** Axial contrast-enhanced T1-weighted MR image of uterus shows heterogeneous enhancement of endometrium (*). Note irregular contour along its right and posterior aspects consistent with myometrial invasion. Subsequent histopathologic assessment revealed well-differentiated endometrioid adenocarcinoma.

21. How is endometrial cancer diagnosed, and what imaging features are considered in staging?
    Endometrial cancer is diagnosed based on histopathology of a specimen from endometrial biopsy, curettage sample, or hysterectomy. Once the diagnosis is established, staging of endometrial cancer with imaging can be performed with PET or MRI, although surgical staging is still considered to be the reference standard. According to the International Federation of Gynecology and Obstetrics (FIGO), staging is based on features including myometrial invasion, cervical involvement, tumor extension into adjacent organs, lymph node involvement, and distant metastasis. Patients with greater than 50% myometrial invasion and cervical invasion are at high risk of recurrence and undergo pelvic lymphadenectomy at the time of tumor resection (Figure 38-10).

22. How is cervical cancer diagnosed, and what tumor features are considered in staging and pretreatment planning?
    Cervical cancer is diagnosed histologically from tissue obtained via a cervical biopsy. Once the diagnosis is made, further workup is required for staging, which may include a combination of physical examination, chest radiography, barium enema examination, intravenous urography, colposcopy, hysteroscopy, cystoscopy, and/or proctoscopy with tissue sampling and histologic confirmation required for additional sites of suspected involvement. The FIGO staging of cervical cancer is clinical, as this allows for uniformity of staging in low-resource countries around the world. That is, tomographic imaging findings from CT, MRI, and PET imaging are not utilized to stage cervical cancer, although they are commonly used for delineation of disease sites and lesion sizes for pretreatment planning purposes. As such, clinical staging is less accurate than surgical staging.
    MRI can be helpful for pretreatment planning by identifying parametrial involvement, invasion of the upper two thirds of the vagina, tumor extension into the adjacent structures, lymphadenopathy, and distant metastases (Figure 38-11). Parametrial invasion is an important criterion that determines whether a tumor is operable or not. A tumor without parametrial invasion can be resected, whereas a tumor with parametrial invasion is generally treated nonsurgically with radiation therapy and chemotherapy. Visualization of the hypointense inner cervical stroma on T2-weighted images indicates preservation of the parametrium, whereas disruption of this stromal ring by a lesion of intermediate-high signal intensity suggests parametrial invasion. PET is particularly useful to detect lymphadenopathy and distant metastatic disease that may not be evident on MRI.

23. What are the major imaging features that suggest presence of an ovarian neoplasm?
    An ovarian mass that may be completely solid, partially solid, or completely cystic, with variable presence of calcification, cystic change, necrosis, hemorrhage, wall thickening, internal septations, mural nodules, or papillary projections. Larger size and documented growth over time favor malignancy. Enhancement of solid components on CT or MRI and blood flow on color and spectral Doppler US also favor malignancy. Associated findings of peritoneal spread of tumor may be seen when ovarian malignancy is present, including complex ascites; peritoneal, mesenteric, or omental masses or infiltrative soft tissue implants; and diffuse peritoneal thickening and enhancement. Lymphadenopathy and distant metastases also may be present.

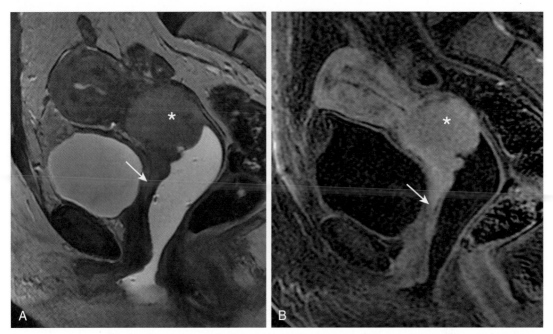

**Figure 38-11.** Cervical cancer on MRI. **A,** Sagittal T2-weighted and **B,** Sagittal contrast-enhanced T1-weighted MR images of uterus show large mass (*) replacing normal cervix with extension into upper third of anterior vaginal wall (*arrow*).

24. **What are the most common perineal cystic lesions seen in the female patient?**
    Several types of perineal cystic lesions can be seen in the female patient arising from the urethra, vagina, labia, or ischiorectal fossa. The more common periurethral cystic lesions include urethral diverticula and Skene's duct cysts. The most common vaginal and labial cysts include Gartner's duct cysts and Bartholin's gland cysts, respectively.
       Urethral diverticula are usually located at the level of the midurethra, whereas Skene's duct cysts are located lateral to the external urethral meatus and inferior to the pubic symphysis. Gartner's duct cysts are found in the anterolateral vagina down to the level of the inferior margin of the pubic symphysis. Bartholin's gland cysts are found at the posterolateral introitus medial to the labium. MRI is very helpful for diagnosis because of its excellent soft tissue contrast. Accurate localization of the palpable abnormality is one of the major keys to diagnosis, and location of origin will markedly narrow the differential diagnosis.

25. **In a patient with cervical motion tenderness and suspected pelvic inflammatory disease (PID), what is the role of imaging?**
    PID is typically a clinical diagnosis, although imaging can assist in early diagnosis and in identifying potential complications. Transvaginal US is the initial imaging study of choice in most cases and can be helpful in establishing a diagnosis of PID. A thickened appearance of the tubal walls seen on US is the most useful diagnostic clue with high (>90%) specificity and with sensitivity ranging from 30% to 100%. Tubo-ovarian abscess (TOA) is identified on US as a nonspecific complex adnexal mass. CT also plays a role in visualizing pyosalpinx, TOA, and right upper quadrant peritonitis related to Fitz-Hugh-Curtis syndrome (Figure 38-12). Although the overall sensitivity of CT signs for diagnosis of acute PID is limited, it can help confirm a suspected diagnosis of PID. The most specific CT imaging finding is thickening of the fallopian tubes. Subtle infiltration or haziness of the pelvic mesenteric fat is one of the earliest findings of PID that may be encountered on CT or MRI.

26. **In a multiparous patient with stress urinary incontinence, vaginal bulging, incomplete defecation, and suspected pelvic organ prolapse, what is the role of imaging?**
    In patients with suspected pelvic organ prolapse, dynamic cine MRI can be obtained to assess pelvic floor function. Patients are imaged dynamically before and after Valsalva and other maneuvers that can potentially confirm diagnosis in patients with suspected pelvic organ prolapse. Sometimes rectal and vaginal contrast is used in combination with Valsalva maneuvers to try to reproduce the patient's symptoms (Figure 38-13). Imaging can quantify the degree of pelvic organ prolapse in all three compartments (anterior, middle, and posterior) during Valsalva. Proposed MRI organ prolapse grading systems utilize reference lines drawn between normal anatomic structures on sagittal images (e.g., the pubococcygeal line [PCL] drawn from the inferior margin of the pubic symphysis to the last horizontal sacrococcygeal joint, the H line drawn from the inferior pubic symphysis to the posterior anorectal junction which demarcates the urogenital hiatus; and the M line drawn from the posterior end of the H line to (and perpendicular to) the PCL which serves as a reference for the pelvic floor descent) to estimate the degree of organ dysfunction. However, physical examination staging with the pelvic organ prolapse quantification (POP-Q) system (which uses the

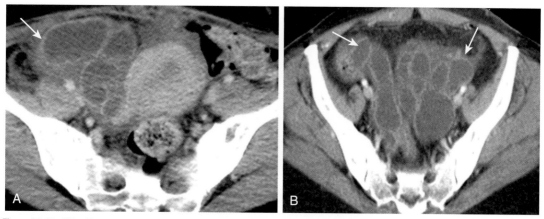

**Figure 38-12.** PID with extensive bilateral pyosalpinges on CT. **A** and **B,** Axial contrast-enhanced CT images of pelvis demonstrate markedly dilated bilateral fallopian tubes (arrows) with wall thickening, enhancement, and surrounding fat stranding.

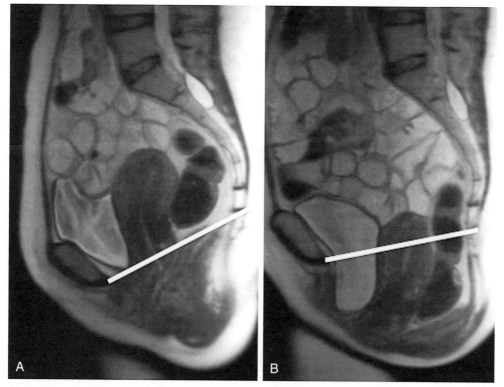

**Figure 38-13.** Multiorgan pelvic prolapse on MRI. **A,** Sagittal T2-weighted MR image shows bladder, uterus, and rectum at rest. Note PCL (*white line*) for reference. **B,** Sagittal T2-weighted MR image during Valsalva maneuver demonstrates laxity of pelvic floor muscles and multiorgan prolapse involving bladder, uterus, and rectum as evidenced by inferior descent of these organs below PCL (*white line*).

vaginal hymen as a point of reference) has become the clinical reference standard for evaluating patients with organ prolapse because of its interobserver and intraobserver reliability. Fluoroscopic imaging studies (such as with voiding cystourethrography [VCUG], double balloon urethrography, and defecography) were used more frequently in the past, although MRI and US are now used more commonly in conjunction with physical examination and other functional urodynamic imaging techniques.

27. **In a female patient with postvoid dribbling, dysuria, dyspareunia, and recurrent urinary tract infections, what is the differential diagnosis?**
Although clinical presentation can be highly variable, the classic triad of postvoid dribbling, dysuria, and dyspareunia is associated with the diagnosis of urethral diverticulum. MRI is the preferred study of choice for identifying a suspected urethral diverticulum. Typical imaging features include a round or oval structure arising from the posterolateral wall of

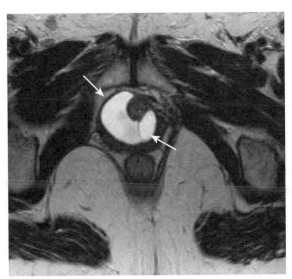

**Figure 38-14.** Urethral diverticulum on MRI. Axial T2-weighted MR image through urethra in female patient shows horseshoe-shaped very high signal intensity fluid-filled cystic lesion (*arrows*) nearly completely surrounding midurethra.

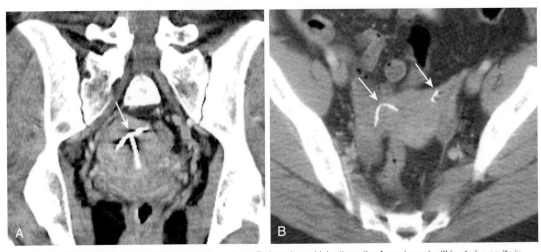

**Figure 38-15.** IUDs on CT. **A,** Coronal CT image of uterus shows T-shaped very high attenuation focus (*arrow*) within uterine cavity in keeping with copper IUD. **B,** Axial CT image of uterus in different patient demonstrates bilateral curvilinear very high attenuation foci (*arrows*) within proximal fallopian tubes in keeping with Essure devices.

the midurethra at the level of the pubic symphysis demonstrating T2-weighted hyperintensity (Figure 38-14). A direct connection between the urethra and diverticulum is not typically seen, although the diagnosis is based on location and morphology. Complications of diverticula include stone formation and intradiverticular neoplasms such as adenocarcinoma, transitional cell carcinoma, and squamous cell carcinoma. For these reasons, urethral diverticula are often surgically resected.

28. What are the imaging features of intrauterine devices (IUDs)?
    Multiple imaging modalities are used to visualize IUDs including radiography, hysterosalpingography, US, CT, and MRI. The most commonly used IUDs are copper, hormonal, and intratubal devices. A copper IUD is seen on US as a hyperechoic T-shaped device in the uterine cavity and a radiopaque T-shaped device on radiography and CT (Figure 38-15, *A*). A hormonal IUD such as the Mirena is less echogenic and therefore may be difficult to visualize on US. Instead, US can be used to demonstrate the echogenic string attached to a hormonal IUD. On radiography and CT, a hormonal IUD is seen as a radiopaque T-shaped device. An intratubal device such as the Essure (Bayer Healthcare) contains a stainless steel inner coil that appears echogenic on US. If correctly positioned, two curvilinear echogenic structures can be identified on US between the proximal fallopian tube and the border between the myometrium and endometrium. On radiography and CT, Essure devices are identified as radiopaque curvilinear structures (Figure 38-15, *B*). If a patient with an IUD presents with pelvic pain, migration of the IUD should be suspected (Figure 38-16).

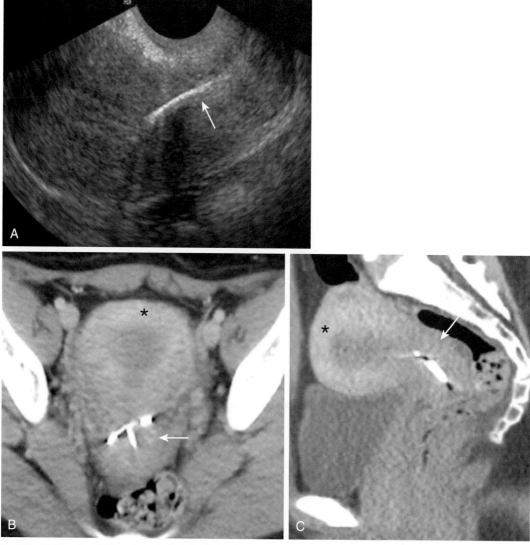

**Figure 38-16.** Migration of IUD on US and CT. **A,** Sagittal US image of uterus shows linear echogenicity (*arrow*) of copper IUD within endocervical canal. **B** and **C,** Axial and sagittal CT images of uterus demonstrate very high attenuation T-shaped copper IUD in endocervical canal (*arrow*) instead of in uterine cavity. Note location of uterine fundus (*).

29. **What is the recommended imaging study in a pregnant patient with right lower quadrant pain?**
    Transabdominal US is the imaging modality of choice for suspected appendicitis in pregnant women. If transabdominal US is negative or equivocal, MRI of the abdomen and pelvis can be obtained for further evaluation. In order to limit fetal exposure to ionizing radiation, US and MRI are preferred over CT.

**KEY POINTS**

- US is the imaging modality of choice for evaluation of the female pelvis. MRI is often utilized when US findings are inconclusive, whereas CT is typically reserved for the emergent setting, and CT and PET are used to evaluate patients with known cancer.
- Septate uterus is the most common type of congenital uterine anomaly.
- Leiomyoma, or fibroid, is the most common neoplasm of the female genitourinary tract and is most often encountered in the uterus.
- Presence of fat within an ovarian mass is diagnostic of a mature teratoma.
- Subtle infiltration or haziness of the pelvic mesenteric fat is one of the earliest findings of PID that may be encountered on CT or MRI.

## BIBLIOGRAPHY

Lee SI, Catalano OA, Dehdashti F. Evaluation of gynecologic cancer with MR imaging, 18F-FDG PET/CT, and PET/MR imaging. *J Nucl Med.* 2015;56(3):436-443.

Yoo RE, Cho JY, Kim SY, et al. A systematic approach to the magnetic resonance imaging-based differential diagnosis of congenital Mullerian duct anomalies and their mimics. *Abdom Imaging.* 2015;40(1):192-206.

Corwin MT, Gerscovich EO, Lamba R, et al. Differentiation of ovarian endometriomas from hemorrhagic cysts at MR imaging: utility of the T2 dark spot sign. *Radiology.* 2014;271(1):126-132.

Kang SK, Giovanniello G, Kim S, et al. Performance of multidetector CT in the evaluation of the endometrium: measurement of endometrial thickness and detection of disease. *Clin Radiol.* 2014;69(11):1123-1128.

Lourenco AP, Swenson D, Tubbs RJ, et al. Ovarian and tubal torsion: imaging findings on US, CT, and MRI. *Emerg Radiol.* 2014;21(2):179-187.

Romosan G, Valentin L. The sensitivity and specificity of transvaginal ultrasound with regard to acute pelvic inflammatory disease: a review of the literature. *Arch Gynecol Obstet.* 2014;289(4):705-714.

Sala E, Rockall AG, Freeman SJ, et al. The added role of MR imaging in treatment stratification of patients with gynecologic malignancies: what the radiologist needs to know. *Radiology.* 2013;266(3):717-740.

Singla P, Long SS, Long CM, et al. Imaging of the female urethral diverticulum. *Clin Radiol.* 2013;68(7):e418-e425.

Surabhi VR, Menias CO, George V, et al. Magnetic resonance imaging of female urethral and periurethral disorders. *Radiol Clin North Am.* 2013;51(6):941-953.

Behr SC, Courtier JL, Qayyum A. Imaging of mullerian duct anomalies. *Radiographics.* 2012;32(6):E233-E250.

Duigenan S, Oliva E, Lee SI. Ovarian torsion: diagnostic features on CT and MRI with pathologic correlation. *AJR Am J Roentgenol.* 2012;198(2):W122-W131.

Graupera B, Hereter L, Pascual MA, et al. Normal and abnormal images of intrauterine devices: role of three-dimensional sonography. *J Clin Ultrasound.* 2012;40(7):433-438.

Lee TT, Rausch ME. Polycystic ovarian syndrome: role of imaging in diagnosis. *Radiographics.* 2012;32(6):1643-1657.

Reiner JS, Brindle KA, Khati NJ. Multimodality imaging of intrauterine devices with an emphasis on the emerging role of 3-dimensional ultrasound. *Ultrasound Q.* 2012;28(4):251-260.

Bell DJ, Pannu HK. Radiological assessment of gynecologic malignancies. *Obstet Gynecol Clin North Am.* 2011;38(1):45-68, vii.

Coutinho A Jr, Bittencourt LK, Pires CE, et al. MR imaging in deep pelvic endometriosis: a pictorial essay. *Radiographics.* 2011;31(2):549-567.

Jung SI, Kim YJ, Park HS, et al. Acute pelvic inflammatory disease: diagnostic performance of CT. *J Obstet Gynaecol Res.* 2011;37(3):228-235.

Takeuchi M, Matsuzaki K. Adenomyosis: usual and unusual imaging manifestations, pitfalls, and problem-solving MR imaging techniques. *Radiographics.* 2011;31(1):99-115.

Chaudhari VV, Patel MK, Douek M, et al. MR imaging and US of female urethral and periurethral disease. *Radiographics.* 2010;30(7):1857-1874.

Iyer VR, Lee SI. MRI, CT, and PET/CT for ovarian cancer detection and adnexal lesion characterization. *AJR Am J Roentgenol.* 2010;194(2):311-321.

Levine D, Brown DL, Andreotti RF, et al. Management of asymptomatic ovarian and other adnexal cysts imaged at US: Society of Radiologists in Ultrasound Consensus Conference Statement. *Radiology.* 2010;256(3):943-954.

Saba L, Guerriero S, Sulcis R, et al. Mature and immature ovarian teratomas: CT, US and MR imaging characteristics. *Eur J Radiol.* 2009;72(3):454-463.

Chang HC, Bhatt S, Dogra VS. Pearls and pitfalls in diagnosis of ovarian torsion. *Radiographics.* 2008;28(5):1355-1368.

Chou CP, Levenson RB, Elsayes KM, et al. Imaging of female urethral diverticulum: an update. *Radiographics.* 2008;28(7):1917-1930.

Chiou SY, Lev-Toaff AS, Masuda E, et al. Adnexal torsion: new clinical and imaging observations by sonography, computed tomography, and magnetic resonance imaging. *J Ultrasound Med.* 2007;26(10):1289-1301.

Del Frate C, Girometti R, Pittino M, et al. Deep retroperitoneal pelvic endometriosis: MR imaging appearance with laparoscopic correlation. *Radiographics.* 2006;26(6):1705-1718.

Kanso HN, Hachem K, Aoun NJ, et al. Variable MR findings in ovarian functional hemorrhagic cysts. *J Magn Reson Imaging.* 2006;24(2):356-361.

Whitten CR, DeSouza NM. Magnetic resonance imaging of uterine malignancies. *Top Magn Reson Imaging.* 2006;17(6):365-377.

Tamai K, Togashi K, Ito T, et al. MR imaging findings of adenomyosis: correlation with histopathologic features and diagnostic pitfalls. *Radiographics.* 2005;25(1):21-40.

Sam JW, Jacobs JE, Birnbaum BA. Spectrum of CT findings in acute pyogenic pelvic inflammatory disease. *Radiographics.* 2002;22(6):1327-1334.

Nalaboff KM, Pellerito JS, Ben-Levi E. Imaging the endometrium: disease and normal variants. *Radiographics.* 2001;21(6):1409-1424.

Outwater EK, Siegelman ES, Hunt JL. Ovarian teratomas: tumor types and imaging characteristics. *Radiographics.* 2001;21(2):475-490.

Woodward PJ, Sohaey R, Mezzetti TP Jr. Endometriosis: radiologic-pathologic correlation. *Radiographics.* 2001;21(1):193-216, questionnaire 88-94.

Patel MD, Feldstein VA, Chen DC, et al. Endometriomas: diagnostic performance of US. *Radiology.* 1999;210(3):739-745.

Reinhold C, Tafazoli F, Mehio A, et al. Uterine adenomyosis: endovaginal US and MR imaging features with histopathologic correlation. *Radiographics.* 1999;19(Spec No):S147-S160.

Ferrazzi E, Torri V, Trio D, et al. Sonographic endometrial thickness: a useful test to predict atrophy in patients with postmenopausal bleeding. An Italian multicenter study. *Ultrasound Obstet Gynecol.* 1996;7(5):315-321.

Hall AF, Theofrastous JP, Cundiff GW, et al. Interobserver and intraobserver reliability of the proposed International Continence Society, Society of Gynecologic Surgeons, and American Urogynecologic Society pelvic organ prolapse classification system. *Am J Obstet Gynecol.* 1996;175(6):1467-1470, discussion 70-71.

Merz E, Miric-Tesanic D, Bahlmann F, et al. Sonographic size of uterus and ovaries in pre- and postmenopausal women. *Ultrasound Obstet Gynecol.* 1996;7(1):38-42.

Granberg S, Wikland M, Karlsson B, et al. Endometrial thickness as measured by endovaginal ultrasonography for identifying endometrial abnormality. *Am J Obstet Gynecol.* 1991;164(1 Pt 1):47-52.

# CHAPTER 39

# IMAGING OF THE MALE PELVIS

*Drew A. Torigian, MD, MA, FSAR, and Parvati Ramchandani, MD, FACR, FSAR*

## PROSTATE GLAND AND SEMINAL TRACT

1. What is the normal anatomy and imaging appearance of the prostate gland and seminal tract on ultrasonography (US), computed tomography (CT), and magnetic resonance imaging (MRI)?

   The prostate gland is an extraperitoneal fibromuscular gland surrounding the prostatic urethra at the bladder base. It is separated into a peripheral zone posteriorly, and a central zone and transitional zone more anteriorly. These zones constitute 70%, 25%, and 5% of the prostate gland, respectively. The transitional zone surrounds the proximal prostatic urethra, whereas the central zone surrounds the transitional zone and ejaculatory ducts. The prostate gland is also divided craniocaudally into the prostate base (superiorly), mid gland, and apex (inferiorly). The anterior fibromuscular stroma is a thick layer of nonglandular tissue that forms the anterior surface of the prostate gland, and the paired neurovascular bundles, responsible for erectile function, are located within the periprostatic fat posterolateral to the prostate gland at the 5 o'clock and 7 o'clock positions.

   The central and transitional zones are not well demarcated on cross-sectional imaging and are collectively referred to as the central gland. On US, the peripheral zone is homogeneous and hyperechoic, whereas the central gland is more heterogeneous and hypoechoic, a differentiation that becomes more marked as the prostate ages and undergoes changes of benign prostatic hyperplasia (BPH). On CT, the peripheral zone is homogeneous and hypoattenuating relative to the more heterogeneously enhancing central gland. However, CT is not generally used for primary evaluation of the prostate gland and seminal tract, given its suboptimal soft contrast resolution. On T1-weighted MR images, the peripheral zone and central gland have low-intermediate signal intensity relative to skeletal muscle and are not well demarcated. On T2-weighted MR images, the peripheral zone has predominantly high signal intensity with thin linear low signal intensity fibrous septa, whereas the central gland has low-intermediate signal intensity relative to skeletal muscle. The anterior fibromuscular stroma has low T1-weighted and T2-weighted signal intensity (Figure 39-1).

   The seminal vesicles are extraperitoneal paired accessory sex glands that are located superior and posterior to the prostate gland. They are essentially long tubes that are convoluted to become approximately 3 cm in length and 1.5 cm in width. The seminal vesicles narrow inferomedially to form the seminal vesicle ducts. On US, the seminal vesicles appear as elongated hypoechoic septated cystic structures. On CT, they are seen as fluid-containing structures with a bow tie configuration. On T1-weighted MR images, the seminal vesicles have intermediate signal intensity. On T2-weighted images, the multiple tubular convolutions are well seen and contain very high signal intensity fluid surrounded by low signal intensity walls (see Figure 39-1).

   The paired vasa deferentia are continuations of the epididymal tails, which ascend from the scrotum within the spermatic cords and into the pelvis via the deep inguinal rings, course posteriorly along the lateral pelvic walls, cross over the ureters, and then curve along the superomedial aspect of the seminal vesicles, where they become more dilated with thicker walls to form the ampullary portions. These then join with the paired seminal vesicle ducts to form the ejaculatory ducts, which are 1 to 2 mm in width, and extend inferiorly through the central zone of the prostate gland to drain into the prostatic urethra on both sides of the verumontanum.

   The paired Cowper (bulbourethral) glands are pea-sized structures that are located within the urogenital diaphragm on either side of the membranous urethra. They each have a single duct that extends through the corpus spongiosum to drain into the bulbar urethra. Given their small size, they are not well visualized on cross-sectional imaging studies.

2. What are the clinical indications for cross-sectional imaging of the prostate gland and seminal tract?

   The most common clinical indication is staging of known prostate cancer diagnosed by previous biopsy, where prostate MRI is used most frequently for this purpose. Other indications include evaluation of patients who have hematospermia or male infertility.

   Transrectal ultrasonography (TRUS) and MRI are most often utilized for evaluation of the prostate gland and seminal tract. CT is not very useful for this purpose given its inferior soft tissue contrast resolution compared to TRUS and MRI.

3. What is the normal size of the prostate gland?

   Prostate gland volume is estimated by multiplying the anteroposterior, transverse, and craniocaudal prostate gland dimensions and 0.52 (an approximation for $\pi/6$). Prostate gland volume normally increases with increasing age, and the prostate gland is generally considered to be enlarged when its volume is >40 ml.

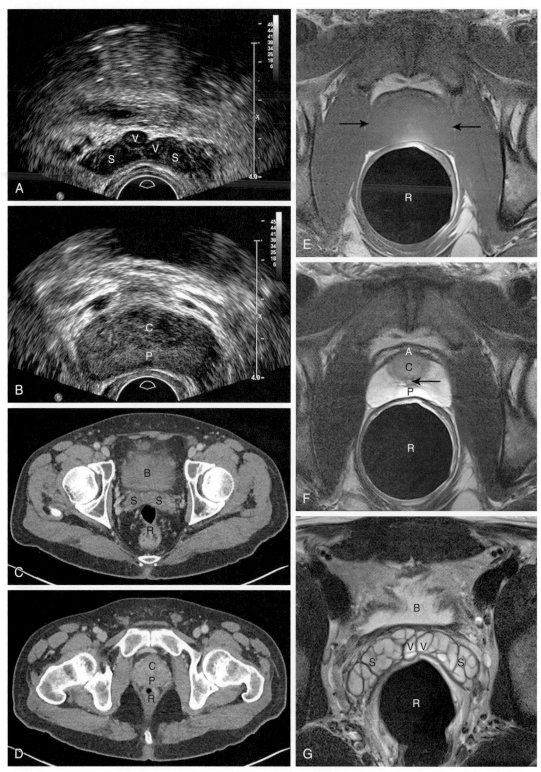

**Figure 39-1.** Normal prostate gland and seminal tract on US, CT, and MRI. **A and B,** Transverse TRUS images through pelvis show seminal vesicles (*S*), ampullary portions of vasa deferentia (*V*), and peripheral zone (*P*) and central gland (*C*) of prostate gland. **C and D,** Axial contrast-enhanced CT images through pelvis demonstrate seminal vesicles (*S*) along with peripheral zone (*P*) and central gland (*C*) of prostate gland and their relationships to urinary bladder (*B*) and rectum (*R*). **E,** Axial T1-weighted MR image through pelvis reveals prostate gland (*between arrows*) anterior to rectum (*R*). Note that peripheral zone and central gland are not well demarcated. **F and G,** Axial T2-weighted MR images through pelvis show high signal intensity peripheral zone (*P*), low-intermediate signal intensity central gland (*C*), and low signal intensity anterior fibromuscular stroma (*A*) of prostate gland, prostatic urethra (*arrow*) within posterior aspect of central gland, seminal vesicles (*S*), and ampullary portions of vasa deferentia (*V*) and their relationships to urinary bladder (*B*) and rectum (*R*).

4. **What is hematospermia, and what are its major causes?**

Hematospermia is the presence of blood in the seminal fluid. The majority of cases of transient hematospermia in men <40 years of age are benign and self-limited and are not due to significant underlying disease processes. These patients are treated with conservative management. In men ≥40 years of age, or in those with other associated symptoms or signs of disease such as persistent hematospermia, TRUS or MRI can be used to evaluate for underlying pathologies including prostate cancer.

Major causes of hematospermia include:
- Idiopathic (the most common cause).
- Prior biopsy.
- Cysts, calculi, or calcification in the prostate gland or ejaculatory tract.
- Calculi or calcification.
- Benign prostatic hyperplasia (BPH).
- Inflammation or infection.
- Prostate cancer.

5. **What does hemorrhage in the prostate gland and seminal tract typically look like on MRI?**

Hemorrhage in the prostate gland and seminal tract typically has high T1-weighted signal intensity, along with variably low T2-weighted signal intensity on MRI (Figure 39-2). Such hemorrhage is very commonly seen on staging MRI following prostatic biopsy.

6. **What is the significance of calcification of the vas deferens?**

Calcification of the vas deferens usually indicates the presence of diabetes mellitus and tends to be bilateral, symmetric, and in the walls of the vasa deferentia.

Chronic inflammation or prior infection may also lead to dystrophic calcification in the vas deferens; in these situations, the calcification is more often unilateral, segmental, and intraluminal in location.

7. **What kinds of cysts occur in the prostate gland and seminal tract?**
- Utricular cysts are congenital and endodermal in origin and arise from the utricle. These are seen within the midline of the prostate gland, do not extend above the superior aspect of the prostate gland, and may communicate with the posterior urethra or ejaculatory duct.
- Müllerian duct cysts are congenital and mesodermal in origin and arise from the caudal ends of the fused müllerian ducts. These are seen within the midline of the prostate gland, often have a teardrop shape, and may extend above the superior aspect of the prostate gland but do not communicate with the urethra or ejaculatory duct.
- Ejaculatory duct cysts are usually acquired secondary to partial obstruction of the ejaculatory duct and are seen in a paramedian location along the course of the ejaculatory duct.
- Seminal vesicle cysts are typically located laterally in one or both seminal vesicles. They are associated with ipsilateral genitourinary anomalies such as renal agenesis, congenital absence of the vas deferens, and ectopic ureteral insertion into mesonephric duct derivatives such as the seminal vesicle or ejaculatory duct. Seminal vesicle cysts may also occur in patients with autosomal dominant polycystic kidney disease (ADPKD).

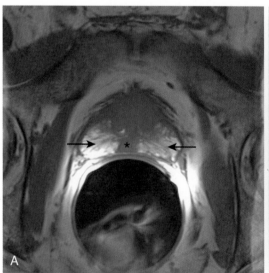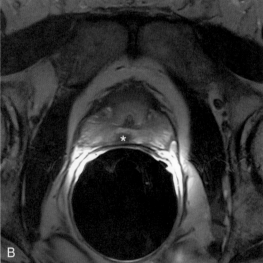

**Figure 39-2.** Hemorrhage and prostate adenocarcinoma on MRI. **A,** Axial T1-weighted MR image through pelvis demonstrates high signal intensity hemorrhage in peripheral zone (*arrows*) along with low-intermediate signal intensity tumor (*) in peripheral zone. **B,** Axial T2-weighted MR image through pelvis reveals tumor (*) has low signal intensity (*) relative to peripheral zone. Note lack of extracapsular spread of tumor from prostate gland.

- Cowper's gland cysts are usually encountered in children and rarely in adults. These are typically located posterior or posterolateral to the bulbomembranous portion of the posterior urethra within the urogenital diaphragm.
- Retention cysts are usually secondary to obstruction of glandular components in the prostate gland and may occur anywhere in the prostate gland, usually off midline.
- Although cysts in the prostate gland and seminal tract are often asymptomatic, they may sometimes cause irritative or obstructive lower urinary tract symptoms secondary to compression/obstruction of the prostatic urethra or ducts and may result in hematospermia. Cysts may also get infected, and calculi or calcifications may form in the cysts.

8. What is prostatitis, and what are its cross-sectional imaging features?

Prostatitis is inflammation or infection of the prostate gland. It is one of the most common urologic diseases in the United States and may be acute or chronic in clinical presentation. In men <35 years old, acute bacterial prostatitis (most often by Gram negative organisms) is most common, whereas in older men, nonbacterial prostatitis is most common.

On TRUS, focal, multifocal, or diffuse areas of decreased echogenicity may be seen. On MRI, both T1-weighted and T2-weighted images demonstrate low signal intensity foci in the peripheral zone, usually without associated contour deformity. There may be associated findings in acute prostatitis such as enlargement of the prostate gland, increased enhancement on CT and MRI, increased blood flow on Doppler US, and periprostatic inflammatory changes.

Granulomatous infections such as tuberculosis may lead to seminal vesiculitis, which manifests on imaging as wall thickening, loss of convolutions, or atrophy of the seminal vesicles. Calcifications may be seen in the prostate gland, vasa deferentia, and seminal vesicles in patients with granulomatous infection.

9. Which patients are at risk for developing a prostatic abscess, and what are its cross-sectional imaging features?

Prostatic abscesses are encountered in up to 2.5% of patients who are hospitalized for prostatitis and are secondary to Gram negative organisms in 90% to 95% of cases, most often *Escherichia coli*. Risk factors include diabetes mellitus, chronic dialysis, immunosuppression, chronic urinary catheterization, and recent urethral manipulation. Treatment is typically with antimicrobial drugs and percutaneous or transurethral drainage.

On cross-sectional imaging, a prostatic abscess appears as a heterogeneous multiloculated complex cystic lesion with complex fluid, internal septations, thick rim enhancement on CT and MRI, and peripherally increased blood flow on Doppler US. Ill-defined focal enlargement of the prostate gland may be seen prior to liquefaction into an abscess. The presence of internal gas is highly specific for this diagnosis. Additional findings of coexistent acute prostatitis and seminal vesiculitis may also be seen (Figure 39-3).

10. What is benign prostatic hyperplasia (BPH), and what are its cross-sectional imaging features?

BPH is an aging phenomenon in the prostate gland, seen in up to 90% of men of advanced age. It is caused by enlargement of the transitional zone.

On cross-sectional imaging, heterogeneous nodular enlargement of the central gland is seen, leading to overall enlargement of the prostate gland. The enlarged central gland is hypoechoic on US and has increased attenuation and enhancement on CT. On T2-weighted MR images, glandular and cystic foci of BPH have high signal intensity, whereas stromal-dominant foci of BPH have low signal intensity. There may be associated compression of the peripheral zone, extension into the peripheral zone, mass effect upon the bladder base, or findings of chronic bladder outlet obstruction such as bladder wall thickening, trabeculation, or diverticulum formation (Figure 39-4).

11. What is the major differential diagnosis for a focal prostatic lesion?

For the answer, see Box 39-1.

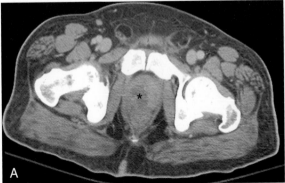
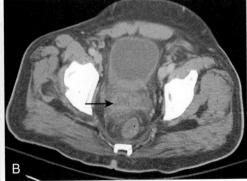

**Figure 39-3.** Prostatic abscess and seminal vesiculitis on CT. **A,** Axial contrast-enhanced CT image through pelvis shows ovoid cystic lesion (*) in prostate gland with rim enhancement. **B,** Axial contrast-enhanced CT image more superiorly through pelvis demonstrates dilation of right seminal vesicle (*arrow*) along with thickening of its walls and surrounding inflammatory infiltration.

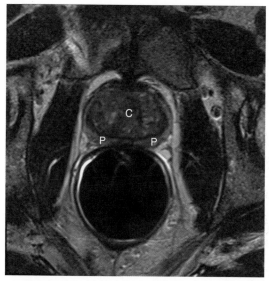

**Figure 39-4.** BPH on MRI. Axial T2-weighted MR image through pelvis reveals moderate nodular enlargement and heterogeneous signal intensity of central gland (*C*) with associated compression of peripheral zone (*P*).

---

**Box 39-1.** Major Differential Diagnosis for Focal Prostatic Lesions

- Cyst (congenital or acquired)
- Hematoma
- Abscess
- Focal prostatitis
- BPH nodule

- Carcinoma
- Sarcoma
- Lymphoma
- Metastasis

---

12. **What is prostate cancer?**

Prostate cancer is the most common noncutaneous cancer in men (with a 1 in 6 lifetime risk) and the second most deadly cancer in men (with lung cancer being the deadliest). It most often occurs in older men and is rare before age 40. The tumor biology is quite variable and is often difficult to predict in advance. In many men, the disease behavior is indolent, whereas in others, it is aggressive and sometimes lethal.

Ninety-five percent of prostate cancers are due to adenocarcinomas, 3% are urothelial (transitional cell) carcinomas, and 2% are related to other tumor types such as neuroendocrine tumor, sarcoma, lymphoma, and metastasis.

Treatment may involve radical prostatectomy (involving resection of the prostate gland and seminal vesicles), radiation therapy, androgen deprivation therapy, focal ablative therapy, or active surveillance (involving close monitoring of the disease course in patients with very low risk disease).

13. **What is the Gleason score?**

The Gleason score is the histologic grading system of choice for prostate cancer, which is important for determining patient prognosis. A Gleason score of ≤6 corresponds to a well-differentiated tumor, which portends a good prognosis; a Gleason score of 7 corresponds to a moderately differentiated tumor, which is associated with an intermediate prognosis; and a Gleason score of 8 to 10 corresponds to a poorly differentiated or undifferentiated tumor, which is associated with a worse prognosis.

14. **What is the role of cross-sectional imaging in the evaluation of patients with prostate adenocarcinoma?**

TRUS is most often used for biopsy guidance, usually in the setting of an abnormal digital rectal exam (DRE) or elevated serum prostate specific antigen (PSA) levels. MRI is also used for biopsy guidance but is most commonly used for disease staging and pretreatment planning (particularly in patients with an intermediate-high risk of extracapsular spread of disease), active surveillance, and detection of tumor recurrence following therapeutic intervention. CT is most often utilized for assessment of regional lymphadenopathy (N stage) and distant metastatic disease (M stage) during staging assessment as well as for response assessment following therapeutic intervention.

15. **What are the cross-sectional imaging features of prostate adenocarcinoma?**

Prostate adenocarcinoma arises most commonly from the peripheral zone (70%) and less commonly from the transitional zone (20%) and central zone (10%). It appears as a focal mass in the prostate gland. On US, it is

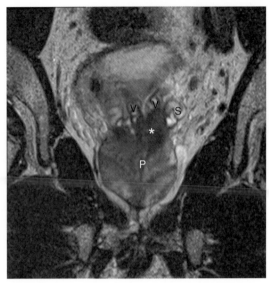

**Figure 39-5.** Extracapsular spread of prostate adenocarcinoma on MRI. Coronal T2-weighted MR image through pelvis shows low signal intensity mass (*) in left base of prostate gland (*P*) which invades left seminal vesicle (*S*) and vasa deferentia (*V*).

hypoechoic or, less often, isoechoic relative to surrounding prostate gland tissue and sometimes has increased blood flow on Doppler US. On CT, it is usually not well visualized but may sometimes be seen as a focal soft tissue attenuation enhancing mass, particularly when large in size or extending into surrounding structures. On MRI, it typically has low-intermediate T1-weighted and low T2-weighted signal intensity relative to normal peripheral zone (see Figure 39-2), restricts diffusion on diffusion-weighted images, and enhances early with subsequent rapid washout.

16. What are the cross-sectional imaging features that suggest extracapsular spread of prostate adenocarcinoma?

A focal irregular prostatic capsular bulge, obliteration of a rectoprostatic angle, soft tissue within the periprostatic fat contiguous with the prostate gland, asymmetry of the neurovascular bundles, and direct tumor invasion of adjacent organs (e.g., seminal vesicles, bladder, rectum) indicate local extracapsular spread of tumor (Figure 39-5). Presence of regional lymphadenopathy (to internal iliac, external iliac, obturator, or sacral lymph nodes), sclerotic osseous metastases (which are high in attenuation on CT and low in signal intensity on MRI), or uncommonly distant metastases to other sites (most often nonregional lymph nodes, lungs, and liver) are also indicators of extraprostatic spread of tumor.

17. Summarize the American Joint Committee on Cancer (AJCC) tumor node metastasis (TNM) staging system for prostate adenocarcinoma.

For the answer, see Box 39-2.

The management of prostate cancer is in rapid evolution. Any T3 lesion (i.e., primary tumor extending beyond the prostate capsule) indicates at least stage III prostate cancer, and any T4 lesion (i.e., primary tumor invading adjacent structures other than the seminal vesicles), N1 lesion (i.e., presence of regional nodal metastasis), or M1 lesion (i.e., presence of distant metastasis) indicates stage IV prostate cancer. Currently, stage I and II prostate adenocarcinomas are usually treated with local therapy such as radical prostatectomy or radiation therapy, whereas stage III and IV prostate adenocarcinomas are usually treated with nonsurgical multimodal therapy including systemic and radiation therapies.

## TESTICLES, EPIDIDYMIDES, AND SCROTUM

18. What is the normal anatomy and imaging appearance of the testicles on US, CT, and MRI?

The testicles are composed of densely packed seminiferous tubules that each converge posteriorly into large ducts and drain into the rete testis at the testicular hilum (also known as the mediastinum testis). Testicles are normally 2 to 3 cm wide and 3 to 5 cm long. In the rete testis, 15 to 20 efferent ductules converge to form the epididymal head superiorly and then converge into a single convoluted tubule in the epididymal body and tail inferiorly. The tubules emerge at an acute angle from the epididymal tail to form the vas deferens.

On US, the testicles have a homogeneous echotexture, are surrounded by a thin curvilinear echogenic tunica albuginea, and have symmetric blood flow on Doppler US. A linear band of echogenicity, representing the mediastinum testis, and an anechoic or hypoechoic focus containing small cystic or tubular structures, representing the rete testis, may be seen posteriorly at the testicular hilum. On CT, they have homogeneous soft tissue attenuation and enhancement, although CT is not used for primary evaluation of testicular disorders given the exposure to ionizing

## Box 39-2. AJCC TNM Staging System of Prostate Adenocarcinoma

### T = Primary Tumor

**Clinical**

TX  Primary Tumor cannot be assessed

T0  No evidence of primary tumor

T1  Clinically inapparent tumor neither palpable nor visible by imaging

    T1a  Tumor incidental histologic finding in 5% or less of tissue resected

    T1b  Tumor incidental histologic finding in more than 5% of tissue resected

    T1c  Tumor identified by needle biopsy (for example, because of elevated PSA)

T2  Tumor confined within prostate[1]

    T2a  Tumor involves one-half of one lobe or less

    T2b  Tumor involves more than one-half of one lobe but not both lobes

    T2c  Tumor involves both lobes

T3  Tumor extends through prostate capsule[2]

    T3a  Extracapsular extension (unilateral or bilateral)

    T3b  Tumor invades seminal vesicle(s)

T4  Tumor is fixed or invades adjacent structures other than seminal vesicles such as external sphincter, rectum, bladder, levator muscles, and/or pelvic wall

**Pathologic (pT)[3]**

pT2  Organ confined

    pT2a  Unilateral, one-half of one side or less

    pT2b  Unilateral, involving more than one-half of side but not both sides

    pT2c  Bilateral disease

pT3  Extraprostatic extension

    pT3a  Extraprostatic extension or microscopic invasion of bladder neck[4]

    pT3b  Seminal vesicle invasion

pT4  Invasion of rectum, levator muscles, and/or pelvic wall

### N = Regional Lymph Nodes

**Clinical**

NX  Regional lymph nodes were not assessed

N0  No regional lymph node metastasis

N1  Metastasis in regional lymph node(s)

**Pathologic**

pNX  Regional nodes not sampled

pN0  No positive regional nodes

pN1  Metastases in regional node(s)

### M = Distant Metastasis[5]

M0  No distant metastasis

M1  Distant metastasis

    M1a  Non-regional lymph node(s)

    M1b  Bone(s)

    M1c  Other site(s) with or without bone disease

### Anatomic Stage/Prognostic Groups[6]

| Group | T | N | M | PSA | Gleason |
|---|---|---|---|---|---|
| I | T1a–c | N0 | M0 | PSA <10 | Gleason ≤6 |
| | T2a | N0 | M0 | PSA <10 | Gleason ≤6 |
| | T1–2a | N0 | M0 | PSA X | Gleason X |
| IIA | T1a–c | N0 | M0 | PSA <20 | Gleason 7 |
| | T1a–c | N0 | M0 | PSA ≥10<20 | Gleason ≤6 |
| | T2a | N0 | M0 | PSA ≥10<20 | Gleason ≤6 |
| | T2a | N0 | M0 | PSA <20 | Gleason 7 |
| | T2b | N0 | M0 | PSA <20 | Gleason ≤7 |
| | T2b | N0 | M0 | PSA X | Gleason X |
| IIB | T2c | N0 | M0 | Any PSA | Any Gleason |
| | T1–2 | N0 | M0 | PSA ≥20 | Any Gleason |
| | T1–2 | N0 | M0 | Any PSA | Gleason ≥8 |
| III | T3a–b | N0 | M0 | Any PSA | Any Gleason |
| IV | T4 | N0 | M0 | Any PSA | Any Gleason |
| | Any T | N1 | M0 | Any PSA | Any Gleason |
| | Any T | Any N | M1 | Any PSA | Any Gleason |

[1]Tumor found in one or both lobes by needle biopsy, but not palpable or reliably visible by imaging, is classified as T1c.

[2] Invasion into the prostatic apex or into (but not beyond) the prostatic capsule is classified not as T3 but as T2.

[3] There is no pathologic T1 classification.

[4] Positive surgical margin should be indicated by an R1 descriptor (residual microscopic disease).

[5] When more than one site of metastasis is present, the most advanced category is used. pM1c is most advanced.

[6] When either PSA or Gleason is not available, grouping should be determined by T stage and/or either PSA or Gleason as available.

*(From Edge SB, Byrd DR, Compton CC, et al. AJCC Cancer Staging Manual. New York: Springer; 2010.)*

radiation and suboptimal soft tissue contrast resolution. On MRI, the testicles have homogeneous intermediate T1-weighted signal intensity and high T2-weighted signal intensity relative to skeletal muscle, are surrounded by a smooth thin curvilinear low signal intensity tunica albuginea, and homogeneously enhance. Thin low signal intensity septa radiating toward the mediastinum testis are often seen within the testicles on T2-weighted images. The mediastinum testis appears as a linear band of low signal intensity at the posteriorly located testicular hilum, whereas the rete testis has high T2-weighted signal intensity due to fluid within the seminiferous tubules (Figure 39-6).

The epididymides are posterolateral to the testicles. On US, they are isoechoic/slightly hyperechoic relative to the testicles and have symmetric blood flow on Doppler US. On CT, they have soft tissue attenuation. On MRI, the epididymides have low-intermediate T1-weighted and low T2-weighted signal intensity relative to the testicles (see Figure 39-6).

The testicular arteries arise from the abdominal aorta near the level of the renal vessels and extend to the scrotum to supply the testicles. The right gonadal vein drains into the inferior vena cava, whereas the left gonadal vein drains into the left renal vein. Normal scrotal skin thickness varies between 2 to 8 mm.

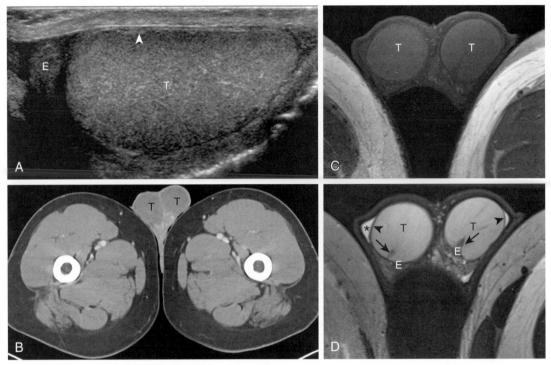

**Figure 39-6.** Normal testicles and epididymides on US, CT, and MRI. **A,** Longitudinal US image through scrotum demonstrates homogeneous echotexture of testicle (*T*) and epididymal head (*E*) along with thin echogenic tunica albuginea (*arrowhead*). **B,** Axial contrast-enhanced CT image through scrotum reveals homogeneous soft tissue attenuation of testicles (*T*). **C,** Axial T1-weighted MR image through scrotum shows homogeneous intermediate signal intensity of testicles (*T*). **D,** Axial T2-weighted MR image through scrotum demonstrates high signal intensity of testicles (*T*) along with low signal intensity linear septa that radiate toward mediastinum testis (*arrows*), low signal intensity epididymides (*E*), thin low signal intensity tunica albuginea (*arrowheads*), and physiologic fluid (*) between visceral and parietal layers of tunica vaginalis.

19. What is cryptorchidism, and what are its cross-sectional imaging features?
    Cryptorchidism occurs when there is incomplete descent of one or both testicles into the scrotum and is seen in 3% of neonates and in 1% of infants (since many testicles descend by age one) and adults. The ectopic testicle is most commonly found in or below the inguinal canal but may less commonly be found elsewhere in the abdomen or pelvis.
    MRI is superior to US for localization of a cryptorchid testicle, especially when located in the abdomen. On US, the cryptorchid testicle is usually small and hypoechoic relative to the normal testicle and has an echogenic mediastinum. On MRI, the cryptorchid testicle is usually small relative to the normal testicle and has increased T2-weighted signal intensity relative to skeletal muscle, similar to the normal testicle.

20. What are the potential complications of cryptorchidism?
    - Development of testicular malignancy (most often seminoma).
    - Infertility.
    - Spermatic cord torsion.
      As such, treatment with orchidopexy or orchidectomy is typically performed.

21. What is the most important question to clarify when imaging a palpable scrotal abnormality?
    Is the mass located in the testicle? The reason is that most intratesticular masses are malignant, whereas most extratesticular scrotal masses are benign.

22. What is the most common cause of a scrotal mass?
    A spermatocele or an epididymal cyst is the most common cause of a scrotal mass. Spermatoceles contain spermatozoa, whereas epididymal cysts do not. However, these are indistinguishable on imaging. On US, a well-circumscribed anechoic cystic lesion with posterior acoustic enhancement is seen in the epididymis, without blood flow on Doppler US. On CT and MRI, a nonenhancing well-circumscribed cystic lesion is seen in the epididymis. Internal septations or complex fluid may sometimes be present (Figure 39-7).
    Tubular ectasia of the rete testis is associated with spermatoceles and epididymal cysts, as well as with advancing age and a history of prior vasectomy. It is secondary to partial or complete obliteration of the efferent ductules. On cross-sectional imaging, multiple tubular cystic structures are seen in the region of the mediastinum

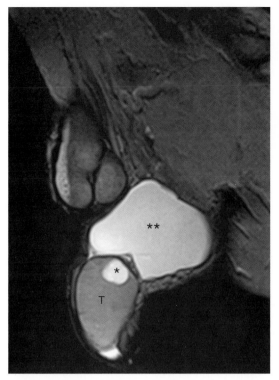

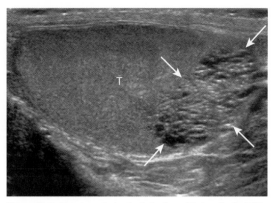

**Figure 39-8.** Tubular ectasia of rete testis on US. Longitudinal US image through testicle shows multiple tubular anechoic cystic structures (*between arrows*) within testicle (*T*) adjacent to mediastinum testis.

**Figure 39-7.** Epididymal cyst and testicular cyst on MRI. Sagittal T2-weighted MR image through scrotum reveals well-circumscribed unilocular very high signal intensity lesion (*) in testicle (*T*) along with similar-appearing lesion (**) superior to testicle within epididymal head.

---

**Box 39-3.** Major Differential Diagnosis for Focal Testicular Lesions

- Tubular ectasia of rete testis
- Cyst
- Epidermal inclusion cyst
- Hematoma
- Abscess
- Infarct
- Fibrosis
- Focal orchitis
- Intratesticular varicocele
- Adrenal rest
- Splenogonadal fusion
- Leydig cell hyperplasia
- Germ cell tumor
- Lymphoma
- Leukemia
- Metastasis

---

testis, often within both testicles, without mass effect. No blood flow is seen on Doppler US, and no enhancement is seen on CT or MRI (Figure 39-8).

Testicular cysts can also occur, which have similar cross-sectional imaging features as those of spermatoceles and epididymal cysts except for having a location within the testicle. They are benign, are more commonly encountered with increasing age, and are typically seen near the mediastinum testis (see Figure 39-7).

23. **What is the major differential diagnosis for a focal testicular lesion?**
   For the answer, see Box 39-3.

24. **What is the major differential diagnosis for multiple intratesticular masses?**
   - Leydig cell hyperplasia.
   - Adrenal rests.
   - Sarcoidosis.
   - Tuberculosis.
   - Lymphoma.
   - Leukemia.
   - Metastases.
   - Bilateral germ cell tumors.

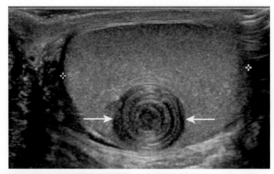

**Figure 39-9.** Testicular epidermoid inclusion cyst on US. Longitudinal US image through testicle demonstrates small well-circumscribed lesion (*arrows*) within testicle containing alternating low and high echogenicity rings with characteristic lamellated "onion-skin" appearance.

25. What is a testicular adrenal rest, and what are its cross-sectional imaging features?

An adrenal rest is a rare benign lesion that is composed of hyperplastic ectopic adrenal gland tissue. It is typically seen in patients with a history of congenital adrenal hyperplasia secondary to elevation of adrenocorticotropic hormone (ACTH) levels. Appropriate corticosteroid replacement therapy can lead to regression of adrenal rests.

On cross-sectional imaging, multiple bilateral oblong-shaped lesions are seen in the testicles, usually in the region of the mediastinum testis. On US, these are usually hypoechoic or sometimes hyperechoic relative to testicular parenchyma, and they have spoke-like vascularity on Doppler US. On MRI, these have intermediate/slightly high T1-weighted and low T2-weighted signal intensity relative to testicular parenchyma, along with mild enhancement.

26. What is splenogonadal fusion, and what are its US imaging features?

Splenogonadal fusion is a rare anomaly where accessory splenic tissue is found in the scrotum, more commonly on the left than right side, which may be fused to the testicle or other surrounding structures. In some cases, a connection with the spleen is maintained via a cord of splenic or fibrous tissue.

On US, a homogeneous hypoechoic testicular lesion is usually seen, which is generally indistinguishable from a testicular neoplasm. A pattern of central blood flow with peripheral branching on Doppler US may suggest this particular diagnosis. A definitive diagnosis may be established through use of a technetium-99m ($^{99m}$Tc) heat-denatured red blood cell (RBC) scan or a $^{99m}$Tc sulfur colloid scan, as the splenic tissue will demonstrate uptake of these radiotracers.

27. What is Leydig cell hyperplasia, and what are its cross-sectional imaging features?

Leydig cell hyperplasia is a rare benign condition that is characterized by the presence of hyperplastic Leydig cells within the testicle. Multiple 1- to 6-mm testicular nodules are characteristically visualized, often involving the testicles bilaterally.

On US, these nodules are usually hypoechoic and may demonstrate increased blood flow on Doppler US. On MRI, they have low T2-weighted signal intensity relative to testicular parenchyma and demonstrate mild enhancement.

28. What is a testicular epidermoid inclusion cyst, and what are its cross-sectional imaging features?

A testicular epidermoid inclusion cyst is a benign lesion of germ cell origin, which consists of desquamated keratinized epithelium and keratin debris (ectodermal elements) surrounded by a fibrous wall. Treatment is with enucleation (rather than with radical orchiectomy for testicular cancer).

On cross-sectional imaging, it appears as a 1- to 3-cm focal well-circumscribed intratesticular lesion without blood flow or enhancement that has alternating low and high echogenicity/T2-weighted signal intensity rings with a characteristic lamellated "onion-skin" appearance. It can also have a "target" appearance with a hyperechoic or low T2-weighted signal intensity center and a hypoechoic or high T2-weighted signal intensity periphery (Figure 39-9).

29. What is testicular microlithiasis, and what is its significance?

Testicular microlithiasis is an asymptomatic abnormality found on testicular US, in which calcifications are seen within the seminiferous tubules of the testicles. Its presence alone in the absence of other risk factors is not worrisome, but follow-up evaluation with US is suggested in patients at risk for development of testicular tumors, such as those with testicular maldescent, prior history of germ cell tumor, atrophic testicles, and Klinefelter syndrome, although this is controversial.

On US, testicular microlithiasis is present when ≥5 punctate echogenic foci are seen in the testicle (Figure 39-10). It is not well visualized on MRI.

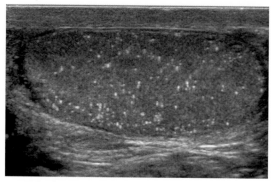

**Figure 39-10.** Testicular microlithiasis on US. Longitudinal US image through testicle reveals multiple ≥5 punctate echogenic foci in testicle.

30. **What is the most common cancer of young men?**
    Testicular cancer is the most common cancer of men between the ages of 15 and 35 years and typically presents clinically as a painless testicular mass. Testicular cancers are often curable, even in patients with metastatic disease at initial presentation, with an overall survival of >90%.

31. **What types of testicular malignancy may occur?**
    95% of testicular cancers are secondary to germ cell tumors.
    - Forty percent to 50% of germ cell tumors are seminomas (the most common pure histologic subtype). These occur in a slightly older age group (average age of 40), are radiosensitive, and are associated with a better prognosis. Serum alpha feto-protein (AFP) levels are not elevated. Treatment generally involves radical orchiectomy, sometimes along with adjuvant radiation therapy or chemotherapy.
    - The remainder of germ cell tumors are nonseminomatous tumors, which include embryonal cell tumor, choriocarcinoma, yolk sac tumor, teratoma, and mixed subtypes. The mixed subtype is the most common histologic subtype of germ cell tumor overall and contains elements of multiple subtypes of germ cell tumor, including nonseminomatous tumors and seminoma. Nonseminomatous tumors occur in a slightly younger age group (average age of 30), are more aggressive in behavior, are less radiosensitive, and are associated with a worse prognosis. Serum AFP levels may be elevated, which is indicative of the presence of a nonseminomatous tumor. Treatment generally involves radical orchiectomy, sometimes with retroperitoneal lymph node dissection or chemotherapy.
    The other 5% of testicular cancers are secondary to non–germ cell tumors, including sex cord stromal tumors (which are benign in 90%), gonadoblastoma, lymphoma, and metastatic disease to the testicle.

32. **Which type of testicular tumor is hormonally active?**
    Leydig cell tumor, the most common subtype of testicular sex cord stromal tumor, is hormonally active in 30% of cases with secretion of androgens or estrogens.

33. **What are some risk factors for testicular cancer?**
    - Intratubular germ cell neoplasia (ITGCN) (where 50% of patients develop invasive tumors in 5 years).
    - Testicular microlithiasis.
    - Cryptorchidism.
    - Klinefelter syndrome.
    - Positive family history of testicular cancer.
    - Contralateral testicular cancer.

34. **What is the role of cross-sectional imaging in patients with testicular cancer?**
    US is most often used for initial detection and diagnosis, whereas MRI is often used as a second-line problem-solving modality. CT and MRI are most often used for staging assessment as well as for response assessment following therapeutic intervention.

35. **What are the cross-sectional imaging features of testicular cancer?**
    On cross-sectional imaging, an intratesticular mass is seen with increased blood flow on Doppler US and enhancement on CT and MRI. Seminoma is typically homogeneous, with hypoechogenicity on US and intermediate T1-weighted and low T2-weighted signal intensity on MRI relative to testicular parenchyma (Figure 39-11). In contradistinction, nonseminomatous germ cell tumor is typically heterogeneous in appearance with variable echogenicity and signal intensity secondary to hemorrhage, cystic change, necrosis, fat, calcification, and/or fibrosis (Figure 39-12). Extratesticular extension and invasion of adjacent structures may sometimes be seen with testicular cancer. Regional

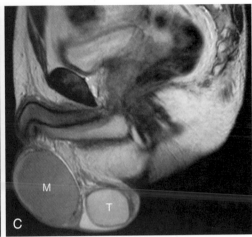

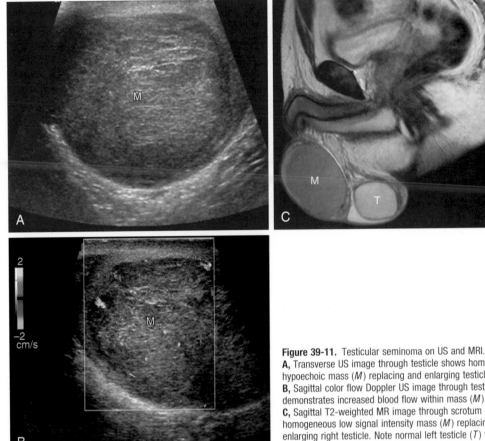

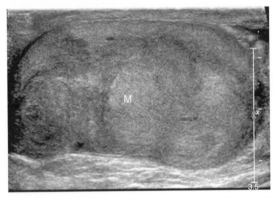

**Figure 39-11.** Testicular seminoma on US and MRI.
**A,** Transverse US image through testicle shows homogeneous hypoechoic mass (*M*) replacing and enlarging testicle.
**B,** Sagittal color flow Doppler US image through testicle demonstrates increased blood flow within mass (*M*).
**C,** Sagittal T2-weighted MR image through scrotum reveals homogeneous low signal intensity mass (*M*) replacing and enlarging right testicle. Note normal left testicle (*T*) for comparison.

**Figure 39-12.** Testicular nonseminomatous germ cell tumor on US. Longitudinal US image through testicle shows heterogeneous mass (*M*) replacement and enlarging testicle. Histopathologic analysis revealed mixed subtype of tumor containing embryonal cell carcinoma and seminoma components.

lymphadenopathy and distant metastatic disease (most often to nonregional lymph nodes, lung, liver, brain, and bone marrow) may also be present.

36. Describe the routes of lymphatic spread of testicular cancer.
   The lymphatic drainage of the testicles follows the gonadal venous drainage, with the left side draining to the pre-aortic or left para-aortic retroperitoneal lymph nodes near the renal hilum and the right side draining to the

aortocaval or pericaval retroperitoneal lymph nodes. As such, testicular cancer tends to first spread via the lymphatics to these regional lymph nodes, skipping the pelvic lymph nodes.

Epididymal lymphatic drainage not only follows the gonadal venous drainage to the retroperitoneum, but also goes to the external iliac nodes. Lymphatic drainage from the scrotal skin is typically to the inguinal nodes. Therefore, pelvic lymphadenopathy may occur when there is tumor invasion of the epididymis or scrotal wall or when there has been prior scrotal or inguinal surgery.

37. Which germ cell tumor has a tendency for early hematogenous metastatic spread?

Choriocarcinoma tends to be associated with early hematogenous metastases, most often to the lungs, brain, and liver, and are often hemorrhagic. As such, it has the worst prognosis of any of the germ cell tumor types.

38. List the stages of testicular cancer.

Stage I: Local disease confined to the scrotum.
Stage II: Regional lymphadenopathy (in the retroperitoneum).
Stage III: Distant metastatic disease.

39. Are there findings that are more suggestive of testicular lymphoma rather than testicular germ cell tumor?

Yes. Testicular lymphoma, which is almost always secondary to B cell non-Hodgkin's lymphoma, usually occurs in men >50 years of age, and it is the most common testicular neoplasm in men >60 years of age.

On cross-sectional imaging, a nonspecific focal or diffuse homogeneous testicular mass is seen with increased blood flow on Doppler US and enhancement on CT and MRI. However, features that are more suggestive of lymphoma include tumor invasion of the epididymis or spermatic cord, indistinct tumor margins, preservation of a normal testicular contour, and bilateral testicular involvement.

40. How often do extratesticular malignancies metastasize to the testicle?

Metastatic disease to the testicle is uncommon, occurring in <1% of patients with extratesticular malignancy, and is generally associated with a poor clinical outcome. The most common primary tumors that spread to the testicle are prostate cancer, lung cancer, melanoma, colorectal cancer, and renal cell carcinoma.

41. What is the most common extratesticular scrotal tumor?

Spermatic cord lipoma is the most common extratesticular scrotal tumor. On US, it is echogenic, and it does not have increased blood flow on Doppler US. On CT and MRI, it has attenuation and signal intensity properties similar to those of fat elsewhere in the body.

The major differential diagnostic consideration for a spermatic cord lipoma is a fat-containing inguinal hernia.

42. What is an adenomatoid tumor, and what are its cross-sectional imaging features?

Adenomatoid tumor is the second most common extratesticular scrotal tumor. It is benign in nature and arises most often from the epididymis and less commonly from the tunica vaginalis or spermatic cord.

On cross-sectional imaging, a small well-circumscribed extratesticular mass is typically seen, which has variable echogenicity, soft tissue attenuation, and low T2-weighted signal intensity relative to testicular parenchyma, with enhancement after contrast administration.

43. What is a varicocele, and what are its cross-sectional imaging features?

A varicocele is an abnormal enlargement of the pampiniform plexus of veins in the scrotum, and it is encountered in ≈15% to 20% of men. Primary varicoceles result from incompetence of the valves in the gonadal vein, leading to retrograde venous blood flow. These are most often encountered on the left side (85%) or bilaterally (15%). Secondary varicoceles occur secondary to extrinsic compression of the gonadal vein, portacaval venous shunting (from portal hypertension), or thrombosis of the gonadal vein, renal vein, or inferior vena cava. A secondary varicocele should be suspected when an isolated right-sided varicocele is encountered.

On cross-sectional imaging, dilated (>2 to 3 mm) serpentine veins are seen, usually located superior and lateral to the testicle. Rarely, intratesticular varicoceles may be encountered. On US, varicoceles are anechoic in appearance and demonstrate increased blood flow and flow reversal during the Valsalva maneuver on Doppler US. On CT and MRI, these demonstrate venous phase enhancement.

44. What are the complications of a varicocele?

Complications of a varicocele include male infertility, pain, and testicular atrophy. Varicocele is the most common and treatable cause of male infertility.

45. What is the significance of asymmetric prominence and enhancement of the spermatic cord vessels?

Asymmetric prominence and enhancement of the spermatic cord vessels is a highly sensitive indicator for the presence of ipsilateral scrotal pathology. When detected, further evaluation of the scrotum with clinical examination and/or additional cross-sectional imaging is warranted.

46. In a patient who presents with an acutely painful scrotum, what is the initial diagnostic imaging test of choice, and what is the major differential diagnosis?

In patients with an acutely painful scrotum, US is the initial diagnostic imaging test of choice. Major differential diagnostic considerations include:
- Acute epididymo-orchitis.
- Spermatic cord torsion.
- Torsion of a testicular appendage.
- Testicular neoplasm.
- Scrotal trauma.
- Inguinal hernia.

47. What is acute epididymo-orchitis, and what are its cross-sectional imaging features?

Acute epididymo-orchitis is inflammation of the epididymis and testicle, and it is most often secondary to bacterial infection. It typically presents clinically with fever and scrotal pain and is treated with antimicrobial drugs. US is the initial diagnostic imaging test of choice.

On cross-sectional imaging, key findings may include increased epididymal or testicular size with increased epididymal and testicular blood flow on Doppler US. The testicles may be heterogeneous in echotexture, signal intensity, or enhancement and may have a striated appearance. There may be scrotal skin thickening, a reactive hydrocele or pyocele, and enlargement and increased enhancement of the ipsilateral spermatic cord vessels (Figure 39-13). Sometimes, the process may be focal, potentially mimicking a testicular neoplasm.

Subsequently, testicular atrophy may occur, along with scarring that manifests as geographic hypoechoic or low T2-weighted signal intensity areas with normal blood flow on Doppler US, sometimes in association with areas of capsular retraction.

48. What is the most common cause of isolated orchitis?

Isolated orchitis is most commonly secondary to mumps virus infection.

49. What is a pyocele, and what are its cross-sectional imaging features?

A pyocele is a collection of pus within the scrotum adjacent to the testicle located between the visceral and parietal layers of the tunica vaginalis. It may occur as a complication of trauma, surgery, or epididymo-orchitis.

On cross-sectional imaging, increased echogenicity, increased attenuation, or variably increased T1-weighted and variably decreased T2-weighted signal intensity of the fluid may be seen. Internal septations, fluid-debris levels, and/or

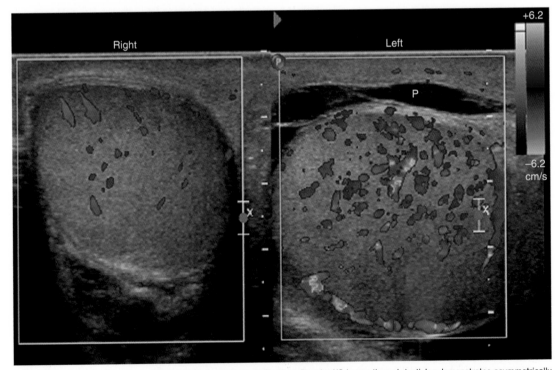

**Figure 39-13.** Left acute epididymo-orchitis on US. Transverse color flow Doppler US image through testicles demonstrates asymmetrically increased blood flow to left testicle. Increased blood flow to left epididymis (*not shown*) was also present. Also note increased fluid surrounding left testicle which contains internal septations representing pyocele (*P*).

foci of gas (with increased echogenicity, dirty posterior acoustic shadowing, and reverberation artifacts on US; very low attenuation on CT; and very low signal intensity on MRI) may also be visualized within the fluid (see Figure 39-13). A thickened wall with increased blood flow on Doppler US and increased enhancement on CT or MRI may also be visualized.

50. What is a hydrocele, and what are its cross-sectional imaging features?

A hydrocele is a collection of fluid within the scrotum adjacent to the testicle located between the visceral and parietal layers of the tunica vaginalis. It is the most common cause of scrotal enlargement.

On cross-sectional imaging, a hydrocele appears as fluid within the scrotum surrounding the testicle that is anechoic and has posterior acoustic enhancement on US, fluid attenuation (0 to 20 HU) on CT, and low T1-weighted and very high T2-weighted signal intensity on MRI.

51. List some causes of a hydrocele.

Ascites (when there is a congenital patent processus vaginalis peritonei), testicular tumor, acute epididymo-orchitis, trauma, surgery, spermatic cord torsion, or idiopathic.

52. What is torsion of a testicular appendage, and what are its US imaging features?

Torsion of a testicular appendage is the leading cause of an acute scrotum in children. The appendix testis (a remnant of the müllerian or paramesonephric duct) and the appendix epididymis (a remnant of the wolffian or mesonephric duct) are testicular appendages that may undergo twisting, leading to ischemia, infarction, and surrounding inflammatory change. Patients with torsion of a testicular appendage are generally treated conservatively.

On US, imaging findings may include: a ≥5-mm spherical paratesticular nodule along the superior aspect of the testicle or epididymal head; normal testicular blood flow and increased periappendiceal blood flow on Doppler US; scrotal wall thickening; and reactive hydrocele.

53. What is spermatic cord torsion, and what are its US imaging features?

Spermatic cord torsion (sometimes given the misnomer of testicular torsion) is a surgical emergency. It is secondary to twisting of the spermatic cord between 90° and 720°, which leads to venous obstruction followed by arterial obstruction, potentially leading to testicular infarction. In most cases, the testicles are viable if treated within 6 hours with detorsion and subsequent orchiopexy.

Intravaginal torsion occurs in 90% of cases and is predisposed by the congenital "bell-clapper" deformity (found in ≈10% of males) where the tunica vaginalis completely surrounds the testicle and epididymis. The testicle and epididymis are then not anchored posteriorly and can freely rotate around their vascular pedicle within the tunica vaginalis. Intravaginal torsion typically occurs in adolescents and young adults, most often during the second decade of life.

Extravaginal torsion, which is much less common, occurs at the level of the inguinal ring and is typically seen in neonates.

Doppler US is the major diagnostic imaging test used for detection and diagnosis of this condition, and it has a sensitivity of ≈90%. On US, the key diagnostic feature is decreased or absent testicular and epididymal blood flow on Doppler US, although blood flow may be preserved with partial, early, or transient torsion, or may even be increased with detorsion and reactive hyperemia. Other imaging findings may include: increased testicular and epididymal size; homogeneous testicular echotexture early on, which is a predictor of testicular viability; increased testicular heterogeneity over time, which is suggestive of necrosis; visualization of a twisted spermatic cord with a "cord knot" or swirling "whirlpool" appearance; and a reactive hydrocele (Figure 39-14).

54. What cross-sectional imaging findings may be encountered in testicular trauma?

Testicular trauma is most often secondary to blunt trauma, usually in the setting of a sports-related injury. Cross-sectional imaging findings of testicular trauma may include testicular contusion, hematoma, laceration/fracture,

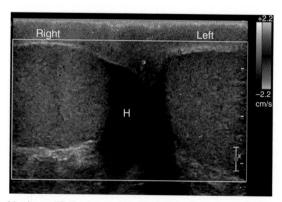

**Figure 39-14.** Right spermatic cord torsion on US. Transverse color flow Doppler US image through testicles reveals asymmetrically absent blood flow to right testicle. Also note increased anechoic fluid surrounding right testicle representing reactive hydrocele (*H*).

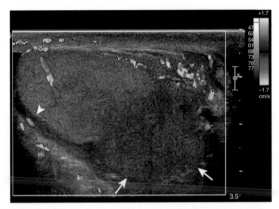

**Figure 39-15.** Testicular rupture on US. Longitudinal color flow Doppler US image through testicle shows bulge along testicular contour (*arrows*) where tunica albuginea is not well visualized. (Note normal echogenic tunica albuginea [*arrowhead*] for comparison.) Also note geographic region of hypoechogenicity in testicle with absent blood flow representing segmental testicular infarction.

rupture, infarction, dislocation, and avulsion. Ancillary imaging findings may include hydrocele, hematocele (hemorrhage within the scrotum adjacent to the testicle located between the visceral and parietal layers of the tunica vaginalis), soft tissue hematoma, scrotal laceration, and post-traumatic epididymitis.

Testicular rupture occurs when there is disruption of the tunica albuginea with associated extrusion of testicular parenchyma. When testicular rupture has occurred, this is considered to be a surgical emergency. US imaging features of testicular rupture include a linear hypoechoic focus in the testicle (representing a laceration/fracture), discontinuity of the tunica albuginea, an ill-defined testicular contour, and a bulge along the testicular contour. Associated findings of testicular hematoma and infarction are also commonly seen (Figure 39-15). If surgery is performed within 3 days of injury, up to 90% of injured testicles can be salvaged.

55. What are the US and MR imaging findings of testicular hematomas?

On US, acute hematomas are isoechoic or hyperechoic relative to testicular parenchyma and may be difficult to detect, whereas subacute hematomas are more heterogeneous and hypoechoic relative to testicular parenchyma. Testicular hematomas do not have increased blood flow on Doppler US.

On MRI, acute hematomas have low signal intensity on T1-weighted and T2-weighted images, whereas subacute hematomas have high T1-weighted signal intensity and variable T2-weighted signal intensity. Testicular hematomas do not enhance with contrast administration.

Hematomas will generally decrease in size over time.

56. What are the US and MR imaging findings of segmental testicular infarction?

On US, segmental testicular infarcts appear as geographic rounded or wedge-shaped hypoechoic areas in the testicle with absent blood flow on Doppler US (see Figure 39-15).

On MRI, they appear as geographic rounded or wedge-shaped areas with intermediate T1-weighted and low T2-weighted signal intensity relative to testicular parenchyma, sometimes with areas of high T1-weighted signal intensity when there is associated hemorrhage. These typically lack enhancement, although some peripheral enhancement may be present.

## PENIS

57. What is the normal anatomy and imaging appearance of the penis on US, CT, and MRI?

The penis is composed of three cylindrical cavernous structures: the paired dorsal corpora cavernosa and the single ventral corpus spongiosum. The crura of the corpora cavernosa are the most proximal portions, which diverge laterally to attach to the ischiopubic rami. The corpus spongiosum extends and enlarges distally to form the glans penis and proximally to form the bulb of the penis, and it contains the anterior portion of the urethra. The tunica albuginea is a thin layer of fibrous tissue that surrounds each of the corpora cavernosa and the corpus spongiosum. The deep (Buck's) fascia is just superficial to the tunica albuginea and surrounds the corpora cavernosa in a dorsal compartment and the corpus spongiosum in a separate ventral compartment.

The cavernosal arteries are terminal branches of the internal pudendal arteries located within the paired corpora cavernosa. They give off the helicine arteries, which provide the primary source of blood for erectile function. The paired dorsal arteries and deep dorsal vein are located deep to the deep (Buck's) fascia and superficial to the tunica albuginea along the dorsal aspect of the penis. The deep dorsal vein provides the primary venous drainage for the corpora cavernosa, whereas the paired dorsal arteries supply blood flow to the glans penis and penile skin.

On US, the tunica albuginea and deep (Buck's) fascia together appear as a thin echogenic border surrounding the homogeneous and hypoechoic corpora. In addition, the cavernosal arteries appear as punctate central foci of echogenicity within the corpora cavernosa. On unenhanced CT, the tunica albuginea and deep (Buck's) fascia appear as higher soft tissue attenuation curvilinear foci surrounding the relatively lower soft tissue attenuation corpora. On MRI, the tunica albuginea and deep (Buck's) fascia are inseparable and appear as a single low signal intensity border surrounding the intermediate T1-weighted and high T2-weighted signal intensity corpora. In addition, the cavernosal arteries appear as punctate central foci of low signal intensity within the corpora cavernosa, and the urethra appears as a flat band of low signal intensity within the corpus spongiosum when viewed in cross-section on T2-weighted images. On both CT and MRI, following intravenous contrast administration, the corpus spongiosum enhances early whereas the corpora cavernosa enhance gradually in a centrifugal fashion given the central location of the cavernosal arteries (Figure 39-16).

58. What congenital abnormality of the penis is associated with bladder exstrophy?
Epispadias is a rare congenital abnormality in which there is ectopic location of the urethral meatus along the dorsal aspect of the penis, along with variable degrees of absence of the dorsal covering of the penis. It is highly associated with bladder exstrophy, a congenital anomaly caused by failure of midline closure of the infraumbilical abdominal wall, since closure of the bladder and urethra during development occurs in the craniocaudal direction. In bladder exstrophy, the anterior bladder wall is absent, the pubic symphysis is widened, the edges of the posterior bladder walls are fused to the skin surface, and the bladder is often small and everted upon the open abdominopelvic wall.

59. When the penile meatus is located more ventrally and proximally than expected, what is this congenital abnormality called, and what is an associated finding?
Hypospadias is a congenital abnormality in which there is ectopic location of the urethral meatus along the ventral aspect of the penis. A dilated utricle is an associated finding, and in general, the more proximally located the hypospadias is, the larger the utricle is.

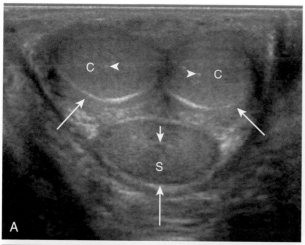

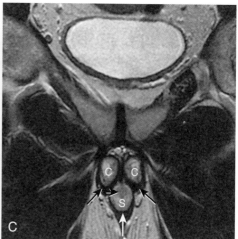

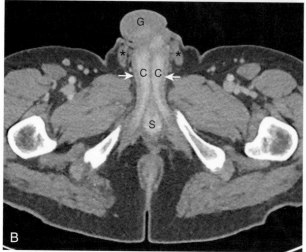

**Figure 39-16.** Normal penis on US, CT, and MRI. **A,** Transverse US image through penile shaft demonstrates hypoechoic corpora cavernosa (*C*) and corpus spongiosum (*S*) surrounded by echogenic tunica albuginea (*long arrows*) along with deep (Buck's) fascia. Also note echogenic cavernosal arteries (*arrowheads*) within corpora cavernosa, and anterior urethra (*short arrow*) within corpus spongiosum. **B,** Axial contrast-enhanced CT image through pelvis reveals enhancement of corpora cavernosa (*C*) with surrounding tunica albuginea and deep (Buck's) fascia (*arrows*), along with enhancement of corpus spongiosum (*S*) at bulb of penis proximally. Also note glans penis (*G*) distally as well as spermatic cords (*). **C,** Coronal T2-weighted MR image through penile shaft shows high signal intensity corpora cavernosa (*C*) and corpus spongiosum (*S*) surrounded by low signal intensity tunica albuginea and deep (Buck's) fascia (*long arrows*). Also note anterior urethra (*short arrow*) within corpus spongiosum.

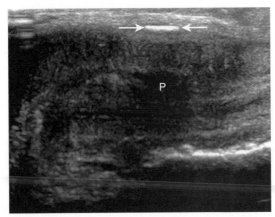

**Figure 39-17.** Peyronie's disease on US. Longitudinal US image through penile shaft reveals focal echogenic calcification (*between arrows*) in tunica albuginea of dorsal penis (*P*).

60. What is Peyronie's disease, and what are its cross-sectional imaging features?

Peyronie's disease results from plaque formation on the tunica albuginea of the penis, usually along its dorsal aspect, leading to painful erections with shortening and curvature of the penis.

On US and MRI, focal echogenic or low signal intensity thickening or calcification of the tunica albuginea is seen (Figure 39-17). On CT, very high attenuation calcification can sometimes be visualized.

61. What is a Cowper duct syringocele, and what are its cross-sectional imaging features?

A Cowper duct syringocele is a cystic dilation of the duct of the Cowper (bulbourethral) gland and is usually encountered in the pediatric age group.

On cross-sectional imaging, a unilocular or multilocular cystic lesion is seen adjacent to the proximal bulbar urethra and urogenital diaphragm. Associated mass effect upon the bulbar urethra and upstream urethral dilation may sometimes also be seen.

62. What cross-sectional imaging findings may be encountered in penile trauma?

Penile trauma is uncommon, but most often occurs from injury to the erect penis during sexual intercourse. The spectrum of injuries that may be visualized on cross-sectional imaging include penile contusion, hematoma, fracture, cavernosal thrombosis, and urethral injury. Visualization of discontinuity of the tunica albuginea indicates presence of a penile fracture.

US is most often used for initial evaluation of suspected penile trauma, followed by MRI as needed, whereas CT is most often used for the initial evaluation of the torso in patients with traumatic injury. Surgical repair is indicated when there is a penile fracture (a surgical emergency) or presence of a urethral injury.

63. If a patient presents with erectile dysfunction, what can one assess on Doppler US to evaluate for potential causes?

Doppler US can be used to assess the blood flow within the cavernosal arteries of the penis. Following administration of a vasodilator to induce erection, the normal average peak systolic velocity (PSV) is >30 cm/second, and no diastolic blood flow is seen. If the cavernosal arterial PSV is <25 cm/second, then arterial insufficiency may be the underlying cause. If the cavernosal arterial diastolic velocity is >5 cm/second, then venous insufficiency is suggested as the underlying cause.

64. What is the most common malignancy of the penis, and what are some of its risk factors?

Squamous cell carcinoma is the most common cancer of the penis, although penile cancer is rare overall. Patients most often present in the sixth to seventh decades of life. Risk factors include infection with human papillomavirus (HPV) types 16 or 18, as well as lack of circumcision.

65. What is the role of cross-sectional imaging in patients with penile cancer?

US and MRI are most often used to evaluate the characteristics and spatial extent of the primary tumor mass (T stage), whereas CT and MRI are most often used to assess for presence of regional lymphadenopathy (N stage) and distant metastatic disease (M stage) as well as for response assessment following therapeutic intervention. Presence of regional lymphadenopathy or distant metastatic disease portends a worse clinical outcome.

66. What are the cross-sectional imaging features of penile cancer?

A heterogeneous enhancing soft tissue penile mass is seen, most commonly occurring in the glans penis. Tumor invasion of subepithelial connective tissue indicates T1 stage disease. Tumor invasion of the corpora may occur, indicating T2 stage disease, which is best detected by loss of the normal low T2-weighted signal intensity tunica albuginea on MRI. Tumor invasion of the urethra or of adjacent organs may also be seen, indicating T3 and T4 stage

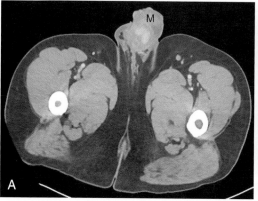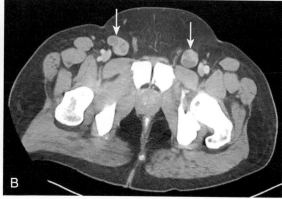

**Figure 39-18.** Penile squamous cell carcinoma on CT. **A,** Axial contrast-enhanced CT image through pelvis shows heterogeneously enhancing exophytic mass (*M*) of glans penis. **B,** Axial contrast-enhanced CT image more superiorly through pelvis demonstrates bilaterally enlarged centrally necrotic inguinal lymph nodes (*arrows*) secondary to metastatic disease.

disease, respectively. Regional lymphadenopathy, involving the inguinal or iliac nodal stations, and distant metastases, most commonly involving the lungs, liver, bone marrow, and nonregional lymph nodes, may also be visualized on CT or MRI (Figure 39-18).

67. **If a patient with known cancer presents with priapism, what diagnosis must be considered?**
Metastatic disease to the penis is extremely rare but may result in a persistent nonsexual erection lasting >4 hours, known as malignant priapism, which is the initial clinical presentation in 20% to 50% of cases. This occurs most commonly with prostate and bladder cancers and less commonly with colorectal cancer and other cancers. Unfortunately, patients with metastatic disease to the penis generally have a very poor clinical outcome.

On cross-sectional imaging, enhancing penile nodules or diffuse infiltration of the corpora cavernosa by tumor may be seen. Cavernosal thrombosis may also be present, which manifests as decreased or absent blood flow on Doppler US, increased T1-weighted and decreased T2-weighted signal intensity on MRI, partial or complete lack of enhancement of one or both corpora cavernosa, and expansion of one or both corpora cavernosa with mass effect upon adjacent structures.

## KEY POINTS

- Extracapsular spread of prostate adenocarcinoma generally indicates nonsurgical disease.
- Testicular cancer is the most common cancer of men between the ages of 15 to 35 years.
- Torsion of a testicular appendage is the leading cause of an acute scrotum in children.
- Most intratesticular masses are malignant, whereas most extratesticular scrotal masses are benign. Spermatoceles and epididymal cysts are the most common causes of a scrotal mass.
- Penile fracture, spermatic cord torsion, and testicular rupture are considered to be surgical emergencies.

## BIBLIOGRAPHY

Coursey Moreno C, Small WC, Camacho JC, et al. Testicular tumors: what radiologists need to know—differential diagnosis, staging, and management. *Radiographics*. 2015;35(2):400-415.
Parker RA 3rd, Menias CO, Quazi R, et al. MR Imaging of the penis and scrotum. *Radiographics*. 2015;35(4):1033-1050.
Suh CH, Baheti AD, Tirumani SH, et al. Multimodality imaging of penile cancer: what radiologists need to know. *Abdom Imaging*. 2015;40(2):424-435.
Avery LL, Scheinfeld MH. Imaging of penile and scrotal emergencies. *Radiographics*. 2013;33(3):721-740.
Torigian DA, Kitazono MT. *Netter's correlative imaging: abdominal and pelvic anatomy*. Philadephia: Elsevier; 2013:1-499.
Yusuf GT, Sidhu PS. A review of ultrasound imaging in scrotal emergencies. *J Ultrasound*. 2013;16(4):171-178.
Philips S, Nagar A, Dighe M, et al. Benign non-cystic scrotal tumors and pseudotumors. *Acta Radiol*. 2012;53(1):102-111.
Wasnik AP, Maturen KE, Shah S, et al. Scrotal pearls and pitfalls: ultrasound findings of benign scrotal lesions. *Ultrasound Q*. 2012;28(4): 281-291.
Pano B, Sebastia C, Bunesch L, et al. Pathways of lymphatic spread in male urogenital pelvic malignancies. *Radiographics*. 2011;31(1): 135-160.
Verma S, Rajesh A. A clinically relevant approach to imaging prostate cancer: self-assessment module. *AJR Am J Roentgenol*. 2011;196(3 suppl):S11-S14.
Edge SB, Byrd DR, Compton CC, et al. *AJCC cancer staging manual*. 7th ed. New York: Springer; 2010.
Lakhani P, Papanicolaou N, Ramchandani P, et al. Asymmetric spermatic cord vessel enhancement and enlargement on contrast-enhanced MDCT as indicators of ipsilateral scrotal pathology. *Eur J Radiol*. 2010;75(2):e92-e96.

Bertolotto M, Pavlica P, Serafini G, et al. Painful penile induration: imaging findings and management. *Radiographics.* 2009;29(2):477-493.

Gupta E, Torigian DA. MRI of the prostate gland. *PET Clin.* 2009;4(2):139-154.

Kim B, Kawashima A, Ryu JA, et al. Imaging of the seminal vesicle and vas deferens. *Radiographics.* 2009;29(4):1105-1121.

Lin EP, Bhatt S, Rubens DJ, et al. Testicular torsion: twists and turns. *Semin Ultrasound CT MR.* 2007;28(4):317-328.

Stewart VR, Sidhu PS. The testis: the unusual, the rare and the bizarre. *Clin Radiol.* 2007;62(4):289-302.

Torigian DA, Ramchandani P. Hematospermia: imaging findings. *Abdom Imaging.* 2007;32(1):29-49.

Alivizatos G, Skolarikos A, Sopilidis O, et al. Splenogonadal fusion: report of a case and review of the literature. *Int J Urol.* 2005;12(1):90-92.

Barwick TD, Malhotra A, Webb JA, et al. Embryology of the adrenal glands and its relevance to diagnostic imaging. *Clin Radiol.* 2005;60(9):953-959.

Fernandez-Perez GC, Tardaguila FM, Velasco M, et al. Radiologic findings of segmental testicular infarction. *AJR Am J Roentgenol.* 2005;184(5):1587-1593.

Carucci LR, Tirkes AT, Pretorius ES, et al. Testicular Leydig's cell hyperplasia: MR imaging and sonographic findings. *AJR Am J Roentgenol.* 2003;180(2):501-503.

Avila NA, Premkumar A, Merke DP. Testicular adrenal rest tissue in congenital adrenal hyperplasia: comparison of MR imaging and sonographic findings. *AJR Am J Roentgenol.* 1999;172(4):1003-1006.

Moore EE, Malangoni MA, Cogbill TH, et al. Organ injury scaling VII: cervical vascular, peripheral vascular, adrenal, penis, testis, and scrotum. *J Trauma.* 1996;41(3):523-524.

# VII
# NEURORADIOLOGY

# CHAPTER 40

# BRAIN IMAGING: ANATOMY, TRAUMA, AND TUMORS

*Hailey H. Choi, MD, Linda C. Kelahan, MD, Ann K. Jay, MD, and Laurie A. Loevner, MD*

1. Identify the normal parts of the brain labeled 1 through 6 in Figure 40-1.
   For the answer, see the figure legend.

2. What imaging modalities can be used to evaluate the brain?
   The two major noninvasive cross-sectional imaging modalities used in neuroimaging are computed tomography (CT) and magnetic resonance imaging (MRI). Catheter angiography, also known as digital subtraction angiography (DSA) or conventional angiography, is reserved for the detection of intracranial vascular processes such as aneurysms and intracranial vasculitis. The advantage to catheter angiography is the potential for intervention at the time of diagnosis, such as coiling of an aneurysm. Myelography involves the injection of contrast material into the subarachnoid space by lumbar puncture, allowing for visualization of the spinal cord and nerve roots which are seen as "filling defects" within the contrast-opacified cerebrospinal fluid (CSF). Myelography (usually followed by postmyelography CT) is reserved for patients with contraindications to MRI (e.g., patients with noncompatible pacemakers or severe claustrophobia), patients with surgical hardware that may cause significant artifact obscuring the spinal canal on MRI, patients with equivocal MRI findings, and obese patients who exceed weight limits for MRI scanners.

3. What are the clinical indications for obtaining CT and MRI of the brain?
   A CT scan can be a good initial examination for evaluating the brain in many acute settings, including trauma. It can assess for acute intracranial hemorrhage, mass effect, hydrocephalus, or stroke. CT is superior to MRI for evaluation of the bony structures. MRI provides greater soft tissue contrast and is often complementary to the CT examination. MRI can better characterize neoplasms (primary or secondary), neurodegenerative disorders, inflammatory diseases, and infectious processes. Diffusion-weighted imaging (DWI) is the most sensitive MRI technique for identifying acute ischemic infarcts. MRI can also better detect acute and chronic intracranial hemorrhage, nonhemorrhagic brain injury, and brainstem injury, and it is often performed in acute or subacute settings when neurologic findings are unexplained by CT findings.

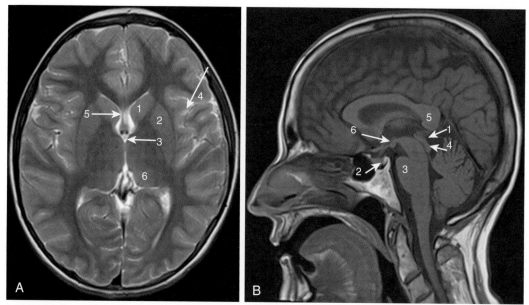

**Figure 40-1.** Normal brain anatomy on MRI. **A,** Axial T2-weighted MR image of brain at level of basal ganglia (*1,* caudate head; *2,* putamen; *3,* third ventricle; *4,* insular cortex; *5,* septum pellucidum; *6,* thalamus). **B,** Sagittal T1-weighted image of brain at midline (*1,* pineal gland; *2,* posterior lobe of pituitary gland ("pituitary bright spot"); *3,* pons; *4,* tectal plate; *5,* splenium of corpus callosum; *6,* mamillary body).

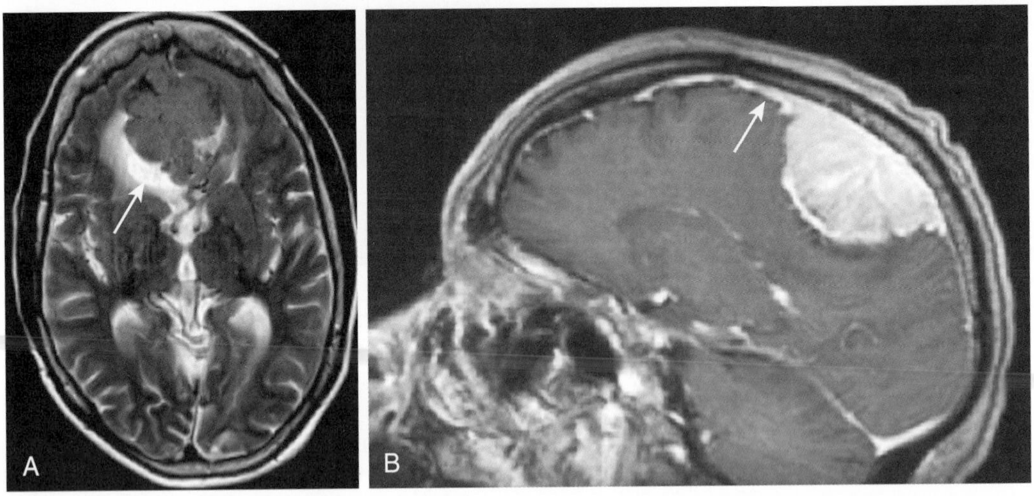

**Figure 40-2.** Intracranial meningioma on MRI. **A,** Axial T2-weighted image shows large mass in midline frontal region. Note CSF cleft (*arrow*), indicating extra-axial site of origin. **B,** Sagittal contrast-enhanced T1-weighted image shows homogeneous enhancement of mass with dural tail (*arrow*) characteristic of meningioma.

4. What are contraindications for performing MRI of the brain?

Contraindications include ferromagnetic implanted electronic devices, such as certain pacemakers, neurostimulator devices, non–MRI-compatible vascular clips, ferromagnetic metallic implants, and foreign bodies in the eye. If history is unavailable, prior imaging studies or radiography can evaluate for the presence of foreign bodies. A major change in device safety relates to advancements in cardiac implantable electronic devices. There are now FDA-approved, "MR conditional" pacemakers on the market, and MRI can be performed if the manufacturer's guidelines are followed. In addition, however, a few academic institutions are safely performing MRI studies on patients with non-MR conditional pacemakers after careful evaluation by a physician. MRI can be performed on patients with aneurysm clips if the model and type is documented to be safe. Most aneurysm clips used after 1995 are made of titanium and are MRI-compatible. Severe claustrophobia is a relative contraindication, and, if necessary, most patients with this condition can successfully undergo MRI with sedation.

5. Define the terms "intra-axial" and "extra-axial", which are commonly used to localize intracranial pathologic conditions.

An intra-axial lesion arises from the brain parenchyma. An extra-axial lesion is one that arises outside of the brain substance, and it may be pial, dural, subdural, epidural, or intraventricular in origin. The most common extra-axial mass is a meningioma (Figure 40-2). In adults, the most common solitary intra-axial masses are primary brain tumors and metastatic disease. An intra-axial mass lesion expands the brain, resulting in gyral swelling and effacement of the cerebral sulci. The gray-white matter interface may be blurred. An extra-axial mass lesion is characterized by obtuse margins and results in crowding of the underlying sulci. Additional features include a cleft of CSF (see Figure 40-2, *A*), dura, or small vessel between the mass and brain, as well as bony remodeling of the skull.

6. What is the Glasgow Coma Scale (GCS), and how is it used?

The GCS provides a reliable, objective way of determining a patient's conscious state and is most often used in the setting of head injuries. Responsiveness and awareness is measured by evaluating eye opening response, verbal response, and motor response. A score between 3 and 15 is assigned. Scores of 13 to 15 correspond to mild closed head injury; 9 to 12 correspond to moderate head injury; and 8 or less correspond to severe brain injury. The GCS does not correlate with survival outcome in cases of severe head trauma with coma.

7. What is the imaging modality of choice in the setting of acute head trauma?

The imaging modality of choice in the setting of acute head trauma is an unenhanced brain CT scan. CT is a readily available, fast, and accurate method for detecting acute intracranial hemorrhage. On CT, acute hemorrhage is hyperattenuating relative to brain and may display mass effect. Emergency physicians and neurosurgeons want to know the exact cause of clinical symptoms in a trauma patient. Specifically, the most significant concern is whether there is a treatable lesion. CT plays a primary role in evaluating the extent of trauma and in determining appropriate management. It is sensitive in distinguishing brain contusions from extra-axial hematomas (subdural and epidural). CT is also excellent for detecting facial and calvarial fractures. When diffuse axonal shear injury is suspected, MRI is more sensitive and can be obtained when the patient is clinically able to tolerate this examination. CT is also useful when foreign bodies (such as bullet fragments) are suspected, and MRI is contraindicated.

8. **What is the role of imaging after concussion or other minor head trauma?**

   The need for a head CT in a patient with minor head trauma, classically defined as having a normal or near-normal (13 to 15) GCS and loss of consciousness, disorientation, or memory loss, is controversial. The majority of the time, these CT scans are found to be normal. The Canada CT Head Rule is a set of guidelines developed with the goal of providing evidence-based clinical decision support. In this set of guidelines, any one of the following "high-risk" clinical criteria were found to be 100% sensitive for a positive head CT (demonstrating injury requiring neurosurgical intervention): GCS <15 at 2 hours after injury, suspected open skull or skull base fracture, greater than 2 episodes of vomiting, or age greater than 65 years old. Sensitivity was reported to be 98% with the following "medium-risk" criteria: amnesia less than 30 minutes prior to impact or a dangerous mechanism of injury. More recent criteria were developed based on the New Orleans Criteria (NOC) trial. These criteria differ from the Canada Head CT rule because they only apply to patients with a GCS of 15 and define a positive head CT as having evidence of any acute injury—not necessarily an injury requiring neurosurgical intervention. The NOC recommends a noncontrast head CT in the following settings: headache, vomiting, age older than 60, intoxication, post-traumatic seizure, physical evidence of trauma above the clavicles, and short-term memory deficits. The NOC are considered 98% to 99% sensitive for identification of any intracranial injury.

9. **What are the advantages and drawbacks of MRI in assessing a trauma patient?**

   MRI is more sensitive in distinguishing different ages of hemorrhage (hyperacute, acute, subacute, and chronic), in detecting diffuse axonal shear injury, and in assessing injury in the posterior fossa and undersurfaces of the frontal and temporal lobes. However, MRI scan times are significantly longer, and performing MRI in patients on ventilators and other monitoring devices can be cumbersome. MRI is less sensitive in detecting fractures. In addition, MRI is contraindicated in some patients with foreign bodies (for example, near the orbit). CT, on the other hand, is readily available and fast; it remains the imaging modality of choice in the setting of trauma.

10. **How does one differentiate a subdural hematoma from an epidural hematoma?**

    An epidural hematoma is usually caused by an arterial injury (most commonly, the middle meningeal artery is injured as a result of a fracture of the temporal bone through which it courses) (Figure 40-3, *A*). An epidural hematoma is extra-axial, runs between the periosteum of the inner table of the skull and the dura, and is confined by the lateral sutures (especially the coronal sutures) where the dura inserts. As a result, an epidural hematoma is usually lenticular in shape and can cross the midline. Prompt surgical clot evacuation is typically performed for large epidural hematomas to prevent brain herniation and its associated complications.

    In contrast, a subdural hematoma is usually caused by injury to the bridging cortical veins (Figure 40-3, *B*). A subdural hematoma runs between the dura and the pia-arachnoid meninges on the surface of the brain and is not confined by the lateral sutures. As a result, subdural hematomas are usually crescentic in shape. In the midline, the dural reflection is attached to the falx cerebri, however. Subdural hematomas (in contrast to epidural hematomas) do not cross the midline, but rather track in the interhemispheric fissure. Subdural hematomas are commonly seen in patients with closed head trauma; elderly patients with minor head trauma; and patients with rapid decompression of hydrocephalus and extra-axial hematomas, where abrupt changes in intracranial pressure make the bridging cortical veins vulnerable. They may also be seen in pediatric patients in the setting of nonaccidental trauma (child abuse).

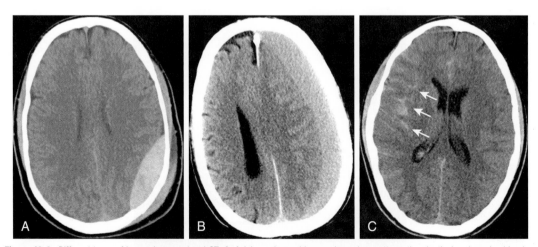

**Figure 40-3.** Different types of hemorrhage on head CT. **A,** Axial unenhanced image shows hyperattenuating, lenticular-shaped epidural hematoma in left parietal region. Note small overlying scalp hematoma. **B,** Axial unenhanced image shows left hemispheric subdural hematoma that crosses coronal and lambdoid sutures but does not cross midline. **C,** Axial unenhanced image shows hyperattenuating hemorrhage (*arrows*) between sulci of right cerebral hemisphere, in keeping with acute subarachnoid hemorrhage.

11. What is the CT appearance of subarachnoid hemorrhage (SAH)?

   SAH appears as areas of hyperattenuation in the subarachnoid space (Figure 40-3, *C*). The subarachnoid space has a serpentine appearance in areas where it dips in between the gyri of the brain. SAH in the setting of trauma usually indicates the presence of superficial cortical contusions but may alternatively be due to a ruptured aneurysm. Vasospasm may ensue, potentially leading to areas of brain infarction.

12. What are the five patterns of brain herniation and herniation syndromes?

   The brain is encased by a rigid skull and further compartmentalized by inelastic dural attachments (falx cerebri, falx cerebelli, and tentorium). Brain swelling, tumor, or hemorrhage can force brain tissue from one compartment into another. If untreated, this herniation can result in further brain damage and vascular injury. Five patterns of brain herniation are as follows:

   - **Subfalcine herniation:** The cingulate gyrus is displaced across the midline, under the falx cerebri. The septum pellucidum is shifted from the midline. This can lead to compression of the ipsilateral lateral ventricle. It may also lead to obstruction of the contralateral foramen of Monro and cause enlargement of the contralateral lateral ventricle. Subfalcine herniation can compress the ipsilateral anterior cerebral artery, leading to infarction.
   - **Uncal (downward transtentorial) herniation:** The medial temporal lobe is displaced medially over the tentorium. On imaging, there will be focal effacement of the ambient and suprasellar cisterns. This can lead to compression of the ipsilateral posterior cerebral artery, cranial nerve III, contralateral posterior cerebral artery, cerebral peduncle, and aqueduct of Sylvius. Clinically, patients may have medial temporal/occipital lobe infarcts, a blown pupil, hemiparesis, or obstructive hydrocephalus.
   - **Ascending transtentorial herniation:** Mass effect from the posterior fossa displaces the cerebellar vermis and hemispheres superiorly through the tentorial incisura. Imaging demonstrates flattening or reversal of the quadrigeminal cistern. Complications are similar to those of uncal herniation.
   - **Tonsillar herniation:** The cerebellar tonsils herniate inferiorly through the foramen magnum. This may cause vascular injury to the posterior inferior cerebellar artery.
   - **Extracranial herniation:** Brain parenchyma herniates through a skull defect.

13. What are Duret hemorrhages?

   Duret hemorrhages occur in the midbrain and upper pons from uncal (downward transtentorial) herniation (Figure 40-4). The downward herniation causes stretching injury to the perforating branches of the basilar artery. It is seen in patients with severe herniation and is usually fatal.

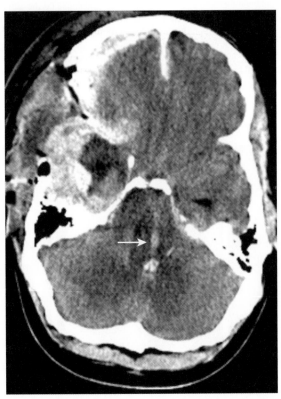

**Figure 40-4.** Duret hemorrhage on CT. Axial unenhanced image shows severe diffuse cerebral edema with transtentorial herniation resulting in high attenuation Duret hemorrhage in pons (*arrow*) due to stretching injury to perforating branches of basilar artery.

14. **What are the imaging manifestations of a brain contusion?**

Contusions are parenchymal bruises of the brain with associated petechial hemorrhage usually related to direct trauma to the head. The most common locations are the inferior, anterior, and lateral surfaces of the frontal and temporal lobes, owing to direct impact of the brain against the rough edges of the inner table of the skull along the floor of the anterior cranial fossa, the sphenoid wing, and the petrous ridges. Additional injuries on the opposite side of the skull (contrecoup injury) may be present as well. On CT, hemorrhagic contusions appear as focal areas of hyperattenuation (blood) with surrounding hypoattenuation (edema) in characteristic anatomic locations of the brain. On T2-weighted MR images, acute hemorrhagic contusions are hypointense in signal intensity with surrounding high signal intensity edema. On susceptibility-weighted (SW) MR images, these lesions are detected with increased sensitivity as areas of low signal intensity.

15. **What are the imaging manifestations of diffuse axonal injury (DAI)?**

DAI is commonly associated with coma, immediate cognitive decline, and poor outcome in patients with significant closed head injury. The stress induced by rotational acceleration/deceleration movement of the head causes differential motion to occur between the neuronal body and axon, which is the area of greatest density difference in the brain. This motion causes axonal stretching and disruption. The sites most commonly involved include the body and splenium of the corpus callosum, brainstem, superior cerebellar peduncle, internal capsule, and gray-white junction of the cerebrum. On CT, DAI may not be initially detected and the striking paucity of findings belies the severity of clinical symptoms. On MRI, rounded or elliptic T2-weighted hyperintense foci are seen in characteristic locations. The majority of lesions are not hemorrhagic; however, if present, microhemorrhages are best seen on SW MR images. DAI lesions can also be hyperintense on DWI.

16. **What is the most common primary intra-axial brain tumor in adults? What cell line does it arise from?**

The most common primary brain tumor in adults is glioblastoma multiforme. It is the most malignant form of astrocytoma and carries a grave prognosis with median survival of about 15 months. Glioblastoma multiforme arises from glial cells. Gliomas account for 35% to 45% of all intracranial tumors. Glioblastoma multiforme accounts for 50% to 60% of gliomas. Other tumors that arise from glial cells include oligodendroglioma, ependymoma, and choroid plexus tumors.

17. **What is the most common extra-axial tumor in adults?**

The most common extra-axial tumor in adults is meningioma. This tumor commonly affects middle-aged women, arises from the arachnoid of the meninges, and is most often benign. The most common locations are the parasagittal dura of the falx, the cerebral convexities, the sphenoid wing, the olfactory groove, and the planum sphenoidale. Other locations include the tuberculum sella and orbit, the cerebellopontine angle, and the cavernous sinus. On unenhanced CT, most meningiomas are slightly hyperattenuating compared to normal brain tissue, with calcifications present in approximately 20%. There may be associated osseous hyperostosis of the adjacent bone. On MRI, meningiomas are isointense to slightly hyperintense relative to gray matter on T2-weighted images. Meningiomas enhance intensely and homogeneously (see Figure 40-2, *B*). A CSF cleft between the mass and the brain is often present (see Figure 40-2, *A*), confirming its extra-axial location. Although the presence of a dural tail is typical of a meningioma, it may not be seen in 30% of cases (see Figure 40-2, *B*).

18. **What are the most common neoplasms arising in the corpus callosum?**

The corpus callosum is the largest white matter tract and connects the two cerebral hemispheres in the midline. The most common tumors that affect the corpus callosum are glioblastoma multiforme and lymphoma. The extension of a neoplasm from one hemisphere to the other via the corpus callosum produces the so-called butterfly pattern (Figure 40-5). Other nonneoplastic white matter diseases that commonly involve the corpus callosum include demyelinating disease (especially multiple sclerosis) and trauma (DAI).

19. **What are the most common neoplasms that metastasize to the brain?**

Breast cancer, lung cancer, and melanoma most commonly spread hematogenously to the brain. Hemorrhagic brain metastases are common with melanoma, choriocarcinoma, thyroid cancer, and renal cell carcinoma. However, because breast and lung cancer are so much more common, it is more likely that a hemorrhagic metastasis is related to one of these latter cancers. Calcified metastases may be seen with mucinous adenocarcinomas (arising from the lung, colon, stomach, ovary, or breast) and bone cancers (osteosarcoma and chondrosarcoma).

20. **What are the most common primary brain tumors that calcify?**

Oligodendroglioma, ependymoma, astrocytoma, craniopharyngioma, and ganglioglioma are the primary central nervous system tumors that most commonly calcify.

21. **What is the imaging appearance of leptomeningeal carcinomatosis or subarachnoid seeding?**

Subarachnoid seeding or leptomeningeal spread of tumor is characterized by tiny nodules of tumor implanted on the surface of the brain, spinal cord, or both. There is "sugar-coating" of the subarachnoid spaces by tumor. Contrast-enhanced T1-weighted images are best for showing this nodular enhancement, particularly in the basilar cisterns, over the cerebral convexities, and along the cranial nerves (Figure 40-6). Communicating hydrocephalus may result from obstruction of the arachnoid villi.

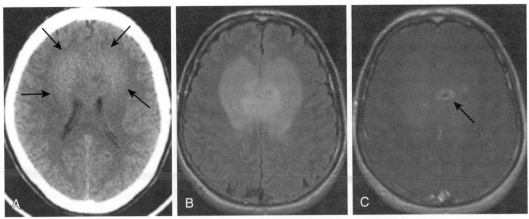

**Figure 40-5.** Glioblastoma multiforme on CT and MRI. **A,** Axial unenhanced CT image shows mildly hyperattenuating mass (*arrows*) involving bilateral frontal lobes and genu of corpus callosum. Hyperattenuation indicates cellularity of this tumor. **B,** Axial fluid attenuation inversion recovery (FLAIR) MR image shows infiltrative nature of this mass which involves both gray and white matter. **C,** Axial contrast-enhanced FLAIR MR image shows heterogeneous enhancement (*arrow*) of mass which crosses corpus callosum to involve bilateral frontal lobes in pattern characteristic of "butterfly" glioma.

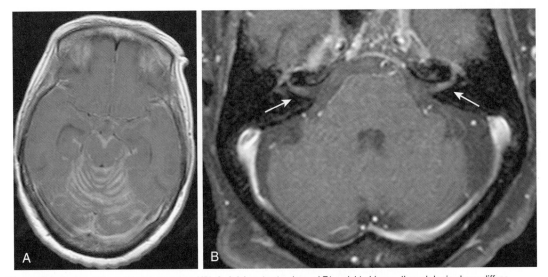

**Figure 40-6.** Leptomeningeal disease spread on MRI. **A,** Axial contrast-enhanced T1-weighted image through brain shows diffuse abnormal leptomeningeal enhancement, predominantly in skull base and cerebellum, which may be seen with leptomeningeal spread of lymphoma or neurosarcoidosis. **B,** Axial contrast-enhanced T1-weighted image in different patient shows abnormal leptomeningeal enhancement of cranial nerves VII and VIII at bilateral cerebellopontine angles (arrows).

22. What are the most common tumors that produce subarachnoid seeding in adults?
    Many primary central nervous system tumors seed the subarachnoid spaces (e.g., glioblastoma multiforme, oligodendroglioma, and ependymoma). Metastatic tumors that commonly spread to the CSF or leptomeninges include breast cancer, lung cancer, melanoma, and hematologic malignancies (lymphoma and leukemia).

23. Why would a mass appear hyperattenuating on an unenhanced CT scan of the head?
    Masses may be hyperattenuating because of the presence of acute hemorrhage, calcification, dense cellularity (lymphoma, meningioma, medulloblastoma, and germinoma), or proteinaceous material.

24. What is the most common tumor in the cerebellopontine angle cistern?
    The most common tumor in the cerebellopontine angle cistern is a vestibular schwannoma (Figure 40-7). Other less common tumors include meningiomas and epidermoid tumors. Nonneoplastic lesions such as vertebrobasilar artery aneurysms or arachnoid cysts may also occur. Vestibular schwannomas are located in the internal auditory canal (IAC) and enhance homogeneously. Large tumors may be heterogeneous due to necrosis or cystic change. Vestibular schwannomas can expand the porus acousticus (the opening of the IAC). Meningiomas also enhance homogeneously

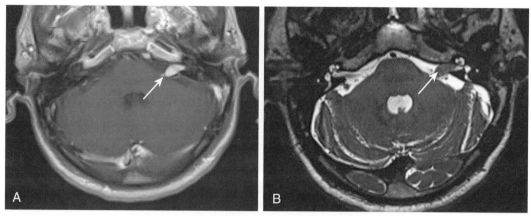

**Figure 40-7.** Vestibular schwannoma on MRI. **A,** Axial contrast-enhanced T1-weighted image shows avidly enhancing mass (*arrow*) in left cerebellopontine angle extending into internal auditory canal. **B,** Axial T2-weighted image shows hypointense mass in left cerebellopontine angle extending into internal auditory canal and mildly expanding porus acousticus (*arrow*).

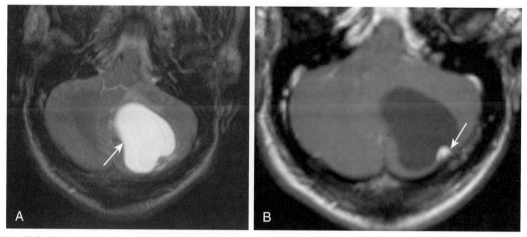

**Figure 40-8.** Hemangioblastoma on MRI. **A,** Axial T2-weighted image shows hyperintense, cystic, left cerebellar mass (*arrow*). There is associated mass effect and mild surrounding edema. **B,** Axial contrast-enhanced T1-weighted image shows small enhancing mural nodule (*arrow*), whereas cystic portion is hypointense and nonenhancing.

but rarely involve the IAC; there is usually associated dural enhancement. It is important for the radiologist to try to distinguish schwannoma from meningioma because this information can affect the surgical approach for resection of these lesions.

25. What is the most common clinical presentation of a vestibular schwannoma?

The most common clinical presentation of a vestibular schwannoma is unilateral sensorineural hearing loss. Adults with unilateral sensorineural hearing loss should be evaluated with contrast-enhanced MRI. Conductive hearing loss is usually evaluated with temporal bone CT to assess for an abnormality of the ossicles and middle ear. In children, temporal bone CT is commonly the first imaging modality used to assess sensorineural and conductive hearing loss because the sensorineural hearing loss in pediatric patients is often related to congenital malformations easily detected on CT.

26. What is the most common posterior fossa/infratentorial mass in adults?

The most common infratentorial neoplasm in adults is a metastasis. A metastasis appears as a well-defined, enhancing mass at the gray-white junction which may have surrounding vasogenic edema. The most common primary posterior fossa tumor in adults is a hemangioblastoma. The typical imaging findings of hemangioblastoma are a cystic mass with an enhancing mural nodule (Figure 40-8). The mural nodule is highly vascular. Solidly enhancing hemangioblastomas can also be seen, however. Multiple hemangioblastomas are associated with von Hippel-Lindau disease.

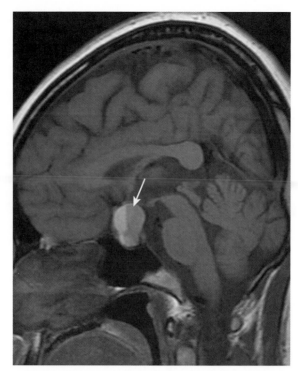

**Figure 40-9.** Pituitary apoplexy on MRI. Sagittal contrast-enhanced T1-weighted image shows lobulated, expansile mass with fluid-fluid level (*arrow*) related to sedimentation of blood products. This patient presented with acute onset of severe headache and visual disturbance.

27. What is pituitary apoplexy?

Pituitary apoplexy is a clinical syndrome that results from hemorrhage and/or infarction of the pituitary gland. Patients can present with headache, visual field deficits, ophthalmoplegia, and mental status change. It commonly occurs in patients with preexisting pituitary adenomas. Additional predisposing factors include pregnancy (Sheehan syndrome), medical treatment of a prolactinoma, prior radiation, and trauma and surgery (high stress situations). On CT, the hemorrhagic pituitary mass can be hyperattenuating. MRI demonstrates high T1-weighted signal intensity blood products (Figure 40-9). Restricted diffusion on DWI in solid infarcted components may also be seen.

28. What is a pituitary microadenoma? What is a pituitary macroadenoma?

The pituitary gland is composed of an anterior lobe and a posterior lobe. The anterior lobe, or adenohypophysis, is divided into the pars tuberalis, pars intermedia, and pars distalis. The posterior lobe, or neurohypophysis, is composed of the posterior pituitary lobe, infundibular stalk, and median eminence of the hypothalamus. Microadenomas are the most common intrasellar neoplasms in adults and, by definition, are less than 10 mm. They are hypointense relative to the pituitary gland on unenhanced and enhanced T1-weighted MR images. In about 75% of cases, microadenomas have associated hormonal abnormalities. Macroadenomas are larger than 10 mm, enlarge the sella turcica, and commonly spread outside of the sella into the suprasellar cistern (commonly referred to as a "snowman" sign) or into the cavernous sinus (Figure 40-10). The differential diagnosis for a pituitary mass also includes Rathke cleft cyst and craniopharyngioma.

29. What visual symptoms can pituitary adenomas cause? What is the most common type of pituitary adenoma?

Pituitary macroadenomas can compress the optic chiasm superiorly and cause bitemporal hemianopsia. The most common type of pituitary adenoma is a prolactinoma.

30. Name advanced imaging techniques that help differentiate brain tumors from other pathologies.

These techniques include magnetic resonance spectroscopy (MRS), perfusion MRI, and DWI. Functional MRI (fMRI) is used for preoperative localization of eloquent brain cortex before surgery.

31. Pineal region masses are associated with what visual disturbance?

Pineal region masses may cause paresis of upward gaze (Parinaud syndrome) from compression of the tectal plate. The clinical manifestations of pineal region masses depend on their size and location near critical anatomic structures—the aqueduct of Sylvius, the tectal plate, and the vein of Galen/internal cerebral veins. Obstructive hydrocephalus results from compression of the aqueduct. Pineal region tumors are categorized into tumors of germ cell origin (60%) and tumors of pineal cell origin. Germ cell tumors are usually germinomas, are seen in males, and

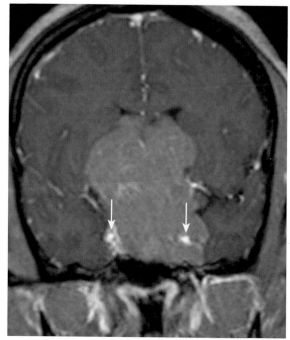

**Figure 40-10.** Pituitary macroadenoma on MRI. Coronal contrast-enhanced T1-weighted image shows large mass centered within pituitary sella and extending into suprasellar space with characteristic "snowman" appearance. Despite its large size, it is not compressing adjacent bilateral carotid arteries (*arrows*).

present with precocious puberty. Intrinsic pineal cell tumors (pineocytoma and pineoblastoma) are seen in male and female patients equally. CSF seeding is common. Because pineal tumors are commonly hypercellular, they appear hyperattenuating on unenhanced CT and have intermediate signal intensity on T1-weighted and T2-weighted MR images.

## KEY POINTS

- The imaging modality of choice in the setting of acute head trauma is an unenhanced brain CT scan.
- An epidural hematoma has a biconvex lenticular shape, is contained by dural sutures, is associated with temporal bone or other skull fractures, and is treated promptly with clot evacuation for large hematomas to prevent brain herniation and its associated complications.
- A subdural hematoma is crescentic in shape, is not contained by dural sutures but does not cross the falx or tentorium, and may or may not be associated with a skull fracture.
- The most common primary intra-axial brain tumor in adults is glioblastoma multiforme. The most common posterior fossa/infratentorial neoplasm in adults is a metastasis. The most common extra-axial tumor in adults is meningioma.

### BIBLIOGRAPHY

Aquino C, Woolen S, Steenburg SD. Magnetic resonance imaging of traumatic brain injury: a pictorial review. *Emerg Radiol.* 2015;22(1):65-78.

Castillo M. History and evolution of brain tumor imaging: insights through radiology. *Radiology.* 2014;273(suppl 2):S111-S125.

Wang LL, Leach JL, Breneman JC, et al. Critical role of imaging in the neurosurgical and radiotherapeutic management of brain tumors. *Radiographics.* 2014;34(3):702-721.

Expert Panel on MRS, Kanal E, Barkovich AJ, et al. ACR guidance document on MR safe practices: 2013. *J Magn Reson Imaging.* 2013;37(3):501-530.

Fakhran S, Yaeger K, Alhilali L. Symptomatic white matter changes in mild traumatic brain injury resemble pathologic features of early Alzheimer dementia. *Radiology.* 2013;269(1):249-257.

Kolias AG, Guilfoyle MR, Helmy A, et al. Traumatic brain injury in adults. *Pract Neurol.* 2013;13(4):228-235.

Omuro A, DeAngelis LM. Glioblastoma and other malignant gliomas: a clinical review. *JAMA.* 2013;310(17):1842-1850.

Strain J, Didehbani N, Cullum CM, et al. Depressive symptoms and white matter dysfunction in retired NFL players with concussion history. *Neurology.* 2013;81(1):25-32.

Cunliffe CH, Fischer I, Parag Y, et al. State-of-the-art pathology: new WHO classification, implications, and new developments. *Neuroimaging Clin N Am.* 2010;20(3):259-271.

Dahiya S, Perry A. Pineal tumors. *Adv Anat Pathol.* 2010;17(6):419-427.

Smith AB, Rushing EJ, Smirniotopoulos JG. From the archives of the AFIP: lesions of the pineal region: radiologic-pathologic correlation. *Radiographics.* 2010;30(7):2001-2020.

Provenzale J. CT and MR imaging of acute cranial trauma. *Emerg Radiol.* 2007;14(1):1-12.

Haydel MJ. Clinical decision instruments for CT scanning in minor head injury. *JAMA.* 2005;294(12):1551-1553.

Johnson PL, Eckard DA, Chason DP, et al. Imaging of acquired cerebral herniations. *Neuroimaging Clin N Am.* 2002;12(2):217-228.

Nelson SJ, McKnight TR, Henry RG. Characterization of untreated gliomas by magnetic resonance spectroscopic imaging. *Neuroimaging Clin N Am.* 2002;12(4):599-613.

Young RJ, Destian S. Imaging of traumatic intracranial hemorrhage. *Neuroimaging Clin N Am.* 2002;12(2):189-204.

Stiell IG, Wells GA, Vandemheen K, et al. The Canadian CT Head Rule for patients with minor head injury. *Lancet.* 2001;357(9266):1391-1396.

Udstuen GJ, Claar JM. Imaging of acute head injury in the adult. *Semin Ultrasound CT MR.* 2001;22(2):135-147.

Haydel MJ, Preston CA, Mills TJ, et al. Indications for computed tomography in patients with minor head injury. *N Engl J Med.* 2000;343(2):100-105.

Ricci PE. Imaging of adult brain tumors. *Neuroimaging Clin N Am.* 1999;9(4):651-669.

Smirniotopoulos JG. The new WHO classification of brain tumors. *Neuroimaging Clin N Am.* 1999;9(4):595-613.

# CHAPTER 41

# BRAIN IMAGING: INFLAMMATORY, INFECTIOUS, AND VASCULAR DISEASES

*Gul Moonis, MD, and Laurie A. Loevner, MD*

1. **How is multiple sclerosis (MS) diagnosed?**
   MS is the most common cause of acquired demyelinating disorders. The disease has a characteristic relapsing-remitting course and usually manifests between the third and fifth decades of life with a female predominance. On magnetic resonance imaging (MRI), the demyelinating lesions of MS are ovoid and hyperintense (bright) in signal intensity on T2-weighted images and occur predominantly in the white matter, especially in the periventricular location (usually perpendicular to the ventricular surface) (Figure 41-1). The corpus callosum, white matter around the temporal horns of the lateral ventricles, and middle cerebellar peduncles are other favored locations of MS plaques. There may be enhancement of the plaques (ringlike or solid) that denotes active disease. Occasionally, MS plaques can be large and masslike (tumefactive MS), in which case differentiation from a tumor may be difficult.

2. **What is the differential diagnosis of MS based on imaging findings?**
   The diagnosis of MS is a clinical one (neurologic symptoms spaced over time and in multiple distributions), with supporting radiologic findings. The diagnosis cannot be made on imaging findings alone because other inflammatory and vascular processes can manifest with similar imaging findings. White matter lesions similar to MS can be seen with a spectrum of inflammatory conditions, including Lyme disease, sarcoidosis, and vasculitis.

3. **What are the clinical and imaging features of acute disseminated encephalomyelitis (ADEM)?**
   ADEM is an acute monophasic demyelinating disease seen most commonly in the pediatric population. It is characterized by acute demyelination following a recent viral infection or vaccination. The white matter lesions in the brain are bilaterally asymmetric and usually demonstrate enhancement (Figure 41-2). Involvement of the basal ganglia,

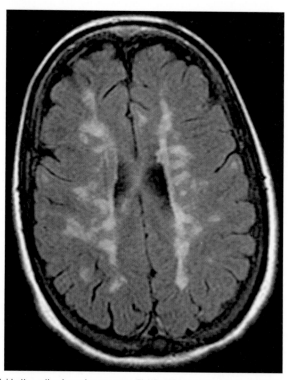

**Figure 41-1.** MS on MRI. Axial fluid attenuation inversion recovery (FLAIR) MR image through head shows numerous ovoid periventricular lesions characteristic of MS plaques. These are oriented along perivascular spaces, and this appearance has been referred to as "Dawson's fingers."

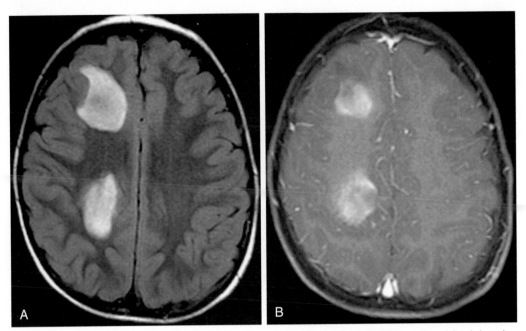

**Figure 41-2.** ADEM in a 6-year-old boy with recent history of viral infection on MRI. **A,** Axial FLAIR MR image through head shows large subcortical white matter lesions in right frontal and parietal lobes. **B,** Axial contrast-enhanced fat-suppressed T1-weighted image reveals enhancement in these lesions.

brainstem, and spinal cord may also occur. Tumefactive MS can mimic this entity radiologically although the diffuse bilateral pattern of involvement with lesions in the gray matter (basal ganglia) and preferential involvement of the subcortical white matter in ADEM may help distinguish the two entities.

4. What are the causes of intracranial abscesses?

Infectious agents gain access to the central nervous system (CNS) by direct spread from a contiguous focus of infection, such as sinusitis, otitis media, mastoiditis, orbital cellulitis, or dental infection. Infection from these locations may also spread to the intracranial compartment by retrograde venous reflux. Hematogenous spread of infection can also occur from a distant nidus of infection, such as the lung. Polymicrobial infection is common with brain abscesses. Four stages have been described in abscess evolution: early cerebritis, late cerebritis, early capsule formation, and late capsule formation. A mature abscess is characterized by a "ring-enhancing" lesion on cross-sectional imaging.

5. What is the imaging differential diagnosis of a ring-enhancing lesion in the brain?

The following disease processes can have an imaging presentation identical to brain abscess: metastatic disease, primary CNS glioma, resolving hematoma, and demyelinating disease. Interpretation of the radiologic findings in conjunction with the clinical history is usually helpful to differentiate between these possible etiologies.

6. What advanced MRI techniques may be useful in distinguishing brain abscess from neoplasm?

Differentiating a subclinical brain abscess from a cystic or necrotic tumor with conventional computed tomography (CT) or MRI can be difficult. [1]H magnetic resonance spectroscopy and diffusion-weighted imaging (DWI) can be useful in this regard (Figure 41-3). Typically, on DWI, an abscess is hyperintense (bright) due to presence of pus.

7. What anatomic location in the brain is preferentially involved by herpes simplex encephalitis?

In adults, type 1 herpes simplex virus is responsible for fulminant, necrotizing encephalitis. The virus preferentially involves the temporal lobes, but involvement of the frontal lobes (especially the cingulate gyrus) is common. Often, there is bilateral temporal lobe involvement, although this is usually asymmetric. On MRI, there is T2-weighted hyperintensity in the temporal and frontal lobes with enhancement (Figure 41-4). Clinically, the patient presents with acute confusion, disorientation, or seizures progressing to stupor and coma. Most cases are a result of reactivation of dormant virus in the trigeminal ganglion. There is commonly asymmetric temporal lobe involvement. Hemorrhage in the affected area is also common.

8. What is the differential diagnosis of an intracranial mass in a patient with human immunodeficiency virus (HIV) infection?

It is crucial to determine whether the cause of HIV-related brain mass is neoplastic or infectious, because these entities are managed differently. Among infectious etiologies, toxoplasmosis and brain abscesses secondary to fungal

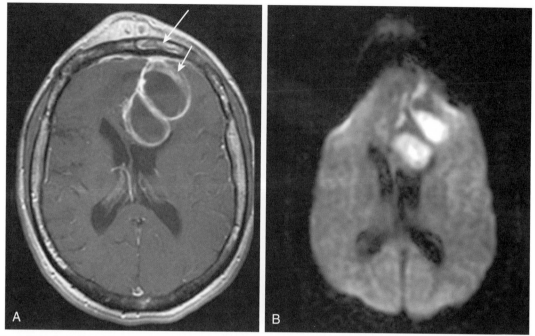

**Figure 41-3.** Frontal lobe brain abscess secondary to frontal sinusitis on MRI. **A,** Axial contrast-enhanced T1-weighted MR image through head shows two ring-enhancing lesions in left frontal lobe (*short arrow*) and enhancing soft tissue (*long arrow*) within and anterior to frontal sinus. **B,** Axial diffusion-weighted MR image reveals restricted diffusion (high signal intensity) within these lesions in keeping with abscesses.

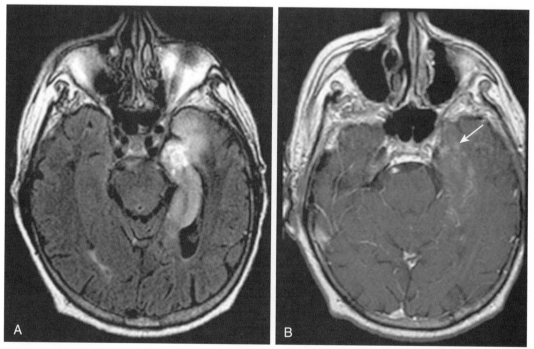

**Figure 41-4.** Herpes simplex encephalitis on MRI. **A,** Axial FLAIR MR image through head shows abnormal hyperintensity in left medial temporal lobe involving gray and white matter. **B,** Axial contrast-enhanced T1-weighted MR image shows mild patchy enhancement (*arrow*) in this location consistent with cerebritis.

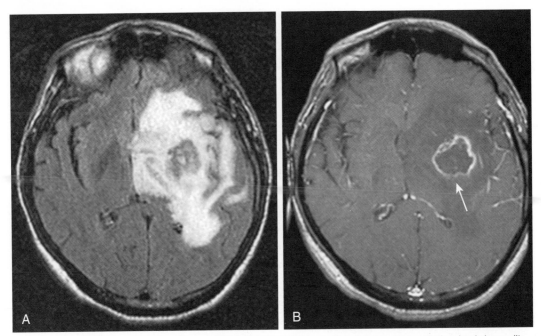

**Figure 41-5.** Toxoplasmosis in HIV-positive patient on MRI. **A,** Axial FLAIR MR image through head shows extensive signal abnormality involving left basal ganglia and adjacent frontal and temporal lobes with mass effect. **B,** Axial contrast-enhanced T1-weighted MR image shows rim-enhancing lesion in center of left basal ganglia (*arrow*) with extensive surrounding low signal intensity edema and midline shift from left to right.

or bacterial etiologies have to be considered. The major neoplastic consideration is primary CNS lymphoma. Toxoplasmosis is the leading cause of focal CNS disease in acquired immunodeficiency syndrome (AIDS) and results from infection by the intracellular parasite *Toxoplasma gondii*. It is usually caused by reactivation of old CNS lesions or by hematogenous spread of a previously acquired infection. On imaging, single or multiple ring-enhancing lesions in the white matter or basal ganglia or both with mass effect may be observed. A single lesion favors the diagnosis of lymphoma over toxoplasmosis (Figure 41-5). Occasionally, progressive multifocal leukoencephalopathy (PML), a demyelinating disease caused by a viral infection, may result in ring-enhancing lesions. PML is caused by a virus that infects the oligodendrocytes in immunocompromised patients.

9. What is a stroke?
   A stroke occurs when the blood supply to a vascular territory of the brain is suddenly interrupted (ischemic stroke), or when a blood vessel in the brain ruptures, spilling blood into the spaces surrounding the brain cells (hemorrhagic stroke). Ischemic stroke is the more common form, responsible for approximately 80% of vascular accidents. In adults, these blockages are usually associated with two conditions: atherosclerosis-related occlusion of vessels (60%) and cardiac embolism (20%).

10. What are the common causes of stroke that one must consider in children and young adults?
    Only 3% of cerebral infarctions occur in patients younger than 40 years old. The most common causes of stroke in young patients are cardiac disease, hematologic diseases (hypercoagulable states), and vascular dissection (from trauma or disease of the vessel wall). Other causes include CNS vasculitis, fibromuscular dysplasia, and venous sinus thrombosis.

11. What are the imaging manifestations of ischemic stroke in the acute stage?
    Commonly, in the acute setting, a CT scan of the head may be normal. The earliest signs (within 6 hours) of an acute infarct on CT are loss of the gray-white differentiation with obscuration of the lateral lentiform nucleus. There may be linear or curvilinear high attenuation noted in the proximal middle cerebral artery, representing acute thrombus or calcified embolus; this is referred to as the "hyperdense artery" sign (Figure 41-6, *A*). Within 12 to 24 hours, there is low attenuation in the appropriate vascular distribution, with increasing mass effect. Mass effect peaks between 3 to 5 days. Findings of acute ischemia are detected earlier on MRI. With the use of DWI, acute ischemic changes can be seen within minutes of onset of the ictus. High signal intensity is noted within the involved vascular territory on T2-weighted images, with characteristic restricted diffusion (also hyperintense in signal intensity) on DWI (Figure 41-6, *B* and *C*). Swelling of the involved cortex and arterial enhancement are noted early in the time course.

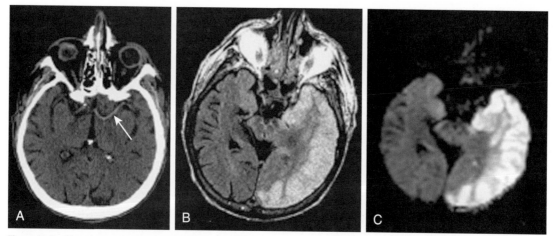

**Figure 41-6.** "Hyperdense artery" sign and acute ischemic stroke on CT and MRI. **A,** Axial unenhanced CT image through head reveals curvilinear hyperattenuation in proximal left middle cerebral artery (*arrow*) in keeping with acute thrombus. **B,** Axial FLAIR MR image shows diffuse hyperintensity involving gray and white matter in left middle cerebral artery vascular territory, characteristic of stroke. **C,** Diffusion-weighted MR image demonstrates restricted diffusion (high signal intensity) in similar distribution, in keeping with acute ischemia.

12. How can one differentiate acute from chronic stroke on imaging?

    Chronic stroke is manifested by encephalomalacic change in the involved vascular territory with accompanying dilation of the sulci and cisterns. There is also ex vacuo dilation of the ipsilateral ventricle. There is absence of mass effect. If it is difficult to distinguish the age of a stroke on CT, MRI that includes DWI can be invaluable.

13. What are watershed infarctions?

    Also known as "border zone infarcts," watershed infarctions occur in the vascular watersheds (the distal most arterial territory with connection between the major arterial branches). In severe hypotension or shock, the systemic blood pressure is insufficient to pump arterial blood to the end arteries. In the cerebrum, not enough blood gets to the "watershed zones" between the anterior and middle cerebral artery territories or between the middle and posterior cerebral artery territories, and in those areas infarcts are likely to develop. Some other causes of cerebral watershed infarcts include heart failure, decreased systemic perfusion pressure, and low blood pressure in the setting of a high-grade stenosis of a major artery (internal carotid artery) supplying the brain.

14. What are lacunar infarctions?

    Lacunar infarctions are small infarcts caused by occlusion or disease of the perforating arteries (arteriolar lipohyalinosis). Initially, these are slightly hypoattenuating on CT. By 4 weeks, sharply circumscribed, cystic lesions develop. These lesions are most commonly seen in the deep gray matter (basal ganglia, thalami), brainstem, internal capsule, and corona radiata. These small infarctions are usually 1 cm or smaller.

15. What are the risk factors for venous sinus thrombosis and venous infarction?

    Venous sinus thrombosis is associated with many systemic conditions, including acute dehydration, hypercoagulable states, chemotherapeutic agents (L-asparaginase), sinusitis and mastoiditis, hematologic malignancies, pregnancy, and trauma. Unenhanced CT reveals the presence of high attenuation and enlargement of the dural venous sinuses (Figure 41-7, *A*). The diagnosis of venous thrombosis is improved significantly with MRI. On unenhanced T1-weighted images, high signal intensity thrombus is noted within the venous sinuses. The "empty delta" sign, which refers to enhancement around the clot in a dural venous sinus, may also be present on contrast-enhanced CT or contrast-enhanced MR images (Figure 41-7, *B*). There may be associated venous infarction. Venous infarctions have a high rate of hemorrhagic transformation compared with arterial infarctions.

16. What is the most common cause of nontraumatic subarachnoid hemorrhage (SAH)?

    Aneurysm rupture is the most common cause of nontraumatic SAH. An aneurysm is a focal dilation of an artery, most commonly encountered at branching points in the intracranial vasculature. Aneurysms are usually due to a congenital weakness in the media and elastica of the arterial wall, but can be acquired in the setting of trauma or mycotic infections. The approximate relative frequency of aneurysm formation in the intracranial vasculature is as follows: anterior communicating artery (30%), distal internal carotid artery and posterior communicating artery (30%), middle cerebral artery (25% to 30%), and the posterior vertebral-basilar circulation (10% to 15%). Multiple aneurysms are seen in approximately 15% of cases. There is increased incidence of intracranial aneurysms in patients with polycystic kidney disease, Marfan's syndrome, and fibromuscular dysplasia (as well as in other rarer entities including moyamoya disease, Ehlers-Danlos syndrome, and Takayasu arteritis).

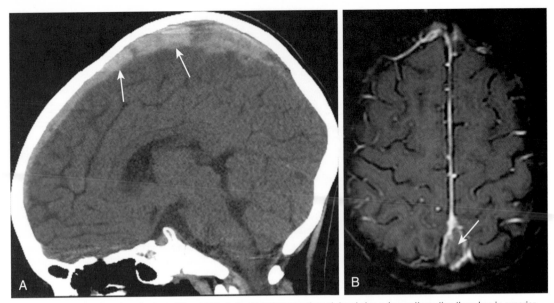

**Figure 41-7.** Venous sinus thrombosis on CT and MRI. **A,** Sagittal CT image through head shows hyperattenuating thrombus in superior sagittal sinus (*arrows*). **B,** Axial contrast-enhanced T1-weighted MR image shows acute thrombus in superior sagittal sinus. Note characteristic "empty delta" sign (*arrow*) that represents nonenhancing clot within superior sagittal sinus.

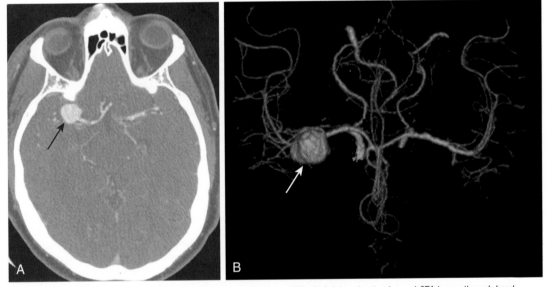

**Figure 41-8.** Right middle cerebral artery (MCA) bifurcation aneurysm on CTA. **A,** Axial contrast-enhanced CTA image through head demonstrates large round enhancing structure (*arrow*) that is contiguous with right MCA at its bifurcation in keeping with aneurysm. **B,** Coronal volume-rendered (VR) contrast-enhanced CTA image shows similar findings confirming cerebral artery aneurysm (*arrow*).

17. **What is the workup of a patient presenting with SAH?**

If a patient presents with the classic history of "the worst headache of my life," an unenhanced CT scan should be obtained to look for SAH followed by CT angiography (CTA) for aneurysm detection (Figure 41-8).

If the results of the CT scan or CTA are negative, but there is high clinical suspicion for SAH, then a lumbar puncture should be performed to look for red blood cells or xanthochromia or both in the cerebrospinal fluid (CSF). If CSF analysis is positive for subarachnoid blood, a diagnostic conventional catheter angiogram is the next step to find the aneurysm, providing an anatomic road map for the neurosurgeon.

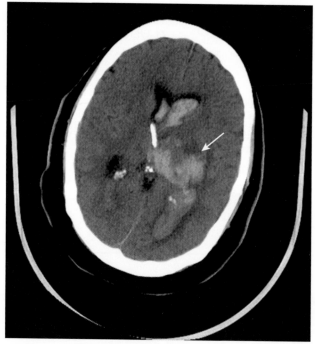

**Figure 41-9.** Left thalamic hypertensive hemorrhage on CT. Axial unenhanced CT image through head shows large focus of hyperattenuating hemorrhage centered in left thalamus (*arrow*) with extension into ventricular system and associated hydrocephalus.

18. If multiple aneurysms are seen on catheter angiography in a patient with SAH, which one most likely bled?

If multiple aneurysms are identified, greater suspicion falls on the aneurysm that is the largest in size, on the aneurysm with a lobulated contour ("nipple" sign), or on the aneurysm closest to the largest clot on CT. Extravasation of intravenous contrast material from the aneurysm is rarely seen, but is diagnostic.

19. What are common locations for hypertensive intraparenchymal hemorrhages?

In adults who present with nontraumatic intraparenchymal hemorrhage in the brain, hypertension is the most common etiologic factor. The arteries in the brain injured by chronic hypertension are typically the perforating arteries, which supply the basal ganglia, thalami, and pons (Figure 41-9). Other areas that may also be affected by hypertensive bleeds include the centrum semiovale and, occasionally, the cerebellum.

20. What is amyloid angiopathy?

Amyloid angiopathy results from deposition of amyloid in the media and adventitia of small and medium-sized vessels of the superficial layers of the cortex and leptomeninges. Amyloid deposition increases with age. Pathologically, there is loss of elasticity and increased fragility of the vessels that cause hemorrhages, which are usually lobar and most often in the frontal and parietal lobes. These parenchymal hemorrhages may be associated with subdural hemorrhage (SDH) and SAH. The usual course is multiple hemorrhagic incidents spaced over time.

21. Review the MRI signal intensity characteristics of intracranial hemorrhage.

For the answers, see Table 41-1.

22. What are the imaging features of cerebral hypoxia/anoxia?

Hypoxia refers to a deficiency of oxygen supply to the cerebral hemispheres, and anoxia refers to absence of oxygen supply to the cerebral hemispheres. Hypoxia/anoxia can have a multifactorial etiology, including drowning, asphyxiation from smoke inhalation, severe hypotension, strangulation, perinatal hypoxic insult, cardiac arrest, and carbon monoxide poisoning. On MRI, increased T2-weighted signal intensity is seen in the perirolandic and occipital cortex and in the basal ganglia (Figure 41-10). The watershed zones between major vascular territories and the hippocampi are also prone to hypoxic-ischemic damage. Layers three, four, and five of the cortex are sensitive to global hypoxia-ischemia and may become necrotic and hemorrhagic (laminar necrosis).

**Table 41-1.** MRI Signal Intensity Characteristics of Intracranial Hemorrhage

| AGE AND COMPOSITION | | T1-WEIGHTED IMAGES | T2-WEIGHTED IMAGES |
|---|---|---|---|
| Hyperacute | Hours old, mainly oxyhemoglobin with surrounding edema | Hypointense | Hyperintense |
| Acute | Days old, mainly deoxyhemoglobin with surrounding edema | Hypointense | Hypointense, surrounded by hyperintense margin of edema |
| Early subacute | Weeks old, predominantly intracellular methemoglobin | Hyperintense | Hypointense |
| Late subacute | Weeks old, predominantly extracellular methemoglobin | Hyperintense | Hyperintense |
| Chronic | Years old, hemosiderin slit or hemosiderin margin surrounding fluid-filled cavity | Hypointense | Hypointense slit or hypointense margin surrounding hyperintense fluid-filled cavity |

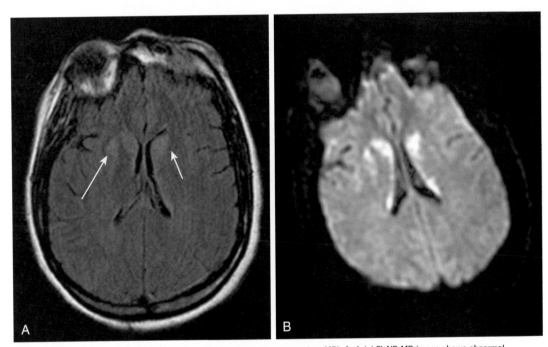

**Figure 41-10.** Acute hypoxic-ischemic injury in patient with respiratory arrest on MRI. **A,** Axial FLAIR MR image shows abnormal hyperintensity in bilateral caudate heads (*left one identified by short arrow*) and right putamen (*long arrow*). **B,** Axial diffusion-weighted MR image shows restricted diffusion (high signal intensity) in similar distribution in keeping with acute hypoxic-ischemic injury.

---

**KEY POINTS**

- MS is the most common acquired demyelinating disorder in adults between 30 and 50 years old, with a female predominance. On MRI, the demyelinating lesions of MS are ovoid and hyperintense on T2-weighted images and occur predominantly in the white matter, especially in the periventricular location (usually perpendicular to the ventricular surface).
- ADEM is an acute monophasic demyelinating disease seen most commonly in the pediatric population. It is characterized by acute demyelination following a recent viral infection or vaccination. The white matter lesions in the brain are bilaterally asymmetric and usually demonstrate enhancement. ADEM lesions are larger than MS, are bilaterally asymmetric, and may involve the gray matter.

## KEY POINTS *(Continued)*

- Aneurysm rupture is the most common cause of nontraumatic SAH. An aneurysm is a focal dilation of an artery, most commonly encountered at branching points in the intracranial vasculature. The most common locations for aneurysm formation are as follows: anterior communicating artery (30%), distal internal carotid artery and posterior communicating artery (30%), middle cerebral artery (25% to 30%), and the posterior vertebral-basilar circulation (10% to 15%).
- The most common locations for hypertensive hemorrhage in the brain are the basal ganglia, thalami, and pons.
- Diffusion-weighted imaging (DWI) is the most sensitive MRI sequence for detection of acute stroke.

## BIBLIOGRAPHY

Vachha B, Rojas R, Prabhu SP, et al. Magnetic resonance imaging in viral and prion diseases of the central nervous system. *Top Magn Reson Imaging.* 2014;23(5):293-302.

Dubey P, Pandey S, Moonis G. Acute stroke imaging: recent updates. *Stroke Res Treatment.* 2013;2013:1-6.

Hsueh CJ, Kao HW, Chen SY, et al. Comparison of the 2010 and 2005 versions of the McDonald MRI criteria for dissemination-in-time in Taiwanese patients with classic multiple sclerosis. *J Neurol Sci.* 2013;329(1-2):51-54.

Mangla R, Kolar B, Almast J, et al. Border zone infarcts: pathophysiologic and imaging characteristics. *Radiographics.* 2011;31(5):1201-1214.

Callen DJ, Shroff MM, Branson HM, et al. Role of MRI in the differentiation of ADEM from MS in children. *Neurology.* 2009;72(11):968-973.

Huang BY, Castillo M. Hypoxic-ischemic brain injury: imaging findings from birth to adulthood. *Radiographics.* 2008;28(2):417-439, quiz 617.

Pagani E, Bizzi A, Di Salle F, et al. Basic concepts of advanced MRI techniques. *Neurol Sci.* 2008;29(suppl 3):290-295.

Leach JL, Fortuna RB, Jones BV, et al. Imaging of cerebral venous thrombosis: current techniques, spectrum of findings, and diagnostic pitfalls. *Radiographics.* 2006;26(suppl 1):S19-S41, discussion S2-S3.

Srinivasan A, Goyal M, Al Azri F, et al. State-of-the-art imaging of acute stroke. *Radiographics.* 2006;26(suppl 1):S75-S95.

Polman CH, Reingold SC, Edan G, et al. Diagnostic criteria for multiple sclerosis: 2005 revisions to the "McDonald Criteria." *Ann Neurol.* 2005;58(6):840-846.

Leuthardt EC, Wippold FJ 2nd, Oswood MC, et al. Diffusion-weighted MR imaging in the preoperative assessment of brain abscesses. *Surg Neurol.* 2002;58(6):395-402, discussion.

Hynson JL, Kornberg AJ, Coleman LT, et al. Clinical and neuroradiologic features of acute disseminated encephalomyelitis in children. *Neurology.* 2001;56(10):1308-1312.

Leonard JR, Moran CJ, Cross DT 3rd, et al. MR imaging of herpes simplex type 1 encephalitis in infants and young children: a separate pattern of findings. *AJR Am J Roentgenol.* 2000;174(6):1651-1655.

# CHAPTER 42

# ADVANCED NEUROSPINAL IMAGING

*Linda J. Bagley, MD, and Laurie A. Loevner, MD*

1. Identify parts of the spine labeled in Figure 42-1.
   For the answer, see the figure legend.

2. What imaging modalities are most often used in the evaluation of spine pathology?
   Radiography, computed tomography (CT), magnetic resonance imaging (MRI), myelography, discography, magnetic resonance angiography (MRA), computed tomographic angiography (CTA), and conventional angiography are utilized for spinal imaging.

3. Describe the strengths, weaknesses, and most appropriate uses of CT in spinal imaging.
   Radiography is often the initial imaging examination used to evaluate the spine. Pathologic conditions of the osseous spine, including fractures, degenerative changes, tumors, infections, and congenital anomalies (including transitional vertebrae), may be detected with radiographs. However, multidetector CT provides superior evaluation of the bony anatomy and of pathologic conditions. Images may be acquired rapidly and reconstructed at narrow intervals (0.6 to 1 mm) with edge-enhancing algorithms. Multiplanar and three-dimensional images can subsequently be created. In the setting of acute spinal trauma, CT has been shown to be more time efficient and significantly more sensitive than radiography for fracture detection. CT, in contrast to radiography, also allows excellent evaluation of retropulsed bone into the spinal canal. However, a higher radiation dose is associated with CT scanning compared with radiography. Dual-energy CT may also be employed in patients with spinal instrumentation to reduce artifacts related to metallic hardware. As a result, CT is often used to image traumatic and nontraumatic osseous spinal pathologic conditions. Although CT is inferior to MRI in its contrast resolution of the soft tissues within the spinal canal, including the spinal cord, nerve roots, epidural compartment, and subdural compartment, it does provide some information about these structures and is certainly superior to radiography.

4. Describe the strengths and drawbacks of MRI.
   MRI provides the best and most direct evaluation of the contents within the spinal canal, including the spinal cord, nerve roots, and epidural and subdural compartments. MRI also provides the most detailed evaluation of the soft tissues, including the intervertebral discs, ligaments, and musculature. Optimal resolution is obtained at high field strengths using phased-array surface coils. Numerous safety concerns arise, however, with the use of MRI. Patients undergoing this examination must be screened for implantable devices and/or retained objects, because many are not MR compatible. Ferromagnetic objects may become projectiles within the magnetic field and injure patients or health

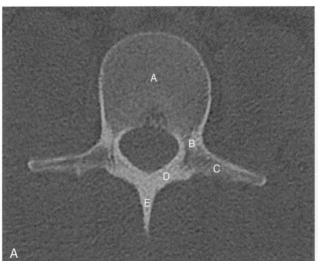
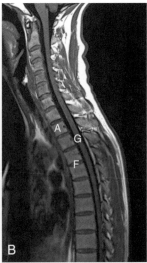

**Figure 42-1.** Normal spine anatomy. **A,** Axial unenhanced CT image of normal vertebra. **B,** Sagittal T1-weighted MR image of spine. *A* = vertebral body; *B* = pedicle; *C* = transverse process; *D* = lamina; *E* = spinous process; *F* = intervertebral disc; *G* = spinal cord.

care providers. When MRI is performed in critically ill patients, MRI-compatible ventilators and monitoring devices must be used. When patients with spinal cord injuries are imaged, spinal precautions must be maintained, and fixation devices must be MRI-compatible. MRI of patients with prior spinal surgery is often of reduced diagnostic value because of artifacts arising from metallic hardware. Use of imaging sequences optimized for metal suppression, however, may mitigate these artifacts. MRI is also time-consuming and requires patient cooperation (i.e., remaining motionless) to obtain high-quality studies.

5. In patients with contraindications to MRI, what imaging study can be used to assess the contents within the spinal canal?
In patients with suspected spinal cord or nerve root compression who cannot be evaluated with MRI, myelography is an alternative, although invasive, technique that may be used to evaluate the spinal canal contents. Myelography is performed most often in patients with contraindications to MRI or who have nondiagnostic MRI studies. Nonionic contrast material is instilled into the subarachnoid space of the spinal canal, typically via lumbar puncture. Risks of this procedure are low, but include headache, allergic reaction to the contrast material, infection, hematoma formation, neural damage, and seizure. The contrast material in the subarachnoid space outlines the spinal cord and nerve roots. Impressions on the contrast column and displacement of neural structures are findings indicative of a pathologic condition (Figure 42-2). Myelography is often complementary with CT, which is performed after myelography for improved delineation of anatomy and spinal pathology.

6. What is discography, and what are its indications?
Discography involves the injection of contrast material into the nucleus pulposus of the intervertebral disc, usually followed by CT scanning of the injected disc. This test is usually performed in patients with multilevel disc disease, axial back pain, or both, in an attempt to reproduce the patient's symptoms and identify the "culprit" disc. Patients with axial back pain, T2-weighted hypointense discs of reduced height, and concordant findings on discography have been reported to have improved outcomes following interbody and combined spinal fusion procedures. Patterns of contrast diffusion may suggest annular degeneration, fissures, or both, although imaging findings must be correlated with patient symptoms (Figure 42-3).

7. What is the primary role of catheter angiography of the spine?
Conventional spinal catheter angiography is primarily used for the detection, characterization, and possible endovascular treatment of spinal vascular malformations.

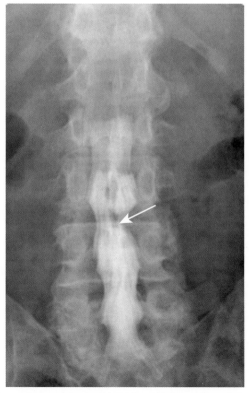

**Figure 42-2.** Disc protrusion on lumbar myelogram. Anteroposterior radiographic image demonstrates extradural impression on thecal sac at L3-4 (*arrow*) with decreased opacification of L3 nerve root sleeve.

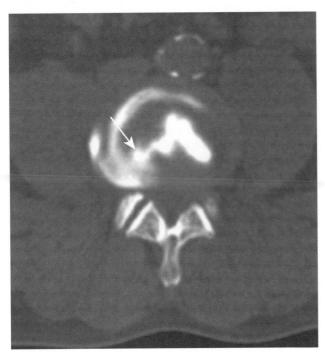

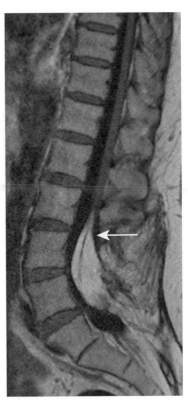

**Figure 42-3.** Degenerative disc disease on CT discography. Note diffuse disc bulge with right lateral disc protrusion. Contrast material extends to outer annular fibers at 7 o'clock position (*arrow*) indicative of radial tear.

**Figure 42-4.** Tethered spinal cord on MRI. Sagittal T1-weighted image reveals abnormally low position of termination of spinal cord at L3 where it is tethered to lipoma (*arrow*).

8. What is spinal dysraphia?

   Spinal anomalies with incomplete midline closure of mesenchymal, osseous, and neural structures are grouped under the term **spinal dysraphia**. Most defects occur in the lumbosacral region.

9. Differentiate between open and occult forms of spinal dysraphia.

   Myeloceles and myelomeningoceles are two types of open spinal dysraphia. Neural tissue (the neural placode, with or without associated meninges) protrudes through the spinal canal and soft tissue defects. Associated abnormalities include Chiari II malformation, hydrocephalus, syringohydromyelia, spinal lipomas, dermoid and epidermoid inclusion cysts, agenesis of the corpus callosum, diastematomyelia, and abnormal spinal curvature. In the occult form of spinal dysraphia, the defects are covered by skin, and no neural tissue is exposed. Occult dysraphias include meningoceles, dorsal dermal sinuses (epithelial-lined tubes connecting the spinal cord and skin), and fat-containing lesions (lipomyelomeningoceles, filum terminale lipomas, and intradural lipomas). Midline cutaneous stigmata (dimples, nevi, and hairy patches) are often present.

10. What are the clinical findings and imaging features of a tethered spinal cord?

    The conus medullaris in adults normally terminates at approximately the L1-L2 level. With a tethered spinal cord/thick filum terminale syndrome (Figure 42-4), the conus medullaris is identified at L2 or below, and the filum terminale is greater than 2 mm in thickness. Associated anomalies (lipomas, diastematomyelia, and myelomeningoceles) are common. Patients typically present in childhood or young adulthood with pain, dysesthesias, bowel or bladder dysfunction, spasticity, and/or kyphoscoliosis.

11. List and describe caudal spinal anomalies.

    Caudal spinal anomalies are malformations of the distal spine, spinal cord, and meninges associated with disorders of the hindgut, kidneys, urinary bladder, and genitalia. Caudal spinal anomalies include the following:

    - **Caudal regression syndrome**: Varying degrees of lumbosacral agenesis with renal and anogenital anomalies and possible fusion of the lower extremities (Figure 42-5).
    - **Terminal myelocystocele**: Cystic dilation of the distal spinal cord, which is tethered, associated with partial sacral agenesis or spina bifida.
    - **Anterior sacral meningocele**: A cerebrospinal fluid (CSF) filled sac that protrudes into the pelvis anterior to the sacrum.

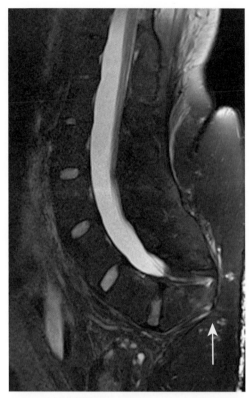

**Figure 42-5.** Caudal regression syndrome on MRI. Sagittal fat-suppressed T2-weighted image reveals partial agenesis of sacrum (*arrow*).

- **Occult intrasacral meningocele**: A mild dural developmental anomaly, a meningeal-lined cyst communicating with the remainder of the thecal sac via a narrow channel, with associated remodeling of the sacrum.
- **Sacrococcygeal teratoma**: The most common presacral mass in children, containing tissue from all three germ layers (endoderm, mesoderm, and ectoderm) and often cystic and solid.

12. What are the split notochord syndromes?

Persistent midline adhesions between endoderm and ectoderm can result in splitting of the notochord. With this split, paired hemicords (diastematomyelia) may result. Persistent endodermal-ectodermal adhesions or communications may produce dorsal enteric fistulas and neuroenteric cysts.
- **Diastematomyelia** predominantly occurs in female patients. In 85% of cases, the split occurs between T9 and S1. The cord is split by a fibrous, osseous, or osteocartilaginous septum, and the hemicords may or may not share a dural sac. Associated neurologic and orthopedic anomalies are common (Figure 42-6).
- **Dorsal enteric fistulas** are very rare and extend from the mesenteric surface of the gut through the prevertebral tissues, vertebrae, and spinal cord to the dorsal skin surface.
- **Neuroenteric cysts** are most often intradural, extramedullary cystic masses in the thoracic region. Vertebral anomalies are seen in less than half of the cases.

13. What are Tarlov cysts?

Tarlov cysts are CSF-filled dilations of sacral nerve root sleeves (Figure 42-7). They are common generally incidental findings detected on spinal CT and MRI scans. They may reach large proportions and may be associated with osseous remodeling/expansion of neural foramina. They originate at the level of the dorsal root ganglion and may result from trapping of CSF. They are rarely symptomatic, but on occasion may compress the adjacent nerve root. Dural ectasia, Tarlov cysts, other perineural cysts, and spinal meningoceles may be seen in association with systemic diseases including connective tissue disorders (such as Marfan's syndrome and Ehlers-Danlos syndrome) as well as phakomatoses such as neurofibromatosis type I (NF-1).

14. What is arachnoiditis?

Arachnoiditis refers to inflammation of the nerve roots of the cauda equina with adhesion of the nerve roots to each other, to the thecal sac, or both. Causes of arachnoiditis include prior surgery, prior intraspinal hemorrhage, inflammatory conditions such as sarcoidosis, prior intrathecal therapy (e.g., chemotherapeutic agents), and prior myelography, particularly with pantopaque. Patients may present with nonspecific back pain, paresthesias, or both. The key imaging features of this diagnosis are abnormal morphologic features and distribution of nerve roots, which

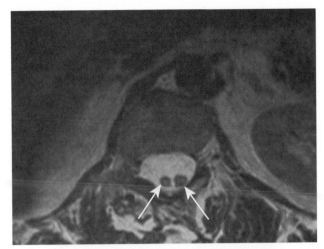

**Figure 42-6.** Diastematomyelia on MRI. Axial T2-weighted image demonstrates two spinal cords within thecal sac (*arrows*).

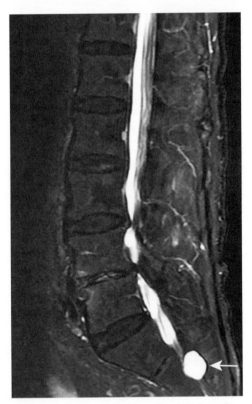

**Figure 42-7.** Tarlov cyst on MRI. Sagittal fat-suppressed T2-weighted image is notable for cystic nerve root sleeve dilation (i.e., Tarlov cyst) at S2 level (*arrow*).

may or may not enhance. Three imaging patterns have been described. The nerve roots may be centrally clumped, appearing as a "pseudocord" within the thecal sac. Alternatively, the nerve roots may be adherent to the periphery of the thecal sac (i.e., the "empty sac" appearance) (Figure 42-8). Uncommonly, the nerve roots may clump together to form a large, mildly enhancing mass, which fills the thecal sac.

15. What are the CT and MR imaging and clinical features of hydrosyringomyelia?
Patients with hydrosyringomyelia may present with sensory disturbances (particularly with respect to pain and temperature and often in a capelike distribution), weakness, spasticity, diminished deep tendon reflexes, and/or bowel and bladder dysfunction. Scoliosis may be present.

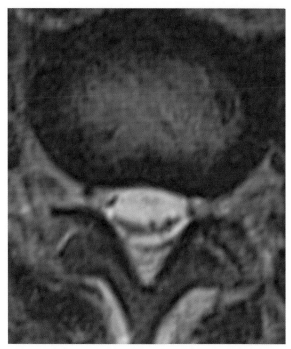

**Figure 42-8.** Arachnoiditis on MRI. Axial T2-weighted image is notable for "empty sac" appearance. Nerve roots are clumped together and displaced to periphery of thecal sac.

This condition may be congenital or acquired and is likely related to abnormal CSF flow dynamics. Common etiologies include Chiari malformations, prior trauma, compressive lesions, and intramedullary neoplasms.

These lesions are best demonstrated on MRI. The cord typically appears expanded with central or slightly eccentric fluid-filled cavity (Figure 42-9). In benign conditions, no enhancement should be seen. On CT, a hypoattenuating lesion may be seen within the spinal cord.

16. **Review the epidemiologic factors of spinal trauma.**
Approximately 30,000 injuries to the spinal column occur in the United States each year. Most injuries are secondary to blunt trauma (most commonly motor vehicle accidents and falls). Penetrating trauma accounts for approximately 10% to 20% of cases. Roughly 2% to 3% of victims of blunt trauma are affected, with a higher incidence of spinal injuries seen in patients with significant craniofacial trauma. Approximately 40% to 50% of spinal injuries produce a neurologic deficit, which is often severe and sometimes fatal. Survival is inversely correlated with patient age. Mortality during initial hospitalization is approximately 10%. Because most patients with spinal trauma are young, the costs of lifetime care and rehabilitation are extremely high, often exceeding $1 million per individual.

17. **What are the appropriate indications for obtaining imaging of the spine in the setting of blunt trauma?**
Pain, neurologic deficit, distracting injuries, altered consciousness (owing to head injury, intoxication, or pharmaceutical intervention), and high-risk mechanism of injury have been shown to be appropriate clinical indications for spinal imaging. The NEXUS and C-spine RULE studies have validated the clinical clearance of approximately 10% to 15% of all trauma patients.

18. **What are the roles of CT and MRI in spinal trauma?**
Fractures and malalignment of the spine are best evaluated with thin-section CT with coronal and sagittal reformatted images. CT is the preferred initial imaging modality in patients with suspected spinal injuries, as it is significantly more sensitive than radiography for detection of fractures and has been shown to be both more time efficient and cost-effective. Spinal cord injuries and other traumatic sequelae within the spinal canal (e.g., disc protrusions, disc extrusions, and subdural and epidural hematomas) are best evaluated with MRI and should be suspected when there are focal neurologic deficits, or when neurologic symptoms are disproportionate to the findings detected on radiographs and CT scans. MRI has a significant role in the evaluation of spinal trauma in the pediatric population, as the incidence of spinal cord injury without radiographic abnormality (SCIWORA) is higher in children than adults. Children (given ligamentous laxity, disproportionate head size, underdeveloped musculature, and immature skeletons) are more likely to suffer soft tissue injuries, and radiation dose considerations are of greater importance.

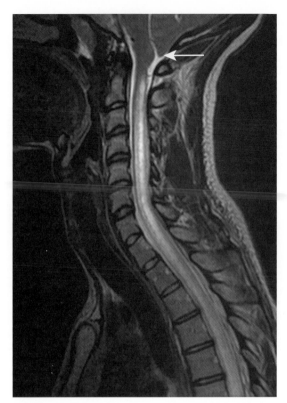

**Figure 42-9.** Hydrosyringomyelia on MRI. Sagittal T2-weighted image demonstrates spinal cord expansion and hyperintense signal intensity due to syrinx in this patient with Chiari I malformation. Note peg-like cerebellar tonsils (*arrow*) that protrude beneath foramen magnum.

19. Describe types of spinal cord injuries.

    Cord contusions are generally seen as hyperintense intramedullary lesions on T2-weighted MR images. The cord may also be expanded (Figure 42-10). The presence of hemorrhage within a contusion is associated with a worse prognosis and may alter the signal intensity characteristics of the lesion. Spinal cord transections are devastating injuries with resultant complete loss of sensory and motor function caudal to the injured level. These lesions are most often seen with penetrating trauma and distraction injuries, as the spinal cord is quite intolerant to stretching (Figure 42-11). MRI may also characterize many compressive lesions, such as epidural and subdural hematomas, disc abnormalities, and osteophytes.

20. What additional structures may be injured in association with cervical spinal trauma that may not be detected on radiographs or CT scans?

    It is always important to consider ligamentous and vascular (especially vertebral artery) injuries in patients with significant trauma to the cervical spine. If there is significant subluxation or dislocation involving the cervical spine on radiographs or CT, ligamentous injury is most likely present. In the absence of subluxation/dislocation, ligamentous injuries may be inapparent, however. Special MRI sequences such as fat-suppressed T2-weighted or short tau inversion recovery (STIR) images usually detect ligamentous injury, including frank disruption, edema, or both. In "high risk" subgroups of patients suffering blunt trauma, the frequency of vascular injury has been reported to be as high as 30%. CTA, MRI, and MRA may be used to evaluate for associated vascular injuries (dissections, occlusions, pseudoaneurysms) that may accompany spinal trauma (Figure 42-12). Conventional angiography is most often reserved for patients requiring endovascular therapy, such as those with active hemorrhage, expanding pseudoaneurysms, and arteriovenous fistulas. In particular, cervical spine fractures involving a transverse process, a foramen transversarium (the osseous canal where the cervical portion of the vertebral artery resides), or both are at higher risk of vertebral artery injury.

21. Name the most common sites of infection in the spine.

    Infections may occur within the vertebra (most commonly the vertebral body [osteomyelitis]), within the disc space (discitis), within the epidural space (abscess), within the meninges (meningitis), and within the paraspinal soft tissues.

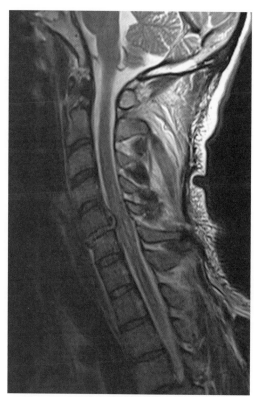

**Figure 42-10.** Spinal cord contusion on MRI. Sagittal T2-weighted image demonstrates mild, grade 1 anterolisthesis of C5 upon C6 with traumatic disc extrusion compressing cervical spinal cord. There is associated contusion of spinal cord seen as spinal cord signal abnormality and expansion extending from C4 through C6-7.

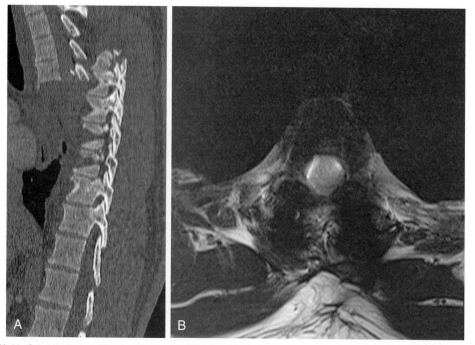

**Figure 42-11.** Spinal fracture on CT and spinal cord transection on MRI. **A,** Sagittal reformatted CT image demonstrates fracture dislocation of midthoracic spine with complete disruption of spinal canal. **B,** Axial T2-weighted MR image obtained following surgical realignment and fixation is notable for complete absence of spinal cord tissue within thecal sac at this midthoracic level. The spinal cord had been transected.

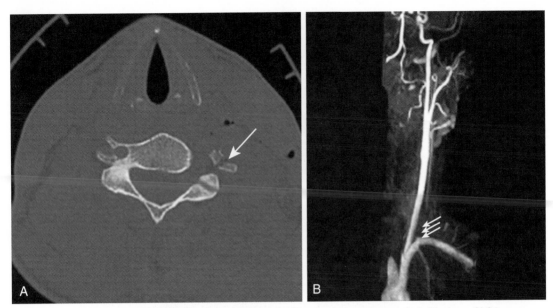

**Figure 42-12.** Traumatic vertebral artery injury on CT and MRI. **A,** Axial CT image demonstrates comminuted fractures of left transverse process adjacent to expected course of left vertebral artery (foramen transversarium) (*arrow*) with extensive soft tissue swelling and subcutaneous emphysema in left neck. **B,** Contrast-enhanced 3D MRA of cervical vasculature reveals no flow in proximal left vertebral artery (*arrows*) secondary to dissection.

22. **What patient populations are particularly prone to the development of infectious spondylodiscitis?**
   Infectious spondylodiscitis most commonly occurs in elderly patients and diabetic patients and in men more often than women. Other groups particularly susceptible to this disorder include intravenous drug abusers, dialysis patients, alcoholics, and immunocompromised individuals.

23. **What is the most common infectious agent responsible for spondylodiscitis?**
   The infecting organism may be bacterial, fungal, or parasitic. The most common cause of discitis is *Staphylococcus aureus*.

24. **What is the typical clinical presentation of discitis?**
   Patients may present with back pain, fever, focal neurologic deficits, leukocytosis, and/or elevated erythrocyte sedimentation rate (ESR) and/or C-reactive protein (CRP).

25. **What are the typical imaging findings of spondylodiscitis?**
   On radiographs and CT, end-plate irregularity/destruction and demineralization may be apparent. The disc space may be narrowed. These findings commonly occur in the later stages of infection, however. Spondylodiscitis may be detected earlier with MRI. The finding of increased signal intensity within the intervertebral disc on T2-weighted images in the appropriate clinical setting should raise suspicion. Loss of disc height with end-plate irregularity or destruction and abnormal signal intensity in the vertebral bone marrow consistent with edema or osteomyelitis can be late imaging findings. Paravertebral soft tissue swelling, fluid collections, and/or abscesses may be present. Typically, enhancement is seen within the bone marrow and disc space. Epidural phlegmon may demonstrate solid enhancement, and the presence of peripheral or "rim" enhancement is usually indicative of abscess formation (Figure 42-13).

26. **Describe the imaging appearance of spondylodiscitis caused by atypical organisms such as tuberculosis.**
   With granulomatous infections such as tuberculosis and fungal infections, there may be relative sparing of the disc space and end plates until late in the infectious course. Earlier involvement of the vertebral bodies is common. Tuberculosis is typically associated with anterior subligamentous involvement, resulting in infection of multiple contiguous levels of the spine.

27. **List noninfectious disorders that can have imaging findings similar to infectious spondylodiscitis.**
   • Degenerative disease or instability
   • Neuropathic arthropathy

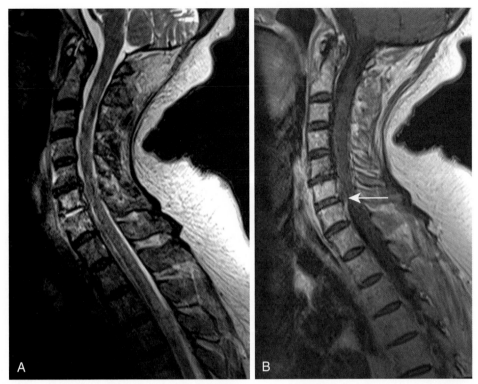

**Figure 42-13.** Spinal discitis/osteomyelitis on MRI. **A,** Sagittal T2-weighted image demonstrates bone marrow edema secondary to osteomyelitis within C6 and C7 vertebral bodies, markedly increased signal intensity within C6-7 intervertebral disc space due to discitis, as well as mild prevertebral soft tissue swelling. **B,** Sagittal contrast-enhanced T1-weighted MR image reveals small peripherally enhancing fluid collection due to abscess (*arrow*) in anterior epidural space. Bone marrow of C6 and C7 as well as prevertebral soft tissue also enhance.

- Dialysis-related arthropathy (amyloid deposition)
- Postoperative changes
- Richter's syndrome (lymphomatous transformation of chronic lymphocytic leukemia)

28. What is the most common inflammatory disorder that affects the spinal cord?

Multiple sclerosis is the most common inflammatory disorder that affects the spinal cord. Patients typically have symptoms of numbness, weakness, or urinary incontinence that wax and wane. Other inflammatory and infectious conditions that involve the spinal cord include neuromyelitis optica (NMO), acute disseminated encephalomyelitis (ADEM), autoimmune disorders including systemic lupus erythematosus, sarcoidosis, Behçet syndrome, paraneoplastic syndromes, and various viral, bacterial, fungal, and parasitic infections including human immunodeficiency virus (HIV) and syphilis.

29. What are the classic imaging findings of multiple sclerosis affecting the spinal cord?

The imaging findings of inflammatory and infectious disorders are often nonspecific. All of these processes produce intramedullary lesions that are hyperintense on T2-weighted MR images. These lesions sometimes enhance and may be associated with cord expansion. More specific diagnoses are often made through correlation of imaging findings with clinical and laboratory data.

The spinal cord is commonly involved in patients with multiple sclerosis. The lesions of multiple sclerosis are often ill-defined, multiple, and located in the dorsolateral white matter of the cord (they are commonly small, but some lesions may extend over several spinal segments) (Figure 42-14). In the active phase of demyelination, the plaques may expand the cord and typically enhance. Chronic lesions lead to focal or generalized cord atrophy.

30. What is the typical MRI appearance of spinal sarcoidosis? How can its appearance, combined with the clinical history, distinguish it from other inflammatory disorders?

The typical MRI appearance of spinal sarcoidosis is extensive leptomeningeal enhancement on the surface of the spinal cord. In sarcoidosis, a long segment of the cord may be expanded with abnormal signal intensity. With sarcoidosis, in contrast to many of the other inflammatory conditions, there typically is pronounced enhancement of the leptomeninges on the surface of the cord. Foci of intramedullary enhancement may also be present.

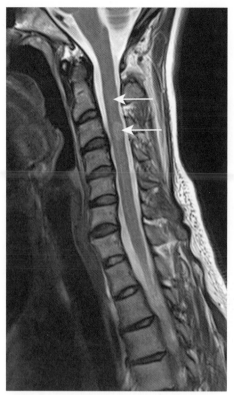

**Figure 42-14.** Demyelinating disease on MRI. Sagittal T2-weighted image reveals foci of hyperintensity within cervical spinal cord (at C2 and C3 levels) (*arrows*).

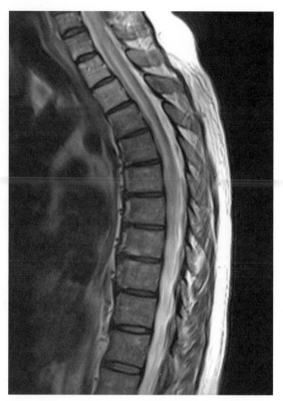

**Figure 42-15.** Radiation myelitis on MRI. Sagittal T2-weighted image demonstrates expansion and edema of upper thoracic spinal cord in patient previously treated with radiation therapy for thymoma. Note uniform fatty replacement of marrow of upper thoracic vertebral bodies also caused by prior radiation therapy.

31. What is the typical time course for the development of radiation myelitis after irradiation for treatment of tumor?

Radiation myelitis generally manifests within 6 months to 3 years after treatment, but may present almost immediately following the completion of therapy or many years following therapy. It occurs within the treatment portal, and the bone marrow of the vertebrae within the port typically is fatty replaced. On MRI, the spinal cord usually has T2-weighted hyperintensity, is expanded, and may enhance (Figure 42-15).

32. Which disorders commonly affect the dorsal spinal cord?

Syphilis has a predilection for the dorsal columns of the spinal cord. With syphilitic infection, enhancement may be seen along the pial surface of the cord and nerve roots. Vasculitis may accompany the infection and lead to cord infarctions. Vacuolar myelopathy occurs in approximately 15% to 30% of patients with acquired immunodeficiency syndrome (AIDS) and more commonly affects the posterolateral cord. Pathologically, vacuoles and lipid-laden macrophages are seen in the white matter. The imaging findings of $B_{12}$ deficiency (spinal cord expansion with signal abnormality in the dorsal columns) may mimic those of syphilis.

33. Name the two most common vascular disorders of the spinal cord.

The two most common vascular disorders of the spinal cord are spinal cord infarcts and vascular malformations.

34. What is the arterial vascular supply to the spinal cord?

The anterior spinal artery is the main arterial supply to the spinal cord. Additional supply is through paired posterior spinal arteries. The anterior spinal artery is located in the midline. In the cervical and upper thoracic cord, contributions to the anterior spinal artery are from the vertebral, cervical, and superior intercostal arteries. A small component of supply to the midthoracic cord arises from the midthoracic intercostal arteries. The predominant contribution to the anterior spinal artery in the lower thoracic and lumbar regions (otherwise known as the artery of Adamkiewicz) most often arises from thoracic intercostal or lumbar arteries, usually on the left, generally between T8 and L2 (Figure 42-16).

35. What are the typical clinical characteristics and imaging findings of spinal cord infarcts?

Spinal cord infarcts most often occur in elderly patients with atherosclerotic vascular disease. Patients undergoing thoracoabdominal aneurysm repair are particularly at risk. Lower thoracic intercostal or upper lumbar arteries are often

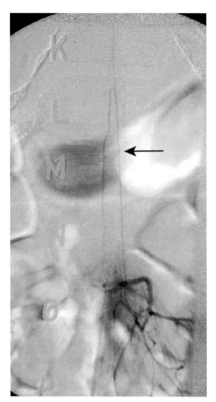

**Figure 42-16.** Anterior spinal artery on conventional angiography. Anteroposterior radiograph from spinal angiogram demonstrates anterior spinal artery (*arrow*) making its classic "hairpin" turn.

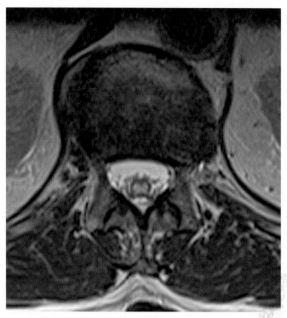

**Figure 42-17.** Spinal cord infarct on MRI. Axial T2-weighted image reveals central hyperintensity of spinal cord.

sacrificed with aneurysm repair procedures, jeopardizing the artery of Adamkiewicz. Patients with spinal cord infarction experience sudden onset of paraplegia, often associated with pain. On MRI, signal abnormality is seen within the central gray matter (Figure 42-17).

36. List types of spinal vascular malformations, and describe their clinical and imaging characteristics.
    - **Dural arteriovenous fistulas** are the most common of the spinal vascular anomalies seen in adults. They typically affect middle-aged and older men, who present with chronic, progressive motor and sensory deficits, usually in the lower extremities. Bowel, bladder, and sexual dysfunction also often occur. These are acquired lesions, most often occurring in the lower thoracic and upper lumbar spine. Arterial supply is from the dural arteries, arising from radicular branches. MRI is notable for diffuse enlargement and signal abnormality within the cord, generally involving the conus. Large vessels, representing dilated veins, are seen within the thecal sac. Enhancement may be present within the cord. The diagnosis is confirmed with spinal angiography (Figure 42-18). Treatment consists of embolization or surgery or both.
    - **Arteriovenous malformations** are seen in younger patients (often teenagers) and often present acutely secondary to intramedullary and/or subarachnoid hemorrhage. The arteriovenous malformation nidus is located within or on the surface of the cord and is supplied by the anterior or posterior spinal arteries (Figure 42-19). In the juvenile variant, the nidus also involves the vertebral column. Therapeutic options for these lesions are limited, often carry greater risks, and include embolization, surgery, and radiosurgery.
    - **Arteriovenous fistulas** are uncommon. They are direct intradural fistulous connections from the anterior or posterior spinal arteries to the pial veins. These lesions typically occur in the thoracic and lumbar regions. Patients with these lesions may have a slowly progressive myelopathy or radiculopathy or may present with subarachnoid hemorrhage. These lesions usually manifest in the second to fourth decades of life. Treatment options again include embolization and surgery.
    - **Aneurysms** of the anterior and posterior spinal arteries are most often seen in association with arteriovenous malformations. Rarely, they may be seen as isolated entities. Patients with these lesions may present with back pain, paralysis, and/or subarachnoid hemorrhage.

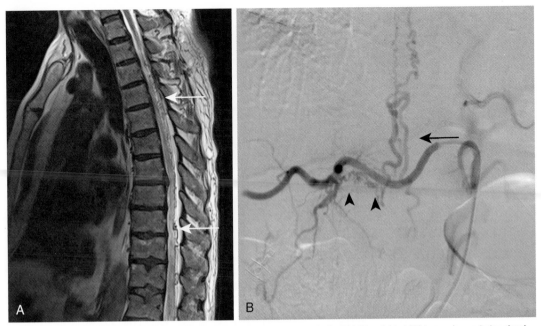

**Figure 42-18.** Dural arteriovenous fistula on MRI and conventional angiography. **A,** Sagittal T2-weighted MR image demonstrates signal abnormality with expansion of thoracic cord with serpentine flow voids along its dorsal surface (*arrows*). Degenerative changes of spine including disc protrusions and Schmorl's nodes are also present. **B,** Frontal projection angiographic image obtained during contrast injection of right intercostal artery reveals prominent radicular branch supplying fistula (*arrowheads*) within right nerve root sleeve. Enlarged pial veins (*arrow*) are also demonstrated within spinal canal.

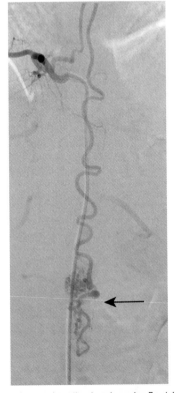

**Figure 42-19.** Spinal cord arteriovenous malformation on conventional angiography. Frontal projection angiographic image obtained during contrast injection of right intercostal artery demonstrates enlarged anterior spinal artery supplying arteriovenous malformation nidus within spinal cord (*arrow*).

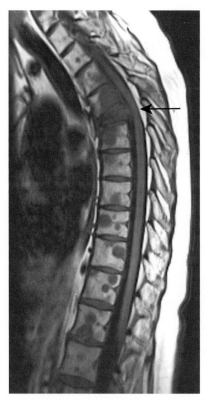

**Figure 42-20.** Spinal metastatic disease with spinal cord compression on MRI. Sagittal T1-weighted image of cervical and thoracic spine is notable for heterogeneous bone marrow signal intensity with multiple rounded hypointense lesions, prominent replacement of upper thoracic vertebral body, and pathologic compression fracture with resultant compromise of spinal canal with cord compression (*arrow*).

- **Cavernomas** may occur anywhere in the spinal cord. They may manifest at any age, chronically or acutely (secondary to hemorrhage). Back pain is often reported. On imaging studies, they are often well-demarcated intramedullary lesions with a surrounding hemosiderin ring (hypointense in signal intensity on T2-weighted MR images). Surrounding signal abnormality due to edema or gliosis may be present, and these lesions may be calcified. Symptomatic lesions are treated with surgical excision.

37. How are spinal lesions classified anatomically?
    - Extradural
    - Intradural-extramedullary
    - Intramedullary

38. Describe the clinical and imaging features of neural compression.
    Cross-sectional imaging, in particular MRI, optimizes detection of spinal cord or nerve root compression (Figure 42-20). Lesions producing spinal cord and/or nerve root compression are most commonly epidural in location, but may be located in the intradural extramedullary compartment. As above, etiologies may be benign or malignant, and presentations may be chronic, subacute, or acute. Patients with benign chronic conditions such as discogenic disease, spondylosis deformans, and spinal canal stenosis may present with a chronic and progressive myelopathy. Imaging studies will often demonstrate distortion of the spinal cord with associated cord atrophy and signal abnormality (myelomalacia). In the settings of malignancy, acute trauma (displaced fractures, malalignment, acute disc protrusion or extrusion), and infection (discitis/osteomyelitis with epidural phlegmon/abscess), patients are more likely to present acutely with pain and loss of sensory, motor, and/or bowel/bladder/sexual function. Such cases must be treated emergently. Neurologic outcomes have been shown to be improved when decompression occurs within 24 hours.

39. What is the most common epidural spinal tumor in adults?
    Metastases are the most common neoplasms involving the epidural space. Epidural involvement is usually related to direct extension from an adjacent vertebral bone metastasis, although involvement of the epidural space in the absence of bone involvement on imaging can occur (most often with lymphoma, leukemia, Ewing sarcoma, breast cancer, and lung cancer). On radiography and CT, metastases may appear as lytic or sclerotic lesions. Pathologic compression fractures may result. Typically, metastases demonstrate increased uptake of radiotracer on bone scintigraphy and $^{18}$F-fluorodeoxyglucose (FDG) positron emission tomography (PET). MRI is the most sensitive structural

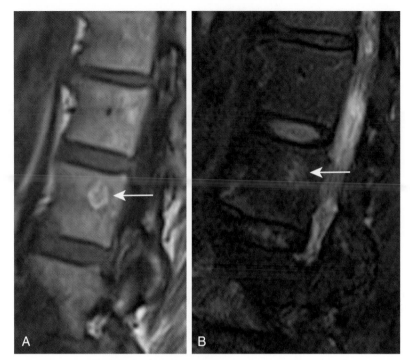

**Figure 42-21.** Spinal hemangioma on MRI. **A,** Sagittal T1-weighted image of lumbar spine and **B,** Sagittal fat-suppressed T2-weighted image of lumbar spine demonstrate mildly heterogeneous well-circumscribed, partially fat-containing, rounded lesion within vertebral body (*arrow*).

imaging modality for the detection of osseous metastases, which appear as foci of signal abnormality within the marrow space, typically hypointense on T1-weighted images and hyperintense on fat-suppressed T2-weighted images relative to skeletal muscle with variable enhancement characteristics (see Figure 42-20). Metastatic lesions are also associated with abnormal diffusion restriction on diffusion-weighted MR images.

40. What is the most common benign osseous lesion involving the spine?

Usually an incidental finding, hemangiomas are benign, present in approximately 11% of patients, and have a characteristic appearance on MRI. They are typically markedly hyperintense on T2-weighted images, and, because they contain internal fat, are also hyperintense on T1-weighted images (Figure 42-21). On CT, they characteristically appear as well-circumscribed geographic lytic lesions with fat attenuation and thickened trabeculae leading to a characteristic "corduroy" appearance (in the sagittal or coronal plane) or a "polka-dot" appearance (in the axial plane). Rarely, these lesions may have extraosseous extension and/or may be symptomatic.

41. What is the differential diagnosis for an intradural-extramedullary neoplasm?

The most common intradural-extramedullary neoplasms are benign and include meningiomas and neural neoplasms (neurofibromas and schwannomas). Meningiomas most commonly occur in the midthoracic region and are much more common in women than in men. Nerve sheath tumors typically enhance avidly and extend along or envelop a nerve root. These tumors may have intradural and extradural components. These tumors are often slow-growing, and bony remodeling, neural foraminal expansion, and vertebral body scalloping are common secondary imaging findings (Figure 42-22). Malignant lesions in the differential diagnosis include metastases, lymphoma, and malignant nerve sheath tumors.

42. What neoplasms are associated with leptomeningeal seeding of tumor?

Leptomeningeal metastatic disease may occur with primary central nervous system neoplasms and with systemic malignancies. Medulloblastoma, ependymoma, glioblastoma multiforme, and other high-grade astrocytomas are the primary central nervous system tumors that are most often associated with leptomeningeal seeding. This phenomenon may also occur, however, with choroid plexus tumors, other glial tumors (including pilocytic astrocytomas), germ cell tumors, retinoblastomas, and primary spinal tumors.

Systemic tumors, including lymphoma, may directly invade the subarachnoid space or may disseminate via lymphatic or hematogenous means. On MRI, leptomeningeal tumor often produces enhancement along the surface of the spinal cord that may be nodular and diffuse and is most prominent along the lumbar nerve roots and cauda equina (Figure 42-23). There may be associated edema (seen as T2-weighted hyperintensity) within the spinal cord. Imaging of the brain may be notable for communicating hydrocephalus. Adequate CSF sampling (up to three high-volume lumbar punctures) remains more sensitive than imaging for the detection of leptomeningeal disease.

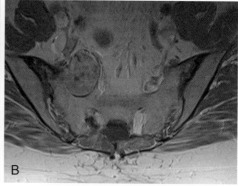

**Figure 42-22.** Neural foraminal schwannoma on MRI. **A,** Axial T1-weighted and **B,** Axial contrast-enhanced T1-weighted MR images through sacrum reveal oval, heterogeneous, well-demarcated mass, expanding right sacral foramen.

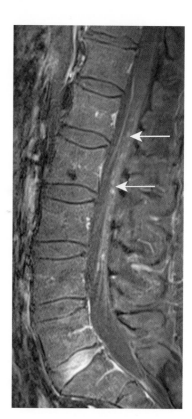

**Figure 42-23.** Leptomeningeal spread of tumor. Sagittal contrast-enhanced fat-suppressed T1-weighted image of lumbosacral spine in patient with widely metastatic lung cancer demonstrates multiple small enhancing nodules (*arrows*) along nerve roots representing leptomeningeal metastases.

43. List the most common intramedullary spinal tumors.
    - Ependymoma
    - Astrocytoma
    - Hemangioblastoma
    - Metastasis

44. Describe the distinguishing clinical and imaging features of intramedullary spinal tumors.
    - **Ependymomas** occur in all age groups, are the most common intramedullary neoplasms in adults, and are slightly more common in men. Ependymoma is the most common primary tumor of the lower spinal cord, conus medullaris, and filum terminale. Imaging findings include bony remodeling (spinal canal expansion, vertebral body scalloping, or pedicle erosion), spinal cord expansion, centrally located mass within the conus or filum, and heterogeneous signal intensity and enhancement, often with hemorrhage or hypercellularity (Figure 42-24).
    - **Astrocytomas** most often occur in the thoracic cord in young adults and children. On MRI, the spinal cord is typically expanded with decreased T1-weighted and increased T2-weighted signal intensity. These tumors are most often eccentric in location and enhance. Cysts may be seen within or adjacent to the lesions.

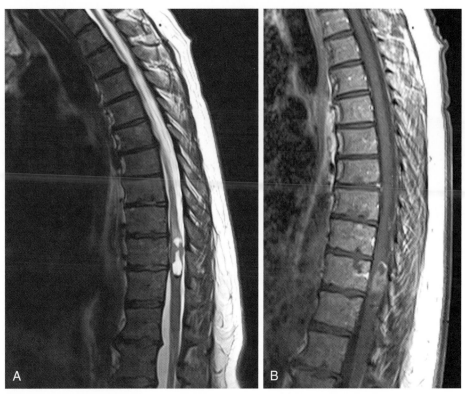

**Figure 42-24.** Spinal cord ependymoma on MRI. **A,** Sagittal T2-weighted image of thoracic spine demonstrates ovoid, lobulated, partially cystic and likely partially hemorrhagic intramedullary lesion. **B,** Sagittal contrast-enhanced T1-weighted image shows heterogeneous enhancement within mass.

- **Hemangioblastomas** are the third most common of the primary intramedullary tumors, but account for less than 5% of such tumors. These tumors are commonly seen in patients with von Hippel-Lindau disease. Hemangioblastomas are most often solitary, are located in the thoracic region, enhance avidly, and are commonly associated with cysts. Because these tumors are often vascular, enlarged vessels may be seen within the spinal canal. Although most are intramedullary, hemangioblastomas may also be intradural-extramedullary or extradural in location.
- **Intramedullary metastases** are less common and are typically found in patients with widespread metastatic disease. They are typically associated with extensive spinal cord edema. The most common primary tumor to metastasize to the spinal cord is lung cancer. Spinal cord metastases may also be seen with breast cancer, melanoma, lymphoma, colon cancer, and renal cell carcinoma.

## KEY POINTS

- With regards to imaging evaluation of the spine:
  - Radiography is used to evaluate for fractures, degenerative changes, and alignment.
  - CT is used to evaluate for osseous pathologic conditions, especially fractures.
  - MRI is the best modality for evaluating the spinal cord, bone marrow, soft tissues including the discs and ligaments, and epidural and subdural compartments.
  - Myelography is reserved largely for symptomatic patients who cannot undergo MRI examination and for those with poor quality or nondiagnostic MRI examinations.
  - Spinal catheter angiography is used primarily for spinal vascular malformations.
- Extradural spinal lesions are located outside the thecal sac. These include intervertebral disc pathology, metastasis, primary osseous abnormalities, epidural abscess, and epidural hematoma.
- Intradural-extramedullary spinal lesions are located inside the thecal sac but outside the spinal cord. These include nerve sheath tumors (neurofibroma, schwannoma), meningioma, metastasis, lymphoma, sarcoidosis, lipoma, arachnoid cyst, and dural vascular malformation.
- Intramedullary spinal lesions are located inside the spinal cord. These include neoplasms (astrocytoma, ependymoma, hemangioblastoma, metastasis), demyelinating processes, infectious and inflammatory myelitis, metabolic disorders, spinal cord ischemia, arteriovenous malformation, cavernoma, and syrinx.

## BIBLIOGRAPHY

Burlew CC, Biffl WL, Moore EE, et al. Blunt cerebrovascular injuries: redefining screening criteria in the era of noninvasive diagnosis. *J Trauma Acute Care Surg.* 2012;72(2):330-335, discussion 6-7, quiz 539.

Fehlings MG, Vaccaro A, Wilson JR, et al. Early versus delayed decompression for traumatic cervical spinal cord injury: results of the Surgical Timing in Acute Spinal Cord Injury Study (STASCIS). *PLoS ONE.* 2012;7(2):e32037.

Yousem DM, Zimmerman RD, Grossman RI. *Neuroradiology: the requisites.* 3rd ed. Philadelphia: Mosby Elsevier; 2010.

Atlas SW. *Magnetic resonance imaging of the brain and spine.* 4th ed. Philadelphia: Lippincott Williams & Wilkins; 2009.

Stiell IG, Wells GA, Vandemheen KL, et al. The Canadian C-spine rule for radiography in alert and stable trauma patients. *JAMA.* 2001;286(15):1841-1848.

Hoffman JR, Mower WR, Wolfson AB, et al. Validity of a set of clinical criteria to rule out injury to the cervical spine in patients with blunt trauma. National Emergency X-Radiography Utilization Study Group. *N Engl J Med.* 2000;343(2):94-99.

# CHAPTER 43

# HEAD AND NECK IMAGING, PART 1

*Deepak Mavahalli Sampathu, MD, PhD, Mary H. Scanlon, MD, FACR, and Laurie A. Loevner, MD*

1. **The hyoid bone divides the neck into what two distinct regions?**
   The hyoid bone divides the neck into the **suprahyoid neck** (extending from the skull base to the hyoid bone) and the **infrahyoid neck** (extending from the hyoid bone to the cervicothoracic junction) (Figure 43-1). The hyoid bone is a logical dividing point because its fascial attachments functionally cleave the neck into these two distinct anatomic regions.

2. **Which imaging modalities are used to evaluate lesions in the suprahyoid and infrahyoid neck?**
   Magnetic resonance imaging (MRI) without and with intravenous gadolinium contrast material is the study of choice for the evaluation of lesions in the suprahyoid neck. The superior soft tissue contrast of MRI enables detailed evaluation of the skull base and evaluation for intracranial extension of disease from direct growth and/or perineural spread. In the infrahyoid neck, where there is abundance of fat and less complex anatomy, computed tomography (CT) with intravenous iodinated contrast material is the imaging study of choice.

3. **What are the three anatomic subdivisions of the pharynx?**
   The three subdivisions of the pharynx are the nasopharynx, oropharynx, and hypopharynx (see Figure 43-1). The **nasopharynx** extends from the base of the skull to the superior surface of the soft palate. The **oropharynx** extends from the soft palate to the hyoid bone. The **hypopharynx** extends from the hyoid bone to the inferior aspect of the cricoid cartilage. The oral cavity is a separate anatomic compartment distinct from the pharynx. The oral cavity is located anterior to the oropharynx, from which it is anatomically demarcated by a ring of structures that include the circumvallate papillae of the tongue, the anterior tonsillar pillars, and the soft palate (Figure 43-2).

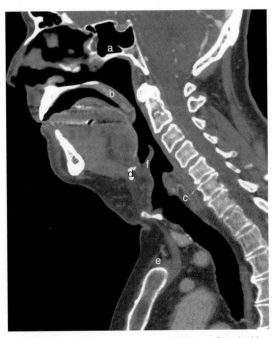

**Figure 43-1.** Normal neck anatomy on CT. Midline sagittal contrast-enhanced CT image. Suprahyoid neck extends from skull base (*a*) to hyoid bone (*d*), and infrahyoid neck extends from hyoid bone bone (*d*) to cervicothoracic junction (*e*). Nasopharynx extends from skull base (*a*) to superior surface of soft palate (*b*). Oropharynx extends from soft palate (*b*) to hyoid bone (*d*). Hypopharynx extends from hyoid bone (*d*) to inferior cricoid cartilage (*c*). Larynx (comprised of supraglottis, glottis, and subglottis) also extends from hyoid bone (*d*) to inferior cricoid cartilage (*c*). Epiglottis (*f*) is part of supraglottic larynx.

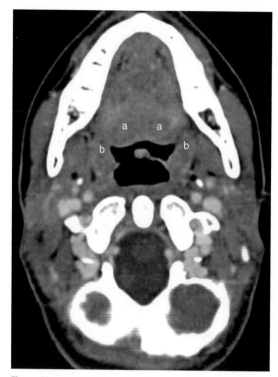

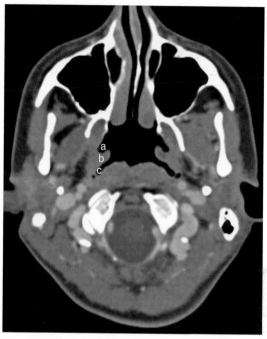

**Figure 43-3.** Normal nasopharynx anatomy on CT. Axial contrast-enhanced CT image. *a* = opening of eustachian tube, *b* = torus tubarius, and *c* = lateral nasopharyngeal recess (also known as fossa of Rosenmüller; most common site of origin of nasopharyngeal cancers).

**Figure 43-2.** Normal oral cavity anatomy on CT. Axial contrast-enhanced CT image. *a* = circumvallate papillae, *b* = anterior tonsillar pillars, which along with soft palate separate oral cavity anteriorly from oropharynx posteriorly.

4. Name the parts of the nasopharynx.
   The nasopharynx is divided into three subsites: the posterior-superior wall (which includes the adenoids and overlying mucosa), the lateral recess (also known as the "fossa of Rosenmüller") present bilaterally, and the anterior-inferior wall (which is the superior surface of the soft palate). The torus tubarius, which is located bilaterally, serves as the cartilaginous opening of the eustachian tube (Figure 43-3).

5. Name the parts of the oropharynx.
   The oropharynx includes the posterior third of the tongue (base of tongue), the paired valleculae, the palatine tonsils, and the tonsillar fossae, as well as the soft palate and uvula.

6. What is Waldeyer's ring?
   Waldeyer's ring is an annular configuration of lymphoid tissue in the nasopharynx and oropharynx, including the adenoids, palatine tonsils, and lingual tonsillar tissue at the tongue base.

7. The piriform sinuses are in what part of the aerodigestive tract?
   The paired piriform sinuses are the lateral boundaries of the hypopharynx. The hypopharynx also has a postcricoid region inferiorly and a posterior wall.

8. What structures are parts of the oral cavity?
   The oral cavity includes the lips, the anterior two thirds of the tongue (oral tongue), the buccal mucosa, the gingiva, the hard palate, the retromolar trigone, and the floor of the mouth.

9. What are the three anatomic subsites of the larynx?
   The supraglottis, glottis, and subglottis are the anatomic subsites of the larynx. The soft tissues of the larynx are supported by a cartilaginous framework that includes the cricoid, thyroid, and arytenoid cartilages.

10. What are the boundaries of the supraglottic larynx?
    The superior extent of the supraglottis is the tip of the epiglottis, and inferiorly the supraglottis extends to the laryngeal ventricle which separates the false vocal folds (part of the supraglottic larynx) from the true vocal cords (part of the glottic larynx) (Figure 43-4). The supraglottis includes the epiglottis, the paired aryepiglottic folds, the paired arytenoid cartilages, and the paired false vocal cords. The aryepiglottic folds separate the medially situated supraglottic airway from the laterally situated piriform sinuses of the hypopharynx.

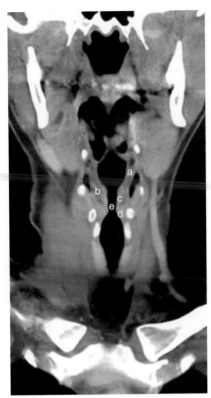

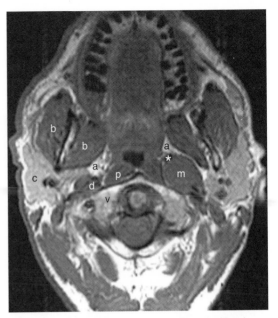

**Figure 43-5.** Normal extramucosal spaces of suprahyoid neck on MRI. Axial T1-weighted MR image shows normal extramucosal spaces on right side of neck: parapharyngeal space (*a*), masticator space (*b*), parotid space (*c*), carotid space (*d*), prevertebral space (*p*), and vertebral space (*v*). On left side of neck, note carotid space mass (*m*) with characteristic anterior displacement of fat in parapharyngeal space (*a*). Retropharynx is a "potential space" that sits anterior to prevertebral space (*p*), and posterior to pharyngeal constrictor muscles. Anterior displacement of internal carotid artery (*) places this mass in carotid space (*d*).

**Figure 43-4.** Normal supraglottic larynx anatomy on CT. Coronal contrast-enhanced CT image. Supraglottis extends from tip of epiglottis superiorly (not shown) to laryngeal ventricle (*e*). Laryngeal ventricle separates false vocal cords (*c*) of supraglottis from true vocal cords (*d*) of glottis. Aryepiglottic folds (*a*) separate supraglottic airway from lateral piriform sinuses of hypopharynx. Tumor can spread transglottically in fat of submucosal paraglottic space (*b*). Mucosal surfaces of paraglottic space may also serve as conduits of spread of laryngeal cancer from one part of larynx to another (i.e., supraglottic cancer may spread to glottis and subglottis).

11. What structures comprise the glottis?
    The glottis includes the paired true vocal cords, the paired vocal ligaments, the anterior commissure, and the posterior commissure.

12. Where is the subglottis located?
    The subglottis is the region of the larynx that extends from the undersurface of the true vocal cords to the inferior surface of the cricoid cartilage.

13. Name and identify the extramucosal spaces of the head and neck in Figure 43-5.
    Lateral to the pharyngeal airway are the prestyloid parapharyngeal space (PPS), the masticator space (MS), the parotid space (PS), and the carotid space (CS). Posterior to the pharyngeal airway are the retropharyngeal space (RPS) and the perivertebral space (PVS). The PPS is the central, primarily fat-containing space around which the other extramucosal spaces are located. The PPS contains fat, lymphatics, nerves, and minor salivary gland rests. The MS contains the muscles of mastication (lateral pterygoid, medial pterygoid, masseter, and temporalis muscles), the ascending ramus of the mandible, and the third branch (V3) of the trigeminal nerve. The PS includes the parotid gland, the facial nerve (VII), the retromandibular vein, the external carotid artery branches, and the intraparotid lymph nodes. The CS includes the internal carotid artery, the internal jugular vein, and cranial nerves IX through XII. Note that the sympathetic nerve plexus and lymph nodes of the deep cervical chain are closely associated with the CS. The RPS includes predominantly fat and lymph nodes. The PVS includes the prevertebral muscle complex (longus colli and longus capitis muscles), the paraspinal muscles, the vertebral bodies, the neurovascular structures exiting the spinal canal, and the brachial plexus. The transverse processes of the vertebral bodies demarcate the PVS into the prevertebral space anteriorly and the paraspinal component posteriorly. If one can localize a mass to the correct extramucosal space, and if the anatomic components of that space are known (Table 43-1), then a short, concise differential diagnosis can be easily formulated.

**Table 43-1.** Extramucosal Spaces of the Head and Neck and Their Contents

| EXTRAMUCOSAL SPACE | CONTENTS |
| --- | --- |
| Parapharyngeal space (PPS) | Fat, lymphatics, nerves, minor salivary gland tissue |
| Masticator space (MS) | Muscles of mastication, ascending ramus of mandible, third branch (V3) of the trigeminal nerve |
| Parotid space (PS) | Parotid gland, facial nerve (VII), retromandibular vein, external carotid artery branches, intraparotid lymph nodes |
| Carotid space (CS) | Internal carotid artery, internal jugular vein, cranial nerves IX through XII (sympathetic nerve plexus and lymph nodes closely associated with CS) |
| Retropharyngeal space (RPS) | Fat, lymph nodes |
| Perivertebral space (PVS) | Prevertebral muscle complex, paraspinal muscles, vertebrae, neurovascular structures in the spinal canal, brachial plexus |

14. Describe how displacement of the fat in the PPS helps to localize lesions or masses to their correct anatomic subsite in the extramucosal compartment.
    The PPS is the central, primarily fat-containing, space that is surrounded by the MS anteriorly, the CS posteriorly, the PS laterally, and the pharyngeal mucosal space medially. Deviation of the fat in the PPS can help localize large masses to one of these four spaces. A large lesion in the MS displaces the PPS fat posteromedially, a mass in the PS displaces it medially, a CS mass displaces the PPS fat anteriorly, and submucosal extension of a pharyngeal mucosal mass displaces the fat laterally (see Figure 43-5).

15. Displacement of the prevertebral muscle complex helps differentiate masses in what two extramucosal spaces?
    Displacement of the longus colli/longus capitis prevertebral muscle complex helps differentiate masses in the RPS and PVS. If the muscles are displaced posteriorly, then the mass arises either from the pharyngeal mucosal space or from the RPS. If the muscles are elevated anteriorly off of the spine, then the mass arises from the PVS (usually from the bone).

16. Displacement of the cervical internal carotid artery helps differentiate masses in what two extramucosal spaces?
    Displacement of the cervical internal carotid artery helps differentiate masses in the PPS (prestyloid parapharyngeal space) and CS (also known as the post-styloid parapharyngeal space). Masses in the PPS, when large enough, displace the adjacent internal carotid artery posteriorly, whereas masses in the CS displace the internal carotid artery anteriorly (because the nerves from which many of the masses in this space arise sit behind the internal carotid artery) (see Figure 43-5).

17. What are the imaging criteria for diagnosis of a pathologic cervical lymph node?
    Imaging criteria for pathologic cervical lymph nodes are based on nodal size and architecture. Any lymph node, regardless of size, that exhibits central necrosis or cystic change is pathologic until proven otherwise (Figure 43-6). The size criteria used to diagnose a pathologic cervical lymph node depend on nodal location. The cervical nodes are anatomically classified by location (levels I to VII) as follows:
    - Level I nodes are the submental and submandibular nodes.
    - Level II, III, and IV nodes are in the internal jugular chain; level II nodes are located from the base of the skull to the inferior margin of the hyoid bone, level III nodes are located between the inferior margin of the hyoid bone and inferior margin of the cricoid cartilage, and level IV nodes are located below the cricoid cartilage.
    - Level V nodes are posterior to the posterior margin of the sternocleidomastoid muscle.
    - Level VI nodes are in the deep visceral chain medial to the internal carotid arteries between the hyoid bone and sternal notch.
    - Level VII nodes are in the superior mediastinum.
        Level I nodes and the jugulodigastric nodes (the only named level II node) are considered pathologic if they are >1.5 cm in size. Otherwise, the upper limit of normal size for level II to VII nodes is 1 cm.

18. What is the best cross-sectional imaging study to identify pathologic nodes?
    If the only clinical question is whether there are pathologic lymph nodes in the neck, neck CT with intravenous contrast administration is the study of choice. Due to its higher spatial resolution, contrast-enhanced CT is more accurate than MRI in detecting nodal necrosis, especially in nodes that are normal in size.

19. What is the most common cause of a calcified cervical lymph node?
    In an adult, the most common cause is metastatic papillary thyroid carcinoma. In a child, metastatic neuroblastoma is the most common cause of calcified lymph nodes. Other less common causes of calcified

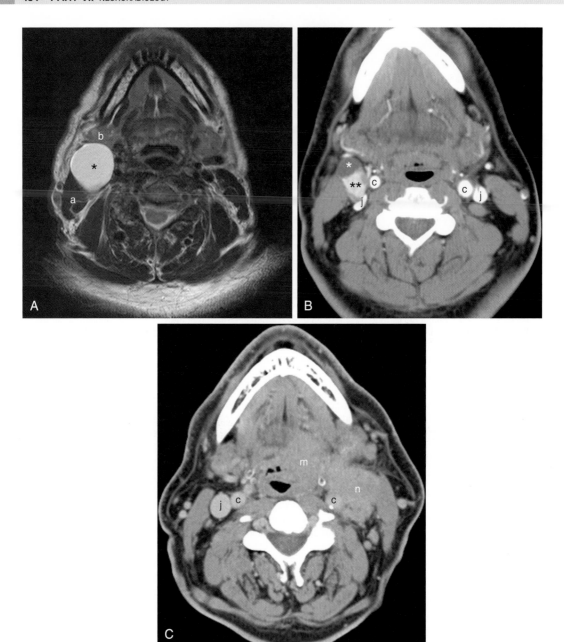

**Figure 43-6.** Pathologic lymph nodes resulting from metastatic thyroid cancer and metastatic head and neck cancer on MRI and CT. **A,** Axial T2-weighted MR image through suprahyoid neck demonstrates high signal intensity cystic lymph node (*) with barely perceptible wall located anteromedial to sternocleidomastoid muscle (a) and posterior to submandibular gland (b), proven to be secondary to metastatic papillary thyroid cancer. In children, cystic mass behind angle of mandible is most likely a branchial cleft cyst. In adults, cystic neck mass is a pathologic lymph node until proven otherwise, where differential diagnosis includes metastatic papillary thyroid cancer and metastasis from oropharyngeal squamous cell carcinoma arising from base of tongue or tonsil. **B,** Axial contrast-enhanced CT image through suprahyoid neck in different patient reveals complex right cervical lymph node from metastatic papillary thyroid carcinoma. Note cystic component anteriorly (*) and solid enhancing component posteriorly (**). Node compresses right internal jugular vein (j). Note normal internal carotid arteries (c) and left internal jugular vein (j). **C,** Axial contrast-enhanced CT image through suprahyoid neck in different patient shows solid conglomerate left cervical lymph node mass (n). Left internal jugular vein is not visualized, indicating compression or invasion of vein. Note primary neoplasm in left base of tongue (m), and internal carotid arteries (c) and contralateral internal jugular vein (j).

lymph nodes include tuberculosis, nontuberculous granulomatous infections, sarcoidosis, and treated lymphoma and other cancers.

20. What is the most common cause of a cystic mass in the lateral neck of an adult?
Metastatic lymphadenopathy is the most common cause of a cystic mass in the lateral neck of an adult. Causes of such metastases include papillary thyroid cancer and squamous cell carcinoma (see Figure 43-6). Carcinoma of the base of the tongue and tonsillar carcinoma (which are both oropharyngeal carcinomas) are the most common primary head and neck carcinomas that result in cystic nodal metastases. Metastatic cancer should always be the primary consideration of a cystic neck mass in adults. Branchial cleft cysts are usually diagnosed in young patients. They are most often found near the angle of the jaw, anteromedial to the sternocleidomastoid muscle, posterior to the submandibular gland, and lateral to the CS.

21. What are the most common causes of cervical lymph node metastases in an adult?
In 85% of patients older than 40 years, lymph node metastases from squamous cell carcinoma of the head and neck are most common. In patients 20 to 40 years old, the major differential diagnosis includes metastatic squamous cell carcinoma, metastatic thyroid cancer, and inflammatory lymphadenitis.

22. In patients with head and neck cancer, how does the presence of metastatic lymphadenopathy affect prognosis?
The presence of metastatic lymph nodes reduces the 5-year survival of patients with squamous cell carcinoma. It follows the rule of 50%. The presence of a single lymph node reduces the 5-year survival by 50%. If the nodes are bilateral, 5-year survival is reduced by another 50%. If there is nodal fixation or extracapsular extension of tumor, expected survival goes down yet again. Fixation of nodes is probably best determined clinically (via nonmobility on palpation). Extranodal spread can be suggested on CT or MRI by the demonstration of shaggy irregular margins of nodes, the presence of soft tissue stranding in the neck fat around the nodes, and enlarging nodal size. The presence of nodal necrosis is also associated with an increased risk of extracapsular spread.

23. What risk factors are associated with the development of head and neck cancer?
Alcohol use and tobacco use (chewing or smoking) are major risk factors and likely play a synergistic role. Viral infections, particularly Epstein-Barr virus (EBV), human papilloma virus (HPV), human immunodeficiency virus (HIV), and herpes simplex virus (HSV), have an established relationship with an increased risk of head and neck cancer. EBV is a primary etiologic agent in the pathogenesis of nasopharyngeal carcinoma, and HPV is strongly associated with oropharyngeal carcinomas. HIV and HSV are less strongly correlated with development of head and neck cancer. Other risk factors for head and neck cancer include occupational exposures (e.g., dry-cleaning agent perchloroethylene, asbestos, pesticides, etc.), radiation exposure, and betel nut chewing (which is widespread in regions of Asia).

24. What major epidemiologic factor accounts for the increasing rate of head and neck cancer in adults younger than 40 years old?
HPV infection has been linked to the increased incidence of oropharyngeal carcinomas (especially in the base of tongue and palatine tonsils) in young adults in recent decades. This is despite the overall decrease in incidence of laryngeal, hypopharyngeal, and oral cavity cancers that has been observed beginning in the late 1980s, which has been attributed to a gradual decrease in smoking. The vast majority of HPV-related head and neck cancers are squamous cell carcinomas. Immunohistochemical positivity for p16 is a marker for HPV-associated neoplasms. HPV-associated carcinomas have a propensity for cystic nodal metastases. Patients with HPV-associated oropharyngeal cancer have a better prognosis compared with those whose cancer is HPV-negative.

25. What is the role of the radiologist in the evaluation and staging of head and neck cancer?
The clinician and radiologist must work together as a team. The clinician/endoscopist can accurately assess the mucosa of the aerodigestive tract. The radiologist, with cross-sectional imaging, sees the submucosal structures. When clinical and radiologic data are combined, there is 85% accuracy in staging patients. The radiologist is best at assessing submucosal spread of neoplasm, identifying necrosis in normal-sized nodes, and identifying retropharyngeal nodes (which are generally clinically occult).

26. What treatment modalities are used for head and neck cancer?
The treatment of head and neck cancer includes surgical and nonsurgical (chemotherapy and radiation therapy) approaches. The goal is to cure patients, preserve function, and maintain quality of life. While conventional open surgical approaches have been associated with significant morbidities (including speech/swallowing dysfunction and cosmetic deformities), transoral robotic surgery (TORS), alone or coupled with de-intensified radiation therapy, is emerging as a minimally invasive surgical technique for small or medium-sized tumors of the oropharynx and for some tumors of the larynx and hypopharynx with excellent oncologic and functional outcomes. When TORS is being considered, the radiologist must make note of the course of the ipsilateral internal carotid artery. A retropharyngeal course of the internal carotid artery is a contraindication to robotic lateral oropharyngectomy (Figure 43-7), because this involves cutting through the constrictor muscles, putting the artery at risk.

27. What are the most common neck masses in a child?
Inflammatory/infectious lymphadenitis and congenital mass lesions (e.g., lymphatic malformation/cystic hygroma, branchial cleft cysts, hemangiomas) are the two most common causes of neck masses in children. Malignancy is the

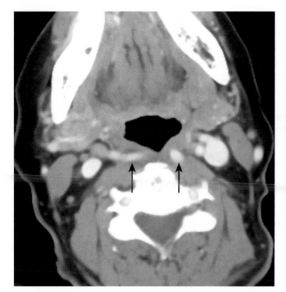

**Figure 43-7.** Retropharyngeal internal carotid arteries on CT. Axial contrast-enhanced CT image demonstrates retropharyngeal course of internal carotid arteries (*arrows*) posterior to pharyngeal constrictor muscles.

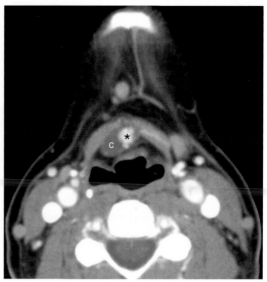

**Figure 43-8.** Thyroglossal duct cyst on CT. Axial contrast-enhanced CT image through infrahyoid neck reveals cyst (*c*) embedded deep to strap muscles. Note solid enhancing nodule (*) in medial aspect of cyst, reflecting coexistent focus of papillary thyroid cancer, seen in approximately 1% of thyroglossal duct cysts. Presence of solid tissue or calcification within thyroglossal duct cyst is usually indicative of coexistent papillary thyroid cancer.

third most common cause. Lateral neck masses include lymphatic malformations, branchial cleft cysts, inflammatory/infectious lymphadenitis, and lymphoma. Midline masses include thyroglossal duct cysts, hemangiomas, and dermoids/epidermoids.

Among the most common congenital neck masses is the thyroglossal duct cyst. It can occur anywhere along the developmental descent of thyroid tissue along the thyroglossal duct, from the foramen cecum at the base of the tongue to the usual location of the thyroid gland. Most are located in the infrahyoid neck (65%), but can occur at the level of the hyoid bone (15%) or in a suprahyoid location (20%). Seventy-five percent are located in the midline (Figure 43-8). The more inferior the cyst, the more likely it is to be off-midline.

Thyroid carcinoma, usually papillary in subtype, arises in less than 1% of thyroglossal duct cysts. The presence of a nodule or calcification associated with the cyst is usually indicative of the presence of carcinoma (see Figure 43-8).

## KEY POINTS

- MRI is the modality of choice for evaluating suprahyoid neck lesions, whereas infrahyoid neck lesions are imaged first with CT.
- Displacement of fat in the parapharyngeal space helps to localize a neck mass to the correct extramucosal space in the suprahyoid neck and to formulate a differential diagnosis.
- The most common cause of a cystic neck mass in an adult is metastatic lymphadenopathy.

### BIBLIOGRAPHY

Loevner LA, Learned KO, Mohan S, et al. Transoral robotic surgery in head and neck cancer: what radiologists need to know about the cutting edge. *Radiographics*. 2013;33(6):1759-1779.

Corey AS, Hudgins PA. Radiographic imaging of human papillomavirus related carcinomas of the oropharynx. *Head Neck Pathol*. 2012; 6(suppl 1):S25-S40.

Gor DM, Langer JE, Loevner LA. Imaging of cervical lymph nodes in head and neck cancer: the basics. *Radiol Clin North Am*. 2006;44(1): 101-110, viii.

Branstetter BF 4th, Weissman JL. Infection of the facial area, oral cavity, oropharynx, and retropharynx. *Neuroimaging Clin N Am*. 2003;13(3):393-410, ix.

Henrot P, Blum A, Toussaint B, et al. Dynamic maneuvers in local staging of head and neck malignancies with current imaging techniques: principles and clinical applications. *Radiographics*. 2003;23(5):1201-1213.

Mack MG, Balzer JO, Herzog C, et al. Multi-detector CT: head and neck imaging. *Eur Radiol*. 2003;13(suppl 5):M121-M126.

Som PM, Curtin HD, Mancuso AA. Imaging-based nodal classification for evaluation of neck metastatic adenopathy. *AJR Am J Roentgenol*. 2000;174(3):837-844.

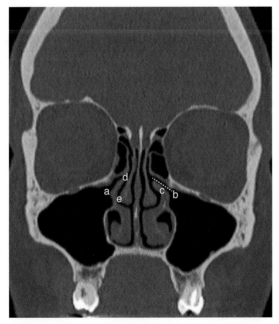

# CHAPTER 44

# HEAD AND NECK IMAGING, PART 2

*Deepak Mavahalli Sampathu, MD, PhD, Mary H. Scanlon, MD, FACR, and Laurie A. Loevner, MD*

1. What is the drainage pathway for the maxillary, frontal, and anterior ethmoid air cells?

   The ostiomeatal complex is the common drainage pathway for the paranasal sinuses. It refers to the uncinate process, a small bone, and the spaces around it through which mucus and secretions drain, including the maxillary sinus ostium, the infundibulum, the hiatus semilunaris, and the middle meatus (Figure 44-1). The frontal sinuses, maxillary sinuses, and anterior ethmoid air cells drain into the middle meatus. The sphenoid sinuses and posterior ethmoid air cells drain via the sphenoethmoidal recess into the superior meatus. Only the nasolacrimal duct drains into the inferior meatus (Table 44-1). The diagnosis of acute sinusitis is clinical and is typically treated medically. Imaging is reserved for patients who have chronic symptoms despite maximal medical therapy. Unenhanced computed tomography (CT) of the paranasal sinuses should not be performed during acute infection, but rather after 4 to 6 weeks of maximal medical therapy. Delineation of the anatomy of the ostiomeatal complex anatomy and the identification of any anatomic variants that narrow this common drainage pathway are important for the ear, nose, and throat surgeon (otorhinolaryngologist) to plan possible correction via endoscopic sinonasal surgery.

2. In which paranasal sinus does malignancy most commonly arise?

   The most common site involved is the maxillary sinus, followed by the ethmoid air cells. It is rare to have a malignancy arise within the frontal or sphenoid sinus. The role of the radiologist is not to make a histologic diagnosis, but rather to

**Figure 44-1.** Normal paranasal sinus anatomy on CT. Coronal unenhanced CT image at level of ostiomeatal complex shows maxillary sinus ostium (*a*), infundibulum (*b, dotted line*), uncinate process (*c*), hiatus semilunaris (*d*), and middle meatus (*e*).

| Table 44-1. Drainage Pathways of Paranasal Sinuses and Nasolacrimal Duct | |
|---|---|
| **DRAINAGE** | **STRUCTURES** |
| Superior meatus | Sphenoid sinuses, posterior ethmoid air cells |
| Middle meatus | Frontal sinuses, anterior ethmoid air cells, and maxillary sinuses |
| Inferior meatus | Nasolacrimal duct |

map the extent of disease so that the surgeon can plan his or her surgical approach. Of sinonasal malignancies, 80% are squamous cell carcinomas. The hallmark of squamous cell carcinoma is osseous destruction. Another 10% are adenocarcinomas and adenoid cystic carcinomas arising from minor salivary gland rests. Other cell types include melanoma and olfactory neuroblastomas (esthesioneuroblastoma).

3. **On an unenhanced CT scan, what are common causes of hyperattenuating material within the paranasal sinuses?**
   The three main causes are inspissated proteinaceous secretions, mycetoma (fungus ball), and blood. Inspissated proteinaceous secretions resulting from chronic sinusitis are the most common of these entities. These dense secretions may also be seen within chronic polyps of the sinonasal cavity, and in sinonasal polyposis, there is associated expansion and bony remodeling. The increased attenuation on CT is due to high protein content. Blood within a paranasal sinus usually shows an air-fluid-hemorrhage level and is most commonly seen in the setting of acute facial fractures.

4. **What classic imaging finding supports the diagnosis of acute sinusitis in the appropriate clinical setting (facial pain, nasal drainage, fever)?**
   An air-fluid level in a paranasal sinus, in the absence of trauma or sinus irrigation, is a characteristic imaging finding of acute sinusitis.

5. **What are the three major salivary glands and the ducts that drain them?**
   The three major salivary glands are the parotid, submandibular, and sublingual glands.
   - The parotid gland is drained by the Stensen duct, which courses from the parotid gland and passes over the masseter muscle to pierce the buccinator muscle at the level of the second maxillary molar tooth.
   - The submandibular gland is drained by the Wharton duct, which drains on either side of the frenulum in the floor of the mouth (Figure 44-2).
   - The sublingual glands consist of 12 to 18 small, paired glands located in the sublingual space in the floor of the mouth. The sublingual glands have many draining ducts, known as the ducts of Rivinus, which drain into the floor of the mouth. If there is a dominant sublingual duct opening into the Wharton duct, it is called the duct of Bartholin.

6. **Which salivary gland has the highest incidence of calculi/stones, and why?**
   By a ratio of 4:1, it is more common to have calculi/stones in the submandibular gland (see Figure 44-2) than in the parotid gland. The submandibular gland is more prone to stone formation because of its more alkaline and viscous secretions. In addition, its draining duct is wider, has a narrower orifice, and takes an upward course. On thin-section unenhanced CT, more than 75% of these stones are radiodense. Obstruction of the duct can result in sialoadenitis (see Figure 44-2).

7. **Which salivary gland contains lymphoid tissue? What is the significance of this tissue?**
   The parotid gland is the first salivary gland to form and the last to encapsulate. As such, it is the only salivary gland to contain lymphoid tissue. For this reason, it is the only salivary gland that has the potential for developing

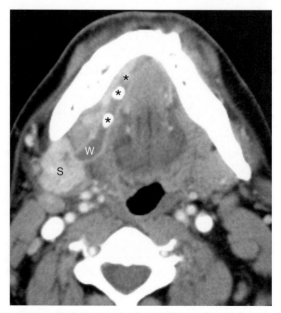

**Figure 44-2.** Sialolithiasis and sialoadenitis on CT. Axial contrast-enhanced CT image through floor of mouth demonstrates multiple radiodense calculi (*'s) in dilated submandibular (Wharton) duct (*w*). Right submandibular gland (*s*) is enlarged and diffusely enhances, consistent with sialoadenitis secondary to obstruction.

lymphadenopathy from systemic diseases (e.g., rheumatoid arthritis, Sjögren's syndrome, human immunodeficiency virus [HIV] infection), metastases to intraglandular nodes (usually from skin cancer of the scalp), lymphoma, and Warthin tumors. A major lymphatic drainage pathway of the scalp is to the lymph nodes in the parotid gland.

8. What is the most common benign tumor of the salivary glands?
The most common benign tumor of the salivary glands is pleomorphic adenoma (benign mixed tumor), which is seen most often in the parotid gland, where it represents ≈80% of all parotid masses. Parotid gland masses follow the 80% rule: 80% are benign, 80% are pleomorphic adenomas, 80% occur in the superficial lobe, and ≈80% of untreated pleomorphic adenomas remain benign (20% may undergo malignant degeneration into squamous cell carcinoma).

9. What are the most common malignancies of the salivary glands?
The most common malignant neoplasm of the parotid gland is mucoepidermoid carcinoma. In the submandibular, sublingual, and minor salivary glands, the most common malignancy is adenoid cystic carcinoma.

10. How is the size of the salivary gland related to the likelihood of a mass in the gland being malignant?
In an adult, the rule is that the larger the salivary gland, the lower the likelihood that a mass within it is malignant. The reverse is true in pediatric patients. In an adult, a parotid mass has a rate of malignancy of 15% to 20%; a submandibular gland mass, 40% to 50%; and a sublingual gland mass, greater than 50%.

11. What imaging features distinguish a benign thyroid mass from a malignant thyroid mass?
There is nothing specific about the appearance of an intrathyroidal mass itself on CT or magnetic resonance imaging (MRI) (e.g., calcification, low attenuation, or hemorrhage) that distinguishes a benign nodule from a malignant nodule (Figure 44-3). Findings on cross-sectional imaging that suggest that a thyroid mass is malignant include the presence of pathologic lymph nodes in the neck, extension of the thyroid mass outside of the thyroid capsule, and vascular invasion (spread into the adjacent internal jugular vein) (see Figure 44-3, C). Of thyroid carcinomas, 80% to 90% are papillary in subtype. Other malignant tumors of the thyroid gland include anaplastic carcinoma, follicular cancer, medullary carcinoma, and primary lymphoma. Rarely, metastatic disease to the thyroid gland occurs (from primary lung, breast, and renal cell carcinomas).

Thyroid nodules are common (seen on 16% of CT/MRI studies that include the thyroid gland, and on 40% to 50% of thyroid ultrasound studies), but the vast majority are benign. Thyroid nodules/masses identified on CT/MRI may be further evaluated by ultrasonography (US). While there is no single consensus statement regarding which thyroid nodules identified on CT/MRI should be worked up by US, one approach involves further workup based on a patient's risk category. In the high-risk category (e.g., fluorodeoxyglucose [FDG]-avid nodules on positron emission tomography [PET], presence of pathologic lymph nodes, a mass with extrathyroidal spread or associated with vocal cord paralysis, or presence of lung metastases), US workup should be strongly considered for any thyroid nodule. For an indeterminate thyroid nodule/mass in an adult younger than 35 years, US should be considered for nodules ≥1.0 cm, and in patients older than 35 years, US should be considered for nodules ≥1.5 cm. US features which are associated with a higher risk of malignancy include microcalcifications, irregular/lobulated margins, marked hypoechogenicity, and taller-than-wide shape in the transverse plane, although these features are not highly sensitive. Tissue for cytology is usually obtained by fine needle aspiration in the physician's office for palpable lesions and under US guidance in the radiology department for lesions that are nonpalpable.

12. What is the most common cause of proptosis in an adult?
Graves' disease is the most common cause of unilateral or bilateral proptosis secondary to increased orbital fat and enlargement of the extraocular muscles. The extraocular muscle bellies are typically involved with characteristic sparing of the tendon insertions (Figure 44-4). In contrast, the pattern of involvement with orbital pseudotumor (the second most common cause of proptosis) includes the tendons. Patients do not have to be hyperthyroid to have Graves' ophthalmopathy. It may occur before, during, or after treatment. The key clinical feature of orbital pseudotumor is eye pain associated with the proptosis. Ocular lymphoma and metastatic disease are other common causes of proptosis.

13. Which metastatic lesion to the orbit is classically associated with enophthalmos?
Intraorbital, retrobulbar (behind the globe) metastatic breast carcinoma is commonly associated with enophthalmos. This association is related to the frequent scirrhous reaction of breast carcinoma that results in retraction of adjacent tissues, similar to what is commonly seen in the breast (retraction and dimpling of the skin).

14. What is the most common primary ocular malignancy in a child and in an adult?
- In a child, retinoblastoma is the most common malignant tumor, and 95% of these masses are calcified. CT is best for detection of calcification (which can be difficult to see with MRI), whereas MRI is best for detection of intracranial extension.
- In an adult, the most common primary ocular malignancy is melanoma, although overall, the most common intraocular malignancy in an adult is a metastasis. The uveal tract is involved by both. Melanomas may grow along the optic nerve and into the subarachnoid space, with resultant dissemination throughout the neural axis.

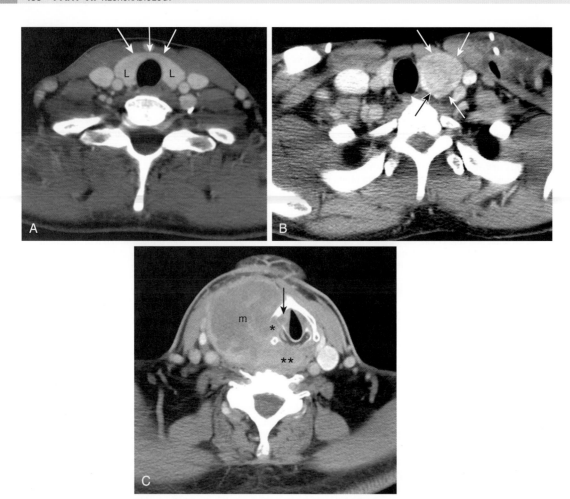

**Figure 44-3.** Normal thyroid gland and thyroid masses on CT. **A,** Axial contrast-enhanced CT image through neck reveals normal right and left lobes of thyroid gland (*L*) and isthmus (*arrows*). **B,** Axial contrast-enhanced axial CT image through neck in different patient shows heterogeneous 2.7-cm mass in left thyroid lobe (*arrows*), which is nonspecific regarding benign etiology (i.e., goiter or adenoma) versus malignancy (thyroid cancer). **C,** Axial contrast-enhanced CT image through neck in different patient demonstrates large heterogeneous mass (*m*) in right lobe of thyroid with direct invasion through thyroid cartilage (*) into paraglottic space (*arrow*). Posteromedially, mass extends into right tracheoesophageal groove (**). Only secondary findings of extension of thyroid mass outside thyroid capsule and into adjacent soft tissues, trachea, larynx, or vessels in carotid sheath, or presence of pathologic cervical lymph nodes are indicative of malignant mass. CT and MRI features of isolated mass in thyroid gland are themselves not indicative of benign versus malignant thyroid pathology.

In children and adults, malignant masses are commonly associated with a retinal detachment. Whenever a nontraumatic retinal detachment is identified, there must be careful evaluation for the presence of an associated intraocular mass.

15. What key clinical and imaging features distinguish an optic nerve glioma from an optic nerve meningioma? How do they differ in appearance from optic neuritis?

The age of the patient and appearance of the optic nerve distinguish an optic nerve glioma from an optic nerve meningioma. Meningiomas occur in middle-aged adults, whereas optic nerve gliomas occur in children (mean age 8 to 9 years). On MRI, optic nerve gliomas manifest as tubular enlargement of the nerve with variable enhancement, whereas thickening and enhancement of the optic nerve sheath is characteristic of a meningioma. On CT, meningiomas may demonstrate calcifications with a "tram-track" appearance. Meningiomas straighten the optic nerve because they arise from the surrounding dura of the optic nerve sheath complex, whereas gliomas kink the nerve as the tumor arises from the nerve itself. With meningiomas, the mass can be separated from the optic nerve. Both can occur in children with neurofibromatosis, but optic nerve gliomas are more common.

Optic neuritis, which is best evaluated by MRI, is characterized by focal or segmental signal abnormality of the optic nerve on T2-weighted images, sometimes with mild enlargement of the nerve, usually to a lesser degree than with gliomas. Enhancement is seen in >90% of cases of optic neuritis and indicates active demyelination. Fifty percent to 60% of patients with optic neuritis eventually develop multiple sclerosis.

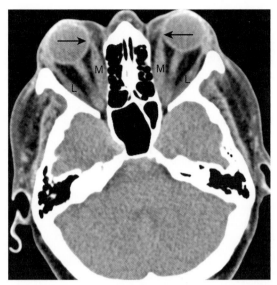

**Figure 44-4.** Proptosis secondary to Graves' disease on CT. Axial unenhanced CT image through orbits reveals bilateral enlargement of medial rectus muscles (*M*) and, to a lesser extent, of lateral rectus muscles (*L*). Note characteristic pattern of involvement in Graves' disease: enlargement of muscle bellies with sparing of tendinous insertions (*arrows*). This imaging feature helps to distinguish Graves' disease from orbital pseudotumor. Clinical presentation is also important, as pseudotumor typically manifests with eye pain.

16. Hearing loss is classified into what two major subtypes?

The two major subtypes of hearing loss are sensorineural and conductive. MRI is the best imaging study to evaluate unilateral or asymmetric sensorineural hearing loss in an adult. The most common neoplasm associated with this hearing loss is a vestibular schwannoma, and thin-section MRI with intravenous contrast administration is obtained through the internal auditory canal and cerebellopontine angle. The remainder of the acoustic pathway, including the cochlear nuclear complex, medulla, and thalami, and the temporal lobes are also evaluated. High-resolution, thin-section unenhanced CT of the temporal bones is the best imaging study for sensorineural hearing loss in patients younger than 15 years because congenital anomalies or atresias involving the otic capsule, the semicircular canals, and the vestibular aqueduct are commonly the cause. CT is the study of choice in patients with conductive hearing loss at any age because it is best for showing the sequela of chronic otitis media or cholesteatoma.

17. What are the types of tinnitus, and how are they subcategorized?

Tinnitus is classified as pulsatile or nonpulsatile. Pulsatile tinnitus is divided further into subjective (patient hears beating) and objective (patient hears beating and so does the physician with a stethoscope). Pulsatile tinnitus is most often secondary to a vascular problem, including masses, malformations, or an anomaly. Causes include glomus tumor, dural arteriovenous fistula, aberrant internal carotid artery, or a high-riding jugular bulb. In subjective pulsatile tinnitus, CT is the first imaging study to perform. In objective pulsatile tinnitus, one may perform MRI, although patients are often assessed with conventional catheter angiography because the most concerning potential diagnosis is dural arteriovenous fistula (AVF). The most common cause of pulsatile tinnitus reported in the neurologic literature is benign intracranial hypertension (pseudotumor cerebri). Tinnitus without a pulsatile quality may be an early symptom of a vestibular schwannoma or otosclerosis. Other causes include cholesteatomas, noise damage, and old age. Relatively rare causes include multiple sclerosis and Chiari I malformation.

18. Cholesteatoma is a "pearly white" mass seen in the middle ear on otoscopic examination. What is a cholesteatoma?

Cholesteatomas can be acquired or congenital. Acquired cholesteatomas are basically ingrowths of skin through a perforation in the tympanic membrane (TM). Patients have a history of chronic otitis media with TM rupture, and often have a history of myringotomy tube placements. Ingrowth of skin results in the accumulation of squamous and keratin debris in the ear cavity. The presence of associated osseous erosions on CT imaging is a hallmark of the diagnosis. One must be familiar with the normal anatomy of this region (Figure 44-5). In the absence of such erosions, a cholesteatoma can look exactly like chronic granulation tissue or chronic otitis media. Most commonly, cholesteatomas occur through a defect superiorly in the pars flaccida portion of the TM. Tissue first fills Prussak space in the epitympanum and erodes the scutum, then the ossicles, and may eventually progress to erode through the roof of the epitympanum (the tegmen tympani) or undergo fistulization to the lateral semicircular canal or facial canal. Less commonly, cholesteatomas occur through a defect inferiorly in the pars tensa portion of the TM.

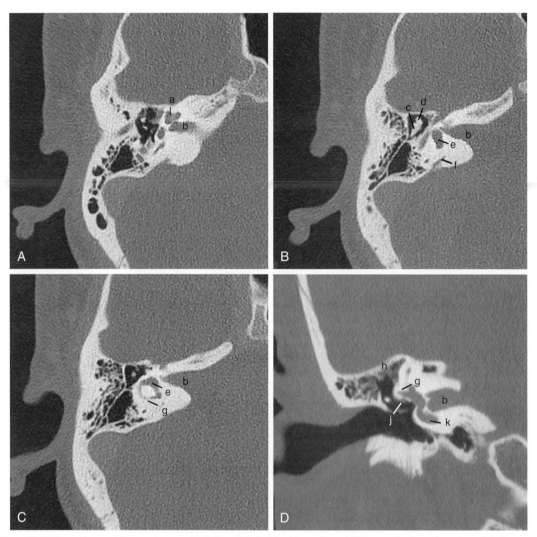

**Figure 44-5.** Normal temporal bone anatomy on CT. **A, B, and C,** Serial axial unenhanced CT images. **D,** Coronal unenhanced CT image. *a* = cochlea, *b* = internal auditory canal, *c* = body of incus, *d* = head of malleus, *e* = vestibule, *f* = vestibular aqueduct, *g* = lateral semicircular canal, *h* = tegmen tympani, *j* = tympanic portion of facial nerve, *k* = basal turn of cochlea.

19. What neoplasms occur in the jugular foramen?

    Glomus tumors, neural neoplasms (schwannoma), meningioma, and metastatic disease occur in the jugular foramen. Glomus jugulare tumors are the most common. They arise from Arnold nerve, a branch of cranial nerve X, which resides in the pars vascularis compartment of the jugular foramen. The jugular foramen is composed of two parts separated by a bony spur, the jugular spine. Anteriorly is the pars nervosa, which contains cranial nerve IX; posteriorly is the pars vascularis, which contains the internal jugular vein and cranial nerves X and XI. Glomus tumors, when large, erode the jugular spur and cause permeative bony changes (in contrast to the smooth osseous scalloping seen with schwannomas). In addition, in contrast to the other masses in this location that may compress the internal jugular vein, glomus tumors commonly grow directly into the jugular vein (Figure 44-6).

20. Unilateral middle ear fluid in an adult should trigger the search for what lesion?

    Unilateral middle ear fluid in an adult should raise suspicion for nasopharyngeal carcinoma, which most often arises from the lateral wall of the nasopharynx (fossa of Rosenmüller). Infiltration of the levator veli palatini muscle leads to eustachian tube dysfunction and serous otitis media. Nasopharyngeal carcinomas can infiltrate widely in all directions. Superiorly, they can extend into the clivus, the sphenoid sinus, and the neural foramina of osseous structures of the skull base.

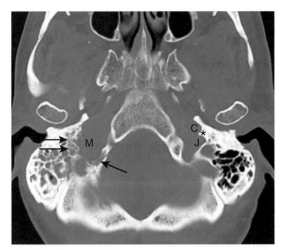

**Figure 44-6.** Normal and abnormal jugular foramina on CT. Axial unenhanced CT image through skull base shows normal left jugular foramen. Internal carotid artery canal (*C*) and pars vascularis (*J*) are separated by a thin bony spur (jugular spine) (*). Right jugular foramen is expanded by mass (*M*) with permeative bony changes (*arrows*), and erosion of jugular spine. These findings are most suggestive of glomus tumor. Metastasis can also have this appearance.

## KEY POINTS

- The best predictor of acute sinusitis in the appropriate clinical setting (facial pain, nasal drainage, fever) is the presence of an air-fluid level on a CT scan.
- CT is the imaging modality of choice for conductive hearing loss.
- MRI is the imaging modality of choice in adult-onset sensorineural hearing loss.

### BIBLIOGRAPHY

Hoang JK, Grady AT, Nguyen XV. What to do with incidental thyroid nodules identified on imaging studies? Review of current evidence and recommendations. *Curr Opin Oncol.* 2015;27(1):8-14.

Loevner LA, Kaplan SL, Cunnane ME, et al. Cross-sectional imaging of the thyroid gland. *Neuroimaging Clin N Am.* 2008;18(3):445-461, vii.

Frates MC, Benson CB, Charboneau JW, et al. Management of thyroid nodules detected at US: Society of Radiologists in Ultrasound consensus conference statement. *Radiology.* 2005;237(3):794-800.

Moonis G. Imaging of sinonasal anatomy and inflammatory disorders. *Crit Rev Computed Tomog.* 2003;44(4):187-228.

Okahara M, Kiyosue H, Hori Y, et al. Parotid tumors: MR imaging with pathological correlation. *Eur Radiol.* 2003;13(suppl 4):L25-L33.

Shah GV, Fischbein NJ, Patel R, et al. Newer MR imaging techniques for head and neck. *Magn Reson Imaging Clin N Am.* 2003;11(3):449-469, vi.

# VIII
# MUSCULOSKELETAL IMAGING

# CHAPTER 45

# IMAGING OF EXTREMITY TRAUMA

*Woojin Kim, MD*

1. **What is the role of radiography, computed tomography (CT), and magnetic resonance imaging (MRI) in the evaluation of extremity trauma?**

   Radiography remains the mainstay for the assessment of acute skeletal trauma with the exception of cervical spine trauma, which is now usually evaluated with CT. Properly positioned radiographs allow for accurate characterization of a large variety of appendicular skeletal injuries. Comparison radiographs of the asymptomatic side can be obtained with ease and may be useful, such as in pediatric cases and for assessment of subtle widening of the acromioclavicular interval. Localization of foreign bodies also remains as one of the important roles of radiography.

   Major indications for CT include diagnosis and evaluation of fractures, particularly when presence of fractures can alter management. CT is superior to radiography in depicting the extent of fractures, the spatial relationship of the fracture fragments, and the presence of intraarticular fragments. Other indications include preoperative planning and evaluation of postoperative complications. Multiplanar reformatted (MPR) images allow for higher diagnostic accuracy than radiography or axial CT images alone. As a result, CT has largely replaced radiography in cervical spine and pelvic fracture evaluations. Its limitations include higher radiation dose and cost, although studies have demonstrated that CT is more cost effective than radiography to clear the cervical spine in high-risk patients. Evaluation of ligamentous injuries is also limited with CT.

   MRI has the advantage of imaging injuries of soft tissue structures, including the labrum, ligaments, muscles, tendons, and cartilage, as well as the lack of radiation dose. It is also useful for the evaluation of occult hip fractures, particularly in older patients with osteoporosis. However, its limitations include higher cost and slower image acquisition.

2. **How are fractures evaluated with radiography?**

   At least two views of the fracture site, taken at 90 degrees to each other, are obtained. Remember, "one view equals no view." The radiographs obtained should include joints immediately above and below the fractured area for evaluation of associated dislocations.

3. **What are imaging features that help distinguish between acute and chronic fractures on radiography, CT, and MRI?**

   On radiographs and CT images, acute fractures demonstrate well-demarcated lucent fracture lines without sclerotic borders. As fractures heal, there is callus formation with fracture lines becoming less visible over time. On MRI, while lack of bone marrow edema associated with fracture deformity on fluid-sensitive sequences (such as T2-weighted and short tau inversion recovery ([STIR] images) is indicative of a chronic etiology, it is important to remember that bone marrow edema can persist for several months and thus is not always indicative of an acute etiology. Associated findings, such as soft tissue hematoma (typically high in signal intensity on T1-weighted images) and lipohemarthrosis (seen as layering fat that arises from the bone marrow and fluid/hemorrhage in the joint space, indicative of an intraarticular fracture), suggest a more acute etiology.

4. **Define the following terms: closed fracture, open fracture, avulsion fracture, comminuted fracture, intraarticular fracture, occult fracture, pathologic fracture, fracture displacement, and fracture angulation.**

   - **Closed fracture** occurs when there is intact skin over the fracture site. If there is communication between the fracture site and the outside environment, it is considered an **open fracture** regardless of how small the overlying skin defect is.
   - **Avulsion fracture** occurs when an osseous fragment is pulled off at the site of insertion of a muscle, ligament, or tendon.
   - **Comminuted fracture** is a fracture with more than two fracture fragments.
   - **Intraarticular fracture** involves the articular surface of a bone adjacent to a joint.
   - **Occult fracture** is a fracture that is not visible on a radiograph.
   - **Pathologic fracture** is a fracture in abnormal bone weakened by a preexisting disease process such as malignancy.
   - **Fracture displacement** describes the offset of the distal fracture fragment relative to the proximal fragment. Both direction and amount of offset (usually described in terms of shaft width) are used for description.
   - **Fracture angulation** describes the direction of distal fracture fragment in relation to the proximal fragment away from expected alignment had the bone not been fractured. Medial angulation can be described as "varus," and lateral angulation can be described as "valgus." Alternatively, angulation can be described in terms of the direction toward which the apex of the angle between the two fracture fragments is pointing. For example, a fracture can either be described as having medial angulation of the distal fracture fragment or lateral apex angulation.

5. What is a stress fracture? What two types may occur?

Stress fractures occur as a result of mismatch between bone strength and mechanical stress upon the bone and are subdivided into fatigue and insufficiency fractures. **Fatigue fractures** are the result of abnormal stresses on normal bone and are commonly seen in athletes. **Insufficiency fractures** are the result of normal stresses on abnormal bone, such as caused by conditions like osteoporosis, osteomalacia, or osteogenesis imperfecta. It should be noted, however, that some authors use the term stress fracture synonymously with fatigue fracture. Common sites for fatigue fractures include: pubic ramus, medial aspect of the femoral neck, tibia, calcaneus, navicular, metatarsal bones, and hallux sesamoid bones. Common sites for insufficiency fractures include: vertebra, sacrum, pubic ramus, femoral neck, and proximal diaphysis of the femur.

6. What is the difference between dislocation and subluxation of a joint?

**Dislocation** is complete loss of contact between the articular surfaces of a joint. **Subluxation** is partial loss of congruity between the articular surfaces of a joint.

7. What are some of the complications of fractures?

Various soft tissue injuries can be associated with fractures, which include neurovascular injuries. When a fracture is allowed to heal in an abnormal position, **malunion** occurs. If the fracture fragments fail to heal and fuse, the resulting complication is termed **nonunion**. If there is injury to the vascular supply to the bone, avascular necrosis can occur, such as from scaphoid waist and talar neck fractures. Osteomyelitis, which is infection of the bone, can also occur after a fracture, especially after an open fracture. **Pseudoarthrosis** refers to nonunion or false joint (as the name suggests), which is a result of failure of fracture healing. **Myositis ossificans** is extraosseous bone formation (heterotopic ossification) that occurs in muscles following trauma.

8. What is an os acromiale?

Os acromiale is an accessory ossification center of the acromion. Although the os acromiale is normally fused by age 25, it can remain unfused in some individuals. It is an important entity to be aware of because it may be misinterpreted as an acromial fracture. In addition, a higher prevalence of subacromial impingement and rotator cuff tears has been associated with os acromiale.

9. Describe type I, II, and III acromioclavicular (AC) separation.

As the term suggests, AC separation is widening of the AC joint space from ligamentous injury.

- **Type I AC separation** is stretching or partial tear of the AC ligament with no displacement seen on a radiograph. One can assess this condition radiographically by obtaining and comparing weight-bearing views of the uninjured shoulder and injured shoulder. This is a stable injury and has excellent prognosis of healing.
- **Type II AC separation** is complete tear of the AC ligament with widening of the AC joint. Most of these injuries heal without surgery.
- **Type III AC separation** is complete disruption of both the AC and coracoclavicular (CC) ligaments, resulting in abnormal widening of the AC and CC intervals. This type of injury requires internal fixation (Figure 45-1).

10. What are the radiographic features of anterior shoulder joint dislocation on an anteroposterior view?

The most common type of shoulder dislocation is anterior. The humeral head is displaced anteromedially and typically rests inferior to the coracoid process. It is also known as infracoracoid dislocation or subcoracoid dislocation (Figure 45-2, *A*).

11. What are Hill-Sachs fracture and Bankart fracture?

Hill-Sachs fracture and Bankart fracture are complications of anterior shoulder dislocation. Hill-Sachs fracture is a defect in the posterolateral aspect of the humeral head. It occurs when there is contact between this region of the humeral head and the anterior-inferior glenoid rim during anterior dislocation. The Bankart fracture is a fracture of the anterior-inferior glenoid rim secondary to this trauma.

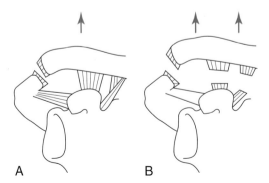

A                                        B

**Figure 45-1. A,** Schematic image of Type II AC joint separation. Only AC ligament is ruptured. **B,** Schematic image of Type III AC joint separation. There is complete tear of AC and coracoclavicular ligaments.

12. What radiographic signs are associated with posterior shoulder dislocation?

Posterior shoulder dislocations are associated with epileptic seizures and electric shocks. Because the humeral head appears almost normally aligned with the glenoid, posterior dislocation of the shoulder can easily be missed on a frontal view radiograph. A "rim" sign refers to widening of the space between the medial border of the humeral head and the glenoid rim. The shoulder is persistently held in internally rotated position, which gives the humeral head a rounded appearance, known as the "light bulb" sign. Therefore, absence of an externally rotated view on a standard shoulder radiographic study should alert the interpreting clinician to the presence of posterior shoulder dislocation. An associated reverse Hill-Sachs fracture, which is impaction fracture of the anteromedial humeral head, seen on the radiograph, is known as the "trough" sign (Figures 45-2, *B-D*).

13. What is pseudosubluxation of the humerus?

With pseudosubluxation of the humerus, there is inferior displacement of the humeral head with widening of the glenohumeral space. This entity is usually caused by hemarthrosis after trauma to the shoulder. As the term suggests, this is not a true dislocation of the glenohumeral joint.

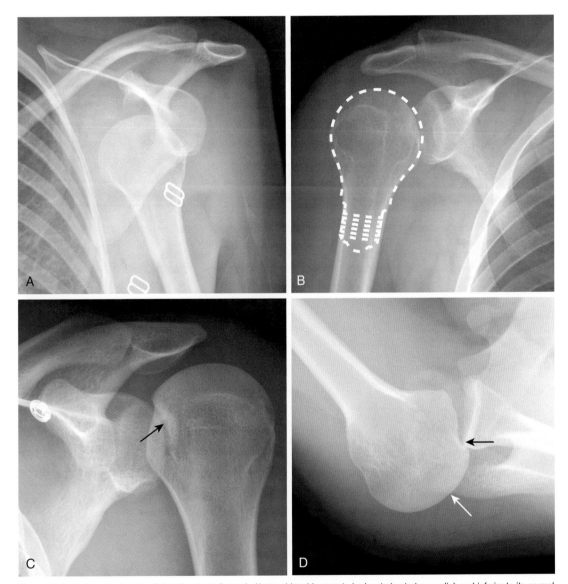

**Figure 45-2. A,** Anterior shoulder dislocation on radiograph. Humeral head is seen to be located anterior, medial, and inferior to its normal location. **B-D,** Posterior shoulder dislocation on radiographs. **B,** Note humerus is persistently held in internal rotation, giving humeral head rounded appearance, known as "light bulb" sign. **C,** Reverse Hill-Sachs fracture, an impaction fracture of the anteromedial humeral head, is seen and known as "trough" sign (*arrow*). **D,** Axillary view of shoulder shows posterior dislocation of humeral head (*white arrow*) relative to glenoid fossa and impaction of humeral head upon posterior glenoid rim, revealing how reverse Hill-Sachs fracture (*black arrow*) occurs.

14. **What are the "posterior fat pad" sign and the "sail" sign in the elbow?**
The "posterior fat pad" and "sail" signs indicate the presence of an intraarticular elbow fracture. Fat is normally present between the synovium and capsule of the elbow joint, which is normally not radiographically visible, with the exception of an occasional normal anterior fat pad that may be seen as a small vertical lucency immediately adjacent to the anterior cortex of the distal humerus. With an intraarticular fracture, subsequent hemarthrosis distends the synovium and causes displacement of this fat. The posterior fat pad becomes visible as a small linear area of radiolucency, and the anterior fat pad is lifted away from the bone as a triangular radiolucency, causing it to resemble a sail.

15. **Describe a Monteggia fracture and its associated finding.**
Monteggia fracture is a fracture of the proximal ulna with radial head subluxation or dislocation. This fracture-dislocation was originally described by Monteggia in 1814. It is important to remember to look for the associated radial head dislocation or subluxation when you see a proximal ulnar fracture because failure to do so can result in radial head necrosis.

16. **Describe a Galeazzi fracture and its associated finding.**
Galeazzi fracture is a fracture of the distal radius with associated distal radioulnar dislocation/subluxation. Galeazzi described this fracture in 1935.

17. **Which carpal bone gets fractured the most often?**
The scaphoid is the carpal bone that is fractured most often. Fracture of the scaphoid should be suspected when there is tenderness in the region of the anatomic snuff box. Scaphoid fractures can be difficult to visualize on radiographs. The blood supply to the scaphoid enters from the waist (middle third) and distal pole by the scaphoid branches of the radial artery. As a result, blood flows proximally from the distal pole. When this is disrupted by a fracture, avascular necrosis of the proximal fracture fragment occurs and can be seen as sclerosis.

18. **What is the "Terry Thomas" sign?**
Scapholunate dissociation results from ligamentous disruption between the scaphoid and lunate bones, leading to rotatory subluxation of the scaphoid. This is manifested by widening of the space between the scaphoid and lunate on the frontal view of the wrist and is known as the "Terry Thomas" sign. Terry Thomas (1911–1990) was a gap-toothed British comic actor.

19. **Define dorsal intercalated segmental instability (DISI) and volar intercalated segmental instability (VISI).**
DISI and VISI describe carpal instability based on the tilt of the lunate bone on the lateral radiograph of the wrist. With DISI, the lunate tilts dorsally; there is also volar tilt of the scaphoid resulting in a scapholunate angle greater than 60° and a capitolunate angle greater than 30°. DISI results from scapholunate dissociation (Figure 45-3, *A*). With VISI, the lunate tilts in a volar direction with dorsal tilt of the capitate. With VISI, the scapholunate angle can either be normal or measure less than 30°. VISI results from lunotriquetral ligament tear, although it can also be seen as a normal variant (Figure 45-3, *B*).

20. **What are the four stages of perilunate instability?**
Perilunate instability results from carpal ligament injuries and can be described in four stages (Figure 45-4).
- Stage I: Scapholunate dissociation
- Stage II: Perilunate dislocation
- Stage III: Midcarpal dislocation
- Stage IV: Lunate dislocation

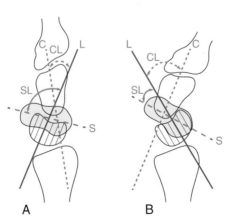

A      B

**Figure 45-3. A,** Schematic image of DISI. Note dorsal tilt of lunate (indicated by solid blue line). There is widening of scapholunate angle. **B,** Schematic image of VISI. Conversely, there is volar tilt of lunate (indicated by solid blue line) with narrowing of scapholunate angle. *SL* = scapholunate angle, *CL* = capitolunate angle.

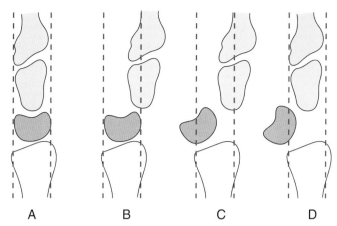

**Figure 45-4. A,** Schematic image of scapholunate dissociation. Normal alignment of lunate with distal radius and capitate is maintained. **B,** Schematic image of perilunate dislocation. Lunate is normally aligned with distal radius whereas remainder of carpus is dislocated. **C,** Schematic image of midcarpal dislocation. Neither lunate nor capitate aligns with distal radius. **D,** Schematic image of lunate dislocation. Lunate is dislocated in volar direction.

21. What is a Stener lesion?

A Stener lesion refers to interposition of the aponeurosis of the adductor pollicis muscle between the bones of the first metacarpophalangeal joint and the torn ulnar collateral ligament (UCL). This prevents healing of the torn UCL, making this a surgical lesion.

22. Match the following fractures with the radiographic images in Figure 45-5.
    • Barton fracture
    • Baseball (mallet) finger
    • Bennett fracture
    • Boxer fracture
    • Colles fracture
    • Smith fracture
    • Triquetral fracture

23. Which is more common, anterior or posterior dislocation of the hip joint?

Posterior hip dislocation is more common. It is manifested by superior displacement of the femoral head. In anterior hip dislocation, the femoral head is displaced anteriorly and medially.

24. What is a Segond fracture?

A Segond fracture is an avulsion fracture of the proximal lateral tibia. The fracture fragment may be very small. Although it may not look severe on a radiograph, it is commonly associated with an anterior cruciate ligament tear and meniscal injury.

25. What is a bipartite patella?

A bipartite patella is another normal anatomic variant that one should not misinterpret as being a fracture. It is a secondary ossification center that is seen in the upper outer quadrant of the patella. It is usually bilateral and has a smooth and sclerotic cortical border.

26. What is a tibial plafond fracture?

A tibial plafond fracture is an intraarticular fracture of the distal tibia caused by impaction of the talus and is often comminuted.

27. What is Böhler's angle?

Böhler's angle (also known as the tuber angle) is formed by the intersection of two lines: (1) a line from highest point of the posterior articular facet to highest point of the posterior tuberosity, and (2) a line from the highest posterior articular facet to the highest point of anterior articular facet. drawn about the calcaneus. The normal value for this angle is between 20 to 40 degrees. A value less than 20 degrees can be seen in calcaneal fracture. However, a normal Böhler's angle does not exclude the presence of a calcaneal fracture.

28. Match the following fractures with the radiographic images in Figure 45-6.
    • Freiberg infraction
    • Jones fracture
    • Lisfranc fracture-dislocation
    • Maisonneuve fracture
    • Segond fracture

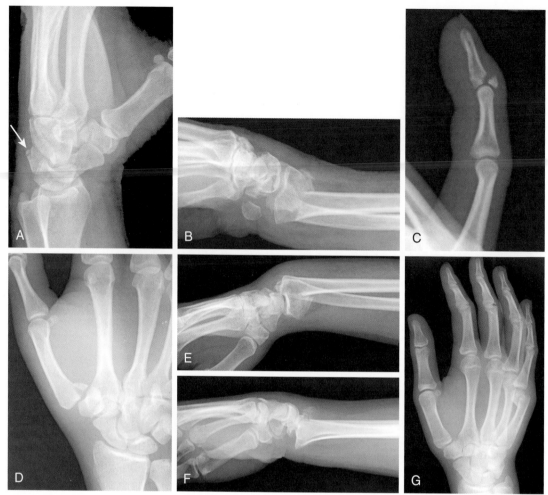

**Figure 45-5.** Various upper extremity fractures on radiographs. **A,** Triquetral fracture. Dorsal avulsion fracture (*arrow*) is best seen on lateral view. **B,** Colles fracture. Nonarticular distal radial fracture with dorsal displacement of distal fracture fragment. **C,** Mallet finger. Avulsion fracture of base of distal phalanx at extensor digitorum tendon insertion site. **D,** Bennett fracture. Intraarticular fracture-dislocation of base of first metacarpal bone. **E,** Smith fracture. Nonarticular distal radial fracture with volar displacement of distal fracture fragment. **F,** Barton fracture. Intraarticular oblique fracture of dorsal aspect of distal radius. **G,** Boxer's fracture. Transverse fracture of distal metacarpal bone(s), in this case the fifth metacarpal bone.

## KEY POINTS

- Radiography is the mainstay for assessment of acute extremity trauma. CT and MRI are often utilized to detect injuries not visualized on radiographs and to depict the full extent of underlying osseous and soft tissue injuries.
- Fatigue fractures are the result of abnormal stresses on normal bone, whereas insufficiency fractures are the result of normal stresses on abnormal bone.
- The most common type of shoulder dislocation is anterior, whereas the most common type of hip dislocation is posterior.
- A fat-fluid level seen in a joint space in the setting of trauma is due to a lipohemarthrosis and is indicative of an intraarticular fracture.

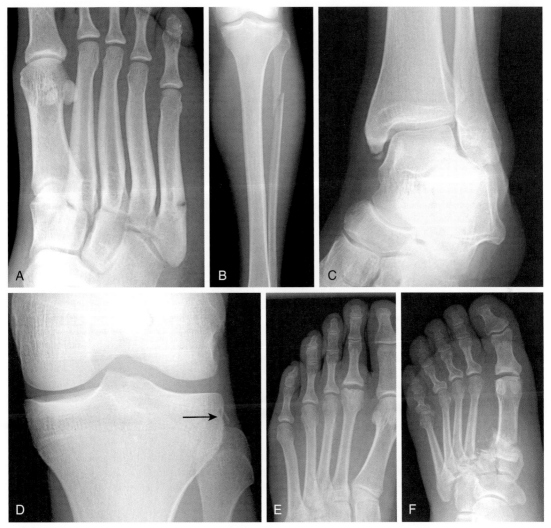

**Figure 45-6.** Various lower extremity fractures on radiographs. **A,** Jones fracture. Transverse fracture of base of fifth metatarsal bone. **B** and **C,** Maisonneuve fracture. Tear of interosseous membrane and fracture of upper third of fibula (**B**) with associated medial malleolus fracture (**C**). **D,** Segond fracture. Small cortical avulsion fracture (*arrow*) of proximal lateral tibia. **E,** Freiberg infraction is osteonecrosis of second or third metatarsal head from subchondral fatigue fracture. **F,** Lisfranc fracture-dislocation represents fracture and dislocation of one or more metatarsal bones from tarsus.

## BIBLIOGRAPHY

Greenspan A, Beltran J. *Orthopedic imaging: a practical approach.* 6th ed. Philadelphia: Wolters Kluwer Health; 2015.
Pope TL Jr, Harris JH Jr. *Harris & Harris' the radiology of emergency medicine.* 5th ed. Philadelphia: Lippincott Williams & Wilkins; 2013.
Guglielmi G, van Kuijk C, Genant HK. *Fundamentals of hand and wrist imaging.* Berlin: Springer-Verlag; 2012.
Ohashi K, El-Khoury GY. Musculoskeletal CT: recent advances and current clinical applications. *Radiol Clin North Am.* 2009;47(3):387-409.
Renner JB. Conventional radiography in musculoskeletal imaging. *Radiol Clin North Am.* 2009;47(3):357-372.
Hunter TB, Peltier LF, Lund PJ. Radiologic history exhibit. Musculoskeletal eponyms: who are those guys? *Radiographics.* 2000;20(3): 819-836.
Schultz RJ. *The language of fractures.* Baltimore, MD: Williams & Wilkins; 1990.

# CHAPTER 46

# IMAGING OF SPINAL TRAUMA

*Woojin Kim, MD*

1. **What are the roles of radiography, computed tomography (CT), and magnetic resonance imaging (MRI) in the evaluation of spinal trauma?**
   When it comes to spinal trauma evaluation, CT has largely replaced radiography given its higher sensitivity for detection of underlying injury. However, radiography is sometimes still obtained for initial evaluation and is widely used to monitor the treatment and healing of spinal injuries. MRI is also widely used to evaluate for presence of ligamentous and muscular injuries as well as spinal cord injuries.

2. **Describe how to interpret a lateral cervical spine radiograph.**
   - Count the vertebral bodies. All seven cervical vertebral bodies and C7-T1 should be visualized.
   - Evaluate for presence of fractures.
   - Evaluate the thickness of prevertebral soft tissue. It should be less than 6-7 mm anterior to C2-C3, and its thickness should be less than 18-21 mm anterior to C6-C7. When the prevertebral soft tissue appears thickened on a lateral radiograph in the setting of acute trauma, this is suggestive of presence of prevertebral edema and/or hemorrhage related to underlying osseous or soft tissue injury.
   - Assess four parallel lines for alignment. From anterior to posterior, these are the anterior vertebral, posterior vertebral, spinolaminar, and posterior spinous lines (Figure 46-1).
   - Examine the atlantoaxial interval, which is the distance between the posterior margin of the anterior arch of C1 (atlas) and the anterior margin of the odontoid process of C2 (axis). This space should not exceed 3 mm in adults and 5 mm in children. This interval should remain constant with flexion and extension in adults. Widening of this space indicates disruption of the transverse ligament of the atlas.
   - Compare the intervertebral disc spaces for widening or narrowing.

3. **What is a swimmer's view?**
   A swimmer's view is obtained when the lower cervical vertebrae cannot be seen on the lateral radiograph, usually because of the patient's inability to cooperate or due to a large shoulder girdle obscuring the spine in this location. This view is obtained by having the patient, in the supine position, raise his or her arm over the head while lowering the opposite arm.

4. **What is the three column concept of the spine?**
   This is a concept that was initially devised by Dr. Francis Denis to describe thoracolumbar spinal injuries. The anterior column of the spine is formed by the anterior longitudinal ligament, anterior annulus fibrosus, and anterior half of the vertebral bodies. The middle column of the spine is formed by the posterior longitudinal ligament, posterior annulus fibrosus, and posterior half of the vertebral bodies. The posterior column of the spine is formed by the posterior arch and interconnecting ligaments. Generally, if two or more spinal columns are involved in an injury, then the spine is considered to be unstable.

5. **What is the difference between compression and burst fractures?**
   Compression fractures are caused by anterior flexion. There is anterior wedging of the affected vertebral body, with the middle vertebral column remaining intact. Because only the anterior vertebral column is affected, this fracture is usually stable. Burst fractures are caused by axial loading injuries. The fracture lines extend through the anterior and posterior cortices of the vertebral body (thus affecting both anterior and middle columns). The posterior displacement of fracture fragments can cause spinal cord injury, and these fractures are considered unstable.

6. **Name some hyperflexion and hyperextension spinal injuries.**
   The most common fracture mechanism involving the spine is hyperflexion, which includes wedge fracture, unilateral interfacet dislocation (UID), bilateral interfacet dislocation (BID), and flexion teardrop fracture. The hyperextension injuries include hangman's fracture and extension teardrop fracture.

7. **Describe a Jefferson fracture and its mechanism of injury.**
   A Jefferson fracture is an unstable burst fracture involving the ring of C1 with lateral displacement of lateral masses and disruption of the transverse ligament of the atlas. This fracture is associated with axial-load injuries.

8. **Describe three different types of odontoid process (also known as dens) fractures.**
   - **Type I fracture** involves the superior tip of the odontoid process. It is extremely rare, and some authorities even argue over its existence.

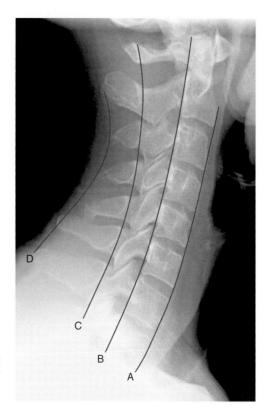

**Figure 46-1.** Normal cervical spine on lateral radiograph. Cervical vertebrae to C7-T1 can be visualized. Four parallel lines used for assessment of alignment are drawn: **A,** anterior vertebral line; **B,** posterior vertebral line; **C,** spinolaminar line; and **D,** posterior spinous line.

- **Type II** is the most common and is characterized by a fracture through the base of the odontoid process. In contrast to the other two types, this fracture is considered mechanically unstable.
- **Type III** fracture involves the body of C2.

9. What is an os odontoideum?

   An os odontoideum describes separation of the dens from the body of C2. It appears as a well-circumscribed ossicle with a smooth, thin cortex that is separated from the adjacent dens by a radiolucent gap. It was originally thought that this entity represented failure of fusion of the secondary ossification center with the remaining dens. Such a congenital anomaly is now known as persistent ossiculum terminale, however, and appears as a small ossicle at the tip of the dens. Most authorities now agree that os odontoideum is more likely an acquired post-traumatic abnormality. Regardless, this entity can be differentiated from an acute odontoid fracture by the presence of a sclerotic cortical margin and occasional hypertrophy of the anterior arch of axis. Os odontoideum can cause atlantoaxial instability. Some studies have shown increased frequency of this entity in patients with Down syndrome.

10. What is a hangman's fracture?

    A hangman's fracture can be seen after a motor vehicle accident in which the chin strikes the dashboard. It is a hyperextension injury with bilateral fractures of the pars interarticularis. This type of fracture can be subtle on radiography and may easily be overlooked (Figure 46-2).

11. What is a flexion teardrop fracture? What is its prognostic significance?

    A flexion teardrop fracture is a severe hyperflexion injury of the cervical spine that results in anterior compression fracture of the vertebral body with disruption of the posterior ligaments. Because of severe kyphotic angulation of the cervical spinal cord at this level, there is usually an associated anterior cervical cord syndrome. The teardrop component is seen as a fracture fragment of the anterior-inferior corner of the involved vertebral body (Figure 46-3). Flexion teardrop fractures are the most severe and unstable spinal fractures. In 1956, Schneider described this fracture as a "teardrop" fracture-dislocation because it reminded him of the tear from a patient after he conveyed the seriousness of the injury.

12. What is an extension teardrop fracture, and how does it differ from the flexion teardrop fracture?

    Similar to the flexion teardrop fracture, an extension teardrop fracture also shows an anterior-inferior fracture fragment on the lateral radiograph. However, this is an avulsion fracture attached to the anterior longitudinal ligament caused by a hyperextension injury.

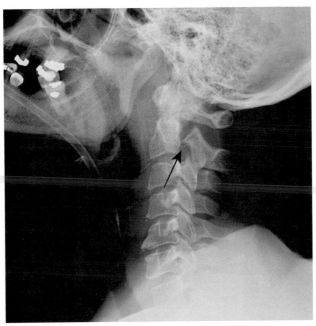

**Figure 46-2.** Hangman's fracture on lateral cervical radiograph. Note fracture of C2 (*arrow*) and offset of spinolaminar line at C2 compared to C3 level.

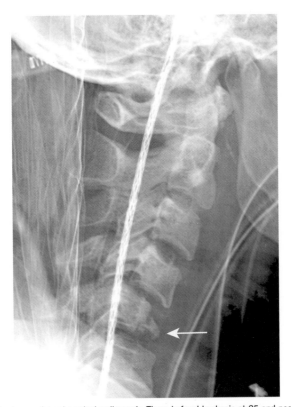

**Figure 46-3.** Flexion teardrop fracture on lateral cervical radiograph. There is focal kyphosis at C5 and posterior displacement of vertebral body along with teardrop fracture fragment (*arrow*) at anteroinferior aspect of C5.

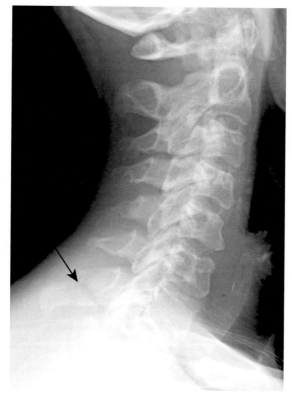

**Figure 46-4.** Clay shoveler's fracture on lateral cervical radiograph. There is minimally displaced acute fracture (*arrow*) of spinous process of C7.

13. **What is a clay shoveler's fracture?**
    A clay shoveler's fracture is a fracture of the spinous process, often seen in the lower cervical spine (Figure 46-4). In the 1930s, numerous men worked as clay shovelers in Australia. This injury occurred as a result of hyperflexion when the worker attempted to throw a shovel full of clay with the shovel stuck in the clay. Currently, this fracture occurs as a result of football and power-lifting injuries.

14. **What is the difference between unilateral and bilateral interfacetal dislocations?**
    Unilateral interfacetal dislocation (UID) (also known as unilateral locked facet injury) is a rotational injury of the cervical spine that results in unilateral facet joint dislocation with associated posterior ligamentous tear. Bilateral interfacetal dislocation (BID) (also known as bilateral locked facet injury) results from extreme hyperflexion, causing anterior dislocation of both facet joints. This is a serious injury that is commonly associated with spinal cord injury.

15. **What types of spinal fractures are considered to be unstable?**
    Of the hyperflexion etiologies, BID, flexion teardrop fracture, and wedge fracture with posterior ligamentous rupture are considered unstable. Of the hyperextension etiologies, dens type II fracture, hangman's fracture, and extension teardrop fracture are considered unstable. Burst fractures are also considered unstable, including the Jefferson fracture.

16. **What is the "reverse hamburger bun" sign?**
    The "reverse hamburger bun" sign refers to the appearance of a dislocated facet joint on axial CT images where there is uncovering of the articular facet. The superior facet of the level below normally constitutes the top bun of the hamburger, the facet joint itself constitutes the meat patty, and the inferior articular facet of the level above constitutes the bottom bun. When there is facet dislocation, the meat patty is exposed without the top bun, also known as the "naked facet" sign.

17. **What is a Chance fracture?**
    There is horizontal splitting of the posterior elements extending anteriorly to involve the vertebral body, intervertebral disc space, or both. It is often associated with tearing of the posterior ligamentous complex. It is also called a seat belt fracture following acute hyperflexion, as it is associated with seatbelt injuries, and most commonly occurs in the upper lumbar spine. Presence of this fracture should alert the clinician to the potential existence of significant intraabdominal injury.

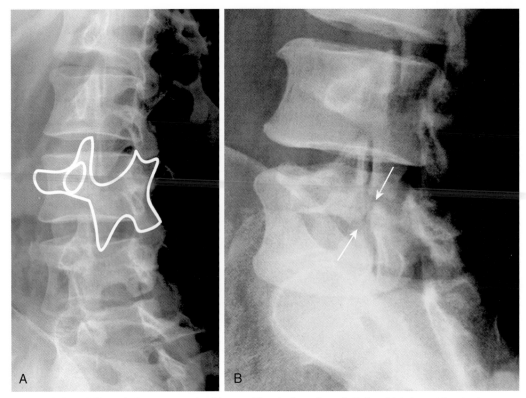

**Figure 46-5. A,** Normal "Scotty dog" appearance of vertebra on oblique lumbar radiograph. **B,** Spondylolysis on oblique lumbar radiograph. Note radiolucent fracture of pars interarticularis (arrows) where "neck" of "Scotty dog" of L5 vertebra is located.

18. What is a "Scotty dog"?

    On an oblique view of the lumbar spine, an outline of what looks like a dog can be seen. The parts of the dog are as follow: the transverse process constitutes the nose; the pedicle, the eye; the superior articular facet, the ear; the pars interarticularis, the neck; the inferior articular facet, the front leg; the lamina, the body; the contralateral superior articular facet, the tail; and the contralateral inferior articular facet, the hind leg (Figure 46-5, *A*).

19. What is spondylolysis?

    Spondylolysis is a defect or fracture of the pars interarticularis. On the "Scotty dog" view, it is seen as a band of radiolucency through the "neck," mimicking a collar (Figure 46-5, *B*). L5 is most commonly involved, and can be unilateral or bilateral.

20. Describe spondylolisthesis and its grading method.

    When spondylolysis involves the bilateral pars interarticularis at a particular vertebral level, it is commonly associated with a condition called spondylolisthesis, which is anterior translation of the involved vertebral body with respect to the more inferiorly located adjacent vertebral body. It is graded I through IV, based on the degree of anterior displacement. If it is displaced anteriorly less than 25% of the vertebral body's anteroposterior dimension, it is considered to be grade I. Displacements of 25% to 50%, 50% to 75%, and greater than 75% constitute grades II, III, and IV, respectively. Its etiology can be congenital, traumatic, degenerative, or pathologic in nature such as from Paget's disease or osteogenesis imperfecta.

**KEY POINTS**

- CT has largely replaced radiography for spinal trauma evaluation given its higher sensitivity for detection of underlying injury. However, radiography is sometimes still obtained for initial evaluation and is widely used to monitor the treatment and healing of spinal injuries. MRI is also widely used to evaluate for ligamentous and muscular injuries as well as spinal cord injuries.
- The three column concept of the spine is useful for spinal assessment. In general, if two or more spinal columns are involved in an injury, then the spine is considered to be unstable.
- Spinal fractures most commonly occur due to hyperflexion injury, but may also occur due to flexion-rotation, hyperextension, axial compression, or multiple complex injuries.

## BIBLIOGRAPHY

Pope TL Jr, Harris JH Jr. *Harris & Harris' radiology of emergency medicine*. 5th ed. Philadelphia: Lippincott Williams & Wilkins; 2013.

Ohashi K, El-Khoury GY. Musculoskeletal CT: recent advances and current clinical applications. *Radiol Clin North Am*. 2009;47(3):387-409.

Renner JB. Conventional radiography in musculoskeletal imaging. *Radiol Clin North Am*. 2009;47(3):357-372.

Hunter TB, Peltier LF, Lund PJ. Radiologic history exhibit. Musculoskeletal eponyms: who are those guys? *Radiographics*. 2000;20(3): 819-836.

Schultz RJ. *The language of fractures*. Baltimore, MD: Williams & Wilkins; 1990.

Denis F. The three column spine and its significance in the classification of acute thoracolumbar spinal injuries. *Spine (Phila Pa 1976)*. 1983;8(8):817-831.

# CHAPTER 47

# IMAGING OF NONTRAUMATIC SPINAL DISORDERS

*Andrew Spencer Wilmot, MD, Drew A. Torigian, MD, MA, FSAR, and Woojin Kim, MD*

1. **What are the indications, advantages, and disadvantages of radiography, computed tomography (CT), and magnetic resonance imaging (MRI) in the evaluation of the spine?**
   Radiography of the spine may be obtained to assess for vertebral alignment, fractures including compression deformities, and degenerative changes and as part of the workup for back pain. It may also be obtained to assess spinal alignment and hardware appearance after spinal fusion surgery. However, radiographs do not show details of the soft tissue structures such as the intervertebral discs, ligaments, spinal cord, and nerves.

   CT of the spine is most commonly used in the setting of acute trauma to assess for fractures. However, when contraindications to MRI are present, CT may be used instead to evaluate for suspected tumor, infection, and spinal cord pathology. Intervertebral discs, spinal canal, and neural foramina are still evaluable on CT, although their visualization is inferior when compared to that on MRI. CT is more sensitive than MRI for detecting calcification, gas, and certain osseous pathologies such as spondylolysis. However, streak artifacts from metallic hardware may obscure portions of the spine in patients who have had prior surgery, leading to limited evaluation.

   MRI of the spine may be obtained to assess for suspected tumor, infection, and spinal cord pathology (all beyond the scope of this chapter). MRI is the modality of choice for assessment of spinal degenerative disease and associated effects upon the spinal canal, neural foramina, ligaments, spinal cord, and nerve roots. It is also useful for evaluation of the surrounding musculature. However, susceptibility artifacts from metallic hardware may obscure portions of the spine in patients who have had prior surgery, also leading to limited evaluation.

2. **Define scoliosis, lordosis, and kyphosis.**
   Scoliosis refers to lateral curvature of the spine in the coronal plane, although abnormal curvature may affect spinal alignment in all dimensions. Dextroscoliosis and levoscoliosis refer to curvature of the spine with convexity toward the right and left, respectively (Figure 47-1). Lordosis (Figure 47-2) and kyphosis (Figure 47-3) refer to convex anterior and posterior curvatures in the sagittal plane, respectively.

3. **What is the most common cause of scoliosis?**
   In most cases, the cause of scoliosis is idiopathic. Adolescent idiopathic scoliosis is diagnosed between age 10 and skeletal maturity and is the most common type of idiopathic scoliosis. There is a heavy predominance in girls. Although idiopathic scoliosis is the most common type of scoliosis, other etiologic factors should be considered before making this diagnosis (Table 47-1).

4. **What is the Cobb angle?**
   The Cobb angle is used to quantify scoliosis. Visually identify the vertebrae at the top and bottom of the curvature on a frontal radiograph of the spine. Draw a line parallel to the superior endplate of the top vertebral body and a line parallel to the inferior endplate of the lower vertebral body. The angle at the intersection of these two lines is the Cobb angle (see Figure 47-1). Scoliosis is generally considered to be present when the Cobb angle is ≥10°.

5. **What is a limbus vertebra?**
   A limbus vertebra is an abnormality of the anterior-inferior corner or anterior-superior corner of a vertebral body secondary to an unfused ring apophysis of the endplate. It appears as a well-corticated ossicle, usually triangular in shape and separated from the rest of the vertebral body by lucent herniated disc material (Figure 47-4).

6. **What is a butterfly vertebra, a hemivertebra, and a block vertebra?**
   These are congenital vertebral anomalies. During development, the vertebral bodies initially form from two chondral centers, side by side, which eventually fuse to form a single vertebral body. If one chondral center fails to form, a hemivertebra results. If the chondral centers fail to fuse in the midline with residual hypoplasia remaining centrally, a butterfly vertebra results (Figure 47-5, *A*). If there is nonsegmentation of these centers from the subjacent chondral centers above or below, a block vertebra may result (Figure 47-5, *B*). These congenital anomalies can result in premature degenerative spinal disease or structural abnormalities such as congenital scoliosis and kyphosis. These anomalies should also raise the possibility of presence of other anomalies in the VACTERL complex (vertebral, anorectal, cardiac, tracheal, esophageal, rectal, and limb anomalies).

7. **What is a transitional vertebra?**
   A transitional vertebra occurs when a vertebra at the junction between spinal morphological segments has features of both segments. A C7 vertebral body with cervical ribs (Figure 47-6, *A*), an L1 vertebral body with ribs (Figure 47-6, *B*),

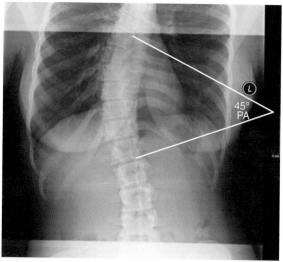

**Figure 47-1.** Dextroscoliosis of thoracolumbar spine on frontal radiograph. Note curvature of thoracolumbar spine with convexity to right and with Cobb angle of 45 degrees.

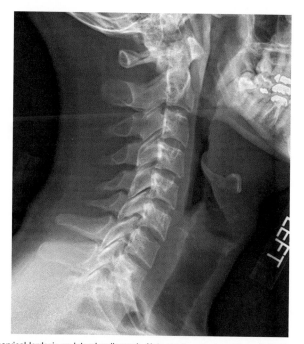

**Figure 47-2.** Normal cervical lordosis on lateral radiograph. Note gentle curvature of cervical spine with anterior convexity.

**Table 47-1.** Etiologic Factors to Consider Before Making the Diagnosis of Idiopathic Scoliosis

| CATEGORY | EXAMPLES |
| --- | --- |
| Congenital* | Block vertebra, hemivertebra, vertebral bar |
| Neuromuscular | Cerebral palsy, muscular dystrophy, spinal cord injury |
| Developmental | Skeletal dysplasia, neurofibromatosis |
| Neoplastic* | Osteoid osteoma, osteoblastoma |
| Traumatic and other | Trauma, postradiation |

*Particularly in otherwise healthy patients, effort should be focused on excluding congenital vertebral segmentation, fusion anomalies, and neoplasms.

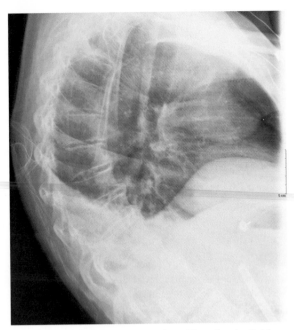

**Figure 47-3.** Kyphosis of thoracic spine on lateral radiograph. Note curvature of thoracic spine that is more exaggerated than normal with posterior convexity.

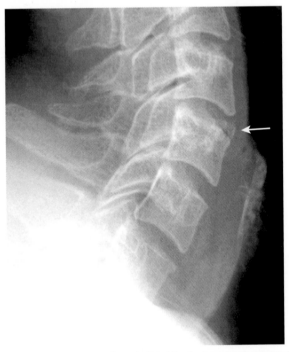

**Figure 47-4.** Limbus vertebra of cervical spine on lateral radiograph. Note triangle-shaped, well-corticated ossicle at anterior-superior endplate of C5 vertebra (*arrow*) that is separated from remainder of vertebral body by linear lucency caused by intervening disc material.

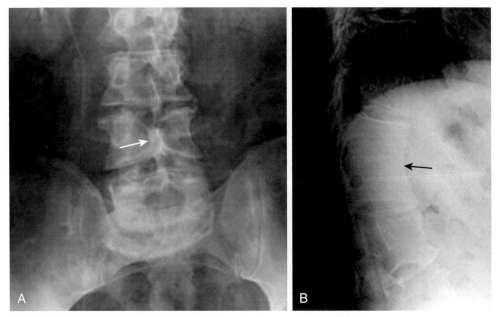

**Figure 47-5. A,** Butterfly vertebra of lumbar spine on frontal radiograph. Note central hypoplasia of L4 vertebral body (*arrow*) leading to shape similar to that of butterflies. **B,** Block vertebra of thoracolumbar spine on lateral radiograph. Note nonsegmentation of two contiguous vertebral bodies (*arrow*) with loss of intervening disc space.

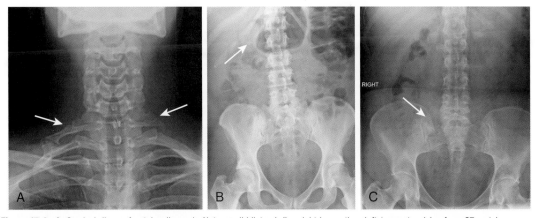

**Figure 47-6. A,** Cervical ribs on frontal radiograph. Note small bilateral ribs, right larger than left (*arrows*), arising from C7 vertebra. **B,** Lumbar rib on frontal radiograph. Note small right rib arising from L1 vertebra (*arrow*). **C,** Transitional vertebra of lumbosacral spine on frontal radiograph. Note partial sacralization of lowest lumbar vertebra (*arrow*) where right transverse process articulates with sacrum and left transverse process of same vertebra is thickened.

and an L5 vertebra with transverse processes that partially or completely fuse to the sacrum (Figure 47-6, *C*) represent cervicothoracic, thoracolumbar, and lumbosacral transitional vertebrae, respectively. Of these, lumbosacral transitional vertebrae are most common.

8. List the imaging features of spinal degenerative disease.
   - Intervertebral disc space narrowing
   - Intervertebral disc extension
   - Vacuum disc phenomenon
   - Osteophyte formation
   - Endplate changes
   - Schmorl's nodes
   - Uncovertebral joint hypertrophy (in the cervical spine)
   - Facet joint hypertrophy
   - Ligamentum flavum hypertrophy
   - Central canal stenosis
   - Neural foraminal stenosis

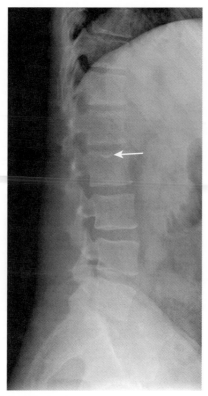

**Figure 47-7.** Schmorl's node of lumbar spine on lateral radiograph. Note lucent indentation along superior endplate of L2 vertebral body with surrounding sclerosis (*arrow*) due to intervertebral disc herniation through vertebral endplate.

9. What is a Schmorl's node?

A Schmorl's node is a herniation of intervertebral disc material through the vertebral endplate, resulting in a lucent area at the endplate with surrounding sclerosis on radiographs and CT, and possibly with surrounding edema on MRI (Figure 47-7).

10. What are Modic changes of the vertebral endplates?

These are MRI findings seen in the bone marrow adjacent to the vertebral endplates associated with degenerative disease in the lumbar spine (Figure 47-8).

- **Modic type I** change refers to a marrow edema–like pattern that histopathologically correlates with subchondral vascularized fibrous tissue and endplate fissures, and which is seen as low signal intensity on T1-weighted images and high signal intensity on fat-suppressed T2-weighted images relative to normal marrow signal.
- **Modic type II** change refers to a fatty marrow change seen as high signal intensity on T1-weighted images and as low signal intensity on fat-suppressed T2-weighted images relative to normal marrow signal.
- **Modic type III** change refers to subchondral sclerosis, which is seen as low signal intensity on both T1-weighted and T2-weighted images relative to normal marrow signal.

11. What terms are used to describe the different types of disc extension beyond the vertebral body margin?

The spectrum includes disc bulge, protrusion, extrusion, and sequestration (Figures 47-9 and 47-10).

- **Disc bulge** is diffuse extension of the intervertebral disc beyond the level of the cortical margin of the adjacent vertebral endplate, which is usually symmetric or slightly eccentric to one side and results from laxity or stretching of the annulus fibrosus. The annulus fibrosus is a ring of sturdy ligament fibers that encases the gel-like nucleus pulposus of the intervertebral disc.
- **Disc protrusion** is a focal disc extension beyond the boundaries of the remainder of the disc, which is still contained within the annulus fibrosus. The neck of the protrusion is the widest portion of the abnormality.
- **Disc extrusion** is a focal disc extension in which its neck is narrower than the extruded portion of the disc, indicating extrusion through an annular fissure. Extrusions often extend superiorly or inferiorly as well along the long axis of the spinal canal.
- **Disc herniation** is a generic term that encompasses both disc protrusion and extrusion.

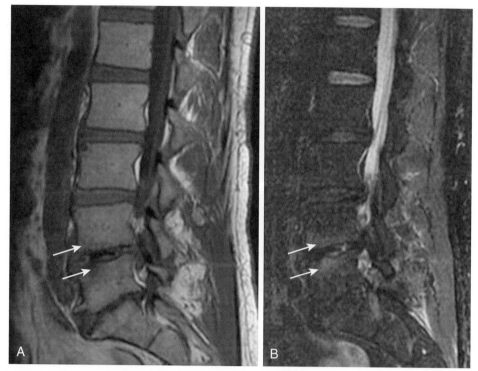

**Figure 47-8.** Modic changes related to degenerative disease of lumbar spine on MRI. **A,** Sagittal T1-weighted and **B,** Sagittal T2-weighted MR images of lumbar spine demonstrate low T1-weighted and high T2-weighted signal intensity changes of vertebral endplates surrounding L4-5 intervertebral disc space (*arrows*) in keeping with Modic type I changes. Also seen is high T1-weighted and low T2-weighted signal intensity in vertebral endplates surrounding L5-S1 intervertebral disc space in keeping with Modic type II changes. Associated loss of disc height and low signal intensity vacuum disc phenomena are also seen at both intervertebral levels due to degenerative disease.

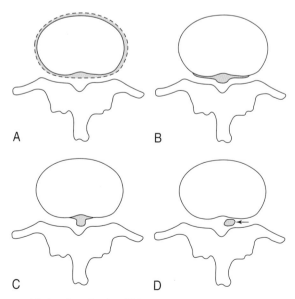

**Figure 47-9.** Illustrations of terms used to describe extension of intervertebral disc beyond margin of vertebral body. **A,** Disc bulge is diffuse and symmetric. **B,** Disc protrusion (in this case central) has focality, and neck is widest part of abnormality. **C,** Disc extrusion (in this case central) also has focality, but neck is narrowest part of abnormality. **D,** Disc sequestrum has lost all connection to parent disc and lies in epidural space.

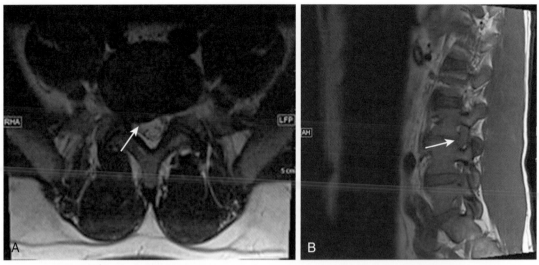

**Figure 47-10.** Disc herniations of lumbar spine on MRI. **A,** Axial T2-weighted image shows right paracentral disc protrusion at L5-S1 which contacts traversing right S1 nerve root (*arrow*). **B,** Parasagittal T1-weighted image demonstrates left neural foraminal disc protrusion at L3-4 which impinges exiting left L3 nerve root.

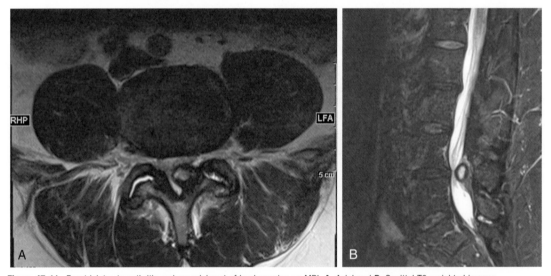

**Figure 47-11.** Facet joint osteoarthritis and synovial cyst of lumbar spine on MRI. **A,** Axial and **B,** Sagittal T2-weighted images demonstrate high signal intensity cyst with low signal intensity rim arising from left facet joint at L4-5 level and extending into epidural space, resulting in spinal canal stenosis. Also note osteophyte formation about facet joints indicating osteoarthritis.

- **Disc sequestrum** or **sequestration** is a free fragment of the intervertebral disc, which has extruded through the annulus fibrosus and separated from the remainder of the disc to lie within the epidural space.
- Location: The location of a disc herniation determines what nerve roots are affected. Central, right central/left central/right paracentral/left paracentral, subarticular, foraminal, and extraforaminal/far lateral describe the location. Right or left central (or paracentral) and subarticular (lateral recess) locations affect the ipsilateral traversing nerve root. The foraminal or extraforaminal disc herniation affects the exiting nerve root.

12. Other than degenerative disc pathology, what other factors commonly contribute to neural foraminal narrowing and spinal canal stenosis?
    Facet joint osteoarthritis, facet joint synovial cysts (Figure 47-11), uncovertebral joint hypertrophy, ligamentum flavum hypertrophy, epidural lipomatosis (Figure 47-12), and spondylolisthesis can all contribute to spinal canal and neural foraminal narrowing. The uncovertebral joints are unique to the C3 through C7 vertebrae of the cervical spine and project superiorly from the posterolateral aspects of the vertebral bodies, helping to maintain anteroposterior alignment.

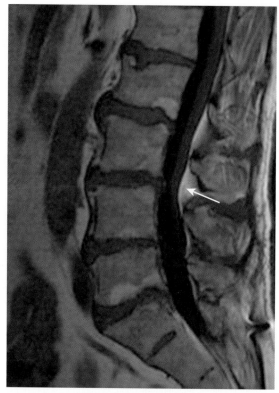

**Figure 47-12.** Epidural lipomatosis of lumbar spine on MRI. Sagittal T1-weighted image demonstrates increased amount of high signal intensity epidural fat (*arrow*) at posterior aspect of spinal canal at L3-4 level, which in combination with posterior disc bulge at L3-4 level results in spinal canal stenosis.

Some patients are born with a narrow spinal canal (often due to pedicles that are short in the anteroposterior dimension). In such patients, a lesser amount of spinal degenerative pathology is necessary to result in spinal canal stenosis (Figure 47-13).

13. **What nerve roots exit the C3-4, C7-T1, T3-4, and L5-S1 neural foramina?**
    In the cervical spine, the C1 nerve roots exit between the occiput and C1, whereas the C8 nerve roots exit at the C7-T1 intervertebral level since there is no C8 vertebra. The cervical nerve roots (with exception of C8) exit above the pedicles of the same-numbered vertebral body (e.g., the C4 nerve roots exit through the C3-4 neural foramina above the pedicles of C4). Because there are eight cervical roots, the relationship switches at the cervicothoracic junction such that in the thoracic and lumbar spine, the nerve roots exit below the pedicles of the same-numbered vertebral body (e.g., the T3 nerve roots exit through the T3-4 neural foramina below the pedicles of T3, and the L5 nerve roots exit through the L5-S1 neural foramina below the pedicles of L5).

14. **What nerve root may be impinged by a right paracentral disc herniation at L5-S1?**
    The nerve roots exit the neural foramina just below the pedicles of the upper vertebral body (i.e., the L5 nerve roots exit just below the L5 pedicles, which are superior to the level of the intervertebral disc space). A right paracentral disc herniation at L5-S1 would therefore not impinge upon the L5 nerve roots because they have already exited, unless large in size or extending cranially into the right neural foramen. Instead, the right S1 nerve root, which descends slightly lateral to the cauda equina in the lateral recess on its way toward the right S1 neural foramen, can be impinged by a right paracentral disc herniation at L5-S1 (see Figure 47-10, *A*).

15. **What nerve root may be impinged by a left foraminal or extraforaminal disc herniation at L3-4?**
    Whereas a central, paracentral, or subarticular disc herniation may impinge the traversing nerve root at a given level, a foraminal or extraforaminal disc herniation may affect the exiting nerve root. At L3-4, the L3 nerve root exits, and therefore the left L3 nerve root may be impinged by a left foraminal or extraforaminal disc herniation at L3-4 (see Figure 47-10, *B*).

16. **What is failed back syndrome? What is the best way to evaluate affected patients?**
    After spinal surgery, 5% to 40% of patients have persistent back or leg pain, and this is referred to as failed back syndrome. Approximately 10% of these patients undergo another operation. Causes of failed back syndrome include: (1) residual or recurrent disc herniation, (2) residual spinal canal, neural foraminal, or lateral recess stenosis,

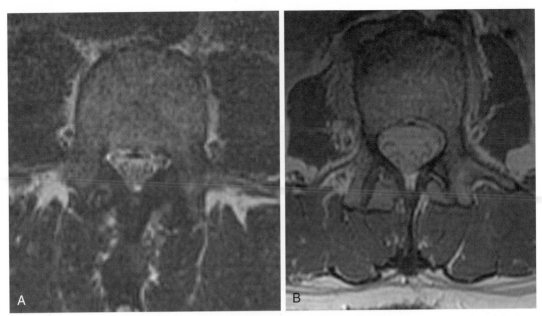

**Figure 47-13.** Congenitally short pedicles of lumbar spine on MRI. **A,** Axial T2-weighted image shows narrowing of spinal canal due to short pedicles, along with ligamentum flavum hypertrophy and facet joint osteoarthropathy. **B,** Axial T2-weighted image reveals patent spinal canal in another patent without congenitally short pedicles for comparison.

(3) formation of scar tissue in the surgical bed, (4) instability, (5) arachnoiditis, (6) surgical error (operation at the wrong level), and (7) surgical complications, including infection, hematoma, and cerebrospinal fluid leak. The best imaging method for evaluating these patients is with MRI before and after intravenous contrast administration, which can help distinguish recurrent disc herniation (nonenhancing) from postoperative fibrosis and granulation tissue formation (avidly enhancing).

17. **What is spondylolisthesis and spondylolysis? Name the two major causes and the key imaging findings.**
Spondylolisthesis is displacement of one vertebral body with respect to the vertebral body below. Anterolisthesis, which is anterior displacement of a vertebral body relative to the one located more inferiorly, is more common than retrolisthesis, which involves posterior displacement. The most common causes are spondylolysis (bilateral fractures through the pars interarticularis of the vertebra) and degenerative facet joint disease. Spondylolysis is recognized by lucency through the pars interarticularis and occurs most commonly at L5. Loss of posterior vertebral body height relative to anterior vertebral body height is also strongly suggestive of bilateral spondylolysis.

18. **What is the "inverted Napoleon hat" sign?**
This is a finding seen on a frontal radiograph of the lumbar spine or pelvis that is associated with spondylolisthesis of L5 upon S1. The anterior-inferior vertebral margin and transverse processes of the severely anteriorly displaced L5 vertebra when superimposed upon S1 have the appearance of Napoleon's hat turned upside down (Figure 47-14).

19. **What is OPLL?**
OPLL stands for ossification of the posterior longitudinal ligament and typically involves the cervical spine. OPLL appears as a longitudinal bony ridge parallel and adjacent to the posterior vertebral margins (Figure 47-15, *A*). It is more common among individuals of Japanese descent and occurs in 50% of patients with diffuse idiopathic skeletal hyperostosis (DISH). OPLL can result in spinal canal stenosis.

20. **What is DISH?**
DISH stands for diffuse idiopathic skeletal hyperostosis (also known as Forestier's disease). DISH has many manifestations throughout the body, including calcification and ossification of ligamentous and tendinous insertion sites, particularly involving the pelvis and patellae (known as "whiskering"), enthesophyte formation on the calcanei and olecranon processes, and paraarticular osteophyte formation, particularly around the hip joints. Its most common manifestation is in the spine, however, where it is associated with calcification and ossification of the anterior longitudinal ligament and large bridging osteophytes anteriorly and laterally, sometimes interrupted by linear lucencies owing to herniation of intervertebral disc material. OPLL can occur in DISH as well (Figure 47-15).

21. **What are three radiographic criteria for the diagnosis of DISH?**
Criteria are: (1) flowing ossification over at least four contiguous vertebrae, (2) minimal loss of disc height relative to ossification formation, and (3) absence of bony ankylosis and sacroiliac joint disease.

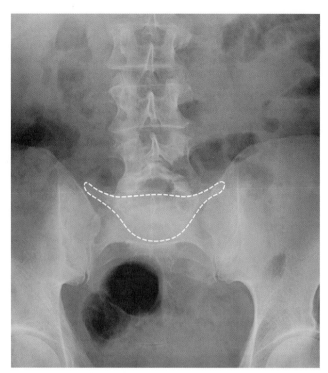

**Figure 47-14.** Anterolisthesis of L5 upon S1 on frontal radiograph. Note "inverted Napoleon hat" sign (*dashed outline*), suggestive of anterolisthesis of L5 upon S1.

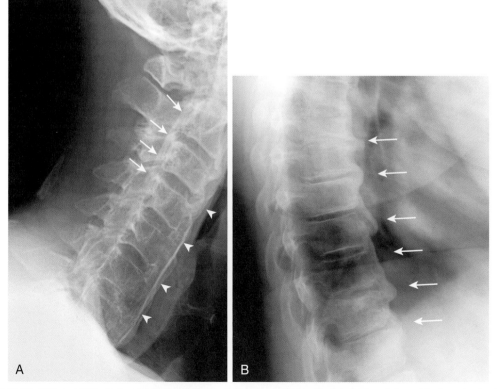

**Figure 47-15.** OPLL and DISH of spine on lateral radiographs. **A,** Note longitudinal ossification along posterior vertebral margins due to OPLL (*arrows*) and flowing ossification over anterior aspect of multiple contiguous vertebrae due to DISH (*arrowheads*) in cervical spine. **B,** Note flowing ossification over anterior aspect of multiple contiguous vertebrae due to DISH (*arrows*) in thoracic spine.

22. **What is the difference between an osteophyte, a syndesmophyte, and an enthesophyte?**
    Osteophytes are thick, triangle-shaped osseous excrescences that form at the site of Sharpey fibers attachment between the annulus fibrosus and the margin of the vertebral body just above or below the endplate margin. Osteophytes typically begin by growing outward. An osteophyte may eventually grow and meet an osteophyte on the other side of the disc space to form a bridging osteophyte.

    Syndesmophytes are thin, gracile ossifications of the annulus fibrosus and are more vertically oriented than osteophytes, attaching right at the endplate margin. Syndesmophytes are typically associated with ankylosing spondylitis.

    Enthesophytes are bony projections that develop at sites of tendon or ligament attachment to bone.

23. **What is Scheuermann's disease?**
    Scheuermann's disease is an osteochondrosis of the thoracic spine, which occurs in adolescents typically 13 to 17 years old, and is a cause of back pain. Osteochondroses affect children and adolescents and involve focal bone necrosis at the epiphysis related to rapid growth and overuse. Scheuermann's disease is characterized by vertebral endplate irregularity, multiple Schmorl's nodes, anterior vertebral wedging, intervertebral disc height loss, and resultant kyphosis. Imaging criteria for diagnosis require three contiguous abnormal vertebrae with at least 5 degrees of anterior wedge deformity.

24. **What is Baastrup's disease?**
    Baastrup's disease (also known as "kissing spines") is due to degenerative change of the spinous processes and interspinous soft tissues of the spine, is a cause of back pain, and occurs with high frequency in the elderly. In this condition, the spinous processes contact one another and may be associated with osteophyte formation, sclerosis, edema, and cyst formation (Figure 47-16).

25. **What is myelofibrosis?**
    Myelofibrosis is a myeloproliferative disorder in which the bone marrow undergoes fibrosis, resulting in diffusely increased density of the bones on radiography and CT due to sclerosis, low signal intensity of the bone marrow on MRI, hepatosplenomegaly, and pancytopenia (Figure 47-17).

26. **What types of nondegenerative arthritides may affect the spine?**
    Ankylosing spondylitis is a seronegative spondyloarthropathy that predominantly affects young males. Thin flowing syndesmophytes result in fusion of the vertebral bodies, leading to a "bamboo spine" (Figure 47-18). Fusion of the facet joints is also common. Patients experience back pain and are at increased risk of spinal fracture.

    Psoriatic and reactive arthritides are two other seronegative spondyloarthropathies, which classically result in bulky asymmetric lateral bridging osteophytes of the spine.

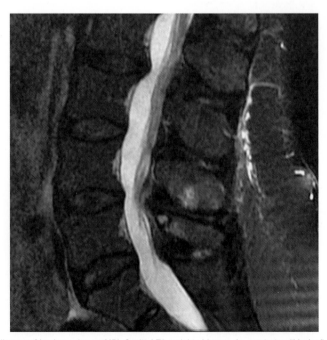

**Figure 47-16.** Baastrup's disease of lumbar spine on MRI. Sagittal T2-weighted image demonstrates "kissing" spinous processes at L4 and L5 with associated high T2-weighted signal intensity bone marrow edema and degenerative cyst formation.

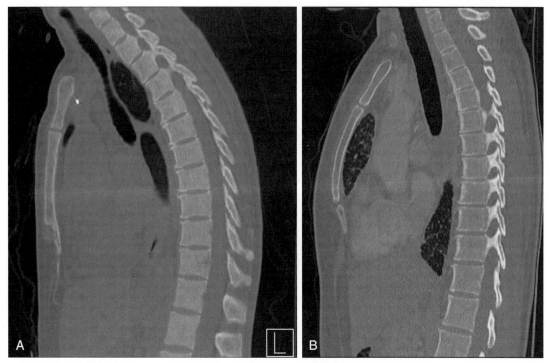

**Figure 47-17.** Myelofibrosis of spine on CT. **A,** Sagittal CT image demonstrates diffuse sclerosis of spinal vertebrae. **B,** Sagittal CT image shows normal appearing thoracic spine for comparison.

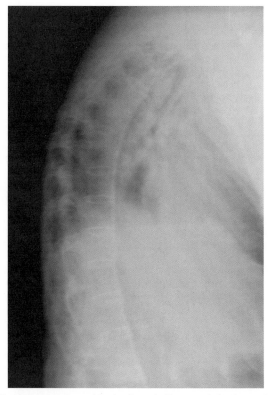

**Figure 47-18.** Ankylosing spondylitis of thoracic spine on lateral radiograph. Note smooth flowing syndesmophytes resulting in "bamboo spine." Also note upper thoracic compression fracture.

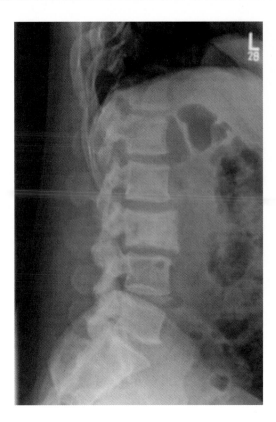

**Figure 47-19.** Paget's disease of lumbar spine on lateral radiograph. Note thickened sclerotic cortices of L3 vertebra resulting in "picture frame vertebra" along with vertebral enlargement and trabecular thickening.

27. **What is Kummel disease?**

Kummel disease is the name for vertebral body collapse due to avascular necrosis caused by preceding trauma. The collapse is delayed and typically occurs approximately 2 weeks after the trauma. On imaging, vertebral body collapse is in association with either an intravertebral vacuum cleft of gas, which has very low density on radiography, very low attenuation on CT, and very low signal intensity on MRI, and/or an intravertebral focus of fluid which has low T1-weighted and high T2-weighted signal intensity on MRI similar to that of other fluid in the body.

28. **What is Paget's disease of bone?**

Paget's disease of bone is a disorder of increased bone turnover that is believed to have a viral etiology, and it is most common in older patients. Spinal involvement is characterized by an enlarged vertebra with thickened sclerotic cortices resulting in a "picture frame" appearance along with trabecular thickening (Figure 47-19).

**KEY POINTS**

- Radiography, CT, and MRI each play an important role in spine imaging. Radiography is used to assess spinal alignment and in the initial workup of back pain. MRI is the best choice when evaluating for presence of spinal canal and neural foraminal stenosis. CT is important in the workup of patients sustaining trauma and as a substitute when MRI is contraindicated.
- *Spinal degenerative disease* is a broad term, which encompasses pathology of the intervertebral discs, vertebral endplates, uncovertebral joints, facet joints, and surrounding soft tissue structures. Spinal degenerative disease can lead to narrowing of the spinal canal and/or neural foramina, which can be symptomatic.
- *Disc bulge*, *protrusion*, *extrusion*, and *sequestration* describe the different patterns in which disc material can extend beyond the vertebral margins. These terms are more specific than the term *disc herniation*.
- A paracentral disc herniation can impinge upon the traversing nerve root, while a neural foraminal or extraforaminal disc bulge can impinge upon the exiting nerve root. Be sure to know which spinal nerves traverse and exit at any given vertebral level.
- Spinal degenerative disease is the most common disorder of the spine, but there are many other nontraumatic spinal disorders to be familiar with, including congenital anomalies and inflammatory spondyloarthropathies.

## BIBLIOGRAPHY

Fardon DF, Williams AL, Dohring EJ, et al. Lumbar disc nomenclature: version 2.0: Recommendations of the combined task forces of the North American Spine Society, the American Society of Spine Radiology and the American Society of Neuroradiology. *Spine J.* 2014; 14(11):2525-2545.

Heuck A, Glaser C. Basic aspects in MR imaging of degenerative lumbar disk disease. *Semin Musculoskelet Radiol.* 2014;18(3):228-239.

Palazzo C, Sailhan F, Revel M. Scheuermann's disease: an update. *Joint Bone Spine.* 2014;81(3):209-214.

Paparo F, Revelli M, Semprini A, et al. Seronegative spondyloarthropathies: what radiologists should know. *Radiol Med.* 2014;119(3):156-163.

Canella C, Schau B, Ribeiro E, et al. MRI in seronegative spondyloarthritis: imaging features and differential diagnosis in the spine and sacroiliac joints. *AJR Am J Roentgenol.* 2013;200(1):149-157.

Amrami KK. Imaging of the seronegative spondyloarthopathies. *Radiol Clin North Am.* 2012;50(4):841-854.

Bogduk N. Degenerative joint disease of the spine. *Radiol Clin North Am.* 2012;50(4):613-628.

Sasiadek MJ, Bladowska J. Imaging of degenerative spine disease–the state of the art. *Advances in clinical and experimental medicine.* 2012;21(2):133-142.

Ihde LL, Forrester DM, Gottsegen CJ, et al. Sclerosing bone dysplasias: review and differentiation from other causes of osteosclerosis. *Radiographics.* 2011;31(7):1865-1882.

Kwong Y, Rao N, Latief K. MDCT findings in Baastrup disease: disease or normal feature of the aging spine? *AJR Am J Roentgenol.* 2011;196(5):1156-1159.

Saetia K, Cho D, Lee S, et al. Ossification of the posterior longitudinal ligament: a review. *Neurosurg Focus.* 2011;30(3):E1.

Kim H, Kim HS, Moon ES, et al. Scoliosis imaging: what radiologists should know. *Radiographics.* 2010;30(7):1823-1842.

Malfair D, Flemming AK, Dvorak MF, et al. Radiographic evaluation of scoliosis: review. *AJR Am J Roentgenol.* 2010;194(3 suppl):S8-S22.

Freedman BA, Heller JG. Kummel disease: a not-so-rare complication of osteoporotic vertebral compression fractures. *J Am Board Fam Med.* 2009;22(1):75-78.

Grimme JD, Castillo M. Congenital anomalies of the spine. *Neuroimaging Clin N Am.* 2007;17(1):1-16.

Modic MT, Ross JS. Lumbar degenerative disk disease. *Radiology.* 2007;245(1):43-61.

Talangbayan LE. The inverted Napoleon's hat sign. *Radiology.* 2007;243(2):603-604.

Rossi A, Gandolfo C, Morana G, et al. Current classification and imaging of congenital spinal abnormalities. *Semin Roentgenol.* 2006;41(4): 250-273.

Smith SE, Murphey MD, Motamedi K, et al. From the archives of the AFIP. Radiologic spectrum of Paget disease of bone and its complications with pathologic correlation. *Radiographics.* 2002;22(5):1191-1216.

Belanger TA, Rowe DE. Diffuse idiopathic skeletal hyperostosis: musculoskeletal manifestations. *J Am Acad Orthop Surg.* 2001;9(4): 258-267.

Lowe TG. Scheuermann's disease. *Orthop Clin North Am.* 1999;30(3):475-487, ix.

# CHAPTER 48

# IMAGING OF METABOLIC BONE DISEASE

*Seong Cheol Oh, MD, and Sung Han Kim, MD*

1. **What is osteoporosis? How does it differ from osteopenia, osteomalacia, and osteosclerosis?**
   - Osteoporosis is characterized by diminished bone density with otherwise normal bone architecture. The main radiographic finding is cortical thinning. Loss of bony trabeculae may also be seen.
   - Osteomalacia is characterized by normal bone density in the setting of abnormal quality of the bone, leading to excess non-mineralized osteoid. In a growing child, this is referred to as rickets.
   - Osteopenia is characterized by diffusely increased lucency of bone as seen on radiography or computed tomography (CT). It is sometimes difficult to distinguish between osteoporosis and osteomalacia radiographically.
   - Osteosclerosis is diffusely increased density of bone as seen on radiography or CT.

2. **What is a DXA scan? How is bone mineral density (BMD) calculated?**
   Dual-energy X-ray absorptiometry (DXA) is the most widely used bone densitometric technique and the examination of choice for diagnosing and following up osteoporosis (Figure 48-1).
   The bone mineral content is assessed by measuring the relative absorption of two distinct energy x-ray beams (usually 70 kVp and 140 kVp). The bone mineral content is then divided by the area measured, yielding bone mineral density (BMD). Note that the unit of measure for BMD is $g/cm^2$ and is technically not a density measurement.

3. **What sites of the skeleton are routinely assessed on a DXA scan?**
   The lumbar spine (L1-L4 or L2-L4) and the proximal femur (femoral neck, trochanteric region, and Ward's triangle) are assessed on a routine DXA scan. (Ward's triangle is the triangular radiolucent area seen on radiography between the primary tensile, primary compressive, and secondary compressive trabeculae in the femoral neck.) If the patient has the diagnosis of hyperparathyroidism, then the forearm is used instead.

4. **What are the World Health Organization (WHO) diagnostic thresholds for normal bone mineral density, osteopenia, and osteoporosis?**
   According to the WHO, it is suggested that the reference data generated from the National Health and Nutrition Examination Survey (NHANES) study be used as a representative sample of the United States population, when using the proximal femur as the measurement site. This normative data was based on Caucasian women aged 20 to 29 years. The T-score is derived when standard deviations (SD) are calculated in relation to the young healthy population.
   Based on measurements from DXA:
   - A normal value for BMD is defined as a T-score greater than or equal to −1 SD.
   - An osteopenia T-score is less than −1 and greater than −2.5 SD.
   - An osteoporosis T-score is less than or equal to −2.5 SD.

5. **What is disuse osteoporosis? When can it be seen? What disease state can it potentially mimic?**
   Disuse osteoporosis results from immobilization and is usually seen in patients after treatment for a fracture. The appearance is different from generalized osteoporosis in that it occurs somewhat rapidly and produces a patchy mottled appearance of the bone. This configuration of the bone can mimic a malignant process such as multiple myeloma. One can differentiate the two processes by observing that in disuse osteoporosis the cortex is being resorbed, while in multiple myeloma the cortex should be solid because it is an intramedullary process.

6. **What are the radiographic findings of hyperparathyroidism?**
   The pathognomonic sign is subperiosteal bone resorption (Figure 48-2, *A*), which is most commonly seen along the radial aspect of the middle phalanges of the hands. Other findings include erosion of the terminal tufts of the distal phalanges, osteosclerosis of spinal vertebrae predominantly next to endplates, leading to a "rugger-jersey" configuration (Figure 48-2, *B*), osteopenia, brown tumors, chondrocalcinosis (i.e., calcification of cartilage), and soft tissue calcification. The frequency of some of these findings is different in primary hyperparathyroidism compared to secondary hyperparathyroidism.

7. **What is renal osteodystrophy? What is a Looser zone fracture?**
   Renal osteodystrophy is a manifestation of secondary hyperparathyroidism due to chronic renal disease combined with osteomalacia, osteoporosis, and soft tissue and vascular calcification. The term is applied to bone disease that is apparent in chronic renal failure patients. These features may become exaggerated or arrested after hemodialysis and renal transplantation.

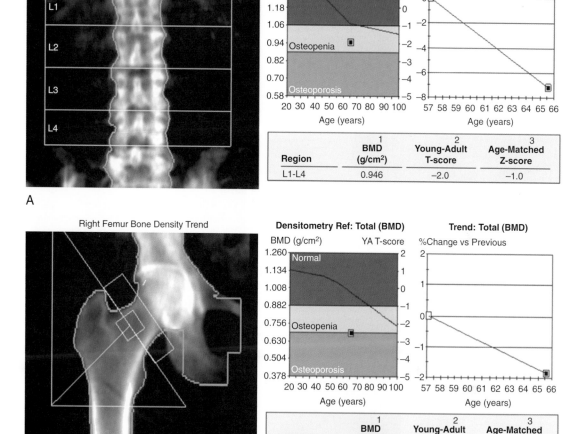

**Figure 48-1.** Osteopenia and osteoporosis on DXA scan. **A,** T-score for lumbar spine is −2.0, in keeping with osteopenia. **B,** T-score for right hip is −2.6, in keeping with osteoporosis.

A Looser zone fracture (Figure 48-3) is a thin transverse band of rarified bone cortex perpendicular to the bone surface. This represents a cortical insufficiency fracture, usually has sclerotic irregular margins, and is pathognomonic for osteomalacia.

8. What is a brown tumor?

A brown tumor is one manifestation of hyperparathyroidism which occurs as a result of excess osteoclastic activity and represents localized accumulation of fibrous tissue and giant cells. Hemosiderin deposition gives the characteristic brown hue to this lesion on gross pathology. It should be noted that this is not a neoplastic lesion. On radiography, one or more lytic foci are seen in the bones.

9. What are the skeletal manifestations of acromegaly?

Acromegaly has various radiographic features including calvarial thickening, enlarged paranasal sinuses, an enlarged sella turcica, and a prognathic jaw. The tufts of the distal phalanges of the hands become hypertrophied and resemble a spade. Thickening of the soft tissue adjacent to the calcaneus is another common feature.

10. What is the difference between metastatic calcification and dystrophic calcification?

Metastatic calcification is related to a disturbance in calcium or phosphorus metabolism and can be seen in a variety of disorders including hypervitaminosis D, hyperparathyroidism, milk-alkali syndrome, multiple myeloma, and skeletal metastatic disease.

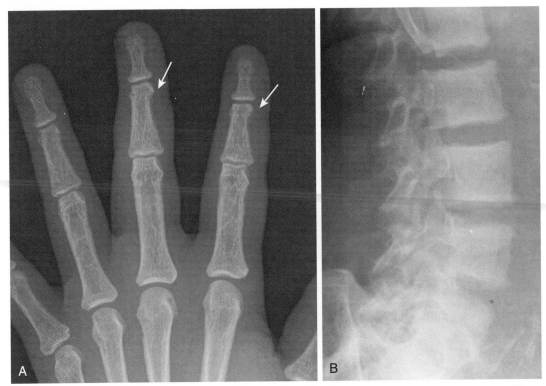

**Figure 48-2.** Hyperparathyroidism on hand and spine radiographs. **A,** Note subperiosteal resorption (*arrows*) of second and third middle phalanges of hand in patient with hyperparathyroidism. **B,** Note "rugger-jersey" appearance of lumbar spine due to osteosclerosis of spinal vertebrae predominantly next to endplates in another patient with hyperparathyroidism.

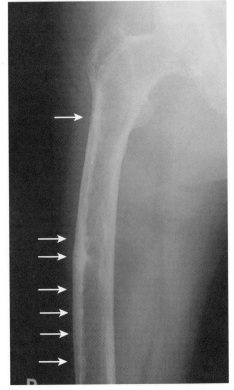

**Figure 48-3.** Osteomalacia on thigh radiograph. Note multiple linear lucent insufficiency fractures of femur perpendicular to lateral cortical surface with surrounding areas of sclerosis (*arrows*), in keeping with Looser zone fractures.

Dystrophic calcification refers to calcium deposition in damaged or devitalized tissue in the absence of a metabolic abnormality.

11. What is tumoral calcinosis?

Tumoral calcinosis is a familial condition characterized by large periarticular calcified masses thought to be secondary to a disorder in phosphate metabolism. Patients usually present in adolescence or early adulthood. Calcified masses around large joints such as the hip, shoulder, and elbow are typical. The diagnosis is one of exclusion.

## KEY POINTS

- Osteoporosis is characterized by diminished bone density with otherwise normal bone architecture, whereas osteomalacia (in adults) or rickets (in children) is characterized by normal bone density in the setting of abnormal quality of bone. Both may manifest as osteopenia (i.e., diffusely increased lucency of bone) on radiography or CT.
- DXA is the most widely used bone densitometric technique and the examination of choice for diagnosing and following up osteoporosis.
- Subperiosteal bone resorption is a pathognomonic radiographic sign of hyperparathyroidism.
- A Looser zone fracture is a pathognomonic radiographic sign of osteomalacia.
- Metastatic calcification is due to alterations in calcium or phosphorus metabolism, whereas dystrophic calcification is due to tissue injury.

## BIBLIOGRAPHY

Boswell SB, Patel DB, White EA, et al. Musculoskeletal manifestations of endocrine disorders. *Clin Imaging.* 2014;38(4):384-396.
Fathi I, Sakr M. Review of tumoral calcinosis: A rare clinico-pathological entity. *World J Clin Cases.* 2014;2(9):409-414.
Adams JE. Advances in bone imaging for osteoporosis. *Nat Rev Endocrinol.* 2013;9(1):28-42.
Lim CY, Ong KO. Various musculoskeletal manifestations of chronic renal insufficiency. *Clin Radiol.* 2013;68(7):e397-e411.
Schneider R. Imaging of osteoporosis. *Rheumatic Dis Clin N Am.* 2013;39(3):609-631.
Link TM. Osteoporosis imaging: state of the art and advanced imaging. *Radiology.* 2012;263(1):3-17.
Guglielmi G, Muscarella S, Bazzocchi A. Integrated imaging approach to osteoporosis: state-of-the-art review and update. *Radiographics.* 2011;31(5):1343-1364.
Lorente-Ramos R, Azpeitia-Arman J, Munoz-Hernandez A, et al. Dual-energy x-ray absorptiometry in the diagnosis of osteoporosis: a practical guide. *AJR Am J Roentgenol.* 2011;196(4):897-904.
Anil G, Guglielmi G, Peh WC. Radiology of osteoporosis. *Radiol Clin North Am.* 2010;48(3):497-518.
Sundaram M. Founders lecture 2007: metabolic bone disease: what has changed in 30 years? *Skeletal Radiol.* 2009;38(9):841-853.
Buckley O, Halpenny D, Torreggiani WC. Role of the radiologist in the preoperative evaluation of primary hyperparathyroidism. *AJR Am J Roentgenol.* 2008;190(1):W82. author reply W3.
Kanis JA, on behalf of the World Health Organization Scientific Group. Assessment of osteoporosis at the primary health-care level. Technical Report. World Health Organization Collaborating Centre for Metabolic Bone Diseases, University of Sheffield, UK 2007:1-337. Available at <www.iofbonehealth.org/sites/default/files/WHO_Technical_Report-2007.pdf>.
Miller PD. Guidelines for the diagnosis of osteoporosis: T-scores vs fractures. *Rev Endocr Metab Disord.* 2006;7(1-2):75-89.
Wittenberg A. The rugger jersey spine sign. *Radiology.* 2004;230(2):491-492.
Jevtic V. Imaging of renal osteodystrophy. *Eur J Radiol.* 2003;46(2):85-95.
Lentle BC, Prior JC. Osteoporosis: what a clinician expects to learn from a patient's bone density examination. *Radiology.* 2003;228(3):620-628.
Reginato AJ, Falasca GF, Pappu R, et al. Musculoskeletal manifestations of osteomalacia: report of 26 cases and literature review. *Semin Arthritis Rheum.* 1999;28(5):287-304.
Cooper KL. Radiology of metabolic bone disease. *Endocrinol Metab Clin North Am.* 1989;18(4):955-976.

# CHAPTER 49

# IMAGING OF ARTHRITIS

*Prashant T. Bakhru, MD*

1. **What kinds of joints exist?**

   Joints can be categorized based upon their structure and function. Fibrous joints such as the skull sutures (synarthrosis) demonstrate minimal to no mobility. Cartilaginous joints such as the intervertebral discs (amphiarthrosis) are slightly more mobile. Synovial joints (diarthrosis) are freely mobile.

2. **What are the advantages and disadvantages of the common imaging modalities used to evaluate arthritis?**

   Conventional radiography is the mainstay for the initial workup of patients with various arthritides. It is a relatively inexpensive imaging technique that allows the radiologist to detect the presence of and characterize the type of arthritis based upon the pattern of observed changes that involve the bones, joints, and soft tissues. However, the pathologic changes that occur early in the disease process may be occult on radiographs, particularly when involving the soft tissue structures. For this reason, magnetic resonance imaging (MRI) is useful to evaluate early changes such as joint effusions, synovitis, cartilage abnormalities, bone marrow edema, osseous erosions, and tendon and ligament abnormalities. Ultrasonography (US) is an imaging technique that may be used to evaluate patients with arthritis. While it is less expensive than MRI, it is operator dependent. Bony erosions that may be occult on radiographs can be visible on gray scale US. US is also useful to evaluate for presence of associated tendon and ligament abnormalities, intraarticular bodies, joint effusions, and extraarticular fluid collections. Color Doppler US is useful to demonstrate synovial hyperemia, which is common in the inflammatory arthropathies. $^{18}$F-fluorodeoxyglucose (FDG) positron emission tomography (PET) is also useful to reveal increased metabolic activity in sites of active arthritis, but it is only currently utilized for research purposes.

3. **What are the radiographic features that are assessed in the evaluation of arthritis?**

   A common technique of radiographic interpretation includes evaluation of the "ABCDs" of arthritis.
   - **A**lignment of joints is assessed, including presence of subluxations and dislocations.
   - **B**ones are carefully assessed for changes in mineralization, presence of erosions, and presence of new bone production (subchondral sclerosis, osteophytes, periostitis).
   - **C**artilage is indirectly evaluated on radiographs. Joint space narrowing and subchondral bony changes imply presence of cartilage disease.
   - **D**istribution (proximal vs. distal, symmetry, involvement of specific joints, regions affected within a joint) of the disease process is assessed to better characterize the specific underlying disease process.
   - **S**oft tissues are evaluated for presence and pattern of swelling and for presence of calcifications.

4. **What are the characteristic imaging findings of osteoarthritis (OA)?**

   Osteophyte formation, subchondral sclerosis, and joint space narrowing are the characteristic features of OA, also known as degenerative joint disease (DJD) (Figure 49-1). OA most commonly affects the distal interphalangeal (DIP) and proximal interphalangeal (PIP) joints of the hands and the major weight-bearing (hip and knee) joints. In addition, the carpal joints at the base of the thumb are commonly affected. Any joint that is damaged by trauma resulting in an irregular articular surface can prematurely be affected by OA as well.

5. **What are some differences between OA and rheumatoid arthritis (RA)?**

   OA is generally secondary to articular cartilage damage from repetitive microtrauma throughout life, whereas RA is an inflammatory arthritis in which inflamed synovium produces erosive changes of the adjacent bones and cartilage. Joint space narrowing in osteoarthritis is usually asymmetric, whereas joint space narrowing in RA is classically symmetric. For example, joint space narrowing tends to occur more superiorly in the hip joint in OA, whereas a more axial (i.e., concentric) distribution of joint space involvement is observed with RA. Subchondral sclerosis and osteophyte formation are reparative responses seen in OA due to chronic wear and tear. These are characteristically absent in RA.

6. **What are some common imaging features of RA?**

   Soft tissue swelling is often present and periarticular in location, usually due to an underlying joint effusion or tenosynovitis. Early in the disease process, this may be the only finding observed. Bone mineral density is typically decreased, particularly within juxtaarticular locations, which is often exacerbated by corticosteroid therapy. Joint space narrowing tends to involve the joint spaces symmetrically. Bony erosions may be present, typically along the margins of the articular surface (i.e., marginal erosions), affecting the "bare areas" of the bones first (Figure 49-2). These areas lack overlying hyaline cartilage, leaving the exposed bone susceptible to the destructive inflammatory process. Overall, the disease process tends to be symmetric in the body. However, asymmetry may be present in early phases of the disease process.

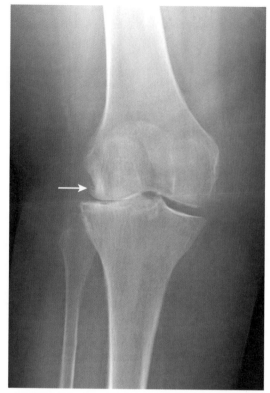

**Figure 49-1.** OA of knee joint on frontal radiograph. Note characteristic osteophyte formation (*arrow*), subchondral sclerosis, and joint space narrowing predominantly involving lateral compartment.

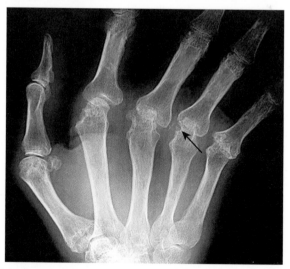

**Figure 49-2.** RA of hand on frontal radiograph. Ulnar deviation of proximal phalanges is noted. A typical marginal erosion involving fourth metacarpal head (*arrow*) is also seen.

7. Which joints in the hand and wrist are usually affected by RA?

RA tends to involve the proximal joints of the hand and wrist. One should pay close attention to the ulnar styloid to evaluate for erosions or subjacent soft tissue swelling, which may indicate presence of tenosynovitis of the extensor carpi ulnaris tendon. Whereas OA commonly involves the DIP joints, RA tends to involve the metacarpophalangeal (MCP) and PIP joints, as well as the radiocarpal and carpal joints. Advanced changes include joint malalignment such as ulnar deviation at the MCP joints (see Figure 49-2). A swan neck deformity may occur due to tendon retraction causing extension at the PIP joint with simultaneous flexion at the DIP joint. The reverse of this (i.e., flexion at the PIP joint and simultaneous extension at the DIP joint) may alternatively be seen, which is the so-called boutonnière (or buttonhole) deformity. End stage disease may present with carpal joint ankylosis (loss of joint spaces with bone fusion).

### 8. What are subchondral cysts?

Subchondral cysts represent areas of synovial fluid entering into the subchondral bone, implying destruction of the overlying articular cartilage. This is a nonspecific finding that is often seen in OA and inflammatory arthritides.

### 9. Does RA affect larger joints?

RA is not uncommon in the knee and hip joints. When present, typical findings include relatively symmetric joint space narrowing with a disproportionate lack of productive bony changes. Protrusio acetabuli is a finding in the hip joint that can be seen in RA (among other etiologies) where there is intrapelvic displacement of the medial wall of the acetabulum. The shoulder joint may be affected by erosive changes at the glenohumeral joint, distal clavicular osteolysis, and a "high-riding" humeral head with a decreased acromiohumeral interval.

### 10. What is erosive (inflammatory) OA?

Erosive OA occurs when there are significant erosive changes and soft tissue swelling in association with OA, potentially mimicking inflammatory arthropathies. However, the disease distribution does not change; there is still a predilection for the DIP joints, and there is generally a lack of bone demineralization. In addition, the erosions involve the subchondral bone centrally along articular surfaces as opposed to the bony margins in RA. When productive bony changes are also present in the periphery, one may observe a characteristic "gull wing" appearance (Figure 49-3). Erosive OA is much more common in women than in men.

### 11. How do the seronegative spondyloarthropathies differ from RA?

Ankylosing spondylitis (AS), psoriatic arthritis (PA), reactive arthritis (Reiter syndrome), and enteropathic arthritis (associated with inflammatory bowel disease) are major types of seronegative spondyloarthropathy. Patients with seronegative spondyloarthropathy usually lack presence of rheumatoid factor (RF) on blood tests (hence the term *seronegative*), whereas RF is characteristically present in RA. The HLA-B27 antigen is frequently present on blood tests in seronegative spondyloarthropathy. In seronegative spondyloarthropathies, involvement of the DIP joints, sacroiliac joints, and spine (with syndesmophyte formation in AS or parasyndesmophyte formation in PA and reactive arthritis) is common, often in association with productive bony changes and enthesopathy. These imaging features are uncommonly seen in RA. With long-standing disease, any patient with seronegative spondyloarthropathy may develop ankylosis of the sacroiliac joints and spine, which is classically associated with AS (Figure 49-4).

### 12. What are the main crystal deposition disorders?

Gout (due to monosodium urate monohydrate deposition), calcium pyrophosphate dihydrate deposition (CPPD) disease, and hydroxyapatite deposition disease (HADD) are the main crystal deposition disorders.

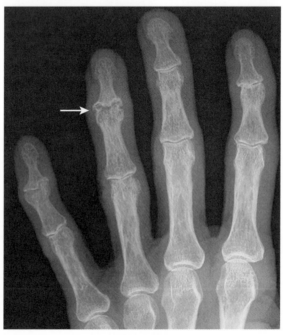

**Figure 49-3.** Erosive OA of DIP joint of hand on frontal radiograph. Note typical "gull wing" appearance of fourth DIP joint due to central erosion and peripheral hypertrophic changes (*arrow*), along with surrounding soft tissue swelling. Similar findings are also seen in fifth DIP joint.

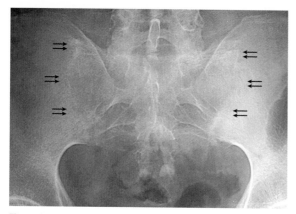

**Figure 49-4.** AS of sacroiliac joints on frontal radiograph. Note fusion (ankylosis) of sacroiliac joints (*arrows*).

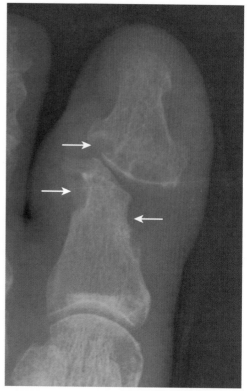

**Figure 49-5.** Gout of first interphalangeal joint on frontal radiograph. Note eccentric "punched out" juxtaarticular erosions (*arrows*) with sclerotic margins and overhanging edges of cortical bone, in association with areas of soft tissue swelling. Also note preservation of bone mineralization and joint space width.

13. **What are the imaging findings in gout?**
    Imaging shows crystal deposition within the periarticular soft tissues, most commonly involving the first metatarsophalangeal (MTP) joints, but also possibly within bones, tendons, and bursae, with an asymmetrical polyarticular distribution most often in the hands and feet. Characteristic changes seen on radiographs occur in the chronic stages of the disease. These include eccentric "punched out" juxtaarticular erosions, which are more marginal than those seen in RA, typically with sclerotic margins and overhanging edges of cortical bone (Figure 49-5). Bone mineralization is normal, and joint spaces are generally preserved until late in the disease course. Earlier findings are nonspecific and include soft tissue swelling, sometimes in a "lumpy bumpy" pattern, and joint effusions. The areas of soft tissue swelling (i.e., tophi) may appear radiodense on radiography due to crystal deposition. Soft tissue calcifications may also be seen and are more often associated with concomitant renal disease. On MRI, tophi usually have low-intermediate T1-weighted signal intensity and variable T2-weighted signal intensity relative to skeletal muscle (Figure 49-6) and enhance.

14. **What is chondrocalcinosis?**
    Chondrocalcinosis refers to soft tissue calcification, usually within hyaline articular cartilage or fibrocartilage. Fibrocartilage is present in structures such as the menisci of the knee, the triangular fibrocartilage of the wrist, the labra of the acetabulum and glenoid, and the symphysis pubis.

15. **Is chondrocalcinosis synonymous with CPPD?**
    No. Chondrocalcinosis may be seen in a variety of disorders including CPPD (Figure 49-7), hyperparathyroidism, hemochromatosis, and OA, as well as with advanced age.

16. **What is pseudogout?**
    Pseudogout is a clinical term reflecting synovitis related to CPPD deposition. This refers to the radiologic diagnosis of calcium pyrophosphate arthropathy (see Figure 49-7). On imaging, the findings appear similar to those of OA but characteristically affect non-weight-bearing joints (wrist, elbow, knee [especially patellofemoral], and shoulder [glenohumeral]), sometimes in association with chondrocalcinosis. In the hand, the MCP joints may be affected,

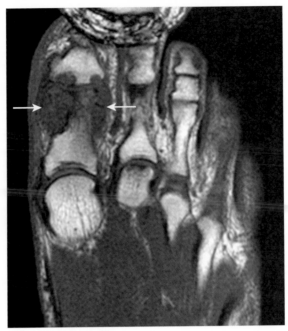

**Figure 49-6.** Gout of first interphalangeal joint on MRI. Coronal T1-weighted image of foot shows low signal intensity tophi (*arrows*) with associated juxtaarticular erosions of first interphalangeal joint.

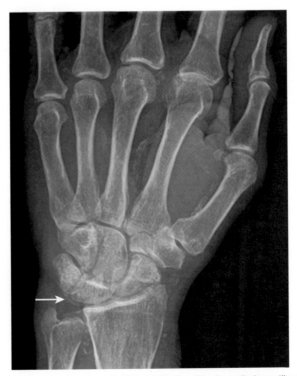

**Figure 49-7.** CPPD arthropathy of wrist on frontal radiograph. Note calcification of hyaline articular cartilage (*arrow*) representing chondrocalcinosis. Also note joint space narrowing and multiple areas of cystic resorption within carpus. Extensive vascular calcifications are also seen, due to known chronic renal disease.

resulting in presence of hooked osteophytes. In the wrist, this disorder can lead to scapholunate dissociation and proximal migration of the capitate bone between the scaphoid and lunate bones, which is called scapholunate advanced collapse (SLAC) or a SLAC wrist.

## KEY POINTS

- Osteophyte formation, subchondral sclerosis, and joint space narrowing are characteristic features of OA, which most commonly affects the DIP and PIP joints of the hands as well as the major weight-bearing (hip and knee) joints.
- Symmetric erosive changes of the MCP and PIP joints of the hands, along with periarticular osteopenia and symmetric joint space loss, are suggestive of RA.
- Eccentric "punched out" juxtaarticular erosions with sclerotic margins and overhanging edges in conjunction with soft tissue tophi are characteristic of gout. Bone mineralization and joint spaces tend to be preserved.

## BIBLIOGRAPHY

Chowalloor PV, Siew TK, Keen HI. Imaging in gout: a review of the recent developments. *Ther Adv Musculoskelet Dis.* 2014;6(4):131-143.
Huang M, Schweitzer ME. The role of radiology in the evolution of the understanding of articular disease. *Radiology.* 2014;273 (suppl 2):S1-S22.
McQueen FM, Doyle A, Dalbeth N. Imaging in the crystal arthropathies. *Rheum Dis Clin North Am.* 2014;40(2):231-249.
Roemer FW, Eckstein F, Hayashi D, et al. The role of imaging in osteoarthritis. *Best Pract Res Clin Rheumatol.* 2014;28(1):31-60.
Schueller-Weidekamm C, Mascarenhas VV, Sudol-Szopinska I, et al. Imaging and interpretation of axial spondylarthritis: the radiologist's perspective—consensus of the Arthritis Subcommittee of the ESSR. *Semin Musculoskelet Radiol.* 2014;18(3):265-279.
Girish G, Glazebrook KN, Jacobson JA. Advanced imaging in gout. *AJR Am J Roentgenol.* 2013;201(3):515-525.
Grainger AJ, Rowbotham EL. Rheumatoid arthritis. *Semin Musculoskelet Radiol.* 2013;17(1):69-73.
Guermazi A, Hayashi D, Eckstein F, et al. Imaging of osteoarthritis. *Rheum Dis Clin North Am.* 2013;39(1):67-105.
Mattar M, Salonen D, Inman RD. Imaging of spondyloarthropathies. *Rheum Dis Clin North Am.* 2013;39(3):645-667.
Vasanth LC, Pavlov H, Bykerk V. Imaging of rheumatoid arthritis. *Rheum Dis Clin North Am.* 2013;39(3):547-566.
Amrami KK. Imaging of the seronegative spondyloarthopathies. *Radiol Clin North Am.* 2012;50(4):841-854.
Brower AC, Fleming DJ. *Arthritis in black and white.* 3rd ed. Philadelphia: Elsevier Saunders; 2012.
Jang JH, Ward MM, Rucker AN, et al. Ankylosing spondylitis: patterns of radiographic involvement—a re-examination of accepted principles in a cohort of 769 patients. *Radiology.* 2011;258(1):192-198.
Narvaez JA, Narvaez J, De Lama E, et al. MR imaging of early rheumatoid arthritis. *Radiographics.* 2010;30(1):143-163, discussion 63-5.
Jacobson JA, Girish G, Jiang Y, et al. Radiographic evaluation of arthritis: degenerative joint disease and variations. *Radiology.* 2008;248(3):737-747.
Jacobson JA, Girish G, Jiang Y, et al. Radiographic evaluation of arthritis: inflammatory conditions. *Radiology.* 2008;248(2):378-389.
Papatheodorou A, Ellinas P, Takis F, et al. US of the shoulder: rotator cuff and non-rotator cuff disorders. *Radiographics.* 2006;26(1):e23.
Chew FS. Radiology of the hands: review and self-assessment module. *AJR Am J Roentgenol.* 2005;184(suppl 6):S157-S168.
Sommer OJ, Kladosek A, Weiler V, et al. Rheumatoid arthritis: a practical guide to state-of-the-art imaging, image interpretation, and clinical implications. *Radiographics.* 2005;25(2):381-398.

# CHAPTER 50

# IMAGING OF MUSCULOSKELETAL INFECTION

*Alexander T. Ruutiainen, MD*

1. **What is the role of imaging in the diagnosis of musculoskeletal infection?**
Imaging examinations can help to diagnose the presence of and delineate the extent of infection involving the soft tissues or bone. However, radiologists rely on correlative clinical findings including history and physical examination findings and laboratory testing results to help establish the diagnosis of infection. The diagnosis of musculoskeletal infection is a collaborative process between radiologists and referring providers.

2. **What imaging modalities are used in diagnosing musculoskeletal infections?**
Most imaging modalities have a role in the diagnosis of infection, and these roles are frequently complementary. These include radiography, computed tomography (CT), magnetic resonance imaging (MRI), ultrasonography (US), and nuclear medicine techniques.

3. **What is the role of US in the diagnosis of musculoskeletal infection?**
In general, musculoskeletal US is an important adjunct to the other modalities. US excels in the evaluation of superficial soft tissues, and benefits from higher spatial resolution than MRI, higher soft tissue contrast than CT, and a lack of ionizing radiation. However, US suffers from poor penetration into deeper structures and is therefore best utilized to evaluate superficial tissues. Additionally, US is optimized for answering a specific clinical question, rather than for the survey of larger anatomic areas such as can be performed with radiography, CT, or MRI.

    In the specific diagnosis of infection, musculoskeletal US can be used to identify fluid collections, particularly pockets of potentially drainable pus in the midst of an extensive cellulitis. US also excels in the identification of nonradiopaque foreign bodies that may act as a nidus for infection.

4. **What is the role of nuclear medicine techniques in the diagnosis of musculoskeletal infection?**
Technetium-99m ($^{99m}$Tc) methylene diphosphonate (MDP) bone scintigraphy ("bone scan"), Indium-111 ($^{111}$In) white blood cell (WBC) scintigraphy ("WBC scan"), and fluorine-18 ($^{18}$F)-fluorodeoxyglucose (FDG) positron emission tomography (PET) are available nuclear medicine techniques that can be used to diagnose musculoskeletal infection. Currently, their use has been largely eclipsed by MRI, although they remain useful for problem-solving applications.

    For example, the diagnosis of periprosthetic infection (osteomyelitis adjacent to orthopedic hardware) is difficult by MRI because of field distortion effects around metal. Similarly, the diagnosis of infection at the site of a recent fracture (when bone marrow edema and soft tissue edema are expected) can be challenging with anatomic imaging techniques. In these and other challenging cases, nuclear medicine techniques can provide valuable diagnostic information.

5. **In general, what is the first-line imaging modality used to diagnose musculoskeletal infection?**
Radiography. It is fast, inexpensive, and frequently the only imaging modality necessary to establish a diagnosis of infection.

6. **Define osteomyelitis, cellulitis, fasciitis, myositis, pyomyositis, phlegmon, and abscess.**
   - **Osteomyelitis**: Infection of bone.
   - **Cellulitis**: Infection of skin and superficial soft tissues.
   - **Fasciitis**: Infection of fascial tissues.
   - **Myositis**: A general term indicating muscle inflammation.
   - **Pyomyositis**: Infection of muscles.
   - **Phlegmon**: A suppurative inflammatory process in the soft tissues.
   - **Abscess**: An organized collection of pus.

7. **What is the clinical significance of an abscess?**
Abscesses are difficult to treat with antimicrobial agents alone, particularly when large in size. They often require drainage for complete treatment. In contradistinction, a phlegmon cannot be drained (because it does not contain an organized pocket of fluid) and therefore is generally treated with antimicrobial agents alone.

8. **Define Brodie abscess, sequestrum, involucrum, cloaca, and sinus tract.**
   - **Brodie abscess**: An organized collection of pus within a bone (i.e., an intraosseous abscess), reflecting subacute osteomyelitis, most often due to *Staphylococcus aureus* infection.
   - **Sequestrum**: A devascularized piece of bone that is seen within an intraosseous abscess.

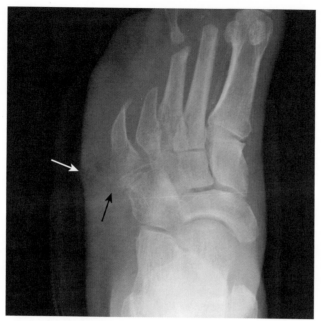

**Figure 50-1.** Acute osteomyelitis on radiography. A radiograph of foot in patient status post amputations for prior bouts of osteomyelitis demonstrates soft tissue ulcer (*white arrow*) on lateral aspect of foot. Just subjacent to ulcer, there is cortical destruction, osteolysis, and osteopenia of base of fifth metatarsal bone (*black arrow*) diagnostic of acute osteomyelitis.

- **Involucrum**: Thickened periosteal new bone formation surrounding a sequestrum, which represents the body's attempt to contain a region of osteomyelitis.
- **Cloaca**: An opening from a sequestrum through the involucrum.
- **Sinus tract**: A connection from a bone to the skin surface, lined with granulation tissue, also called a fistula. It can allow the drainage of pus.

9. What is the first-line modality in the diagnosis of acute osteomyelitis?
   Radiography.

10. What are the primary findings of acute osteomyelitis on radiographs?
    Bone destruction (osteolysis), osteopenia, and periosteal reaction, particularly if located adjacent to a soft tissue ulcer (Figure 50-1).

11. What is the most specific finding of acute osteomyelitis on radiographs?
    Osseous destruction subjacent to a soft tissue ulcer.

12. What differential diagnoses may simulate the appearance of acute osteomyelitis on radiographs?
    Traumatic changes and postsurgical findings are the most common mimickers of osteomyelitis on radiographs. In particular, healing fractures result in periosteal reaction, and surgical defects can simulate the appearance of osteolysis. Comparison studies, and in particular, accurate and pertinent clinical history, can obviate some of these pitfalls.

13. Is radiography sensitive for the detection of acute osteomyelitis in the early clinical setting?
    No. The radiographic findings of acute osteomyelitis take time to develop, typically 1 to 2 weeks, although this depends on the severity of the infection. Therefore, radiographic findings may not be present in early or very low-grade infections.

14. If radiographs are positive for acute osteomyelitis, is there a role for MRI?
    MRI is often unnecessary for the diagnosis of osteomyelitis if this has already been established radiographically. However, MRI excels in delineating the extent of the infection and is often helpful in preoperative planning.

15. If radiographs are negative for acute osteomyelitis, is there a role for MRI?
    Yes, particularly if there is suspicion for early or low-grade osteomyelitis.

16. What are the MRI findings of osteomyelitis?
    On MRI, acute osteomyelitis manifests as bone marrow edema with increased signal intensity on fluid-sensitive sequences such as T2-weighted and short tau inversion recovery (STIR) images with corresponding decreased signal

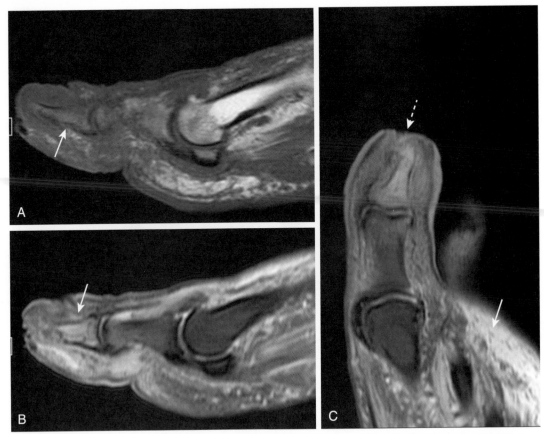

**Figure 50-2.** Acute osteomyelitis on MRI. **A,** Sagittal T1-weighted, **B,** Sagittal fat-suppressed T2-weighted, and **C,** Coronal fat-suppressed T2-weighted images of great toe demonstrate bone marrow edema in distal phalanx as manifested by low T1-weighted signal intensity (*arrow* in **A**) and high T2-weighted signal intensity (*arrow* in **B**). This bone marrow edema is located subjacent to soft tissue ulcer at tip of great toe (*dashed arrow* in **C**). Note associated soft tissue edema in subcutaneous tissues (*solid arrow* in **C**). It is often difficult to determine whether abscess may be present if intravenous contrast material is not administered.

intensity on T1-weighted images (Figure 50-2). The same findings which may be visible radiographically (cortical destruction and periosteal reaction) are also frequently present. Following the administration of intravenous contrast material, there is frequently abnormal enhancement as well.

17. **Is bone marrow edema specific for the diagnosis of acute osteomyelitis?**
    No. Bone marrow edema may be caused by many other processes including traumatic injury, stress reaction, postsurgical change, tumors, and so forth.

18. **What can help establish the diagnosis of acute osteomyelitis on MRI?**
    First, clinical history that is suggestive of infection is useful to make a diagnosis of acute osteomyelitis. Additionally, other findings of infection often are encountered, including skin ulceration, cellulitis, fasciitis, pyomyositis, phlegmon, and abscess. The presence of such findings increases confidence that the bone marrow edema represents acute osteomyelitis. In particular, if a skin ulcer is seen to directly communicate with a bone that demonstrates bone marrow edema, then the diagnosis of osteomyelitis is almost certain.

19. **What are the routes of spread of infection that involve bone?**
    Osteomyelitis is most commonly caused by (1) direct spread from adjacent tissues, particularly through a skin ulcer, but can also be introduced by (2) penetrating trauma, (3) surgical contamination, or (4) hematogenous seeding.

20. **How does the MRI appearance of acute osteomyelitis differ if the source of infection is hematogenous?**
    Many of the ancillary signs that are typically used to establish the diagnosis of acute osteomyelitis will be absent—in particular, a skin ulcer is unlikely to be present. Infection may present only as patchy areas of bone marrow edema. In such cases, clinical history, such as of known bacteremia, is vital for accurate diagnosis. Another suggestive finding is polyostotic involvement (multifocality), although multifocal bone marrow edema can be caused by many other disease processes besides infection.

21. How does the diagnosis of osteomyelitis differ in patients with Charcot arthropathy (neuropathic joint)?
Patients with neuropathic arthropathy of Charcot have preexisting joint space destruction, bony fragmentation, and bone marrow edema—findings that would otherwise raise suspicion for osteomyelitis. However, both Charcot arthropathy and osteomyelitis are often coexistent, particularly in patients with advanced diabetes mellitus. Therefore, the diagnosis of osteomyelitis is particularly challenging in these patients. Radiographs are helpful only if they have highly specific signs of infection (e.g., soft tissue gas) or if they show rapid temporal evolution of the osteolysis. MRI diagnosis relies on identifying a skin ulcer that directly extends to the region of bone marrow edema. That is, bone marrow edema without subjacent ulceration most probably reflects neuropathic arthropathy, whereas bone marrow edema subjacent to a skin ulcer most likely reflects osteomyelitis. In this way, MRI is sometimes only marginally better than a careful physical examination in this patient population.

22. Is intravenous contrast material necessary for the diagnosis of acute osteomyelitis by MRI?
No. In general, the diagnosis is established based on a combination of bone marrow edema, ancillary findings such as skin ulceration, and clinical history. Contrast material can occasionally be helpful in evaluating the pattern of bone marrow enhancement. However, MRI contrast is very useful in the diagnosis of the soft tissue infection that typically accompanies osteomyelitis.

23. What is the role of intravenous contrast material in the diagnosis of soft tissue infection?
Contrast material is helpful to delineate the presence and extent of soft tissue infection. In particular, it is often necessary to diagnose an abscess or other organized fluid collection (Figure 50-3). Although large abscesses or hematomas can be identified on unenhanced images, confident diagnosis is only possible by delineation of a nonenhancing fluid collection that is surrounded by soft tissue enhancement.

24. What imaging study is ordered in a patient with suspected septic arthritis?
None, or at most any cross-sectional imaging study to confirm the presence of a joint effusion. No imaging study has sufficient sensitivity to fully exclude this important diagnosis. If septic arthritis is suspected, then the only way to exclude joint space infection is to proceed with joint aspiration (arthrocentesis). Typically, this can be done in the office or at the bedside (such as of the shoulder, elbow, knee, and ankle joint), although some joints (hip and unusual sites

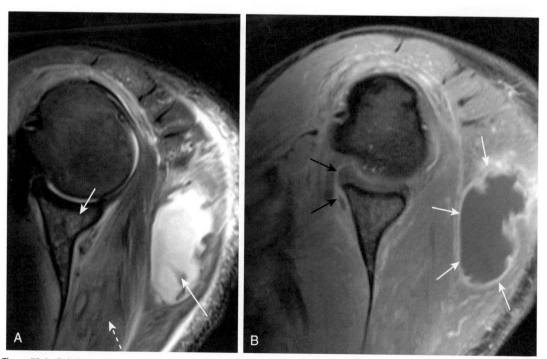

**Figure 50-3.** Soft tissue abscess and other manifestations of advanced infection on MRI. **A,** Axial fat-suppressed T2-weighted and **B,** Axial postcontrast fat-suppressed T1-weighted images of shoulder show large soft tissue loculated fluid collection (*long solid white arrow* in **A**) that demonstrates rim enhancement (*white arrows* in **B**) in keeping with abscess. There is also high T2-weighted signal intensity edema in surrounding musculature including infraspinatus muscle (*dashed white arrow* in **A**) suggestive of pyomyositis. Bone marrow edema in glenoid of scapula (*short solid white arrow* in **A**) likely reflects acute osteomyelitis. Presence of adjacent small shoulder joint effusion with prominent synovial enhancement (*black solid arrows* in **B**) is suspicious for septic arthritis, although diagnosis of joint infection should always be established or excluded by arthrocentesis.

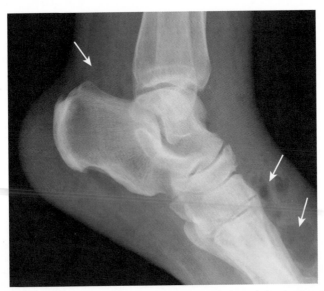

**Figure 50-4.** Necrotizing soft tissue infection on radiography. Lateral radiograph of foot reveals low density soft tissue gas (*arrows*). If patient has not had recent surgical intervention, penetrating trauma, or some other event that could explain presence of gas, then this finding should raise concern for necrotizing infection by gas-forming organisms. This is a surgical emergency and requires prompt diagnosis and treatment.

like the sacroiliac joints) may benefit from an image-guided arthrocentesis using either fluoroscopic, sonographic, or rarely CT guidance.

25. **Are there any imaging findings that are suggestive of septic arthritis?**
Yes. The findings of a large complex joint effusion with thick synovial enhancement and bone marrow edema in the bones surrounding the joint raise suspicion for septic arthritis, particularly when only one joint is involved. Periarticular osteopenia, uniform joint space narrowing, osseous erosions, and soft tissue swelling may also be seen. Nevertheless, the diagnosis should still be confirmed with arthrocentesis to exclude rare mimickers of infection (such as an aggressive inflammatory arthropathy) and, more important, to obtain a microbiological diagnosis to aid in the selection of appropriate antimicrobial therapy.

26. **What is necrotizing fasciitis?**
Necrotizing fasciitis is an aggressive, rapidly progressive, and frequently fatal infection involving the fascial layers of the body, often by polymicrobial organisms, and is a surgical emergency. Its diagnosis, although primarily clinical, also rests on the identification of soft tissue emphysema (i.e., gas in the soft tissues) (Figure 50-4). Large quantities of gas can be easily diagnosed via radiography, while smaller amounts may require the use of CT. Other suggestive imaging features include fascial plane thickening, edema, or enhancement, as well as edema, phlegmon, or abscess formation in subjacent muscles. Whether radiography or CT is used, the imaging test and its interpretation are rapidly provided, and if the clinical and imaging findings support this diagnosis, then the patient is taken to the operating room for debridement and is also treated with antimicrobial agents. Slower imaging modalities such as MRI and US are less often utilized when this diagnosis is suspected.

27. **What is the radiographic and MRI appearance of infectious spondylitis?**
Infectious spondylitis, often called "discitis-osteomyelitis," is infection of the spine. In adults, the appearance is similar to the manifestations of septic arthritis: destruction, enhancement, and an effusion of at least one disc space and findings of acute osteomyelitis of the adjacent vertebral bodies. In children, infection of the intervertebral discs without surrounding osteomyelitis can also occur due to the vascularity of the discs. On radiography, discitis-osteomyelitis manifests as progressive endplate destruction and disc space narrowing. While not infrequently mistaken for advanced degenerative disease on either radiographs or MRI, infection can demonstrate more specific signs on cross-sectional imaging such as paraspinal and psoas abscesses and phlegmon.

28. **What is Pott's disease?**
Pott's disease of the spine is tuberculous spondylitis. Like pyogenic (bacterial) spondylitis, it can affect one or more vertebral bodies. Unlike bacterial discitis-osteomyelitis, however, *Mycobacterium tuberculosis* typically causes less disc space destruction than pyogenic infection, often spreading along the longitudinal ligaments of the spine to affect several vertebral bodies with relative preservation of their intervertebral discs. In advanced stages, tuberculosis causes vertebral destruction and advanced kyphotic deformities. Once common—and even visible on archeological specimens of human skeletons—Pott's disease is now quite uncommon.

**29. What is the significance of unilateral sacroiliitis?**

Sacroiliitis, or inflammation of the sacroiliac joint, can be caused by both inflammatory and infectious processes. When the process is bilateral, it is generally the cause of a rheumatologic disease such as ankylosing spondylitis or inflammatory bowel disease–related spondyloarthropathy (particularly if symmetric) or reactive arthritis or psoriatic arthritis (particularly if asymmetric). Although unilateral sacroiliitis can be caused by one of the asymmetric seronegative spondyloarthropathies (reactive or psoriatic arthritis), it should also raise concern for infection. Therefore, patients with unilateral sacroiliitis often need sacroiliac joint aspiration, typically under fluoroscopic or CT guidance, for definitive diagnosis.

## KEY POINTS

- The accurate diagnosis of musculoskeletal infection requires correlation between a thorough clinical history and physical, laboratory testing, and imaging studies. The imaging workup generally begins with radiography. Subsequent MRI may be used to diagnose early osteomyelitis and the soft tissue components of infection.
- Osteomyelitis manifests as bone marrow edema on MRI, although this appearance is not specific for infection. A correlative clinical history or direct evidence of spread from the adjacent tissues (such as from a skin ulcer) is necessary to support the diagnosis.
- The injection of intravenous contrast material is not necessary for the diagnosis of acute osteomyelitis. However, it is critical for the identification of surrounding soft tissue infection, and in particular for differentiating an abscess from a phlegmon. This distinction is important because the former is drained while the latter is treated with antimicrobial agents alone.
- A large complex joint effusion with thick synovial enhancement and periarticular bone marrow edema raise suspicion for septic arthritis, particularly when only one joint is involved. Periarticular osteopenia, uniform joint space narrowing, osseous erosions, and soft tissue swelling are also suggestive imaging features of septic arthritis. However, whenever this diagnosis is suspected clinically, it should be excluded by joint aspiration.
- Necrotizing fasciitis is a surgical emergency, requiring prompt diagnosis and treatment. Its diagnosis, while primarily clinical, also rests in the identification of soft tissue emphysema. Other suggestive imaging features include fascial plane thickening, edema, or enhancement, as well as edema, phlegmon, or abscess formation in subjacent muscles.

## BIBLIOGRAPHY

Israel O, Sconfienza LM, Lipsky BA. Diagnosing diabetic foot infection: the role of imaging and a proposed flow chart for assessment. *Q J Nucl Med Mol Imaging*. 2014;58(1):33-45.

Pattamapaspong N, Sivasomboon C, Settakorn J, et al. Pitfalls in imaging of musculoskeletal infections. *Semin Musculoskelet Radiol*. 2014;18(1):86-100.

Paz Maya S, Dualde Beltran D, Lemercier P, et al. Necrotizing fasciitis: an urgent diagnosis. *Skeletal Radiol*. 2014;43(5):577-589.

Rowe SP, Cho SY. The role of PET in the evaluation of musculoskeletal infections. *Semin Musculoskelet Radiol*. 2014;18(2):166-174.

Manaster BJ, May DA, Disler DG. *Musculoskeletal imaging: the requisites*. 4th ed. Philadelphia: Elsevier Saunders; 2013.

Palestro CJ. FDG PET in musculoskeletal infections. *Semin Nucl Med*. 2013;43(5):367-376.

Brant WE, Helms CA. *Fundamentals of diagnostic radiology*. 4th ed. Philadelphia: Lippincott Williams & Wilkins; 2012.

Soldatos T, Durand DJ, Subhawong TK, et al. Magnetic resonance imaging of musculoskeletal infections: systematic diagnostic assessment and key points. *Acad Radiol*. 2012;19(11):1434-1443.

Garcia-Arias M, Balsa A, Mola EM. Septic arthritis. *Best Pract Res Clin Rheumatol*. 2011;25(3):407-421.

Hatzenbuehler J, Pulling TJ. Diagnosis and management of osteomyelitis. *Am Fam Physician*. 2011;84(9):1027-1033.

Horowitz DL, Katzap E, Horowitz S, et al. Approach to septic arthritis. *Am Fam Physician*. 2011;84(6):653-660.

Shikhare SN, Singh DR, Shimpi TR, et al. Tuberculous osteomyelitis and spondylodiscitis. *Semin Musculoskelet Radiol*. 2011;15(5):446-458.

Turecki MB, Taljanovic MS, Stubbs AY, et al. Imaging of musculoskeletal soft tissue infections. *Skeletal Radiol*. 2010;39(10):957-971.

Helms CA, Major NM, Anderson MW, et al. *Musculoskeletal MRI*. 2nd ed. Philadelphia: Saunders Elsevier; 2009.

Pineda C, Espinosa R, Pena A. Radiographic imaging in osteomyelitis: the role of plain radiography, computed tomography, ultrasonography, magnetic resonance imaging, and scintigraphy. *Semin Plast Surg*. 2009;23(2):80-89.

Stumpe KD, Strobel K. Osteomyelitis and arthritis. *Semin Nucl Med*. 2009;39(1):27-35.

Russell JM, Peterson JJ, Bancroft LW. MR imaging of the diabetic foot. *Magn Reson Imaging Clin N Am*. 2008;16(1):59-70, vi.

Burrill J, Williams CJ, Bain G, et al. Tuberculosis: a radiologic review. *Radiographics*. 2007;27(5):1255-1273.

Christian S, Kraas J, Conway WF. Musculoskeletal infections. *Semin Roentgenol*. 2007;42(2):92-101.

Stoller DW. *Magnetic resonance imaging in orthopaedics and sports medicine*. 3rd ed. Philadelphia: Lippincott Williams & Wilkins; 2006.

# CHAPTER 51

# IMAGING OF MUSCULOSKELETAL TUMORS

*Judy S. Blebea, MD, and Bradley Lamprich, MD*

1. **What radiographic features are considered when evaluating a suspected bone tumor?**
   When evaluating a suspected bone tumor, morphologic features, location in a bone (epiphysis, metaphysis, diaphysis), distribution within the skeleton (axial vs. appendicular), presence of tumor matrix, periosteal reaction, and/or presence of a soft tissue mass are considered. Morphologic features to consider are the pattern of bone destruction and the size, shape, margins, and zone of transition of the lesion. A geographic lesion with a sharp border suggests a nonaggressive or benign lesion, whereas a poorly defined margin, especially one associated with cortical destruction, favors malignancy. Periosteal reaction reflects the rate of growth of the underlying lesion. Slow-growing lesions may produce a laminated periosteal reaction with uniform, wavy layers. Malignant lesions that grow in spurts can produce an "onion-skin" pattern, whereas aggressive lesions with rapid growth are associated with a "sunburst" or "hair-on-end" periosteal reaction (Figure 51-1). Codman triangle is the uplifting of the periosteum in a triangular configuration and can be seen with benign and malignant lesions.

2. **How do cartilage tumor matrix and neoplastic bone matrix differ?**
   Cartilage matrix is typically ringlike, flocculent, or flecklike in the shape of rings and arcs (Figure 51-2), whereas neoplastic bone matrix is typically cloudlike, amorphous, or ivory-like. The detection of tumor matrix can be helpful in recognizing the etiologic factor of the underlying lesion, that is, whether it is osseous or cartilaginous in origin.

3. **Which imaging study should be ordered first for the evaluation of a suspected musculoskeletal tumor?**
   Radiographs are the first step in detecting and diagnosing a bone tumor. See Box 51-1 for a list of the radiographic features to assess for bone tumors. Radiographs should also be obtained first with suspected soft tissue tumors to identify possible underlying bone involvement or the presence of calcifications.

4. **What is the role of magnetic resonance imaging (MRI) in the evaluation of musculoskeletal tumors?**
   MRI is the most important diagnostic test for local staging and preoperative planning of primary bone and soft tissue tumors. It is also useful for monitoring the response to chemotherapy or radiation therapy and detecting postoperative tumor recurrence. The use of MRI guidance for biopsy may be considered for lesions that cannot be visualized by any other modality such as a suspected bone marrow lesion. With osteosarcoma, MRI is indicated in the initial workup to evaluate for regional or "skip" metastases in the affected bone, which are frequently radiographically occult.

5. **What is the role of intravenous contrast material in MRI of musculoskeletal tumors?**
   Contrast enhancement may be used to help distinguish tumor margins and to assess tumor vascularity. It may also help distinguish malignant viable tissue from inflammatory changes and necrosis for preoperative biopsy planning. For a follow-up or post-therapy MRI evaluation, contrast enhancement may be helpful to assess tumor response to chemotherapy, to determine the presence of a fluid collection, and to detect tumor recurrence.

6. **What are some musculoskeletal tumor features evaluated with MRI? Can MRI be used to distinguish between benign and malignant tumors?**
   The tumor location, extent, and relationship to the neurovascular bundle and the presence of skip lesions and joint involvement are important features that are assessed with MRI, which help to determine the stage of the tumor and to plan a surgical approach. Although MRI may help in the assessment of the aggressiveness of a lesion and in the recognition of certain "pathognomonic" lesions, it cannot be used to reliably distinguish between benign and malignant tumors and is generally nonspecific in determining tumor cell type. Biopsy of the lesion is often required.

7. **What is the role of computed tomography (CT), ultrasonography (US), bone scintigraphy, and positron emission tomography/computed tomography (PET/CT) in the evaluation of musculoskeletal tumors?**
   CT may be helpful to detect the nidus in a suspected osteoid osteoma. CT-guided percutaneous cryoablation has been shown to be an effective treatment of osteoid osteoma. CT is also used for percutaneous image-guided biopsy of bone tumors and in the workup for detection of pulmonary metastases. US offers real-time multiplanar imaging for performing musculoskeletal soft tissue biopsies and can be used to guide the biopsy of a bone lesion with an extraosseous soft tissue component. US may be particularly useful for biopsy of small soft tissue lesions that are difficult to detect on a noncontrast CT and also provides real-time confirmation of needle placement. Technetium-99m ($^{99m}$Tc) methylene diphosphonate (MDP) bone scintigraphy with single photon emission computed tomography (SPECT)

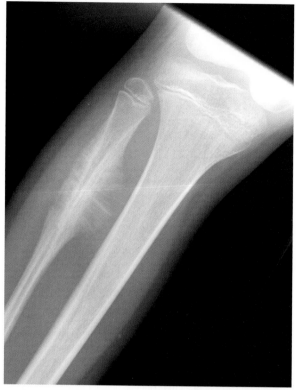

**Figure 51-1.** Osteosarcoma on radiograph. Note aggressive lesion of proximal fibula with sunburst or "hair-on-end" periosteal reaction.

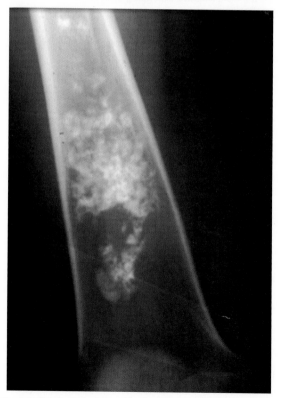

**Figure 51-2.** Enchondroma on radiograph. Note lesion in femur with presence of ringlike, flocculent, or flecklike matrix in shape of rings and arcs indicative of cartilage matrix.

**Box 51-1.** Radiographic Features to Assess for Bone Tumors

- Morphologic features and pattern of bone destruction, including zone of transition
- Periosteal reaction
- Location in the bone and distribution in the skeleton
- Presence of tumor matrix
- Presence of a soft tissue mass

is often utilized for the detection of osseous metastases. $^{18}$F-fluorodeoxyglucose (FDG) PET/CT may also be used for the detection of metabolically active soft tissue neoplasms or osseous malignancies. Some studies indicate that $^{18}$F-sodium fluoride (NaF) PET/CT is a potentially superior imaging technique for the detection of osseous metastases.

8. **Which classification system is used for soft tissue and bone tumors?**
The World Health Organization (WHO) classification system of tumors of soft tissue and bone is commonly used and is based on histologic and genetic typing. The WHO classification system has been adopted by the American Joint Cancer Commission (AJCC) for sarcoma staging.

9. **What is the staging system adopted by the Musculoskeletal Tumor Society, and what three features form the basis of this staging system?**
The Musculoskeletal Tumor Society has adopted the Enneking staging system. Grade, local extent, and presence of metastases are the three features assessed with this system.

10. **What is the most common malignant tumor involving the skeleton?**
Metastases are the most common malignant skeletal tumors.

11. **What are the most common primary neoplasms that metastasize to osseous structures?**
The most common primary cancers that metastasize to osseous structures include prostate, breast, and lung cancers, followed by kidney and thyroid cancers and are remembered by the mnemonic PB (lead) KetTLe (Figure 51-3). The axial skeleton is more frequently involved than the appendicular skeleton because of the presence of red bone marrow. For this reason, it is also rare to have metastases distal to the elbow or knee, but if metastases are seen in these locations, one should consider lung carcinoma as the potential primary tumor. Lytic osseous metastases must have destroyed 30% to 50% of the bone to be seen on radiographs. Sclerotic osseous metastases appear radiodense. Nuclear medicine bone scans are more sensitive than radiographs for the detection of osseous metastatic disease. Common sites for osseous metastatic disease are the vertebrae, pelvis, proximal femurs, and skull.

12. **Which tumors can give rise to lytic, expansile, or "blown-out" osseous metastases?**
Osseous metastases from renal cell carcinoma and thyroid cancer can show this pattern. Osseous metastases from melanoma may be expansile as well.

13. **What is the most common primary malignant bone tumor in adults?**
Multiple myeloma is the most common primary malignant bone tumor in adults, usually occurring in patients older than 40 years of age. Multiple myeloma represents approximately 1% of all malignant diseases and about 10% to 15% of hematologic malignancies. The excessive proliferation of abnormal plasma cells can result in the formation of a single lesion (plasmacytoma) or multiple lesions (multiple myeloma).

14. **If the diagnosis of multiple myeloma is suspected, what radiographic evaluation should be performed?**
A skeletal survey is usually obtained. Approximately 75% of patients with multiple myeloma have positive radiographic findings with characteristic "punched-out" osteolytic lesions that have discrete margins and uniform size (Figure 51-4). Multiple compression fractures can also be seen. MRI is very sensitive for detecting the presence of bone marrow lesions and may help in determining tumor extent. FDG PET/CT may also be useful to diagnose, stage, and monitor therapy of multiple myeloma.

15. **What is the second most common primary bone tumor after multiple myeloma?**
Osteosarcoma is the second most common primary bone tumor after multiple myeloma. About 75% of osteosarcoma lesions occur around the knee and typically arise in the metaphyseal region (Figure 51-5). The peak incidence is in the second and third decades of life, and there is a smaller second peak in patients older than 50 years; this later peak has more pelvic and craniofacial involvement. Osteosarcoma can develop after radiation exposure, with an average latent period of 11 years.

16. **Which primary bone tumors tend to involve the epiphysis most commonly?**
Chondroblastoma and giant cell tumor (GCT) tend to involve the epiphysis most commonly. Chondroblastoma is a benign lesion that is typically well defined and located in the epiphysis (Figure 51-6), most often occurring in children and young adults. Although benign, chondroblastomas can be locally invasive and metastasize to the lungs. A GCT usually arises in the metaphyseal region and extends to involve the epiphysis, most often in young adults. GCTs are eccentrically located lesions with a nonsclerotic zone of transition that occurs after closure of the growth plate. A clear cell chondrosarcoma may also occur in the epiphyseal region (Box 51-2).

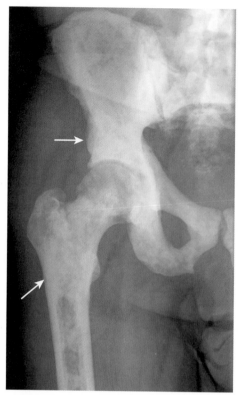

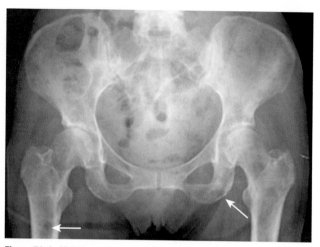

**Figure 51-4.** Multiple myeloma on radiograph. Note multiple "punched out" lytic lesions (*arrows*) in pelvic bones and proximal femurs.

**Figure 51-3.** Osseous metastases from prostate carcinoma on radiograph. Note multiple sclerotic lesions (*arrows*) throughout visualized portions of pelvic bones and right femur.

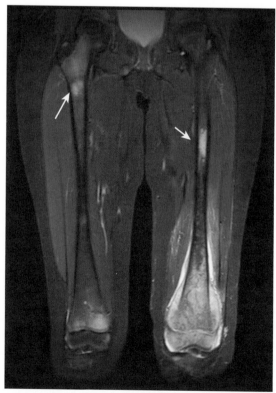

**Figure 51-5.** Osteosarcoma on MRI. Coronal fat-suppressed T2-weighted image shows extent of aggressive bone lesion in distal left femur and presence of associated soft tissue mass. Note skip lesion in mid left femur (*short arrow*) and metastasis in proximal right femur (*long arrow*).

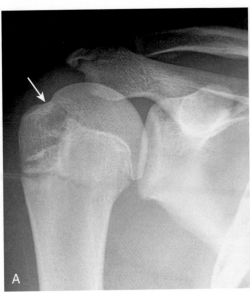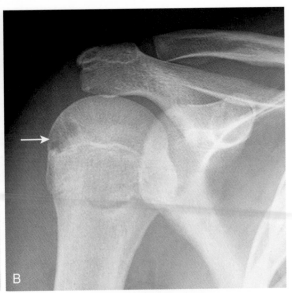

**Figure 51-6.** Chondroblastoma on radiograph. **A** and **B,** Note well-defined lytic lesion within proximal humeral epiphysis (*arrows*).

**Box 51-2.** Primary Bone Tumors in the Epiphyseal Region

- Chondroblastoma
- Giant cell tumor (GCT)
- Clear cell chondrosarcoma

17. Which primary bone tumors tend to involve the diaphysis most commonly?

Multiple myeloma, Ewing's sarcoma, and primary lymphoma of bone tend to involve the diaphyseal region of bones most commonly.

18. Which type of tumor can manifest with bone pain, swelling, fever, and increased erythrocyte sedimentation rate (ESR), mimicking an infection?

Ewing sarcoma is a malignant round cell tumor with a predilection for the long bones and pelvis that can manifest with pain, swelling, fever, and increased ESR. Radiographs may show a permeative or moth-eaten pattern of bone destruction with an onion-skin type of periosteal reaction and an associated soft tissue mass.

19. Which of the following has an increased incidence of skeletal malignancy: high-dose radiation therapy, bone infarction, Paget's disease of bone, or chronic osteomyelitis?

All of these entities have an increased incidence of skeletal malignancy, and osteosarcoma and fibrosarcoma are the most common forms of malignant degeneration.

20. Where do sarcomas most commonly metastasize?

Sarcomas tend to undergo hematogenous spread, most commonly to the lungs.

21. What is the most common benign skeletal neoplasm?

Osteochondroma is the most common benign skeletal neoplasm. This lesion accounts for 20% to 50% of benign bone tumors and 10% to 15% of all bone tumors. Osteochondromas occur most commonly in the first two decades of life, arise from the metaphysis pointing away from the joint, and can be either flattened (sessile) or stalklike (Figure 51-7). There is usually cessation of growth of the osteochondroma after closure of the growth plate. Osteochondromas can occur after radiation therapy in children and may present with pain because of mechanical irritation or fracture.

22. Which clinical and radiographic features suggest malignant degeneration of an osteochondroma?

Features suggesting malignant degeneration include pain, growth after closure of the growth plate, bony destruction, a thickened cartilage cap, and a soft tissue mass. The risk of malignant transformation of a solitary osteochondroma is approximately 1%, whereas the risk with multiple hereditary exostoses is much higher, to 25% to 30%. A sessile lesion is more likely to degenerate, usually undergoing malignant transformation to a chondrosarcoma.

23. What is the most common benign bone tumor of the hand? Where else may these lesions occur, and what are the features of malignant transformation?

An enchondroma is the most common benign bone tumor of the hand. Small, peripheral enchondromas of the hand are usually well-defined lytic lesions that are typically benign, but may be detected as a result of pathologic fracture

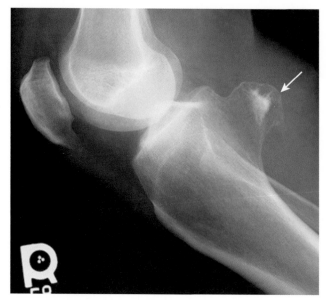

**Figure 51-7.** Osteochondroma on radiograph. Note bony protuberance (*arrow*) arising from posterior tibia.

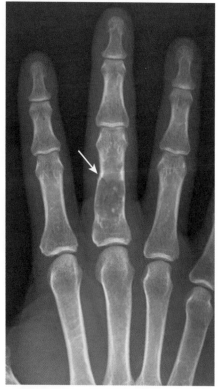

**Figure 51-8.** Enchondroma on radiograph. Note geographic lytic lesion in proximal third phalanx with associated pathologic fracture (*arrow*) through lesion.

(Figure 51-8). Solitary enchondromas can also occur in the long bones, and are usually oval in shape with central calcifications. Features suggestive of malignant degeneration include an enlarging painful lesion with progressive destruction of the chondroid matrix and presence of an expansile soft tissue mass.

24. **Which primary bone tumor has the characteristic history of pain at night that is relieved by aspirin?**

Osteoid osteoma is a benign primary bone tumor that has a characteristic history of pain at night that is relieved by aspirin. The classic radiographic appearance of this lesion is a round or oval lucent lesion, which represents the nidus, typically measuring less than 1 cm and surrounded by a zone of bone sclerosis with cortical thickening (Figure 51-9). If larger than 1 cm, one should consider a Brodie abscess with osteomyelitis as an alternative diagnosis.

25. **What is fibrous dysplasia?**

Fibrous dysplasia is a developmental anomaly of bone that usually manifests as a solitary lesion with focal bone expansion, cortical thinning or thickening, and a ground glass appearance. Patients with fibrous dysplasia may be asymptomatic or present with pathologic fracture. Polyostotic fibrous dysplasia with associated endocrine dysfunction that usually manifests as precocious female sexual development is known as *McCune-Albright syndrome*.

26. **What is a bone island?**

A bone island, or enostosis, is a benign hamartoma that appears radiographically as an oval or round sclerotic focus that may have radiating bone spicules from the center of the lesion. Bone islands are typically asymptomatic, are incidentally discovered, and usually do not show increased radiotracer uptake on a nuclear medicine bone scan. Osteopoikilosis is a benign condition with multiple bone islands.

27. **What is the most common location for a skeletal hemangioma?**

The most common site of involvement is the spine, particularly in the thoracic segment. Most vertebral hemangiomas are small and asymptomatic, with a coarse, vertical trabecular pattern or corduroy appearance in the vertebral body on radiographs or CT. In addition, hemangiomas of the spine often have fat attenuation on CT, fat signal intensity on MRI, and high signal intensity on heavily T2-weighted MR images relative to skeletal muscle.

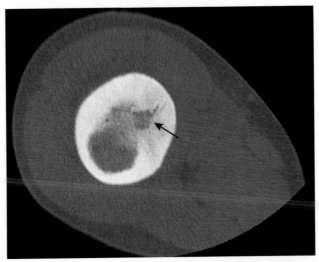

**Figure 51-9.** Osteoid osteoma on CT. Axial CT image shows subcentimeter round lytic nidus (*arrow*) in long bone with surrounding sclerosis and cortical thickening.

## KEY POINTS

- Order a radiograph when first evaluating a patient with a suspected or known bone tumor.
- MRI is useful for staging, pretreatment planning, response assessment, and detection of recurrence of musculoskeletal tumors. US and CT are more often used for image-guided biopsy. CT is also utilized to detect pulmonary metastases, and to identify the nidus of and to guide the percutaneous ablation of an osteoid osteoma.
- Nuclear medicine techniques are often used to detect osseous involvement by multiple myeloma, metastatic disease, and other musculoskeletal malignancies, and have high sensitivity of detection.

### BIBLIOGRAPHY

Costelloe CM, Chuang HH, Madewell JE. FDG PET/CT of primary bone tumors. *AJR Am J Roentgenol*. 2014;202(6):W521-W531.

Ghosh P. The role of SPECT/CT in skeletal malignancies. *Semin Musculoskelet Radiol*. 2014;18(2):175-193.

Kannivelu A, Loke KS, Kok TY, et al. The role of PET/CT in the evaluation of skeletal metastases. *Semin Musculoskelet Radiol*. 2014;18(2):149-165.

Morley N, Omar I. Imaging evaluation of musculoskeletal tumors. *Cancer Treat Res*. 2014;162:9-29.

Steffner R. Benign bone tumors. *Cancer Treat Res*. 2014;162:31-63.

Costelloe CM, Madewell JE. Radiography in the initial diagnosis of primary bone tumors. *AJR Am J Roentgenol*. 2013;200(1):3-7.

Douis H, Saifuddin A. The imaging of cartilaginous bone tumours. II. Chondrosarcoma. *Skeletal Radiol*. 2013;42(5):611-626.

Howe BM, Johnson GB, Wenger DE. Current concepts in MRI of focal and diffuse malignancy of bone marrow. *Semin Musculoskelet Radiol*. 2013;17(2):137-144.

Koppula B, Kaptuch J, Hanrahan CJ. Imaging of multiple myeloma: usefulness of MRI and PET/CT. *Semin Ultrasound CT MR*. 2013;34(6):566-577.

Kransdorf MJ, Bridges MD. Current developments and recent advances in musculoskeletal tumor imaging. *Semin Musculoskelet Radiol*. 2013;17(2):145-155.

Peller PJ. Role of positron emission tomography/computed tomography in bone malignancies. *Radiol Clin North Am*. 2013;51(5):845-864.

Douis H, Saifuddin A. The imaging of cartilaginous bone tumours. I. Benign lesions. *Skeletal Radiol*. 2012;41(10):1195-1212.

Walker RC, Brown TL, Jones-Jackson LB, et al. Imaging of multiple myeloma and related plasma cell dyscrasias. *J Nucl Med*. 2012;53(7):1091-1101.

Wu JS, Hochman MG. *Bone tumors: a practical guide to imaging*. 1st ed. New York: Springer; 2012.

Kim SH, Smith SE, Mulligan ME. Hematopoietic tumors and metastases involving bone. *Radiol Clin North Am*. 2011;49(6):1163-1183, vi.

Motamedi K, Seeger LL. Benign bone tumors. *Radiol Clin North Am*. 2011;49(6):1115-1134, v.

Nichols RE, Dixon LB. Radiographic analysis of solitary bone lesions. *Radiol Clin North Am*. 2011;49(6):1095-1114, v.

Rajiah P, Ilaslan H, Sundaram M. Imaging of primary malignant bone tumors (nonhematological). *Radiol Clin North Am*. 2011;49(6):1135-1161, v.

Davies AM, Sundaram M, James SJ. *Imaging of bone tumors and tumor-like lesions: techniques and applications*. 1st ed. Berlin: Springer; 2009.

Resnick DL. *Diagnosis of bone and joint disorders*. 4th ed. Philadelphia: Saunders; 2002.

# CHAPTER 52

# MRI OF THE SHOULDER

*Angel J. Lopez-Garib, MD, and Sung Han Kim, MD*

1. Describe the imaging planes used for evaluating the shoulder on a magnetic resonance imaging (MRI) examination. How should the patient be positioned in the scanner?

   Oblique coronal, oblique sagittal, and axial planes are routinely used (Figure 52-1). Oblique coronal and sagittal sequences are obtained perpendicular and parallel to the glenoid articular surface, respectively. While the patient is supine on the scanner table, the shoulder should be held in neutral to slightly externally rotated position to ensure that the supraspinatus muscle is parallel to the oblique coronal plane.

2. Name the four muscles of the rotator cuff and their sites of attachment. What is the normal MRI appearance of the tendons?

   From anterior to posterior, the rotator cuff is composed of the subscapularis muscle, which attaches on the lesser tuberosity of the humerus; and the supraspinatus, infraspinatus, and teres minor muscles, which attach on the greater tuberosity (see Figure 52-1). As in other areas of the body, the normal tendons are homogeneously low in signal intensity on all pulse sequences.

3. What are the symptoms of rotator cuff pathology? Which rotator cuff tendon is most commonly torn?

   The most common symptoms of rotator cuff tears include pain, especially at night, and pain and weakness with abduction of the arm. Most rotator cuff tears involve the supraspinatus tendon and usually occur in patients older than 40 years of age.

4. Define shoulder impingement syndrome.

   Shoulder impingement syndrome refers to compression of the supraspinatus tendon and subacromial bursa between the coracoacromial arch and humeral head. It can be secondary to multiple causes, including subacromial spurs, osteoarthritis of the acromioclavicular joint, and an os acromiale, among others. Impingement is thought to precipitate degeneration of the rotator cuff tendons, leading to rotator cuff tears.

5. Describe the MRI findings of rotator cuff pathology.

   Tendinopathy (chronic tendon degeneration) manifests on MRI as mildly increased signal intensity and thickening of the tendon (Figure 52-2). Tendon tears demonstrate increased T2-weighted signal intensity, as bright as fluid, within the tendon. Chronic rotator cuff tears may demonstrate superior displacement of the humeral head ("high riding humeral head"), and fatty change and/or atrophy of the rotator cuff muscles (best evaluated on oblique sagittal T1-weighted images).

6. What is an os acromiale?

   An os acromiale occurs when one of the accessory ossification centers of the acromial process fails to completely fuse. The acromial ossification centers appear by age 15 and usually fuse by 25 years of age. On MRI, it is easiest to identify this on the superior-most images of the axial images. An os acromiale may cause impingement by narrowing the subacromial space.

7. What is the glenoid labrum, and what are the symptoms of a labral tear?

   The glenoid labrum is fibrocartilagenous tissue around the rim of the glenoid. It results in deepening of the glenoid fossa, increasing stability of the inherently unstable shoulder joint, and also serves as a site for ligament attachments. The normal labrum is low in signal intensity on all pulse sequences and is most commonly triangular-shaped in cross-section. Symptoms of labral tear include pain with overhead activities, a locking or popping sensation, decreased range of motion, and a sense of shoulder instability.

8. When should shoulder MR arthrography be performed?

   Shoulder MR arthrography involves distention of the glenohumeral joint by direct injection of gadolinium-based contrast material into the joint space. This procedure increases the sensitivity for detection of subtle intraarticular pathology, such as labral tears, and is usually performed in younger patients.

9. What are the MRI findings of a labral tear?

   A labral tear can be identified on MRI by increased signal intensity within the labral substance. Alternatively, an MR arthrogram will show extension of intraarticular contrast directly into the tear (Figure 52-3).

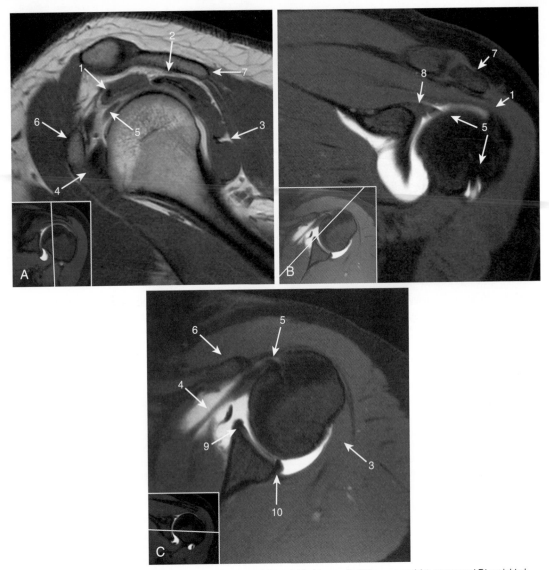

**Figure 52-1.** Normal shoulder MR arthrogram. **A,** Oblique sagittal T1-weighted image. **B,** Oblique coronal fat-suppressed T1-weighted image. **C,** Axial fat-suppressed T1-weighted image. *1* = supraspinatus muscle/tendon, *2* = infraspinatus muscle/tendon, *3* = teres minor muscle/tendon, *4* = subscapularis muscle/tendon, *5* = long head of the biceps tendon, *6* = coracoid process, *7* = acromion, *8* = superior labrum, *9* = anterior labrum, *10* = posterior labrum.

10. What is a paralabral cyst, and what is its clinical significance?

   A paralabral cyst can form around the labrum from extrusion of synovial fluid through a labral tear with a one-way ball-valve mechanism. A cystic structure around or extending from the labrum that is very closely associated with a labral tear is the major finding and should be suspected even if a labral tear is not clearly identified. Furthermore, the exact location of the paralabral cyst must be defined because it can often be the cause of a nerve impingement syndrome.

11. Define glenohumeral instability.

   Glenohumeral instability refers to recurrent subluxation or dislocation of the shoulder joint, most common anteriorly, but can also be posterior or multidirectional.

12. Describe the MRI findings seen with anterior shoulder instability.

   Anterior shoulder instability often results from anterior shoulder dislocation. Classic findings include an impaction fracture of the posterosuperior humeral head (Hill-Sachs deformity) and a tear of the anteroinferior glenoid labrum with associated fracture of the glenoid rim (bony Bankart lesion). These findings are best evaluated on the axial images.

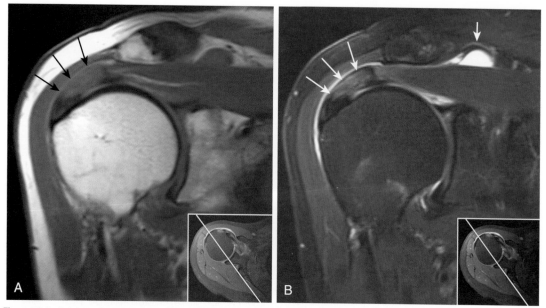

**Figure 52-2.** Rotator cuff tendinopathy on MRI. **A,** Oblique coronal T1-weighted image and **B,** Oblique coronal fat-suppressed T2-weighted image through shoulder show marked thickening of supraspinatus tendon (*long arrows*) along with increased T1-weighted and T2-weighted signal intensity, in keeping with tendinosis. No discontinuous fibers or high T2-weighted signal intensity fluid is noted within the tendon to indicate tear. Note high T2-weighted signal intensity fluid within subacromial/subdeltoid bursa (*short arrow*).

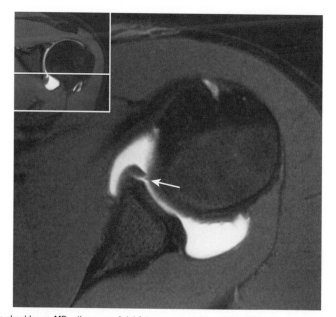

**Figure 52-3.** Labral tear in shoulder on MR arthrogram. Axial fat-suppressed T1-weighted MR arthrogram image shows contrast material extending into torn anterior inferior labrum (*arrow*). No appreciable displacement is seen. This patient had history of shoulder dislocation, and small Hill-Sachs deformity was also present (not shown).

13. What is a SLAP lesion?

SLAP stands for **S**uperior **L**abrum **A**nterior-**P**osterior. A SLAP lesion is a type of labral tear that involves the superior labrum and extends anteriorly and/or posteriorly to variable extents (Figure 52-4, *A*). These types of tears can be seen in the setting of trauma, such as with a fall on an outstretched arm, or in overhead throwing athletes with repetitive injury.

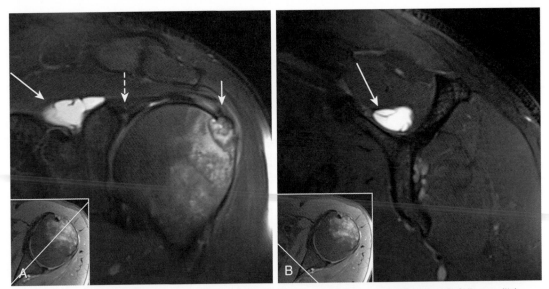

**Figure 52-4.** SLAP lesion and paralabral cyst on MRI. **A,** Oblique coronal fat-suppressed T2-weighted image and **B,** Oblique sagittal fat-suppressed T2-weighted images show large minimally septated paralabral cyst (*long arrows*) extending from SLAP lesion (*dashed arrow*) into suprascapular notch. Such cysts can impinge upon suprascapular nerve and result in supraspinatus and infraspinatus neuropathy. Note minimally displaced fracture of greater tuberosity of humerus (*short arrow*) with associated bone marrow edema.

14. Describe the nerve entrapment syndromes that can occur around the shoulder.
    A paralabral cyst can extend into the suprascapular notch (Figure 52-4) or the spinoglenoid notch and result in suprascapular nerve impingement syndrome. Both the supraspinatus and infraspinatus muscles are affected at the level of the suprascapular notch, whereas only the infraspinatus muscle is affected at the spinoglenoid notch.
    Another common impingement syndrome occurs with the axillary nerve in the quadrilateral space. Usually fibrous tissue compresses the axillary nerve, resulting in neuropathic changes in the teres minor and deltoid muscles.

15. What is Parsonage-Turner syndrome?
    Parsonage-Turner syndrome is a neuritis involving nerves originating from the brachial plexus, with the suprascapular nerve most commonly involved. As with the nerve impingement syndromes, MRI findings include high T2-weighted signal intensity within the muscle (from acute denervation) or fatty atrophy (from chronic denervation) involving one or more of the rotator cuff muscles or deltoid muscles.

16. Describe the clinical and MRI findings of adhesive capsulitis.
    Adhesive capsulitis, commonly called "frozen shoulder," occurs secondary to fibrotic adhesions with thickening and tightening of the joint capsule. Clinically, it is characterized by shoulder pain, stiffness, and decreased range of motion. MRI will demonstrate thickening of the coracohumeral ligament and joint capsule. These changes appear as mildly increased T2-weighted signal intensity within the rotator cuff interval (hiatus between the subscapularis and supraspinatus tendons) and in the inferior axillary pouch.

---

## KEY POINTS

- MRI is useful for detailed evaluation of the soft tissue and osseous structures of the shoulder and for detection and characterization of shoulder pathology.
- MR arthrography increases the sensitivity for detection of subtle intraarticular pathology such as labral tears.
- Most rotator cuff tears involve the supraspinatus tendon.
- A paralabral cyst can form around the labrum from extrusion of synovial fluid through a labral tear with a one-way ball-valve mechanism and can often be the cause of a nerve impingement syndrome.

**BIBLIOGRAPHY**

Pope TL Jr, Bloem HL, Beltran J, et al. *Musculoskeletal imaging.* 2nd ed. Philadelphia: Elsevier Saunders; 2014.
Helms CA, Major NM, Anderson MW, et al. *Musculoskeletal MRI.* 2nd ed. Philadelphia: Saunders Elsevier; 2009.
Stoller DW. *Magnetic Resonance imaging in orthopaedics and sports medicine.* 3rd ed. Philadelphia: Lippincott Williams & Wilkins; 2006.

# CHAPTER 53

# MRI OF THE ELBOW

*Bradley Lamprich, MD, and Judy S. Blebea, MD*

1. Name the labeled structures of the elbow shown on magnetic resonance imaging (MRI) in Figures 53-1 and 53-2.

2. What are the three articulations of the elbow?

   The radiocapitellar, ulnotrochlear, and proximal radioulnar joints. The three articulations are within a common joint capsule and work together as a hinge, allowing flexion/extension at the elbow and supination/pronation of the forearm.

3. What is the common flexor tendon, and where does it originate?

   The common flexor tendon refers to the common origin for the flexor muscles of the forearm including the pronator teres, flexor carpi radialis, palmaris longus, flexor digitorum superficialis, and flexor carpi ulnaris muscles. It originates at the medial epicondyle, which is the bony protuberance at the medial aspect of the distal humerus proximal to the trochlea.

4. What is the common extensor tendon, and where does it originate?

   The common extensor tendon refers to the common origin of the extensor muscles of the forearm including the extensor carpi radialis longus, extensor carpi radialis brevis, extensor digitorum communis, extensor carpi ulnaris, and extensor digiti minimi muscles. It originates from the lateral epicondyle, which is the bony projection of the lateral aspect of the distal humerus proximal to the capitellum. The anconeus and supinator muscles also originate at the lateral epicondyle.

5. What is the function of the ulnar collateral ligament (UCL), and what are its components?

   The UCL, also known as the medial collateral ligament (MCL), is a focal thickening of the medial joint capsule. It stabilizes the medial aspect of the elbow and resists valgus stress. The UCL is comprised of three components: the anterior bundle, posterior bundle, and oblique band (also known as the transverse ligament).

6. Which component of the UCL is the primary restraint to valgus stress?

   The anterior bundle of the UCL, which arises from the inferior aspect of the medal epicondyle and extends to the medial aspect of the coronoid process (known as the sublime tubercle), is the primary restraint to valgus stress at the elbow.

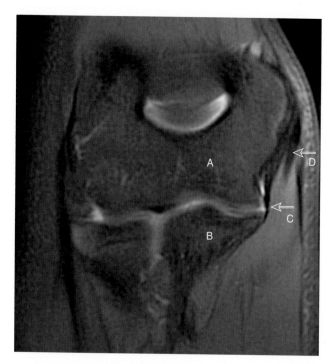

**Figure 53-1.** Normal elbow anatomy on MRI. Coronal fat-suppressed T2-weighted image of elbow shows trochlea (*A*) and ulna (*B*) comprising ulnotrochlear joint. Ulnar collateral ligament (*C*) attaches on inferior aspect of medial epicondyle of humerus and extends to sublime tubercle of ulna. Overlying ulnar collateral ligament is common flexor tendon (*D*).

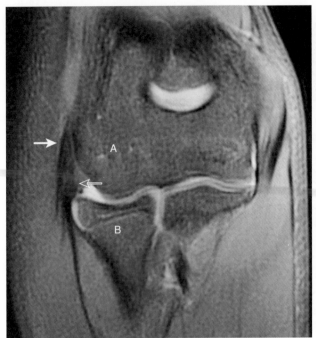

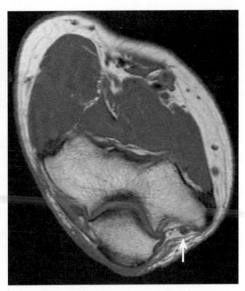

Figure 53-3. Normal cubital tunnel on MRI. Axial T1-weighted image of elbow reveals ulnar nerve in cubital tunnel (*arrow*) posterior to medial epicondyle.

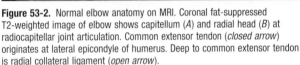

Figure 53-2. Normal elbow anatomy on MRI. Coronal fat-suppressed T2-weighted image of elbow shows capitellum (*A*) and radial head (*B*) at radiocapitellar joint articulation. Common extensor tendon (*closed arrow*) originates at lateral epicondyle of humerus. Deep to common extensor tendon is radial collateral ligament (*open arrow*).

7. What are the three components of the lateral ligament complex of the elbow?
Radial collateral ligament, lateral ulnar collateral ligament (LUCL), and annular ligament. The annular ligament is attached to the ulna and wraps around the radial head, acting as the primary stabilizer of the radioulnar joint and preventing dislocation of the radial head. The radial collateral ligament extends in a fan shape from the lateral epicondyle to the annular ligament. The LUCL arises from the posterior aspect of the lateral epicondyle and extends around the posterior aspect of the radial head and neck to the ulna.

8. What is the importance of the LUCL?
The LUCL acts as a sling that extends around the posterior radial head and neck and is the primary stabilizer to varus stress. Disruption of the LUCL leads to posterolateral rotatory instability. The LUCL is frequently disrupted following posterior elbow dislocations.

9. What structure passes through the cubital tunnel?
The ulnar nerve passes through the cubital tunnel posterior to the medial epicondyle (Figure 53-3).

10. What are the borders of the cubital tunnel?
The cubital tunnel is the channel through which the ulnar nerve passes at the elbow between the medial epicondyle and the olecranon. The roof of the cubital tunnel is formed by the cubital tunnel retinaculum, normally a thin fibrous structure that extends from the olecranon to the medial epicondyle. The floor of the cubital tunnel is comprised of the elbow capsule and the posterior bundle and oblique band of the UCL.

11. What are common indications for MRI of the elbow?
- Bone and cartilage pathology: radiographically occult fractures including stress fractures, bone contusions, tumors, osteochondritis dissecans, and cartilage defects.
- Ligament tears.
- Muscle and tendon pathology: medial epicondylitis, lateral epicondylitis, distal biceps tears, triceps tears, and muscle strains/injury.
- Joint space pathology: effusions, synovitis, and arthropathies.
- Ulnar nerve pathology: neuritis and cubital tunnel syndrome.

12. What are common indications for MR arthrography of the elbow?
An elbow MR arthrogram is performed by injecting dilute contrast material into the joint space before acquisition of MR images. The intraarticular contrast material is best used to evaluate for intraarticular bodies in the joint space, osteochondral lesions, and ligament tears.

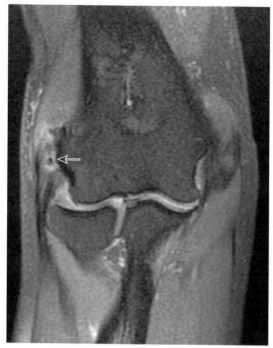

**Figure 53-4.** Lateral epicondylitis (tennis elbow) on MRI. Coronal fat-suppressed T2-weighted image shows high fluid signal intensity at common extensor tendon origin adjacent to lateral epicondyle (*open arrow*).

13. What other imaging modalities are utilized for evaluation of the elbow?
    The initial imaging evaluation should always start with radiography of the elbow. Radiographs will often detect the pathology and provide information about the bones, joint spaces, and soft tissues that may help guide further evaluation if necessary. MRI is the next most commonly utilized modality to evaluate the elbow after radiography. Computed tomography (CT) can provide fine bony detail better than MRI and may be beneficial to further characterize fractures in the setting of trauma. Ultrasonography (US) can be used to evaluate ligament and tendon pathology, the presence of joint effusions, and ulnar nerve pathology.

14. What is the MRI appearance of tendinopathy?
    Normal tendons are low in signal intensity on all MR imaging sequences. With chronic degeneration, microscopic tearing, and repair, the tendons become thickened and increased in signal intensity, giving the appearance of tendinosis on MRI.

15. What is the MRI appearance of a tendon tear?
    A tear can be distinguished from chronic tendinopathy by the presence of fluid signal intensity (high T2-weighted and low T1-weighted signal intensity) within the tendon, disrupted tendon fibers, and/or focal thinning of the tendon.

16. What is "tennis elbow," and what are its causes?
    Tennis elbow is a common term for lateral epicondylitis (Figure 53-4). It is a common source of pain at the lateral elbow and usually occurs with repetitive stress injury caused by repeated contraction of the extensor muscles of the forearm. The stress leads to microtearing, degeneration, immature repair, and subsequent tendinosis. The degenerated tendon is then at risk for acute tears with continued stress. The injury is common in racket sport athletes with repetitive exertion of the extensor tendons during the backhand swing.

17. What is "golfer's elbow," and what are its causes?
    Golfer's elbow is a common term for medial epicondylitis. It is a common source of pain at the medial elbow caused by stress from repetitive contraction of the flexors of the forearm. It is commonly seen in golfers, overhead throwing athletes, bowlers, and racket sport athletes (pain with forehand stroke and serve), but is also seen in carpenters and those with other occupations requiring similar repetitive stress of the forearm flexors.

18. What is the most frequent cause of a distal biceps tendon tear?
    The distal biceps tendon insets onto the proximal radius at the radial tuberosity. Tendon ruptures usually occur with contraction of the biceps against resistance when lifting heavy objects. On MRI, the tendon will be discontinuous and may be retracted proximally with surrounding fluid and edema (Figure 53-5).

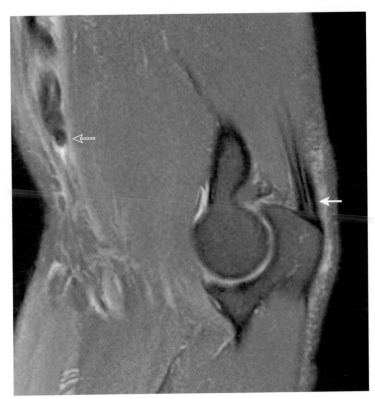

**Figure 53-5.** Distal biceps tendon rupture on MRI. Sagittal fat-suppressed T2-weighted image demonstrates complete tear of distal biceps tendon which is proximally retracted above elbow (*open arrow*). Note that normal triceps tendon is intact inserting on olecranon (*closed arrow*).

19. **What is a ganglion cyst? Where do they occur at in the elbow?**
    A ganglion cyst is a thin-walled cyst filled with mucinous fluid that occurs in soft tissues around a joint. These cysts are frequently caused by repetitive overuse and are seen with osteoarthritis, but are also present with inflammatory conditions or following trauma. They are more frequently seen at the wrist and foot and are uncommon at the elbow. When present, they may become symptomatic if they occur anteriorly and compress the superficial or deep branches of the radial nerve, or in the cubital tunnel with compression of the ulnar nerve.

20. **What are the causes and MRI appearance of olecranon bursitis?**
    Olecranon bursitis is most commonly caused by acute or repetitive trauma and may be associated with tears or tendinosis of the triceps tendon. Other causes include systemic diseases such as rheumatoid arthritis, gout, hydroxyapatite deposition, and calcium pyrophosphate deposition. Approximately 20% of acute olecranon bursitis cases present with infection from a hematogenous source or from direct spread from lacerations or cellulitis. The typical MRI appearance is a high T2-weighted fluid signal intensity collection superficial to the olecranon. When chronic, it may have a more complex appearance mimicking a solid mass.

21. **What is cubital tunnel syndrome, and what are its causes?**
    Cubital tunnel syndrome is ulnar neuropathy occurring from abnormalities in the cubital tunnel. Common causes include thickening of the cubital tunnel retinaculum, an anomalous muscle (anconeus epitrochlearis), thickening or heterotopic calcification in the UCL, and bone spurs.

22. **What ligament is the most commonly injured by the throwing athlete?**
    The UCL (Figure 53-6). Baseball pitchers and other overhead throwing athletes place the elbow under repeated valgus stress, which leads to chronic degeneration and tearing of the anterior bundle of the UCL. Rupture of this ligament leads to instability and accelerated secondary osteoarthritis. Athletes who rupture this tendon frequently require "Tommy John" surgery with reconstruction of the medial elbow stabilizers.

---

**KEY POINTS**

- Initial imaging evaluation of the elbow should begin with radiography. MRI is the next most frequently employed imaging modality and is useful to evaluate most common elbow pathologies. MR arthrography of the elbow is useful to assess for intraarticular bodies, osteochondral lesions, and ligament tears.

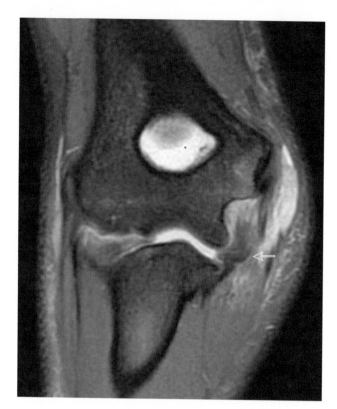

**Figure 53-6.** UCL tear on MRI. Coronal fat-suppressed T2-weighted image of elbow reveals disruption of proximal UCL (anterior bundle). Ligament is thickened and retracted distally (*arrow*) with high fluid signal intensity adjacent to tear proximally. There is also high fluid signal intensity around partially torn common flexor tendon, which may occur with acute trauma.

## KEY POINTS *(Continued)*

- The flexor and extensor muscles of the forearm have common tendon origins on the medial and lateral epicondyle, respectively.
- Tennis elbow (lateral epicondylitis) and golfer's elbow (medial epicondylitis) are due to inflammation of the common extensor and common flexor tendons, respectively.
- Distal biceps tears occur from contraction of the biceps against resistance when lifting heavy objects, and the torn tendon may retract proximal to the elbow.
- Cubital tunnel syndrome is ulnar neuropathy caused by abnormalities in the cubital tunnel, where the ulnar nerve passes posterior to the medial epicondyle.

## BIBLIOGRAPHY

Kancherla VK, Caggiano NM, Matullo KS. Elbow injuries in the throwing athlete. *Orthop Clin N Am.* 2014;45(4):571-585.
Beltran LS, Bencardino JT, Beltran J. Imaging of sports ligamentous injuries of the elbow. *Semin Musculoskelet Radiol.* 2013;17(5):455-465.
Lomasney LM, Choi H, Jayanthi N. Magnetic resonance arthrography of the upper extremity. *Radiol Clin North Am.* 2013;51(2):227-237.
Manaster BJ, May DA, Disler DG. *Musculoskeletal imaging: the requisites.* 4th ed. Philadelphia: Elsevier Saunders; 2013.
Martin S, Sanchez E. Anatomy and biomechanics of the elbow joint. *Semin Musculoskelet Radiol.* 2013;17(5):429-436.
Wenzke DR. MR imaging of the elbow in the injured athlete. *Radiol Clin North Am.* 2013;51(2):195-213.
Hayter CL, Adler RS. Injuries of the elbow and the current treatment of tendon disease. *AJR Am J Roentgenol.* 2012;199(3):546-557.
Stein JM, Cook TS, Simonson S, et al. Normal and variant anatomy of the elbow on magnetic resonance imaging. *Magn Reson Imaging Clin N Am.* 2011;19(3):609-619.
Frick MA, Murthy NS. Imaging of the elbow: muscle and tendon injuries. *Semin Musculoskelet Radiol.* 2010;14(4):430-437.
Hariri S, Safran MR. Ulnar collateral ligament injury in the overhead athlete. *Clin Sports Med.* 2010;29(4):619-644.
Miller TT, Reinus WR. Nerve entrapment syndromes of the elbow, forearm, and wrist. *AJR Am J Roentgenol.* 2010;195(3):585-594.
Sampaio ML, Schweitzer ME. Elbow magnetic resonance imaging variants and pitfalls. *Magn Reson Imaging Clin N Am.* 2010;18(4):633-642.
Simonson S, Lott K, Major NM. Magnetic resonance imaging of the elbow. *Semin Roentgenol.* 2010;45(3):180-193.
Stevens KJ. Magnetic resonance imaging of the elbow. *J Magn Reson Imaging.* 2010;31(5):1036-1053.
Walz DM, Newman JS, Konin GP, et al. Epicondylitis: pathogenesis, imaging, and treatment. *Radiographics.* 2010;30(1):167-184.
Fowler KA, Chung CB. Normal MR imaging anatomy of the elbow. *Radiol Clin North Am.* 2006;44(4):553-567, viii.
Stoller DW. *Magnetic resonance imaging in orthopaedics and sports medicine.* 3rd ed. Philadelphia: Lippincott Williams & Wilkins; 2006.

# CHAPTER 54

# MRI OF THE HAND AND WRIST

*J. Bruce Kneeland, MD*

1. **What are some common indications for performing magnetic resonance imaging (MRI) of the hand and wrist?**

   MRI of the wrist is routinely used to assess a wide variety of osseous and soft tissues abnormalities, including radiographically occult fractures; tendon, ligament, or cartilage injuries; tunnel syndromes; palpable abnormalities; and wrist pain. This chapter will concentrate predominantly on MRI of the wrist.

   MRI of the hand is obtained much less frequently than MRI of the wrist. It is technically demanding, requires special techniques and equipment not widely available, and consistent, high-quality images are more difficult to obtain. Moreover, ultrasonography (US) has emerged as a strong competitor with both higher resolution than MRI and the capacity to image small structures during the passive or active performance of maneuvers. The downside to US is the shortage of both technologists and radiologists qualified to perform and interpret the studies.

   MRI of the hand is occasionally used for the assessment of injury to the flexor and extensor tendons, as well as injury to the complex pulley system used to stabilize the flexor tendons. MRI is also sometimes used to assess injury to periarticular soft tissues such as the joint capsule and collateral ligaments as well as the volar plates (focal thickenings of the joint capsule) of the metacarpophalangeal and interphalangeal joints. The only periarticular structure that is commonly studied with MRI is the ulnar collateral ligament (UCL) of the carpometacarpal joint of the thumb. Other uses of MRI include assessment of either bony or soft tissue infection as well as of soft tissue masses.

2. **What is the anatomy of the hand and wrist?**

   The distal radius and ulna articulate with the proximal row of carpal bones, although the ulna does not articulate directly but is separated by the articular disc of the triangular fibrocartilage complex (TFCC). The proximal carpal row consists of scaphoid, lunate, triquetrum, and pisiform bones. The distal carpal row consists of the trapezium, trapezoid, capitate, and hamate bones.

   The distal carpal row articulates with the bases of the metacarpal bones, which in turn articulate with the proximal phalanges. In the thumb, there are only two (proximal and distal) phalanges joined at the interphalangeal (IP) joint, whereas in the remainder of the digits there are three phalanges (proximal, middle, and distal) joined by the proximal interphalangeal (PIP) and distal interphalangeal (DIP) joints.

   The ligaments of the wrist consist of both the intrinsic ligaments, which extend between the bones of the proximal carpal row, and the extrinsic ligaments, primarily on the volar and dorsal surface of the wrist, which extend over much greater distances, often crossing the radiocarpal and carpometacarpal articulations. The extrinsic ligaments provide the overall stability of the wrist, whereas the intrinsic ligaments maintain the relationship of the bones of the proximal row.

   Multiple tendons cross the dorsal surface of the wrist, contained within six separate compartments. As they extend onto the dorsal surface of the fingers, the tendons divide up in a complex pattern to form the dorsal "hood." The flexor tendons cross the wrist on the volar surface within the carpal tunnel and exit onto the fingers as the deep and superficial flexor tendons, where they are held close to the bone by a series of fibrous pulleys.

3. **What is meant by the term "intercalated segment"?**

   The intercalated segment is the proximal row of carpal bones. The name derives from the fact that there are no tendinous insertions on the proximal carpal bones and that they are inserted ("intercalated") between the radius and the distal carpal row. The use of this term will become evident in the rest of this chapter.

4. **What is ulnar variance?**

   Ulnar variance describes the relationship between the lengths of the radius and ulna as seen at the wrist. Positive ulnar variance refers to the situation in which the ulna is longer than the radius and is associated with degenerative disease of the TFCC. Negative ulnar variance describes the situation in which the ulna is shorter than the radius, and is associated with Kienböck's disease. Both of these entities will be discussed below.

5. **What is the normal MRI appearance of the wrist?**

   The predominant signal intensity of normal bone marrow is the same as that of the subcutaneous fat and is generally bright unless specific measures have been taken to suppress it. Cortical bone has very low signal intensity on all standard imaging sequences. Cancellous bone is seen as a fine network with very low signal intensity within the fatlike signal intensity of the bone marrow. Normal tendons, normal ligaments, and the TFCC demonstrate low signal intensity on all MRI sequences, although small foci of mildly increased signal intensity, believed to represent mild degeneration, are seen with increasing frequency in asymptomatic patients of increasing age. The clinical significance

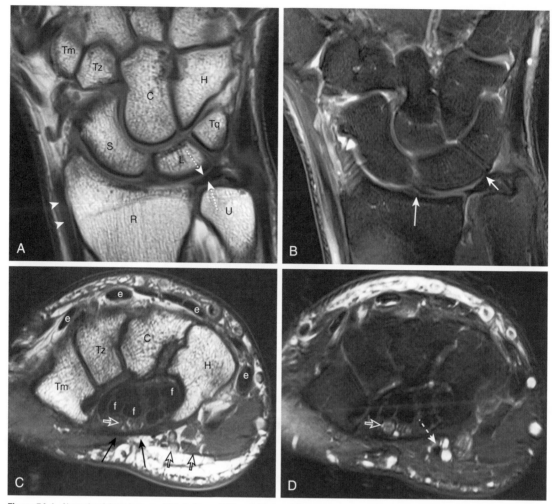

**Figure 54-1.** Normal wrist anatomy on MRI. **A,** Coronal PD-weighted and **B,** coronal fat-suppressed T2-weighted images of wrist. **C,** Axial PD-weighted and **D,** axial fat-suppressed T2-weighted images through carpal tunnel of wrist (volar side faces down). Key: *R* = radius, *U* = ulna, *S* = scaphoid, *L* = lunate, *Tq* = triquetrum, *Tm* = trapezium, *Tz* = trapezoid, *H* = hamate, *C* = capitate; *dotted white arrows* = triangular fibrocartilage, *long white arrow* = scapholunate ligament, *short white arrow* = lunotriquetral ligament, *black arrows* = flexor retinaculum, *hollow white arrows* = median nerve, *hollow black arrows* = superficial fascia of ulnar tunnel, *dashed white arrow* = ulnar nerve, *white arrow heads* = segment of abductor pollicis longus tendon parallel to long axis, *e* = representative extensor tendons in cross-section, *f* = representative flexor tendons in cross-section.

of such foci must be considered in the patient's clinical context. Nerves appear similar to skeletal muscle on T1-weighted and proton density (PD)-weighted images and brighter than skeletal muscle on T2-weighted images, although the degree of brightness on T2-weighted images is variable such that the distinction between normal and abnormal can be problematic (Figure 54-1).

6. What are the boundaries and contents of the carpal tunnel?
   The carpal tunnel is bounded by the bones of the wrist on its deep margin and a taut fibrous band, the flexor retinaculum, on its superficial margin. The major contents are the long flexor tendons of the fingers and thumb, the flexor carpi radialis tendon, and the median nerve (see Figures 54-1, *C*, and 54-1, *D*).

7. What are the boundaries and contents of the ulnar tunnel (Guyon's canal)?
   The ulnar tunnel (Guyon's canal) is located superficial to the carpal tunnel on the ulnar aspect of the wrist and contains the ulnar nerve, artery, and vein. The flexor retinaculum is the floor. The radial surface of the pisiform is the ulnar margin. A superficial fascial layer is the roof (see Figures 54-1, *C*, and 54-1, *D*).

8. What is carpal tunnel syndrome (CTS)?
   CTS is the most common of the peripheral nerve entrapment syndromes and is caused by increased pressure on the median nerve within the carpal tunnel. The clinical presentation is generally pain and paresthesias in the distribution of the median nerve.

9. What is the MRI appearance of CTS?

   MRI findings include enlargement and increased T2-weighted signal intensity of the median nerve proximal to the carpal tunnel, flattening of the nerve within the carpal tunnel, and volar bowing of the flexor retinaculum. In some cases, MRI may indicate a specific cause of CTS such as fractures and/or dislocations of the distal radius or carpal bones, increased fluid or thickening of the tendon sheath of the flexor tendons, soft tissue masses such as neurogenic tumors or cysts, or an anomalous muscle. In general, CTS is diagnosed by clinical examination and confirmed by electromyographic and nerve conduction studies. The accuracy and role of MRI for the diagnosis of CTS are controversial, and MRI is probably best reserved for those cases in which the clinical diagnosis is somewhat obscure.

   In cases of recurrent CTS following surgical division of the flexor retinaculum, MRI may demonstrate either incomplete division of the flexor retinaculum or postoperative fibrosis as low signal intensity fibrous bands on the superficial margin of the carpal tunnel.

10. What is ulnar tunnel syndrome (UTS)?

    Similar findings to CTS on MRI have been described in the much less common UTS in which entrapment of the ulnar nerve is seen within the ulnar tunnel (Guyon's canal). Similar to CTS, the role of MRI is not well defined and is probably most useful for the identification of unusual causes such as a mass lesion, anomalous muscle belly, and ulnar artery aneurysm.

11. What is the MRI appearance of traumatic injuries to the TFCC?

    Traumatic injuries to the TFCC generally appear as the presence of high signal intensity on T2-weighted images extending through the full thickness of normally low signal intensity articular disc of the TFCC close to its attachment to the radius (Figure 54-2). The detection of tears close to its ulnar attachment is more difficult because this portion of the TFCC generally has higher signal intensity on these sequences.

12. What is the MRI appearance of degenerative injuries to the TFCC?

    Either thinning or a full-thickness defect of the TFCC may be seen. There is also thinning of the articular cartilage on both the distal ulna as well as the apposed surface of the lunate, both of which may be hard to visualize. High signal intensity on T2-weighted images representing either bony edema or cyst formation may be visible in the portion of the lunate that abuts the TFCC. The ulna is generally longer than the radius (positive ulnar variance) in this situation, but this is not always the case.

13. What is the MRI appearance of tendon degeneration, tendon tear, and tenosynovitis?

    Degeneration of a tendon is seen as increased signal intensity within the normally low signal intensity tendon and either enlargement or attenuation of the tendon in cross-section. A full-thickness tear is seen as a discontinuity of the tendon with variable degree of separation of the two ends. Partial-thickness tears are seen as a focal attenuation of the tendon, although the distinction between partial-thickness tear and chronic attenuation associated with degeneration can be difficult if not impossible to make with confidence. Tenosynovitis is seen as distention of the surrounding tendon sheath (tenosynovium) by fluid that has low signal intensity on T1-weighted images and high signal intensity on T2-weighted images.

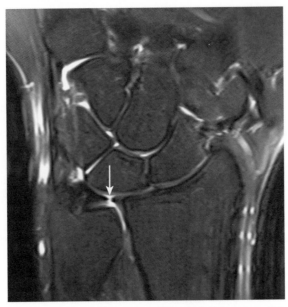

**Figure 54-2.** Full-thickness tear of TFCC on MRI. Coronal fat-suppressed T2-weighted image shows high signal intensity fluid (*arrow*) within focal defect of TFCC.

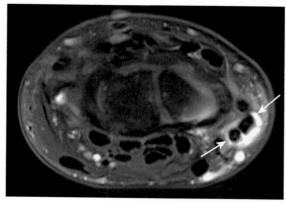

**Figure 54-3.** Early de Quervain's disease on MRI. Axial fat-suppressed T2-weighted image demonstrates high signal intensity fluid within distended sheath (*arrows*) of first extensor compartment surrounding APL and EPB tendons.

14. **What is de Quervain's disease?**
De Quervain's disease is a stenosing tenosynovitis of the abductor pollicis longus (APL) and extensor pollicis brevis (EPB) tendons, which lie in the first extensor compartment at the level of the wrist. In its early stages, it is seen on T2-weighted images as distention of the tendon sheath surrounding both tendons by high signal intensity fluid in the region of the distal radius (Figure 54-3). Increased signal intensity may be seen in the tendons due to the development of associated tendon degeneration. In later stages, the fluid-filled tendon sheath is replaced by surrounding low signal intensity scar tissue that encases the two tendons.

15. **What is intersection syndrome?**
Intersection syndrome is a tenosynovitis of the extensor carpi radialis longus (ECRL) and extensor carpi radialis brevis (ECRB) tendons, located in the second extensor compartment, which occurs where the two tendons from the first compartment (APL and EPB) cross superficial to those of the second compartment, approximately 4 cm proximal to the wrist. Similar to the other disorders that result in tenosynovitis, it is seen as high T2-weighted signal intensity within distended fluid-filled sheaths surrounding the tendons of the second extensor compartment.

16. **What is wrist instability?**
Instability of the wrist is a common cause of wrist pain. Instability in general is defined as the inability of the osseous structures to maintain their normal anatomic relationship under physiologic loading forces. Instability of the wrist is caused by injury to ligaments of the wrist either on a traumatic or an attritional (chronic overload) basis and can be classified using many different schemes. One of the most popular schemes, at least for the proximal wrist, is based on the orientation of the lunate bone. Those cases in which the distal surface of the lunate is angled toward the dorsum are identified as dorsal intercalated segmental instability (DISI). Those cases in which the lunate has a volar angulation are referred to as volar intercalated segmental instability (VISI). The DISI pattern of instability is associated with tears of the (intrinsic) ligament between the scaphoid and lunate (scapholunate ligament), and the VISI pattern of instability is associated with tears of the ligament between the lunate and triquetrum (lunotriquetral ligament). Both ligaments are U-shaped structures in sagittal cross-section between the adjacent bones that "open" distally and have strong components on the distal and volar surface and weak components on the proximal surface. The volar or dorsal tilt of the lunate may be evident on radiographs obtained in the lateral projection, in which case it is referred to as "static" instability and is considered to represent a more severe degree of instability. In some cases, this abnormal tilt of the lunate can be demonstrated by the application of provocative maneuvers, either using fluoroscopy or physical examination, and is referred to as "dynamic" instability, which is considered less severe.

17. **What is the MRI appearance of tears of the scapholunate and lunotriquetral ligaments?**
Tears of these ligaments can be seen as either the absence of the ligament or as the presence of high signal intensity fluid traversing the full thickness of the ligament on T2-weighted images. The characteristic volar or dorsal angulation of the lunate can often be seen with better accuracy on MRI than with radiography, given its nature as a cross-sectional (rather than projectional) imaging technique which avoids superimposition of the carpal bones (Figure 54-4).

18. **What is the role of MR arthrography for evaluation of wrist ligamentous injuries?**
In some cases of ligamentous injury, the ligament may appear thinned rather than discontinuous and there may be no joint fluid present to highlight the defect. In addition, although tears of the mechanically insignificant proximal segment are generally well seen, tears of the much stronger dorsal and volar segments are often harder to detect. In such cases, MR arthrography may be a useful adjunct. MR arthrography consists of the injection of a small amount of dilute gadolinium-based contrast material into the radiocarpal joint under fluoroscopic guidance followed by MRI. The contrast passes through defects in the scapholunate and lunatotriquetral ligaments and can often identify tears that are not seen well on conventional MRI studies, including those in the more mechanically significant dorsal and volar

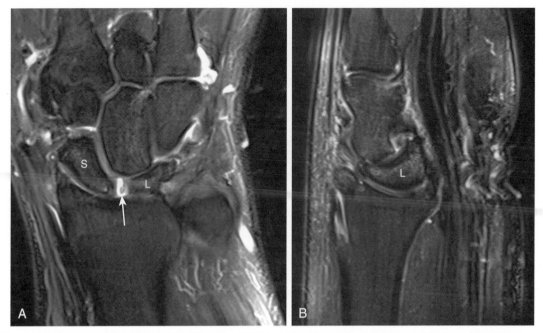

**Figure 54-4.** Tear of scapholunate ligament on MRI. **A,** Coronal fat-suppressed T2-weighted image through wrist shows high signal intensity fluid (*arrow*) replacing ligament in space between scaphoid (*S*) and lunate (*L*) bones. **B,** Sagittal fat-suppressed T2-weighted image through wrist reveals associated dorsal tilt (*toward reader's left*) of distal surface of the lunate (*L*) bone.

components. MR arthrography does have the disadvantages of being mildly invasive with the attendant risks of infection, hemorrhage, and contrast reaction, and of requiring the use of fluoroscopic equipment close to the MRI system.

19. What are the MRI findings of fractures?

MRI is an accurate technique for the identification of fractures in the wrist and hand, even when radiographic findings are normal. On fat-sensitive sequences (e.g., T1-weighted or PD-weighted images), fractures are seen as low signal intensity linear foci with surrounding low signal intensity edema. On fluid-sensitive sequences (e.g., fat-suppressed T2-weighted images), fractures are seen as either high or low signal intensity linear foci with surrounding high signal intensity edema. The fracture lines themselves may be obscured by the surrounding edema and not visible as distinct structures.

20. What is the role of MRI in the evaluation of scaphoid fractures?

The role of MRI in the evaluation of scaphoid fractures is not only for the detection of radiographically occult fractures as in other carpal bones, but also for the diagnosis of osteonecrosis of the proximal pole of the scaphoid bone. The latter entity arises from disruption of the vascular supply that enters through the proximal pole, predisposes to nonunion, and necessitates a change in therapy. The presence of low signal intensity in the proximal pole on all sequences is quite specific for osteonecrosis, but is not seen in all cases. Despite some initial enthusiasm for the use of intravenous contrast material, this probably does not increase the accuracy of MRI for this diagnosis.

21. What is Kienböck's disease?

Kienböck's disease is due to osteonecrosis of the lunate bone and is a cause of ulnar-sided wrist pain. Radiographs often show collapse of the lunate in advanced cases. The ulna is generally shorter than the radius (negative ulnar variance) with this disorder. The role of MRI in patients suspected of having this disorder is the detection of osteonecrosis in early cases in which radiographic findings are normal. Osteonecrosis of the lunate bone is seen as diffuse or heterogeneous low signal intensity on T1-weighted images and as diffuse or heterogeneous high signal intensity on T2-weighted images (Figure 54-5).

22. What is a ganglion cyst?

Ganglion cysts are cystic lesions that arise at multiple locations in the musculoskeletal system, including the wrist. The most common site in the wrist (and in the musculoskeletal system in general) is on its dorsal surface, in particular, on the dorsal surface of the scapholunate ligament. Ganglion cysts are seen on MRI as homogeneous lesions with low signal intensity fluid on T1-weighted images and very high signal intensity fluid on T2-weighted images. In rare cases in which there is a heterogeneous appearance, it may be necessary to give intravenous contrast material to demonstrate the lack of enhancement, thereby confirming the cystic nature of these lesions.

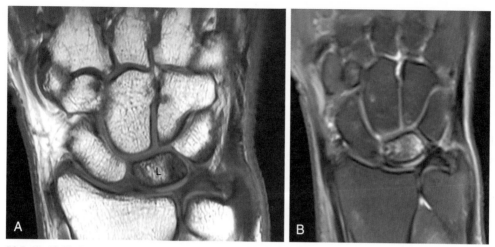

**Figure 54-5.** Kienböck's disease on MRI. **A,** Coronal T1-weighted and **B,** Coronal fat-suppressed T2-weighted images demonstrate heterogeneous abnormal signal intensity in lunate bone without collapse due to osteonecrosis.

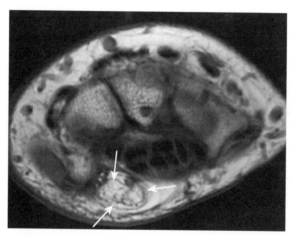

**Figure 54-6.** FLH of median nerve on MRI. Axial T1-weighted image through wrist shows predominantly fat signal intensity enlargement of median nerve (*white arrows*) containing low signal intensity nerve fascicles located in volar aspect of wrist.

23. What is a fibrolipomatous hamartoma (FLH)?

FLH is a benign overgrowth of the nerve consisting of fatty and fibrous tissue. The median nerve in the carpal tunnel is the most common site of such a lesion. It is seen on MRI as fatty infiltration and enlargement of the nerve surrounding lower signal intensity nerve fascicles, often with a coaxial cable-like appearance in cross-section (Figure 54-6).

24. What is "gamekeeper's thumb"?

This refers to a tear of the UCL of the metacarpophalangeal joint of the thumb. Although originally described in gamekeepers on large estates in the United Kingdom who would stress this joint by the repeated use of cervical dislocation to kill small animals, it is more commonly caused in this era by the use of ski poles. Gamekeeper's thumb can generally be diagnosed on clinical grounds.

25. What is a Stener lesion?

The major associated complication of UCL tear is the Stener lesion, in which the torn UCL is proximally retracted, and lies in a location superficial to the adductor pollicis aponeurosis. In this location, the UCL cannot heal and reattach to the proximal phalanx.

The retracted UCL appears on MRI as a curled up, low signal intensity ball. The subjacent adductor aponeurosis appears as a low signal intensity linear focus. The combination of a low signal intensity ball and low signal intensity linear structure has been referred to as a "yo-yo on a string." In this author's experience, the low signal intensity ball is generally seen and the low signal intensity linear focus less so.

## KEY POINTS

- MRI can reliably diagnose a number of disorders of both the bones and soft tissues of the hand and wrist.
- Ligament and tendon injuries are seen as full- or partial-thickness high signal intensity foci in the normally low signal structures on T2-weighted images.
- Radiographically occult abnormalities within the bones of the wrist such as nondisplaced fractures and osteonecrosis can be detected with MRI.

**BIBLIOGRAPHY**

Wolfe SW, Pederson WC, Hotchkiss RN, et al. *Green's operative hand surgery.* 6th ed. Philadelphia: Elsevier Churchill Livingstone; 2011.
Helms CA, Major NM, Anderson MW, et al. *Musculoskeletal MRI.* 2nd ed. Philadelphia: Saunders Elsevier; 2009.
Stoller DW. *Magnetic resonance imaging in orthopaedics and sports medicine.* 3rd ed. Philadelphia: Lippincott Williams & Wilkins; 2006.
Lichtman DM, Alexander AH. *The wrist and its disorders.* 2nd ed. Philadelphia: Saunders; 1997.

# CHAPTER 55

# MRI OF THE HIP

*Elena Taratuta, MD*

1. **What is the basic normal anatomy of the hip?**

   The hip is a ball-and-socket joint formed by the femoral head and the acetabulum, providing a large range of multidirectional motion. The acetabulum is tilted anteriorly, allowing a greater degree of flexion than extension. It covers 40% of the femoral head, and its depth is increased by the acetabular labrum, a horseshoe-shaped fibrocartilagenous structure covering the rim of the posterior, superior, and anterior acetabulum. The proximal femur consists of the head, neck, and lesser and greater trochanters. The mostly spherical femoral head, except for the fovea (an indentation in the medial femoral head), is covered by the articular cartilage, which extends over the epiphyseal part of the head to the head-neck junction. The greater femoral trochanter serves as the site of attachment for the hip abductors and lateral rotators (gluteus medius and minimus, obturator internus and externus, and piriformis muscles). The iliopsoas tendon inserts on the lesser trochanter.

2. **What are the indications for magnetic resonance imaging (MRI) of the hip?**

   Hip MRI is the examination of choice when radiography fails to reveal the cause of hip pain, either traumatic or nontraumatic. Following trauma, some of the common causes of hip pain in patients with normal radiographs are occult proximal femoral (for example, neck or intertrochanteric) fractures, bone contusions, stress or insufficiency fractures, or soft tissue injuries such as labral tears, muscle strains, ligament sprains, and tendon tears. Nontraumatic causes of hip pain include avascular necrosis (AVN), transient osteoporosis, impingement syndromes, bone or soft tissue neoplasms, infection (osteomyelitis, septic arthritis, abscess), and inflammation (bursitis, synovitis, inflammatory arthritis). Most of these entities are typically occult on both radiographs and on computed tomography (CT), whereas MRI is much more sensitive and specific.

3. **What is the proper MRI technique used for the evaluation of hip pain?**

   The exact MR imaging sequence combination depends on the scanner, clinical indication, patient factors, and radiologists' preferences. In the setting of trauma, the entire pelvis and both hips should be included in at least one (coronal and/or axial) plane. For evaluating joint pathology, such as labral tears or cartilage abnormalities, a smaller field of view with a lower slice thickness producing higher spatial resolution images should be used. Both T1-weighted (for anatomic detail) and fluid-sensitive sequences such as fat-suppressed T2-weighted, fat-suppressed proton density (PD)-weighted, or short tau inversion recovery (STIR) images (for detection of bone marrow edema) are necessary.

4. **When should intravenous contrast material be administered for hip MRI?**

   In general, intravenous contrast material is not needed, except to differentiate solid from cystic soft tissue masses or to localize an abscess prior to drainage. Occasionally, it is used in cases of osteonecrosis to differentiate enhancing viable from nonenhancing necrotic bone. Intraarticular contrast for MR arthrography is very useful to assess for presence of labral tears.

5. **What is the significance of the bone marrow edema pattern in the proximal femur?**

   Bone marrow edema, manifested on MRI as hypointensity on T1-weighted images and hyperintensity on fluid-sensitive images, is a nonspecific finding observed in a variety of disease entities, including osteonecrosis, idiopathic transient osteoporosis of the hip (ITOH), transient bone marrow edema syndrome, and infiltrative neoplasms. Somewhat more characteristic and specific patterns of bone marrow edema can be seen in association with fractures, stress injuries, and infectious and inflammatory diseases.

6. **What is AVN of the hip?**

   AVN is a form of osteonecrosis that occurs in the epiphyseal or subchondral region, and in the hip typically involves the anterolateral aspect of the femoral head. Unilateral AVN can be a result of trauma, such as a displaced femoral neck fracture, while bilateral AVN occurs due to nontraumatic causes seen in a large variety of clinical conditions, the more common of which include hemoglobinopathies, corticosteroid use, metabolic and endocrine diseases, and alcoholism. The presumed mechanism is failure to repair necrotic fractured trabeculae.

7. **What is the role of MRI in the diagnosis of the femoral head AVN?**

   MRI is the most sensitive imaging modality for detection of AVN in the early stages, allowing initiation of therapy before the onset of femoral head collapse. Delayed diagnosis and treatment can result in subchondral fracture with collapse of the femoral head, in turn leading to cartilage damage, osteoarthritis, and joint destruction, eventually necessitating arthroplasty. Another use of MRI is assessment of the percentage of bone marrow involvement and evaluation of temporal changes, which can help select appropriate therapy and determine response to treatment.

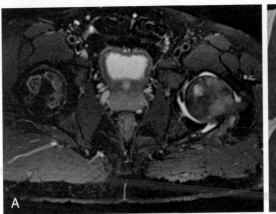
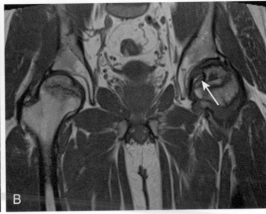

**Figure 55-1.** AVN of hips on MRI. **A,** Axial fat-suppressed T2-weighted image through hips shows characteristic geographic pattern of signal abnormality with serpentine rims in femoral heads, along with left proximal femoral bone marrow edema and associated left hip joint effusion. **B,** Coronal T1-weighted image through hips demonstrates serpentine low signal intensity foci in femoral heads surrounding fat signal intensity regions along with subchondral collapse of left femoral head (*arrow*). This patient was on corticosteroid therapy.

Patients with clinical risk factors for AVN and negative radiographs, who present with classic symptoms of deep throbbing hip, groin, or gluteal pain exacerbated by activity, should undergo MRI.

8. What is the MRI appearance of hip osteonecrosis?

The MRI appearance depends on the stage of disease. In the early stage, AVN presents on MRI as diffuse femoral head bone marrow edema, identical to that seen in ITOH, which can create a diagnostic challenge. Subsequently, the edema becomes more focal in the subchondral anterolateral femoral head, with a characteristic serpentine low signal intensity rim surrounding an area of fatty marrow (Figure 55-1, *A*), which is the most commonly seen geographic pattern. In the later stage, there is loss of the spherical shape of the femoral head due to subchondral fracture, with collapse and sclerosis appearing as an area of low T1-weighted and variable T2-weighted signal intensity (Figure 55-1, *B*). This corresponds to the "crescent sign" seen on radiographs.

9. What is ITOH?

This uncommon self-limited disease, also referred to as transient painful bone marrow edema, primarily affects middle-aged men as well as women in the third trimester of pregnancy. It is usually unilateral, resolves spontaneously in 6 to 8 months, and may recur in the same hip. Although the exact etiology is unknown, vascular causes, hormonal changes, and stress or insufficiency microfractures have been implicated. Patients typically present with severe hip pain without a history of trauma.

10. What are the imaging features of ITOH?

Radiographs are initially negative and may demonstrate osteopenia of the affected hip 3 to 6 weeks after the onset of pain, but MRI can demonstrate bone marrow edema as early as 48 hours after the onset of pain (Figure 55-2). Since the MRI appearance is similar to early AVN, it is important to make a correct diagnosis or at least to include ITOH in the differential diagnosis in order to institute appropriate conservative treatment. Erroneous treatment for early AVN, such as core decompression, can increase the risk of fracture. Some more specific MRI signs that may help distinguish ITOH from other diseases are marrow sparing in the medial and lateral-most femoral head and greater trochanter, homogeneous well-marginated hyperintensity on fluid-sensitive sequences, signal intensity abnormalities extending from the femoral head to the intertrochanteric line, and a small to moderate associated hip joint effusion. If intravenous contrast material is administered, there is prominent heterogeneous enhancement in the affected bone. MRI findings follow the clinical course and resolve with successful treatment.

11. What are the most common types of radiographically occult hip fractures?

Acute nondisplaced femoral neck fractures as well as insufficiency and stress fractures are usually not visible on radiographs or CT. Insufficiency fractures occur in osteoporotic bone with physiologic stresses, whereas stress (or fatigue) fractures occur in normal bone from increased abnormal or repetitive stress and are most common in young athletes. Subcapital femoral fractures (those at the junction of the femoral head and neck) tend to occur in osteoporotic bone. Extracapsular fractures (intertrochanteric and subtrochanteric) affect older patients more often than intracapsular fractures do and are usually caused by direct injury. MRI can also differentiate pathologic fractures from osteoporotic or insufficiency fractures, and fractures from bone contusions.

12. Why is MRI important in the early diagnosis of occult proximal femoral fractures?

MRI is the most sensitive and specific method for early diagnosis of radiographically occult fractures because its superior contrast resolution allows for visualization of the linear fracture signal abnormality and the associated bone marrow edema immediately after the fracture has occurred (Figure 55-3). If there is a strong clinical suspicion of an

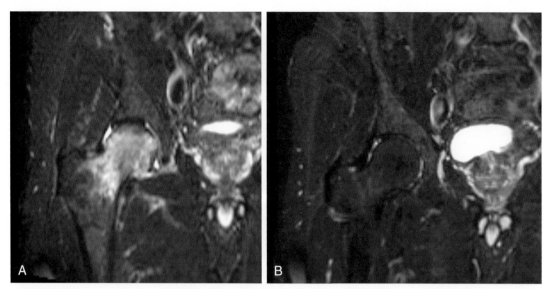

**Figure 55-2.** ITOH on MRI. **A,** Coronal STIR image demonstrates intense high signal intensity bone marrow edema in right femoral head and neck extending to trochanteric line, with small associated hip joint effusion. Of note is absence of other abnormalities such as fracture or edema in subjacent acetabulum. **B,** Coronal STIR image obtained 8 months later demonstrates complete resolution of bone marrow edema confirming clinical diagnosis of ITOH. This patient had originally presented with atraumatic right hip pain.

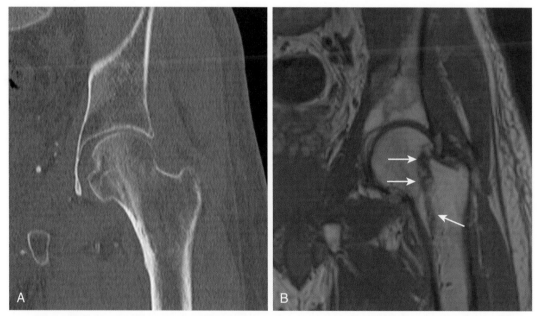

**Figure 55-3.** Occult femoral neck fracture. **A,** Coronal CT image of left hip demonstrates no evidence of fracture. **B,** Coronal T1-weighted image of left hip obtained 2 days later (given worsening of clinical symptoms) shows hypointense linear signal abnormality surrounded by band of bone marrow edema extending from lateral subcapital femur to medial trochanteric line (*arrows*) representing nondisplaced acute fracture. The patient had originally presented with left groin pain after fall.

occult fracture, for example, in an osteoporotic patient with hip pain, MRI should be performed for early diagnosis. Delayed diagnosis and treatment of these injuries can lead to complications such as AVN, progression from incomplete to complete fracture, fracture displacement, and arthritis, which would require more invasive treatment methods, including hip replacement.

13. How are stress and insufficiency fractures diagnosed on MRI?
   The most sensitive MR imaging sequences for demonstrating these injuries are fluid-sensitive ones, in which both stress and insufficiency fractures appear as linear low signal intensity foci surrounded by high signal intensity bone

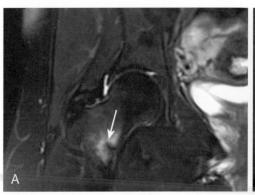
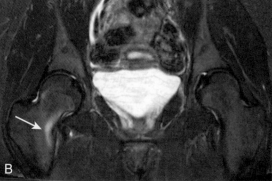

**Figure 55-4.** Stress injuries of hip on MRI. **A,** Coronal STIR image through hip shows linear low signal intensity (*arrow*) surrounded by high signal intensity bone marrow edema in medial (compressive surface) right femoral neck not extending to opposite cortex, representing incomplete stress fracture in patient with medial thigh pain. **B,** Coronal STIR image through hips reveals bone marrow edema along medial aspect of right femoral neck (*arrow*) without linear low-signal abnormality fracture line but with mild adjacent soft tissue edema, representing stress reaction in this runner with 1 month of atraumatic right hip pain.

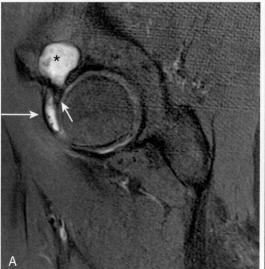
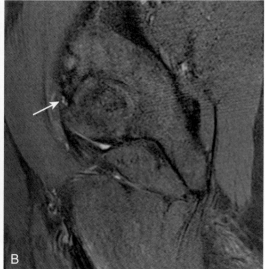

**Figure 55-5.** Paralabral cyst and labral tear of hip on MRI. **A,** Sagittal PD-weighted fat-suppressed image demonstrates anterosuperior labral tear (*short arrow*) and associated extraosseous septated paralabral cyst anteriorly (*long arrow*). There is also full-thickness cartilage defect in superior acetabulum with large subchondral geode (*asterisk*). **B,** Adjacent sagittal MR image shows hyperintense curvilinear neck of paralabral cyst, which connects to labral tear (*arrow*) in this patient with hip pain.

marrow edema (Figure 55-4, *A*). These fractures can be complete (involving the entire circumference of the cortex) or incomplete (involving only one side of the cortex) most commonly along the compressive surface in the medial aspect of the femoral neck. MRI is also highly sensitive for radiographically occult milder or earlier forms of stress injuries, stress reaction, and microtrabecular stress fracture. Stress reactions appear as focal bone marrow edema in the medial femoral neck without linear signal abnormality (Figure 55-4, *B*); microtrabecular stress fractures may in addition demonstrate linear low signal intensity similar to stress fractures but isolated to the spongy bone and not involving the cortices. These injuries are commonly associated with a hip joint effusion and adjacent soft tissue edema, which demonstrate hyperintense signal intensity on fluid-sensitive sequences.

14. What is the differential diagnosis of cystic lesions around the hip joint?
Cystic lesions around the hip joint may occur in both intra- and extraosseous structures and appear as well-marginated smooth or lobulated lesions with or without internal septations demonstrating fluid signal intensity on all imaging sequences. Common intraosseous cystic lesions include paralabral cysts, subchondral cysts or geodes (Figure 55-5, *A*), and synovial herniation pits; extraosseous cystic lesions include paralabral, synovial, or ganglion cysts, as well as bursal fluid collections (e.g., with iliopsoas and greater trochanteric bursitis). It is usually possible to differentiate among these possibilities on MRI by thorough examination of their exact location and relation to other structures and lesions.

15. **What causes a paralabral cyst, and how can MRI help determine if a juxtaarticular cyst is paralabral?**

Paralabral cysts form as a result of a labral tear, either traumatic or degenerative in nature, and may communicate with the tear anywhere along the labrum. The tears most commonly affect the anterior labrum, while the cysts are usually located lateral to the anterosuperior or posterosuperior labrum. The normal labrum in cross-section appears as a triangle of low signal intensity on MRI, and a labral tear is seen as a linear or irregular fluid signal intensity focus extending through the substance of the labrum, or, in cases of labral detachment, as fluid signal intensity between the labrum and the acetabulum (see Figure 55-5, *A*). This abnormal fluid can expand the labrum and extend to its surface and beyond, forming a paralabral cyst. In many cases, a neck of the cyst can be traced to the labral tear (Figure 55-5, *B*), and presence of a paralabral cyst is highly suggestive of a labral tear. These cysts can range in size up to several centimeters, can be simple or septated, and may have an intraosseous component extending into the acetabulum (see Figure 55-5, *A*).

16. **What is femoroacetabular impingement (FAI), and why is it important to recognize?**

FAI is a result of abnormal mechanical contact between the bony prominences of the acetabulum and proximal femur during hip motion, resulting in labral and cartilage tears, and leading to premature osteoarthritis. Multiple developmental and acquired hip disorders, in which there is a mismatch between the femoral head and the acetabulum, are associated with FAI. Two recognized types of FAI related to anatomic variants are the cam (femoral cause) type and pincer (acetabular cause) type. In the cam type, there is an aspherical femoral head with abnormal bony prominence at the lateral femoral head and neck junction (femoral "dysplastic bump"), while in the pincer type, there is focal overcoverage of the femoral head by the superolateral acetabulum. Most patients with FAI demonstrate a combination of both types. Patients are usually young and athletic and typically present with symptoms of groin or trochanteric pain after sports activities, often preceded by awareness of limited hip mobility. Early diagnosis and treatment can prevent or delay the onset of degenerative arthritis.

17. **How does MRI help in evaluation of patients with FAI?**

Although the diagnosis of FAI is based primarily on clinical factors and radiographic evaluation, MRI or MR arthrography can be obtained for early detection of labral and cartilage degeneration and tears (often associated with paralabral cysts), and for demonstration of subtle anatomic variations not visible on radiographs. MRI is also highly sensitive for more specific secondary signs of FAI, including subchondral edema and cysts in the superolateral acetabulum, absent or blunted labral tissue, a femoral "dysplastic bump" and femoral herniation pits (in cam type) (Figure 55-6), and a calcified/ossified labrum and os acetabuli (in pincer type).

18. **What are the causes of greater trochanteric pain syndrome?**

Pain localizing to the lateral aspect of the hip is usually due to greater femoral trochantic bursitis or abductor tendon abnormalities, both often caused by repetitive hip flexion in middle-aged and elderly patients and indistinguishable clinically. MRI findings are more specific than clinical signs, and can differentiate between bursitis and tendon pathology. Bursitis is manifested by increased T2-weighted fluid signal intensity in the trochanteric (subgluteus

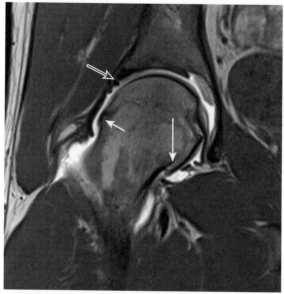

**Figure 55-6.** FAI on MRI. Coronal T1-weighted MR arthrogram image demonstrates femoral "dysplastic bump" (*short arrow*) characteristic of cam type FAI, superolateral labral tear (*hollow arrow*), and femoral head osteophyte (*long arrow*) indicating premature osteoarthritis in this young adult patient with right hip pain.

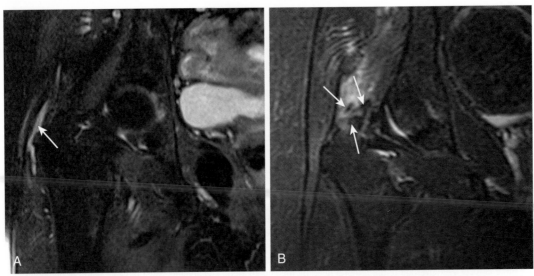

**Figure 55-7.** Greater trochanteric pain syndrome on MRI. **A,** Coronal fat-suppressed PD-weighted image through right hip shows hyperintense fluid collection following contour of right greater femoral trochanter (*arrow*) due to greater trochanteric bursitis. **B,** Coronal STIR image through right hip of different patient demonstrates tear of hypointense adductor tendons with adjacent hyperintense edema and fluid just above greater trochanter (*arrows*).

maximus) bursa paralleling the greater trochanter and interdigitating around the tendons (Figure 55-7, *A*). This fluid can be difficult to visualize on T1-weighted images. Abnormalities of the hip abductor tendons, which attach on the greater femoral trochanter (gluteus medius on the superoposterior facet, gluteus minimus on the anterior facet), include tendonopathy, manifested on MRI as increased signal intensity, and partial- and full-thickness tears, manifested as discontinuity of the tendon fibers (Figure 55-7, *B*). Bursitis and tendinosis often coexist. Although patients with trochanteric pain syndrome always have peritrochanteric T2-weighted signal abnormalities, the converse is not usually true. Presence of increased peritrochanteric T2-weighted signal intensity, especially when of low grade and symmetric, can be seen in asymptomatic patients and does not imply pathology.

## KEY POINTS

- MRI is the examination of choice for evaluation of suspected hip fractures when radiography fails to reveal the cause of hip pain, because it is a highly sensitive and specific modality for detection of radiographically occult fractures and is more sensitive than CT for detection of other possible causes of hip pain such as soft tissue injuries.
- MRI plays a very important role in early diagnosis of occult femoral neck fractures and proximal femoral stress injuries, because delayed diagnosis and treatment of these abnormalities can lead to complications that may require more invasive treatment methods.
- Bone marrow edema in the femoral head and neck is a nonspecific finding that can be seen in a large variety of disease entities, although careful examination of the specific pattern, distribution, and shape of edema can be used to narrow the differential diagnosis.
- Although early AVN of the femoral head and ITOH can look identical on MRI, it is important to include ITOH into the differential diagnosis in the appropriate clinical setting to avoid inappropriate treatment, which can lead to serious complications and preclude recovery.
- Patients with greater trochanteric pain syndrome always have peritrochanteric T2-weighted signal abnormalities, although a small amount of bilaterally symmetric peritrochanteric fluid can be seen in asymptomatic patients and by itself does not imply pathology.

## BIBLIOGRAPHY

LeBlanc KE, Muncie HL Jr, LeBlanc LL. Hip fracture: diagnosis, treatment, and secondary prevention. *Am Fam Physician.* 2014;89(12):945-951.

Magerkurth O, Jacobson JA, Girish G, et al. Paralabral cysts in the hip joint: findings at MR arthrography. *Skeletal Radiol.* 2012;41(10):1279-1285.

DuBois DF, Omar IM. MR imaging of the hip: normal anatomic variants and imaging pitfalls. *Magn Reson Imaging Clin N Am.* 2010;18(4):663-674.

Helms CA, Major NM, Anderson MW, et al. *Musculoskeletal MRI.* 2nd ed. Philadelphia: Saunders Elsevier; 2009.

Sankey RA, Turner J, Lee J, et al. The use of MRI to detect occult fractures of the proximal femur: a study of 102 consecutive cases over a ten-year period. *J Bone Joint Surg Br.* 2009;91(8):1064-1068.

Blankenbaker DG, Ullrick SR, Davis KW, et al. Correlation of MRI findings with clinical findings of trochanteric pain syndrome. *Skeletal Radiol.* 2008;37(10):903-909.

Tannast M, Siebenrock KA, Anderson SE. Femoroacetabular impingement: radiographic diagnosis—what the radiologist should know. *AJR Am J Roentgenol.* 2007;188(6):1540-1552.

Stoller DW. *Magnetic resonance imaging in orthopaedics and sports medicine.* 3rd ed. Philadelphia: Lippincott Williams & Wilkins; 2006.

Oka M, Monu JU. Prevalence and patterns of occult hip fractures and mimics revealed by MRI. *AJR Am J Roentgenol.* 2004;182(2):283-288.

Andrews CL. From the RSNA Refresher Courses. Radiological Society of North America. Evaluation of the marrow space in the adult hip. *Radiographics.* 2000;20(Spec No):S27-S42.

Schnarkowski P, Steinbach LS, Tirman PF, et al. Magnetic resonance imaging of labral cysts of the hip. *Skeletal Radiol.* 1996;25(8):733-737.

Hayes CW, Conway WF, Daniel WW. MR imaging of bone marrow edema pattern: transient osteoporosis, transient bone marrow edema syndrome, or osteonecrosis. *Radiographics.* 1993;13(5):1001-1011, discussion 12.

# CHAPTER 56

# MRI OF THE KNEE

*Sung Han Kim, MD*

1. **What sequences are typically included in a routine magnetic resonance imaging (MRI) examination of the knee?**
   Routine knee MRI typically includes:
   - Sagittal fat-suppressed proton density (PD)-weighted and fat-suppressed T2-weighted images.
   - Coronal T1-weighted and fat-suppressed T2-weighted images.
   - Axial fat-suppressed T2-weighted images.
       Please see Figure 56-1 for some normal knee anatomy on MRI.

2. **Describe the clinical presentation of meniscal injury. What part of the meniscus is most commonly torn?**
   The clinical presentation of a meniscal tear is typically pain and locking of the knee. The posterior horn of the medial meniscus is the primary weight-bearing surface and is most commonly torn. The anterior horn of the lateral meniscus is the most common site for a false-positive diagnosis, where the normal anterior transverse meniscal ligament may mimic a tear.

3. **What is the appearance of the normal menisci on MRI?**
   The menisci are crescent-shaped structures within the joint at the medial and lateral aspects of the superior tibial articular surface. They are composed mainly of fibrocartilage and are low in signal intensity on all imaging sequences. On sagittal images, the menisci appear as bow tie–shaped structures. The posterior horn of the medial meniscus is larger than the anterior horn whereas the posterior and anterior horns of the lateral meniscus are similar in size.

4. **What are the criteria for diagnosing a meniscal tear on MRI?**
   A meniscal tear can be diagnosed using either of these two major criteria:
   - Abnormal meniscal morphology
   - Increased signal intensity within the meniscal tissue which extends to the articular surface on at least two contiguous slices

5. **Describe the common types of meniscal tears.**
   - **Horizontal** or **oblique tear** is the most common type, frequently involving the posterior horn of the medial meniscus (Figure 56-2). This is a degenerative type tear rather than a traumatic type tear.
   - **Longitudinal tear** is a vertically oriented tear that extends parallel to the circumference of the meniscus and is almost always associated with traumatic injury.
   - **Radial tear** occurs in vertical orientation perpendicular to the long axis of the meniscus. This is often seen as a cleft in the meniscus or with a truncated meniscal contour. If the tear is along the imaging plane, the absence of the meniscus on one image can be used to make the diagnosis ("ghost meniscus" sign) (Figure 56-3). A radially torn medial meniscus will often extrude medially, extending beyond the margin of the tibial plateau by greater than 3 mm.
   - **Complex tear** is a tear that extends in more than one plane. This tear has extensive distortion of the meniscal substance and results in multiple flaps.
   - **Bucket handle tear** is a type of a longitudinal tear where the inner edge of the meniscus is displaced. This type of tear can be identified by noting absence of the inner margin of the bow tie as seen on sagittal images. The displaced fragment can lie anterior to the posterior cruciate ligament (PCL) ("double PCL" sign) or may have flipped anteriorly to abut the anterior meniscal horn ("double anterior horn" sign).
   - **Displaced flap tear** occurs when a fragment of the meniscus is displaced away from the site of tear. This most commonly occurs in the medial meniscus where the fragment is displaced into the medial gutter along the tibial plateau. The clinician should be alerted of this finding because it can be overlooked during arthroscopy if the surgeon fails to probe the medial gutter.
   - **Meniscal root tear** is a subtype of radial tear that occurs most frequently at the posterior medial meniscal root. This tear cannot resist hoop stress and often leads to complications such as meniscal extrusion, early secondary osteoarthritis, and subchondral insufficiency fracture.

6. **What is a parameniscal cyst, and what is its significance?**
   A parameniscal cyst can form around the meniscus from extrusion of synovial fluid through a meniscal tear by one-way ball-valve mechanism. A cystic structure around or extending from the meniscus is a finding that is very closely associated with a meniscal tear, and so an underlying meniscal tear should be suspected even if not clearly identified.

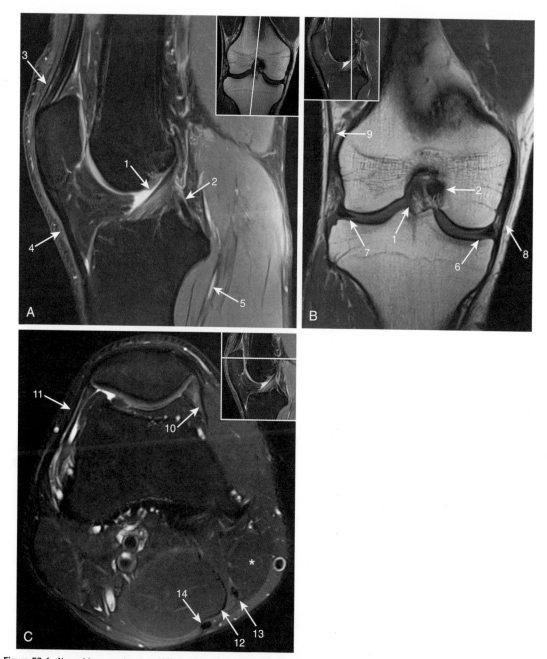

**Figure 56-1.** Normal knee anatomy on MRI. **A,** Midsagittal fat-suppressed PD-weighted image. **B,** Coronal T1-weighted image. **C,** Axial fat-suppressed T2-weighted image. *1* = anterior cruciate ligament (ACL), *2* = posterior cruciate ligament (PCL), *3* = quadriceps tendon, *4* = patellar tendon, *5* = popliteus muscle, *6* = medial meniscus, *7* = lateral meniscus, *8* = medial collateral ligament (MCL), *9* = iliotibial band, *10* = medial patellar retinaculum, *11* = lateral patellar retinaculum, *12* = semimembranosus muscle and tendon, *13* = gracilis tendon, *14* = semitendinosus tendon, * = sartorius muscle and tendon.

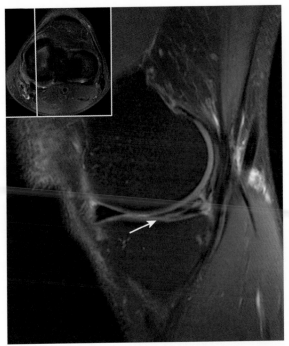

**Figure 56-2.** Meniscal tear on MRI. Sagittal fat-suppressed PD-weighted image shows obliquely oriented increased signal intensity in posterior horn of medial meniscus that extends to inferior articular surface (*arrow*) due to oblique/horizontal tear, which is likely degenerative in nature.

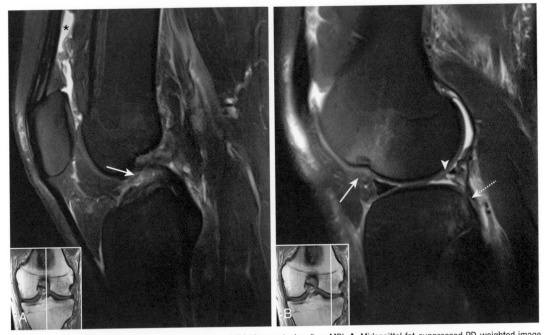

**Figure 56-3.** ACL rupture, radial lateral meniscal tear, and "kissing contusions" on MRI. **A,** Midsagittal fat-suppressed PD-weighted image shows complete rupture of ACL with wavy torn ligament fibers in intercondylar notch (*arrow*). Note associated moderate joint effusion in suprapatellar bursa (*). **B,** Sagittal fat-suppressed PD-weighted image through lateral weight-bearing joint compartment shows feathery high signal intensity bone marrow edema in posterior lateral tibial plateau (*dashed arrow*) and in anterior lateral femoral condyle (*arrow*) due to "kissing contusions" from pivot shift mechanism of injury. Note associated depressed lateral femoral sulcus, which is another indirect sign of ACL rupture. Finally, note absence of normal lateral meniscus (*arrowhead*) in posterior horn representing "ghost meniscus" sign, which indicates radial tear of meniscus along imaging plane.

7. **What is a discoid meniscus, and what is its significance?**
Discoid meniscus is a common variant with morphologic enlargement of the meniscus. Patients usually present with clicking or locking of the knee. As acquired sagittal images can be variable in thickness from scan to scan, this diagnosis can best be made on coronal images. On a coronal MR image through the middle of the femoral condyle, a meniscus that extends centrally beyond the midpoint of the femoral condyle represents a discoid meniscus. The lateral meniscus is more commonly affected, and discoid menisci occur bilaterally in up to 25%.

8. **Describe the anterior cruciate ligament (ACL) and posterior cruciate ligament (PCL) attachment sites.**
The cruciate ligaments arise from the intercondylar notch of the femur, insert on to the tibial plateau, and serve as major stabilizers of the knee joint. The ACL follows a course parallel to the roof of the intercondylar notch arising from the medial surface of the lateral femoral condyle and attaching on the anterior aspect of the tibial spine. The PCL arises from the lateral surface of the medial femoral condyle and attaches at the posterior surface of the tibial plateau. It gently curves between the posterior femur and the posterior tibia.

9. **Describe the MRI appearance of ACL rupture (i.e., tear).**
The most characteristic appearance of ACL rupture is absence or discontinuity of the fibers (see Figure 56-3). Usually, a tear of the ACL is an all-or-none phenomenon where few identifiable fibers are left, or at best an irregular or wavy contour of the ligament remains. Although sagittal images can be used to diagnose the majority of ACL ruptures, the ACL is oriented obliquely relative to routine imaging planes, and therefore should be evaluated on all images in all planes.

Avulsion fracture of the tibial spine is another typical appearance of ACL "tear." This type of injury pattern is classically seen in the pediatric population.

10. **What are some secondary MRI findings of ACL rupture?**
   - Anterior translation of the tibia in relation to the femur by greater than 7 mm.
   - Segond fracture: an avulsion fracture from the lateral tibial plateau by the lateral capsular ligament.
   - "Kissing contusions" in the anterior aspect of the lateral femoral condyle and posterior aspect of the lateral tibial plateau occurring as a result of pivot-shift injury (see Figure 56-3, *B*).
   - "Deep lateral femoral sulcus" sign: depression of the sulcus terminalis portion of the lateral femoral condyle (see Figure 56-3, *B*).

11. **What comprises the medial collateral ligament (MCL)?**
The MCL can be divided into a deep layer and a superficial layer. The deep layer consists of the meniscofemoral and meniscotibial ligaments, and the superficial layer consists of the tibial collateral ligament.

12. **What comprises the lateral collateral ligament (LCL) complex?**
The LCL complex consists of the following from anterior to posterior:
   - Iliotibial band attaching to the Gerdy's tubercle of the tibia
   - Fibular collateral ligament between the lateral femoral condyle and the fibular head
   - Biceps femoris tendon inserting into the fibular head

13. **How is ligamentous injury graded on MRI?**
Ligamentous injury can be graded as I, II, or III.
   - Grade I (sprain): Edema around an intact ligament.
   - Grade II (partial tear): Edema within ligament and in surrounding tissue.
   - Grade III (complete tear): Complete disruption of ligament.

14. **What structures are present at the posterolateral corner of the knee, and why are they important?**
The posterolateral corner structures stabilize the knee from varus and rotatory stresses. They consist of the LCL complex, the popliteus muscle and tendon, the lateral head of the gastrocnemius tendon, as well as the arcuate, fabellofibular, and popliteofibular ligaments.

Posterolateral corner injury is often associated with cruciate ligament tears. Failure of prompt treatment often leads to a poor outcome with early secondary osteoarthritis.

15. **What is O'Donoghue's "unhappy triad"?**
O'Donoghue's "unhappy triad" is a common football and skiing injury that occurs as a result of valgus stress and twisting motion during weight bearing. Classically, MCL injury, ACL tear, and medial meniscal tear constitute this triad.

16. **Describe findings of transient lateral patellar dislocation.**
   - "Kissing contusions" at the medial patellar facet and anterolateral aspect of the lateral femoral condyle from impaction event (Figure 56-4).
   - Patellar and femoral trochlear cartilage injury.
   - Medial patellar retinaculum injury.
   - Knee joint effusion.

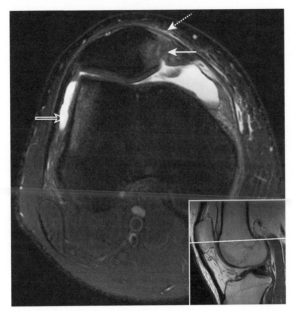

**Figure 56-4.** Transient lateral patellar dislocation on MRI. Axial fat-suppressed T2-weighted image shows feathery high signal intensity bone marrow edema in medial patella (*arrow*) and in anterior lateral femoral condyle (*hollow arrow*). This pattern is in keeping with lateral patellar dislocation with impaction of these surfaces. Depressed fracture of medial patella as seen in this case can also occur with this injury. Sprain of medial retinaculum (*dashed arrow*) is also common in this setting.

17. Describe the MRI findings of patellar tendinitis.

    Patellar tendinitis, also known as jumper's knee, is an overuse syndrome usually seen in young athletes who participate in activities requiring jumping such as basketball or volleyball. In contrast, quadriceps tendon injury is more commonly seen in older populations. The intrasubstance degeneration of the tendon is seen as thickening and increased signal intensity on all pulse sequences. This diagnosis can be easily recognized on sagittal MR images.

18. What is osteochondritis dissecans (OCD)?

    Osteochondritis dissecans refers to a fragmented portion of subchondral bone along an articular surface. The exact etiology is still unknown but repetitive trauma is thought to be at least partially responsible. In the knee, the most common site of involvement is the lateral aspect of the medial femoral condyle along its non-weight-bearing surface. This is most commonly seen in young male patients.

19. What are the MRI features of an unstable OCD fragment?

    MRI is the modality of choice for evaluating these lesions. Signs of an unstable fragment can be seen on T2-weighted images and include the following:
    - A fluid signal intensity rim surrounding the fragment.
    - Cystic foci between the fragment and the host bone.
    - A defect in the overlying cartilage.

20. What is subchondral insufficiency fracture of the knee? Describe its MRI appearance.

    Subchondral insufficiency fracture of the knee is characterized by sudden onset of pain in the absence of trauma. It usually involves the weight-bearing surfaces and most commonly occurs in the central weight-bearing surface of the medial femoral condyle. In contrast to OCD, this entity is more common in elderly women in the sixth or seventh decades of life. It was formerly known as spontaneous osteonecrosis of the knee.

    The typical MRI appearance is a low T1-weighted signal intensity focus just beneath the articular surface with a large amount of bone marrow edema seen on T2-weighted images (Figure 56-5).

21. What is pes anserinus?

    Pes anserinus literally means "goose foot" and is composed of, from anterior to posterior in the medial aspect of the knee, tendons of the sartorius gracilis, and semitendinosus muscles. A common mnemonic for this is "Say grace before tea." There are many small bursae around its insertion which can become inflamed with overuse, resulting in pes anserine bursitis.

22. Where is a popliteal (Baker) cyst located, and what is its significance?

    A popliteal cyst is a bursa that is contiguous with the knee joint in the posterior knee. It usually herniates between the tendons of the medial head of the gastrocnemius muscle and the semimembranosus muscle (Figure 56-6). Rupture of a popliteal cyst can be symptomatic and can often be confused with deep venous thrombosis.

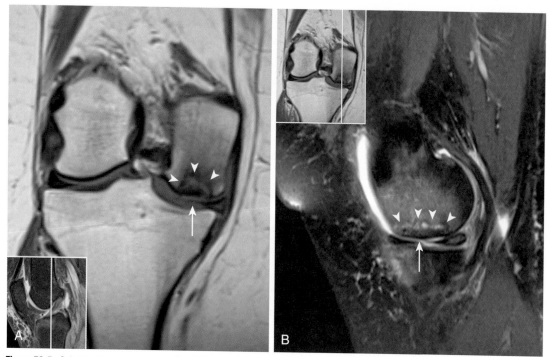

**Figure 56-5.** Subchondral insufficiency fracture of knee on MRI. **A,** Coronal T1-weighted image and **B,** Sagittal fat-suppressed T2-weighted image through central weight-bearing surface of medial joint compartment show bone marrow edema in femoral condyle with subchondral curvilinear signal abnormality (*arrowheads*) typical for this diagnosis. There is associated mild collapse of articular surface (*arrow*) but there is no unstable fragment. In contrast to OCD, this lesion usually occurs on weight-bearing surfaces in middle age or older patients.

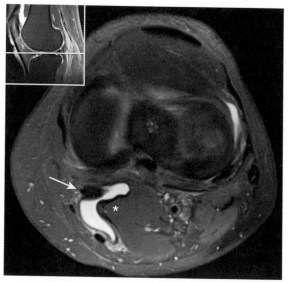

**Figure 56-6.** Popliteal (Baker) cyst on MRI. Axial fat-suppressed T2-weighted image through knee joint shows high signal intensity structure herniating between semimembranosus tendon (*arrow*) and medial head of gastrocnemius (*).

## KEY POINTS

- A meniscal tear is present when either abnormal signal intensity within a meniscus extending to the articular surface on two contiguous slices or abnormal meniscal morphology is visualized.
- Although uncommon, it is important to diagnose meniscal root tears because they often lead to complications such as meniscal extrusion, early secondary osteoarthritis, and subchondral fracture.
- ACL injury often occurs with other associated injuries, including MCL injury, meniscal tear, and "kissing contusions."
- Posterolateral corner injury is an important finding to detect and should be discussed with the clinician as soon as possible to allow for prompt treatment.

**BIBLIOGRAPHY**

Choi JY, Chang EY, Cunha GM, et al. Posterior medial meniscus root ligament lesions: MRI classification and associated findings. *AJR Am J Roentgenol.* 2014;203(6):1286-1292.

Mohankumar R, White LM, Naraghi A. Pitfalls and pearls in MRI of the knee. *AJR Am J Roentgenol.* 2014;203(3):516-530.

Pope TL Jr, Bloem HL, Beltran J, et al. *Musculoskeletal imaging.* 2nd ed. Philadelphia: Elsevier Saunders; 2014.

Zbojniewicz AM, Laor T. Imaging of osteochondritis dissecans. *Clin Sports Med.* 2014;33(2):221-250.

Ciuffreda P, Lelario M, Milillo P, et al. Mechanism of traumatic knee injuries and MRI findings. *Musculoskelet Surg.* 2013;97(suppl 2): S127-S135.

Griffin JW, Miller MD. MRI of the knee with arthroscopic correlation. *Clin Sports Med.* 2013;32(3):507-523.

De Smet AA. How I diagnose meniscal tears on knee MRI. *AJR Am J Roentgenol.* 2012;199(3):481-499.

MacMahon PJ, Palmer WE. A biomechanical approach to MRI of acute knee injuries. *AJR Am J Roentgenol.* 2011;197(3):568-577.

Alatakis S, Naidoo P. MR imaging of meniscal and cartilage injuries of the knee. *Magn Reson Imaging Clin N Am.* 2009;17(4):741-756, vii.

Bining J, Andrews G, Forster BB. The ABCs of the anterior cruciate ligament: a primer for magnetic resonance imaging assessment of the normal, injured and surgically repaired anterior cruciate ligament. *Br J Sports Med.* 2009;43(11):856-862.

Helms CA, Major NM, Anderson MW, et al. *Musculoskeletal MRI.* 2nd ed. Philadelphia: Saunders Elsevier; 2009.

O'Keeffe SA, Hogan BA, Eustace SJ, et al. Overuse injuries of the knee. *Magn Reson Imaging Clin N Am.* 2009;17(4):725-739, vii.

Rosas HG, De Smet AA. Magnetic resonance imaging of the meniscus. *Top Magn Reson Imaging.* 2009;20(3):151-173.

Vinson EN, Major NM, Helms CA. The posterolateral corner of the knee. *AJR Am J Roentgenol.* 2008;190(2):449-458.

Stoller DW. *Magnetic Resonance Imaging in Orthopaedics and Sports Medicine.* 3rd ed. Philadelphia: Lippincott Williams & Wilkins; 2006.

# CHAPTER 57

# MRI OF THE FOOT AND ANKLE

*Mohammed T. Nawas, MD, and Sung Han Kim, MD*

1. **What are the compartments of the ankle joint, and what structures do they contain?**
   The ankle joint contains four compartments: Anterior, medial, lateral, and posterior.
   - Anterior compartment: From medial to lateral, the anterior compartment contains the anterior tibialis tendon, extensor hallucis longus tendon, peroneal nerve, dorsalis pedis artery, and extensor digitorum longus tendon. The tendons in the anterior compartment can be remembered by using the mnemonic "Tom hates Dick."
   - Medial compartment: From medial to lateral, the medial compartment contains the posterior tibialis tendon, flexor digitorum longus tendon, posterior tibial artery, posterior tibial vein, posterior tibial nerve, and flexor hallucis longus tendon. The structures in the medial compartment can be remembered by using the mnemonic "Tom, Dick, and very nervous Harry."
   - Lateral compartment: It contains the peroneal longus and peroneal brevis tendons. The peroneus brevis tendon abuts the bone.
   - Posterior compartment: It contains the Achilles tendon.
        Please see Figure 57-1 for some normal ankle anatomy on MRI.

2. **Which bones form the hindfoot, midfoot, and forefoot?**
   The hindfoot is composed of the calcaneus and talus.
   The midfoot is composed of the navicular, cuboid, and three cuneiforms (medial, middle, and lateral).
   The forefoot is composed of the metatarsals and phalanges (proximal, middle, and distal).

3. **What is the MRI appearance of tendon abnormalities?**
   - Tendinopathy: This refers to degeneration of a tendon, which typically results from overuse. The affected tendon will be intermediate to high in signal intensity on T2 weighted images but not as high in signal intensity as with a tendon tear.

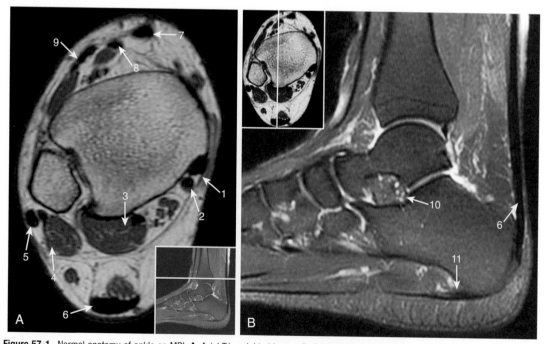

**Figure 57-1.** Normal anatomy of ankle on MRI. **A,** Axial T1-weighted image. **B,** Sagittal fat-suppressed T2-weighted image. *1* = posterior tibialis tendon, *2* = flexor digitorum longus tendon, *3* = flexor hallucis longus tendon and muscle, *4* = peroneus brevis tendon and muscle, *5* = peroneus longus tendon, *6* = Achilles tendon, *7* = tibialis anterior tendon, *8* = extensor hallucis longus tendon, *9* = extensor digitorum longus tendon, *10* = sinus tarsi, *11* = plantar fascia.

- Partial tear: This appears as a linear hyperintense defect within the tendon on T2 weighted images. The signal abnormality is typically very bright, similar to that of fluid.
- Complete tear: This results in discontinuity of the affected tendon. There is often associated retraction of the torn ends of the tendon.
- Paratenonitis: The Achilles tendon does not have a tendon sheath. Instead, it is surrounded by loose connective tissue, which can become inflamed. This condition is referred to as paratenonitis and can be seen as edema in the soft tissue surrounding the tendon. This is often manifested as edema within Kager's fat pad, also known as the pre-Achilles fat pad.
- Tenosynovitis: This refers to an inflammatory process of the tendon sheath. The affected tendon will demonstrate fluid that completely surrounds the circumference of the tendon.

4. **What is the MRI appearance of Achilles tendon rupture?**
Achilles tendon ruptures are commonly seen following sports-related injuries and most frequently seen in men between the ages of 30 and 50. Patients usually report a "pop" during forceful dorsiflexion. On MRI, sagittal images are the most helpful to make this diagnosis. The tendon tear usually occurs in the hypovascular watershed region located 2 to 6 cm proximal to the calcaneal insertion (Figure 57-2). In addition to discontinuity of tendon fibers, a large amount of surrounding edema is typically present in the acute setting. Any gap between the proximal and distal ends of the tendon should be noted because this will impact surgical management.

5. **Which ligaments are injured during ankle inversion?**
The lateral ankle ligaments are injured during ankle inversion. The lateral ankle ligaments are composed of the anterior talofibular ligament, calcaneofibular ligament, and posterior talofibular ligament. The anterior talofibular ligament is the first ligament to tear during ankle inversion and is therefore the most commonly injured ligament. A more severe ankle inversion will next result in a calcaneofibular ligament tear followed by a posterior talofibular ligament tear, although injury involving all three ligaments is rare.

6. **Which ligaments are injured during ankle eversion?**
The medial ankle ligaments are injured during ankle eversion. The medial ankle ligaments are referred to collectively as the deltoid ligament complex, which is composed of superficial and deep components. The lateral ankle ligaments are injured much more commonly than the medial ligaments.

7. **How does an osteochondral lesion occur?**
An osteochondral lesion, previously known as osteochondritis dissecans, occurs secondary to inversion or eversion injuries of the ankle, and is a direct result of the tibia contacting the talar dome. As the name implies, there is injury both to the bone and the overlying hyaline articular cartilage. MRI is useful not only to recognize these lesions, but also to characterize them as stable or unstable (Figure 57-3), using well-studied criteria.

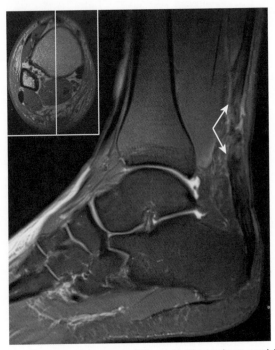

**Figure 57-2.** Achilles tendon rupture on MRI. Sagittal fat-suppressed T2-weighted image shows complete rupture of Achilles tendon in hypovascular watershed region. Note large amount of surrounding soft tissue edema and large gap between torn tendon ends (*arrows*).

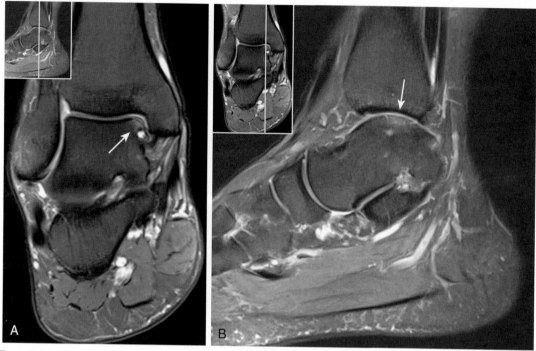

**Figure 57-3.** Osteochondral lesion in ankle on MRI. **A,** Coronal fat-suppressed T2-weighted image and **B,** Sagittal fat-suppressed T2-weighted image show moderate-size osteochondral lesion in medial talar dome (*arrow*). There is fissuring of overlying articular cartilage but no unstable fragment is present. Note small adjacent very high signal intensity subchondral cyst at medial and anterior margin.

The specific MRI findings that suggest that an osteochondral lesion is unstable are:
- Linear high signal intensity surrounding the fragment on fluid sensitive images
- Large cysts deep to the fragment
- Absence of the fragment from the donor site

8. What are the most common sites of avascular necrosis in the ankle?
The three areas in the ankle that are susceptible to avascular necrosis are the talar dome, the second or third metatarsal heads, and the lateral hallux sesamoid.

In the setting of a talar neck fracture, there is often compromise of the quite variable blood supply to the talar dome, which may result in avascular necrosis. This is problematic because it can lead to collapse of the talar dome and accelerated degeneration of the ankle joint.

Characteristic collapse of the second and third metatarsal heads, referred to as Freiberg's infraction, is thought to be a result of avascular necrosis. This appearance is typically seen in the setting of chronic repetitive trauma.

9. What is tarsal coalition, and where does it occur?
Tarsal coalition refers to abnormal congenital bridging between the tarsal bones of the foot. This bridging, or nonsegmentation, can be fibrous, cartilaginous, or osseous. The two most common types of tarsal coalition are the talocalcaneal coalition and the calcaneonavicular coalition. The talocalcaneal coalition occurs on the medial aspect of the joint, and involves the middle facet. MRI will show the bony fusion as well as associated abnormalities, such as edema within the involved bone. Coalition is often discovered during adolescence or young adulthood with symptoms of pain and stiffness in the hindfoot or midfoot. Tarsal coalition occurs bilaterally in 25% of cases. If symptoms are severe, it can be treated surgically.

10. Describe the MRI appearance of plantar fasciitis.
The plantar fascia originates from the calcaneus and is composed of three bands: the medial, central, and lateral bands. The central band is the largest and most commonly involved in the setting of plantar fasciitis. Normally, the plantar fascia is a thin band, which is low in signal intensity on all imaging sequences. Plantar fasciitis can be diagnosed when there is thickening of the origin of the plantar fascia, often with hyperintensity on T2 weighted images due to edema.

11. What is plantar fibromatosis?
Plantar fibromatosis is a benign fibrous proliferation of the plantar fascia, which occurs in all age groups and is bilateral in up to one third of cases. On MRI, there is nodular thickening of the plantar fascia that occurs in the medial or midportion of the fascia. T1-weighted and T2-weighted images typically demonstrate signal intensity that is equal to

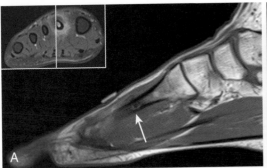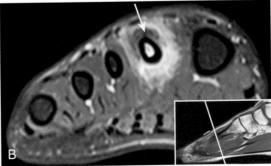

**Figure 57-4.** Stress fracture in foot on MRI. **A,** Sagittal T1-weighted image and **B,** Coronal fat-suppressed T2-weighted image reveal stress fracture through mid shaft of second metatarsal bone. Note low T1-weighted signal intensity fracture line as well as large amount of high T2-weighted signal intensity bone marrow edema and surrounding soft tissue edema. In addition, there is suggestion of callus formation indicative of early healing.

or slightly greater than that of skeletal muscle. Classically, there is avid postcontrast enhancement. This diagnosis can usually be made with confidence given the typical location, morphology, and signal intensity characteristics.

12. **What is a Morton's neuroma, and where does it occur?**
A Morton's neuroma is an abnormality of the plantar digital nerve, which is located between the metatarsal heads, toward the plantar surface of the foot. A Morton's neuroma is not a true neoplasm, but rather represents focal perineural fibrosis, which is often a result of ill-fitting shoes. There is a marked female preponderance, and it typically occurs in the second or third intermetatarsal spaces. Although the enhancement pattern is variable, intense enhancement is common. Morton's neuromas are often associated with inflammation of the bursa between the metatarsal heads, referred to as intermetatarsal bursitis.

13. **What is the tarsal tunnel, and what does it contain?**
The tarsal tunnel is located on the medial aspect of the ankle and contains the flexor tendons (posterior tibial, flexor digitorum longus, flexor hallucis longus) as well as the posterior tibial artery, vein, and nerve. The tunnel begins superiorly at the medial malleolus and extends inferiorly to the navicular bone. It is bordered laterally by the calcaneus and medially by the flexor retinaculum. The abductor hallucis muscle forms its floor.

14. **What is tarsal tunnel syndrome?**
Tarsal tunnel syndrome occurs when there is entrapment neuropathy of the posterior tibial nerve within the tarsal tunnel, which results in pain and paresthesia on the plantar side of the foot. Any process that contributes to impingement or compression of the posterior tibial nerve as it passes through the tarsal tunnel can result in tarsal tunnel syndrome. Common causes include tenosynovitis of the medial compartment tendons, ganglion cysts, nerve sheath tumors, and accessory muscles.

15. **What is the MRI appearance of stress fractures in the foot?**
Stress fractures occur as a result of chronic repetitive injury. The most common locations for stress fractures in the foot are the calcaneus and the metatarsal shafts. Fracture lines will appear as bandlike linear regions of low signal intensity on T1-weighted images. T2 weighted images will demonstrate high signal intensity within the medullary cavity surrounding the fracture, representing bone marrow edema (Figure 57-4). Edema within the periosteum and surrounding soft tissues will also often be present. A "stress reaction" represents a less severe injury with similar imaging findings, except for absence of a low T1-weighted signal intensity fracture line. Stress reactions and stress fractures will typically heal spontaneously after several weeks of reduction in activity.

16. **What is sinus tarsi syndrome?**
The sinus tarsi is a space in the hindfoot between the talus and calcaneus that normally contains fat and neurovascular structures. The sinus tarsi syndrome typically presents with lateral hindfoot pain and a subjective feeling of instability. The most common cause of sinus tarsi syndrome is prior ankle sprain, which over time results in scarring within the tarsal sinus. This scarring can be identified on MRI as replacement of the normal high T1-weighted signal intensity fat with low signal intensity fibrous tissue. Other less common causes of sinus tarsi syndrome include inflammatory arthritis, ganglion cysts, and neoplasms.

**KEY POINTS**

- Ankle inversion occurs much more commonly than ankle eversion and results in injury to the anterior talofibular ligament, calcaneofibular ligament, and posterior talofibular ligament in sequence.
- The sensitivity for detection of stress fractures is significantly higher when utilizing MRI, as compared with radiography or computed tomography (CT).
- MRI can be used to evaluate for and categorize osteochondral lesions, which commonly occur in the talar dome.
- Tarsal coalition is a common cause of foot pain in the younger population.

## BIBLIOGRAPHY

Pope TL Jr, Bloem HL, Beltran J, et al. *Musculoskeletal Imaging.* 2nd ed. Philadelphia: Elsevier Saunders; 2014.

Lawrence DA, Rolen MF, Morshed KA, et al. MRI of heel pain. *AJR Am J Roentgenol.* 2013;200(4):845-855.

Lee SJ, Jacobson JA, Kim SM, et al. Ultrasound and MRI of the peroneal tendons and associated pathology. *Skeletal Radiol.* 2013;42(9): 1191-1200.

Nazarenko A, Beltran LS, Bencardino JT. Imaging evaluation of traumatic ligamentous injuries of the ankle and foot. *Radiol Clin North Am.* 2013;51(3):455-478.

Bae S, Lee HK, Lee K, et al. Comparison of arthroscopic and magnetic resonance imaging findings in osteochondral lesions of the talus. *Foot Ankle Int.* 2012;33(12):1058-1062.

Rios AM, Rosenberg ZS, Bencardino JT, et al. Bone marrow edema patterns in the ankle and hindfoot: distinguishing MRI features. *AJR Am J Roentgenol.* 2011;197(4):W720-W729.

Walker EA, Fenton ME, Salesky JS, et al. Magnetic resonance imaging of benign soft tissue neoplasms in adults. *Radiol Clin North Am.* 2011;49(6):1197-1217, vi.

Donovan A, Rosenberg ZS, Cavalcanti CF. MR imaging of entrapment neuropathies of the lower extremity. Part 2. The knee, leg, ankle, and foot. *Radiographics.* 2010;30(4):1001-1019.

Donovan A, Rosenberg ZS. MRI of ankle and lateral hindfoot impingement syndromes. *AJR Am J Roentgenol.* 2010;195(3):595-604.

Peduto AJ, Read JW. Imaging of ankle tendinopathy and tears. *Top Magn Reson Imaging.* 2010;21(1):25-36.

Pierre-Jerome C, Moncayo V, Terk MR. MRI of the Achilles tendon: a comprehensive review of the anatomy, biomechanics, and imaging of overuse tendinopathies. *Acta Radiol.* 2010;51(4):438-454.

Helms CA, Major NM, Anderson MW, et al. *Musculoskeletal MRI.* 2nd ed. Philadelphia: Saunders Elsevier; 2009.

Bancroft LW, Peterson JJ, Kransdorf MJ. Imaging of soft tissue lesions of the foot and ankle. *Radiol Clin North Am.* 2008;46(6):1093-1103, vii.

Campbell SE, Warner M. MR imaging of ankle inversion injuries. *Magn Reson Imaging Clin N Am.* 2008;16(1):1-18, v.

Crim J. Imaging of tarsal coalition. *Radiol Clin North Am.* 2008;46(6):1017-1026, vi.

Stoller DW. *Magnetic resonance imaging in orthopaedics and sports medicine.* 3rd ed. Philadelphia: Lippincott Williams & Wilkins; 2006.

# IX

# ULTRASONOGRAPHY

# OBSTETRIC ULTRASONOGRAPHY IN THE FIRST TRIMESTER

*Courtney A. Woodfield, MD*

# CHAPTER 58

1. **What are the indications for ultrasonography (US) in the first trimester?**
   First-trimester US is commonly performed for both symptomatic and asymptomatic pregnant patients for a variety of reasons, including:
   - Confirmation, dating, and assessing viability of an intrauterine pregnancy, especially when the last menstrual date is uncertain.
   - Evaluating the etiology of vaginal bleeding, pelvic pain, or a pelvic mass.
   - Measuring embryonic nuchal translucency (NT) as part of screening for fetal chromosomal abnormalities.
   - Early screening of certain fetal anomalies (i.e., anencephaly) in high-risk patients.
   - Imaging guidance for chorionic villus sampling, embryo transfer, and localization and removal of an intrauterine device.

   US in the first trimester may be performed transabdominally and/or transvaginally. Transabdominal US provides an overall view of the pelvis and is typically performed first, even without a full urinary bladder. If a normal intrauterine pregnancy is identified transabdominally, transvaginal imaging may be unnecessary. However, if an intrauterine pregnancy or the adnexa are not well visualized transabdominally, transvaginal US should be performed whenever possible. The transvaginal approach uses a higher-frequency transducer that is placed in closer proximity to the uterus and adnexa, allowing for improved resolution and possibly earlier detection of an intrauterine or ectopic pregnancy. Spectral Doppler imaging should be avoided in the first trimester.

2. **What is typically evaluated during obstetric US in the first trimester?**
   - Presence or absence, and location of a gestational sac.
   - Presence or absence of a yolk sac and of an embryo within a gestational sac.
   - Dating of a gestation based on the mean gestational sac diameter and, when possible, preferably on the embryonic crown-rump length (CRL).
   - Embryonic cardiac activity recorded by two-dimenstional video clip or M-mode imaging.
   - Number of gestations.
   - Other uterine and adnexal masses.
   - Presence or absence of pelvic fluid.

3. **Describe the US features of a normal gestational sac.**
   By 5 weeks of gestational age, the gestational sac is typically visible as a small, round or oval cystic-fluid collection located within the decidua of the thickened and echogenic endometrium along the upper uterine body. The gestational sac grows at a rate of 1.1 mm/day and is typically visible by a serum beta human chorionic gonadotropin (β-hCG) level of 1000 to 2000 mIU/mL. Definitive diagnosis of a pregnancy can only be made once a gestational sac contains a yolk sac and/or embryo. If a suspected gestational sac is seen without a yolk sac or embryo, then follow-up US and/or follow-up serial maternal serum β-hCG levels are performed to ensure accurate diagnosis and management of a potentially viable early pregnancy.

4. **Describe the US features and significance of an abnormal gestational sac.**
   On US examination, an irregularly shaped gestational sac that is low-lying and surrounded by a weakly echogenic and thin rim of decidual reaction is 90% to 100% predictive of an abnormal intrauterine pregnancy. A mean gestational sac diameter that is less than 5 mm greater than the embryonic CRL, which is known as first-trimester oligohydramnios, is also associated with a poor pregnancy outcome. A mean gestational sac size of 16 to 24 mm without an embryo is suspicious for a failed pregnancy. However, a higher cutoff of 25 mm is now recommended as the mean gestation sac size by which an embryo should be seen, before diagnosing a failed pregnancy.

5. **When should a yolk sac and an embryo be visible by US?**
   The yolk sac is usually seen at 5.5 weeks of gestation as a thin, circular structure, measuring between 3 and 5 mm. The embryo develops adjacent to the yolk sac and is usually seen around 6 weeks of gestation. Figure 58-1 depicts the normal early gestational US appearance of an embryo and a yolk sac within a gestation sac.

6. **What are the US findings of an abnormal yolk sac?**
   A yolk sac that is large (76 mm), fragmented, or calcified is suggestive of an abnormal intrauterine pregnancy (Figure 58-2).

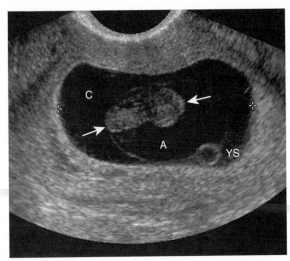

**Figure 58-1.** Normal 9-week intrauterine pregnancy on US. Transvaginal US image demonstrates well-defined embryo (*arrows*) and yolk sac (*YS*) with normal separation of amnionic (*A*) and chorionic (*C*) sacs.

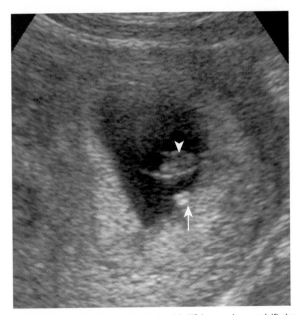

**Figure 58-2.** Early failed intrauterine pregnancy on US. Transabdominal pelvic US image shows calcified yolk sac (*arrow*) and embryonic remnant (*arrowhead*).

7. At what point should embryonic cardiac activity be detected on US?

   Embryonic cardiac activity is usually visible as soon as an embryo is detectable sonographically, often at a CRL as small as 2 mm. The absence of sonographically detectable embryonic cardiac activity by a CRL ≥7 mm is diagnostic of a failed pregnancy, as is the absence of an embryo with a heartbeat ≥2 weeks after an US examination demonstrates a gestational sac without a yolk sac, and absence of an embryo with a heartbeat ≥11 days after an US demonstrating a gestational sac with a yolk sac. Between 5 and 8 weeks, the embryonic heart rate is usually 100 beats/min or greater. From 8 weeks to term, the average heart rate is 140 beats/min (range 120 to 180 beats/min). The thresholds for bradycardia based on embryonic size are listed in Table 58-1.

8. What is the first trimester nuchal translucency (NT) measurement?

   Screening for fetal chromosomal abnormalities can include a sonographic measurement of fetal NT (the anechoic soft tissue posterior to the cervical spine or occipital bone) in the first trimester between a gestational age of 11 to 14 weeks. NT measurements are used in conjunction with maternal serum biochemistry to determine the risk of having a fetal chromosomal abnormality, most commonly Down syndrome. There are strict guidelines for measuring NT to

**Table 58-1.** Thresholds for Bradycardia Based on Embryonic Size

| CROWN RUMP LENGTH (MM) | BRADYCARDIA (BEATS PER MINUTE) |
| --- | --- |
| <5 | <80 bpm |
| 5-9 | <100 bpm |
| 10-15 | <110 bpm |

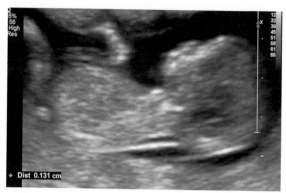

**Figure 58-3.** Nuchal translucency (*NT*) on US. Transabdominal pelvic US image of 11-week gestation fetus reveals normal NT measurement of 1.3 mm as measured in midsagittal plane with fetus in neutral position.

ensure an accurate measurement of the sagittal nuchal thickness with the fetal neck in the neutral position (Figure 58-3). A NT measurement greater than 3 mm from 11 to 14 weeks is considered abnormal.

9. **Describe the first trimester US features of twin gestations.**
   Multigestational pregnancies can result from the fertilization of two or more separate ova (dizygotic or fraternal twins) or a single fertilized ovum that subsequently divides (monozygotic or identical twins). Dizygotic twins each have their own amnions, chorions, and yolk sacs and are therefore dichorionic diamniotic (DC/DA). The chorionicity and amnionicity of monozygotic twins depend on when they divide and can therefore be DC/DA (division within the first 3 days postconception), monochorionic diamniotic (MC/DA) (division between days 4 and 8), or monochorionic monoamniotic (MC/MA) (division after day 8). Amnionicity and chorionicity are easiest to determine in the first trimester at 6 to 9 weeks. The first-trimester ultrasound features of a DC/DA twin gestation are two separate gestational sacs, each surrounded by a chorionic echogenic ring, and each containing a yolk sac and embryo. Later in the first and second trimester, a triangular shaped extension of placental tissue can be seen arising from the placental surface and tapering between the layers of the intertwin membrane. This is referred to as the chorionic peak or "lambda" sign (Figure 58-4). MC/DA twins have a thinner intervening membrane and are seen as two embryos with their own amnions in a single chorion. There are also typically two yolk sacs. MC/MA twins have no intervening membrane, both embryos are within a single chorion and single amnion, and a single yolk sac may be present.

10. **List seven causes of vaginal bleeding in the first trimester.**
    - Implantation bleed.
    - Subchorionic hemorrhage.
    - Embryonic pregnancy/blighted ovum.
    - Embryonic demise.
    - Spontaneous abortion.
    - Ectopic pregnancy.
    - Molar pregnancy.

11. **Name three possible causes of a positive serum β-HCG level and an empty uterus on US.**
    - Early normal intrauterine pregnancy (<5 weeks).
    - Complete spontaneous abortion.
    - Ectopic pregnancy.

12. **Name six types of early pregnancy complications, and describe their US appearances.**
    For the answer, see Table 58-2 and Figure 58-5.

13. **What is an ectopic pregnancy?**
    An ectopic pregnancy refers to a pregnancy located anywhere outside of the endometrial cavity. Ectopic pregnancies occur with a frequency of approximately 14 in 1000 pregnancies. An ectopic pregnancy most commonly occurs in the

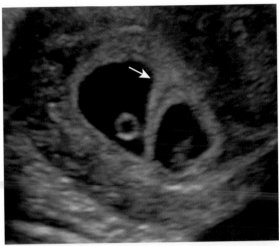

**Figure 58-4.** Dichorionic diamniotic twin gestation on US. Transvaginal US image of 7-week twin gestation demonstrates chorionic peak or "lambda" sign (*arrow*) with thick intertwin membrane separating two gestational sacs.

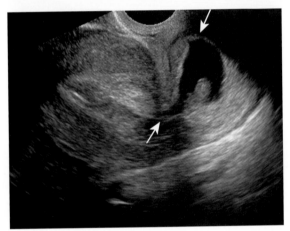

**Figure 58-5.** Abortion in progress on US. Sagittal transvaginal US image shows misshapen and elongated gestational sac containing embryo (*arrows*) positioned within endocervical canal. US examination from one week prior (*not shown*) demonstrated this gestation at normal location along upper uterine body, distinguishing current image from cervical ectopic pregnancy.

**Table 58-2.** US Appearance of Six Types of Early Pregnancy Complications

| TYPE OF ABORTION | DEFINITION | ULTRASOUND FINDINGS |
|---|---|---|
| Threatened abortion | Vaginal bleeding with a closed cervical os | Ranges from live embryo to a small empty gestational sac to a normal empty uterus |
| Abortion in progress | Intrauterine gestation in the process of being expelled | Irregular gestational sac in the lower uterus/cervix ± a live embryo |
| Incomplete abortion | Incomplete passage of gestational tissues | Thickened endometrium ± fluid and debris, and areas of increased endometrial vascularity |
| Complete abortion | Expulsion of all gestational tissues | Normal empty uterus which may be mildly vascular |
| Blighted ovum | Failed or abnormal embryonic development | Empty gestational sac or sac with abnormal yolk sac and no embryo; any abnormal gestational sac development |
| Embryonic demise | Lack of embryonic growth and absent expected cardiac activity | Embryo without cardiac activity |

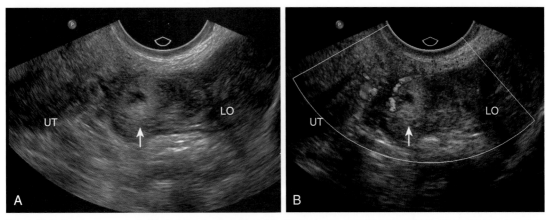

**Figure 58-6.** Ectopic pregnancy on US. **A,** Coronal gray scale and **B,** Doppler transvaginal US images of left adnexa demonstrate ectopic pregnancy (*arrow*) as tubal ring between uterus (*UT*) and left ovary (*LO*). There is also a small amount of adjacent particulate free fluid (*FF*).

fallopian tube (95% to 97% of cases), typically in the isthmic or ampullary portion of the tube. Other sites include the interstitial portion of the fallopian tube (interstitial pregnancy) (2% to 5%), the ovary (1%), the cervix (<0.1%), and the abdominal cavity (<0.1%).

14. Who is at increased risk for an ectopic pregnancy?
    Women with a history of prior ectopic pregnancy, pelvic inflammatory disease, fallopian tube surgery, in vitro fertilization, or use of an intrauterine contraceptive device are at increased risk for an ectopic pregnancy.

15. What is the classic clinical presentation of an ectopic pregnancy?
    Approximately 45% of patients with ectopic pregnancies present with the clinical triad of vaginal bleeding, pelvic pain, and a palpable adnexal mass.

16. List four possible US findings associated with an ectopic pregnancy.
    • Embryo located outside of the uterus (5% to 10% of cases): 100% diagnostic of an ectopic pregnancy.
    • Complex or solid adnexal mass (Figure 58-6): the most common finding.
    • Moderate to large amount of pelvic free fluid, especially if particulate.
    • Empty uterus in conjunction with serum β-hCG level that is above the level at which a gestational sac should be seen.

17. What is a pseudogestational sac?
    In the setting of an ectopic pregnancy, a variable amount of fluid or hypoechoic debris may accumulate within the endometrial cavity, giving rise to a pseudogestational sac of an ectopic pregnancy (Figure 58-7). This collection of fluid and debris may be surrounded by a single, thin, echogenic rim of decidual reaction due to endometrial stimulation by the circulating hormones of an ectopic pregnancy. A pseudogestational sac may be present in 5% of ectopic pregnancies.

18. What is a heterotopic pregnancy?
    A heterotopic pregnancy occurs when there are concurrent intrauterine and extrauterine gestations. The frequency of heterotopic pregnancies in natural conceptions is approximately 1 in 30,000. Patients who are pregnant by in vitro fertilization or the use of ovulation induction have a higher incidence of multiple gestations and are also at increased risk for ectopic and heterotopic pregnancies.

19. What is a molar pregnancy?
    A molar pregnancy is the most common and most benign form of gestational trophoblastic disease and is characterized by proliferation of placental tissue after abnormal fertilization of an empty ovum by one (complete mole, no fetus) or two (partial mole, fetus present) sperm. Patients characteristically present with markedly elevated serum β-hCG levels, an enlarged uterus, hyperemesis gravidarum, preeclampsia, vaginal bleeding, or a combination of these findings.

20. What is the US appearance of a molar pregnancy?
    The edematous placental tissue and prominent chorionic villi of a molar pregnancy classically have a "snowstorm" appearance on US. The endometrial canal is filled with hyperechoic placental tissue with good through-transmission and numerous small cystic villi, which may be too small to visualize (Figure 58-8). A complete mole involves the entire placenta without a fetus. A partial mole involves a portion of the placenta and has an associated fetus, usually with multiple anomalies.

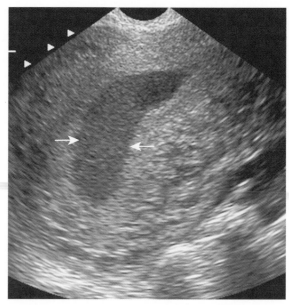

**Figure 58-7.** Pseudogestational sac of ectopic pregnancy on US. Sagittal transvaginal US image shows echogenic material consistent with hemorrhage filling endometrial cavity (*arrows*).

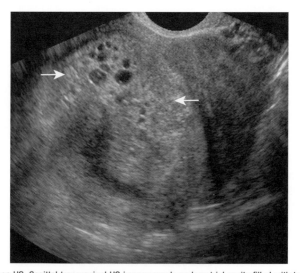

**Figure 58-8.** Molar pregnancy on US. Sagittal transvaginal US image reveals endometrial cavity filled with heterogeneous cystic and solid placental tissue (*arrows*) characteristic of complete molar pregnancy.

## KEY POINTS

- For a viable intrauterine gestation, an embryo should be visible sonographically by a mean gestational sac diameter of 25 mm, and an embryonic heart rate should be detected by a crown-rump length of 7 mm.
- The best time to differentiate the chorionicity and amnionicity of a twin gestation is in the first trimester, between 6 and 9 weeks.
- The most common sonographic finding of an ectopic pregnancy is an adnexal mass.
- Molar pregnancies in the first trimester have a "snowstorm" appearance on US due to edematous placental tissue with small cystic villi.

**BIBLIOGRAPHY**

Doubilet PM, Benson CB, Bourne T, et al. Diagnostic criteria for nonviable pregnancy early in the first trimester. *N Engl J Med.* 2013;369(15):1443-1451.

Levi CS, Lyons EA. The first trimester. In: Rumack CM, Wilson SR, Charboneau JW, et al., eds. *Diagnostic ultrasound.* 4th ed. Philadelphia: Mosby Elsevier; 2011:1072-1118.

Paspulati RM, Turgut AT, Bhatt S, et al. Ultrasound assessment of premenopausal bleeding. *Obstet Gynecol Clin North Am.* 2011;38(1):115-147, viii.

Lin EP, Bhatt S, Dogra VS. Diagnostic clues to ectopic pregnancy. *Radiographics.* 2008;28(6):1661-1671.

Levine D. Ectopic pregnancy. *Radiology.* 2007;245(2):385-397.

Middleton WD, Kurtz AB, Hertzberg BS. The first trimester and ectopic pregnancy. In: *Ultrasound: the requisites.* St. Louis: Mosby; 2004:342-373.

Wagner BJ, Woodward PJ, Dickey GE. From the archives of the AFIP. Gestational trophoblastic disease: radiologic-pathologic correlation. *Radiographics.* 1996;16(1):131-148.

# CHAPTER 59

# OBSTETRIC ULTRASONOGRAPHY IN THE SECOND TRIMESTER

*Courtney A. Woodfield MD*

1. **What are the indications for obstetric ultrasonography (US) in the second (and third) trimester?**
   There are numerous indications for US imaging in the second (and third) trimester, the most common ones including screening evaluation of fetal anatomy; screening for fetal anomalies; estimation of gestational age; and evaluation of fetal growth, fetal well-being, fetal presentation, cervical insufficiency, amniotic fluid status, placental location, and vaginal bleeding. In most circumstances, US in the second and third trimester only requires transabdominal imaging. Transvaginal or transperineal imaging may be required for more detailed evaluation of the cervix and placental position in cases with placenta previa, suboptimal visualization of the cervix, or with a shortened cervix on transabdominal imaging.

2. **List the basic components of a standard (level 1) second trimester US examination.**
   A standard second trimester US examination includes documentation of the following:
   - Fetal number and presentation.
   - Fetal cardiac activity.
   - Estimate of amniotic fluid volume.
   - Location, appearance, and relationship of the placenta to the internal cervical os.
   - Placental location.
   - Gestational age.
   - Fetal weight estimation.
   - Fetal anatomic survey, including head (cerebral ventricles, choroid plexus, midline falx, cerebellum, cistern magna, nose and lips), chest (four-chamber heart, right and left ventricular outflow tracts), abdomen (situs, stomach, kidneys, urinary bladder, fetal umbilical cord insertion site, umbilical cord vessel number), spine (cervical, thoracic, lumbar, sacral), extremities (arms and legs), gender in multiple gestations.
   - Maternal uterus, cervix, and adnexa.

3. **How is gestational age determined in the second trimester?**
   The most accurate estimation of gestational age is in the first trimester based on embryonic crown-rump length. In the second trimester (after 14 weeks gestation), dating is based on a combination of fetal measurements including biparietal diameter (BPD) (measured in the transverse plane at the level of the thalami from the outer edge of the proximal skull to the inner edge of the distal skull), head circumference (HC) (also measured at the level of the thalami), abdominal circumference (AC) (measured at the level of the fetal stomach and junction of the umbilical vein and portal venous sinus), and femoral diaphysis length (FL) (Figure 59-1). These measurements are also used in calculations for estimation of fetal weight. A head-to-abdominal circumference ratio can also be calculated to assess appropriate fetal growth. The HC is normally larger than the AC in the second and early third trimesters, with a reversal of this ratio at term.

4. **How is the amniotic fluid volume measured?**
   Amniotic fluid volume can be assessed qualitatively (by an experienced imager) or measured semiquantitatively. For semiquantitative assessment, the amniotic fluid index (AFI) is calculated by individually measuring and then adding together the deepest vertical empty fluid pockets (no umbilical cord or fetal parts) in each quadrant. A normal AFI is between 8 cm and 24 cm, and each individual fluid pocket should be between 2 cm and 8 cm.

5. **What is oligohydramnios?**
   Oligohydramnios is too little amniotic fluid, defined quantitatively as a single deepest vertical fluid pocket depth less than 2 cm or total AFI of less than 8 cm. A lack of amniotic fluid can impair fetal lung development and result in fetal pulmonary hypoplasia with high fetal morbidity and mortality. Oligohydramnios can result from a variety of etiologies including fetal **d**emise, fetal **r**enal abnormalities, **i**ntrauterine growth retardation (IUGR), **p**remature rupture of membranes, **p**ost dates, and **c**hromosomal abnormalities (mnemonic DRIPPC).

6. **What is polyhydramnios?**
   Polyhydramnios is too much amniotic fluid, defined quantitatively as a single deepest vertical pocket measurement greater than 8 cm or total AFI of greater than 24 cm. Polyhydramnios may be idiopathic (in up to 40%), secondary to maternal factors such as diabetes and hypertension, or secondary to fetal factors including anything that might impair

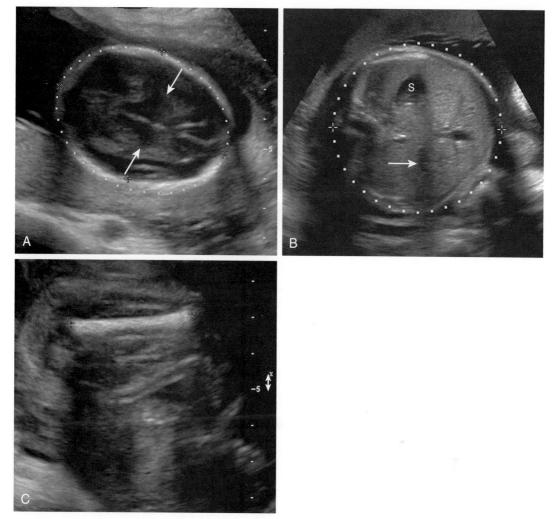

**Figure 59-1.** Fetal measurements for calculating gestational age on US. **A,** Biparietal diameter and head circumference at level of thalami (*arrows*). **B,** Abdominal circumference at level of liver and portal vein (*arrow*), stomach (*s*). **C,** Femur length.

fetal swallowing of amniotic fluid (upper gastrointestinal tract obstruction, chest narrowing or mass, and severe central nervous system abnormalities) and fetal hydrops.

7. **How is cervical incompetence evaluated sonographically?**
Cervical length can first be assessed transabdominally with a partially distended bladder. A fully distended bladder may falsely lengthen the cervix due to mass effect. If the cervix is not well visualized or appears shortened transabdominally, then transvaginal or transperineal imaging should be performed. The normal cervical length is ≥3 cm. A length of 2 to 3 cm is considered borderline shortened, and <2 cm definitively shortened. If the internal os is open (referred to as funneling), the maximal width of the dilated cervical canal should also be measured, and any prolapse of membranes, umbilical cord, and/or fetal parts should be documented (Figure 59-2). The major risk of an incompetent cervix is preterm delivery.

8. **Describe the various types of placenta previa.**
The placenta normally terminates >2 cm above the internal cervical os. Extension of the placental edge within 2 cm of the internal os is referred to as low-lying placenta. Extension of the placenta up to or over the cervix is referred to as placenta previa. Placenta previa can be marginal (at the edge of the internal os) (Figure 59-3), partial (partial coverage of the internal os), or complete (complete coverage of the internal os). Some cases of placenta previa may resolve as the pregnancy progresses, and therefore follow-up imaging is performed in the third trimester. If a placenta previa persists, then plans can be made for a cesarean section.

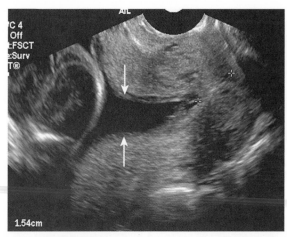

**Figure 59-2.** Cervical incompetence on US. Sagittal transvaginal US image shows cervical length is decreased to 1.54 cm (*between + 's*) and dilation of internal os (*arrows*).

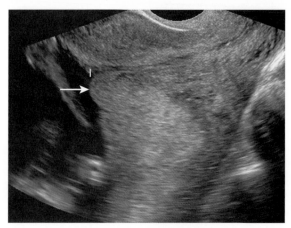

**Figure 59-3.** Marginal placenta previa on US. Sagittal transvaginal US image shows that placenta (*arrow*) extends up to edge of internal os (*I*).

9. **Differentiate the various types of placenta accreta.**
   Invasion of the placenta into the uterine wall is referred to as placenta accreta. Risk factors for placenta accreta include prior placenta previa, prior uterine surgery (cesarean section, myomectomy), prior retained products of conception, and multiparity. Placenta accreta is further defined as accreta vera (also called accreta; the most common type) if the placenta is only adherent to the uterine myometrium, increta if the placenta invades into the myometrium, and percreta if the placenta completely penetrates the myometrium (usually then extending up to/into the bladder). All forms of placenta accreta can be difficult to diagnose sonographically, but suggestive US features include absence of the normal subplacental hypoechoic zone, heterogeneous placental echotexture, subplacental vascular spaces, and placental extension into the bladder wall. The major complication of placenta accreta is massive maternal hemorrhage at delivery.

10. **Does US have a role in assessing second (and third) trimester maternal pain and bleeding?**
    The major consideration in any pregnant patient presenting with pelvic pain or bleeding is placental hemorrhage and placental abruption. Risk factors for placental hemorrhage include maternal hypertension, smoking, alcohol or cocaine use, trauma, and premature rupture of membranes. The role of US is to detect hemorrhage/hematoma associated with the placenta. Hemorrhage is describe as retroplacental if it is located between the placenta and uterine wall, marginal if it is located lateral to the placenta, and intraplacental if it is located within the placenta. Placental abruption occurs if a retroplacental hemorrhage is large enough to separate the placenta from the uterus (Figure 59-4). Placental bleeds can be difficult to detect sonographically if the blood readily decompresses through the vagina rather than building up as a measurable hematoma. Visualization of a retroplacental hematoma on US is associated with a worse outcome for the fetus and mother due to a higher risk of complete placental separation. Depending on the age of the placental bleed, the blood products may range from hypoechoic or completely anechoic in the acute and chronic phases to hyperechoic and heterogeneous in the subacute phase.

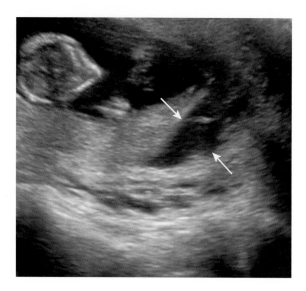

**Figure 59-4.** Placental abruption on US. Sagittal transabdominal US image demonstrates retroplacental hematoma with marginal abruption (*arrows*).

11. How many vessels are in the umbilical cord?

Normally, the umbilical cord is comprised of three vessels (two arteries and one vein). A two-vessel cord (one artery and one vein) in isolation does not always imply a fetal abnormality, and in multiple gestations is a more common normal variant. However, detection of a two-vessel umbilical cord should prompt a search for other fetal structural abnormalities including those related to the heart. A two-vessel cord can also be associated with growth retardation and fetal aneuploidies.

12. Why is the diameter of the fetal lateral ventricle measured during routine second trimester US?

Measurement of the width of the lateral ventricle at the atrium is a standard second trimester fetal measurement used to detect hydrocephalus. Normally, the lateral ventricle diameter is <10 mm (usually 4 to 8 mm). A lateral ventricle measurement >10 mm is indicative of hydrocephalus. A dangling choroid plexus surrounded by fluid in the lateral ventricle is a secondary sign of hydrocephalus. Possible etiologies for fetal hydrocephalus include cerebral acqueductal stenosis, neural tube defect with Chiari malformation, Dandy Walker malformation, hemorrhage, and infection.

13. What is the importance of the fetal cisterna magna measurement during routine second trimester US?

A normal fetal cisterna magna diameter is <10 mm (usually 2 to 8 mm). Effacement of the cisterna magna suggests a possible Chiari II malformation with a meningocele or myelomeningocele. Enlargement of the cisterna magna can be seen with a Dandy Walker malformation, in which case there is also cerebellar vermian hypoplasia or agenesis and communication of a posterior fossa cyst with the fourth ventricle. An enlarged cisterna magna with a normal appearing cerebellum and brain and no communication with the fourth ventricle can be a normal variant known as mega cisterna magna.

14. Describe the US features of anencephaly.

Anencephaly is one of the most common neural tube defects with a frequency of 1 in 1000. The fetal skull and cerebral cortex are absent while the skull base, brainstem, and orbits remain (Figure 59-5). US can depict absence of the calvarium and brain above the orbits as early as 8 weeks gestation, but definitive diagnosis should be reserved for when the calvarium should be ossified at 14 weeks. In some instances, dysmorphic "angiomatous stromal" tissue may be seen above the brainstem.

15. What is the purpose of evaluating the fetal lips on US?

Evaluation of the fetal lips at the time of routine second trimester US can detect a cleft lip, the most common facial anomaly. A cleft lip can be unilateral or bilateral and is associated with a cleft palate in up to 80% of cases. Cleft lip and palate can be isolated or associated with trisomy 13 or 18, amniotic bands, or a limb-body-wall complex, all of which carry a poor prognosis for the fetus.

16. Can US differentiate spina bifida in utero?

During routine second trimester US, the fetal spine is screened for any open or closed spinal defect. Open spina bifida containing only herniated meninges is a meningocele. If the herniated contents also include spinal cord elements, it is a myelomeningocele. On US, these defects usually appear as cystic structures bulging through splayed posterior osseous elements, most commonly in the lumbosacral region. If the contents of the cystic bulge are completely anechoic, this suggests a meningocele. If there are echogenic strands within the cystic bulge, this suggests herniated neural elements as well and therefore a myelomeningocele.

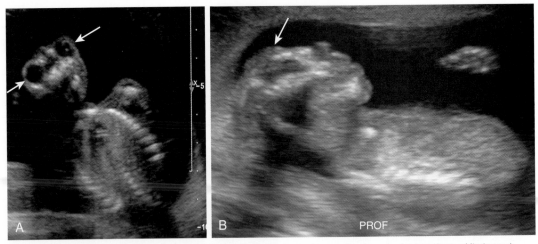

**Figure 59-5.** Anencephaly on US. **A,** Coronal transabdominal US image shows absence of brain and calvarium above orbits (*arrows*). **B,** Sagittal transabdominal US image demonstrates small amount of angiomatous stroma (*arrow*) above orbits.

17. Are there secondary intracranial signs of open spina bifida on US?

    Most cases of open spina bifida are associated with posterior fossa abnormalities (Chiari II malformations) in utero due to downward traction of the spinal cord. This includes downward-curved "C shaped" herniation of the cerebellum (the "banana" sign), effacement of the cisterna magna, flattening of the bilateral frontoparietal bones (the "lemon" sign), and ventriculomegaly (Figure 59-6). The "banana" sign is seen in more than 90% of cases, and the "lemon" sign in up to 98% of cases of open neural tube defects.

18. How many anomalies can be detected on the second trimester US four-chamber heart view?

    With the standard four-chamber heart view alone (Figure 59-7), up to 70% of fetal cardiac anomalies can be detected, including cardiomegaly, cardiac masses (rhabdomyoma), septal defects, endocardial cushion defects, and hypoplastic left heart. With the addition of visualizing the right and left ventricular outflow tracts and a short-axis view of the great vessels at the base of the heart, up to 80% of anomalies may be detected, including tetralogy of Fallot, transposition of the great vessels, and truncus arteriosus.

19. How is fetal pulmonary hypoplasia assessed on US?

    The appearance of a small fetal thorax and low thoracic circumference is suggestive of pulmonary hypoplasia. A fetal thorax-to-head ratio of <1 carries a poor prognosis. The echogenicity of the fetal lungs on US is not a reliable indicator of lung maturity. Pulmonary hypoplasia can be idiopathic or secondary (from oligohydramnios or from mass effect by an intrathoracic mass such as a congenital diaphragmatic hernia (CDH) or congenital cystic adenoid malformation (CCAM) of the lung).

20. What is the most common intrathoracic/extracardiac fetal anomaly?

    Congenital diaphragmatic hernia (CDH) occurs in 1 of every 2000 to 3000 live births. Up to 90% occur on the left side and can occur posterolaterally as a Bochdalek hernia in 90%, or anteromedially as a Morgagni hernia in 10%. CDH is diagnosed on US by the demonstration of abdominal contents (stomach, liver, bowel, mesenteric fat), cystic structures, or solid structures within the thorax. The diagnosis is often first suspected when the stomach and/or bowel is seen adjacent to the heart on a standard four-chamber heart view (Figure 59-8). Other US findings include peristaltic movements in the chest, contralateral cardiac and mediastinal shift, and a small AC. There is an association with polyhydramnios and pulmonary hypoplasia if fetal swallowing and lung development is impaired due to intrathoracic mass effect.

21. Describe the US features of an omphalocele versus gastroschisis.

    Omphalocele and gastroschisis are the most common abdominal wall defects, occurring in up to 1 in 4000 (omphalocele) and 1 in 10,000 (gastroschisis) live births. An omphalocele is a midline anterior abdominal wall defect containing variable herniated abdominal contents including the liver and/or bowel (Figure 59-9, *A*). The umbilical cord inserts on the anterior aspect of the herniation, and the herniation is covered by a thin peritoneal membrane. In contrast, gastroschisis is an isolated, paraumbilical anterior abdominal wall defect of herniated free-floating bowel without an overlying peritoneal membrane (Figure 59-9, *B*). A gastroschisis defect is most commonly to the right of the umbilical cord insertion site on the abdominal wall. Therefore, demonstrating the abdominal cord insertion site on routine second trimester US is critical to detect and differentiate abdominal wall defects. Omphaloceles carry a worse prognosis because up to 90% are associated with additional fetal malformations (including those of the cardiac, thoracic, gastrointestinal, genitourinary, and central nervous systems) and up to 40% are associated with fetal aneuploidy (trisomy 13 and 18). In contrast, gastroschisis is typically an isolated finding not seen in association with other structural abnormalities, but can be complicated by bowel malrotation, atresia, stenosis, and perforation with resulting meconium peritonitis.

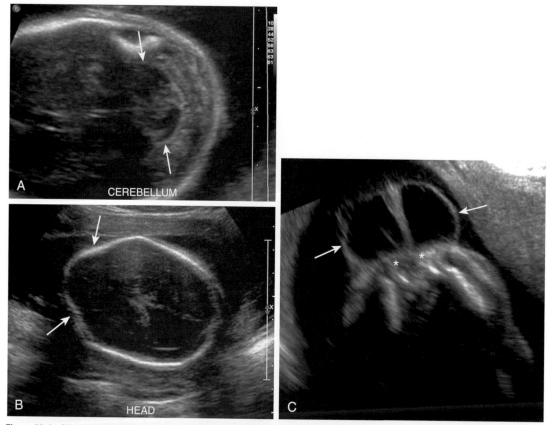

**Figure 59-6.** Chiari II malformation associated with myelomeningocele on US. **A,** Transverse transabdominal US image through posterior fossa demonstrates "banana" sign of inferiorly displaced "C-shaped" cerebellum (*arrows*) with effacement of cisterna magna. **B,** Transverse transabdominal US image through head reveals "lemon" sign of bifrontoparietal calvarial flattening (*arrows*). **C,** Transverse transabdominal US image of lumbosacral spine demonstrates splaying of posterior elements (*) and cystic mass arising posteriorly from spine (*arrows*).

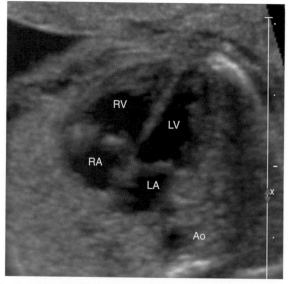

**Figure 59-7.** Normal four-chamber view of heart on US. Transabdominal US image shows normal right ventricle (*RV*), left ventricle (*LV*), right atrium (*RA*), left atrium (*LA*), and aorta (*Ao*).

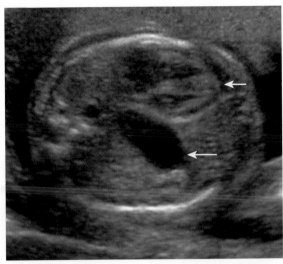

**Figure 59-8.** CDH on US. Transabdominal US image demonstrates stomach (*long arrow*) adjacent to heart (*short arrow*) in thorax.

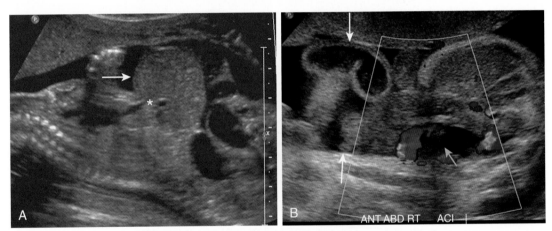

**Figure 59-9.** Omphalocele versus gastroschisis on US. **A,** Sagittal transabdominal US image of omphalocele shows anterior abdominal wall defect with membrane-covered herniated liver (*arrow*) centered on umbilical vein (*\**). **B,** Transverse transabdominal US image of gastroschisis demonstrates anterior abdominal wall defect with herniated free-floating bowel (*long arrows*) to right of umbilical cord insertion site (*short arrow*).

22. When should the urinary bladder be visible on US?

    By 16 weeks gestation, the bladder should be visible sonographically. As the bladder may normally fill and empty during the course of a routine second trimester US, if the bladder is not first visualized, repeat US imaging should be performed every 15 to 20 minutes for 1 hour before determining that the bladder is nonvisible. If the bladder is still not seen after 1 hour of reimaging, nonvisualization may be due to bilateral intrinsic renal impairment, upper urinary tract obstruction, bladder exstrophy, or a systemic cause such as IUGR. Bladder exstrophy is associated with an infraumbilical wall defect.

23. What is the significance of finding dilated bilateral renal pelves on routine second trimester US?

    Prior to 23 weeks gestation, the normal diameter of fetal renal pelves is ≤5 mm, and after 23 weeks, ≤7 mm. Dilated renal pelves can be the result of vesicoureteral reflux, ureteropelvic junction obstruction, posterior urethral valves (where the bladder would also be distended) (Figure 59-10), duplicated renal collecting system, or ureterocele. Pyelectasis is also seen in up to 25% of fetuses with Down syndrome. If dilation of the renal pelves (with or without caliectasis) is detected in utero, postnatal follow-up US is required to assess the degree of any remaining obstruction and renal function.

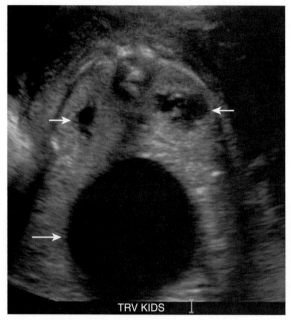

**Figure 59-10.** Posterior urethral valves on US. Transabdominal US image shows findings of lower urinary tract obstruction due to posterior urethral valves in male fetus with markedly distended bladder (*long arrow*) and bilateral hydronephrosis (*short arrows*).

24. **How is IUGR diagnosed sonographically?**
    IUGR is defined as an estimated fetal weight less than the tenth percentile for expected gestational age. It can be due to a variety of etiologies including multiple maternal factors that result in placental insufficiency such as hypertension, smoking, or alcohol or drug use. Fetal causes include chromosomal abnormalities and infection.

25. **The estimated fetal weight (EFW) for a fetus at 34 weeks gestation on US is greater than the ninetieth percentile. What are the potential complications at delivery?**
    An EFW greater than the ninetieth percentile for gestational age is defined as large for gestational age and further defined as macrosomia with a fetal weight >4000 g at birth. Risk factors for an abnormally large fetus include maternal diabetes (most common), maternal obesity, and prolonged pregnancy. Complications for the infant at birth include asphyxia, meconium aspiration, neonatal hypoglycemia, shoulder dystocia, and brachial plexus injury.

26. **When should the umbilical artery systolic to diastolic (S/D) ratio be measured?**
    In any setting of oligohydramnios with intact membranes or in any setting of IUGR, Doppler US imaging of the umbilical artery should be performed as a means to assess for placental insufficiency. Normally, the S/D ratio in the umbilical artery gradually decreases during pregnancy as diastolic flow increases with increasing gestational age. Elevated S/D ratios (>4.0 at 26 to 30 weeks, >3.5 at 30 to 34 weeks, and >3 after 34 weeks) indicate diminished diastolic flow, a sign of increased vascular resistance in the placenta, and are associated with increased risk of perinatal morbidity and mortality. Absent or reversed end diastolic flow in the umbilical artery indicates a particularly poor prognosis and usually prompts immediate delivery.

27. **Describe the ultrasound features of fetal hydrops.**
    Fetal hydrops is excessive fluid accumulation in the fetal body cavities and soft tissues that results in pericardial and pleural effusions, ascites, skin thickening, placental thickening, and polyhydramnios. Causes of fetal hydrops are defined as either immune or nonimmune. Immune hydrops due to maternal and fetus blood group incompatibility is now rare. Nonimmune etiologies include chromosomal anomalies, fetal anatomic defects including cardiac malformations, any mass obstructing venous return to the heart, and maternal-fetal infection.

28. **List the complications that can be associated with a twin gestation.**
    For the answer, see Table 59-1.

29. **What are the ultrasound features of a monochorionic diamniotic twin-to-twin transfusion syndrome (TTTS)?**
    TTTS is a serious complication of monochorionic twins resulting from arteriovenous shunting of blood in a shared placenta. The recipient twin is large, polycythemic, and at risk for high-output cardiac failure which can manifest as hydrops and polyhydramnios. The donor twin is small, anemic, and can develop oligohydramnios, becoming "stuck" against the uterine wall (Figure 59-11). The mortality rate is 40% to 90%, with both twins at risk.

**Table 59-1.** Complications Associated with Twin Gestation

| TWIN TYPE | COMPLICATION |
|---|---|
| All twins | Prematurity<br>IUGR |
| Monochorionicity (due to vascular anastomoses in a shared placenta) | Twin-to-twin transfusion syndrome (TTTS)<br>Twin embolization syndrome (TES)<br>Twin reversed arterial perfusion (TRAP) sequence |
| Monoamnionicity | Conjoined twins<br>Entangled cords |

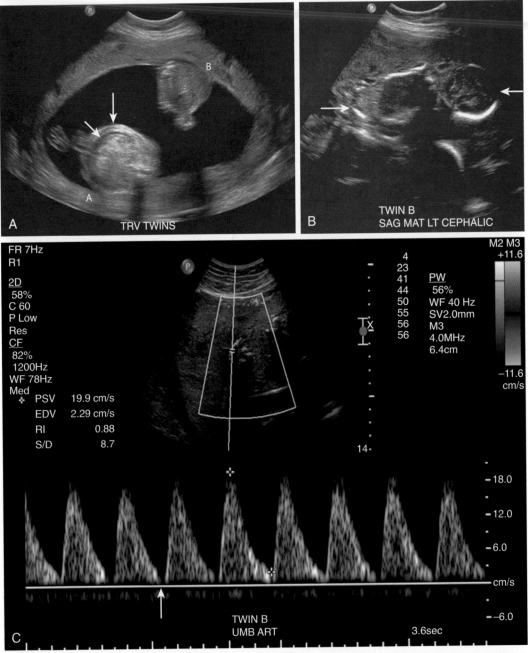

**Figure 59-11.** TTTS on US. **A,** Transabdominal US image shows that twin A, recipient twin, has polyhydramnios and hydrops manifested by skin thickening (*long arrow*) and ascites (*short arrow*). **B,** Transabdominal US image demonstrates that twin B, donor twin (*arrows*), has paucity of amniotic fluid indicative of oligohydramnios. **C,** Doppler US interrogation of umbilical artery of twin B demonstrates lack of diastolic flow (*arrow*) in umbilical artery and elevated S/D ratio of 8.7, indicative of placental insufficiency and poor prognosis for twin B.

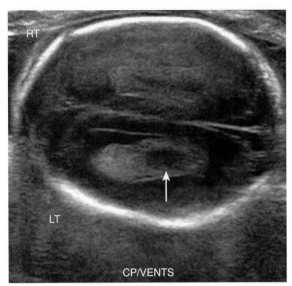

**Figure 59-12.** Choroid plexus cyst on US. Transabdominal US image reveals anechoic ovoid cyst (*arrow*) in choroid plexus, which is "soft" marker for possible fetal aneuploidy.

30. Name seven "soft" ultrasound markers of potential fetal aneuploidy.

There are several markers of fetal aneuploidy that should be searched for and documented during routine second trimester US. These are considered "soft" because they are incidental, nonpathologic findings that may be seen in normal fetuses, but are associated with an increased incidence of chromosomal abnormalities, most commonly Down syndrome. The following markers can be used to screen for or adjust the risk for fetal aneuploidies:

- Choroid plexus cysts (Figure 59-12).
- Increased nuchal thickness (>3 mm first trimester and >6 mm second trimester).
- Echogenic intracardiac focus.
- Echogenic bowel.
- Short long bones (<third percentile for gestational age).
- Mild renal pyelectasis (anterior-posterior diameter of >4 to 5 mm).
- Two-vessel cord, single umbilical artery.

## KEY POINTS

- The required components of a routine second trimester sonographic examination include documentation of fetal age, number, and lie, placental location, fetal heart rate, fetal anatomy, amniotic fluid volume, and maternal uterus and adnexa.
- Transvaginal or transperineal imaging should be performed for a shortened or inadequately visualized cervix on transabdominal imaging.
- Routine second trimester US screens for multiple structural fetal anomalies, some of the more common and severe ones including anencephaly, spina bifida, CDH, omphalocele, gastroschisis, and urinary tract obstruction.
- Routine second trimester US also screens for "soft" markers that may indicate an increased risk for fetal aneuploidy, including choroid plexus cysts, intracardiac echogenic focus, renal pyelectasis, and echogenic bowel.

**BIBLIOGRAPHY**

Sommerfeldt JC, Putnins RE, Fung KF, et al. AIRP best cases in radiologic-pathologic correlation: twin reversed arterial perfusion sequence. *Radiographics*. 2014;34(5):1385-1390.

Sonek J, Croom C. Second trimester ultrasound markers of fetal aneuploidy. *Clin Obstet Gynecol.* 2014;57(1):159-181.

Nguyen D, Nguyen C, Yacobozzi M, et al. Imaging of the placenta with pathologic correlation. *Semin Ultrasound CT MR.* 2012;33(1):65-77.

Bromley B, Benacerraff B. Chromosomal abnormalities. In: Rumack CM, Wilson SR, Charboneau JW, et al., eds. *Diagnostic ultrasound.* 4th ed. Philadelphia: Mosby Elsevier; 2011:1119-1144.

Levine D. Overview of obstetric imaging. In: Rumack CM, Wilson SR, Charboneau JW, et al., eds. *Diagnostic ultrasound.* 4th ed. Philadelphia: Mosby Elsevier; 2011:1040-1060.

Salomon LJ, Alfirevic Z, Berghella V, et al. Practice guidelines for performance of the routine mid-trimester fetal ultrasound scan. *Ultrasound Obstet Gynecol.* 2011;37(1):116-126.

Chalouhi GE, Stirnemann JJ, Salomon LJ, et al. Specific complications of monochorionic twin pregnancies: twin-twin transfusion syndrome and twin reversed arterial perfusion sequence. *Semin Fetal Neonatal Med.* 2010;15(6):349-356.

Elsayes KM, Trout AT, Friedkin AM, et al. Imaging of the placenta: a multimodality pictorial review. *Radiographics*. 2009;29(5):1371-1391.

Middleton WD, Kurtz AB, Hertzberg BS. Part II: obstetrics and gynecology. In: *Ultrasound: the requisites.* St. Louis: Mosby; 2004:303-341, 74-586.

# CHAPTER 60

# ADVANCED FETAL ULTRASONOGRAPHY AND THERAPY

*Steven C. Horii, MD, FACR, FSIIM*

1. What is a "level II" obstetric ultrasound examination, and what elements of fetal anatomy are included?

   A level II obstetric ultrasound examination is a comprehensive real-time ultrasonography (US) evaluation of fetal anatomy to detect fetal anomalies, whereas a level I obstetric ultrasound is a more general evaluation to detect obstetric problems.

   For the elements of fetal anatomy that are included in a level II obstetric ultrasound examination, see Table 60-1.

2. What is a "detailed extended" obstetric ultrasound examination?

   The detailed extended obstetric ultrasound examination involves real-time US maternal evaluation plus detailed fetal anatomic examination. This is used when there is an increased risk of fetal abnormalities. The elements included in the detailed extended obstetric ultrasound examination are more detailed themselves in comparison to those of the level II examination. For the elements of fetal anatomy that are included in a detailed extended obstetric ultrasound examination, see Table 60-2.

   In addition to the fetal anatomic survey elements of a level II obstetric ultrasound examination, a detailed extended obstetric ultrasound examination usually includes:

   - Doppler US evaluation of the umbilical artery, umbilical vein, and ductus venosus.
   - Measurement of the fetal nasal bone length.
   - Documentation of the fetal extremities (includes imaging the forearms and forelegs to show the radius, ulna, tibia, and fibula and detailed imaging of the hands and feet to show five digits).
   - Cardiac outflow tracts.
   - Fetal gender.

     Other anatomy that is evaluated depends on the suspected or detected abnormalities, including:

   - Doppler US evaluation of one or both middle cerebral arteries.
   - Demonstration of the corpus callosum (and pericallosal artery on color flow Doppler US).

**Table 60-1.** Elements of Fetal Anatomy in a Level II Obstetric Ultrasound Examination (Fetal Anatomic Survey)

| Head, Face, and Neck | Chest |
|---|---|
| Cerebral lateral ventricles | Heart |
| Choroid plexus |     Four-chamber view |
| Midline falx |     Left ventricular outflow tract |
| Cavum septi pellucidi |     Right ventricular outflow tract |
| Cerebellum | |
| Cisterna magna | |
| Upper lip | |
| Nuchal fold (≤20 weeks) (not included in the basic elements, but advised if the fetus is ≤20 weeks) | |
| **Abdomen** | **Spine** |
| Stomach (presence, size, situs) | Cervical, thoracic, lumbar, and sacral (in sagittal and |
| Kidneys |     transverse planes) |
| Urinary bladder | |
| Umbilical cord insertion | |
| Umbilical cord number of vessels | |
| **Extremities** | **Gender** |
| Arms and legs | In multiple gestations and when medically indicated |

**Table 60-2.** Elements of Fetal Anatomy in a Detailed Extended Obstetric Ultrasound Examination

| COMPONENT | DETAILED ELEMENTS | COMPONENT | DETAILED ELEMENTS |
|---|---|---|---|
| Head and neck | 3rd ventricle<br>4th ventricle<br>Lateral ventricles<br>Cerebellar lobes, vermis, cisterna magna<br>Corpus callosum<br>Integrity and shape of cranial vault<br>Brain parenchyma<br>Neck | Spine | Integrity of spine and overlying soft tissue<br>Shape and curvature |
| | | Extremities | Number: architecture and position<br>Hands<br>Feet<br>Digits: number and position |
| Face | Profile<br>Coronal face (nose, lips, lens)<br>Palate, maxilla, mandible, tongue<br>Ear position and size<br>Orbits | Genitalia | Sex |
| | | Placenta | Masses<br>Placental cord insertion<br>Accessory/succenturiate lobe with location of connecting vascular supply to primary placenta |
| Chest | Aortic arch<br>Superior vena cava and inferior vena cava<br>3-vessel view<br>3-vessel and trachea view<br>Lungs<br>Integrity of the diaphragm<br>Ribs | | |
| | | Biometry | Cerebellar width<br>Inner and outer orbital diameters<br>Nuchal skin thickness (15-22 weeks)<br>Humerus<br>Ulna/radius<br>Tibia/fibula |
| Abdomen | Small and large bowel<br>Adrenal glands<br>Gallbladder<br>Liver<br>Renal arteries<br>Spleen<br>Integrity of abdominal wall | | |

- Measurement of fetal external ear length.
- Measurement of the cerebellar width and cisterna magna anteroposterior diameter.
- Demonstration of the anterior maxilla and mandible on transverse views.
- Aortic and ductal arch views.
- Cardiothoracic circumference (or area) ratio.
- Pulmonary vein drainage to the left atrium.
- Fetal gallbladder.
- Fetal spleen.
- Fetal adrenal glands.
- Sagittal and transverse kidney images.
- Fetal perineum (showing anal orifice).
- Fetal genitalia.
- Measurement of long bones (all four extremities) as well as foot length.
- Measurement of other skeletal structures such as clavicles, scapulae, and finger lengths.

3. What are the common nonemergent indications to perform a detailed extended obstetric ultrasound study?

Nonemergent indicators of abnormal pregnancy that may prompt use of a detailed extended examination include:

- Abnormal maternal screening. This includes the sequential screen which includes measurement of some combination of maternal serum alpha fetoprotein (AFP), pregnancy-associated plasma protein A (PAPP-A), estriol, human chorionic gonadotropin (hCG), and dimeric inhibin A (DIA). More recent screening involves the cell-free DNA screening test, also referred to as noninvasive prenatal testing (NIPT), which examines the fetal DNA found in maternal blood and can detect trisomy 13, 18, and 21 and Turner syndrome. A patient who has an abnormal result of chorionic villus sampling or amniocentesis would also be a candidate for a detailed extended ultrasound study.
- Size-date discrepancy (includes polyhydramnios and oligohydramnios as causes).

- Changes in fetal movement. This can be an emergency if fetal activity changes from normal to markedly decreased or absent, as it indicates fetal distress at a minimum and fetal demise in the worst case scenario.
- History of previous pregnancy (or pregnancies) resulting in abnormal fetuses or with spontaneous abortions that have shown chromosomal abnormalities.
- Advanced maternal age (i.e., the patient is, or will turn, ≥35 years of age during the pregnancy).
- Family history of congenital anomalies.
- Maternal infections exposure (TORCH-toxoplasmosis, other, rubella, cytomegalovirus, herpes; other includes such known teratogenic virus as parvovirus B19).

4. What is the significance of an elevated maternal serum AFP level?

An elevated maternal serum AFP level may prompt an amniocentesis because an elevated level in the amniotic fluid is strong evidence of a fetal anomaly, usually a neural tube or abdominal wall defect. Maternal serum AFP is usually high in multiple gestations and is normally higher than the overall population average in some ethnic groups.

5. What is the significance of size-date discrepancies?

Size-date discrepancies are frequently the result of errors in dating, usually because of an unknown last menstrual date or irregular menstrual cycles. Implantation bleeding can be mistaken by the patient as a menstrual period and cause a dating error. US is used to check on the fetal size compared with that predicted from dates. This may require sequential US studies to demonstrate a normal growth rate or to show an abnormal one.

Large for dates fetuses can result from maternal diabetes mellitus, either gestational or type II. Assuming that an error in dating has been excluded, a large for dates pregnancy (i.e., when the fundal height measured by the obstetrician is greater than expected) can also mean multiple gestations, high amniotic fluid level (polyhydramnios), or fetal macrosomia. Small for dates fetuses can result from too low of an amniotic fluid level (oligohydramnios), intrauterine growth restriction, or constitutionally small fetus (a diagnosis of exclusion). US is useful for both large and small for gestational age pregnancies to determine the etiology and plan follow-up.

6. A detailed extended obstetric ultrasound examination can take considerably longer than a level II study. What are the safety elements of obstetric US?

Though ultrasound is not ionizing radiation and is generally regarded as safe, use of ultrasound does mean exposing tissues to mechanical energy. The mechanical energy of ultrasound has two basic effects in tissue: heating, and mechanical compressive and shear forces. Heating, or thermal, effects result from the sound energy causing tissues to vibrate. This vibration results in a rise in temperature. Compressive and shear forces can disrupt some tissues and have been shown to cause hemorrhages in bowel and lung (in experimental animal studies). The mechanical forces are much intensified if gas is present (which should not be so in a fetus) or near the edges or surfaces of bone because the reflection from bone can be so strong. The shear forces can also cause cavitation, resulting in the formation and collapse of small bubbles. This exerts tremendous local forces and can disrupt normal tissues. In nonmedical situations, cavitation exerts a powerful enough force to erode metal.

The United States Food and Drug Administration (FDA) has imposed output limits on ultrasound machines because of these thermal and mechanical effects. The maximum output is 720 milliwatts (mW) per square centimeter ($cm^2$). However, for fetal US, the FDA limits output to 94 mW/$cm^2$. This power limit is the reason that an obstetric ultrasound study is performed using the ultrasound machine's "OB" setting. Machines set up the output power limits based on examination type. In agreeing to higher output limits for US machines overall, the FDA required manufacturers to display indices of the output power being used. This is known as the output display standard (ODS) and is the reason for the display on each image of two indices: the thermal index (TI) and the mechanical index (MI) (Figure 60-1).

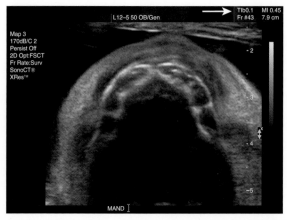

**Figure 60-1.** FDA Output Display Standard (ODS) on US. Transverse image shows normal fetal mandible. Note values of bone-based thermal index (*Tlb*) and mechanical index (*MI*) (*arrow*). The values of 0.1 and 0.45, respectively, are within specification.

7. **Why does the TI have a letter after it?**

The thermal index has three variants depending on the tissue types that will be encountered: TIs for soft tissue, TIb for bone, and TIc for the cranium. The thermal index is the ratio of the power being produced by the machine to the power needed to raise tissue temperature by $1°$ centigrade. The mechanical index can be thought of as the likelihood of causing cavitation. Use of color flow Doppler and spectral Doppler US increases the output power. For documentation of embryonic and fetal cardiac activity, M-mode may be used because it does not require output power greater than regular gray scale B-mode imaging.

8. **What values of TI and MI are recommended for fetal US studies?**

TI and MI recommendations for fetal studies include:
- TIs values are used for first trimester studies.
- TIb values are used for second and third trimester studies.
- TI <0.5 should be used particularly for first trimester studies.
- TI <0.5 may likely be used for extended scan times.
- TI >0.5 and <1.0 should be limited to scan times of less than 30 minutes.
- TI >2.5 should be limited to scan times of less than one minute.
- MI ≤1.9 (the current FDA limit) can be used as needed in the absence of gas bodies.

   In general, as for ionizing radiation, the principle of "as low as reasonably achievable (ALARA)" should be employed for ultrasound, particularly for obstetric studies.

9. **What constitutes fetal therapy?**

Improvements in ultrasound technology have made possible detailed visualization of the fetus and uterus. The real-time aspect also means that ultrasound can be used for guiding therapies. Fetal therapy had its beginnings with fetal transfusion for Rh incompatibilities. The techniques of intraperitoneal blood transfusion and sampling of umbilical vein blood were developed in the 1960s to 1970s and used ultrasound guidance. In the 1980s, ideas about surgery on the fetus were tested in laboratory experiments on animals and eventually brought to human fetuses. The first reported open fetal surgical procedure was performed in 1982 by Harrison and colleagues. They created bilateral ureterostomies in a 21-week fetus that had bilateral hydronephrosis. The procedure was a technical success, but the neonate succumbed to the (at the time) unrecognized problems of renal dysplasia and pulmonary hypoplasia. Through the following decade, fetal surgical treatments were developed, and success rates increased.

   Fetal therapeutic techniques include:
- Open fetal surgery (hysterotomy, performing the surgery, and closing the hysterotomy).
- Interventional techniques (ultrasound-guided shunt placements and fluid aspiration).
- Ex-utero intrapartum therapy (EXIT). This is performed for management of conditions that obstruct the fetal airway or compromise breathing. The fetus is delivered via caesarian section, but the umbilical cord is not ligated. Surgery is then performed on the fetus while still connected to the placenta so that the fetus continues to be supplied oxygenated blood via the placental connection, giving surgeons time to relieve the airway obstruction. Once the airway is established (or the surgical procedure is finished), the delivery is completed.
- Fetal therapy also includes medical management, which is an integral part of treatment of the fetus whether or not the surgical methods are employed. While fetal therapy begins with the mother and fetus, in most instances, treatment is continued for the neonate, so centers that perform fetal therapeutic procedures have the support of neonatal intensive care.

10. **What are the major fetal anomalies for which diagnostic and therapeutic techniques are available?**

Fetal ultrasound evaluation for anomalies is very extensive. Any anomaly that results in anatomic and some physiologic derangements can be evaluated by US. These evaluations typically start with the detailed extended obstetric ultrasound examination and with specific imaging and measurements added for the anomaly and planned intervention. While the number of conditions treated by fetal surgical and interventional techniques is growing, the ones that have established therapies include:
- Spina bifida.
- Lung masses including congenital pulmonary airway malformation (CPAM) (known as congenital cystic adenomatoid malformation [CCAM]), bronchopulmonary sequestration (BPS), and congenital lobar emphysema (CLE).
- Pleural effusion.
- Congenital high airway obstruction syndrome (CHAOS).
- Congenital diaphragmatic hernia (CDH).
- Fetal neck masses.
- Sacrococcygeal teratoma (SCT).
- Bladder outlet obstruction (lower urinary tract obstruction [LUTO]).
- Twin abnormalities including twin to twin transfusion syndrome (TTTS); selective intrauterine growth restriction (sIUGR); twin anemia-polycythemia sequence (TAPS); twin reversed arterial perfusion (TRAP) syndrome; and conjoined twins.

   Therapy for these conditions takes advantage of state-of-the-art surgical and interventional techniques. US and magnetic resonance imaging (MRI) are used routinely to help make specific diagnoses and plan for treatment. For all

US performed for a fetal anomaly, if one is found, the fetal anatomic survey is done to exclude other anomalies as it is not unusual for a fetus to have more than one abnormality. This is also true if an anomaly is detected during an otherwise routine ultrasound study.

11. **How are fetuses with open spina bifida and myelomeningocele (MMC) evaluated?**

A suspicion for a fetal neural tube defect is often raised by the maternal serum screening for AFP level. An open spinal defect in the fetus results in higher levels of AFP in both the amniotic fluid and maternal serum. Because there are nonfetal causes for elevated AFP levels, US is performed to evaluate the fetal spine. In addition to the elements of the detailed extended examination, evaluation for spina bifida with MMC includes:

- Detailed evaluation of the brain, particularly the cerebral ventricles as ventriculomegaly often accompanies an MMC (Figure 60-2).
- Determination of whether Chiari II malformation and hindbrain herniation are present (Figure 60-3).
- Evaluation of the cerebral ventricles for evidence of additional complications, including intraventricular hemorrhage and gray matter heterotopia (often better seen with fetal MRI).
- Determination of the level of the bony defect and the start of the skin defect (Figure 60-4).
- Evaluation of the spine for any associated bony abnormality such as kyphosis or scoliosis. If present, the Cobb angle is measured.
- Determination of whether there is an MMC sac or a myeloschisis (there is an open spina bifida but no membrane covering or surrounding the defect).
- Measurement of the MMC sac (Figure 60-5).

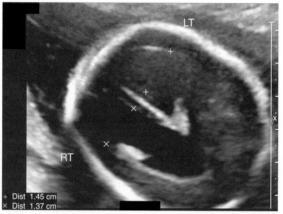

**Figure 60-2.** Fetal ventriculomegaly on US. Transverse image through head of fetus with spina bifida and MMC demonstrates dilated lateral ventricles. Measurements are shown for left (+) and right (×) lateral ventricles performed at, or just posterior to, tip of choroid plexus. Values of 1.45 cm for left and 1.37 cm for right are above normal value of 1 cm.

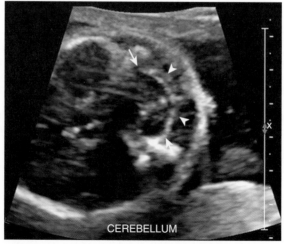

**Figure 60-3.** Fetal hindbrain herniation on US. Transverse image through posterior fossa of infant with MMC and Chiari II malformation reveals near complete effacement of cisterna magna with only trace cerebrospinal fluid (*arrowheads*). Note low-positioned cerebellum of hindbrain herniation (*arrows*).

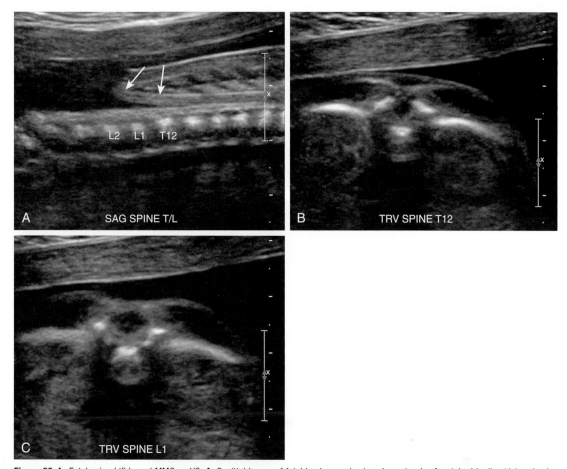

**Figure 60-4.** Fetal spina bifida and MMC on US. **A,** Sagittal image of fetal lumbosacral spine shows levels of vertebral bodies (determined by counting lowest rib-bearing vertebral body as T12) and neural elements (*arrows*) extending into MMC defect. **B,** Transverse image through spine at T12 level demonstrates larger than normal gap in posterior elements. **C,** Transverse image through spine at L1 level reveals definite abnormal widening of posterior elements.

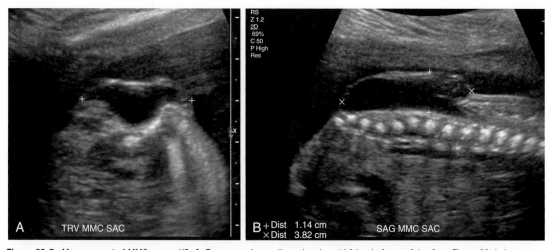

**Figure 60-5.** Measurement of MMC sac on US. **A,** Transverse image through spine at L3 level of same fetus from Figure 60-4 shows MMC sac (+). **B,** Sagittal image of lumbosacral spine shows measurements of MMC sac (+ and X), which extends to S2-S3 level.

- Evaluation of the spinal cord for associated abnormalities such as syringomyelia (Figure 60-6).
- Real-time examination of the lower extremities for movement and exclusion or confirmation of talipes equinovarus (club foot) (Figure 60-7).

12. **What is the therapeutic approach to treatment of fetuses with spina bifida and MMC?**
   The fetal surgical treatment for spina bifida is well established. A multicenter clinical trial, the Management of Myelomeningocele Study (MoMS), showed significantly better outcomes for fetuses that had the myelomeningocele (MMC) repaired in utero compared with those that had the surgical repair post delivery. The surgical treatment involves a hysterotomy for access to the fetus, positioning the fetus to expose the spinal defect, and performing the surgical repair much as would be done for postnatal repairs. The fetus is then replaced in the uterus, fluid is added to replace amniotic fluid lost, and the uterus is closed. The mother is then carefully monitored for the development of complications including premature labor, chorioamniotic membrane separation, and infection. The fetus is then reevaluated at intervals to assess its well-being and to determine if the ventriculomegaly is normalizing.

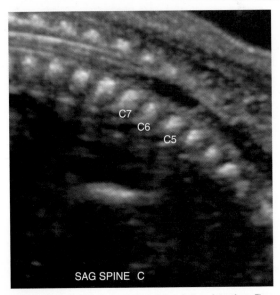

**Figure 60-6.** Fetal syringomyelia on US. Sagittal image through cervical spine of same fetus from Figure 60-4 demonstrates hypoechoic area within spinal canal demarcated by labeled cervical vertebral levels. This represents dilation of central canal complex of spinal cord. Assessment of spinal cord for such abnormalities is routine in ultrasound evaluation of spinal dysraphism.

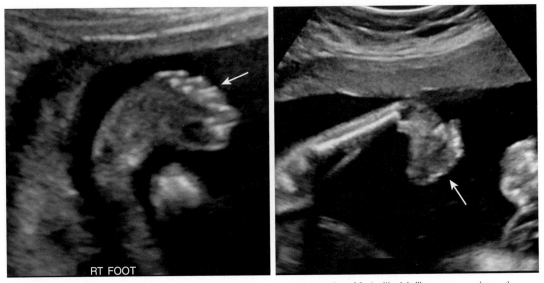

**Figure 60-7.** Fetal talipes equinovarus on US. Note inversion and medial rotation of feet with club-like appearance (*arrows*).

13. **What are the imaging requirements for thoracic and lung abnormalities?**

    In addition to the detailed extended ultrasound examination, evaluation of lung lesions usually includes:
    - Determination of the location of the lung mass, and whether or not there is a mediastinal shift or compression.
    - Measurement of the lung mass; calculation of lung mass volume along with lung mass volume to head circumference (HC) ratio.
    - Measurement of normal lung segments.
    - Determination of lung mass arterial supply and venous drainage.
    - Measurement of macroscopic cysts within lung mass (if present).
    - Determination of pleural effusion volume.

14. **What specific imaging is performed for fetal pleural effusions?**

    Fetal pleural effusions are divided into two main groups: hydropic and nonhydropic. Hydropic pleural effusions result from conditions causing the hydrops itself and are often evident from the history or presence of anomalies known to be associated with hydrops. Nonhydropic pleural effusions can be associated with:
    - Congenital heart defects not causing fetal congestive failure.
    - Lung lesions.
    - CDH.
    - Chromosomal abnormalities (trisomy 18, trisomy 21, and Turner syndrome).
    - Pulmonary lymphangiectasia (which may also result in hydrops).
    - Pulmonary venous atresia.
    - Thoracic wall hamartoma.
    - High output failure due to fetal mass (e.g., SCT) or other noncardiac etiology.

    US for pleural effusions is directed at determining whether or not hydrops is present and in determining the underlying etiology. For nonhydropic effusions, it may be difficult to determine an etiology if the cause is not from an associated cardiac abnormality, lung lesion, or chromosomal abnormality.

    For both treatment decision making and follow-up, estimation of the pleural effusion volume is helpful. Though 3D US has been advocated for such measurements, particularly for follow-up, we have used a simpler measurement. We measure the internal (pleural surface to pleural surface) dimensions of each hemithorax. We then measure the lung on each side and calculate the volumes of each hemithorax and lung using the prolate ellipsoid formula (volume = L × W × D × 0.523). Subtraction of the lung volume from the hemithorax volume gives an estimate of the pleural effusion volume for that side (Figure 60-8).

15. **What are the therapeutic strategies for fetal pleural effusions?**

    The primary treatment is to treat the underlying cause, if possible. Since large pleural effusions can compromise fetal lung development, treatment is warranted. The usual goal, if the effusion is large, is to reduce the volume. If a temporizing treatment is needed (for example, until the therapy for the underlying cause becomes effective), the maternal-fetal medicine physicians may perform an ultrasound-guided fetal thoracentesis. In some instances, this also has a value in determining how rapidly the pleural fluid is accumulating. If, after thoracentesis, the fluid does not reaccumulate, or does so only very slowly, then a longer-term treatment may not be needed. If the effusion reappears

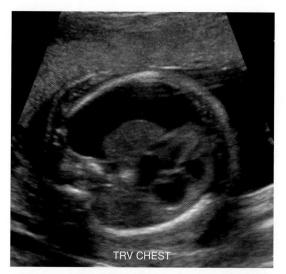

**Figure 60-8.** Fetal pleural effusion on US. Transverse image through fetal thorax at level of four-chamber heart view reveals large anechoic left pleural effusion with heart displacement into right hemithorax and collapsed left lung. Left hemithorax volume was 16.6 mL and left lung volume was 3.5 mL. Difference of 13.1 mL represents estimate of pleural effusion volume.

quickly, then the maternal-fetal medicine physicians may elect to perform an ultrasound-guided pleuroamniotic shunt placement. These shunts are typically double pigtail in type and are placed using interventional techniques and ultrasound guidance.

16. How are fetal lung masses evaluated sonographically?

Aside from determining whether or not a fetal lung mass is present, the type of mass is important. Most CPAM lung lesions are more echogenic than normal lung (Figure 60-9), and many will have cysts. The cysts can vary in size from

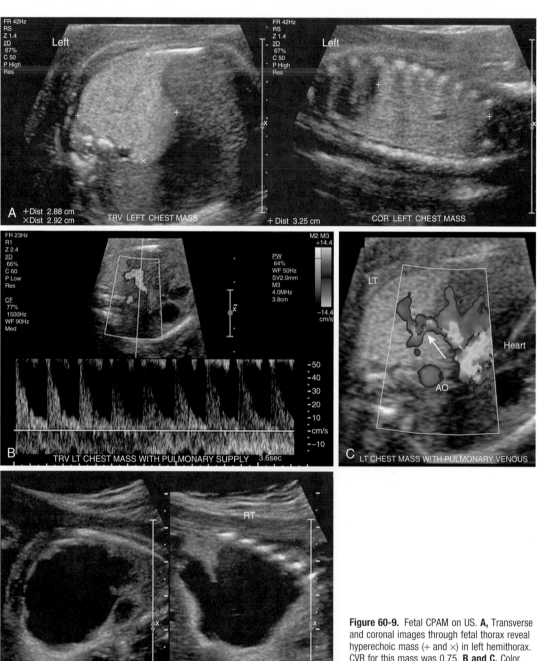

**Figure 60-9.** Fetal CPAM on US. **A,** Transverse and coronal images through fetal thorax reveal hyperechoic mass (+ and ×) in left hemithorax. CVR for this mass was 0.75. **B and C,** Color flow spectral and color flow Doppler images of same mass show pulmonary arterial supply and venous drainage (*arrow*). **D,** Transverse and coronal image through thorax of different fetus show largely anechoic mass in right hemithorax in keeping with macrocystic variety of CPAM.

subcentimeter to several centimeters. The current classification scheme for these masses is based on whether or not the lesions contain macroscopic cysts. Once a mass is identified and the location within the thorax documented, determination of the arterial supply and venous drainage is important. CPAMs have an arterial supply from the pulmonary arteries and venous drainage to the pulmonary veins.

BPS is also usually hyperechoic and by gray scale appearance alone can be difficult to distinguish from a CPAM. The important aspect that can differentiate them is the blood supply (Figure 60-10). BPS always has a nonpulmonary arterial supply, although the source is variable, and may be intralobar (the most common type, contained within the pleura of a lobe) or extralobar (with its own pleural investment). Differentiation between these is aided by the venous drainage. Intralobar BPS drains to the pulmonary circulation, typically to the pulmonary veins of the lobe in which they are located, whereas extralobar BPS drains to the systemic veins. Both the arterial supply and venous drainage of BPS

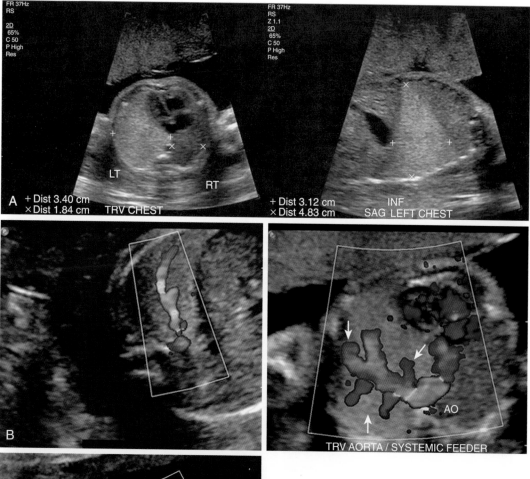

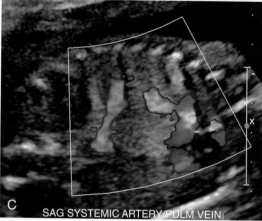

**Figure 60-10.** Fetal BPS on US. **A,** Transverse and sagittal images through fetal thorax demonstrate left lower lobe hyperechoic lung mass (+ on transverse image, + and × on sagittal image). Note similarity in its appearance to mass shown in Figure 60-9. Mass measured 4.8 cm (anteroposterior) × 3.4 cm (transverse) × 3.1 cm (length) with calculated volume of 26.4 mL. Based on head circumference measurement (*not shown*), CVR was ≈1.14. **B,** Color flow Doppler US images of same mass reveal systemic arterial blood supply to mass from thoracic aorta. Right image was acquired with lower velocity range setting for color flow to show branching of aortic feeding vessel (*arrows*). **C,** Sagittal image of same mass shows both aortic supply and pulmonary venous drainage. Lack of pulmonary arterial supply indicates that this mass is due to BPS, and presence of pulmonary venous drainage indicates that it is most likely intralobar.

may be variable. Arterial supply is often from the thoracic aorta but may be from subdiaphragmatic aortic branches. Venous drainage is also variable and depends on location. Extralobar BPS most often occur adjacent to the left hemidiaphragm and have a male predominance. Approximately 10% of extralobar BPS are extrathoracic. Intra-abdominal BPS venous drainage can be to the azygos system, phrenic veins, or other systemic veins. Unlike intralobar BPS, the extralobar type has a higher incidence of associated abnormalities, including CPAM, CDH, and cardiac and spinal anomalies. In rare circumstances, an extralobar BPS that is close to the esophagus or stomach may develop a fistula to these structures or be associated with an esophageal or gastric bronchus.

In some instances, lung masses may have features of both a CPAM and BPS, typically with both a pulmonary and systemic arterial supply. These are termed *hybrid lesions* and are evaluated much like a distinct CPAM or BPS.

For lung lesions, the CPAM or BPS is initially measured by US (and MRI), and a mass volume to HC ratio is calculated. This value, often termed the *CVR* (for CPAM volume ratio), is used for follow-up studies because some of these masses decrease in size as the pregnancy progresses. For those that grow, serial assessment of the CVR is helpful to determine the growth rate. The CVR is also predictive of outcome for CPAM, particularly the development of hydrops, a major complication of CPAM. If the CVR is ≤1.6, the risk for development of hydrops is low compared with those fetuses with a CVR >1.6.

17. What are the therapeutic strategies for treatment of lung masses?

Ten percent to 20% of CPAM lesions will decrease in size as the pregnancy progresses. For BPS, ≈66% will decrease in size. For these reasons, if the fetus does not have hydrops or has a CVR well below 1.6, observation with regular monitoring of the mass volume and CVR may be performed.

For masses that approach the CVR 1.6 threshold (typically 1.5) and do not have hydrops, administration of corticosteroids (e.g., betamethasone) to the mother can moderate CPAM growth or cause a reduction in size.

For those lung masses that are very large and cause fetal hydrops, fetal surgery may be performed to remove the mass. In some instances, when the mass has large cystic components, aspiration of the cystic components or placement of a shunt (cyst to amnion) is performed using interventional techniques rather than open surgery. This reduces the size of the mass and can prevent, or reverse, fetal hydrops. These, along with BPS and CPAM masses that are not removed in utero, are recommended for postdelivery removal because of the potential for infection and malignant transformation.

Lung masses that result in fetal hydrops can also produce the "mirror syndrome" (also known as Ballantyne syndrome) in the mother. In these cases, the mother develops symptoms that mirror those of the fetus. These usually include edema (always present) and proteinuria (usually mild). The mirror syndrome can also result from other fetal conditions that result in fetal hydrops.

If the fetal lung mass causes fetal hydrops close to the time of delivery, a therapeutic option is removal of the mass using EXIT. Delivery at centers that can provide neonatal respiratory support is advised for large CPAM and BPS lesions that do not decrease in size but are below the critical CVR ratio.

18. What is CHAOS, and how is it diagnosed and treated?

Congenital high airway obstruction syndrome (CHAOS) results from obstruction of the trachea above the level of the carina, usually from laryngeal or tracheal stenosis, but it can be from any cause of obstruction or severe stenosis high in the airway. As a result, the lungs become markedly expanded by the secretions normally exhaled by the fetus (Figure 60-11). The hyperexpansion of the lungs flattens or everts the diaphragm and compresses the mediastinal

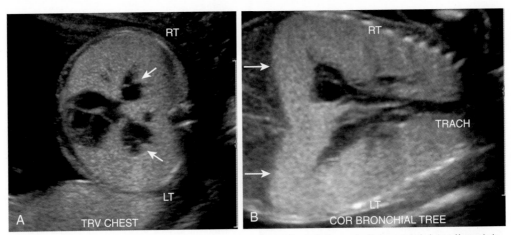

**Figure 60-11.** Fetal CHAOS on US. **A,** Transverse image through fetal thorax demonstrates markedly hyperechoic lungs. Hypoechoic structures (*arrows*) in central aspects of lungs represent dilated bronchi. Heart is near anterior center of thorax and is slightly compressed. **B,** Coronal image through fetal thorax reveals dilated bronchi and trachea (*TRACH*). Also note bilateral diaphragmatic eversion (*arrows*) and hyperexpanded lungs.

structures, restricting venous return and potentially causing hydrops. Diagnostic US features include enlarged hyperechoic lungs, distended bronchi and trachea, and a compressed heart. Polyhydramnios is often present along with other findings of nonimmune hydrops. Fetal MRI may be useful to show the location and length of the atretic tracheal segment.

Treatment makes use of EXIT as for other conditions with airway obstruction. Once the airway is established, the EXIT delivery is completed, and the neonate is cared for by a respiratory care team.

19. **How is the diagnosis of a congenital diaphragmatic hernia (CDH) made sonographically, and what features and measurements are important?**

CDH is suspected if:

* The fetal stomach is not seen in the fetal abdomen and is evident at the level of the heart on a transverse image of the fetal thorax (Figure 60-12).
* The stomach is not at the heart level, but the heart is shifted to one side (usually the right) with bowel in the chest on the other side (usually the left). Most CDH are left-sided, which are 5 to 10 times more common than right-sided hernias.
* CDH is associated with a number of other fetal anomalies, and so the ultrasound examination is also directed to detect any of these. Cardiac abnormalities are the most common association, and if fetal echocardiography is not performed as part of the evaluation of the fetus with anomalies, it is performed if a CDH is found.

Sagittal scans of the fetus can usually depict the defect in the diaphragm, usually posteriorly on the left (a Bochdalek hernia). With color flow Doppler US, the presence of bowel and liver in the chest can be demonstrated with the superior mesenteric artery (SMA), SMA branches, hepatic veins, portal veins directed from or into the chest. An important aspect of CDH evaluation is to determine whether or not part of the liver is intrathoracic in location. Color flow Doppler US is again helpful to show one (or more) of the hepatic veins turning cephalad and above the plane of the diaphragm. Gray scale imaging can show the intrathoracic portion of the liver in continuity with the intra-abdominal portion. Real-time imaging can be helpful to demonstrate peristalsis in the intrathoracic bowel loops.

If a part of the fetal liver is in the thorax, the prognosis is generally worse because presence of an intrathoracic portion of liver is a sign of a large hernia. To quantify the effects of the hernia on the fetal lungs, a metric has been developed that uses measurements of the contralateral lung at the level of the four-chamber heart view. There are several approaches to making this measurement, but the method in widest use is to measure the largest transverse diameter (in mm) of the contralateral lung at the base and parallel with the coronal plane of the fetal chest. An anteroposterior diameter is then measured perpendicular to this (also in mm). The resulting values are multiplied, and then divided by the HC (in mm). This value is known as the lung to head ratio (LHR). Some studies have shown the LHR to be predictive of outcome with high survival rates when the LHR is >1.4. In an attempt to normalize the LHR for fetal lung growth, the LHR of the affected fetus is compared with the LHR of a normal fetus at the same age. Tables of LHR values for both right and left lungs are available, and the observed to expected (O/E) LHR ratio is calculated, which is an index of lung hypoplasia. Studies have shown that O/E LHR ratios <15% have a 100% fetal mortality rate. If the O/E LHR ratio is >45%, the survival rate is above 75%. In between these values, survival rates increase with increasing O/E LHR ratio, with the 50% survival proportion correlated with an O/E LHR ratio of ≈38%.

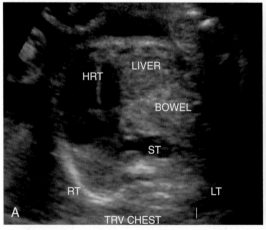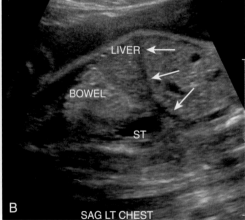

**Figure 60-12.** Fetal CDH on US. **A,** Transverse image through fetal thorax shows abnormal location of stomach (*ST*) at same level as 4-chamber heart view along with posterior positioning. Heart (*HRT*) is displaced into right hemithorax with slight compression of left atrium and ventricle. Portions of liver and bowel (*labeled*) are also seen in left hemithorax. **B,** Sagittal image through left hemithorax and left abdomen with head of fetus toward left side of image. Diaphragm is evident as hypoechoic curved structure (*arrows*). Stomach, bowel, and liver (*labeled*) are seen above diaphragm. Defect in diaphragm is not evident on this image as it was taken medial to site of defect.

20. How is CDH treated?

Fetal open surgery for CDH has shifted to postnatal procedures after stabilization of the neonate. Though open fetal surgery was initially utilized, survival rates were low. Advances in the care of neonates with CDH meant that the survival rate of neonates with CDH was higher than the survival rate of fetuses treated with open fetal surgery. While most CDH fetuses are now treated as neonates, a procedure less invasive than open surgery is being evaluated. It involves the reversible occlusion of the fetal trachea, intentionally creating a CHAOS-like situation. The expanding lungs exert pressure on the herniated abdominal contents. This can push the herniated contents at least partway back into the abdomen. The tracheal occlusion is then reversed so an airway can be established. This procedure is known as fetoscopic tracheal occlusion (FETO). Though FETO is attractive and has some successes, improvements in survival of affected neonates using improved respirators and techniques has also meant that this method may not be superior to postnatal management.

21. How are fetuses with neck masses diagnosed and treated?

Fetal neck masses are generally of the following types:

- Lymphangioma.
- Hemangioma.
- Cystic hygroma.
- Teratoma.

Other masses (hemangioendothelioma, bronchogenic cyst, enlarged thyroid gland, and branchial cleft cyst) are uncommon.

Detection by US is straightforward, but characterization can be more problematic. Cystic hygromas and lymphangiomas can have a similar ultrasound appearance, although cystic hygromas are most often posterior and have a posterior midline septum. Lymphangiomas can be anterior or posterior in location, and color flow Doppler US may demonstrate some internal vascularity (Figure 60-13). Hemangiomas are usually more solid in appearance relative to lymphangiomas and can be anterior or posterior in location. Teratomas can be predominantly cystic but often are more mixed in appearance, and they may be almost entirely solid (Figure 60-14). Approximately 50% of teratomas have internal calcifications, which can help to differentiate a teratoma from a solid-appearing hemangioma.

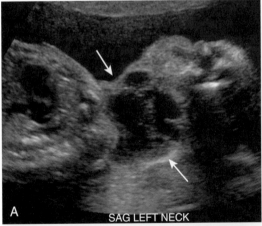

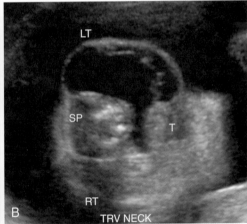

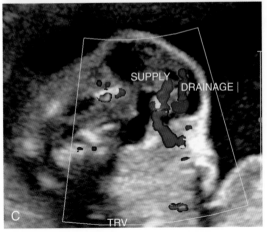

**Figure 60-13.** Fetal neck lymphangioma on US. **A,** Sagittal image through fetal neck demonstrates mass (*arrows*) with cystic spaces and thick septations. **B,** Transverse image through fetal neck reveals left-sided mass crossing anterior to spine (*SP*) and posterior to trachea (*T*). **C,** Transverse color flow Doppler image through fetal neck shows arterial supply (marked SUPPLY) and venous drainage (marked DRAINAGE). Arterial supply was from right carotid artery with some smaller branches (*not shown*) from left external carotid artery.

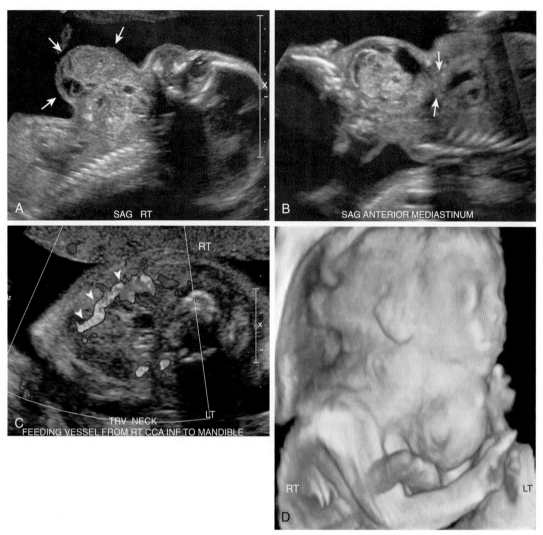

**Figure 60-14.** Fetal neck teratoma on US. **A,** Sagittal image through fetal neck demonstrates predominantly solid anterior neck mass (*arrows*) with some anechoic cystic portions as well. **B,** Coronal image through fetal neck and upper thorax reveals mass extends into anterior superior mediastinum (*arrows*) with some narrowing at thoracic inlet. **C,** Transverse color flow Doppler image through fetal neck shows arterial feeding vessel originating from right common carotid artery (*arrowheads*). **D,** Left posterior oblique coronal 3D image of fetal head to upper thorax demonstrates location of bulk of mass inferior to mandible.

A further division of fetal neck masses is based on anterior and posterior locations. The most important characteristic of a fetal neck mass is whether or not the mass is anterior in location. Anterior masses have the potential to obstruct or narrow the trachea and may also interfere with fetal swallowing, so this determines how these masses are treated (see Figure 60-14).

Therapy for neck masses is surgical removal, although cystic hygromas usually regress spontaneously. If the fetus develops polyhydramnios because of interference with swallowing, amniocentesis for fluid reduction can be performed. For anteriorly located masses, if they obstruct the trachea, then EXIT is usually performed with the goal of establishing an airway.

22. What is involved in the evaluation of sacrococcygeal teratoma (SCT), and how is it treated?
    SCTs are relatively rare tumors that arise at the base of the coccyx. The majority (≈75%) are benign. For US, the imaging is directed to determine:
    • The characteristics of the teratoma: cystic, solid, or mixed.
    • The size and volume of the mass. The volume to HC ratio can also be computed for follow-up purposes.
    • The type of the mass (the American Academy of Pediatrics classification):
       • Type I—external; may be pedunculated or have a small presacral component.
       • Type II—mostly external with a significant intrapelvic component.

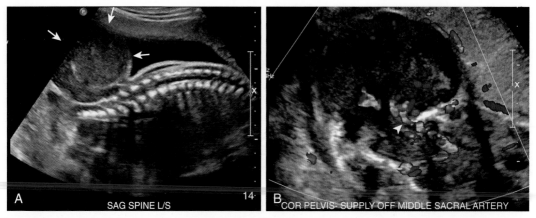

**Figure 60-15.** Fetal SCT with fibrosarcomatous elements on US. **A,** Sagittal image through fetal spine reveals large echogenic sacrococcygeal mass (*arrows*). **B,** Coronal color flow Doppler image through mass shows hypertrophied middle sacral artery as primary arterial feeding vessel (*arrowhead*). With decreased color flow Doppler velocity range, vascularity throughout mass was observed (*not shown*).

- • Type III—mostly intrapelvic with abdominal extension, usually with a small external component.
- • Type IV—entirely internal with abdominal extension.
- The vascular supply and venous drainage.
- Displacement of pelvic structures.
- Extension into the spinal canal.
- Presence of associated hydronephrosis.
- Proximity to the anus.
- Presence of cardiac overload or hydrops.

These findings are important for postnatal surgical treatment, but early evidence of hydrops or other evidence of high output failure could prompt an open surgical approach unless the fetus is mature enough for early delivery. Development of maternal mirror syndrome, other fetal anomalies, multiple gestation, and placentomegaly (placental thickness at cord insertion is >3.5 to 4.0 cm) are all contraindications to open fetal surgery. US can help to plan delivery before high output failure ensues and to assist in postnatal surgical planning (Figure 60-15).

23. What is lower urinary tract obstruction (LUTO) in a fetus, and how is it diagnosed and treated?
LUTO is often the result of posterior urethral valves and affects males much more often than females. In females, posterior urethral valves do not occur, so other etiologies are considered. Ultrasound diagnostic findings include:
- A markedly distended urinary bladder, typically with a "keyhole" shape (Figure 60-16).
- Severe oligohydramnios.
- Hydronephrosis and hydroureter.
- Hyperechoic renal parenchyma (see Figure 60-16) and cysts (evidence of renal dysplasia).
- Male gender.
- Decreased fetal thoracic circumference (evidence of pulmonary hypoplasia).

If the fetus is female, then additional evaluation for other causes (e.g., cloacal abnormality) is undertaken. The oligohydramnios leaves little room for fetal movement including breathing motion, which adversely affects lung development. The cephalad displacement of the diaphragm by the large bladder and abdominal organs is a contributing factor. Assessment of the fetal renal function, either by fetal vesicocentesis and urine electrolyte analysis or fetal cord blood measurement of serum beta$_2$-microglobulin can be used prior to performing an ultrasound-guided vesicoamniotic shunt, the treatment of choice for LUTO.

On occasion, the fetal urinary bladder is distended, but the amniotic fluid volume is normal or near normal. In these instances, US is used to search for the way in which the bladder is emptying. It is sometimes a pressure-dependent phenomenon with the urethra (or urachus) opening when the pressure in the bladder becomes great enough.

24. What are the important ultrasound findings in evaluation of abnormalities in twins, and what are the treatment methods?
Both monochorionic and dichorionic twins are subject to the same anomalies that can affect a singleton fetus. However, for monochorionic twins, the abnormalities peculiar to these twins typically involve a discrepancy in the sizes of the fetuses or their amniotic fluid volumes (or both). For monochorionic twins, because of the risk for developing the complications discussed below, surveillance US studies are advised every two week after 16 weeks. Development of any of the complications will likely necessitate even more frequent follow-up.

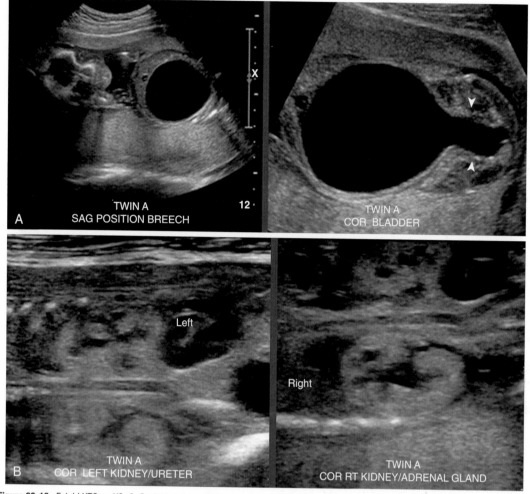

**Figure 60-16.** Fetal LUTO on US. **A,** Sagittal and coronal images through fetus demonstrate markedly distended bladder and low amniotic fluid volume. Note typical "keyhole" shape of bladder with narrow part of keyhole resulting from dilated proximal urethra (*arrowheads*). **B,** Coronal images through fetus reveal markedly increased echogenicity of kidneys (*labeled*) indicating dysplastic change and hydronephrosis. Dilated tubular structure inferior to left kidney represents dilated tortuous left ureter. Dilated right ureter is more difficult to see.

In addition to the elements of the detailed extended obstetric ultrasound examination, evaluation of twins with a discordance in weight or fluid volume includes (where measurements and observations apply to both fetuses):

- If not already done, establish whether the twins are mono- or dichorionic. The complications discussed in the following questions virtually all occur in monochorionic twins.
- Assessment of the placenta: thickness and appearance in addition to location.
- Measurement of the amniotic fluid of the fetuses. An amniotic fluid index (AFI) may be measured for each fetus, but it is not clear that the AFI method is appropriate for twins, so the single deepest vertical pocket is used for fluid volume assessment.
- Assessment of the placental cord insertions and measurement of the distance between them.
- Calculation of estimated fetal weights and the ratio of weights.
- Umbilical artery, umbilical vein, and ductus venosus Doppler US evaluation.
- Middle cerebral artery Doppler US evaluation.
- Evaluation of the fetal bladders for degree of filling and evidence of voiding (cycling of the fetal bladder).
- Evaluation of the fetal heart for cardiomegaly, pericardial effusion, and myocardial thickening.
- Examination for hydropic changes (ascites, pleural or pericardial effusion, scalp edema).
- Determination of locations of potential access to the amniotic sacs (areas free of the placenta)—this may be done by the maternal-fetal medicine physicians prior to treatment.
- Fetal echocardiography for assessment of fetal cardiac function.

For **twin to twin transfusion syndrome (TTTS)**, stages are defined based on the ultrasound findings. Table 60-3 shows the ultrasound findings and corresponding stages. Increasing stage is correlated with more severe TTTS

**Table 60-3.** Stages of Twin to Twin Transfusion Syndrome (TTTS) (adapted from [15]).

| STAGE | POLY/ OLIGOHYDRAMNIOS | ABSENT BLADDER IN DONOR | CRITICALLY ABNORMAL DOPPLER US | ASCITES, PERICARDIAL EFFUSION, SCALP EDEMA, OVERT HYDROPS | DEMISE OF ONE OR BOTH TWINS |
|---|---|---|---|---|---|
| I | + | − | − | − | − |
| II | + | + | − | − | − |
| III | + | + | + | − | − |
| IV | + | + | + | + | − |
| V | + | + | + | + | + |

and urgency for treatment (Figure 60-17). TTTS is believed to result from asymmetry in inter-twin blood flow between the two fetuses. The vascular connections between the two cords on the placental surface can lead one fetus (the "donor") to pump blood into the circulation of the "recipient." This results in one fetus being small with low amniotic fluid and the other being larger with an abundance of amniotic fluid. Left untreated, the donor twin becomes more severely growth restricted with the complications of oligohydramnios while the recipient twin develops hydrops from the volume overload. This can lead to the demise of both fetuses.

Treatment for TTTS is aimed at separating the circulations of the fetuses. If a reasonable plane between the two placental cord insertions can be found, a laser fiber is passed through one channel of a fetoscope and observed through a video camera attached to the other channel. The laser is used to photocoagulate the surface connections between the two fetal placental circulations. This treatment has been very successful with normalization of the criteria used to assess for TTTS. Survival of at least one twin is ≈80%. The survival rate for both fetuses ranges between 60% and 70%. Long-term complications include neurologic abnormalities in 6% to 11%.

**Twin anemia-polycythemia sequence (TAPS)** is a recognized complication of TTTS treatment, although spontaneous occurrences have also been reported. The syndrome resulting from TTTS is believed to be caused by very small residual arteriovenous connections between the twin circulations. These allow a very slow "transfusion" from one fetus to the other. This results in polycythemia in the recipient fetus and anemia in the donor. In spontaneous cases, the cause is believed to be the same, but not the result of previous TTTS treatment (Figure 60-18). The diagnosis is established through Doppler US evaluation of the middle cerebral arteries. In early stages, the middle cerebral artery peak systolic velocity (MCA PSV) is >1.5 multiples of the median (MoM) for the donor and <1.0 MoM for the recipient. Increasing stages are indicated by greater MCA PSV values and onset of hydrops in the donor or development of abnormal umbilical artery, umbilical vein, or ductus venosus Doppler US findings. As with TTTS, the highest stage is the demise of one or both fetuses.

Treatment has been aimed at correcting the anemia through fetal transfusion or prevention through the use of a modified laser photocoagulation technique in treatment of TTTS. The Solomon technique involves extending the laser photocoagulation to create a true separation of the placental circulations, not just eliminating the vascular connections on the fetal surface of the placenta. This process is also known as dichorionization because it effectively creates two placentas. If a separation plane is not clearly visible or the placental portions are very asymmetric, this technique is not applicable because it is likely to result in the demise of the fetus with the smaller placental portion.

**Selective intrauterine growth restriction (sIUGR)** is a complication of monochorionic twins resulting from the twins having unequal portions of the placenta. This might result, for example, from one twin having a placental cord insertion that is central and the other having a cord insertion that is marginal or velamentous. The unequal size twins that result can mimic TTTS, but there are ultrasound characteristics that can help differentiate sIUGR from TTTS. These include:

- Normal amniotic fluid volume in the larger fetus or both fetuses (no polyhydramnios-oligohydramnios; may have normal-normal, or normal-oligohydramnios).
- Both have urinary bladders that cycle (empty and fill) during the study.
- Large weight discordance (typically ≥25%) with the smaller fetus at <10th percentile weight for gestational age and the other in the normal weight range.

Evaluation of the umbilical artery with Doppler US is critical for staging. In Type I sIUGR, the smaller fetus has positive end-diastolic flow in the umbilical artery; in Type II sIUGR, the smaller fetus has persistently absent or persistently reversed end-diastolic flow in the umbilical artery; and in Type III sIUGR, the smaller fetus has intermittently absent or reversed end-diastolic flow in the umbilical artery. Stage III sIUGR carries a poor prognosis with demise of the smaller twin and potential neurologic sequelae (or demise) of the larger twin. Treatment for type I is usually expectant management with weekly or twice-weekly ultrasound evaluation for growth and umbilical artery assessment. For types II and III, the laser photocoagulation therapy used for TTTS will not work for sIUGR because of the marked differences in placental proportions. To prevent the neurologic complications for the larger fetus, the usual

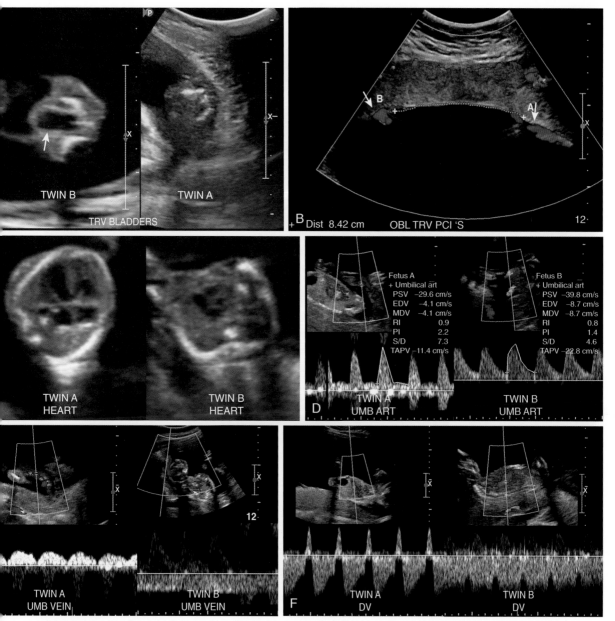

**Figure 60-17.** TTTS on US. **A,** Images through fetal urinary bladders demonstrate donor fetus "A" has no urine in the bladder (persistent throughout study), whereas recipient fetus "B" has mildly distended bladder (persistent throughout study). Note also that fetus "A" appears "stuck" to side of uterus, and intertwine membrane is not visible as it is closely apposed to fetus, whereas fetus "B" has large amount of amniotic fluid. These findings are in keeping with stage II TTTS. **B,** Color flow Doppler image through placenta of same fetuses reveals placental cord insertions (labeled A and B with arrows) as well as distance measurement between them. This measurement is useful in planning treatment as close spacing (<5 cm) warrants caution in planning laser separation. **C,** Transverse images through fetal hearts of different set of twins show recipient fetus "A" has cardiomegaly, whereas donor fetus "B" has normal-sized heart (and smaller thoracic size). **D,** Color flow spectral and color flow Doppler images through umbilical arteries demonstrate low diastolic flow evidenced by high systolic to diastolic (S/D) ratio in fetus "A" and normal blood flow in fetus "B." **E,** Color flow spectral and color flow Doppler images through umbilical veins reveal abnormal pulsatile blood flow in fetus "A" and normal monophasic blood flow in fetus "B." **F,** Color flow and spectral Doppler images through ducti venosi show markedly abnormal Doppler waveform with reversed flow during atrial systole in fetus "A" and normal blood flow in fetus "B." Other findings in this set of twins included polyhydramnios of fetus "A," oligohydramnios of fetus "B," and no urine in bladder of fetus "B." These findings are in keeping with stage III TTTS.

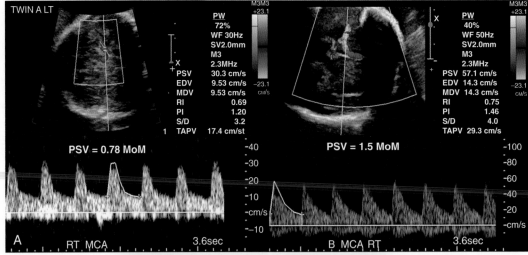

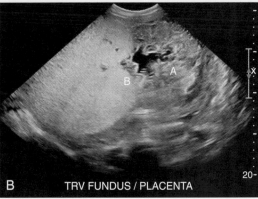

**Figure 60-18.** TAPS on US. **A,** Color flow spectral and color flow Doppler images through fetal middle cerebral arteries demonstrate low MCA PSV of 0.78 MoM in polycythemic recipient fetus "A" and high MCA PSV of 1.5 MoM in anemic donor fetus "B." **B,** Image through placenta reveals markedly different appearance of portions of placenta (marked "A" and "B"). Portion associated with fetus "B" is abnormally thickened and hyperechoic—a finding seen with fetal anemia. Portion associated with fetus "A" is of normal thickness and shows some mature changes consistent with gestational age of 29 weeks. There was also fluid discordance with fetus "A" exhibiting polyhydramnios and fetus "B" exhibiting low normal amniotic fluid volume (not shown). This set of monochorionic diamniotic twins had not undergone any TTTS therapy.

treatment for types II and III is cord coagulation of the smaller twin. This results in demise of the smaller twin but reduces the risk of neurologic problems for the larger twin.

In the **twin reversed arterial perfusion (TRAP) sequence,** either fetus dies early in development, or succumbs to severe anomalies. Because of the vascular connections between the placental circulations of monochorionic twins, the normal fetus ("pump twin") can pump blood into the abnormal (acardiac or parabiotic) twin. The acardiac twin, as the term suggests, has no intrinsic cardiac activity (although we have seen a case with an "acardiac" twin that had cardiac activity, but with severe bradycardia and maldevelopment). Blood flow becomes reversed in the umbilical artery and vein of the acardiac twin. Because the oxygenated blood is entering the acardiac fetus via the umbilical arteries, the most oxygenated blood circulates first through the pelvis and lower extremities. This likely accounts for the appearance of most acardiac fetuses with more lower than upper body development. Ultrasound diagnosis is not difficult, but aspects are important for therapy planning. The ultrasound examination includes:

- Evaluation of the umbilical cords of both fetuses; the acardiac fetus usually has a single umbilical artery. It is important to determine how the cords insert on the placenta because this may affect later treatment.
- Documentation of reversed flow in the umbilical artery and vein of the acardiac twin (Figure 60-19).
- Measurement of the acardiac twin to estimate the weight. There are formulae to estimate the weight based on the length, but we use a method of measuring the major elements (body and whatever limbs are present) and adding the individual volumes estimated from the prolate ellipsoid formula (see Figure 60-19). An assumption of 1 mL of tissue weighing 1 gram is used for conversion of volume to weight.
- Evaluation of the pump twin for any evidence of cardiac decompensation (development of hydrops); an echocardiogram is also usually done.
- Evaluation of the pump twin for any anomalies; anomalies of the pump twin have been reported in up to 9% of the "normal" twins.

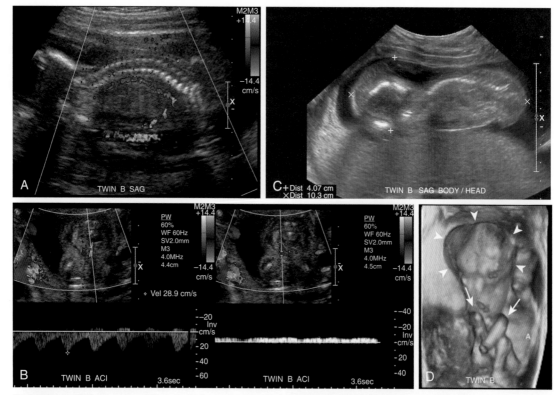

**Figure 60-19.** TRAP sequence on US. **A,** Sagittal color flow Doppler image through twin B shows reversed flow in aorta. No cardiac activity was present (*not shown*) indicating acardiac twin. **B,** Color flow spectral and color flow Doppler images through umbilical vessels of twin B demonstrate single umbilical artery with reversed blood flow toward fetus (*left image*) and abnormal umbilical venous blood flow away from fetus (*right image*). Note that color flow scale is not inverted (flow toward ultrasound transducer is red) but spectral Doppler is inverted (positive flow direction is below baseline). **C,** Sagittal image through twin B reveals severe edematous/hygromatous changes and maldeveloped appearance of skull (+ and ×). There were no upper extremities (not shown). **D,** Coronal 3D image of twin B shows edge of skin swelling around skull (*arrowheads*). Lower extremities are shown (*arrows*), and normal twin A (labeled A) is in background.

Because the acardiac twin cannot survive on its own and continuing to allow the pump twin to supply blood to it can result in cardiac overload, treatment is usually occlusion of the umbilical cord of the acardiac fetus. This was initially done by ligation, but more recently is performed using radiofrequency ablation via a fetoscope.

25. What is the role of US for conjoined twins?

Conjoined twins constitute a rare (about 1 per 200,000 live births in the United States) complication of twinning in which the dividing zygote that would result in separate embryos fails to divide completely.

The chief role of US is to determine the type of conjoined twins, what anatomic structures are shared or connected, and the nature of the vascular anatomy. The precise description of conjoined twins is complex, but a simple designation based on where the fetuses are joined includes: craniopagus (joined at the head), thoracopagus (joined at the thorax), omphalopagus (joined at the abdomen), and ischiopagus (joined at the pelvis). Combinations of these (e.g., thoraco-omphalopagus) can occur. An example of thoraco-omphalopagus conjoined twins is shown in Figure 60-20.

From US and MRI studies, the fetal therapy team can determine if separation of the fetuses is possible and if such separation can result in a single, or two, live neonate(s). Separation surgery is always postnatal.

## KEY POINTS

- There are well-established reasons for performing second and third trimester ultrasound studies, and guidelines are available that describe what the examination should include, the facility, and the training requirements for these examinations.
- Although US is considered safe, there are potential bioeffects, so use on fetuses should be governed by the ALARA principle.
- Fetal therapy uses US for diagnosis, treatment planning, therapeutic procedure guidance, and management of follow-up.
- Fetal therapeutic procedures, whether open surgical, EXIT, postnatal surgical, or minimally invasive interventional, have shown improvements in survival and quality of life for affected fetuses and neonates.

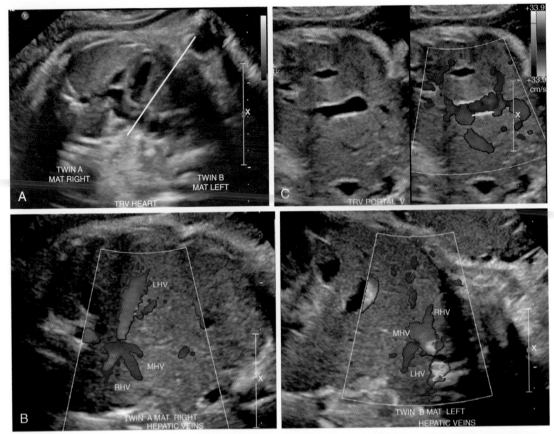

**Figure 60-20.** Conjoined twins on US. **A,** Transverse image through fetal thorax demonstrates fetuses are joined at thorax and abdomen (thoraco-omphalopagus). Note complex heart which appears to be two four-chambered hearts, although it was not certain if they were fused along plane shown by line. **B,** Transverse color flow Doppler images through fetal abdomen reveal joined liver where each portion of liver has a set of hepatic veins (*labeled*). **C,** Transverse gray scale (*left*) and color flow Doppler (*right*) images through fetal abdomen show single main portal vein that had right and left branches at either end and in each segment of liver. These twins were subsequently successfully separated, and their hearts turned out to have separate pericardial sacs.

## Acknowledgment

Images used for the figures in this chapter were taken by sonographers: Maryann Giannone, Olga Gitman, Suzanne Iyoob, Devon Looney, and Kate Weir.

## BIBLIOGRAPHY

ACR-ACOG-AIUM-SRU Practice Guideline for the Performance of Obstetric Ultrasound. <http://www.acr.org/~/media/f7bc35bd59264e7cbe648f6d1bb8b8e2.pdf>; 2014:1-14.

Wax J, Minkoff H, Johnson A, et al. Consensus report on the detailed fetal anatomic ultrasound examination: indications, components, and qualifications. *J Ultrasound Med.* 2014;33(2):189-195.

Oliver ER, Coleman BG, Goff DA, et al. Twin reversed arterial perfusion sequence: a new method of parabiotic twin mass estimation correlated with pump twin compromise. *J Ultrasound Med.* 2013;32(12):2115-2123.

Adzick NS, Thom EA, Spong CY, et al. A randomized trial of prenatal versus postnatal repair of myelomeningocele. *N Engl J Med.* 2011;364(11):993-1004.

Bianchi DW, Crombleholme TM, D'Alton ME, et al. Myelomeningocele. In: *Fetology: diagnosis and management of the fetal patient.* New York: McGraw-Hill; 2010:151-165.

Deprest JA, Flake AW, Gratacos E, et al. The making of fetal surgery. *Prenatal Diagn.* 2010;30(7):653-667.

Nelson TR, Fowlkes JB, Abramowicz JS, et al. Ultrasound biosafety considerations for the practicing sonographer and sonologist. *J Ultrasound Med.* 2009;28(2):139-150.

Fowlkes JB. Bioeffects Committee of the American Institute of Ultrasound in M. American Institute of Ultrasound in Medicine consensus report on potential bioeffects of diagnostic ultrasound: executive summary. *J Ultrasound Med.* 2008;27(4):503-515.

Jani J, Nicolaides KH, Keller RL, et al. Observed to expected lung area to head circumference ratio in the prediction of survival in fetuses with isolated diaphragmatic hernia. *Ultrasound Obstet Gynecol.* 2007;30(1):67-71.

Goldstein RB. The thorax. In: Nyberg DA, McGahan JP, Pretorius DH, et al., eds. *Diagnostic imaging of fetal anomalies.* Philadelphia: Lippincott Williams & Wilkins; 2003:381-420.

Hedrick HL. Ex utero intrapartum therapy. *Semin Ped Surg.* 2003;12(3):190-195.

National Institute for Health and Clinical Excellence (NICE) Interventional Procedure Guidance [IPG198]. Interventional procedure overview of intrauterine laser ablation of vessels for the treatment of twin to twin transfusion syndrome. Overview. 336. <http://www.nice.org.uk/guidance/ipg198/evidence/overview-306073693>; 2003:1-23.

Sebire NJ, Sepulveda W, Jeanty P, et al. Multiple gestations. In: Nyberg DA, McGahan JP, Pretorius DH, et al., eds. *Diagnostic imaging of fetal anomalies*. Philadelphia: Lippincott Williams & Wilkins; 2003:777-814.

Coleman BG, Adzick NS, Crombleholme TM, et al. Fetal therapy: state of the art. *J Ultrasound Med*. 2002;21(11):1257-1288.

Crombleholme TM, Coleman B, Hedrick H, et al. Cystic adenomatoid malformation volume ratio predicts outcome in prenatally diagnosed cystic adenomatoid malformation of the lung. *J Pediatr Surg*. 2002;37(3):331-338.

Quintero RA, Morales WJ, Allen MH, et al. Staging of twin-twin transfusion syndrome. *J Perinatol*. 1999;19(8 Pt 1):550-555.

Consensus Conference. The use of diagnostic ultrasound imaging during pregnancy. *JAMA*. 1984;252(5):669-672.

Harrison MR, Golbus MS, Filly RA, et al. Fetal surgery for congenital hydronephrosis. *N Engl J Med*. 1982;306(10):591-593.

# CHAPTER 61

# NECK ULTRASONOGRAPHY

*Jill E. Langer, MD*

1. **What is the basic normal anatomy and sonographic imaging appearance of the thyroid gland?**

   The thyroid gland is a butterfly-shaped organ located in the anterior neck, just below the thyroid cartilage and anterior to the trachea. It extends posteriorly to the esophagus and laterally to the carotid sheath, and consists of two lateral conically shaped lobes and the isthmus, a narrow band of midline tissue that connects the lateral lobes. The thyroid gland also has a pyramidal lobe, a superior extension of thyroidal tissue of variable length which is a vestigial remnant of the thyroglossal tract that arises from the isthmus and ascends toward the hyoid bone (Figure 61-1). The normal thyroid gland has relatively homogeneous, bright parenchymal echogenicity with a smooth overlying capsule (Figure 61-2). The dimensions of the thyroid gland vary with body habitus, but the general values for an adult are 15 to 20 mm in anteroposterior diameter, 20 to 30 mm in lateral width, and 40 to 60 mm in craniocaudal length, and the anteroposterior diameter of the isthmus is usually 6 mm. On ultrasonography (US) examination, the pyramidal lobe is quite small, but when hypertrophied, for example in the setting of Graves' disease, it can be imaged and may be discontinuous from the isthmus.

2. **What is the basic normal anatomy and sonographic imaging appearance of the parathyroid glands?**

   The parathyroid glands are typically four in number and occur as a superior pair and an inferior pair. Supernumerary glands are seen approximately in 3% to 13% of patients, and fewer than four glands can occur. The superior glands are derived from the fourth branchial pouch along with the lateral lobes of the thyroid. The superior glands tend to be more consistent in location, with most (>90%) located on the posterior surface of the thyroid, toward the upper pole (Figure 61-3). Infrequently, they may be located above the lateral lobe of the thyroid or rarely in the retropharyngeal (1%) or retroesophageal (1%) space or in the thyroid gland itself (0.2%). The inferior glands arise from the third branchial pouch along with the thymus gland and their location is more variable. Sixty percent can be found posterior to the thyroid gland at the lower pole, and 25% are located inferior to the thyroid gland along a migratory path that extends into the superior mediastinum including within the thymus. The inferior glands may fail to descend and may be located above the superior glands. Ectopic parathyroid glands are not unusual and may be found within the carotid sheath, within the aorticopulmonary window, posterior to the carina, within the pericardium, or within the posterior triangle of the neck. Most parathyroid glands individually measure 3 mm in anteroposterior diameter, 1 mm in lateral width, and 5 mm in craniocaudal length, and due to their small size are infrequently identified on neck US.

3. **What is the basic normal anatomy and US imaging appearance of cervical lymph nodes?**

   The American Joint Committee on Cancer (AJCC) classification system of nodal location is recommended when reporting nodal location on imaging exams because it more accurately corresponds with surgical and pathology reporting (Figure 61-4). This classification system divides the neck into three compartments, the central compartment and the paired lateral compartments, each having multiple nodal levels. The distinction of the lateral and central compartments is very important for surgical planning, because abnormal nodes in the lateral neck cannot be accessed from the central compartment and vice versa. The lateral compartment nodes (levels I through V) are found in the submental region (level I), along the jugulocarotid vascular bundle (levels II through IV) and posterior to the sternocleidomastoid muscle (V). The jugulocarotid or anterior cervical nodes are further classified as follows: level II lymph nodes are located above the level of the hyoid bone to the base of the skull; level III nodes are between the levels of the hyoid bone and the cricoid cartilage; and level IV nodes are below the level of the cricoid cartilage extending to the clavicle. Level V nodes are in the posterior neck, posterior to the lateral border of the sternocleidomastoid muscle. The central compartment contains the thyroid and parathyroid glands, is bordered laterally by the carotid sheaths, and extends superiorly to the hyoid bone and inferiorly into the upper mediastinum. The central compartment level VI nodes are located anterior to the thyroid gland (prelaryngeal nodes), posterior and inferior to the thyroid gland, and adjacent to the trachea (paratracheal nodes). Central compartment nodes that are below the level of the suprasternal notch are level VII nodes.

   Normal lymph node morphology is characterized by a hypoechoic outer cortex with densely packed lymphocytes and a central hyperechoic hilum containing lymphatic sinuses and vessels. The size of normal lymph nodes may vary depending on the neck region, with submandibular or level II lymph nodes tending to be larger, perhaps due to reactive hyperplasia from repeated oral cavity inflammation, with a long axis up to 2 cm. The short axis diameter varies less and is typically less than 8 mm in level II and less than 5 mm in the other cervical regions (Figure 61-5).

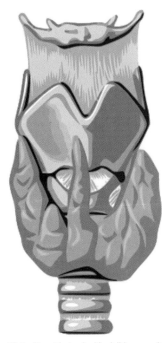

Figure 61-1. Thyroid gland with visible pyramidal lobe. (*See online version of the book for full color image.*)

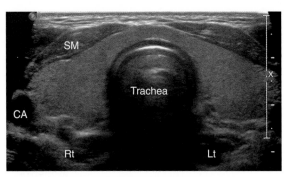

**Figure 61-2.** Normal thyroid gland on US. Note position of thyroid overlying trachea and homogeneously bright appearance of parenchyma relative to strap muscles of neck. *CA* = carotid artery; *SM* = strap muscles.

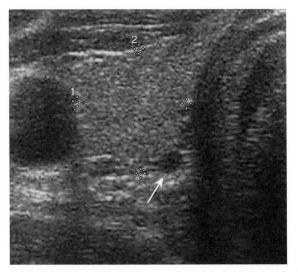

**Figure 61-3.** Normal parathyroid gland on US. Normal-appearing 3-mm parathyroid gland (*arrow*) is seen along posterior surface of thyroid gland at its midpole, likely a superior parathyroid gland.

4. **What are the indications for US of the thyroid gland, parathyroid glands, and neck lymph nodes?**

   US of the neck is commonly used to both characterize and localize palpable neck lesions, and to guide fine needle aspiration (FNA). Specifically, US of the thyroid gland can be used to (1) determine the echotexture of the gland and assess for the presence of a nodule, (2) assess nodule characteristics to determine the need for FNA, (3) follow up thyroid nodule size, (4) screen for occult thyroid cancer in high risk patients, and (5) guide FNA of thyroid nodules. Sonographic evaluation of cervical lymph nodes is commonly performed to detect metastatic disease in patients with a history of malignancy, and to examine palpable nodes for malignant features and guide FNA of abnormal-appearing nodes.

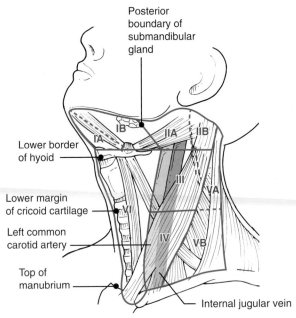

**Figure 61-4.** The AJCC classification system of nodal location. *(From Woo SB. Oral Pathology, 2/e. A Comprehensive Atlas and Text, In Press.)*

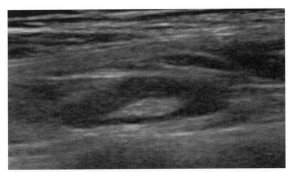

**Figure 61-5.** Normal cervical lymph node on US. Note that this midlateral, level III, cervical lymph node has hypoechoic outer cortex that is relatively symmetric in thickness and central echogenic hilum.

Primary hyperparathyroidism is the most frequent indication for performing US of the parathyroid glands. This condition leads to accelerated bone destruction, renal stone formation, and elevated serum calcium levels and is most commonly diagnosed in the fifth through seventh decades of life. Most cases of primary hyperparathyroidism are caused by a single parathyroid adenoma (89%). Other causes include hyperplasia of all four glands (6%), double adenomas (4%), and, rarely, parathyroid carcinoma. In most instances, parathyroid adenomas are sporadic. There is an increased incidence of parathyroid hyperplasia in patients with multiple endocrine neoplasia (MEN) syndromes.

5. What is a thyroid goiter?
Thyroid goiter refers to an enlarged thyroid gland of any cause and may occur in the setting of autoimmune thyroid disease or as a result of one or more focal lesions in the gland. The thyroid gland may also be enlarged due to nonthyroid conditions such as during pregnancy or in the setting of chronic renal disease.

6. What is chronic lymphocytic (Hashimoto's) thyroiditis?
This is the most common diffuse thyroid disease. It affects as many as 5% to 10% of the adult population, with a strong female predominance, and is the most common cause of hypothyroidism in children and adults. This autoimmune thyroid disease is pathologically characterized by a lymphocytic infiltrate and glandular fibrosis.

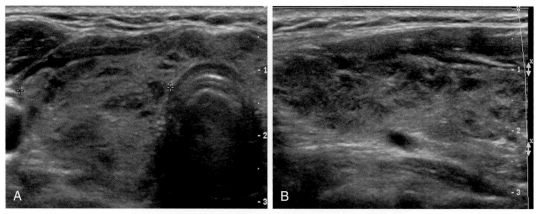

**Figure 61-6.** Hashimoto's thyroiditis on US. **A,** Axial and **B,** Sagittal images show geometrically shaped, hypoechoic patchy regions throughout thyroid gland, interspersed with more normal-appearing regions. Note scattered linear bright lines and irregular capsule of thyroid, representing fibrosis, a prominent feature of this autoimmune disease.

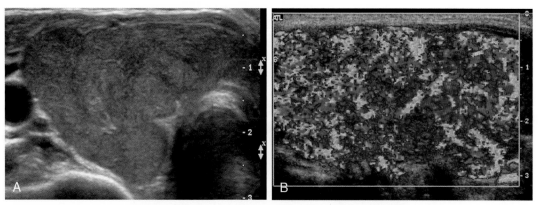

**Figure 61-7.** Graves' disease on US. **A,** Axial image shows diffusely enlarged and hypoechoic thyroid gland, with smoothly lobulated surface. **B,** Color Doppler sagittal image shows vascularity throughout entire gland, characteristic of Graves' disease.

The thyroid gland may have a variety of appearances ranging from patchy, ill-defined, or geographic, hypoechoic regions superimposed on a normal background parenchyma to a diffusely hypoechoic gland with scattered linear echogenicities and an irregular capsule reflecting intraglandular fibrosis (Figure 61-6). The gland is usually enlarged, less commonly normal or small in size, and may have either increased or decreased vascularity depending on the degree of disease activity.

7. What is Graves' disease?

Graves' disease is also an autoimmune thyroid disease and is pathologically characterized by cellular hyperplasia of the thyroid follicles as a result of circulating antibodies stimulating the thyroid to produce excess thyroid hormone. On US, the most characteristic appearance is that of an enlarged, hypoechoic, and very vascular gland with a smoothly lobulated surface and little or no fibrosis (Figure 61-7).

8. How good is US for detecting thyroid abnormalities?

US is very sensitive for identifying nonpalpable thyroid abnormalities. When a focal abnormality is noted in the thyroid parenchyma, it is called a nodule (Figure 61-8). Screening studies have shown that thyroid nodules are extremely common, especially those less than 1 cm, are more prevalent in women than men, and occur with increasing frequency with advancing age. Up to 67% of senior adults will have focal thyroid lesions when evaluated by US. The vast majority of focal nodules in the thyroid gland prove to be hyperplastic regions containing nonneoplastic cells in which the orderly follicular architecture is disrupted by regions of larger and irregularly shaped follicles, often with abundant colloid and cystic appearance on US.

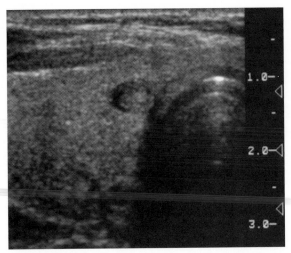

**Figure 61-8.** Incidental 5-mm thyroid nodule on US. Due to excellent resolution of US, small benign nodules such as this are commonly detected in adults. The vast majority of small incidentally detected thyroid nodules are benign.

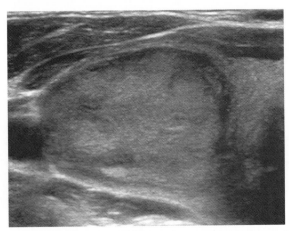

**Figure 61-9.** Follicular adenoma of thyroid gland on US. 2.5-cm solid nodule with partial capsule is noted. Biopsy was performed for confirmation because some thyroid cancers can also have this appearance.

9. **What proportion of focal thyroid nodules are neoplastic?**

Approximately 20% of all focal nodules that are biopsied are neoplastic, with the majority due to benign follicular adenomas and the minority due to thyroid malignancy. Follicular adenomas are much more common in women and are usually incidentally detected when the patient is undergoing imaging of the thyroid for another reason. On US, follicular adenomas may be entirely solid or have internal cystic regions, have a well-defined capsule, and tend to have marked vascularity throughout the nodule (Figure 61-9). They are not considered to pose a risk of malignancy although a small percentage may become hyperfunctioning and lead to hyperthyroidism (Figure 61-10).

10. **What types of thyroid cancer are there?**

Most thyroid cancers are well differentiated and have an excellent prognosis after surgical removal. Papillary cancer is the most common type, accounting for 80%, and pure follicular cancer is the second most common type, accounting for 10% to 15%. Medullary thyroid carcinomas arise from the parafollicular or C cells of the thyroid gland, account for approximately 5% of thyroid cancers, and are most likely to occur sporadically although they are seen with increased frequency in patients with MEN IIB syndrome. The more aggressive thyroid cancers, such as poorly differentiated and anaplastic cancers, are the least common and have a poor prognosis.

11. **How is US useful to determine which thyroid nodules warrant FNA?**

US has relatively high specificity for identifying papillary thyroid cancers based on imaging features (Box 61-1). If extension of a lesion beyond the thyroid capsule or if metastatic lymph nodes are present, a thyroid malignancy can be diagnosed (Figures 61-11 and 61-12). Current imaging guidelines require evaluation of the lateral cervical nodes in all patients undergoing neck US because the detection of metastatic thyroid cancer to the lateral cervical lymph nodes may aid in the definitive preoperative diagnosis of malignancy in nodules with indeterminate cytologic results and alter

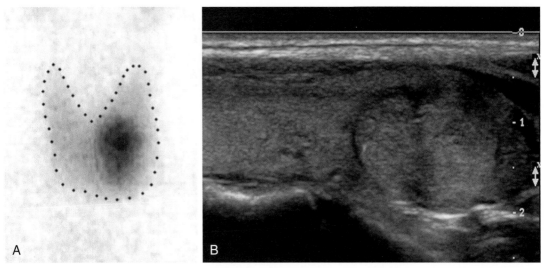

**Figure 61-10.** Functioning adenoma of thyroid gland on thyroid scintigraphy and US. **A,** [123]I scan performed in hyperthyroid patient demonstrated autonomously functioning nodule with radiotracer uptake seen in lower pole of left lobe of thyroid gland. **B,** Longitudinal view of left lobe of thyroid gland shows 2.2-cm predominantly solid nodule.

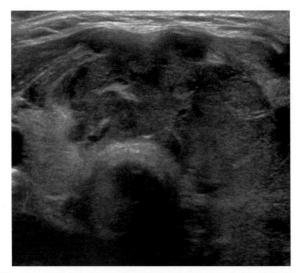

**Figure 61-11.** Anaplastic thyroid cancer on US. Note large solid and hypoechoic mass replacing much of thyroid gland in this patient with history of rapidly growing neck mass. At surgery, this mass extended beyond thyroid gland into adjacent soft tissues of neck and trachea.

---

**Box 61-1.** Imaging Features Associated with Thyroid Malignancy

- Invasion of adjacent structures
- Lymphadenopathy
- Microcalcifications
- Large, coarse calcifications
- Marked hypoechogenicity
- Infiltrative or microlobulated margins
- Taller-than-wide shape

---

the surgical approach to patients with known nodal disease. Specific imaging features that have a high correlation with thyroid malignancy include presence of microcalcifications, coarse and dystrophic calcifications, marked hypoechogenicity, infiltrative and/or microlobulated margins, and taller-than-wide shape (Figures 61-11, 61-12, and 61-13). However, not all malignancies demonstrate these features, such that their absence cannot reliably exclude a malignancy. Additionally, there is overlap in the appearance of benign follicular adenomas and follicular cancers. Both may appear as predominantly solid noncalcified vascular lesions, often with an identifiable capsule or halo (Figures 61-9 and 61-14).

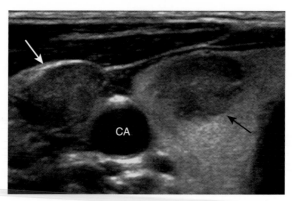

**Figure 61-12.** Papillary thyroid cancer on US. Note solid hypoechoic nodule (*black arrow*) with microcalcifications and microlobulated border in right lobe of thyroid gland, suspicious for papillary thyroid cancer. Also seen is abnormal-appearing lateral cervical node (*white arrow*) due to metastatic tumor. *CA* = carotid artery.

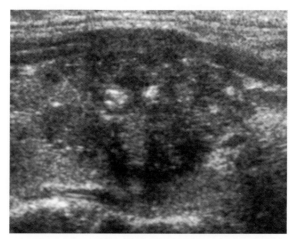

**Figure 61-13.** Medullary thyroid cancer on US. Note solid, hypoechoic thyroid gland lesion with coarse dystrophic calcifications, along with extracapsular extent anteriorly.

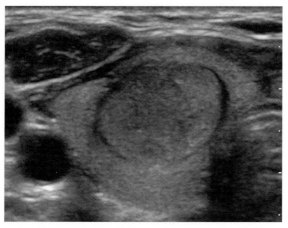

**Figure 61-14.** Follicular thyroid cancer on US. Note solid, nearly isoechoic lesion with defined capsule, similar in appearance to that of benign follicular adenoma.

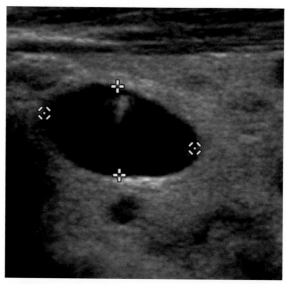

**Figure 61-15.** Cystic thyroid nodule on US. Note nearly entirely cystic nodule due to hyperplastic nodule with abundant colloid and little or no identifiable parenchyma. Such nodules are considered benign and usually do not need biopsy or follow-up imaging.

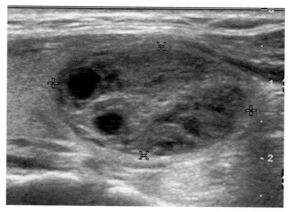

**Figure 61-16.** Spongiform thyroid nodule on US. This appearance is associated with very low risk of malignancy, under 1% in nodules under 2 cm.

There are some sonographic features that correlate with a very high likelihood that a thyroid nodule is benign, due to a hyperplastic focus rather than a neoplasm. Nodules that are nearly entirely cystic without an identifiable solid component (Figure 61-15) or have a spongiform appearance, defined as interspersed cystic spaces without marked vascularity, calcifications, or irregular margins (Figure 61-16), are two features of thyroid nodules that indicate a very low (less than 1%) risk of malignancy. Small spongiform nodules are not typically biopsied when under 2 cm in size but when larger in size may be followed by serial US to assess for the development of suspicious features or a rapid growth pattern.

Sonographic features therefore play an important role in determining which thyroid nodules warrant FNA. Other factors that also influence the need for FNA include the patient's overall health, risk factors for thyroid malignancy such as a history of head and neck irradiation as a child or a known predisposing genetic risk, and the method of discovery of the nodule including rapid growth or detection by [18]F-fluorodeoxyglucose (FDG) positron emission tomography (PET). When multiple nodules are present in the thyroid gland, the decision about which nodules would need FNA is based on the sonographic features of each nodule rather than nodule size alone.

12. **What is the most common congenital anomaly of the neck?**
The most common congenital anomaly of the neck is a thyroglossal duct cyst. The thyroglossal tract arises from the foramen cecum at the junction of the anterior two thirds and posterior one third of the tongue and runs to the level of the thyroid gland, along the embryologic migratory path of the thyroid gland. Any part of the tract can persist, causing a sinus, fistula, or cyst. The most common location for a thyroglossal duct cyst is midline or slightly off midline, between the isthmus of the thyroid gland and the hyoid bone or just above the hyoid bone (Figure 61-17). These are

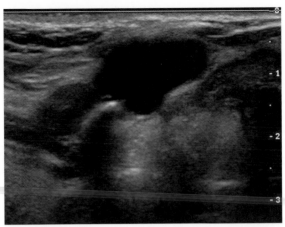

**Figure 61-17.** Thyroglossal duct cyst on US. Note characteristic relationship of anechoic cystic lesion with posterior acoustic enhancement to echogenic hyoid bone with posterior acoustic shadowing in patient with palpable neck lesion.

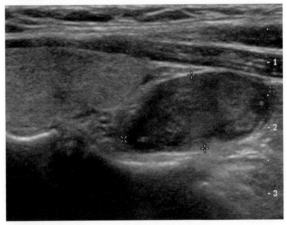

**Figure 61-18.** Parathyroid adenoma on US. Sagittal image shows enlarged, oval inferior parathyroid gland just below left lobe of thyroid gland.

most commonly noted in children as a palpable lesion but can occur at any age and might not become evident until adult life. Mucinous clear secretions may collect within these cysts, causing them to appear as spherical masses or fusiform lesions, rarely larger than 2 to 3 cm in diameter. Superimposed infection may convert these lesions into abscess cavities, and rarely, a cancer may develop in the cyst.

13. What are some parathyroid gland pathologies that may occur?
Parathyroid adenomas cause the affected parathyroid gland to appear solid and homogeneously hypoechoic as a result of compact cellularity and usually measure between 1 to 2 cm in greatest dimension (Figure 61-18). They are usually oval or bean shaped, but larger adenomas can be multilobulated and have cystic areas, and rarely calcifications. Color and power Doppler US imaging commonly show a characteristic extrathyroidal feeding vessel (typically a branch of the inferior thyroidal artery), which enters at one of the poles and travels around the periphery of the gland, resulting in a characteristic arc or rim of vascularity (Figure 61-19), an important distinguishing feature from lymph nodes, which have a central vascular supply. The sensitivity and specificity of US in localizing a solitary parathyroid adenoma are quite variable, ranging from 70% to 90%. The wide range of sensitivities is likely due to a variety of factors including patient size, quality of probe used, size and location of adenoma, concomitant thyroid disease, and, perhaps most important, the skill and experience of the sonographer (Figure 61-20). The specificity of US in locating parathyroid adenomas, on the other hand, is much more consistent and ranges from 92% to 97%.

The appearance of both hyperplastic parathyroid glands and parathyroid carcinoma can overlap with a parathyroid adenoma. In general, hyperplastic parathyroid glands are only minimally enlarged (Figure 61-21). Some consider the visualization of a parathyroid gland by neck US to be abnormal, reflecting a change from the high adipose content in a normal gland which blends in with the fibrofatty connective tissue of the neck and is difficult to visualize to a gland with hypercellular composition and visible hypoechogenicity. The patient is often not yet hypercalcemic at

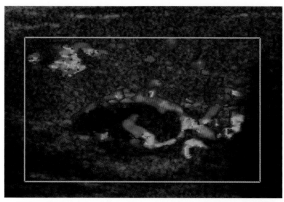

**Figure 61-19.** Parathyroid adenoma on color Doppler US. Note rim flow pattern, which helps to differentiate enlarged parathyroid gland from other neck lesions such as enlarged cervical lymph nodes.

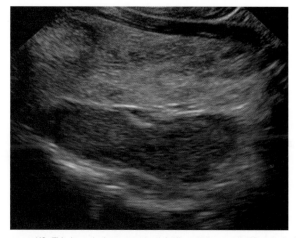

**Figure 61-20.** Parathyroid adenoma on US. This large lesion was not originally noted on neck US as typically performed with high-frequency linear transducers. Repeat examination with lower-frequency probe and large field of view was necessary for visualization of lesion in this patient with large body habitus.

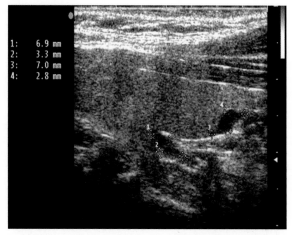

**Figure 61-21.** Parathyroid hyperplasia on US. Longitudinal image shows minimal enlargement of two right parathyroid glands. All four parathyroid glands were minimally enlarged in this patient with primary hyperparathyroidism.

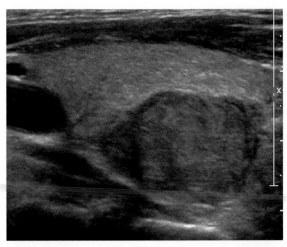

**Figure 61-22.** Parathyroid cancer on US. Note large parathyroid mass with irregular margins.

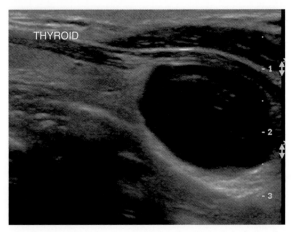

**Figure 61-23.** Parathyroid cyst on US. Note anechoic lesion seen just below thyroid gland. Aspiration demonstrated presence of clear fluid.

---

**Box 61-2.** Imaging Features Associated with Malignant Cervical Lymphadenopathy

- Round shape
- Loss of the echogenic hilum
- Eccentric cortical hypertrophy
- Cystic change
- Calcification
- Peripheral vascularity
- Reticular pattern (suggestive of lymphoma)

---

this stage but may become so in the future. Parathyroid cancers are relatively uncommon but should be suspected when a lesion demonstrates irregular margins or size over 2 cm (Figure 61-22). Parathyroid cysts may also be seen as anechoic lesions with posterior acoustic enhancement in the expected location of the parathyroid gland (Figure 61-23).

14. **What are some causes of cervical lymphadenopathy?**
Cervical lymphadenopathy is common in patients with metastatic head and neck cancer or lymphoma and is also commonly found in patients with upper respiratory infections and systemic diseases. Although computed tomography (CT) and magnetic resonance imaging (MRI) are also used to evaluate cervical lymph nodes, the internal architecture of small lymph nodes and the presence of subtle findings such as small calcifications and peripheral vascularity are better assessed by US (Box 61-2). US is also commonly used to guide FNA of abnormal-appearing nodes.

15. **What imaging features may be useful to distinguish benign from malignant lymph nodes?**
Nodal size is one of the criteria used to differentiate reactive from malignant lymph nodes. Although larger nodes tend to have a higher incidence of malignancy, reactive nodes can be as large as malignant nodes, and therefore the use of a size threshold alone will lead to many false positive and false negative results. Most inflammatory diseases, except for granulomatous infections such as by tuberculosis, involve lymph nodes diffusely and homogeneously, generally

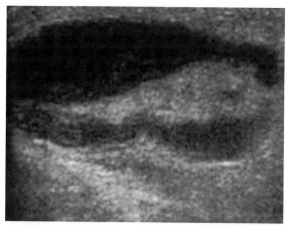

**Figure 61-24.** Reactive cervical lymph node on US. Although this node was quite large, it proved to be reactive due to cat scratch fever. Note preservation of oval shape.

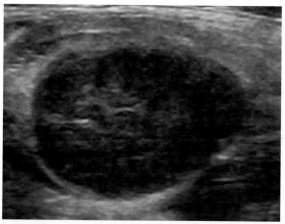

**Figure 61-25.** Malignant cervical lymph node on US. Note minimally enlarged round node without echogenic central hilum. Also note scattered linear echogenic foci, forming a reticular pattern, which is relatively specific for lymphoma. This patient had Hodgkin's lymphoma.

preserving their oval shape (Figure 61-24). Malignant lymph nodes tend to be round in shape with a short-to-long axis ratio (S/L ratio) >0.5, whereas reactive or benign lymph nodes are more likely to have an S/L ratio <0.5. Although a round shape helps to identify a malignant lymph node, it should not be used as the sole criterion and is more specific when disruption of the normal nodal architecture is also evident. In the normal neck, about 90% of nodes with a maximum transverse diameter greater than 5 mm will have echogenic hilum visible on high-resolution US. Malignant lymph nodes usually do not show an echogenic hilum, which may be an important clue to detect disease involvement of nodes that are normal in size and shape. However, identification of a normal-appearing hilum cannot reliably exclude the presence of a small burden of metastatic disease, especially when occurring in the periphery of the node. Visualization of an internal reticular echo pattern of lymph nodes may also be encountered and is relatively specific for lymphoma (Figure 61-25).

Most nodal metastases appear as hypoechoic or heterogeneous regions within nodes, but papillary thyroid cancer may appear very echogenic, likely due to follicular formation. Irrespective of size, eccentric cortical hypertrophy, which is due to focal tumor infiltration within the lymph node, is a useful sign to identify metastatic nodes (Figure 61-26). Other features that are suspicious for metastatic involvement include cystic change related to liquefactive necrosis, a common finding in squamous cell carcinoma metastases, or to the presence of colloid in the setting of metastatic papillary thyroid cancer (Figure 61-27). Calcification within cervical lymph nodes is uncommon but is most commonly due to metastatic papillary thyroid carcinoma (Figure 61-28). Therefore, when calcified and/or cystic cervical nodes are noted, especially in children and young adults, a primary papillary tumor in the thyroid gland should be suspected. Often, the nodal metastases from papillary thyroid cancer are quite large, whereas the primary lesion may be quite small or even invisible. Nodal calcifications can also be due to medullary thyroid carcinoma, treated lymphoma, and granulomatous disease. Normal and reactive lymph nodes usually show hilar vascularity, with a vessel pattern tapering toward the periphery of the node, or may be avascular. Peripheral vascularity, especially when focal, is uncommon in benign nodes and is another useful indicator of malignancy (Figure 61-29).

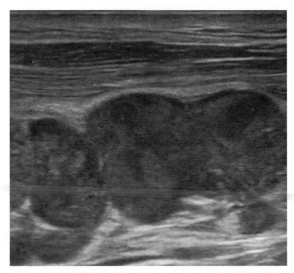

**Figure 61-26.** Malignant cervical lymph nodes on US. Note chain of lateral cervical nodes with rounded shape and hypoechoic regions in patient with metastatic lung cancer.

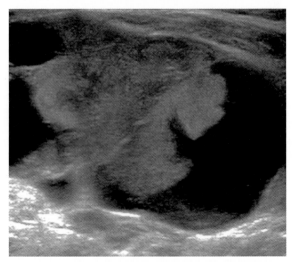

**Figure 61-27.** Cystic cervical lymph node on US. Note large node with cystic change due to metastatic papillary thyroid cancer.

**KEY POINTS**

- Lymph node location on imaging exams should be reported according to the AJCC classification system. The most important aspect is correctly identifying nodes that are located in the central compartment of the neck versus those in the lateral compartment when surgical resection is planned.
- US is a very sensitive technique that identifies focal abnormalities or nodules in the thyroid gland in a large percentage of adults, many of which are clinically occult and the majority of which are benign. The sonographic appearance of these abnormalities is very important in deciding which nodules warrant fine needle aspiration.
- Sonographic features of thyroid nodules that are associated with a higher risk of malignancy include microcalcifications, coarse and dystrophic calcifications, marked hypoechogenicity, infiltrative and/or microlobulated margins, and taller-than-wide shape.
- Sonographic features associated with a very low risk of malignancy are a nearly entirely cystic nodule and a spongiform appearance in a nodule under 2 cm without marked vascularity, calcifications, or irregular margins.
- Features suspicious for malignant cervical lymphadenopathy include round shape, eccentric cortical hypertrophy, cystic change, calcifications, and peripheral vascularity.

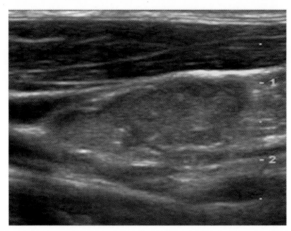

**Figure 61-28.** Calcified cervical lymph node on US. Note replacement of normal nodal architecture by echogenic solid tissue with scattered punctate echogenic calcifications in patient with metastatic papillary thyroid cancer.

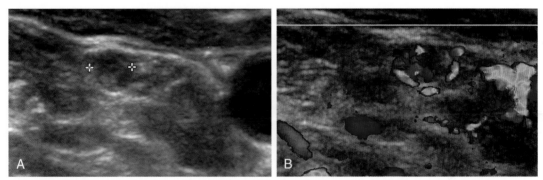

**Figure 61-29.** Normal-sized malignant cervical lymph node on US. **A,** Gray scale image shows 5-mm round node with questionable visualization of echogenic hilum. **B,** Color Doppler image shows abnormal peripheral flow in node that proved to harbor small focus of metastatic papillary thyroid cancer.

## BIBLIOGRAPHY

AIUM practice guideline for the performance of ultrasound examinations of the head and neck. *J Ultrasound Med.* 2014;33(2):366-382.

Langer JE, Mandel SJ. Thyroid nodule sonography: assessment for risk of malignancy. *Imaging Med.* 2011;3(5):513-524.

Anderson L, Middleton WD, Teefey SA, et al. Hashimoto thyroiditis: part 1, sonographic analysis of the nodular form of Hashimoto thyroiditis. *AJR Am J Roentgenol.* 2010;195(1):208-215.

American Thyroid Association Guidelines Taskforce on Thyroid N, Differentiated Thyroid C, Cooper DS, et al. Revised American Thyroid Association management guidelines for patients with thyroid nodules and differentiated thyroid cancer. *Thyroid.* 2009;19(11):1167-1214.

Johnson NA, Tublin ME, Ogilvie JB. Parathyroid imaging: technique and role in the preoperative evaluation of primary hyperparathyroidism. *AJR Am J Roentgenol.* 2007;188(6):1706-1715.

Frates MC, Benson CB, Charboneau JW, et al. Management of thyroid nodules detected at US: Society of Radiologists in Ultrasound consensus conference statement. *Radiology.* 2005;237(3):794-800.

Frasoldati A, Valcavi R. Challenges in neck ultrasonography: lymphadenopathy and parathyroid glands. *Endocr Pract.* 2004;10(3):261-268.

Ahuja A, Ying M. Sonography of neck lymph nodes. Part II: abnormal lymph nodes. *Clin Radiol.* 2003;58(5):359-366.

Khati N, Adamson T, Johnson KS, et al. Ultrasound of the thyroid and parathyroid glands. *Ultrasound Q.* 2003;19(4):162-176.

Ying M, Ahuja A. Sonography of neck lymph nodes. Part I: normal lymph nodes. *Clin Radiol.* 2003;58(5):351-358.

Reeder SB, Desser TS, Weigel RJ, et al. Sonography in primary hyperparathyroidism: review with emphasis on scanning technique. *J Ultrasound Med.* 2002;21(5):539-552, quiz 53-4.

Solbiati L, Osti V, Cova L, et al. Ultrasound of thyroid, parathyroid glands and neck lymph nodes. *Eur Radiol.* 2001;11(12):2411-2424.

Som PM, Curtin HD, Mancuso AA. Imaging-based nodal classification for evaluation of neck metastatic adenopathy. *AJR Am J Roentgenol.* 2000;174(3):837-844.

Bruneton JN, Balu-Maestro C, Marcy PY, et al. Very high frequency (13 MHz) ultrasonographic examination of the normal neck: detection of normal lymph nodes and thyroid nodules. *J Ultrasound Med.* 1994;13(2):87-90.

Ralls PW, Mayekawa DS, Lee KP, et al. Color-flow Doppler sonography in Graves disease: "thyroid inferno." *AJR Am J Roentgenol.* 1988;150(4):781-784.

# CHAPTER 62

# ABDOMINAL ULTRASONOGRAPHY

Courtney A. Woodfield, MD

1. List some of the most common indications for abdominal ultrasonography (US).
   - Abdominal, flank, and/or back pain.
   - Abnormal laboratory values (e.g., abnormal liver function tests).
   - Palpable abdominal mass.
   - Signs or symptoms referred from abdomen (e.g., jaundice or hematuria).

2. What is the sonographic appearance of the liver?
   The liver is normally homogeneous in echotexture, equal to or slightly more echogenic than the renal cortex, and hypoechoic compared to the spleen and pancreas. Along the midhepatic line, the liver is normally <15.5 cm in length. The hepatic veins are readily visible sonographically and help define hepatic anatomy. The right hepatic vein divides the right hepatic lobe into anterior and posterior segments. The middle hepatic vein separates the anterior segment of the right hepatic lobe and the medial segment of the left hepatic lobe. The gallbladder also separates the anterior segment of the right lobe and the medial segment of the left lobe. The left hepatic vein divides the left hepatic lobe into medial and lateral segments (Figure 62-1). The ligamentum teres also separates the medial and lateral segments of the left hepatic lobe.

3. How are the hepatic veins and portal veins differentiated on US?
   Portal veins travel with hepatic arteries and bile ducts (the portal triad). A connective sheath surrounds this portal triad with resulting echogenicity of the portal vein walls. In contrast, the hepatic veins travel in isolation and have almost imperceptible walls (see Figure 62-1).

4. What is the most common cause of increased hepatic echogenicity?
   Increased hepatic echogenicity is detected when the liver is considerably more echogenic than the kidney. The most common cause is hepatic steatosis. Other sonographic features of hepatic steatosis include finer and more compact echotexture and decreased transmission of sound waves such that the deeper aspect of the liver is difficult to visualize, as are the adjacent diaphragm and intrahepatic vessels. There are numerous causes of hepatic steatosis, including obesity, alcohol abuse, diabetes mellitus, corticosteroid use, malnutrition, and chemotherapy.

5. Describe the US appearance of acute hepatitis.
   Acute hepatitis can result in liver edema, which manifests on US as diffusely decreased hepatic echogenicity with increased echogenicity of the portal triads (the "starry sky" sign). There can be associated hepatomegaly and gallbladder wall thickening.

6. Name and describe the US appearance of common benign and malignant focal hepatic lesions.
   For the answer, see Table 62-1, Figure 62-2, and Figure 62-3.

7. Describe the US appearance of a target lesion in the liver and its significance.
   A target lesion on US is characterized as a hepatic lesion with an echogenic center and a peripheral hypoechoic rim (see Figure 62-3). This appearance has a high association with malignancy, including metastatic disease, hepatocellular carcinoma, and lymphoma. In contrast, lesions with a reverse target appearance (an isoechoic to hypoechoic center and a hyperechoic rim) are more commonly associated with a benign etiology, such as a hemangioma.

8. What are the sonographic features of cirrhosis?
   The liver may be increased in size in the early stages of cirrhosis and later become small with relative enlargement of the caudate and/or left hepatic lobe. The liver has a nodular contour and a more echogenic and heterogeneous echotexture. Associated features of portal hypertension may be seen, which include ascites, splenomegaly, recanalization of the paraumbilical vein, and portal vein enlargement.

9. What is the appearance of gallstones on US?
   US is the modality of choice for detecting gallstones. Gallstones appear as rounded echogenic structures in the gallbladder lumen with posterior acoustic shadowing. Stones smaller than 5 mm may not shadow but will still appear echogenic. Gallstones are also typically mobile. Gallstones may also be seen in association with biliary sludge, which appears as dependent, low-level layering echogenic material in the gallbladder (Figure 62-4).

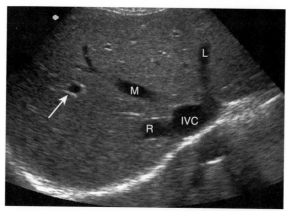

**Figure 62-1.** Normal liver on US. Transverse US image of liver shows right (*R*), middle (*M*), and left (*L*) hepatic veins joining at inferior vena cava (*IVC*). The right hepatic vein divides right hepatic lobe into anterior and posterior segments. The middle hepatic vein separates anterior segment of right hepatic lobe from medial segment of left hepatic lobe, and left hepatic vein divides left hepatic lobe into medial and lateral segments. Note imperceptible walls of hepatic veins compared to echogenic walls of portal vein (*arrow*).

**Table 62-1.** US Appearance of Common Focal Hepatic Lesions

| LESION | US APPEARANCE | ADDITIONAL FEATURES |
|---|---|---|
| Cyst | Anechoic, well-demarcated thin wall, well-defined back wall, posterior acoustic enhancement | Cysts complicated by hemorrhage or infection can develop a thick wall, internal echoes, and/or septations |
| Hemangioma | Well-defined, homogeneously hyperechoic (most common), hypoechoic center with echogenic border (less common) | More common in women, up to 10% are multiple |
| Focal nodular hyperplasia (FNH) | Similar echogenicity to adjacent liver, central scar variably seen as hypoechoic center | More common in women, subtle benign lesion |
| Adenoma | Variable appearance from hypoechoic to hyperechoic (with hemorrhage) | Associated with oral contraceptive agents, and with increased risk of hemorrhage and malignant degeneration |
| Focal hepatic steatosis | Region of increased echogenicity compared to normal liver background | Can change rapidly, no mass effect, most commonly anterior to portal vein at porta hepatis |
| Focal fatty sparing | Region of decreased echogenicity compared to abnormal echogenic liver background | Most commonly anterior to portal vein at porta hepatis, or adjacent to gallbladder fossa |
| Hepatocellular carcinoma (HCC) | Variable appearance; when small (<5 cm) hypoechoic, with time and increasing size more complex and inhomogeneous due to necrosis, fibrosis, or fatty change, sometimes with peripheral hypoechoic halo | May be a solitary nodule, multiple nodules, or diffuse infiltration, sometimes with portal vein invasion |
| Metastasis | Variable appearance from echogenic, hypoechoic, target, calcified, or cystic; hypoechoic halo | More commonly multiple, with variably sized liver masses |
| Abscess | Complex cystic appearance with variable luminal echogenicity from anechoic to highly echoic, fluid-fluid levels, septations, debris, variable wall thickness, or gas | Most commonly secondary to seeding from intestinal sources |

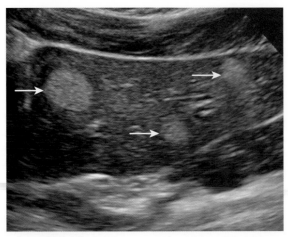

**Figure 62-2.** Hepatic hemangiomas on US. Sagittal US image through left hepatic lobe reveals three ovoid, well-circumscribed echogenic lesions, typical of hepatic hemangiomas (*arrows*).

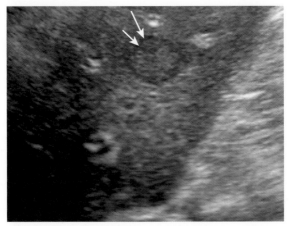

**Figure 62-3.** Hepatic target lesion on US. Sagittal US image through liver illustrates target lesion with echogenic center (*short arrow*) and hypoechoic rim (*long arrow*), in this case due to metastatic breast cancer.

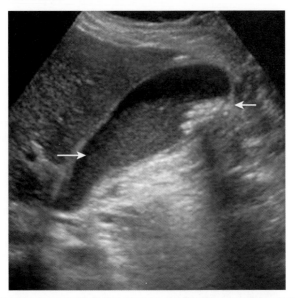

**Figure 62-4.** Gallstones and gallbladder sludge on US. Sagittal US image of gallbladder demonstrates clustered, subcentimeter, layering, echogenic stones (*short arrow*) with posterior acoustic shadowing at gallbladder fundus. There is also a large amount of layering, low-level echogenicity material (*long arrow*) due to gallbladder sludge.

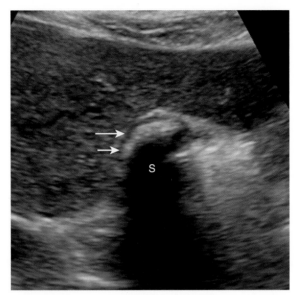

**Figure 62-5.** Gallstone on US. Transverse US image through gallbladder fossa illustrates "wall-echo-shadow" (WES) sign comprised of hypoechoic gallbladder wall (*long arrow*), leading edge of echogenic gallstone(s) (*small arrow*), and posterior acoustic shadowing (*S*).

10. **What is the "wall-echo-shadow" sign?**
    The "wall-echo-shadow" (WES) sign is the result of the gallbladder being filled with small stones, or a single giant stone. The hypoechoic nondependent gallbladder wall is first visualized (wall), followed by echogenic gallstones (echo), and then posterior acoustic shadowing (shadow), which obscures the remainder of the gallbladder (Figure 62-5). The WES sign can be differentiated from air or calcification in the gallbladder wall, as in these cases, the normal hypoechoic gallbladder wall is not seen, only gallbladder fossa echogenicity with posterior acoustic shadowing.

11. **Can tumefactive sludge and gallbladder polyps be differentiated from gallstones sonographically?**
    When sludge consolidates to form a mass, so-called tumefactive sludge, it is still typically mobile and avascular, which differentiates it from a polyp, and it does not shadow, which differentiates it from a gallstone. Gallbladder polyps can be as echogenic as are small gallstones, but they are nonmobile and do not shadow. Color Doppler flow can also sometimes be detected in a polyp.

12. **Name possible causes of gallbladder wall thickening.**
    Normally, the gallbladder wall measures 3 mm or less in thickness. There are multiple etiologies for gallbladder wall thickening including generalized edematous states (congestive heart failure, renal failure, hypoalbuminemia, cirrhosis), gallbladder inflammation (cholecystitis or secondary inflammation from acute hepatitis), neoplasm (gallbladder adenocarcinoma, metastasis), and adenomyomatosis (Figure 62-6).

13. **Describe the US appearance of adenomyomatosis.**
    Gallbladder adenomyomatosis is a benign condition consisting of dilation of the Rokitansky-Aschoff sinuses in the gallbladder wall with associated smooth muscle proliferation. There is resultant thickening of and cystic space formation in the gallbladder wall. This process can be focal or diffuse, and the sonographic appearance includes thickening of the gallbladder wall with cystic spaces, and more characteristically tiny echogenic foci in the gallbladder wall with dirty ring down ("comet tail") artifact (Figure 62-7).

14. **What is the significance of gallbladder wall calcification?**
    Calcification of the gallbladder wall is referred to as **porcelain gallbladder**. It is a rare entity with an unknown etiology but is associated with gallstone disease, female gender, and age >60 years. There is also a higher incidence of gallbladder carcinoma with a porcelain gallbladder such that prophylactic removal of the gallbladder is commonly recommended. On US, wall calcification appears as a hyperechoic wall with variable posterior acoustic shadowing.

15. **How does acute cholecystitis manifest on US?**
    The sonographic features of acute cholecystitis include gallbladder distention (>4 cm), gallbladder wall thickening (>3 mm) and hyperemia, gallstones (especially if impacted at the gallbladder neck or in the cystic duct), pericholecystic fluid, and a positive sonographic Murphy's sign (focal tenderness over the gallbladder when compressed by the US transducer). The combination of gallstones and a positive Murphy's sign has a positive predictive value of 92% and a negative predictive value of 95% for acute cholecystitis.

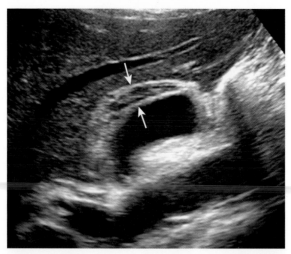

**Figure 62-6.** Gallbladder wall edema on US. Sagittal US image through gallbladder reveals gallbladder wall edema and thickening (*arrows*), in this case due to hepatitis.

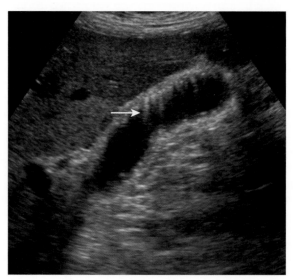

**Figure 62-7.** Gallbladder adenomyomatosis on US. Sagittal US image of gallbladder demonstrates characteristic echogenic foci in gallbladder wall with dirty ring down ("comet tail") artifact (*arrow*).

16. Name four complications of cholecystitis and their appearance on US.
    Complications of cholecystitis include gallbladder gangrene, hemorrhage, perforation, and emphysema. Gangrenous cholecystitis is diagnosed on US by visualizing nonlayering bands of echogenic tissue in the lumen due to sloughed membranes and blood. The gallbladder wall also becomes more irregular with small wall collections due to abscesses or hemorrhage. The sonographic Murphy's sign is also usually absent with gangrene. Hemorrhagic cholecystitis is also a gangrenous process wherein there is bleeding into the gallbladder wall and lumen with resultant low-level echoes to heterogeneous echoes filling the gallbladder lumen. Gallbladder perforation may be directly detected as a focal defect in the gallbladder wall or via secondary signs of gallbladder collapse and pericholecystic fluid collection. Emphysematous cholecystitis is a rare but potentially fatal condition, which is more commonly seen in diabetics and may occur in the absence of gallstones. Gas in the gallbladder wall and lumen appears as echogenic lines with dirty posterior acoustic shadowing.

17. Can US differentiate between benign and malignant gallbladder polypoid lesions (polyps)?
    There are both benign (cholesterol, inflammatory) and malignant (gallbladder adenocarcinoma, metastases [most commonly melanoma]) gallbladder polyps. Benign polyps are very common and are typically multiple, oval, and less than 10 mm in size. In contrast, malignant polyps are more commonly single, sessile, and greater than 10 mm in size. Other risk factors for a malignant polypoid include age >60, gallstone disease, and rapid change in size.

18. Describe the US appearances of gallbladder carcinoma.

    Gallbladder carcinoma can appear as a mass in the gallbladder fossa with obliteration of the gallbladder (the most common finding), can present as focal or diffuse irregular gallbladder wall thickening, or can appear as an intraluminal polypoid gallbladder mass (typically >1 cm in size with prominent internal vascularity). Contiguous hepatic invasion is the most common initial route of spread.

19. What is the normal caliber of the extrahepatic bile duct?

    The normal caliber of the extrahepatic bile duct is ≤7 mm. In older patients (>60 years) and in patients who have had previous cholecystectomy, the extrahepatic bile duct may measure up to 10 mm in caliber. In general, a diameter >7 mm without cholecystectomy should at least prompt correlation with serum liver function test parameters to determine if there is cholestasis.

20. List four possible causes of biliary obstruction.

    • Choledocholithiasis.
    • Congenital biliary disease (choledochal cysts, Caroli's disease).
    • Cholangitis with stricture formation (such as with pyogenic, helminthic, or HIV infection or with sclerosing cholangitis).
    • Neoplastic disease (cholangiocarcinoma, metastatic disease).

21. What is the normal sonographic appearance of the pancreas?

    On US, the pancreas is normally homogeneous in echotexture and isoechoic to hyperechoic compared to the normal liver. Aging and obesity can result in fatty change and resultant increased echogenicity of the pancreas. The pancreatic duct is visualized on US in up to 86% of patients and normally has a diameter of <3 mm.

22. Does US have a role in evaluating acute pancreatitis?

    In the early and milder forms of pancreatitis, the pancreas may appear normal on US. Alternatively, the pancreas may be obscured by gas from a secondary adynamic ileus in the acute setting. Therefore, the primary role of US in acute pancreatitis is to determine whether or not gallstones or stones in the common bile duct are the cause of pancreatitis. When visible, the sonographic appearance of acute pancreatitis is focal or diffuse hypoechoic enlargement of the pancreas.

23. What are the sonographic features of pancreatic adenocarcinoma?

    Most commonly, pancreatic adenocarcinoma appears sonographically as an ill-defined, hypoechoic pancreatic mass. Dilation of the main pancreatic duct upstream to the mass is also commonly seen. When the mass is located in the pancreatic head, both the main pancreatic duct and the extrahepatic bile duct may be dilated (the "double-duct" sign), which is an ominous indication of an obstructive pancreatic adenocarcinoma (Figure 62-8). The differential diagnosis for a focal hypoechoic pancreatic mass includes focal pancreatitis, peripancreatic lymph nodes, ampullary carcinoma, pancreatic lymphoma, and metastatic disease to the pancreas.

24. Can the two main cystic neoplasms of the pancreas be differentiated sonographically?

    Serous, or microcystic, cystadenoma is a multilocular cystic lesion comprised of cystic foci measuring from <1 mm up to 2 cm. There can be a central scar with or without calcification. The sonographic appearance can vary depending on the size of the cystic foci from a slightly echogenic solid-appearing mass when all the cystic foci are small to a

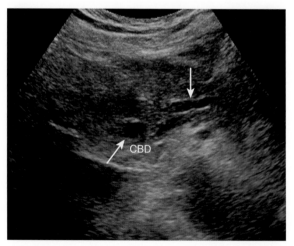

**Figure 62-8.** "Double-duct" sign on US. Transverse US image at level of pancreas illustrates dilated common bile duct (*arrow with CBD*), and dilated main pancreatic duct (*arrow*). Subsequent CT examination through abdomen (*not shown*) confirmed obstructing pancreatic head mass.

solid-appearing mass with cystic spaces. The central scar is echogenic on US. This lesion is benign, is most commonly seen in women >60 years, and most commonly occurs within the pancreatic tail.

Mucinous, or macrocystic, cystadenomas and cystadenocarcinomas are unilocular or multilocular cystic lesions with occasional papillary projections or calcifications. The cystic foci are usually >2 cm in size and fewer than 6 in number. On US, these cystic lesions are typically well circumscribed, with variable wall thickness and variable cystic foci size and contents (anechoic fluid, echogenic debris, mural vegetations, or solid components). These lesions are malignant or potentially malignant, are most commonly seen in middle-aged women, and most commonly occur in the pancreatic body or tail.

25. What is the normal sonographic appearance of the kidney?
The adult kidney usually measures 9 to 13 cm in length. The renal cortex is normally isoechoic to hypoechoic compared to the liver and hypoechoic compared to the spleen. Renal medullary pyramids are hypoechoic relative to the renal cortex. The renal sinus is predominantly composed of fat and is hyperechoic.

26. Does US have a role in evaluating pyelonephritis?
Sonographic imaging of the kidneys is usually reserved for refractory rather than acute cases of pyelonephritis, in order to search for potential complications such as renal abscess formation. Most patients with acute pyelonephritis have normal-appearing kidneys on US. When present, sonographic features that can be seen with pyelonephritis include increased renal size, compression of the renal sinus, variable change in renal echotexture (hypoechoic to hyperechoic), poorly marginated foci, loss of corticomedullary differentiation, focal or diffusely decreased renal perfusion, and/or renal parenchymal gas.

27. What are the US findings of urinary obstruction?
US is often the first imaging study of choice in patients with newly diagnosed renal dysfunction in order to exclude an underlying mechanical obstruction. Diagnosing urinary obstruction sonographically is based on the detection of hydronephrosis. Sonographically, the dilated renal collecting system appears as multiple anechoic structures conforming to the expected location of the renal calyces in contiguity with a centrally dilated renal pelvis (Figure 62-9). Bilateral hydronephrosis is usually due to obstruction at the level of the bladder. However, the cause of unilateral hydronephrosis due to obstruction of the ureter at or above the bladder can be difficult to delineate on US as the midureter is often not visible sonographically. Detection of hydronephrosis should prompt imaging of the bladder and visible ureter for the underlying cause of obstruction. The bladder should also be imaged with color Doppler technique to search for ureteral jets. The presence of a ureteral jet excludes complete urinary tract obstruction.

28. What is the US appearance of renal calculi?
Renal calculi are very common and one of the most common causes of urinary tract obstruction. Renal calculi are detected sonographically as echogenic foci with posterior acoustic shadowing. In addition, most urinary tract calculi demonstrate a twinkling artifact with color and power Doppler imaging, which is the presence of color behind a strongly reflecting interface without real flow. Calculi <5 mm in size may be sonographically occult.

29. Describe the various appearances and management of renal cysts detected sonographically.
Renal cysts are extremely common and are typically incidental. Simple cysts are round or ovoid with anechoic fluid contents, well-demarcated back walls, and posterior acoustic enhancement. Simple cysts do not need any further

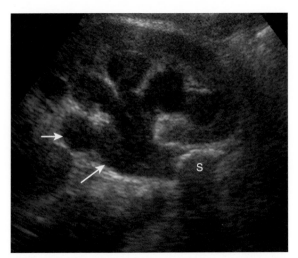

**Figure 62-9.** Hydronephrosis on US. Sagittal US image of kidney shows hydronephrosis with dilated calyces (*short arrow*) joining dilated renal pelvis (*long arrow*). In this case, the cause of hydronephrosis is evident sonographically as echogenic shadowing stone (*S*) in proximal right ureter.

follow-up. Minimally complicated cysts with a few thin internal septations, small peripheral thin calcification, or internal echoes can be managed with short-term (6-month) follow-up US. In contrast, any cystic lesion with a thickened wall, mural nodularity, multiple or thickened internal septations, or thick, irregular, or amorphous calcification is suspect for a cystic renal neoplasm and may be further evaluated with dedicated contrast-enhanced computed tomography (CT) or magnetic resonance imaging (MRI) of the kidneys.

30. Name four diseases associated with renal cysts and their extrarenal manifestations.
    - Autosomal dominant polycystic kidney disease (ADPKD) is a genetic disorder resulting in enlarged kidneys with multiple cysts of variable size and echogenicity. Cysts are also seen in multiple additional organs including the liver and pancreas. In addition, there is also an association with cerebral berry aneurysms, but not an increased risk of renal cell carcinoma (RCC) if not on dialysis.
    - Acquired cystic kidney disease (ACKD) manifests as 3 to 5 small cysts per kidney in patients on dialysis. The kidneys are otherwise small and echogenic, and there is an increased risk of RCC. There are no specific extrarenal associations.
    - Von Hippel-Lindau (VHL) syndrome is an autosomal dominant genetic condition associated with multiple renal cysts up to 3 cm in size and an increased risk of multifocal RCC. Extrarenal manifestations include central nervous system (CNS) hemangioblastomas, pheochromocytomas, retinal angiomatosis, and pancreatic cysts and neoplasms.
    - Tuberous sclerosis (TS) is an autosomal dominant genetic condition also associated with multiple variably sized renal cysts up to 3 cm, as well as renal angiomyolipomas (AMLs), and an increased risk of RCC. Extrarenal manifestations include mental retardation, seizures, adenoma sebaceum, central nervous system (CNS) tumors, cardiac rhabdomyomas, and pulmonary lymphangiomyomatosis.

31. Renal US detects a 3-cm hypoechoic solid mass in the right kidney of a 57-year-old man with hematuria. What is the most likely diagnosis?
    RCC is the most common solid renal mass and the most likely diagnosis for a solid renal mass on US. Most RCCs are isoechoic to hypoechoic to the kidney. However, smaller ones (<3 cm) may be echogenic. Other associated features include calcification, necrosis, or hemorrhage. Less commonly, RCCs are cystic lesions. Detection of a solid renal mass should prompt evaluation of the ipsilateral renal vein and inferior vena cava for possible tumor invasion.

32. Is it possible to differentiate AMLs and RCCs sonographically?
    AMLs are benign renal neoplasms composed of varying amounts of fat, smooth muscle, and blood vessels. An AML is typically hyperechoic compared to the renal parenchyma on US (Figure 62-10). However, this hyperechoic appearance is not completely diagnostic for an AML, because small (<3 cm) RCCs may also be hyperechoic. The presence of posterior acoustic shadowing without calcification is suggestive of an AML, whereas presence of internal calcification or cystic regions favors an RCC. However, in most cases, CT or MRI is indicated to further characterize a hyperechoic renal mass.

33. What is the significance of increased renal echogenicity on US?
    When the right kidney is more echogenic than the normal liver and the left kidney is isoechoic or more echogenic than the normal spleen, the kidneys can be characterized as being abnormally echogenic (Figure 62-11). Increased renal echogenicity is an indication of parenchymal disease but is nonspecific for the type of parenchymal disease, which may include acute or chronic glomerulonephritis, acute interstitial nephritis, diabetes mellitus, systemic lupus erythematosus, HIV nephropathy, and amyloidosis. Percutaneous renal biopsy is therefore frequently required for a definitive diagnosis.

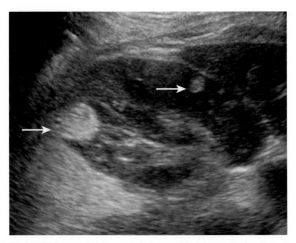

**Figure 62-10.** Renal AML on US. Sagittal US image of kidney reveals two ovoid, circumscribed, echogenic masses (*arrows*), typical of AMLs, although US alone cannot completely exclude RCCs.

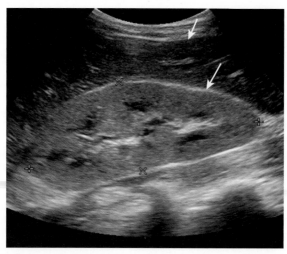

**Figure 62-11.** Renal parenchymal disease on US. Sagittal US image of right kidney (*long arrow*) shows it to be abnormally more echogenic than adjacent normal liver (*short arrow*). In this case, HIV nephropathy is the underlying etiology.

---

### KEY POINTS

- The most common etiology for increased hepatic echotexture on US is hepatic steatosis.
- US is the imaging modality of choice for detecting gallstones.
- Dilation of both the main pancreatic duct and the common bile duct (the "double duct" sign) is an ominous sign of a potentially obstructing pancreatic head carcinoma.
- Both AMLs and RCCs can be echogenic on US. Therefore, an incidental echogenic renal lesion on US typically requires further evaluation with renal CT or MRI.

### BIBLIOGRAPHY

Khalili K, Wilson SR. The biliary tree and gallbladder. In: Rumack CM, Wilson SR, Charboneau JW, et al., eds. *Diagnostic ultrasound.* 4th ed. Philadelphia: Mosby Elsevier; 2011:172-215.

Ralls P. The pancreas. In: Rumack CM, Wilson SR, Charboneau JW, et al., eds. *Diagnostic ultrasound.* 4th ed. Philadelphia: Mosby Elsevier; 2011:216-260.

Tublin M, Thurston W, Wilson SR. The kidney and urinary tract. In: Rumack CM, Wilson SR, Charboneau JW, et al., eds. *Diagnostic ultrasound.* 4th ed. Philadelphia: Mosby Elsevier; 2011:317-391.

Wilson SR, Withers CE. The liver. In: Rumack CM, Wilson SR, Charboneau JW, et al., eds. *Diagnostic ultrasound.* 4th ed. Philadelphia: Mosby Elsevier; 2011:78-145.

Kono Y, Mattrey RF. Ultrasound of the liver. *Radiol Clin North Am.* 2005;43(5):815-826, vii.

Bennett GL, Balthazar EJ. Ultrasound and CT evaluation of emergent gallbladder pathology. *Radiol Clin North Am.* 2003;41(6):1203-1216.

# CHAPTER 63

# MUSCULOSKELETAL ULTRASONOGRAPHY

*Barry Glenn Hansford, MD, and Corrie M. Yablon, MD*

1. **What are some benefits of ultrasonography (US) for musculoskeletal applications?**
   There are multiple benefits and unique advantages that US offers in musculoskeletal imaging. US does not involve the use of ionizing radiation, which is especially attractive when imaging pediatric and pregnant patients, and there are no absolute contraindications to diagnostic US. In addition, US has a higher spatial tissue resolution than magnetic resonance imaging (MRI) and computed tomography (CT), and it allows for real-time dynamic examination of anatomic sites with suspected abnormality. US can effectively be used to image patients with surgical hardware that leads to artifacts on CT and MRI, and Doppler US can provide important physiologic information about tissue blood flow. In particular, US is useful to distinguish whether a lesion is cystic or solid and to guide biopsies and therapeutic injections.

2. **What are the common indications for musculoskeletal US?**
   Musculoskeletal US may be used for a wide range of indications. Some of the most common indications include evaluation for tendon pathology in the rotator cuff, quadriceps, patellar, Achilles, and elbow common flexor/extensor tendons. It is also commonly used to assess for ligamentous injury in the anterior talofibular ligament of the ankle, medial and lateral collateral ligaments of the knee, and ulnar collateral ligament (UCL) of the thumb. Additional common indications include the evaluation of bursal abnormalities (Baker cyst, subacromial-subdeltoid bursitis/calcific bursitis), muscle injury or hematoma, and joint effusions. US can be used to evaluate palpable masses and is also extremely useful for real-time interventional guidance, allowing direct visualization of the needle within the target.

3. **When is musculoskeletal US not utilized?**
   Musculoskeletal US is significantly limited for the evaluation of internal joint derangement and is not used as the sole modality to evaluate for deep ligamentous injury (e.g., the anterior and posterior cruciate ligaments), labral pathology, cartilage injury, and meniscal injury. US is also not utilized to evaluate bone tumors because the ultrasound beam cannot effectively penetrate deep structures or cortical bone.

4. **How are images oriented in musculoskeletal US?**
   The convention in musculoskeletal US imaging is to have the notch of the transducer directed to the patient's head or the patient's left side. Images are described as being in "long axis" or "short axis" to the structure being imaged, corresponding to "longitudinal" and "transverse" planes in body imaging. When describing the orientation of the transducer to a tendon, the terms *long axis* and *short axis* are preferred, because tendons and ligaments travel obliquely around the joints. For example, if one is imaging the posterior tibialis tendon in the ankle, which courses vertically proximal to the medial malleolus but then travels anteriorly distal to the medial malleolus, the transducer would be oriented longitudinally with respect to the body, and then transversely as it follows the tendon distally. Meanwhile, the tendon is being imaged in "long axis" the entire time.

5. **What are the commonly used transducers in musculoskeletal US?**
   The transducer frequency is one important determinant of image quality. The higher the frequency, the greater the spatial resolution of the images and the lower the degree of tissue penetration. It is important to select the transducer with the highest frequency that still allows penetration to the depth of the structure being imaged. Linear probes are preferable to curved probes for musculoskeletal US because the ultrasound waves are propagated parallel to the transducer surface, limiting artifacts during evaluation of linear structures such as tendons. The linear 12-5 MHz is the workhorse transducer for musculoskeletal US, while the linear 17-5 MHz transducer may be used for the evaluation of more superficial structures. The compact or "hockey stick" linear transducer is ideally suited for the evaluation of small joints and guiding procedures performed on the distal extremities where sharp contours allow for limited contact with the probe surface. The 5-9 MHz curvilinear transducer is less commonly used in musculoskeletal US but has a role in the evaluation of deep structures or patients with larger body habitus.

6. **What is anisotropy, and how can this be used to differentiate among soft tissue structures?**
   Anisotropy refers to the variation of ultrasound interaction with fibrillar tissues and is primarily observed when evaluating tendons and ligaments. For example, when the ultrasound beam is directed perpendicular to a structure such as a tendon, the typical hyperechoic fibrillar appearance is generated. The tendon will appear speckled and hyperechoic in the short axis and striated and hyperechoic in the long axis (Figure 63-1). Upon slight angulation of the transducer probe from this perpendicular plane, the hyperechoic appearance of the tendon will become hypoechoic. This artifact may be confused for pathology as tendon and ligament abnormalities are often hypoechoic. Therefore, when evaluating a tendon or ligament, it is important to focus on the segment that is perpendicular to the ultrasound

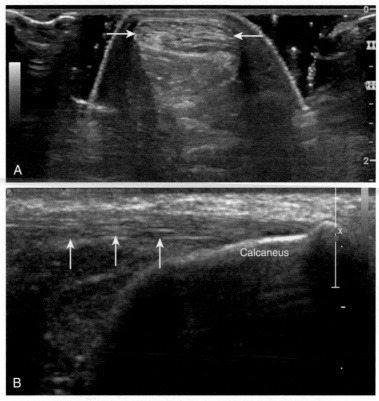

**Figure 63-1.** Normal appearance of Achilles tendon on US. **A,** In short axis, tendon appears speckled (*arrows*). **B,** In long axis, tendon appears fibrillar or striated (*arrows*).

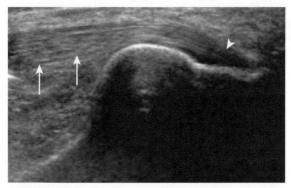

**Figure 63-2.** Anisotropy of Achilles tendon on US. Note that tendon perpendicular to ultrasound beam appears fibrillar and echogenic (*arrows*), whereas tendon insertion obliquely oriented with respect to ultrasound beam appears hypoechoic (*arrowhead*).

beam to exclude anisotropy as the cause of a focal hypoechoic defect. Anisotropy can be helpful in differentiating among normal soft tissue structures, especially in the ankle or wrist, where a hyperechoic tendon or ligament is often surrounded by hyperechoic soft tissues. Toggling or "heel-toeing" the transducer along the tendon or ligament will cause the structure to become hypoechoic, providing greater contrast from a background of hyperechoic fat which does not possess anisotropy (Figure 63-2).

7. **What is the normal sonographic appearance of various soft tissues (skin, subcutaneous fat, fascia, cortical bone, hyaline cartilage, fibrocartilage, and muscle)?**
The epidermis and dermis of the skin typically appear as a thin hyperechoic layer. Subcutaneous fat is hypoechoic with thin linear echogenic septations paralleling the skin surface. Fascia appears as a thin, linear hyperechoic layer with variable thickness. Cortical bone is very hyperechoic with posterior acoustic shadowing. Hyaline cartilage, which covers the articular surface of bone, is uniformly hypoechoic. This is in contrast to the fibrocartilaginous labrum and meniscus, which are hyperechoic (Figure 63-3). Normal muscle tissue appears relatively hypoechoic with interspersed

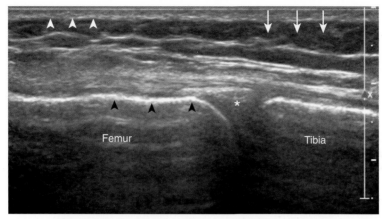

**Figure 63-3.** Normal appearance of soft tissues of medial knee on US. On this longitudinal image, skin appears uniformly thin and echogenic (*white arrowheads*) compared to underlying subcutaneous fat (*white arrows*), which is hypoechoic and traversed by thin echogenic septa. Cortical bone (*black arrowheads*) is thin and echogenic. Fibrocartilagenous meniscus (*) is echogenic.

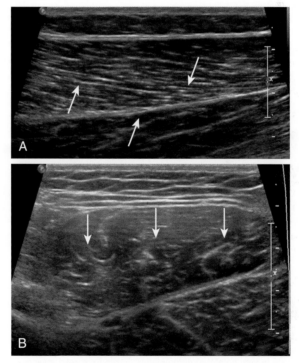

**Figure 63-4.** Normal appearance of muscle on US. **A,** In long axis, muscle has characteristic pennate appearance (*arrows*). **B,** In short axis, muscle has hypoechoic, loosely speckled, or "starry sky," appearance (*arrows*).

hyperechoic fibroadipose septa; in long axis, normal muscle has a pennate, or featherlike, appearance. In short axis, muscle demonstrates a characteristic "starry sky" appearance (Figure 63-4).

8. What is the normal echotexture of tendons and ligaments?
Normal tendons are hyperechoic with a signature fibrillar echotexture. Ligaments are also hyperechoic but can be differentiated from tendons due to their more compact, finely striated echotexture. Additionally, ligaments may be discerned from tendons as they connect two osseous structures (Figure 63-5).

9. What is the normal echotexture of peripheral nerves?
Peripheral nerves demonstrate a fascicular appearance in which individual nerve fascicles are hypoechoic. The hypoechoic fascicles are surrounded by hyperechoic connective tissue referred to as epineurium. Large peripheral nerves will often be surrounded by a rim of hyperechoic fat. Short axis imaging is often helpful to clarify that an

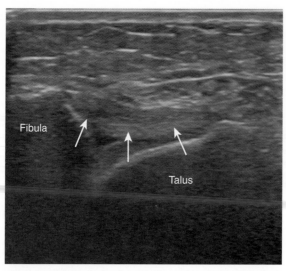

**Figure 63-5.** Normal appearance of anterior talofibular ligament on US. Ligament (*arrows*) is fibrillar and echogenic. Note that ligament fibers are more compact than tendon fibers shown in Figure 63-1.

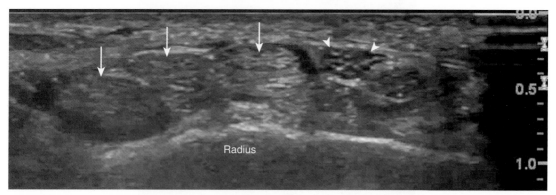

**Figure 63-6.** Normal appearance of median nerve and flexor tendons on US. At volar aspect of wrist, median nerve in short axis (*arrowheads*) appears as speckled or "honeycomb" hypoechoic structure, in contrast to adjacent flexor tendons (*arrows*), which appear hyperechoic.

interrogated structure indeed represents a nerve, because peripheral nerves display a characteristic speckled or honeycomb appearance in short axis (Figure 63-6).

10. **Which soft tissue masses can be diagnosed on US?**
    Although US findings are often nonspecific for the characterization of soft tissue masses, there are several instances in which US is diagnostic. US is very helpful at differentiating cystic from solid masses. A simple cyst should appear anechoic on US with increased through transmission and thin, nearly imperceptible walls. A mass is solid appearing with heterogeneous or homogeneous hypoechoic internal echotexture. The borders of a mass may be irregular or ill-defined. While a mass may be partially cystic, it should not be diffusely anechoic as with a simple cyst. In the case of a partially cystic mass, there is often irregular or nodular thickening of the walls or internal septations. Finally, a simple cyst should not have vascularity upon color or power Doppler imaging. Masses will often have increased blood flow either diffusely/centrally or at regions of septal/wall thickening. Masses that can frequently be diagnosed under US include: ganglion cyst, parameniscal cyst, lipoma, fat necrosis, peripheral nerve sheath tumor (PNST), and giant cell tumor of the tendon sheath (GCTTS).

11. **How can US differentiate between a ganglion cyst and a bursa?**
    Ganglion cysts associated with a tendon sheath (or joint) may appear unilocular or multilocular with multiple internal septations, and this appearance is not uncommon about the ankle, foot, wrist, and hand tendons (Figure 63-7). This unilocular appearance of a ganglion cyst may be differentiated from a bursa by dynamic compression with the transducer. Ganglion cysts are normally not compressible, and they should not arise at the expected location of a bursa. Bursae are easily compressible.

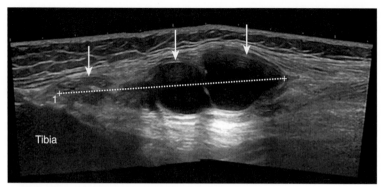

**Figure 63-7.** Ganglion cyst of proximal tibiofibular joint of knee on US. Note lobulated septated lesion (*arrows*) with both anechoic fluid distally and echogenic debris proximally, along with increased through transmission deep to anechoic part of cyst.

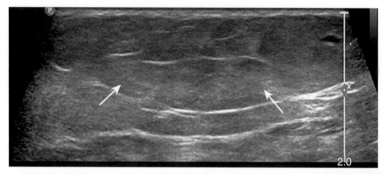

**Figure 63-8.** Lipoma on US. Note well-circumscribed lesion (*arrows*) that appears isoechoic to surrounding fat, which contains thin echogenic linear septations paralleling skin surface.

12. How can a ganglion cyst be differentiated from a parameniscal cyst on US?

Ganglion cysts may have a variety of appearances at US, but are noncompressible, are in close proximity to a tendon or joint, and do not have vascularity on Doppler imaging. Large ganglion cysts, defined as greater than 10 mm, often demonstrate the classic anechoic mulilobulated or multiloculated appearance with increased through transmission. However, small ganglion cysts, defined as less than 10 mm, often do not appear as simple cystic lesions but instead are hypoechoic without posterior acoustic enhancement. When attempting to differentiate a ganglion cyst from a cyst arising from fibrocartilage (paralabral or parameniscal), location is the key. Fibrocartilage cysts should be in contact with the labrum or menisci, while ganglion cysts are often located at the sinus tarsi in the ankle, superficial to the scapholunate ligament or near the radial artery in the wrist, or within Hoffa's (infrapatellar) fat pad of the knee.

13. What is the sonographic appearance of a lipoma?

Soft tissue lipomas may arise anywhere including within muscle, between tissue planes, or in subcutaneous fat. A lipoma residing in the subcutaneous tissue should be oval and homogeneously isoechoic or minimally hyperechoic. It is important to keep in mind that a simple lipoma does not have blood flow on Doppler imaging (Figure 63-8). With gentle transducer pressure, the lipoma should be soft and compressible, a finding of diagnostic value which is uniquely interrogated with sonographic evaluation. Intramuscular lipomas are generally seated more deeply and therefore are more difficult to fully evaluate with US. Although somewhat nonspecific appearing, an intramuscular lipoma is relatively hyperechoic to background muscle. Given the difficulty in evaluating the margins of an intramuscular lipoma and because a deep lipomatous tumor is more likely to be malignant than a superficial one, contrast-enhanced MRI is often obtained to confirm the diagnosis of an intramuscular lipoma.

14. What is an angiolipoma?

An angiolipoma is a vascular lipoma or hamartoma variant that one should consider when a small hyperechoic mass is present within the subcutaneous tissues. It is usually a small, slow-growing lesion that is most common in young men and may be painful and multiple approximately 50% of the time.

15. What is fat necrosis?

Subcutaneous fat necrosis is a benign process that often presents as a palpable subcutaneous nodule on the extremities or torso with or without an antecedent event. Two typical sonographic appearances have been ascribed to fat necrosis located within the subcutaneous soft tissues. The first is a well-defined isoechoic mass with a hypoechoic halo; the second is an ill-defined hyperechoic region.

16. What are the sonographic characteristics of a PNST?

When a solid mass is found to be contiguous with a peripheral nerve, one can confidently offer the diagnosis of a peripheral nerve sheath tumor. Given the high resolution of US, it is often used to definitively demonstrate peripheral nerve continuity with a mass. On US, a PNST is usually well defined, round/ovoid, and hypoechoic with scattered low-level internal echoes. While increased through transmission may initially lead one to mistake a PNST for a simple cyst, the presence of flow on color or power Doppler imaging is diagnostic of a solid mass. Finally, focal transducer pressure over the lesion will often elicit radicular symptoms, increasing the diagnostic accuracy of the US exam.

17. What is the sonographic appearance of a GCTTS?

GCTTS, or localized pigmented villonodular synovitis, has a characteristic appearance and location on US. This lesion is most often associated with the flexor tendon sheath of the finger and is at least partially in close contact with a tendon sheath; however, the lesion characteristically does not move with the tendon as the tendon is flexed and extended, because the mass is attached to the tendon sheath as opposed to the tendon itself. GCTTS is usually a solid-appearing, homogeneous and hypoechoic mass with detectable blood flow on Doppler imaging. Although this constellation of findings is commonly observed with GCTTS, these lesions may go on to soft tissue biopsy for a histologic diagnosis, especially if symptomatic.

18. When should a soft tissue mass detected on US be referred for MRI?

There are multiple indications for obtaining an MRI for further characterization of a soft tissue mass detected on US, including, but not limited to, those instances in which the lesion cannot be definitively diagnosed as a ganglion cyst or lipoma; does not definitively arise from a joint or synovial space; is greater than 5 cm in size; is very deep; demonstrates vascularity on Doppler imaging; is hypoechoic; shows complex echogenicity with irregular borders; invades fascial planes; or has soft tissue calcifications.

19. What is the appearance of a hematoma on US? How should hematomas be followed up?

A hematoma may have a variety of appearances on US depending on when it is imaged. If imaged acutely, a hematoma often appears as an ill-defined but predominantly hyperechoic collection. A subacute hematoma becomes more hypoechoic, although a heterogeneous appearance is common. A hematoma starts to resorb from the periphery inward, becoming smaller and more echogenic. In the end, a residual anechoic fluid collection or seroma may persist indefinitely. If a lesion demonstrates the typical sonographic features of a hematoma, follow-up is indicated if the lesion substantially enlarges or becomes symptomatic. A 6-week follow-up study is often obtained to document that the hematoma is resolving, because soft tissue tumors may present initially with intramuscular hemorrhage, which may mask the underlying lesion.

20. Describe the sonographic appearance of rotator cuff tendon pathology on US.

The spectrum of tendon pathology on US includes tendinosis, partial tear, full-thickness tear, and tenosynovitis, not just in the rotator cuff of the shoulder joint but in other sites as well. In the following examples, pathology of the supraspinatus tendon will be discussed. The normal supraspinatus tendon is demonstrated in Figure 63-9. Tendinosis indicates a degenerative process that may be focal or diffuse. Tendinosis is characterized by a swollen, hypoechoic tendon, with loss of the normal fibrillar architecture. There may be hyperemia on color Doppler imaging (Figure 63-10). It is important to distinguish tendinosis from anisotropy by making sure the portion of the tendon that is being evaluated is perpendicular to the ultrasound beam.

Partial-thickness tears may demonstrate a variety of appearances on US and often occur on a background of tendinosis. The most common appearance is a well-defined hypoechoic or anechoic cleft that partially disrupts the

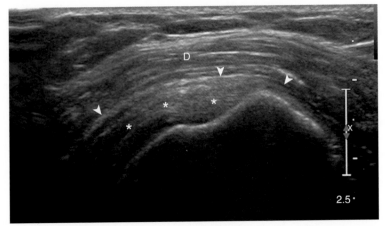

**Figure 63-9.** Normal supraspinatus tendon on US. Deltoid muscle (*D*) is seen deep to skin and subcutaneous fat. Subacromial-subdeltoid bursa is thin, curvilinear hypoechoic structure separated from overlying deltoid muscle by thin layer of echogenic bursal fat (*arrowheads*). Supraspinatus tendon (*) is seen in long axis deep to subacromial-subdeltoid bursa and inserts on greater tuberosity of humerus.

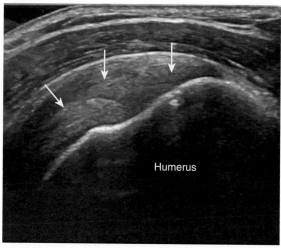

**Figure 63-10.** Tendinosis of supraspinatus tendon on US. Long axis image shows supraspinatus tendon to be thickened and hypoechoic (*arrows*). Compare this appearance to that of normal supraspinatus tendon in Figure 63-9.

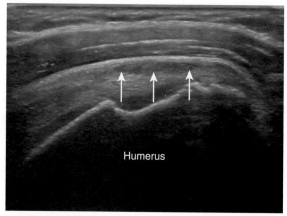

**Figure 63-11.** Partial-thickness tear of supraspinatus tendon on US. Long axis image demonstrates volume loss of supraspinatus tendon with hypoechoic defect (*arrows*) at bursal aspect of distal tendon at insertion on greater tuberosity.

tendon fibers. Types of partial-thickness tears include intrasubstance or delaminating tears, intrasubstance tearing at the tendon footprint, partial bursal sided tears, and partial articular sided tears (Figure 63-11). Full-thickness tears demonstrate full-thickness disruption of fibers with a fluid-filled gap. There may be retraction of the tendon fibers if the tear is large (Figure 63-12). There may also be hemorrhage or synovial hypertrophy filling the tendon gap.

Tenosynovitis is often mechanical or traumatic in nature and may be associated with underlying tendon pathology. Inflammatory/infectious etiologies may also result in tenosynovitis. On US, synovial tissue and/or fluid surrounds the tendon within the tendon sheath. The synovial tissue may appear isoechoic to hyperechoic to the adjacent tendon. A peripheral rim of hyperemia may be observed on Doppler imaging (Figure 63-13).

21. **What is the accuracy of US in the diagnosis of rotator cuff tears?**
    The diagnostic accuracy of US in evaluation of both partial- and full-thickness rotator cuff tears is comparable with MRI and highly correlates with arthroscopy, with a sensitivity and specificity of up to 95% when utilized by experienced operators.

22. **How is dynamic imaging useful in US?**
    One of the unique advantages US provides is the ability to image dynamically, resulting in real-time functional information regarding certain pathologies, which may only be confirmed upon performing provocative movements during sonographic examination. Several circumstances in which dynamic evaluation is crucial include, but are not limited to: subacromial impingement, biceps subluxation, snapping iliopsoas tendon, differentiation of partial from complete tears of the Achilles tendon, UCL tears in the elbow, UCL tears in the thumb including evaluation for a Stener lesion, and impingement of hardware on tendons (i.e., evaluation of a fixation plate and screws in the wrist or ankle).

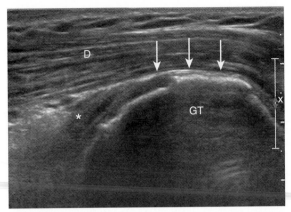

**Figure 63-12.** Full-thickness tear of supraspinatus tendon on US. Note tendon stump of supraspinatus tendon (*) retracted from footprint at greater tuberosity (*GT*) of humeral head. Humeral head directly contacts subacromial-subdeltoid bursa (*arrows*). Deltoid muscle (*D*) overlies subacromial-subdeltoid bursa.

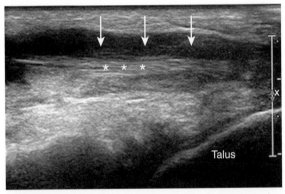

**Figure 63-13.** Tenosynovitis of extensor digitorum longus (EDL) tendon on US. Tendon sheath of EDL is distended with mixed echogenicity fluid and synovial hypertrophy (*arrows*). Fibrillar structure of EDL (*) can be seen.

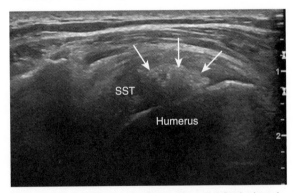

**Figure 63-14.** Calcific tendinosis of distal supraspinatus tendon on US. Amorphous ill-defined echogenic calcium deposit (*arrows*) is seen within supraspinatus tendon (*SST*).

23. What is the sonographic appearance of calcific tendinosis?

Calcific tendinopathy, or calcific tendinosis, is an extremely painful condition caused by the deposition of calcium hydroxyapatite within or around a tendon. Calcium hydroxyapatite on radiographs appears as amorphous calcific densities. On US, calcium hydroxyapatite appears echogenic. It may be either amorphous or well defined, with or without posterior shadowing (Figure 63-14). It most commonly occurs around the shoulder but can occur anywhere a tendon inserts on bone.

24. **What is the sonographic appearance of ligament pathology?**

Normal ligaments should appear hyperechoic with compact fibrillar fibers. A sprain or partial-thickness tear of a ligament appears as hypoechoic swelling and heterogeneity of the ligament, but without complete ligament fiber disruption. An acute full-thickness tear is characterized by discontinuity or nonvisualization of the ligament. In the expected location of the ligament, one will find heterogeneous or hyperechoic tissue that represents the torn ligament and hemorrhage. In cases for which differentiation of partial- from full-thickness tears is difficult, dynamic imaging may be employed to look for ligament fragments or joint widening. A chronic ligamentous injury may appear as either an abnormally attenuated or thickened, hypoechoic ligament that appears intact but then demonstrates laxity upon dynamic evaluation.

25. **What is the sonographic appearance of musculoskeletal infection?**

Infection of the superficial soft tissues, or cellulitis, has a variety of sonographic appearances depending on the time course of imaging. In the acute setting, cellulitis appears as swollen, hyperechoic subcutaneous tissue with hyperemia on color Doppler imaging (Figure 63-15). As time goes on, cellulitis may appear hypoechoic with the development of anechoic branching channels and distortion of soft tissue. In the setting of cellulitis, the observation of perifascial fluid and hyperechoic foci of gas with associated dirty shadowing and/or comet tail artifact may represent necrotizing fasciitis, a surgical emergency.

An abscess may have a variety of appearances on US but typically presents as a fairly well-defined hypoechoic, heterogeneous fluid collection with increased posterior acoustic enhancement and peripheral hyperemia on Doppler imaging (Figure 63-16). It is not uncommon to observe central foci/pockets of gas and a thickened, echogenic hyperemic abscess wall. The use of transducer pressure to induce the swirling of internal contents is helpful to differentiate an abscess from a seroma. Additionally, changing scanning parameters such as increasing the field of view and depth may make posterior acoustic enhancement through a suspected abscess appear more conspicuous compared to adjacent background structures.

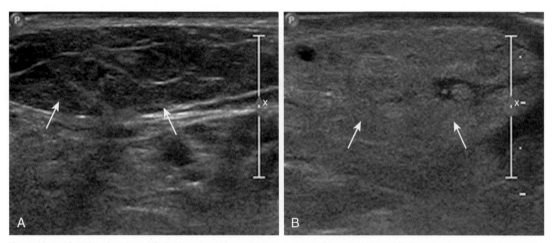

**Figure 63-15.** Cellulitis of ankle on US. **A,** Note normal hypoechoic fat (*arrows*) of normal ankle and **B,** Swollen hyperechoic subcutaneous fat (*arrows*) in contralateral cellulitic ankle.

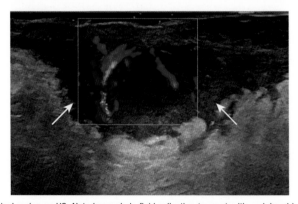

**Figure 63-16.** Abscess of inguinal region on US. Note hypoechoic fluid collection (*arrows*) with peripheral hyperemia on color Doppler imaging.

Septic bursitis refers to the involvement of a bursa by infection. On US, septic bursitis may appear as synovitis and complex fluid within a bursa. Rarely, foci of gas with associated comet tail artifact may be identified. When attempting to differentiate septic bursitis from an abscess, the most important thing to consider is location. Septic bursitis will occur in the location of a known bursa and often appear more well defined than an abscess. Infectious myositis may appear as an enlarged hypoechoic muscle with associated hyperemia. It is important to look for intramuscular fluid collections to exclude pyomyositis.

If the soft tissue infection is located adjacent to bone, osteomyelitis may be present. If US demonstrates cortical irregularity or erosions, it is important to consider osteomyelitis, which may be more fully characterized with MRI. Septic arthritis may appear identical to inflammatory arthritis upon US examination. If infection cannot be definitively excluded, direct sampling of joint fluid is indicated. In the setting of septic arthritis, fluid is identified distending a joint recess. Unfortunately, the appearance of the fluid (i.e., hypoechoic versus hyperechoic) and associated hyperemia is not useful in discerning between infection and inflammation.

26. **What are some common artifacts seen in musculoskeletal US?**

It is important to be aware of common artifacts that are often seen with musculoskeletal US, not only to avoid misinterpreting a finding, but also because artifacts may provide valuable diagnostic clues about underlying pathology. Posterior acoustic shadowing is present when the ultrasound beam is refracted, reflected, or absorbed, resulting in an anechoic region deep to a structure or interface. Several entities that may result in posterior acoustic shadowing include gas, bone, calcification, and even some foreign bodies. Posterior acoustic shadowing behind bone and calcifications is often referred to as "clean" shadowing and appears uniformly anechoic due to the majority of the ultrasound beam being absorbed (Figure 63-17). Posterior acoustic shadowing caused by gas is often referred to as "dirty" shadowing and results in multiple low-level echoes due to the degree of reflection at gas/tissue interfaces.

When comparing solid and fluid-containing structures, the ultrasound beam is gradually attenuated to a greater extent by a solid structure than by one containing fluid. Therefore, the strength of the ultrasound beam is greater after passing through fluid and results in stronger reflections which appear brighter than the reflections from the same interface located deep to solid tissues. This artifact is known as increased through transmission or posterior acoustic enhancement, and it appears on the image as a bright band extending deep to an object (see Figure 63-7). This artifact may be useful in distinguishing between cystic and solid masses, but it is important to understand that some solid masses (i.e., nerve sheath tumors) may attenuate sound less than the adjacent soft tissues, resulting in increased through transmission of a solid mass.

Reverberation is another commonly observed artifact in musculoskeletal US. Reverberation occurs when the ultrasound beam reflects off of a smooth and flat interface (i.e., bone, metal implant, etc.) and back to the transducer multiple times, resulting in a series of linear echoes extending deep to the smooth, flat interface. If the reflected echoes appear continuous deep to the flat interface, the term *ring down* is often used (Figure 63-18). This artifact makes US an important modality to evaluate soft tissues/structures adjacent to surgical hardware because ring down artifact occurs deep to the hardware and will not obscure superficial regions of interest.

Comet tail artifact is another form of reverberation which appears as a short trail of posterior bright echoes that narrow as they extend from the source of the artifact. This is often seen with soft tissue gas and allows for ease of identification.

Refraction is often seen as shadowing at the edge of a curved surface such as those typically present in cystic structures. Ultrasound waves oriented at a tangential angle to a cyst wall or curved surface are scattered and refracted, resulting in the appearance of a linear shadow due to a lack of echoes returning to the transducer from the lateral cyst wall and anything in a direct path posterior to it. Occasionally, this artifact may confuse the unwary into

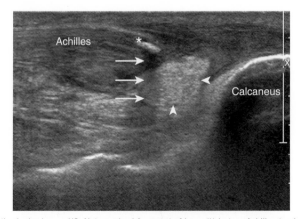

**Figure 63-17.** Posterior acoustic shadowing on US. Note avulsed fragment of bone (*) in torn Achilles tendon with associated posterior acoustic shadowing (*arrows*). Also note echogenic hemorrhage at site of Achilles tear (*arrowheads*).

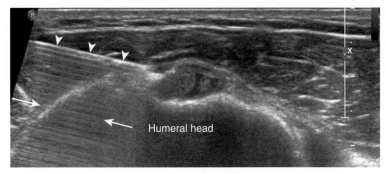

**Figure 63-18.** Reverberation artifact during biceps tendon sheath injection on US. As ultrasound beam bounces back and forth from echogenic needle (*arrowheads*) to transducer, reverberation artifact (*arrows*) results.

assuming a cystic structure has a defect within it. This spurious assumption is easily corrected by changing the angle of the ultrasound beam.

27. How is carpal tunnel syndrome diagnosed on US?

There are a variety of ways to evaluate for carpal tunnel syndrome with US. One of the most accurate methods is to calculate the difference between the cross-sectional area of the median nerve at the carpal tunnel and at the level of the pronator quadratus muscle. The most accurate diagnostic discrimination is achieved by using a change in cross-sectional area threshold of 2 mm, which has been reported to result in a sensitivity of 99% and specificity of 100% for the diagnosis of carpal tunnel syndrome.

## KEY POINTS

- The benefits of US include: absence of ionizing radiation; the ability to image patients who are not candidates for CT or MRI; high spatial resolution; dynamic imaging capability; functional assessment capability with Doppler imaging; and the ability to image patients with hardware.
- Anisotropy occurs when the ultrasound beam is not perpendicular to a fibrillar structure. This artifact can be corrected by toggling or "heel-toeing" the probe.
- Common indications for US include the evaluation of tendons and ligaments, muscles, bursae, and soft tissue masses.
- It is important to be aware of artifacts commonly seen in musculoskeletal US.
- US is useful for differentiating a cyst from a solid mass.

**BIBLIOGRAPHY**

Jacobson JA. *Fundamentals of musculoskeletal ultrasound.* 2nd ed. Philadelphia: Elsevier Saunders; 2013.
Wagner JM, Lee KS, Rosas H, et al. Accuracy of sonographic diagnosis of superficial masses. *J Ultrasound Med.* 2013;32(8):1443-1450.
Yablon CM, Bedi A, Morag Y, et al. Ultrasonography of the shoulder with arthroscopic correlation. *Clinics Sports Med.* 2013;32(3):391-408.
Adhikari S, Blaivas M. Sonography first for subcutaneous abscess and cellulitis evaluation. *J Ultrasound Med.* 2012;31(10):1509-1512.
Jamadar DA, Robertson BL, Jacobson JA, et al. Musculoskeletal sonography: important imaging pitfalls. *AJR Am J Roentgenol.* 2010;194(1):216-225.
Feldman MK, Katyal S, Blackwood MS. US artifacts. *Radiographics.* 2009;29(4):1179-1189.
Klauser AS, Halpern EJ, De Zordo T, et al. Carpal tunnel syndrome assessment with US: value of additional cross-sectional area measurements of the median nerve in patients versus healthy volunteers. *Radiology.* 2009;250(1):171-177.
Tuite MJ. Musculoskeletal ultrasound: its impact on your MR practice. *AJR Am J Roentgenol.* 2009;193(3):605-606.
Nazarian LN. The top 10 reasons musculoskeletal sonography is an important complementary or alternative technique to MRI. *AJR Am J Roentgenol.* 2008;190(6):1621-1626.
Walsh M, Jacobson JA, Kim SM, et al. Sonography of fat necrosis involving the extremity and torso with magnetic resonance imaging and histologic correlation. *J Ultrasound Med.* 2008;27(12):1751-1757.
del Cura JL, Torre I, Zabala R, et al. Sonographically guided percutaneous needle lavage in calcific tendinitis of the shoulder: short- and long-term results. *AJR Am J Roentgenol.* 2007;189(3):W128-W134.
Wang G, Jacobson JA, Feng FY, et al. Sonography of wrist ganglion cysts: variable and noncystic appearances. *J Ultrasound Med.* 2007;26(10):1323-1328, quiz 30-1.
Middleton WD, Patel V, Teefey SA, et al. Giant cell tumors of the tendon sheath: analysis of sonographic findings. *AJR Am J Roentgenol.* 2004;183(2):337-339.
Reynolds DL Jr, Jacobson JA, Inampudi P, et al. Sonographic characteristics of peripheral nerve sheath tumors. *AJR Am J Roentgenol.* 2004;182(3):741-744.

# CHAPTER 64

# VASCULAR ULTRASONOGRAPHY

*Courtney A. Woodfield, MD*

1. List some of the most common indications for vascular ultrasonography (US).
   Vascular ultrasound is commonly used to evaluate the following:
   - Extremity deep venous thrombosis.
   - Carotid artery stenosis.
   - Abdominal aortic aneurysm.
   - Renal artery stenosis.
   - Hepatic vasculature in the setting of cirrhosis and after transjugular intrahepatic portosystemic shunt (TIPS) placement.
   - Pseudoaneurysm and arteriovenous fistula.

2. How is vascular flow assessed with US?
   Flow within vessels is detected and displayed with the use of color and spectral Doppler imaging. Color Doppler US with pulsed spectral display allows for the presence or absence of flow to be displayed (as a color) as well as the direction, velocity, and character of the blood flow. The Doppler spectral display is the waveform in a vessel that depicts both the speed and direction of blood flow (i.e., velocity). By convention, the waveform for blood flowing toward the transducer is depicted above the zero velocity baseline, and the color in the vessel is displayed as red. In contrast, the waveform for blood flowing away from the transducer is displayed below the baseline, and the color in the vessel is displayed as blue.

3. What information can be obtained from the spectral Doppler waveform of a vessel?
   A spectral Doppler waveform of a vessel contains both quantitative and qualitative information regarding blood flow in the interrogated vessel. Quantitative measurements include absolute velocities (peak systolic velocity (PSV), end diastolic velocity [EDV]), velocity ratios, and acceleration times. Qualitative measurements include the shape of the waveform and spectral broadening (a sign of turbulent flow; when normal blood flow is disturbed, blood has a wider range of velocities).

4. How does spectral Doppler US detect vascular stenosis?
   Velocity measurements in a vessel help to detect stenosis. As a vessel narrows, the velocity in the vessel increases at the point of stenosis in order to maintain the same rate of blood flow through the stenosed region. The degree of vessel stenosis correlates best with the PSV measurement when the stenosis is >50%, such that the greater the degree of stenosis the higher the PSV in the waveform. Another measure of stenosis or resistance in a vascular bed is the resistive index (RI): $RI = (S-D)/S$, where S is the PSV of blood flow in a vessel and D is the EDV. PSV and EDV can both be used to evaluate blood flow in a vessel when the direction of flow can be clearly identified (i.e., in the carotid artery), whereas RI is more commonly used when the direction of flow cannot be identified (e.g., with renal transplant vascularity). Table 64-1 outlines the characteristic changes of an arterial waveform in relation to a stenosis.

5. Describe the normal spectral Doppler waveform in a low-resistance artery.
   Flow within arteries supplying organs that require constant perfusion include arteries to the brain, liver, and kidneys. The waveforms in these arteries will have continuous monophasic forward flow toward the organ throughout diastole. They have broad systolic peaks, gradual transition between systole and diastole, and persistent diastolic flow (Figure 64-1). Low-resistance vessels will also have low RIs.

6. Describe the normal spectral Doppler waveform in a high-resistance artery.
   Flow within arteries supplying structures with variable flow demands, such as the extremities at rest and the bowel during fasting, have higher resistance triphasic waveforms. These waveforms are characterized by narrow systolic

**Table 64-1.** Arterial Stenosis Spectral Doppler Waveform Changes

| LOCATION | PSV | DIASTOLIC FLOW | OTHER |
|---|---|---|---|
| Proximal to stenosis | Decreased | Decreased | |
| At stenosis | Increased | Increased | Turbulence with spectral broadening |
| Distal to stenosis | Decreased | Decreased | Decreased acceleration time; tardus parvus |

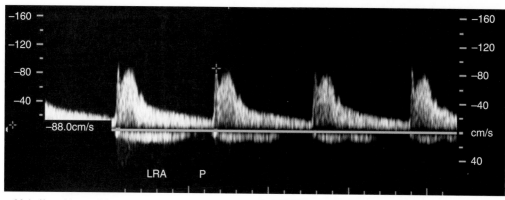

**Figure 64-1.** Normal low-resistance spectral Doppler waveform of main renal artery with broad systolic peak, gradual transition between systole and diastole, and persistent forward diastolic flow.

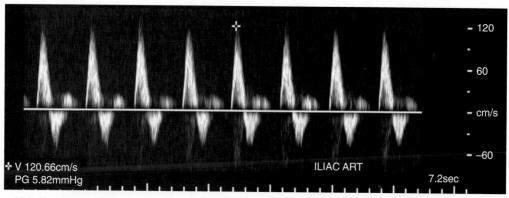

**Figure 64-2.** Normal high-resistance spectral Doppler waveform of external iliac artery with narrow systolic peak, abrupt transition between systole and diastole, transient reversal of diastolic flow, and return of low-level forward flow during rest of diastole.

peaks, followed by an abrupt transition between systole and diastole with transient reversal of diastolic flow, and then a return of low-level forward flow during the rest of diastole (Figure 64-2).

7. **Describe the normal spectral Doppler waveform in a vein.**
   Veins typically have low-level monophasic waveforms. There can be some pulsatility of the waveform in veins closer to the heart, such as the hepatic veins. A normal vein in the extremity will also have some respiratory and cardiac waveform variability.

8. **How is extremity deep vein thrombosis diagnosed sonographically?**
   US is the initial imaging study of choice for evaluating suspected upper or lower extremity deep vein thrombosis (DVT). In symptomatic patients, the sensitivity and specificity of US for DVT is at least 95% and 98%, respectively. The most important sonographic feature used to diagnose DVT is venous compressibility. Normally, the deep extremity veins are fully compressible (Figure 64-3). In contrast, thrombosed veins will not fully compress (Figure 64-4). The gray scale luminal echogenicity of the vein is less reliable, because normal veins can have artifactual low-level echoes and intraluminal clot can be hypoechoic or anechoic. Color Doppler US depicts venous thrombus as a filling defect or absence of flow.

   Additional color Doppler features that can be assessed include spontaneous and phasic venous flow in response to augmentation. A venous waveform that lacks normal respiratory phasicity can indicate venous obstruction superior to that site. Similarly, compression of veins inferior to the vein being examined normally increases flow on spectral display. Lack of increased flow with augmentation indicates venous obstruction somewhere in between the site of compression and the Doppler site.

9. **Can US differentiate between acute and chronic deep vein thrombosis?**
   US with color spectral Doppler imaging cannot reliably differentiate between acute and chronic DVT, because in both cases the vein is not fully compressible. However, in general, as acute thrombus ages, it reorganizes and retracts. Sonographically, this can appear as irregular wall thickening, calcified retracted thrombus, decreased vein diameter, and presence of collateral veins.

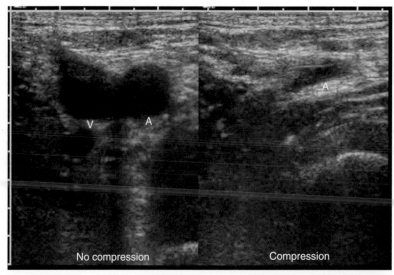

**Figure 64-3.** Normal venous compression on US. Transverse gray scale US image of left common femoral artery (*A*) and vein (*V*) without compression and with compression. The normal vein completely collapses with compression.

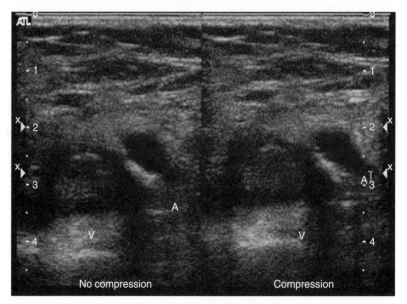

**Figure 64-4.** Acute deep venous thrombosis on US. Transverse gray scale US images of left common femoral artery (*A*) and vein (*V*) without compression and with compression demonstrate lack of compressibility of vein with echogenic luminal thrombus.

10. How is venous insufficiency evaluated sonographically?

Venous insufficiency is most commonly due to valvular damage from a DVT. In the lower extremities, venous insufficiency is best assessed sonographically with the patient in the upright position with provocative maneuvers (i.e., Valsalva and calf squeezing). Color spectral Doppler waveforms are obtained of both deep and superficial veins to the level of the knee. Normally, after calf squeezing, flow in the veins is antegrade with a very short period of flow reversal as returning blood closes the first competent venous valve. In contrast, insufficient veins will have a longer and greater degree of flow reversal (i.e., >2 sec). The time used to quantify abnormal flow reversal is institution dependent and needs to be validated at each institution.

11. Name the common indications for carotid artery US.
- Evaluation of patients with transient ischemic attacks or cerebrovascular accident.
- Evaluation of carotid bruit or pulsatile neck mass.
- Follow-up for known carotid artery stenosis or dissection.
- Follow-up after carotid endarterectomy or stenting.
- Preoperative screening prior to major vascular surgery.

12. How are the extracranial carotid arteries evaluated sonographically?

Sonographic evaluation of the carotid arteries in the neck involves gray scale imaging to detect wall thickening, plaque, and the degree of luminal narrowing. Color spectral Doppler imaging is used to demonstrate the presence and direction of blood flow as well as the velocity of blood flow. Normally, the internal carotid artery (ICA) has low-resistance flow, whereas the normal external carotid artery (ECA) has high-resistance flow, and the common carotid artery (CCA) is a hybrid waveform of the ICA and ECA.

13. What are the sonographic criteria for diagnosing extracranial carotid artery stenosis?

The presence and amount of carotid plaque, the PSV in the ICA and CCA, the EDV in the ICA, and the ratio of the ICA PSV to the CCA PSV are all used to detect and quantify the degree of carotid artery stenosis. Greater than 50% narrowing of the ICA is considered a stenosis, and greater than 70% narrowing is typically associated with symptoms where carotid endarterectomy is considered. The ultrasound criteria for 50% stenosis of the ICA is an ICA PSV >125 cm/sec and/or an ICA/CCA PSV ratio >2.0 (Figure 64-5). The ultrasound criteria for 70% to 99% stenosis is an ICA PSV >230 cm/sec and/or an ICA/CCA PSV ratio >4.0. All of these sonographic grading criteria are based on the North American Symptomatic Carotid Endarterectomy Trial (NASCET). Distal to a high-grade stenosis, there may be a tardus parvus waveform.

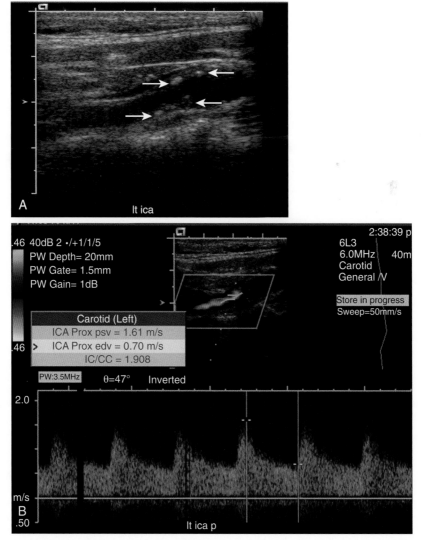

**Figure 64-5.** Internal carotid artery (ICA) stenosis on US. **A,** Sagittal gray scale US image of proximal left ICA shows moderate mixed soft and calcified plaque (*arrows*). **B,** Sagittal color spectral Doppler image demonstrates peak systolic velocity in left proximal ICA of 161 cm/ sec corresponding to 50% to 69% stenosis based on NASCET criteria.

14. **Define the carotid artery "string" sign.**

Severe narrowing of the ICA such that only a small amount of residual flow is seen along the almost completely occluded (>95% stenosis) artery lumen is referred to as the "string" sign. Such a high-grade ICA stenosis needs to be distinguished from a completely occluded ICA because a patient with a high-grade stenosis is still a surgical candidate for endarterectomy, whereas a patient with complete ICA occlusion is not an endarterectomy candidate. Strict attention to sonographic technique is required so as not to mistake subtotal ICA occlusion with slow flow from complete ICA occlusion.

15. **Can US detect subclavian steal syndrome?**

A routine component of the carotid artery US examination is demonstration of the patency, direction of flow, and waveform of the vertebral arteries in the neck. Normally, the vertebral arteries demonstrate monophasic antegrade flow toward the head. Biphasic or complete reversal of flow away from the head in the vertebral artery is an indication of subclavian artery stenosis proximal to the origin of the vertebral artery. In this case, the subclavian artery "steals" blood from the ipsilateral vertebral artery with retrograde flow down the vertebral artery supplying the subclavian artery distal to the point of subclavian stenosis.

16. **Is there a role for US in evaluating abdominal aortic aneurysms (AAAs)?**

US is often used as a screening tool for patients at increased risk for an AAA or to monitor patients with a known AAA. Sonographically, the proximal, mid, and distal abdominal aorta are imaged, and their greatest outer diameters are measured in the sagittal and transverse planes. Similar to cross-sectional imaging, an outer abdominal aorta diameter >3.0 cm is considered to indicate an aneurysm. Normally, the abdominal aorta waveform is triphasic, becoming lower resistance with dilation. US can also evaluate the presence and extent of mural thrombus along the abdominal aorta. If intervention is planned for an AAA, computed tomographic angiography (CTA) or magnetic resonance angiography (MRA) is also typically performed to obtain precise measurements regarding the size of the abdominal aorta and iliac arteries, relationship of the AAA to the renal arteries, as well as the patency of abdominal aorta branch vessels.

17. **What is the role of US in diagnosing renovascular hypertension?**

Patients with difficult to control severe hypertension are the group most likely to have hypertension on the basis of main renal artery stenosis (RAS). RAS only accounts for up to 5% of all patients with hypertension but is a potentially curable cause of hypertension. US can be used as an initial screening test for main RAS. It has the advantage of being relatively less expensive and not requiring intravenous contrast material to image the main renal arteries as compared to CTA or MRA of the kidneys. However, it has the disadvantages of a higher technical failure rate due to high operator dependence. The normal main renal artery has a rapid systolic upstroke and continuous diastolic flow. Color spectral Doppler findings of main RAS are a PSV in the main renal artery >200 cm/sec and/or a main renal/aortic PSV ratio >3.5. Detection of a parvus tardus waveform (small-amplitude waveform with a prolonged systolic rise) in more distal intrarenal arteries also suggests more proximal main RAS (Figure 64-6).

18. **What is the role of vascular US in evaluating renal transplants?**

US with color spectral Doppler imaging is the preferred initial study of choice for screening transplanted kidneys for vascular complications, as potentially nephrotoxic contrast agents are not required as in the case of CT or MR imaging. In addition to detecting main RAS in the transplant kidney, vascular US also screens for direct and indirect signs of main renal vein thrombosis. In the immediate post-transplant period, acute tubular necrosis and acute transplant rejection can both result in elevated RIs and low or absent diastolic flow in the intrarenal arteries. Elevated RIs in the late post-transplant period are most commonly due to chronic rejection or cyclosporine toxicity.

19. **Describe the normal hepatic spectral Doppler waveforms.**

The normal hepatic artery has a rapid systolic upstroke and continuous diastolic flow. The normal portal veins have continuous hepatopedal (toward the liver) flow with mild phasicity due to respiratory and cardiac activity. Normal portal vein velocity is approximately 20 cm/sec. Due to proximity to the heart, the normal hepatic veins have multiphasic waveforms secondary to transmitted cardiac pulsation with prominent antegrade systolic and diastolic waves, with small retrograde waves after both systole and diastole reflecting right atrial overfilling against a closed tricuspid valve after systole and atrial contraction after diastole.

20. **What various vascular complications can be detected with color spectral Doppler imaging of the liver?**

Similar to renal transplants, US is commonly the first study of choice for detecting vascular complications following liver transplantation. US can detect hepatic artery stenosis as a PSV >200 to 300 cm/sec in the artery. More distally, an intrahepatic tardus parvus waveform may be detected. Portal hypertension in both the native and transplant liver results in progressively slower flow and eventually hepatofugal (away from the liver) flow in the portal vein (Figure 64-7). The main portal vein may also increase in diameter (>13 mm) with portal hypertension. Portal vein thrombosis with absence of color spectral Doppler flow is also readily detected with US. Alterations of the normal hepatic venous waveform can also reflect both cardiac (i.e., tricuspid regurgitation, congestive heart failure) and hepatic parenchymal disease (i.e., cirrhosis, steatosis).

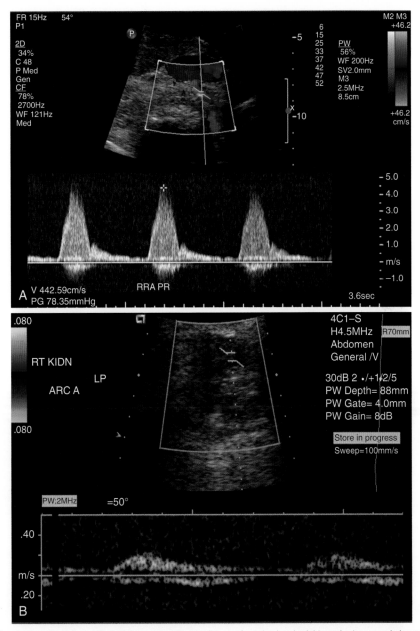

**Figure 64-6.** Renal artery stenosis on US. **A,** Color spectral Doppler image of proximal main right renal artery reveals increased peak systolic velocity of 443 cm/sec. **B,** Color spectral Doppler image of more distal right intrarenal artery shows diminished amplitude tardus parvus waveform.

21. When and how should US be used to evaluate a transjugular intrahepatic portosystemic shunt (TIPS)?

Color spectral Doppler US is the initial study of choice for evaluating a TIPS used to treat portal hypertension. The TIPS procedure consists of placing a stent between the higher pressure portal system and the lower pressure hepatic veins. A TIPS is most commonly placed between the right portal vein and the right hepatic vein, with resulting hepatopedal flow in the main and right portal veins, but hepatofugal flow in the left portal vein and the anterior and posterior branches of the right portal vein, as all the portal veins now flow toward the TIPS (Figure 64-8). The most common complication of TIPS is stent stenosis. US is used to routinely monitor TIPS and detect early stent stenosis to allow for stent recanalization before clot matures and the stent fully occludes, which would necessitate a second TIPS. Normal flow in a patent TIPS is turbulent, with mean PSV of 95 to 120 cm/sec but potentially up to 190 cm/sec. Higher and lower PSV in the stent or a significant change in stent PSV (i.e., >40 to 60 cm/sec change) compared to a prior

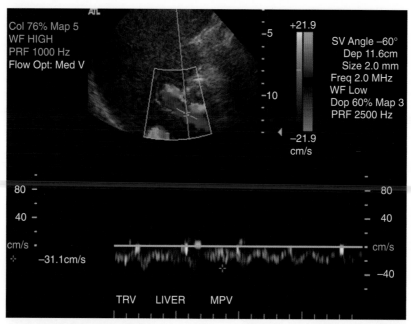

**Figure 64-7.** Portal hypertension on US. Color spectral Doppler image of main portal vein illustrates abnormal reversal of blood flow (below baseline) in portal vein away from liver (hepatofugal).

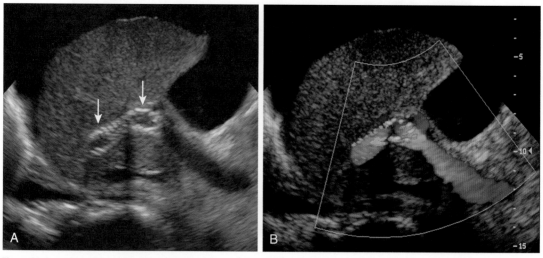

**Figure 64-8.** Transjugular intrahepatic portosystemic shunt (TIPS) on US. **A,** Transverse gray scale US image of liver demonstrates TIPS (*arrows*). **B,** Color Doppler image shows flow throughout shunt directed toward heart.

ultrasound examination also suggests a stent stenosis. A late sign of TIPS stenosis is a change in the direction of flow in the portal veins from toward the stent (hepatofugal) to away from the stent (hepatopedal).

22. **What are the ultrasound features of an arteriovenous fistula (AVF)?**
An AVF can occur anywhere in the body but most commonly occurs in the groin following arterial puncture of the femoral artery for a cardiac catheterization procedure or in the kidney following renal biopsy. Direct visualization of the fistula may be difficult, and therefore diagnosis typically relies on identifying color spectral Doppler changes to the arterial and venous waveforms proximal to the puncture site. Direct communication between an artery and vein results in a high-velocity, low-resistance (increased diastolic flow) waveform in the feeding artery and turbulent, pulsatile flow in the draining vein (Figure 64-9). Color Doppler may also demonstrate perivascular vibration, due to turbulent blood flow, as a mix of random red and blue color in the soft tissues around the fistula site.

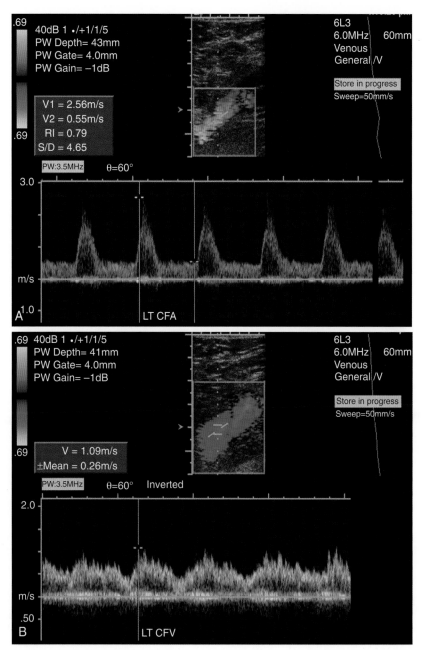

**Figure 64-9.** Common femoral AVF on US. **A,** Color spectral Doppler image of feeding common femoral artery shows high-velocity, low-resistance (increased diastolic flow) waveform. **B,** Color spectral Doppler image of draining common femoral vein shows turbulent and pulsatile flow.

23. How is a pseudoaneurysm diagnosed sonographically?

A pseudoaneurysm results from laceration of an artery, again most commonly seen in the groin following femoral artery puncture and in the kidney following percutaneous renal biopsy. On gray scale imaging, a pseudoaneurysm typically appears as an ovoid, hypoechoic collection adjacent to the artery. Color Doppler imaging then further distinguishes this hypoechoic collection from a more common postprocedural hematoma. A hematoma will have no detectable color Doppler flow, whereas a pseudoaneurysm demonstrates a characteristic "yin-yang" appearance of intraluminal swirling blood as blood flows into the pseudoaneurysm along one side and out along the other. Thus, one half of the pseudoaneurysm lumen is red and the other half is blue on color Doppler imaging. The characteristic spectral Doppler waveform of a pseudoaneurysm is a "to-and-fro" flow pattern at the pseudoaneurysm neck, as blood enters the pseudoaneurysm sac during systole and exits during diastole (Figure 64-10).

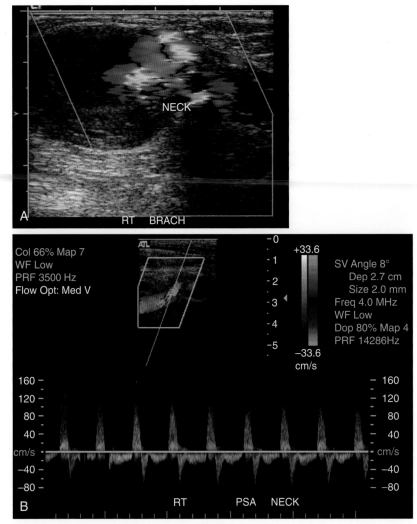

**Figure 64-10.** Pseudoaneurysm on US. **A,** Color Doppler image demonstrates partially thrombosed pseudoaneurysm of brachial artery with "yin-yang" flow. **B,** Color spectral Doppler image of common femoral artery in different patient illustrates classic "to-and-fro" flow waveform detected at neck of pseudoaneurysm.

24. **Can US be used to treat pseudoaneurysms?**
    There are two main nonsurgical means of treating a pseudoaneurysm, both based on US. Ultrasound-guided direct transcutaneous pressure can be held over the neck of the pseudoaneurysm to thrombose and close off the neck. However, this can be a time-consuming and painful method with variable success rates. A more popular method now used is ultrasound-guided direct injection of thrombin into the pseudoaneurysm with a success rate of up to 90%.

## KEY POINTS

- The most important sonographic feature for diagnosing deep venous thrombosis is lack of or incomplete venous compressibility.
- Sonographic criteria for quantifying the degree of extracranial internal carotid artery stenosis is based on the North American Symptomatic Carotid Endarterectomy Trial (NASCET) criteria.
- US is often the first study of choice to evaluate the hepatic and renal vasculature in the settings of renal or liver transplantation, renal hypertension, and cirrhosis with portal hypertension or after TIPS placement.
- Classic secondary US signs of an arteriovenous fistula (which are often hard to directly visualize) are a high-velocity, low-resistance (increased diastolic flow) waveform in the feeding artery and turbulent, pulsatile flow in the draining vein.
- US can be used to both diagnose and treat pseudoaneurysms.

## BIBLIOGRAPHY

Bluth El, Carroll BA. The extracranial cerebral vessels. In: Rumack CM, Wilson SR, Charboneau JW, et al., eds. *Diagnostic ultrasound*. 4th ed. Philadelphia: Mosby Elsevier; 2011:948-997.

Ettore AS, Lewis BD. The peripheral veins. In: Rumack CM, Wilson SR, Charboneau JW, et al., eds. *Diagnostic ultrasound*. 4th ed. Philadelphia: Mosby Elsevier; 2011:1023-1039.

Polak JF, Alessi-Chinetti JM. The peripheral arteries. In: Rumack CM, Wilson SR, Charboneau JW, et al., eds. *Diagnostic ultrasound*. 4th ed. Philadelphia: Mosby Elsevier; 2011:998-1022.

Wood MM, Romine LE, Lee YK, et al. Spectral Doppler signature waveforms in ultrasonography: a review of normal and abnormal waveforms. *Ultrasound Q*. 2010;26(2):83-99.

Arger PH, DeBari-Iyoob S. *The complete guide to vascular ultrasound*. 1st ed. Philadelphia: Lippincott Williams & Wilkins; 2004.

Grant EG, Benson CB, Moneta GL, et al. Carotid artery stenosis: gray-scale and Doppler US diagnosis—Society of Radiologists in Ultrasound Consensus Conference. *Radiology*. 2003;229(2):340-346.

# PATIENT SEDATION AND PAIN MANAGEMENT

*Charles T. Lau, MD, MBA, and S. William Stavropoulos, MD*

# CHAPTER 65

1. **What is the purpose of sedation and pain management during an interventional radiology procedure?**
   The purpose is to enable a patient to tolerate a potentially painful procedure yet still maintain satisfactory cardiopulmonary function and the ability to cooperate with verbal commands and tactile stimuli.

2. **What is the difference between analgesia and anesthesia?**
   Analgesia is the relief of pain without alteration of a patient's state of awareness. Anesthesia is the state of unconsciousness.

3. **What is the difference between anxiolysis and amnesia?**
   Anxiolysis is the relief of fear or anxiety without alteration of awareness. Amnesia is the loss of memory.

4. **What capabilities should the patient maintain during conscious sedation?**
   The patient should:
   - Remain responsive and cooperative.
   - Maintain spontaneous ventilation.
   - Be able to protect the airway.
   - Maintain protective reflexes.

5. **Describe the levels of patient sedation.**
   The levels of patient sedation exist along a continuum: light sedation, moderate sedation, deep sedation, and general anesthesia. A patient under light sedation can respond to stimuli and maintains intact airway reflexes. A patient under moderate sedation should maintain spontaneous ventilation and be able to protect the airway. A patient under deep sedation can respond to vigorous stimuli but may lack airway reflexes. A patient under general anesthesia has no response to stimuli and lacks all protective reflexes.

6. **List the details that should be included in the presedation evaluation of a patient.**
   - Patient medical history.
   - Previous adverse experience to sedation or anesthesia.
   - Current medication use and drug allergies.
   - Time and nature of last oral intake.
   - History of alcohol or substance abuse.
   - Focused physical examination including heart, lungs, and airway.
   - Pertinent clinical laboratory findings.

7. **How long should a patient typically fast before undergoing conscious sedation?**
   A patient should not have solid foods for 6 to 8 hours and clear liquids for 2 to 3 hours before undergoing sedation.

8. **The physical status of a patient is often measured on a 6-point scale, known as the American Society of Anesthesiologists (ASA) Physical Status (PS) classification. Describe this scale.**
   - ASA I: Normal healthy patient.
   - ASA II: Patient with mild systemic disease, without substantive functional limitations.
   - ASA III: Patient with severe systemic disease, with substantive functional limitations.
   - ASA IV: Patient with severe systemic disease that is life-threatening.
   - ASA V: Moribund patient with a poor chance for survival without surgery.
   - ASA VI: Declared brain-dead patient whose organs are being removed for donor purposes.

9. **Commonly, conscious sedation is administered by the provider (e.g., interventional radiologist) with patient monitoring provided by a qualified nurse. What patient factors should influence a provider to consider consulting an anesthesiologist to administer conscious sedation?**
   Patient factors should include:
   - ASA PS classification of III, IV, or V.
   - Obesity.
   - Pregnancy.
   - Mental incapacity.
   - Extremes of age.

10. **What patient factors must be monitored during conscious sedation?**
Level of consciousness, ventilation, oxygenation, and blood pressure should be monitored, along with continuous cardiac monitoring.

11. **What equipment must be present when administering conscious sedation to a patient?**
A patient undergoing conscious sedation should be under direct observation until recovery is complete. Equipment needed to monitor oxygenation; blood pressure; and heart rate, rhythm, and waveform should be present. Pharmacologic antagonists and commonly used agents, supplemental oxygen, a defibrillator, and appropriate equipment to establish airway and provide positive-pressure ventilation need to be readily available.

12. **What pharmacologic agents are commonly used for patients undergoing conscious sedation? What is their reversal agent?**
Benzodiazepines are typically used to provide conscious sedation. Common benzodiazepines include midazolam, lorazepam, and diazepam. Flumazenil is used as a reversal agent for benzodiazepines. The effect of flumazenil is usually visible in 2 minutes, with peak effects at 10 minutes.

13. **What are the usual effects of benzodiazepines?**
Benzodiazepines produce sedation and amnesia but do not provide analgesia. Significant adverse effects of benzodiazepines include respiratory and cardiovascular depression. Paradoxic reactions can occur with benzodiazepines and are more common in the elderly.

14. **What pharmacologic agents are commonly used for pain control? What is their reversal agent?**
Opiates are commonly used to provide pain control. Commonly used opiates include fentanyl, morphine, and meperidine. Naloxone is used as a reversal agent for opiates and is typically administered intravenously. The effect of naloxone is usually visible in 2 to 3 minutes. However, its duration of action may be substantially shorter than many long-acting opiates, and repeated dosing may be necessary.

15. **What are the typical effects of opiates?**
Opiates provide systemic analgesia, mild anxiolysis, and mild sedation. Opiates do not induce amnesia.

16. **What pharmacologic agent used for pain control is contraindicated in patients taking a monoamine oxidase (MAO) inhibitor?**
Meperidine administered to patients taking MAO inhibitors can cause various undesirable and potentially lethal side effects and is contraindicated. Side effects include agitation, fever, and seizures progressing in some instances to coma, apnea, and death. The narcotic analgesic of choice for patients taking MAO inhibitors is morphine.

17. **What are the strategies to manage a patient who has a known hypersensitivity to iodinated contrast material?**
Adverse reactions to iodinated contrast material range from nuisance side effects such as hives and emesis to potentially lethal reactions such as anaphylaxis and laryngeal edema. Patients with a history of even a minor hypersensitivity reaction to iodinated contrast material may be at increased risk for a severe reaction, and special precautions should be exercised when administering iodinated contrast material to these patients. Premedication of the patient with oral corticosteroids and the use of low-osmolar contrast agents may reduce the risk of minor reactions, but no randomized controlled clinical trials have shown that these protect against severe life-threatening adverse reactions to iodinated contrast material. Alternative contrast agents, such as gadolinium-based agents, $CO_2$, or both, may be used in patients with a history of severe iodinated contrast material reactions. If iodinated contrast material must be used in a patient with a history of bronchospasm, laryngeal edema, or anaphylaxis, it may be prudent to have an anesthesiologist standing by.

18. **List possible options for the management of an acute vasovagal reaction.**
Normal saline, lactated Ringer's solution, or atropine may be given intravenously.

19. **What is the basic life support sequence of steps for patient resuscitation?**
Advanced Cardiac Life Support (ACLS) guidelines provide a series of algorithms regarding distressed patients in various clinical settings. The basic life support sequence of steps for resuscitation is a core part of these algorithms. Intervention in a patient with an unstable condition begins with the assessment of **C**irculation (heart rate and blood pressure), establishment of an **A**irway, followed by assessment of **B**reathing (ventilation). This C-A-B sequence was introduced in 2010 to emphasize the importance of starting chest compressions as soon as possible and represents a change from the original A-B-C (Airway, Breathing, Circulation) sequence.

20. **Describe the management of acute hypotension.**
During conscious sedation, an overdose of either a benzodiazepine or an opiate may cause respiratory depression that manifests as acute hypotension. Vigorous stimulation (sternal rub) may remedy the situation. If not, pharmacologic reversal may be needed. If hypoxia is not the etiology of the hypotension, evaluation of a patient's heart rate provides a simple algorithm for treating acute hypotension. A vasovagal reaction should be suspected if the patient is bradycardic, and treatment should proceed accordingly. If the patient is tachycardic, one should immediately evaluate for a source of blood loss. A fluid challenge with normal saline may help determine whether a patient has intravascular

volume depletion. Pharmacologic intervention with epinephrine or dopamine may be indicated if the patient fails to respond to the fluid challenge. A complete algorithm for treating hypotension can be found in the ACLS guidelines.

21. List possible options for the management of an acute hypertensive crisis.
During a procedure, pain and anxiety may precipitate hypertension. A benzodiazepine such as midazolam, mixed with an opiate such as fentanyl, is likely to decrease the blood pressure of an uncomfortable or anxious patient. To treat a patient in true hypertensive crisis, further pharmacologic intervention may be needed. Intravenous labetalol often normalizes blood pressure. Sublingual nitroglycerin and intravenous furosemide are other agents that may also be useful in this setting.

22. How is acute pulmonary edema managed?
Pulmonary edema interferes with the ability to oxygenate blood. Therapy consists of securing an airway, providing supplemental oxygen, and administering intravenous furosemide or other agents to induce diuresis.

23. Describe the immediate options for management of an anaphylactic reaction.
An anaphylactic reaction can be rapidly fatal. An airway should be secured immediately, and oxygen should be administered. The mainstay of therapy consists of epinephrine. Additional therapy may include intravenous fluid resuscitation for pressure support, diphenhydramine, methylprednisolone, and dopamine. Cardiopulmonary resuscitation may also be required.

24. Describe the immediate options for management of acute laryngeal edema.
Laryngeal edema may lead to airway obstruction and death. An airway should be established, oxygen is provided, and epinephrine is administered immediately.

25. Describe the immediate options for management of bronchospasm.
The patient should be monitored closely, and oxygen should be administered by nasal cannula or face mask. Pharmacologic treatment may include albuterol or epinephrine. In severe cases, intubation may be required.

26. What are possible options for the management of generalized urticaria?
A patient with generalized urticaria can be treated with either diphenhydramine or epinephrine. Vital signs should be obtained, and the patient should be observed to ensure that a more severe reaction is not evolving. The reaction should be documented in the patient's medical record.

---

## KEY POINTS

- Proper equipment and qualified personnel should be readily available prior to administration of conscious sedation to any patient.
- A patient under moderate sedation should maintain spontaneous ventilation and be able to protect the airway.
- Flumazenil is used as a reversal agent for benzodiazepines, whereas naloxone is used as a reversal agent for opiates.
- The basic life support sequence of steps for patient resuscitation (C-A-B) includes assessment of **C**irculation (heart rate and blood pressure), establishment of an **A**irway, and assessment of **B**reathing (ventilation).
- The main medication used to treat an anaphylactic reaction is epinephrine. Other therapies may include fluid resuscitation, diphenhydramine, methylprednisolone, and dopamine.

**BIBLIOGRAPHY**

John-Nwankwo J. *ACLS provider manual: study guide for advanced cardiovascular life support.* 1st ed. North Charleston, SC: CreateSpace Independent Publishing Platform; 2016.

ASA Physical Status Classification System. American Society of Anesthesiologists, 2014. Available at: <http://www.asahq.org/~/media/sites/asahq/files/public/resources/standards-guidelines/asa-physical-status-classification-system.pdf#search=%22physical%20classification%22>.

ACR Manual on Contrast Media, Version 9. ACR Committee on Drugs and Contrast Media, 2013. Available at: <http://www.acr.org/~/media/ACR/Documents/PDF/QualitySafety/Resources/Contrast%20Manual/2013_Contrast_Media.pdf>.

Sinz E, Navarro K, Soderberg ES. *Advanced cardiovascular life support: provider manual.* Dallas, TX: American Heart Association; 2011.

Wojtowycz M. *Handbook of interventional radiology and angiography.* 2nd ed. St Louis: Mosby; 1995.

# CHAPTER 66

# EQUIPMENT, TERMS, AND TECHNIQUES IN INTERVENTIONAL RADIOLOGY

*Jeffrey A. Solomon, MD, MBA, and S. William Stavropoulos, MD*

1. **What are the characteristics of a diagnostic catheter?**

   Catheters may be selected for a specific application based on many characteristics (Figure 66-1). Although there are numerous catheters, experience and personal preference play a large role in the selection process.

   - **Length:** Catheters are available in various lengths, the most common being 65 cm and 100 cm. The appropriate length is based on the access site and desired application. From a femoral approach, a 100-cm-long catheter may be used for a cerebral arteriogram, whereas a 65-cm-long catheter would suffice for a renal arteriogram.
   - **Tip configuration:** Tip configuration describes the curve on the leading edge of the catheter. Various curves are available that are designed to select branch vessels that originate at different angles. Common catheter curves include Cobra, Simmons, and Berenstein.
   - **Outer diameter:** Most diagnostic catheters used today are 4 or 5 French (Fr), meaning that they are less than 2 mm in diameter.

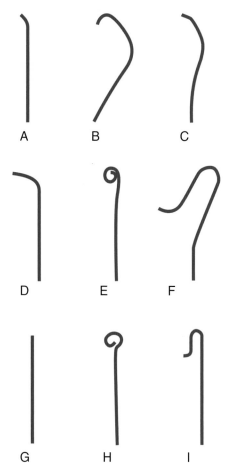

**Figure 66-1.** Types of catheters. *A* = Berenstein; *B* = Cobra; *C* = H1H; *D* = multipurpose-A; *E* = pigtail; *F* = Simmons; *G* = straight; *H* = tennis racket; *I* = SOS.

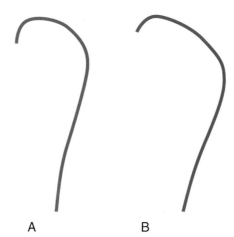

**Figure 66-2.** Difference between Cobra 1 and Cobra 2 catheters. Radius of secondary curve on Cobra 1 catheter in **A** is smaller than that of Cobra 2 catheter in **B,** although overall configuration of catheters is similar.

- **Inner diameter:** This describes the inner channel of the catheter. Most catheters are designed to accommodate guidewires that are either 0.035 inches or 0.038 inches in diameter. It is important to match the inner diameter of the catheter with the devices (wire or coil) that are placed through it.
- **Coating:** Some catheters have a hydrophilic coating that becomes very slippery when wet. This may facilitate crossing a stenosis.
- **Stiffness:** Some catheters may contain braided fibers within the shaft. Braiding of polymers increases the stiffness of the catheter. Some clinical applications are better suited to stiffer catheters, whereas others are better served by floppier ones.

2. What is the difference between Cobra 1, Cobra 2, and Cobra 3 catheters?
   A Cobra 1 catheter and a Cobra 2 catheter have the same general shape except that the radius of the secondary curve of the catheter is greater for the Cobra 2 (Figure 66-2). A Cobra 3 catheter has the same general "cobra" shape, but the secondary curve is even greater still. The same nomenclature applies to Simmons catheters and others as well.

3. What is a French? What is a gauge?
   A French (Fr) is a unit of measure of diameter that is often applied to catheters. 1 Fr is equal to one third of a millimeter. A 6 Fr catheter is therefore 2 mm in diameter. A gauge is also a unit used to measure diameter where higher gauge values are associated with smaller diameters. Although it can be used to measure catheters, it is frequently used for needles. For example, a 21-gauge needle is approximately 0.03 inches in outer diameter, whereas an 18-gauge needle is 0.05 inches in outer diameter.

4. What are the two general categories of stents? How do they differ?
   Improvements in biomedical engineering and metallurgy have helped expand the clinical applications for noncoronary stents. Although various commercial stents are available, they can be classified as either balloon-expandable or self-expandable. The characteristics of each type vary, making one type more suitable for certain clinical applications than the other. There is significant overlap for uses of both types of stents, and user preference plays a role in selection.

5. How is a balloon-expandable stent deployed?
   The Palmaz stent is the prototypic balloon-expandable stent. Such stents come packaged either individually or premounted on a balloon. When the balloon is inflated, the stent expands to the diameter of the balloon. As the stent expands, it changes very little in length. The relatively constant size and method of delivery/deployment of this type of stent allow for precise and predictable placement. Balloon-expandable stents are the stents of choice for treating renal artery stenosis. Because they are made of laser-cut stainless steel, these stents may cause significant artifact on magnetic resonance imaging (MRI) examinations. Balloon-expandable stents may be permanently deformed by extrinsic compression and should not be used in situations in which they could be subject to these forces.

6. What two materials are used to make self-expandable stents?
   There are two broad categories of self-expandable stents: stents made from woven Elgiloy wires and stents laser-cut from nitinol tubes. Self-expandable stents exert a continuous outward force, resist deformation, and are preferable to balloon-expandable stents in regions potentially subject to external compressive forces. To ensure full expansion, self-expandable stents are dilated with a balloon of appropriate diameter after deployment.

7. How do woven Elgiloy and nitinol self-expandable stents differ?
   Woven stents, such as the Wallstent, have several unique characteristics. They are very radiopaque and can be easily seen on fluoroscopy, even in obese patients. The stents are reconstrainable, meaning that they can be almost entirely

deployed, recaptured, moved, and then redeployed in a different location. The tradeoff, however, is that the length of the stent depends on its fully expanded diameter. These stents may shorten significantly as they expand over time, uncovering a region of pathology. Alternatively, if the stent does not expand to the degree expected, the stent may remain too long. Woven stents are available in large sizes (up to 24 mm in diameter) and are often used to create transjugular intrahepatic portosystemic shunts (TIPS) or to stent large central veins.

Laser-cut self-expandable stents are not reconstrainable. Because the stents are constructed of rings linked together, they are subject to significant foreshortening and remain at a relatively stable length regardless of diameter. Nitinol is less radiopaque then Elgiloy, and these stents may be difficult to see, especially in obese patients.

8. **What is nitinol?**
Nitinol was developed by the U.S. Navy and stands for nickel titanium alloy. This metal is particularly useful for medical applications because it has thermal memory. This property allows stents to be made at a certain diameter, cooled, and then compressed onto a delivery system. When the stent is deployed at body temperature, the stent attempts to regain its original configuration and diameter. A nitinol stent that is slightly oversized (by approximately 20%) with regard to the vessel exerts an outward force to keep the vessel open as the stent attempts to regain its original diameter.

9. **What do the terms** *hoop strength*, *chronic outward force*, **and** *radial resistive force* **mean?**
Hoop strength is a measure of a stent's ability to avoid collapse and withstand the radial compressive forces of a vessel after dilation.

Chronic outward force is the continuing radial expansion force that a self-expandable stent exerts on a vessel as it tries to expand to its original diameter.

Radial resistive force is the force that a self-expandable stent exerts as it resists radial compression by a vessel.

10. **What is a sheath?**
A sheath is a device that may be placed into a vessel at the site of percutaneous access. Sheaths permit rapid exchanges of guidewires and catheters while maintaining intravascular access. Sheaths are sized based on the diameter of the catheter or device that they allow to pass. A 7-Fr sheath accepts devices up to 7 Fr in outer diameter. A 7-Fr sheath is in fact closer to 8 or 9 Fr in diameter.

11. **What is a guiding catheter?**
A guiding catheter is a special type of catheter that does not taper at its tip to the diameter of the guidewire. This configuration allows the passage of devices of large diameter through the catheter. When used in this manner, a guiding catheter functions similarly to a long sheath. In contrast to sheaths, guiding catheters lack a side port and hemostatic valve. Guiding catheters are sized based on the outer diameter. A 7-Fr guiding catheter fits through a 7-Fr sheath, but a 7-Fr device does not fit through a 7-Fr guiding catheter. Guiding catheters are available with various tip configurations.

12. **What is an up-and-over sheath?**
Sometimes called a Balkin sheath, an up-and-over sheath is a U-shaped sheath (Figure 66-3). It is designed to facilitate interventions in which arterial access is via one femoral artery and the lesion to be treated is in the contralateral extremity. A catheter and guidewire are placed into the aorta, and the contralateral iliac artery is selected. The sheath is placed over the wire. The preshaped "U" curve assists passage over the aortic bifurcation. After angioplasty or stenting, arteriography can be performed by injecting contrast material through the side arm of the sheath.

13. **Explain the Trojan horse technique.**
The original balloon-expandable stents came from the manufacturer packaged in a small box. To use the stent, an appropriate balloon was selected, and the stent was hand-crimped onto the balloon by the operator. If not mounted properly, stents had the tendency to slip on the balloon when being advanced across a tight stenosis. The Trojan horse technique minimizes this risk. Instead of pushing the stent across the lesion, the lesion is crossed with a sheath or guiding catheter (Figure 66-4). The balloon-mounted stent is advanced through the catheter or sheath to the desired location, and then the sheath or catheter is withdrawn to expose the stent in the proper location. In this way, complications related to stent slippage are minimized. This is just one example of how the Trojan horse technique is used. The term applies to the technique in general and can be used to deliver any device in this manner, not just a balloon-expandable stent.

14. **What are the defining characteristics of guidewires?**
Guidewires are available in numerous configurations. The selection of wire type depends on the intended application. Defining characteristics include the following:
- **Length:** Wires are available in lengths from 70 cm to more than 300 cm. Short wires may be used for obtaining vascular access or placing drains. Longer 300-cm wires are used in catheter exchanges or to perform procedures at a great distance from the access site.
- **Diameter:** The most commonly used wires are 0.035 inch, 0.038 inch, or 0.018 inch in diameter. Wires 0.010 inch are available for special applications, such as cerebral interventions. The size of the wire should be selected based on the catheter used and the intended application.

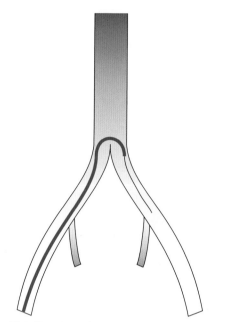

**Figure 66-3.** Up-and-over (Balkin) sheath. "Up-and-over" design allows diagnostic angiography and interventional procedures to be performed in lower extremity via access site in contralateral lower extremity.

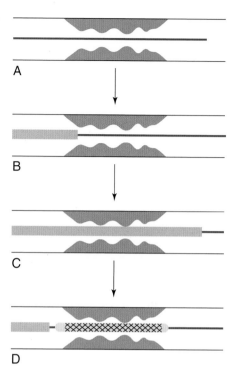

**Figure 66-4.** Trojan horse technique. **A,** Lesion is crossed with wire. **B,** Sheath or guiding catheter is used to cross lesion. **C,** Stent is advanced through sheath or guiding catheter and centered over lesion. **D,** Guiding catheter or sheath is withdrawn, exposing stent.

- **Stiffness:** Wires vary from very floppy to extremely stiff.
- **Coating:** Some wires may have a hydrophilic coating. When wet, these wires become very slippery, which may facilitate the crossing of tight stenoses.
- **Tip configuration:** Wires have specialized tips that have been engineered for specific applications. Some wires have preformed angles to assist in the selection of vessels. Other wires have floppy or atraumatic tips to prevent vascular injury. Some specialized wires have tips that can be shaped during a procedure to accomplish a specific task.

15. What is an exchange-length wire? How long does it have to be?
    An exchange-length wire is long enough to perform a catheter exchange without having to withdraw the wire. Most wires are 150 cm long and are paired with catheters that are either 65 or 100 cm long. If a catheter needs to be exchanged over a wire, the wire needs to be at least twice as long as the catheter to make the exchange without having to pull the wire back and risk losing access. This is easy to remember: If a 100-cm-long catheter is advanced all the way into a vessel, a 200-cm wire would be needed to exchange the catheter; 100 cm of the wire would be used before the tip of the wire comes out of the catheter, and another 100 cm of wire is needed so that the catheter can be pulled out without moving the wire.

16. What is a Cope loop?
    Dr. Constantin Cope is one of the pioneers of interventional radiology and is credited with some of the field's most ingenious inventions. One of these is the Cope loop, which is a pigtail catheter with a locking mechanism to prevent accidental displacement. A small string runs through the center of the catheter and is fixed to the distal curved end. The other end of the string exits the hub of the catheter. The curl on the catheter is straightened out as it is advanced over a guidewire. After the wire is removed, the string is pulled and tied, which causes the end of the catheter to curl and lock. The fixed diameter of the locked coil prevents migration. To remove the catheter, the hub and string are cut, releasing the distal lock.

17. What is the origin of the term "stent"?
    The word "stent" derives from the surname of nineteenth-century English dentist Stent. He developed gums and resins used to make models of jaws, and the verb "to stent" came to mean "to hold tissue in place." The term "stent" was later adopted by surgeons to describe a device or material used to prop open a space.

18. **What does it mean to "Dotter" a lesion?**
    Dr. Charles Dotter was an early pioneer in interventional radiology. Before the availability of angioplasty balloons, he described a technique in which stenoses were treated by passing dilators of successively larger diameter through them.

19. **What is a micropuncture set?**
    A micropuncture set is used to obtain vascular access. It contains a 21-gauge single-wall needle, an 0.018-inch wire, and a dilator. The dilator is tapered to the 0.018-inch wire to allow for easy placement. The inner portion of the dilator can be removed along with the wire to allow the dilator to accept a standard 0.035-inch wire. This set can be used as an alternative to double-wall needles. Some prefer this set for gaining access for thrombolysis because it uses the single-wall technique.

20. **What is the difference between the single-wall and the double-wall technique?**
    To perform a single-wall technique, only the ventral wall of the vessel is punctured to gain entry to the vessel. A double-wall puncture (Seldinger technique) is performed by puncturing the dorsal and ventral walls of the vessel and subsequently withdrawing the needle. When pulsatile blood is encountered, the tip of the needle is in an intraluminal position, and a guidewire can be placed safely.

21. **What are the advantages and disadvantages of a single-wall puncture?**
    The single-wall technique is preferred for bypass grafts and for patients at risk for puncture site hemorrhage, such as patients undergoing thrombolysis. The disadvantage is an increased risk for access site vascular dissection.

22. **What is a snare?**
    A snare is a device that may be used to remove intravascular foreign bodies such as wires or coils (Figure 66-5). A snare consists of a wire with a nitinol loop at the end. The plane of the loop is oriented perpendicular to the long axis of the wire. The snare is advanced through a catheter. Under fluoroscopic guidance, the loop is used to engage a free edge of the foreign body. The wire and loop are retracted into the catheter. This locks the foreign body between the snare loop and catheter. The snare, loop, and foreign body are then removed in unison.

23. **What is a reverse curve catheter?**
    A reverse curve catheter is one in which the tip of the catheter doubles back on itself to form a partial loop (Figure 66-6). Because of the loop at the end, special maneuvers must often be done to form the loop when the catheter is inside the patient. After the loop is formed, the catheter is pulled down to select a branch vessel. When the tip of the catheter engages the orifice of the vessel, the use of the catheter may be slightly counterintuitive. The presence of the

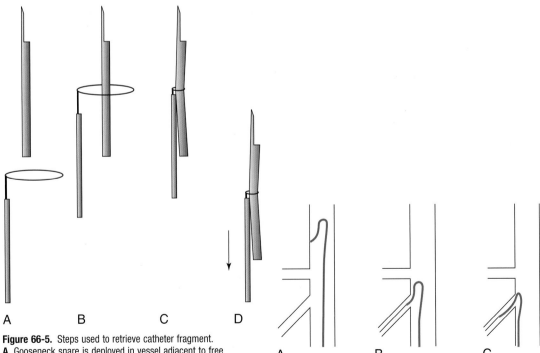

**Figure 66-5.** Steps used to retrieve catheter fragment. **A,** Gooseneck snare is deployed in vessel adjacent to free end of fragment. **B,** Free end of catheter fragment is engaged by loop of snare. **C,** Snare is pulled back into its outer catheter to grasp catheter fragment tightly. **D,** Snare, outer catheter, and catheter fragment are withdrawn in unison.

**Figure 66-6.** Steps for using reverse curve catheter. **A,** Catheter is formed in aorta. **B,** Vessel is selected. **C,** As catheter is pulled out, its tip moves farther into vessel.

loop at the end of the catheter causes the tip of the catheter to advance distally in the selected vessel if the catheter is pulled out. This is exactly opposite what happens with a conventional catheter. One must push a reverse curve catheter inward to deselect a branch vessel. Reverse curve catheters often provide stable access to vessels because of the way they behave. The Simmons catheter is the prototypic reverse curve catheter.

24. **What are the different ways to form a Simmons catheter?**
One way is first to place a wire over the aortic bifurcation and then form the catheter by placing the tip over the bifurcation and pushing up. The catheter may also be formed in the thoracic aorta where the diameter is sufficiently large. A technique commonly used at the Hospital of the University of Pennsylvania involves anchoring a suture with a wire in the tip of the catheter. The loop is formed by gently pulling on the string while advancing the catheter.

25. **What is a Waltman loop?**
The distal tip of any catheter can be looped back to form a reverse curve catheter. A Waltman loop is the configuration of a standard catheter when the distal end has been formed into a reverse curve loop. The simplest technique to do this involves selection of an aortic branch vessel. The tip is maintained in a constant position as wire and catheter are advanced in unison. This creates a large reverse curve that can stabilize access and facilitate difficult catheterizations.

26. **What is "road mapping"?**
"Road mapping" is an imaging technique present on many modern fluoroscopy units. An arteriogram is performed first. When the road map function is selected, the fluoroscopy monitor displays a static subtracted angiographic image from this prior run. When fluoroscopy is performed, a real-time subtracted fluoroscopic image is superimposed on the static angiogram. In effect, the vessels are highlighted with everything but the motion of the catheter and guidewire subtracted out. This technique facilitates selection of small or tortuous vessels.

27. **How do you select the proper injection rate for an arteriogram?**
The easiest way to select the proper rate is to give a test injection of contrast agent by hand to estimate the rate of flow. The injection rate should approximate the intrinsic rate of flow of the vessel. Giving a test injection is always prudent to ensure that the catheter is in the appropriate location. Accidental power injection into the subintimal space or a tiny branch vessel may occur if this recommendation is not followed.

28. **What is meant by an injection of "20 for 40"?**
One must dictate the rate and volume for a power-injected run of contrast material. The term "20 for 40" means that the injection rate is 20 mL/second for a total volume of 40 mL. This would therefore be a 2-second-long injection.

29. **What is a rate rise?**
A rate rise is another way that a power injection of contrast material can be modified and describes the time in seconds that it takes from the beginning of the injection to reach the desired injection rate. For an injection of "20 for 40" with no rate rise, the velocity of contrast agent in the catheter immediately jumps from 0 to 20 mL/s. That is, no rate rise implies a step function. If a rate rise of 0.6 second is used, it takes 0.6 second for the injection to reach maximum velocity. Rate rises are used to minimize the recoil of the catheter during rapid injections.

30. **What is a Hickman catheter?**
A Hickman catheter is a device used for long-term intravenous access, most commonly for chemotherapy or total parenteral nutrition. The line is available in single-lumen, double-lumen, or triple-lumen models. It is ideally placed in the internal jugular vein, with the exit site tunneled several centimeters away. The catheter has an antimicrobial cuff on its surface.

31. **What is a PermaCath?**
PermaCath is a brand name and should not be used to describe the device in general terms. It is one type of tunneled dialysis catheter.

32. **What is a Medcomp?**
Medcomp is also a brand name and should not be used as a generic reference. It is one type of nontunneled dialysis catheter.

## KEY POINTS

- Balloon-expandable stents are the stent of choice for renal arteries because they can be placed with greater accuracy.
- Self-expandable stents are indicated when there may be an extrinsic compressive force acting on the stent.
- The best way to determine the appropriate injection rate of contrast material for a given vessel is to give a test injection by hand and then to approximate the intrinsic rate of flow.

## BIBLIOGRAPHY

Mauro MA, Murphy KPJ, Thomson KR, et al. *Image-guided interventions: expert radiology series.* 2nd ed. Philadelphia: Saunders; 2014.
Valji K. *Vascular and interventional radiology.* 2nd ed. Philadelphia: Saunders; 2006.
Duda SH, Wiskirchen J, Tepe G, et al. Physical properties of endovascular stents: an experimental comparison. *J Vasc Interv Radiol.* 2000;11(5):645-654.

# CHAPTER 67

# INFERIOR VENA CAVA FILTERS

*S. William Stavropoulos, MD*

1. **What is an inferior vena cava (IVC) filter?**
   An IVC filter is a device inserted percutaneously into the IVC designed to prevent pulmonary emboli (PE) originating from lower extremity deep vein thrombosis (DVT) and to maintain caval patency.

2. **What are some common indications for IVC filter placement?**
   For patients with lower extremity DVT, accepted indications include:
   - A contraindication to anticoagulation.
   - Recurrent thromboembolic disease despite adequate anticoagulation.
   - Significant bleeding complication while undergoing anticoagulation.
   - Inability to achieve anticoagulation.

3. **List relative indications for IVC filter placement.**
   - Thromboembolic disease with limited cardiopulmonary reserve.
   - Poor compliance with anticoagulation therapy.
   - Chronic PE with pulmonary hypertension.
   - Prophylaxis in the setting of prolonged immobilization.
   - Large clot burden or free-floating pelvic/IVC thrombus.

4. **What is a prophylactic IVC filter?**
   A prophylactic IVC filter is placed in patients who are at an increased risk for, but do not currently have, DVT or PE. These filters are most commonly placed in patients who face prolonged immobilization. This population primarily consists of trauma patients with long bone or pelvic fractures and neurosurgical patients with transient or permanent motor deficits. Prophylactic filters may also be placed in patients with DVT risk factors before having surgery.

5. **What is Virchow's triad?**
   Virchow's triad is a basis for understanding the factors that contribute to thrombosis, including:
   - A hypercoagulable state, such as caused by malignancy, nephrotic syndrome, or oral contraceptives.
   - Vascular stasis resulting from shock, heart failure, venous obstruction, extrinsic compression, or other causes.
   - Vascular injury secondary to various causes, such as trauma, inflammation, surgery, or central lines.

6. **What are absolute contraindications to IVC filter placement?**
   Although rare, absolute contraindications include a lack of venous access; complete thrombosis of the IVC; or a severe, uncorrectable coagulopathy.

7. **What are relative contraindications to IVC filter placement?**
   The decision to place a permanent medical device should be made on a case-by-case basis and only after careful deliberation of the patient's history. One relative contraindication to filter placement is septic emboli or active bacteremia because of the theoretic risk of infectious seeding of the filter. IVC filters are not routinely placed in adolescents or pregnant women. A severe hypercoagulable state or a history of IVC thrombus may preclude filter placement because of the risk of complete IVC thrombosis.

8. **How many PE originate from the lower extremities?**
   Of PE, 75% to 90% originate from the lower extremities. The remainder originate from the right atrium and upper extremities and likely account for some of the cases of recurrent PE after IVC filter placement.

9. **When would a superior vena cava (SVC) filter be placed?**
   Filters are rarely placed in the SVC because the small clot burden in the upper extremities is rarely thought to lead to clinically significant PE. SVC filters are indicated in the unique setting of symptomatic PE that can be traced with a high degree of certainty to upper extremity clot.

10. **Why is a vena cavogram performed before IVC filter placement?**
    A vena cavogram is performed to evaluate the size, anatomy, and patency of the IVC. It is important to know the diameter of the IVC because each filter can be safely placed in vessels up to a certain size. Most IVC filters can be placed in a cava up to 28 mm in diameter, whereas a bird's nest filter can be used in a cava up to 40 mm. Filters can migrate into the heart or pulmonary arteries if they are not sized appropriately. Ideally, the tip of the filter should rest in the infrarenal IVC. A vena cavogram is helpful in identifying the location of the renal veins and variant anatomy that may affect filter placement. The presence of a nonocclusive clot in the cava may change the approach used to place the filter or its location. A jugular approach may be used when there is a large clot low in the IVC to help prevent

pushing the clot centrally. To be effective, a filter needs to be placed above any clot in the IVC; this may warrant suprarenal placement.

11. How is a vena cavogram performed before IVC filter placement?

A vena cavogram can be performed via access from a jugular vein, femoral vein, or arm vein. A 5-Fr pigtail catheter with radiopaque markers is recommended so that accurate measurements of the IVC can be taken. The tip of the catheter is placed just above the confluence of the iliac veins, and an injection rate is chosen that causes contrast material to flow down the left and right common iliac veins. Identifying both iliac veins excludes the existence of a duplicated IVC, a normal anatomic variant that alters filter placement. Patients should perform a Valsalva maneuver to distend the IVC maximally during the contrast material injection so that the caval diameter can be accurately measured, preventing caval migration. A radiopaque ruler can be placed underneath the patient to be used as a landmark to facilitate accurate filter placement.

12. What do the renal veins look like on a cavogram?

Usually, the renal veins are not opacified by contrast material injected into the IVC because the opacified blood in the cava flows preferentially back to the right atrium. The location of the renal veins can be determined, however, because unopacified blood from the renal veins mixes with and dilutes opacified blood in the cava. The location of the renal veins can be inferred from inflow defects in the stream of contrast material in the IVC. If there is doubt about their locations, a selective injection of the renal veins may be performed.

13. Can a cavogram be performed if the patient is allergic to iodinated contrast material or has an elevated creatinine level?

If iodinated contrast material cannot be used because of an elevated creatinine level or a severe contrast agent allergy, a cavogram can be performed using intravenous $CO_2$ or gadolinium-based contrast material as an alternative contrast agent. If available, intravascular ultrasonography (IVUS) can also be utilized.

14. What common venous anomalies are seen on a cavogram?

In interpreting a cavogram, one should be familiar with the common venous anomalies, including circumaortic renal vein, retroaortic left renal vein, caval duplication, and left-sided IVC.

15. How common is IVC duplication? What does it look like on a cavogram?

IVC duplication occurs in 0.2% to 0.3% of patients. In a patient with a duplicated IVC, the left common iliac vein does not join with the right common iliac vein but instead extends cranially to join the left renal vein. Simultaneous injections of the right and left femoral veins reveal two IVCs. The one on the right extends from the right common iliac vein into the right atrium. The one on the left extends from the left common iliac vein and joins with the left renal vein, which then empties into the right-sided IVC. If one understands this anatomy, one can appreciate why refluxing contrast material down both common iliac veins during a cavogram excludes the presence of a duplicated IVC.

16. What should be done in a patient with duplicated IVC who needs an IVC filter?

Failure to recognize the presence of a duplicated IVC may lead to the placement of a single filter in the right-sided cava. A filter in this position would leave the entire left leg and left pelvis "unprotected" because a clot could bypass the filter by traveling from the left leg, up the left-sided cava to the left renal vein, and then to the heart and lungs. If the left-sided cava is recognized, a filter could be placed in each cava, or a single suprarenal filter could alternatively be placed.

17. What are the characteristics of a left-sided IVC?

Left-sided IVC occurs in 0.2% to 0.5% of patients. This vessel usually crosses to the right side of the abdomen at the level of the left renal vein and suprarenally continues in the position of the normal right-sided cava.

18. What are the characteristics of a circumaortic left renal vein? How common is this anatomic variant?

A circumaortic left renal vein is an anatomic variant in which the left renal vein forms a ring around the abdominal aorta. It has a prevalence of 1.5% to 8.7%. The anterior segment of the ring connects with the IVC at the expected level of the left renal vein, and the posterior segment connects with the IVC below the level of insertion of the anterior segment.

19. Where should a filter be placed in a patient with a circumaortic left renal vein?

If unrecognized, a circumaortic left renal vein may provide a collateral pathway for a clot to circumnavigate a filter and embolize to the lungs. If the filter is placed above the posterior segment, a clot may travel up the posterior segment to the anterior segment that is above the filter and then pass on to the lungs. The filter should therefore be placed below the lowest renal vein. This placement ensures that a clot would encounter the filter as it travels centrally.

20. What is a retrievable IVC filter?

A retrievable or optional IVC filter can be left in place permanently or can be removed if it is no longer needed.

21. What patients could benefit from a retrievable IVC filter?

Patients who could benefit from a retrievable IVC filter are those who only need short-term protection from DVT. This might include trauma patients who cannot be anticoagulated acutely but are expected to recover, surgical patients with a short-term increased risk for PE, surgical patients who need to be off of their anticoagulation for a short term during the perioperative time frame, and patients with a temporary contraindication to anticoagulation.

22. Can patients with an IVC filter still get PE?

Yes. There are several ways for patients with a filter to get PE. A patient may have had an anatomic variant that was not recognized during filter placement that permitted a clot to bypass the filter. Even in the absence of such variants, a filter would not protect a patient from PE originating in every part of the body. A filter would not offer protection from a clot originating in the upper extremities or right atrium. Similarly, a clot from an ovarian vein that embolizes to the renal vein and then centrally would not be stopped by an infrarenal filter. Small clots may pass through a filter, and large clots may propagate through a filter as pieces break off and embolize centrally. Overall, the rate of recurrent PE in patients with caval filters ranges from 3% to 5%. These rates are based on clinical findings and imaging studies performed in patients to detect symptomatic PE. The rates of asymptomatic PE after IVC filter placement are largely unknown.

23. Where in the IVC should the filter be placed, and why?

It is preferable that the filter be placed immediately below the lowest renal vein. With the apex of the filter sitting just below the renal veins, any clot caught by the filter is subject to high blood flow from the renal veins and may be more likely to lyse. Theoretically, this may help maintain caval patency over the lifetime of the patient. Placement below the renal veins also decreases the risk of renal vein thrombosis if the filter is subject to a large clot burden. Suprarenal IVC filters are relatively safe but have a theoretic increased risk of renal vein thrombosis and should be reserved for instances in which there is thrombus in the infrarenal IVC.

24. What complications are related to IVC filter placement?

Complications of filter placement can be related to the access site and include hematoma, venous thrombosis, and accidental arterial puncture. Complications related to the device include filter migration, malposition, fracture, infection, IVC perforation, failed deployment, and caval occlusion. IVC filter migration into the right atrium and pulmonary artery has been reported and can be fatal. IVC filters can be dislodged by wires or catheters placed during venous access performed at a later time. A potential complication for house staff may occur during central line placement. If the wire is inserted too far down the IVC in a patient with a filter, it may become entrapped. Attempts to pull the wire out may pull the filter with it and lacerate the cava. If you are placing a central line and the wire feels like it is "stuck," check the patient's record to see whether he or she has a filter. If the patient has a filter, you may want to call the interventional radiologist who can help remove the wire under fluoroscopic guidance.

25. How often does IVC occlusion occur after IVC filter placement?

IVC occlusion after filter placement can be due to either trapped thrombus in the filter or primary IVC thrombosis. Rates of symptomatic IVC occlusion are 2% to 10% according to reports in the literature.

---

## KEY POINTS

- IVC filters prevent ≈97% of symptomatic PE that originate from the lower extremities.
- A cavogram before IVC filter placement is essential.
- Retrievable IVC filters may be removed when they are no longer needed.
- In most cases, IVC filters should be placed below the lowest renal vein when possible.
- When fishing with a wire in a patient with a filter, be careful! You might actually "catch" something.

---

**BIBLIOGRAPHY**

Kinney TB. Update on inferior vena cava filters. *J Vasc Interv Radiol.* 2003;14(4):425-440.

Schutzer R, Ascher E, Hingorani A, et al. Preliminary results of the new 6F TrapEase inferior vena cava filter. *Ann Vasc Surg.* 2003;17(1):103-106.

Stavropoulos SW, Itkin M, Trerotola SO. In vitro study of guide wire entrapment in currently available inferior vena cava filters. *J Vasc Interv Radiol.* 2003;14(7):905-910.

Asch MR. Initial experience in humans with a new retrievable inferior vena cava filter. *Radiology.* 2002;225(3):835-844.

Rousseau H, Perreault P, Otal P, et al. The 6-F nitinol TrapEase inferior vena cava filter: results of a prospective multicenter trial. *J Vasc Interv Radiol.* 2001;12(3):299-304.

Streiff MB. Vena caval filters: a comprehensive review. *Blood.* 2000;95(12):3669-3677.

Cho KJ, Greenfield LJ, Proctor MC, et al. Evaluation of a new percutaneous stainless steel Greenfield filter. *J Vasc Interv Radiol.* 1997;8(2):181-187.

Neuerburg JM, Gunther RW, Vorwerk D, et al. Results of a multicenter study of the retrievable Tulip Vena Cava Filter: early clinical experience. *Cardiovasc Intervent Radiol.* 1997;20(1):10-16.

Wojtowycz MM, Stoehr T, Crummy AB, et al. The Bird's Nest inferior vena caval filter: review of a single-center experience. *J Vasc Interv Radiol.* 1997;8(2):171-179.

Winchell RJ, Hoyt DB, Walsh JC, et al. Risk factors associated with pulmonary embolism despite routine prophylaxis: implications for improved protection. *J Trauma.* 1994;37(4):600-606.

Crochet DP, Stora O, Ferry D, et al. Vena Tech-LGM filter: long-term results of a prospective study. *Radiology.* 1993;188(3):857-860.

Ferris EJ, McCowan TC, Carver DK, et al. Percutaneous inferior vena caval filters: follow-up of seven designs in 320 patients. *Radiology.* 1993;188(3):851-856.

Rogers FB, Shackford SR, Wilson J, et al. Prophylactic vena cava filter insertion in severely injured trauma patients: indications and preliminary results. *J Trauma.* 1993;35(4):637-641, discussion 641-642.

Becker DM, Philbrick JT, Selby JB. Inferior vena cava filters. Indications, safety, effectiveness. *Arch Intern Med.* 1992;152(10):1985-1994.

Molgaard CP, Yucel EK, Geller SC, et al. Access-site thrombosis after placement of inferior vena cava filters with 12-14-F delivery sheaths. *Radiology.* 1992;185(1):257-261.

Grassi CJ. Inferior vena caval filters: analysis of five currently available devices. *AJR Am J Roentgenol.* 1991;156(4):813-821.

Millward SF, Marsh JI, Peterson RA, et al. LGM (Vena Tech) vena cava filter: clinical experience in 64 patients. *J Vasc Interv Radiol.* 1991;2(4):429-433.

Huisman MV, Buller HR, ten Cate JW, et al. Unexpected high prevalence of silent pulmonary embolism in patients with deep venous thrombosis. *Chest.* 1989;95(3):498-502.

Tobin KD, Pais SO, Austin CB. Femoral vein thrombosis following percutaneous placement of the Greenfield filter. *Invest Radiol.* 1989;24(6):442-445.

Golueke PJ, Garrett WV, Thompson JE, et al. Interruption of the vena cava by means of the Greenfield filter: expanding the indications. *Surgery.* 1988;103(1):111-117.

Katsamouris AA, Waltman AC, Delichatsios MA, et al. Inferior vena cava filters: in vitro comparison of clot trapping and flow dynamics. *Radiology.* 1988;166(2):361-366.

Dorfman GS, Cronan JJ, Tupper TB, et al. Occult pulmonary embolism: a common occurrence in deep venous thrombosis. *AJR Am J Roentgenol.* 1987;148(2):263-266.

Friedell ML, Goldenkranz RJ, Parsonnet V, et al. Migration of a Greenfield filter to the pulmonary artery: a case report. *J Vasc Surg.* 1986;3(6):929-931.

# CHAPTER 68

# IMAGE-GUIDED PERCUTANEOUS NEEDLE BIOPSY

*Ana S. Kolansky, MD*

1. **What are the major indications for image-guided percutaneous needle biopsy?**

   Image-guided percutaneous needle biopsy (IPNB) is an established, effective nonsurgical procedure that is performed in selected patients to obtain a pathologic diagnosis or to guide appropriate patient management. Indications for percutaneous needle biopsy include:
   - To determine if a lesion is benign or malignant.
   - To obtain material for microbiological analysis in suspected infection.
   - To stage disease in patients with known or suspected malignancy.
   - To obtain material for biomarker, protein, or genotype analysis to subsequently guide targeted therapies in select patients.
   - To determine the primary cell type in patients with metastatic disease and an unknown primary tumor.
   - To diagnose certain diffuse parenchymal diseases (e.g., in the liver and kidneys).

2. **What are the available imaging modalities for IPNB?**

   Image guidance for percutaneous needle biopsy is provided to precisely localize a lesion that is not palpable and, therefore, requires imaging for localization. IPNB can be performed using fluoroscopy, ultrasonography (US), computed tomography (CT), or magnetic resonance imaging (MRI), and the use of these modalities is dependent on the target organ, the type of lesion, and patient parameters. Lesions that can be easily seen on a radiograph may be biopsied fluoroscopically, including large lung lesions and some bone lesions. To ensure proper needle placement, fluoroscopic equipment must be able to provide complex angle imaging. Fluoroscopy is less desirable due to increased radiation exposure to personnel during the procedure. Its use for lung biopsies has decreased over time, as CT is able to detect and provide needle guidance of small lung lesions.

   US is perhaps the most versatile modality for IPNB. It is a safe and accurate method that uses real-time imaging to guide needles into abdominal and pelvic organs and masses. It is also typically used to sample thyroid and breast lesions. Its advantage over CT-guided biopsies is that it can be done portably, is less expensive, and does not use ionizing radiation. However, some lesions are not visualized sonographically because of size or location. US is typically used to sample lesions within superficial lymph nodes (Figure 68-1), liver (Figure 68-2), and kidneys, but has little role in sampling lesions in the chest unless the lesion is in the pleura or chest wall.

   CT allows for biopsy of lesions not seen fluoroscopically or sonographically and provides the most accurate visualization of anatomy for accurate and safe access to lesions, avoiding transgression of vital structures. It is used for sampling of lesions in the neck, lung, pleura, mediastinum (Figure 68-3), abdomen, and pelvis, including deep retroperitoneal and pelvic lymph nodes (Figure 68-4).

   Some lesions can only be visualized by MRI, which can also be utilized on rare occasion. MRI has limited use because of expense, difficulty in accessing the patient within the magnet, and difficulties with use of ferromagnetic instruments within the magnetic field.

3. **What are the contraindications for percutaneous biopsy?**

   There are no absolute contraindications for IPNB. Consideration of performance of a biopsy must be carefully weighed against the risks of the procedure. There are several relative contraindications, which in some cases may preclude the performance of a percutaneous biopsy. Relative contraindications for percutaneous needle biopsy include:
   - Coagulopathy that cannot be adequately corrected.
   - Hemodynamic instability or severely compromised cardiopulmonary function.
   - Patient inability to cooperate or to be adequately positioned for the procedure.
   - Lack of a safe pathway through tissues to the lesion.
   - Pregnancy (when image guidance requires exposure to ionizing radiation).

4. **What criteria are used to determine whether or not a lesion is amenable to IPNB?**

   When contemplating IPNB, there are several things to consider. For a lesion to be amenable to IPNB, it must be visible on one of the imaging modalities discussed above. Additionally, there must be a safe route to access the lesion without likely damage to vital organs or vascular structures. Vascular lesions should not undergo percutaneous needle biopsy. If a lesion is considered amenable to IPNB, patients must then be assessed to make sure they are candidates for this procedure.

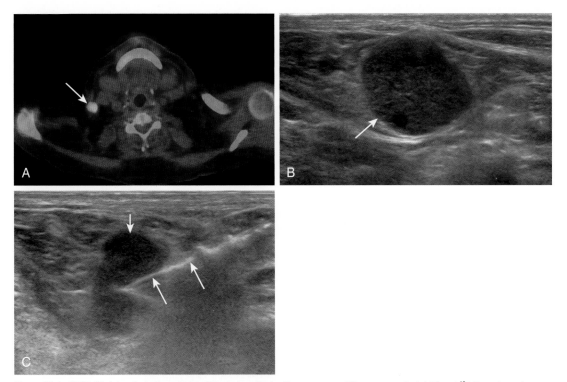

**Figure 68-1.** IPNB of indeterminate thoracic lymph node in patient with squamous cell lung cancer. **A,** Axial fused $^{18}$F-fluorodeoxyglucose (FDG) positron emission tomography/computed tomography (PET/CT) image shows enlarged FDG-avid right supraclavicular lymph node (*arrow*). **B,** US image redemonstrates hypoechoic 1.6 × 2-cm right supraclavicular node (*arrow*). **C,** US-guided coaxial needle biopsy of lymph node (*short arrow*) obtained both cytologic and histologic samples, confirmed metastatic disease to lymph node, and facilitated targeted therapy. Note echogenic biopsy needle (*long arrows*).

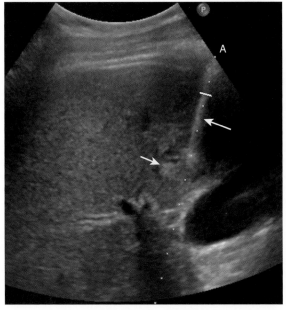

**Figure 68-2.** IPNB of indeterminate liver mass in patient with melanoma. US-guided core biopsy with 18-G coaxial needle confirmed metastatic melanoma in 3-cm echogenic left hepatic lobe mass (*short arrow*). Note echogenic biopsy needle (*long arrow*).

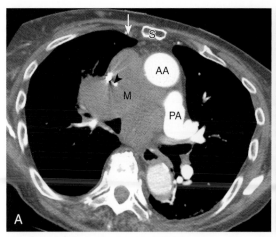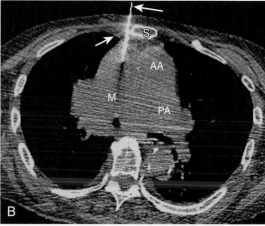

**Figure 68-3.** IPNB of indeterminate mediastinal mass in patient with superior vena cava (*SVC*) syndrome and history of prior tobacco use. **A,** Axial contrast-enhanced CT image through chest shows large soft tissue mediastinal mass (*M*), which encases and obliterates SVC (*arrowhead*) and is suspicious for malignancy such as by lymphoma or lung cancer. Note ascending aorta (*AA*), pulmonary artery (*PA*), sternum (*S*), and right internal mammary vessels (*arrow*). **B,** CT-guided FNA and core biopsy of mass with 20-G needle (*long arrow*) via right parasternal approach avoided inadvertent injury to lung, internal mammary vessels, and large vessels. Histopathologic analysis revealed small cell lung cancer as cause of mass. Again note ascending aorta (*AA*), pulmonary artery (*PA*), sternum (*S*), and right internal mammary vessels (*short arrow*).

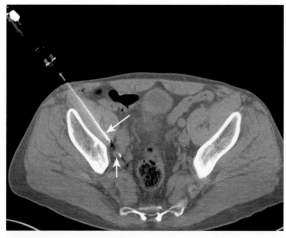

**Figure 68-4.** IPNB of indeterminate pelvic lymph node in patient with prostate cancer, lung cancer, and melanoma. CT-guided coaxial core biopsy of enlarged right obturator lymph node (*short arrow*) using 20-G coaxial core needle (*long arrow*). Histopathologic analysis revealed reactive inflammatory lymph node.

5. **How effective is percutaneous needle biopsy?**
   Percutaneous biopsy is a very effective procedure with high diagnostic yield. Low false-positive and false-negative results are achieved in most organs. The success of IPNB is affected by multiple variables, including the number of samples obtained, the size and location of the target lesion, the type of needle used, the availability of an on-site cytologist, and the experience of the performing physician and the pathology staff. The reported overall success rate of IPNB ranges between 70% and 96% among all organs.

6. **What patient preparation is necessary prior to percutaneous biopsy?**
   Percutaneous biopsy requires special attention to coagulation indices. While there are varying opinions about the safe values of these indices, which may depend upon the particular target lesion and organ to be sampled along with local practices, the following parameters can serve as a general guide:
   - Platelet count >50,000/mm$^3$ (values between 50,000 and 100,000/mm$^3$ are used).
   - International normalized ratio (INR) <1.4.
   - Normal prothrombin time (PT) and partial thromboplastin time (PTT).
   - Cessation of anticoagulants to attain normal indices.
   - Cessation of antiplatelet agents such as aspirin may also be required.
      If sedation is anticipated, patients should remain NPO for 4 to 6 hours prior to the procedure.

7. **What type of anesthesia is used for IPNB?**

Biopsies in the chest, abdomen, and pelvis can be performed under local anesthesia using 1% lidocaine, often with mild analgesia using fentanyl, and at times with use of conscious sedation such as midazolam hydrochloride. The type of anesthesia used should be assessed on a case-by-case basis. Monitoring of vital signs, including blood pressure, heart rate, cardiac rhythm, and oxygen saturation is required during such procedures.

8. **What is the difference between fine-needle aspiration (FNA) and core biopsy?**

Percutaneous needle biopsy includes two basic techniques for obtaining tissue samples: FNA and core biopsy. NA refers to sampling using thin hollow needles (20 gauge [G] and smaller) that extract loose cells for cytologic evaluation. Core biopsy refers to the use of hollow needles (20 G and larger) with a cutting mechanism that extracts a thin cylinder of tissue, usually 1 to 2 cm long, for histologic evaluation. The size of the needle and the use of aspiration or core biopsy depend on the target organ and the type of lesion that requires sampling. Most cancers can be diagnosed by cytologic analysis, but certain lesions require assessment of histopathologic architecture of tissue for diagnosis. In most cases, needle aspirations are adequate for differentiating benign from malignant disease and can serve to stage patients with cancer. However, the majority of patients do not undergo surgical resection, and specimens obtained for therapeutic planning purposes should allow for extended diagnoses, including the determination of biomarker profiles. In the current era of personalized medicine and targeted chemotherapies, molecular studies of biopsy samples is increasingly necessary, and evaluation for these markers often requires core biopsy specimens. Both types of biopsies can be performed during a single procedure, if needed, thus obtaining both cytologic and histologic specimens. Which type of biopsy to perform is determined by the type of tumor suspected, the size and location of the lesion, and what information is necessary for treatment planning.

9. **What is the difference between the single-needle technique and the coaxial needle technique of percutaneous biopsy?**

Biopsy procedures can be performed with a single-needle technique, using a fine needle for obtaining the sample. Alternatively, a coaxial needle technique can be used, whereby an introducer needle is placed in or near the lesion and through which a smaller caliber biopsy needle is advanced to the target. This procedure allows the operator to obtain several samples, including simultaneous fine-needle and core biopsies, through single-needle localization. The disadvantage of this technique is that it requires the use of a larger caliber introducer, which may be more traumatic, especially in the lung, and is associated with a higher rate of bleeding complications.

10. **How does one decide whether to use a percutaneous approach or a bronchoscopic approach to biopsy a lung nodule?**

Lung nodules and masses may be biopsied by bronchoscopy or by IPNB. Generally, lesions close to the hilum (central lesions) are accessed by bronchoscopy, whereas peripheral lesions are accessed percutaneously (Figure 68-5). With the new use of navigational endobronchial ultrasonography (EBUS), bronchoscopy may allow access to more peripheral lesions, as long as there is a visible bronchus leading to the lesion. However, bronchoscopy requires anesthesia, which carries a higher risk in patients with compromised respiratory status.

11. **What are the indications for liver biopsy, and what is the best way to biopsy the liver?**

Liver biopsy is used for diagnosis of liver masses and of diffuse acute or chronic liver disease (Figure 68-6). The liver can be biopsied with image guidance using US, CT, or endoscopic ultrasonography (EUS) via the gastrointestinal tract. The most common imaging modality utilized for liver biopsy is US. CT is generally reserved for tissue sampling of focal hepatic lesions that are not accessible by US. Transjugular liver biopsy (TJLB), where access is obtained via the internal jugular vein and sampling is done via the hepatic veins, is an alternative to percutaneous liver biopsy in patients with diffuse liver disease, coagulopathy, morbid obesity, and ascites. In TJLB, the risk of hemorrhage is reduced, because bleeding from the biopsy will drain into the hepatic veins. TJLB is utilized when hemodynamic evaluation is also indicated as part of the diagnostic workup or in patients who are also undergoing a transjugular intrahepatic portosystemic shunt (TIPS) procedure.

12. **What are the indications for renal biopsy, and what is the best way to biopsy the kidney?**

Renal biopsy is a safe technique used to establish a diagnosis of focal renal lesions not characterized by diagnostic imaging or to assess nonfocal renal disease (nephropathy) or renal transplant rejection. With a high positive predictive value of renal biopsy for the diagnosis of renal cell carcinoma, malignancy can be confirmed prior to percutaneous ablation, when surgical removal is not anticipated. Complicated cystic lesions can also be safely biopsied to differentiate benign renal cysts from cystic renal cell carcinoma. Nonfocal renal biopsies can be used to diagnose a wide spectrum of nephropathies affecting native kidneys and renal transplants (Figure 68-7).

The kidney is biopsied percutaneously under US or CT guidance, with some operators preferring US guidance for nonfocal renal disease and CT for biopsy of focal renal masses. Renal transplants are most often biopsied by US, given their superficial location in the pelvis. Generally, core biopsy samples are obtained.

13. **What are the complications of percutaneous biopsy?**

Percutaneous needle biopsies are safe procedures, and the risk of serious complications is low. Complications can be stratified as minor and major complications. Major complications result in hospital admission for therapy, an unplanned increase in the level of care, prolonged hospitalization, permanent adverse sequelae, or death. Minor complications result in no sequelae, require little or no therapy, or require a short hospital stay for observation. Major complications

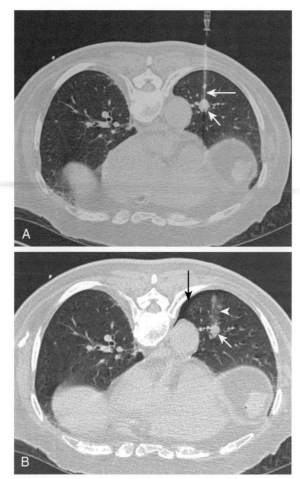

**Figure 68-5.** IPNB of indeterminate new lung nodule in patient with squamous cell tongue cancer. **A,** CT-guided FNA of left lower lobe lung nodule (*short arrow*) with patient in prone position. Note high-attenuation biopsy needle (*long arrow*). **B,** Postbiopsy CT image shows new tiny pneumothorax (*long arrow*) and expected minimal hemorrhage (*arrowhead*) in biopsy tract in lung. Again note lung nodule (*short arrow*). Cytologic analysis confirmed metastatic disease to lung.

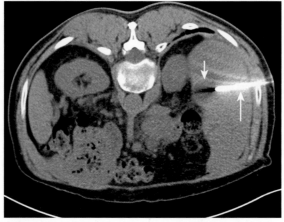

**Figure 68-6.** IPNB of indeterminate liver lesion in patient with history of hepatic abscesses following liver transplantation for hepatitis C–induced cirrhosis and hepatocellular carcinoma. CT-guided core biopsy with 18-G coaxial system (*long arrow*) of hypoattenuating hepatic lesion (*short arrow*) revealed hepatic abscess.

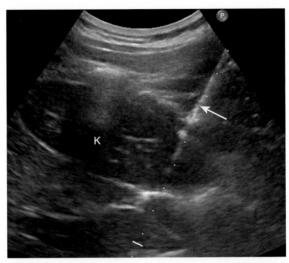

**Figure 68-7.** IPNB of kidney in patient with systemic lupus erythematosus (SLE) and deteriorating renal function. US-guided core needle biopsy of right kidney (*K*) confirmed presence of lupus nephritis. Note echogenic biopsy needle (*arrow*).

of percutaneous biopsy include bleeding that requires transfusion or intervention, infection, or organ or nerve injury. Major bleeding is infrequent and may be affected by needle size, use of cutting needles (core biopsy), and lesion vascularity. A very rare major complication includes seeding of the needle tract with tumor (<0.5% in all organs).

Following renal biopsy, bleeding can result in hematuria or a perinephric (retroperitoneal) or intrarenal hematoma. Hemorrhage requiring transfusion occurs in less than 0.5% to 6% of patients, depending on needle size, and renal loss is seen in less than 0.1% of cases. Renal arteriovenous fistula (AVF) formation, renal arterial pseudoaneurysm formation, infection, and adjacent organ injury can occur but are all rarely reported complications. The risk of tumor seeding after biopsy of a renal cancer is extremely low, with only a few reported cases in the literature.

Major bleeding in liver biopsies ranges from 0.3% to 3% and may result in subcapsular hematoma, hemoperitoneum, or hemobilia. Infection as the result of liver biopsy is rare. Damage to the target organ or nearby organ, such as with development of a pneumothorax, hepatic arterial pseudoaneurysm, or AVF, is also a rare complication.

Pneumothorax is the most common complication of lung biopsy, occurring in approximately one fourth of lung biopsies (see Figure 68-5). Thoracostomy tube placement is necessary in 2% to 15% of patients with biopsy-related pneumothoraces. A pneumothorax occurring with a lung or mediastinal biopsy is considered as a minor complication when it does not require intervention or when thoracostomy tube placement results in a brief hospitalization (<48 hours). A pneumothorax following lung or mediastinal biopsy is considered as a major complication (in 1% to 2% of biopsies) when it results in prolonged hospitalization (>48 hours), placement of multiple thoracostomy tubes, or pleurodesis. Minor hemoptysis may occur after lung biopsy, but hemoptysis requiring hospitalization or intervention is a rare complication (in 0.5% of biopsies). The most serious and very rare complication of lung biopsy is air embolism, where air enters the heart or vessels, which is reported in 0.06% to 0.07% of cases.

14. What are some factors that increase the risk of pneumothorax following percutaneous biopsy?
    Factors that increase the risk of pneumothorax include larger needle size, type of needle used, increased number of pleural punctures, lung lesion size <2 cm, increased depth of lesion location in the lung, relative inexperience of the performing radiologist, older patient age, presence of emphysema, and presence of pulmonary fibrosis.

15. How does one manage an air embolus encountered after percutaneous biopsy?
    Air embolism is a rare but life-threatening complication of lung biopsy, which can result in severe cardiac and neurologic events and death (Figure 68-8). Some postulate that air embolism occurs more frequently than suspected but goes undetected in asymptomatic patients. Air embolism should be suspected in patients with unexpected neurologic or cardiac events during a lung biopsy. Patients are placed on 100% oxygen via a nonrebreather mask or intubation, and supportive measures are implemented. Patient positioning remains controversial, where some practitioners advocate for placing the patient in a Trendelenburg (i.e., supine position with the feet more elevated than the head) and left lateral decubitus position to prevent gas from reaching the left ventricular outflow tract and the cerebral and coronary circulation. Others advocate for keeping patients supine to minimize movement and further migration of the gas. The most efficacious rescue therapy is the use of hyperbaric oxygen, which has been reported as successful by reducing intravascular bubble size, increasing oxygen diffusion into tissues, and decreasing the nitrogen content of the bubbles, facilitating the eventual resorption of the air.

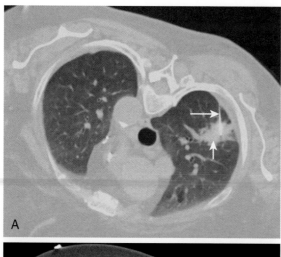

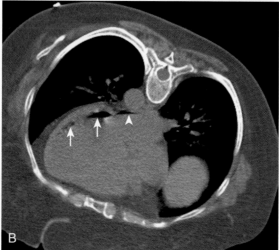

**Figure 68-8.** IPNB of indeterminate new lung nodule in patient with history of tobacco use and multiple myeloma. **A,** CT-guided FNA of 2.5-cm right upper lobe nodule (*short arrow*) with patient in prone position using 22-G needle (*long arrow*). Cytologic analysis revealed chronic granulomatous inflammation. **B,** Postbiopsy CT image demonstrates very low attenuation air within left atrium (*arrowhead*) and left ventricle (*arrows*) indicative of air embolism. Patient was placed in Trendelenburg position, received supportive measures, and was treated with hyperbaric oxygen, resulting in full recovery.

### 16. How are patients managed after percutaneous biopsy?

Following biopsy, patients are observed for a period of time prior to discharge to ensure the absence of complications. The time of postprocedure observation will vary depending on the organ biopsied. If indicated, follow-up imaging or laboratory studies to evaluate for acute complications may also be performed. For example, following renal biopsies, patients are monitored with assessment of vital signs (pulse, blood pressure, and peripheral oxygen saturation level), serial complete blood count (CBC), and observation for pain or hematuria, with follow-up imaging also routinely performed in some practices. Following lung biopsy, patients are monitored for pneumothorax with one or two postbiopsy chest radiographs over a course of 2 to 4 hours. Patients with stable, small, and asymptomatic pneumothoraces can be discharged, while larger or symptomatic pneumothoraces are admitted for observation or treated with thoracostomy tubes and either admitted or discharged with a Heimlich valve. Appropriate discharge instructions for all biopsies should include a contact number that patients can call with any questions or concerns that they may have.

### 17. How are biopsy specimens handled?

Proper handling of the biopsy specimen is key to a successful procedure and outcome. Availability of an on-site cytologist facilitates a preliminary assessment of the biopsy aspirate. On-site cytologists can help direct whether additional sampling is needed and whether a core biopsy is recommended. They can also suggest if microbiology specimens should be obtained. Cytologic specimens are placed in cytofixative, while histologic specimens are placed in formalin or fresh saline. In the workup of hematologic malignancies, specimens are placed in fresh saline for appropriate processing. Microbiology specimens are placed in sterile preservative-free saline.

## KEY POINTS

- IPNB is an effective nonsurgical procedure for the diagnosis of malignant and other lesions, which has a high diagnostic yield and a low complication rate.
- Imaging for percutaneous needle biopsy may be performed with fluoroscopy, US, CT, or MRI.
- Unresolved coagulopathy is a contraindication to percutaneous needle biopsy.
- Appropriate monitoring for postprocedure complications is important after any biopsy procedure.

## BIBLIOGRAPHY

ACR-SIR-SPR Practice Parameter for the Performance of Image-Guided Percutaneous Needle Biopsy (PNB), Amended 2014 (Resolution 39). Available at: <http://www.acr.org/~/media/ACR/Documents/PGTS/guidelines/PNB.pdf>. In, 2014:1-19.

Guimaraes MD, Marchiori E, Hochhegger B, et al. CT-guided biopsy of lung lesions: defining the best needle option for a specific diagnosis. *Clinics.* 2014;69(5):335-340.

Behrens G, Ferral H. Transjugular liver biopsy. *Semin Intervent Radiol.* 2012;29(2):111-117.

Lorenz J. Systemic air embolism. *Semin Intervent Radiol.* 2011;28(2):267-270.

Gupta S, Wallace MJ, Cardella JF, et al. Quality improvement guidelines for percutaneous needle biopsy. *J Vasc Interv Radiol.* 2010;21(7):969-975.

Uppot RN, Harisinghani MG, Gervais DA. Imaging-guided percutaneous renal biopsy: rationale and approach. *AJR Am J Roentgenol.* 2010;194(6):1443-1449.

Hatfield MK, Beres RA, Sane SS, et al. Percutaneous imaging-guided solid organ core needle biopsy: coaxial versus noncoaxial method. *AJR Am J Roentgenol.* 2008;190(2):413-417.

Myers RP, Fong A, Shaheen AA. Utilization rates, complications and costs of percutaneous liver biopsy: a population-based study including 4275 biopsies. *Liver Int.* 2008;28(5):705-712.

Hiraki T, Fujiwara H, Sakurai J, et al. Nonfatal systemic air embolism complicating percutaneous CT-guided transthoracic needle biopsy: four cases from a single institution. *Chest.* 2007;132(2):684-690.

Maturen KE, Nghiem HV, Caoili EM, et al. Renal mass core biopsy: accuracy and impact on clinical management. *AJR Am J Roentgenol.* 2007;188(2):563-570.

Tomiyama N, Yasuhara Y, Nakajima Y, et al. CT-guided needle biopsy of lung lesions: a survey of severe complication based on 9783 biopsies in Japan. *Eur J Radiol.* 2006;59(1):60-64.

Anderson JM, Murchison J, Patel D. CT-guided lung biopsy: factors influencing diagnostic yield and complication rate. *Clin Radiol.* 2003;58(10):791-797.

Geraghty PR, Kee ST, McFarlane G, et al. CT-guided transthoracic needle aspiration biopsy of pulmonary nodules: needle size and pneumothorax rate. *Radiology.* 2003;229(2):475-481.

# CHAPTER 69

# ADVANCED PROCEDURES IN INTERVENTIONAL RADIOLOGY

*Jeffrey A. Solomon, MD, MBA, and S. William Stavropoulos, MD*

## ENDOVASCULAR ANEURYSM REPAIR (EVAR)

1. **What is the basic composition of a stent graft?**
   A stent graft is composed of a metallic stent structure covered by a medical-grade fabric. The stents are typically made from stainless steel or nitinol (nickel titanium alloy), and the fabric is either Dacron (polyester) or expanded polytetrafluoroethylene (ePTFE). A stent graft comes compressed and loaded in a delivery catheter. Stent graft designs include straight tubes and bifurcated "pant leg" designs to accommodate the iliac branch. Bifurcated designs can either be unibody (one piece) or modular (multiple pieces).

2. **Who is at risk for abdominal aortic aneurysm (AAA), and what are the major complications of AAA?**
   The incidence of AAA increases after age 50 and peaks in the eighth decade of life, when the frequency rate of AAA ranges from 0.5% to 3% in autopsy studies. The prevalence of AAA is higher in older men with risk factors (4.5%) and lower in older women with risk factors (1%). The main risk factors for AAA include male gender and age older than 65, smoking history, atherosclerosis, hypertension, and family history. Major complications of AAA include rupture, thromboembolic disease, and compression of adjacent organs when large in size. There are more than 15,000 deaths annually due to AAA rupture (the thirteenth leading cause of death in the U.S.).

3. **What is the natural history of AAA, and when is intervention indicated?**
   Aneurysms grow over time. Increased expression and activity of matrix metalloproteinases (MMPs) and decreased activity of their inhibitors result in the loss of aortic wall structural integrity, which leads to AAA formation and expansion. The rate of growth is generally 1 to 4 mm per year for aneurysms less than 4 cm in diameter, 4 to 5 mm per year for aneurysms 4 to 6 cm, and 7 to 8 mm per year for aneurysms greater than 6 cm. Intervention is typically indicated when the aneurysm reaches 5.5 cm, although many clinicians will intervene at the 5-cm threshold. The risk of rupture increases as the aneurysm grows: diameter greater than 5 cm = 20% eventual, 4% annual; diameter greater than 6 cm = 40% eventual, 7% annual; diameter greater than 7 cm = 50% eventual, 20% annual. Given that aneurysms grow, studies are ongoing to determine the benefit of earlier intervention when aneurysm diameters are smaller and patients are relatively healthier.

4. **How are most AAAs detected, and what is the role of screening?**
   Symptomatic aneurysms manifest with back, abdominal, buttock, groin, testicular, or leg pain. Most AAAs are asymptomatic, however. AAAs can be easily detected via ultrasonography (US), which has been shown to be cost-effective in targeted, high-risk patients. If AAA ruptures, the mortality rate is greater than 85%, and the morbidity rate and cost are significant for patients who survive. Elective repair of aneurysms is associated with low rates of mortality and morbidity, so aneurysmal disease is well suited to screening. Many hospitals and private, mobile screening companies offer aneurysm screening, often in conjunction with screening for other conditions such as peripheral and carotid arterial disease. The U.S. Congress passed the SAAAVE Act (Screen Abdominal Aortic Aneurysms Very Efficiently) in late 2005. Medicare-funded AAA screening is limited to male ever-smokers and to men and women with a positive family history of AAA.

5. **In general, when is endovascular aneurysm repair (EVAR) favored over open surgical repair?**
   EVAR is preferred over operative repair when the surgical operative risk is higher because of comorbidities and older age. EVAR has been shown in studies to have lower short-term rates of death and complications, although the survival curves merge in the long term. Generally, open surgical repair is preferred for younger, healthier patients, in whom longer term durability is a primary concern. EVAR versus open repair is essentially a matter of proper patient selection based on physiologic and anatomic risk factors and is often a matter of patient preference for less invasive therapy.

6. **Describe briefly the traditional open surgical repair of AAA.**
   With the patient under general anesthesia, a vascular surgeon makes an incision in the abdominal wall and exposes the aorta and the aneurysm. The incision is either down the center of the abdomen from immediately below the sternum to below the umbilicus or across the abdomen from underneath the left arm across to the center of the abdomen and down to below the umbilicus. Clamps are placed above and below the aneurysm to arrest blood flow;

the surgeon then butterflies the aneurysm and removes blood clots and plaque. A surgical tube graft is sewn to the healthy sections of the aorta connecting both ends of the aorta together. The clamps are removed, the wall of the aneurysm is wrapped around the graft, and the incision is closed. Recovery from AAA surgery is typically 7 to 10 days.

7. Name some findings on preprocedure imaging of AAA that may preclude a patient from undergoing EVAR.

A major preclusion to EVAR is proximal neck complexity or lack of a suitable landing zone just below the renal arteries to ensure fixation and seal of the stent graft. A short neck is defined as one that is less than 10 cm from immediately below the renal arteries to the beginning of the aneurysmal zone. An angulated neck is defined as greater than 45 degrees from immediately below the renal arteries to the beginning of the aneurysmal zone. A wide neck is greater than 32 mm. A neck that flares immediately below the renal arteries or an aneurysm that extends into and above the renal arteries (juxtarenal) would also preclude safe landing of a stent graft. Another contraindication is complex iliac arteries. The arteries may be tortuous or calcified, precluding passage of the delivery catheter, or they may be aneurysmal in which case it may be difficult to achieve fixation and seal of the iliac "legs" of a bifurcated stent graft. Lower profile delivery systems, branched and fenestrated grafts, and more flexible and conformable designs are under development to attempt to solve some of these contraindications to EVAR.

8. What is an endoleak? What are the different types of endoleaks, and how are they treated?

An endoleak is persistent blood flow into the aneurysmal sac after placement of a stent graft. A type I endoleak results from poor attachment to the vessel wall. It can be caused by poor apposition of the stent graft to the aortic or iliac wall, often owing to tortuosity, angulation, or disease (e.g., thrombus or calcification). Stent graft undersizing and aortic neck dilation are also causes of type I leaks. Type I leaks are typically treated with balloon dilation or the placement of an additional stent graft or balloon-expandable stent. Type II endoleaks are not caused by the graft itself but rather by retrograde flow into the aneurysm sac from collateral arterial branches such as lumbar arteries or the inferior mesenteric artery. Type II endoleaks sometimes resolve spontaneously or are monitored to see if they contribute to sac expansion or pressurization. If intervention is indicated, they are treated using coils or embolic glues. Type III endoleaks are caused by modular disconnections of stent graft pieces or by graft or metal fatigue causing tears in the fabric. This type of endoleak was more common in the early days of EVAR but is now decreasing in incidence because of more durable designs and more overlap of stent graft pieces in the initial procedure. Type IV endoleaks are transgraft endoleaks caused by fabric porosity or microabrasion caused by graft or metal fatigue. Type III and type IV endoleaks are treated by placement of additional stent graft pieces or through open repair. Type V endoleaks (also called endotension) occur when there is continued aneurysm sac expansion without evidence of a leak site and are poorly understood. Treatment with additional endoluminal components or with open surgical repair may be performed as needed.

9. What follow-up imaging tests do patients treated with EVAR undergo?

Patients require lifelong imaging surveillance to monitor for endoleak, aneurysm expansion, and graft integrity. Imaging follow-up after EVAR is usually performed by periodic contrast-enhanced computed tomography (CT). The typical regimen is a baseline CT study at 1 month, with a follow-up study at 6 months and annually thereafter. To reduce the need for expensive, radiation-exposing serial CT scans, some experts advocate for follow-up via color flow duplex US scanning in the absence of endoleak.

10. What are some of the complications related to EVAR?

Complications of EVAR include endoleak, continued enlargement or pressurization of the aneurysm sac without endoleak, delayed aneurysm rupture, graft migration, graft limb occlusion, graft infection, stent-graft structural breakdown, and groin or access complications.

11. What are the major studies that have looked at the outcomes of EVAR?

The major randomized controlled studies include (1) the Dutch Randomized Endovascular Aneurysm Management (DREAM) trial, (2) the EVAR versus open repair in patients with abdominal aortic aneurysm randomized controlled trial (EVAR trial 1), and (3) the EVAR and outcome in patients unfit for open repair of abdominal aortic aneurysm randomized controlled trial (EVAR trial 2). Major registry data include the European EUROSTAR database, the U.S.-based Lifeline Registry of Endovascular Aneurysm Repair, and the Medicare matched cohort data published in the *New England Journal of Medicine*. Short-term and long-term data from Investigational Device Exemption (IDE) studies from all U.S. Food and Drug Administration (FDA)-approved stent grafts are available at the respective manufacturers' websites.

12. What are the results of the major EVAR studies?

The EVAR 1 trial showed a 3% lower initial mortality for EVAR, with a persistent reduction in aneurysm-related death at 4 years. Improvement in overall late survival was not shown. Similarly, the DREAM trial observed an initial mortality advantage for EVAR, but overall 1-year survival was equivalent in both groups. The EVAR 2 trial did not show a survival advantage of EVAR with respect to nonoperative management, although the design of this trial has been heavily debated. The Medicare matched cohort study concluded that, compared with open repair, endovascular repair of AAA is associated with lower short-term rates of death and complications. The survival advantage was more durable among older patients. In the Lifeline Registry, patients receiving endovascular grafts were older and had more cardiac comorbidities compared with surgical controls (e.g., open repair), but there was no difference in the primary end points of all-cause mortality, AAA death, or aneurysm rupture between the endovascular graft and surgical control groups up to 3 years.

13. **What devices are currently commercially available in the United States for EVAR, and how do they differ?**

Current FDA-approved devices include the Cook Zenith, the Endologix Powerlink, the Gore Excluder, the Medtronic AneuRx, and the Medtronic Talent. Except for the unibody Powerlink platform, all platforms are modular in design. Each manufacturer offers a slightly different range of widths and lengths, including tapered and flared iliac extensions. The Zenith and the Excluder are equipped with tiny hooks or barbs to aid in fixation of the graft to the aortic wall. Some stent grafts are suprarenal, meaning they have uncovered stent structures that extend across and above the renal arteries. The Zenith and the Talent are suprarenal stent grafts. The AneuRx and the Excluder are infrarenal stent grafts. The Powerlink offers infrarenal and suprarenal aortic cuffs and is the only graft that is designed to "sit" on the iliac bifurcation. All stent grafts are self-expanding, but each has a different delivery catheter and actuator mechanism.

14. **What advantages will future generations of stent grafts have over ones that are currently available?**

Currently approved stent grafts have catheter delivery profiles ranging from 20 to 24 Fr. New designs currently in clinical trials have profiles ranging from 14 to 18 Fr, which would decrease access complications and significantly improve the ability to treat patients (especially women) with complex and narrow iliac arteries, for which EVAR is currently contraindicated. Patients with complex proximal aortic necks and juxtarenal aneurysms would benefit from branched and fenestrated grafts that permit endovascular repair, while preserving renal patency. More durable fixation methods (e.g., endostapling) and more flexible stent graft designs would expand the applicability of EVAR further.

15. **What are advantages of EVAR over traditional open surgical repair?**

The advantages of EVAR are that it is less invasive than open surgery, has a lower surgical morbidity and mortality rate, and reduces the length of postoperative hospital stays. The disadvantages of EVAR are the initial cost of the devices, the need for lifelong follow-up imaging, and the question of long-term durability.

## TRANSARTERIAL CHEMOEMBOLIZATION (TACE)

16. **What is meant by transarterial chemoembolization (TACE)?**

TACE is a procedure that involves blocking (embolizing) the arterial blood supply to a tumor and injecting chemotherapeutic drugs directly into the artery that feeds the tumor. A catheter is placed in the femoral artery and used to select the hepatic artery. The catheter in the hepatic artery is used for delivery of the embolic agent and drugs. The catheter is removed immediately after treatment.

17. **What types of hepatic malignancies can be treated with TACE?**

TACE is most often used for liver tumors. The most common tumors treated with chemoembolization are hepatocellular carcinoma (HCC) and hepatic metastatic lesions from colon cancer. Other tumors include metastatic hepatic lesions from carcinoid tumors and other neuroendocrine tumors, breast cancer, islet cell tumors of pancreas, ocular melanomas, and sarcomas. Benign tumors such as hepatic adenomas can also be treated with chemoembolization.

18. **What is a typical mixture used to perform TACE?**

There is no standard mixture of chemotherapy drugs or embolic agents that is widely used for TACE.

19. **What is the purpose of ethiodized oil (Ethiodol) in the TACE mixture?**

Ethiodol is used during TACE because it is selectively retained by tumor cells, is radiopaque, and can be seen under fluoroscopy during chemoembolization as well as on CT.

20. **What types of patients should be considered candidates for TACE?**

TACE is a liver-directed therapy for liver tumors. It works best in HCC when the tumor has not spread to extrahepatic sites. The best therapy for HCC is often liver transplantation. TACE is used to control HCC while the patient is on the transplant list awaiting liver transplantation. For patients who are not transplant candidates, TACE offers a noncurative treatment for HCC. For metastatic lesions to the liver, TACE is best used when disease outside the liver is well controlled, and the metastatic lesions to the liver represent the biggest threat to the patient's health.

21. **How are patients followed after TACE, and when is retreatment indicated?**

Patients are generally admitted for 1 night in the hospital after TACE. Patients receive a post-TACE CT or magnetic resonance imaging (MRI) examination and are seen in an outpatient interventional radiology clinic 1 month after TACE. Additional clinic visits and imaging with MRI or CT of the liver are done every 3 months to evaluate the success or failure of the procedure. Retreatment can be performed and is usually indicated if follow-up imaging shows new masses in the liver or recurrent disease at the site of the treated tumor.

22. **What is the typical imaging and clinical workup prior to TACE?**

Before TACE, patients are seen in the interventional radiology clinic, and a full history and physical examination are performed. MRI or CT is obtained within 1 month of the planned TACE. Within 1 week of the procedure, blood work is performed that includes complete blood count, international normalized ratio (INR), serum creatinine, and liver function tests.

23. What is postembolization syndrome?

Nearly all patients get postembolization syndrome after TACE. This condition includes low-grade fever, nausea, abdominal pain, and fatigue. It is worst in the first 24 to 48 hours after the procedure and usually resolves within 1 week after TACE.

24. What medications are patients typically treated with after TACE?

After TACE, patients are given powerful antibiotics to lessen the chance of infection and intravenous medications to control nausea and pain while they are in the hospital. When they are sent home, patients receive a 5-day course of an oral antibiotic and oral medications for nausea and pain.

25. What is the major risk factor for hepatic abscess formation secondary to TACE?

Hepatic abscess is always mentioned as a risk after TACE, but the risk increases greatly if the patient does not have a competent sphincter of Oddi. This can occur because of biliary stent placement or because of a biliary bypass procedure. Bacteria from the intestines can then colonize the biliary tree, leading to an increased risk of hepatic abscess formation after TACE.

26. What tumor markers are used to follow HCC? What about metastatic colon cancer?

For HCC, the most reliable tumor marker is serum alpha fetoprotein (AFP). For colon cancer, the tumor marker commonly used is serum carcinoembryonic antigen (CEA).

27. What laboratory values are checked when determining candidacy for TACE?

Within 1 week of the procedure, blood work is performed, which includes complete blood count, INR, serum creatinine, and liver function tests. If the patient has an elevated INR, bilirubin, aspartate aminotransferase (AST), or alanine aminotransferase (ALT), this may indicate that the patient has some degree of liver failure. Preexisting liver failure increases the risk of TACE and may be a reason not to perform the procedure.

28. How can the liver tolerate embolization of the hepatic artery without undergoing infarction?

The liver can tolerate TACE because it receives its blood supply from two sources: the hepatic artery and the portal vein. Liver tumors derive most of their blood supply from the hepatic artery, whereas the normal portion of the liver receives most of its blood supply from the portal vein. Before the TACE agents are delivered, an arteriogram is done to confirm patency of the portal vein. If the portal vein is completely occluded, the risk of liver failure and infarction after TACE increases significantly. An occluded portal vein may be reason not to perform TACE.

29. What does one look for on follow-up imaging to evaluate the success of a TACE procedure?

After TACE, MRI or CT of the abdomen is performed with intravenous contrast material. The intravenous contrast material causes the tumors to enhance if they are still viable. If a tumor is successfully treated, it is necrotic and will not enhance after contrast material administration. In patients who had elevated tumor markers prior to treatment, a subsequent decrease in tumor marker levels after treatment would also be an indication of successful TACE.

# RADIOFREQUENCY ABLATION (RFA)

30. What is radiofrequency ablation (RFA), and how does it work?

RFA is a technique for generating heat in living tissues through alternating electrical currents. The alternating currents result in agitation of ions and frictional heat, which can result in coagulation necrosis of tissue. This technology has been applied to the treatment of many conditions, including liver, kidney, bone, and lung tumors. A metal probe can be placed percutaneously in the tumor using US or CT guidance and is attached to the RF machine. RFA results in tumor death via thermal energy.

31. What characteristics of hepatic lesions are considered treatable by RFA? What are the characteristics of renal lesions treatable by RFA?

RFA is best done when there are three or fewer tumors to treat in the liver or kidney. Liver or kidney tumors 3 cm or smaller in size respond best to RFA. Larger tumors can be treated, but results are not usually as good.

32. What is the major CT and MR imaging characteristic of a lesion successfully treated with RFA?

MRI or CT is performed with intravenous contrast material 1 month after RFA to evaluate the success of the treatment. The intravenous contrast material causes tumors to enhance if they are still viable. If a tumor is successfully treated, it is necrotic and will not enhance after contrast material administration on CT or MRI.

33. How are patients followed after RFA procedures?

Patients usually have CT or MRI performed 1 month after the procedure and then at 3- to 6-month intervals as determined by the tumor type and institutional protocols.

34. What subset of patients with renal lesions is best treated with RFA?

Currently, RFA is usually reserved for patients who are not surgical candidates because of comorbid medical conditions or renal insufficiency or who have refused surgical resection of the kidney mass. As more long-term studies of RFA in renal masses are performed, more patients may be considered as candidates for this therapy.

35. What are complications of RFA?

Complications after RFA include bleeding, infection, injury to the organ being treated, and injury to surrounding organs including bowel.

# UTERINE FIBROID EMBOLIZATION (UFE)

36. What are typical symptoms of uterine fibroids?

Symptoms can be diverse bur may include menorrhagia (abnormal bleeding with menses), dysmenorrhea (painful menses), and bulk symptoms such as pain and pressure. Other symptoms include infertility, urinary urgency and incontinence, and constipation.

37. What clinical workup is required before undergoing uterine fibroid embolization (UFE)?

Workup should include a thorough history focusing on the presence of symptoms compatible with uterine fibroids. A physical examination is performed directed at evaluating the fibroid uterus. Laboratory evaluation includes a Pap smear and endometrial biopsy depending on symptoms, complete blood count, serum creatinine, and coagulation factors.

38. What imaging is required before UFE?

Cross-sectional imaging is performed before UFE. This can be either with US or preferably with contrast-enhanced MRI. The purpose of imaging is to evaluate fibroid size and location and to determine the possibility of adnexal disease that may alter management of the patient. Knowledge of the size and location of fibroids is important because submucosal fibroids are usually associated with bleeding and are at risk for being expelled after embolization. Large intracavitary fibroids may be a relative contraindication because of the risk of infection. The presence of fatty or hemorrhagic/red degeneration of a fibroid, which is seen as increased T1-weighted signal intensity on pretreatment MRI, is a negative predictor of successful treatment after UFE. MRI is also useful to detect the presence of ovarian arterial collateral supply to the uterus, which may lead to UFE treatment failure.

39. How is a patient followed after undergoing UFE?

Patients are followed closely in the immediate postembolization period to help manage pain. Usually MRI is obtained 3 to 6 months after the procedure to ascertain the degree of fibroid infarction and to correlate imaging findings with changes in symptoms.

40. What are the risks associated with UFE?

Aside from the risks that are common to any angiographic procedure, such as bleeding and reaction to intravenous contrast material, complications associated with UFE include infection or infarction of the uterus that might result in hysterectomy, fibroid expulsion, or premature menopause.

41. What are the alternatives to UFE?

Medical management consisting of hormonal therapy exists, but most patients presenting for UFE have already failed this treatment. Myomectomy is an option for patients seeking therapy for infertility. Hysterectomy is an option for patients with fibroids when pregnancy is not a consideration.

42. How do symptoms typically respond to UFE?

There is a success rate of 85% to 90% in controlling bleeding and bulk symptoms. Urinary symptoms may not respond as well.

43. Are there any other indications for UFE other than fibroids?

Uterine embolization can be used to treat bleeding emergencies such as postpartum hemorrhage, uterine atony, and cervical ectopic pregnancy. Uterine embolization may also be used for other conditions such as adenomyosis, although its success may not be as durable as with the treatment of fibroids.

44. What type of embolic agent is typically used?

Polyvinyl alcohol (PVA) particles or trisacryl particles (Embosphere) have been shown to have the best success to date for UFE. Absorbable gelatin sponge (Gelfoam) has been shown to work when used for treatment of acute bleeding.

45. Is there a correlation between postprocedure pain and clinical outcomes?

There is no correlation between degree of pain and clinical outcomes. Patients usually return to normal activities within 1 to 2 weeks after UFE.

46. What is a typical analgesia protocol for patients undergoing UFE?

Patients receive intravenous ketorolac tromethamine (Toradol) periprocedurally and are managed with fentanyl (Fentora) and midazolam (Versed) during the procedure. Postprocedure, a patient-controlled analgesia pump with morphine or hydromorphone (Dilaudid) along with an oral nonsteroidal anti-inflammatory drug (NSAID) is used to control pain. Some authorities advocate the use of epidurals during hospitalization. Patients are discharged with an oral narcotic such as oxycodone with acetaminophen and an NSAID such as ibuprofen.

47. What are the indications for discharge from the hospital after UFE?

Patients may be discharged when they are able to tolerate oral intake, and pain is controlled with oral medications.

48. Describe the vascular anatomy relevant to UFE.

Although anatomic variations exist, the paired uterine arteries are typically the first branches of the anterior division of the internal iliac arteries. Embolization is usually performed with the tip of the catheter in the horizontal segment of the uterine artery that is past the cervical-vaginal branch. The ovarian arteries usually arise from the abdominal aorta and can also supply the uterus in a small proportion of patients.

49. What is the risk of premature menopause related to UFE?

The risk is low for patients younger than 45 years old and increases after this age. The rate of premature menopause may be 40% in patients older than 51 years.

50. Is pregnancy possible after UFE?

Yes, although the incidence of placental location abnormalities, such as placenta previa, may be increased. There may also be a higher rate of miscarriage, but it is uncertain if this is related to a history of UFE or the higher maternal age in this specific patient population.

## KEY POINTS

- AAA rupture is often fatal; AAAs must therefore be detected, monitored, and treated prior to rupture. Intervention is typically indicated when the aneurysm reaches 5.5 cm, although many clinicians treat at the 5-cm threshold.
- There are two primary treatment options for AAAs: EVAR and open surgical repair. EVAR is preferred when the operative risk is higher because of comorbidities and older age. Open repair is preferred for younger, healthier patients, in whom longer-term durability is a primary concern.
- EVAR is less invasive than open surgery, has a lower surgical morbidity and mortality rate, and reduces the length of postoperative hospital stays. EVAR complications include endoleak, continued enlargement or pressurization of the aneurysm sac without endoleak, delayed aneurysm rupture, graft migration, graft limb occlusion, graft infection, stent-graft structural breakdown, and groin or access complications.
- TACE is a liver-directed therapy for liver tumors, including HCC, hepatic metastases, and occasionally hepatic adenomas.
- RFA is a technique for generating heat and subsequent coagulation necrosis in living tissues through alternating electrical currents and is used to treat many conditions, including liver, kidney, bone, and lung tumors.

## BIBLIOGRAPHY

Sieghart W, Hucke F, Peck-Radosavljevic M. Transarterial chemoembolization: modalities, indication and patient selection. *J Hepatol.* 2015;62(5):1187-1195.

Clark ME, Smith RR. Liver-directed therapies in metastatic colorectal cancer. *J Gastrointest Oncol.* 2014;5(5):374-387.

Kim YS, Lim HK, Rhim H, et al. Ablation of hepatocellular carcinoma. *Best Pract Res Clin Gastroenterol.* 2014;28(5):897-908.

Klatte T, Kroeger N, Zimmermann U, et al. The contemporary role of ablative treatment approaches in the management of renal cell carcinoma (RCC): focus on radiofrequency ablation (RFA), high-intensity focused ultrasound (HIFU), and cryoablation. *World J Urol.* 2014;32(3):597-605.

Kolbeck KJ, Farsad K. Catheter-based treatments for hepatic metastases from neuroendocrine tumors. *AJR Am J Roentgenol.* 2014;203(4):717-724.

LeFevre ML, Force USPST. Screening for abdominal aortic aneurysm: U.S. Preventive Services Task Force recommendation statement. *Ann Intern Med.* 2014;161(4):281-290.

Xing M, Kooby DA, El-Rayes BF, et al. Locoregional therapies for metastatic colorectal carcinoma to the liver—an evidence-based review. *J Surg Oncol.* 2014;110(2):182-196.

Lencioni R, Petruzzi P, Crocetti L. Chemoembolization of hepatocellular carcinoma. *Semin Intervent Radiol.* 2013;30(1):3-11.

Mahnken AH, Pereira PL, de Baere T. Interventional oncologic approaches to liver metastases. *Radiology.* 2013;266(2):407-430.

Minami Y, Kudo M. Therapeutic response assessment of transcatheter arterial chemoembolization for hepatocellular carcinoma: ultrasonography, CT and MR imaging. *Oncology.* 2013;84(suppl 1):58-63.

Bulman JC, Ascher SM, Spies JB. Current concepts in uterine fibroid embolization. *Radiographics.* 2012;32(6):1735-1750.

Iannuccilli JD, Dupuy DE, Mayo-Smith WW. Solid renal masses: effectiveness and safety of image-guided percutaneous radiofrequency ablation. *Abdom Imaging.* 2012;37(4):647-658.

Toor SS, Jaberi A, MacDonald DB, et al. Complication rates and effectiveness of uterine artery embolization in the treatment of symptomatic leiomyomas: a systematic review and meta-analysis. *AJR Am J Roentgenol.* 2012;199(5):1153-1163.

Aggarwal S, Qamar A, Sharma V, et al. Abdominal aortic aneurysm: a comprehensive review. *Exp Clin Cardiol.* 2011;16(1):11-15.

Kirby JM, Burrows D, Haider E, et al. Utility of MRI before and after uterine fibroid embolization: why to do it and what to look for. *Cardiovasc Intervent Radiol.* 2011;34(4):705-716.

Bashir MR, Ferral H, Jacobs C, et al. Endoleaks after endovascular abdominal aortic aneurysm repair: management strategies according to CT findings. *AJR Am J Roentgenol.* 2009;192(4):W178-W186.

Schermerhorn ML, O'Malley AJ, Jhaveri A, et al. Endovascular vs. open repair of abdominal aortic aneurysms in the Medicare population. *N Engl J Med.* 2008;358(5):464-474.

Steward MJ, Warbey VS, Malhotra A, et al. Neuroendocrine tumors: role of interventional radiology in therapy. *Radiographics.* 2008;28(4):1131-1145.

Leurs LJ, Buth J, Harris PL, et al. Impact of study design on outcome after endovascular abdominal aortic aneurysm repair. A comparison between the randomized controlled DREAM-trial and the observational EUROSTAR-registry. *Eur J Vasc Endovasc Surg.* 2007;33(2):172-176.

Stavropoulos SW, Charagundla SR. Imaging techniques for detection and management of endoleaks after endovascular aortic aneurysm repair. *Radiology.* 2007;243(3):641-655.

Kroencke TJ, Scheurig C, Kluner C, et al. Uterine fibroids: contrast-enhanced MR angiography to predict ovarian artery supply—initial experience. *Radiology.* 2006;241(1):181-189.

Blankensteijn JD, de Jong SE, Prinssen M, et al. Two-year outcomes after conventional or endovascular repair of abdominal aortic aneurysms. *N Engl J Med.* 2005;352(23):2398-2405.

EVAR Trial Participants. Endovascular aneurysm repair and outcome in patients unfit for open repair of abdominal aortic aneurysm (EVAR trial 2): randomised controlled trial. *Lancet.* 2005;365(9478):2187-2192.

EVAR Trial Participants. Endovascular aneurysm repair versus open repair in patients with abdominal aortic aneurysm (EVAR trial 1): randomised controlled trial. *Lancet.* 2005;365(9478):2179-2186.

Kitamura Y, Ascher SM, Cooper C, et al. Imaging manifestations of complications associated with uterine artery embolization. *Radiographics.* 2005;25(suppl 1):S119-S132.

Lifeline Registry of EPC. Lifeline registry of endovascular aneurysm repair: long-term primary outcome measures. *J Vasc Surg.* 2005;42(1):1-10.

Pelage JP, Cazejust J, Pluot E, et al. Uterine fibroid vascularization and clinical relevance to uterine fibroid embolization. *Radiographics.* 2005;25(suppl 1):S99-S117.

Greenhalgh RM, Brown LC, Kwong GP, et al. Comparison of endovascular aneurysm repair with open repair in patients with abdominal aortic aneurysm (EVAR trial 1), 30-day operative mortality results: randomised controlled trial. *Lancet.* 2004;364(9437):843-848.

Prinssen M, Verhoeven EL, Buth J, et al. A randomized trial comparing conventional and endovascular repair of abdominal aortic aneurysms. *N Engl J Med.* 2004;351(16):1607-1618.

# PERIPHERAL ARTERIAL DISEASE DIAGNOSIS AND INTERVENTION

*Jeffrey I. Mondschein, MD, and Jeffrey A. Solomon, MD, MBA*

# CHAPTER 70

1. **What is the appropriate landmark for a femoral artery puncture?**

   Some risks of arteriography can be minimized by properly selecting the puncture site. Above the inguinal canal, the common femoral artery becomes the external iliac artery and dives posteriorly. Punctures above the inguinal canal may be problematic for several reasons. Because the artery is deep in relation to the puncture site, manual compression may be difficult, leading to a hematoma or arterial pseudoaneurysm. In the event of an access site complication that requires surgical intervention, the surgical approach for puncture above the inguinal ligament is more involved. A puncture that is too low may result in an arteriovenous fistula (AVF). The inguinal crease is a landmark that is commonly used for femoral artery puncture, but this is a very inaccurate estimate for the location of the inguinal ligament, especially in obese patients. The best landmark is the middle of the medial third of the femoral head identified fluoroscopically (Figure 70-1). Ultrasonography (US) may also be used to guide access.

2. **If the femoral artery cannot be accessed, what are other options to obtain access for an arteriogram?**

   Multiple options for access may exist in any given patient. The appropriate access site depends on the patient's symptoms, intended procedure, prior surgical history, known sites of arterial occlusion, and clinical setting. A brachial artery approach may be used if a femoral approach is impossible. Other access options include direct puncture of bypass grafts, direct translumbar aortic puncture, radial artery access, and retrograde popliteal or dorsalis pedis access.

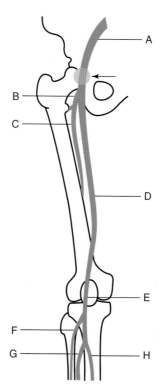

**Figure 70-1.** Leg arterial vascular anatomy. The arrow and blue circle indicate the preferred site for percutaneous access to common femoral artery, over middle third of femoral head. *A* = external iliac artery, *B* = femoral bifurcation, *C* = deep femoral artery, *D* = superficial femoral artery, *E* = popliteal artery, *F* = anterior tibial artery, *G* = peroneal artery, *H* = posterior tibial artery.

3. If a brachial approach must be used, is the right or left arm used?

A left brachial approach is preferred. A catheter placed from the left arm passes the left vertebral artery origin but not that of the left common carotid artery; this may reduce the risk of stroke.

4. What are some complications unique to brachial access?

There is a small risk of stroke associated with brachial access. The arm cannot tolerate large hematomas, and bleeding after removal of a catheter or sheath may result in a compartment syndrome. If a hematoma does develop, it must be followed up carefully to ensure that neurovascular compromise does not occur. Surgical evacuation of the hematoma may be required to prevent a neurologic deficit. In recent years, many practitioners have shifted to radial access, because there is theoretically less risk of limb ischemia and upper extremity neurologic complications.

5. What is claudication?

Claudication is derived from the Latin verb *claudicare*, which means "to limp." Claudication describes exercise-induced leg pain secondary to peripheral arterial disease (PAD). Patients with claudication typically complain of a burning or aching sensation in the thigh or calf, which starts after walking a predictable distance and remits with rest. With advanced disease, there may be progression to rest pain, skin ulceration, and tissue loss.

6. What are the risk factors for PAD and claudication?

Risk factors include hypertension, diabetes mellitus, high cholesterol levels, cigarette smoking, and advanced age. Claudication is also more likely in individuals who already have atherosclerosis in other arteries, such as the coronary or carotid arteries.

7. Does the location of leg pain suggest the location of arterial stenosis?

Leg pain usually occurs downstream from hemodynamically significant stenoses. For example, calf pain may result from disease of the superficial femoral artery, whereas thigh or buttock pain may be caused by iliac arterial disease.

8. Why is it important to identify patients with claudication?

PAD affects more than 10 million Americans, and its prevalence is increasing. PAD is an important marker for many other serious conditions, including coronary artery disease, cerebrovascular disease, aneurysms, diabetes mellitus, and hypertension. Patients with PAD have a 4- to 6-fold increased cardiovascular mortality compared to age-matched controls. The mortality rate for patients with claudication may be 75% at 15 years after diagnosis of PAD. Early diagnosis of the disease gives patients the chance to modify their atherosclerotic risk factors and to reduce their risk of coronary and carotid artery disease.

9. What is the Fontaine classification?

The Fontaine classification is a widely used classification system for lower extremity ischemia. It describes four stages based on signs and symptoms.
- Stage 1 is asymptomatic disease.
- Stage 2a is intermittent claudication when walking more than 200 m.
- Stage 2b is intermittent claudication when walking less than 200 m.
- Stage 3 is rest pain.
- Stage 4 is tissue necrosis or gangrene.

10. What is the Rutherford-Becker classification system?

This is another classification system for chronic limb ischemia. It is popular in the United States and is based on clinical and objective criteria (Table 70-1).

11. What are the clinical categories of acute limb ischemia?

For the answer, see Table 70-2.

12. What is the ankle-brachial index (ABI)?

The ABI is an essential component used for risk stratification for PAD. The ABI is used to screen for hemodynamically significant disease and to help define its severity. With the patient in the supine position, bilateral brachial blood pressures are obtained. A blood pressure cuff is placed on the calf of each leg, and an ankle systolic pressure is obtained. Determining ankle systolic pressure may require the use of Doppler US. The ABI is calculated by dividing the ankle systolic pressure by the highest systolic pressure from either arm.

13. How is the ABI interpreted?

A normal ABI is slightly greater than 1. A significant obstruction to blood flow to the lower extremities reduces the ankle pressure and the ABI. The risk of PAD and other cardiovascular disease as well as symptoms increases as the ABI decreases (Tables 70-3 and 70-4).

14. What can cause a falsely elevated ABI?

The ability to determine the systolic blood pressure accurately is predicated by the ability to compress the artery and obstruct blood flow. Diabetes mellitus may cause significant calcification of peripheral vessels, making them difficult to compress; this would elevate the observed cuff pressure and the calculated ABI and could create false-negative tests.

**Table 70-1.** Clinical Categories of Chronic Limb Ischemia (Rutherford Becker Classification System)

| GRADE | CATEGORY | CLINICAL DESCRIPTION | OBJECTIVE CRITERIA |
|---|---|---|---|
| 0 | 0 | Asymptomatic, not hemodynamically significant | Normal treadmill/stress test |
| I | 1 | Mild claudication | Completes treadmill test, ankle pressure after exercise <25-50 mm Hg less than blood pressure |
| | 2 | Moderate claudication | Between categories 1 and 3 |
| | 3 | Severe claudication | Cannot complete treadmill test, ankle pressure after exercise <50 mm Hg |
| II | 4 | Ischemic rest pain | Resting ankle pressure <40 mm Hg, flat or barely pulsatile ankle or metatarsal pulse volume recording, toe pressure <30 mm Hg |
| | 5 | Minor tissue loss: nonhealing ulcer, focal gangrene with diffuse pedal edema | Resting ankle pressure <60 mm Hg, flat or barely pulsatile ankle metatarsal pulse volume recording, toe pressure <40 mm Hg |
| III | 6 | Major tissue loss: extending above transmetatarsal level, functional foot no longer salvageable | Same as category 5 |

**Table 70-2.** Clinical Categories of Acute Limb Ischemia

| CATEGORY | DESCRIPTION | CAPILLARY RETURN | MUSCLE WEAKNESS | SENSORY LOSS | ARTERIAL DOPPLER SIGNAL | VENOUS DOPPLER SIGNAL |
|---|---|---|---|---|---|---|
| Viable | Not immediately threatened | Intact | None | None | Audible (ankle pressure >30 mm Hg) | Audible |
| Threatened | Salvageable if promptly treated | Intact, but slow | Mild, partial | Mild, incomplete | Inaudible | Audible |
| Irreversible | Major tissue loss, amputation indicated regardless of treatment | Absent (marbling) | Profound, paralysis (rigor) | Profound, anesthetic | Inaudible | Inaudible |

**Table 70-3.** Ankle-Brachial Index (ABI) by Symptoms

| ABI | SYMPTOMS |
|---|---|
| 1-1.10 | Normal |
| 0.3-0.9 | Claudication |
| ≤0.5 | Rest pain |
| ≤0.2 | Tissue loss |

15. **What is meant by the terms** *inflow* **and** *outflow*?

At least two criteria must be met for an artery to remain patent. There must be sufficient flow of blood into the vessel. With respect to the femoral artery, inflow vessels include the aorta, common iliac artery, and external iliac artery. A stenosis of any of these vessels constitutes an inflow lesion. Even with perfect inflow, there also must be flow out of a vessel for it to remain patent. With respect to the femoral artery, the popliteal, peroneal, anterior tibial, and posterior tibial arteries constitute outflow vessels.

**Table 70-4.** Ankle-Brachial Index (ABI) by Cardiovascular Risk

| ABI | CARDIOVASCULAR RISK CATEGORY |
|---|---|
| >1.40 | Noncompressible arteries (increased risk) |
| 1.00-1.40 | Normal (no/low risk) |
| 0.91-0.99 | Borderline (probably normal; no/low risk) |
| 0.70-0.89 | Abnormal (low/moderate risk) |
| 0.50-0.69 | Abnormal (moderate/high risk) |
| <0.49 | Abnormal (high risk) |

16. What are the basic steps in performing an angioplasty procedure?

A thorough diagnostic arteriogram is performed first. This is important so that the lesion can be sized and an appropriate angioplasty balloon can be selected. The patient is then given heparin. It is important to give heparin before crossing the lesion to prevent thrombosis. The next step involves crossing the lesion with a catheter and guidewire. The lesion is then dilated with an angioplasty balloon. After the balloon is removed, an arteriogram is performed with the wire across the lesion to evaluate the result of the angioplasty. It is important to leave the wire in place until the follow-up arteriogram is performed in case a complication, such as a flow-limiting dissection or arterial rupture, occurs.

17. What constitutes a technically successful angioplasty?
- Restoration of luminal diameter with <30% residual stenosis.
- A pressure gradient <5 mm Hg across the lesion.
- Absence of a flow-limiting dissection or vessel rupture.
- Relative reduction in the number and caliber of collateral vessels seen on angiography.

18. What are the complications of angioplasty?

The types and incidence of complications vary with the location and morphology of the lesion. Complications include spasm, flow-limiting dissection, plaque embolization, vessel rupture, access site trauma, renal dysfunction, or allergic reaction to iodinated contrast material, and rarely death.

19. What are the indications for stenting?

Primary indications for stenting include failed angioplasty caused by a flow-limiting dissection or elastic recoil of the stenosis. The lumen of a stented segment will narrow somewhat over time due to pseudointimal proliferation. Therefore, stents work better in larger caliber arteries. However, recent studies have demonstrated that stents may also be useful for limb salvage in smaller vessels, and there is limited evidence that suggests that drug-eluting stents may further aid patency.

20. What constitutes a hemodynamically significant arterial stenosis?

A stenosis is generally considered significant if the luminal diameter is reduced by 50%, and the systolic pressure gradient is greater than 10 mm Hg across the lesion. A lumen that is diminished by 50% would have a corresponding 75% reduction in cross-sectional area, which would likely reduce flow to a clinically significant level. In patients with claudication and lesions that are equivocal based on the aforementioned criteria, provocative testing may be performed. One may stimulate arterial dilation with a prolonged inflation of a blood pressure cuff above the systolic pressure on the limb proximal to the level of stenosis, a technique called reactive hyperemia. A gradient greater than 20 mm Hg after vasodilation is considered significant. Nitroglycerin can also be used as a pharmacologic vasodilator. One should remember to treat the patient and not the arteriographic or pressure findings. The clinical history is also important in deciding whether a lesion is significant. Treating an entirely asymptomatic lesion is almost never indicated.

21. What is the kissing balloon technique?

This technique is most commonly used to perform angioplasty of the common iliac arteries (Figure 70-2). Often, stenoses of the proximal common iliac arteries are associated with large, eccentric, calcified plaques. Sequential, as opposed to simultaneous, angioplasty may displace the plaque and lead to compromise of the contralateral iliac artery. The kissing balloon technique mitigates this risk through the use of simultaneous angioplasty. This requires bilateral retrograde femoral artery access. If stents are being placed bilaterally, sequential placement of one stent may result in prolapse of its proximal portion across the origin of the contralateral common iliac artery, effectively "jailing" the other side. Therefore, the kissing balloon technique may also be useful with balloon expandable stents in this situation. The kissing balloon technique may be used for the dilation of complex bifurcation stenosis in other locations as well.

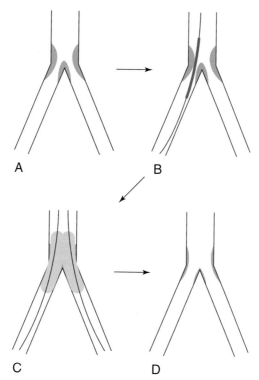

**Figure 70-2.** Kissing balloon technique. **A,** Bifurcation lesion. **B,** Sequential angioplasty risks occlusion of contralateral unprotected vessel. **C,** Simultaneous angioplasty prevents plaque displacement. **D,** Desired result following angioplasty.

22. If a wire cannot be passed through the lumen of a vessel because of chronic total occlusion, what techniques may be used to allow for endovascular treatment?

    Subintimal recanalization may be performed. This is a technique that uses a catheter and hydrophilic guidewire to traverse the intima of the vessel adjacent to the site of occlusion and then tunnel through the subintimal space within the vessel wall. At the other side of the occluded segment, the catheter is used to redirect the wire back into the true lumen of the vessel. Angioplasty and stenting can then be performed, allowing the vessel lumen proximal and distal to the occlusion to be bridged through a newly created lumen in the subintimal space. The most difficult step of subintimal recanalization is re-entry into the vessel lumen from the subintimal space. Several crossing devices have been introduced to facilitate this step.

23. What is an atherectomy device, and what types of lesions might it be useful for?

    Atherectomy devices are endovascular tools that cut or ablate atherosclerotic plaque away from the wall of the diseased artery in an effort to expand the flow lumen. There are currently four types of atherectomy devices: directional, rotational, orbital, and laser. There is currently little evidence to support widespread use of the technique, and no benefit over angioplasty and stenting has been definitively proven. However, atherectomy is being used in clinical practice, and continued evaluation is ongoing. Theoretically, the technique may facilitate treatment of long segment and heavily calcified lesions as well as eccentric atherosclerotic plaque at risk for embolization during intervention.

24. What are the basic principles in performing a thrombolysis procedure?

    Catheter-directed pharmacologic thrombolysis therapy consists of the delivery of a lytic agent directly into a thrombosed vessel or graft. The catheter is largely responsible for instilling the lytic agent only within the thrombosed segment so that relatively small overall doses of a lytic agent can achieve high local concentration within the clot. In this way, significant local effects can be achieved while minimizing systemic effects, thereby decreasing the risk of bleeding at other sites. The immediate goal of the procedure is to lyse an unwanted clot while preventing a systemically lytic state to minimize bleeding complications. The secondary goal of a thrombolysis procedure is to uncover the cause of the thrombosis. Commonly, bypass grafts and native vessels thrombose because of stenoses in inflow vessels, anastomoses, or outflow vessels. Unless the underlying cause for the thrombosis is treated, thrombosis is likely to recur. Less commonly, there are instances in which grafts or vessels thrombose without underlying stenoses. Embolic disease, diminished cardiac output, and noncompliance with anticoagulation therapy are some causes of thrombosis in the absence of an underlying stenosis.

25. In general, how is a thrombolysis procedure performed?

A thorough history and physical examination of the patient are performed. Particular attention should be given to any prior surgeries described in the history. Understanding the patient's vascular anatomy is of paramount importance for planning access and intervention. Prior arteriograms, if available, should be reviewed. These may also help in the planning of the access site and in determining an appropriate end point for the procedure. Comparison to a baseline physical examination is essential for monitoring the patient's progress or deterioration during the procedure. After laboratory findings are reviewed and patient informed consent has been obtained, a thorough diagnostic arteriogram is performed. The patient is given heparin, and a sheath is placed. The thrombosed segment is crossed with a wire, and an infusion catheter is placed across the clot. Lytic agents are infused continuously through the catheter, and the patient is sent to the intensive care unit for monitoring. Every 12 to 24 hours, the patient is brought back to the interventional suite for a follow-up arteriogram. Sometimes, mechanical thrombolysis devices are also used to help remove the clot. When the clot has resolved, the underlying lesion is treated.

26. What is the guidewire traversal test?

The guidewire traversal test is an attempt to pass a guidewire across a thrombosed vessel before lysis. If the wire can be successfully passed across the occlusion, the clot is more likely to be acute and will probably lyse. If the guidewire traversal test fails, the occlusion is more likely to be chronic and less responsive to lytic agents. An end-hole catheter, positioned proximal to the clot, may be used to deliver lytic agents and soften the clot to facilitate wire traversal. When a wire has been passed, an infusion catheter can be placed. Placement of an infusion catheter within the bulk of the clot helps lend specificity to the lysis procedure and may reduce the overall time required for lysis.

27. List the contraindications to thrombolysis.

- Absolute contraindications include active internal bleeding, known intracranial pathology, stroke within the past 6 months, craniotomy in the past 2 months, irreversible limb ischemia, and infected bypass graft.
- Relative contraindications include uncontrollable hypertension, history of gastrointestinal bleeding, bacterial endocarditis, diabetic retinopathy, coagulopathy, pregnancy, recent major surgery, recent major trauma, and recent cardiopulmonary resuscitation.

    In patients with relative contraindications, it is imperative to analyze the potential risk-to-benefit ratio carefully in each case.

28. What is a PVR examination?

PVR stands for **pulse volume recording**, which is a noninvasive method to evaluate arteries of the lower extremity. A brachial pressure and arterial waveform are obtained as reference standards. The process is repeated at different stations, including the high thigh, low thigh, calf, ankle, and foot. The segmental pressures and waveforms are analyzed to identify the level and severity of possible stenoses. Arterial waveforms provide especially useful information in the setting of a calcified vessel. This test is one way that surveillance may be performed after a vascular intervention. It can also be used to plan an intervention in a symptomatic patient. It is particularly useful in patients who have renal insufficiency, because their kidney function may limit the ability to safely use diagnostic tests that require vascular contrast administration, such as CT angiography (CTA).

29. What is Leriche syndrome?

Leriche syndrome is a set of symptoms and signs due to chronic lower extremity ischemia resulting from aortoiliac obstruction. It is characterized by intermittent buttock claudication, absent femoral pulses, and sexual impotence.

30. What is an ACT measurement?

ACT stands for **activated clotting time**. It is a clotting test that may be performed in the interventional suite and is commonly used to monitor the effect of heparin. A small sample of whole blood is placed in the testing machine, and a result is available in less than 5 minutes. The reference range varies considerably, but it is usually 70 to 180 seconds. Although it can be obtained quickly, ACT is less precise than partial thromboplastin time and can be affected by a host of factors including ambient temperature, platelet count, and hemodilution.

31. How are groin pseudoaneurysms managed?

Pseudoaneurysms resulting from femoral artery puncture can be managed in several ways, based on the patient's clinical status and the anatomy of the lesion. The first step is to recognize that the complication has occurred. A postprocedure groin check may reveal a pulsatile mass or ecchymosis. The patient may complain of groin pain. US can be used to diagnose or exclude the injury. If a pseudoaneurysm is found, several options exist. Manual or US-guided compression may cause the pseudoaneurysm to thrombose. Direct thrombin injection can also be performed if the anatomy of the lesion is suitable. Surgical intervention is also an option if other techniques fail.

32. What are the major pathways of collateral circulation to supply the lower extremities in a patient with known aortic occlusion?

A simple way to help remember the collateral supply is to divide it into anterior, middle, and posterior pathways (Figure 70-3).

- Anterior pathway: Subclavian artery through the internal mammary artery to the superior epigastric artery, to the inferior epigastric artery, and then to the external iliac artery. This is known as the pathway of Winslow.

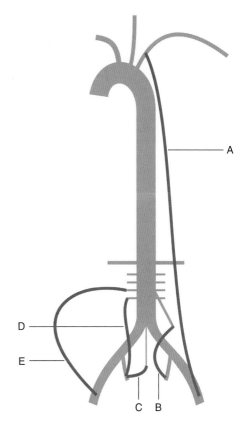

**Figure 70-3.** Collateral vascular pathways in aortic occlusion. Anterior supply: Left subclavian artery to left external iliac artery, via internal mammary and inferior epigastric arteries (*A*). Middle supply: Inferior mesenteric artery to internal iliac artery (*B*). Posterior supply: Median sacral artery to internal iliac artery (*C*). Lumbar artery to internal iliac artery (*D*). Lumbar artery to external iliac artery (*E*).

- Middle pathway: Superior mesenteric artery to the inferior mesenteric artery, via the arc of Riolan and the marginal artery of Drummond, to the superior and inferior hemorrhoidal arteries, to the internal iliac arteries, and then to the external iliac arteries.
- Posterior pathway: Lumbar arteries to the internal iliac arteries via retroperitoneal collaterals and then to the external iliac arteries by way of the iliolumbar and circumflex iliac arteries.

## KEY POINTS

- Asymptomatic arterial lesions rarely require treatment.
- Patients rarely die from PAD, but this disease serves as a marker for other, potentially life-threatening processes, such as cerebrovascular disease and coronary artery disease.
- PAD can cause significant morbidity due to claudication, rest pain, poor wound healing, and potential need for amputation.
- PAD is underdiagnosed, especially in women.
- Outflow is a key determinant for the long-term patency of angioplasty.

## Bibliography

Mauro MA, Murphy KPJ, Thomson KR, et al. *Image-guided interventions: expert radiology series*. 2nd ed. Philadelphia: Saunders; 2014.

Kim ES, Wattanakit K, Gornik HL. Using the ankle-brachial index to diagnose peripheral artery disease and assess cardiovascular risk. *Cleve Clin J Med*. 2012;79(9):651-661.

Diehm C, Allenberg JR, Pittrow D, et al. Mortality and vascular morbidity in older adults with asymptomatic versus symptomatic peripheral artery disease. *Circulation*. 2009;120(21):2053-2061.

Pentecost MJ, Criqui MH, Dorros G, et al. Guidelines for peripheral percutaneous transluminal angioplasty of the abdominal aorta and lower extremity vessels. A statement for health professionals from a Special Writing Group of the Councils on Cardiovascular Radiology, Arteriosclerosis, Cardio-Thoracic and Vascular Surgery, Clinical Cardiology, and Epidemiology and Prevention, the American Heart Association. *J Vasc Interv Radiol*. 2003;14(9 Pt 2):S495-S515.

Sacks D, Bakal CW, Beatty PT, et al. Position statement on the use of the ankle brachial index in the evaluation of patients with peripheral vascular disease. A consensus statement developed by the Standards Division of the Society of Interventional Radiology. *J Vasc Interv Radiol*. 2003;14(9 Pt 2):S389.

# CHAPTER 71

# EMBOLIZATION TECHNIQUES AND APPLICATIONS

*Sara Chen Gavenonis, MD, and S. William Stavropoulos, MD*

1. **Describe embolotherapy and some of its indications.**
   Embolotherapy is temporary or permanent vascular occlusion induced by the intravascular administration of materials via a percutaneous route. Embolization has various clinical applications, including control of bleeding; treatment of vascular malformations; and tumor or organ ablation for curative, palliative, or preoperative purposes.

2. **What materials are most commonly used for embolization?**
   Various embolic materials are commercially available. The most widely used embolic materials are absorbable gelatin sponge (Gelfoam), a temporary agent; metallic coils; and polyvinyl alcohol (PVA) particles. Specific clinical situations may warrant the use of other agents, such as absolute ethanol, synthetic microspheres, or liquid "glues."

3. **What is Gelfoam, and how is it prepared and delivered?**
   Gelfoam is a reabsorbable gelatin that is most widely used in its sheet form. Wedges (1 to 2 mm) of Gelfoam are divided from the larger sheets. The Gelfoam can be injected as "torpedoes" through a catheter placed in a blood vessel, or the Gelfoam can be suspended in a contrast/saline slurry, which can be injected.

4. **How does Gelfoam work, and when is it used?**
   Gelfoam causes vascular occlusion by mechanically obstructing vessels, serving as a matrix for thrombus formation, and causing endothelial inflammation that incites further thrombus formation. Gelfoam is reabsorbed in 5 to 6 weeks, during which time vessel recanalization is anticipated. Clinical situations in which temporary vascular occlusion is preferred include pelvic arterial hemorrhage after trauma, priapism, peripartum hemorrhage, and some cases of upper gastrointestinal (GI) bleeding. The rationale for using Gelfoam in these situations is based on the belief that use of a temporary agent would minimize long-term ischemic effects on the end organ.

5. **What are metallic coils?**
   Metallic coils are made of either stainless steel or platinum. Dacron fibers are woven into some coils to promote thrombosis. Coils are available in a wide variety of shapes, sizes, and configurations. Special wires are used to push the coils through catheters that have been placed into the vessel intended to be embolized. Coils occlude vessels by causing mechanical obstruction, inducing clot formation, and provoking an inflammatory reaction.

6. **When are coils preferred?**
   One way to classify embolic materials is based on whether they cause permanent or temporary occlusion. Another way is based on the size (diameter) of the vessel where the occlusion occurs. Coils cause vascular occlusion in vessels that are 1 to 2 mm in diameter and larger. Coils are preferred in clinical situations in which permanent occlusion is intended in vessels of this size. This includes the treatment of arteriovenous fistulas (AVFs), GI bleeding, aneurysms, endoleaks after endovascular repair of abdominal aortic aneurysm (AAA), and traumatic vascular injuries in the proper clinical settings. Coils should not be used if occlusion is desired in vessels smaller than 1 mm, including situations in which the target of embolization is an organ. When embolizing the uterus or performing chemoembolization of the liver, coils are not used. PVA particles or ethanol can be used to cause microvascular thrombosis, depending on the specific clinical situation.

7. **What happens when coils are the wrong size?**
   When coils are undersized, they can remain mobile after they are pushed out of the catheter and continue to travel with the flow of blood until they embolize to a vessel that is smaller than the diameter of the coil. If this happens while a venous embolization is being performed, the coils travel back toward the right heart and often through the pulmonary artery before lodging in a small vessel. The lungs are also a likely final destination for coils that inadvertently pass through an AVF. When deployed in an artery, coils that are too small can migrate into distal branches or into another vascular distribution. This migration may result in nontarget embolization and decreased efficacy of the intended embolization. Coils that are too large can partially recoil into the parent vessel or cause the catheter to back out of the proper vessel. Retrievable coils are now available and allow optimization of positioning, configuration, and sizing before full deployment.

8. **When are PVA particles used?**
   PVA particles range in size from 50 to 2000 μm. Their mechanism of action is to obstruct vessels physically and incite extensive granulation tissue formation. PVA particles result in permanent occlusion. The size of the particle used is

based on the location of desired thrombosis. The smaller the particles are, the more distal the embolization. Particle selection is often based on the experience of the operator. If the particles selected are too small, end-organ ischemia and necrosis may occur. If the particles are too large, collateral vessels may quickly reconstitute blood flow to the target organ, significantly decreasing the efficacy of the procedure. The smallest particles are reserved for tumor embolization or preoperative devascularization of other tissues because they can cause significant tissue ischemia via occlusion down to the capillary level.

9. When performing an embolization procedure, why is it always recommended to place a vascular sheath at the access site?

A vascular sheath assists in catheter exchanges during the procedure. More importantly, the sheath maintains vascular access in the event the embolic agent clogs the delivery catheter, and the catheter needs to be removed.

10. What is postembolization syndrome?

Postembolization syndrome is an expected set of symptoms and signs, including pain, fever, nausea, vomiting, and leukocytosis, that patients may experience after an embolization. The cause is likely secondary to organ ischemia/infarction. Prophylactic antibiotics to prevent superinfection of ischemic tissue and pain control and antiemetic agents are helpful in treating postembolization syndrome. The syndrome is transient and should resolve within 3 to 5 days after the procedure.

11. How can nontarget embolization be minimized?

Meticulous preembolization diagnostic angiography can ensure proper selective catheterization of the desired vessel.

12. When performing an embolization procedure for an upper GI bleed, what information from the endoscopy report is essential?

Because clinically significant upper GI bleeding may be intermittent or too slow to be identified angiographically, arteriograms performed in this setting often display normal results. Empiric embolizations are commonly performed even when arteriograms have normal results. Embolization of an arteriographically "normal" vessel can be performed safely because of the redundant collateral supply to the stomach and duodenum. Ischemic complications of such embolizations are rare unless the patient has a compromised network of collaterals from previous surgery. Before the procedure, it is necessary to know exactly where the patient is bleeding. If the source is duodenal, the gastroduodenal artery is embolized. If the source is gastric, the left gastric artery is embolized.

13. Can a lower GI bleed be treated with empiric embolization?

The colon and small bowel lack the extensive collateral network present in the stomach and duodenum. Empiric embolization of a vascular distribution would cause extensive ischemia and bowel necrosis. The approach to lower GI bleeds is therefore much different. To perform an embolization, the site of bleeding must be identified on the angiogram. Nuclear medicine scans to detect bleeding are often performed before an arteriogram. These scans are noninvasive and can detect intermittent bleeding and hemorrhage that is much slower than that which can be detected on an arteriogram. If the nuclear medicine scan shows negative results, it is of virtually no value to perform an arteriogram. If the nuclear medicine scan shows positive results, and the site of hemorrhage can be identified on the arteriogram, embolization can be attempted.

14. In the setting of pelvic trauma or peripartum hemorrhage in a patient with an unstable condition, is superselective embolization always indicated?

In emergent settings, with a patient with an unstable condition, the goal is efficient hemostasis and stabilization of the patient's condition. Embolization of the entire internal iliac artery, if necessary, can be performed, usually with Gelfoam. The time saved by avoiding further catheterization may be lifesaving. If the patient's condition is stable, selective embolization may be performed to reduce ischemic complications (Figure 71-1).

15. Name some clinical indications for arteriography in patients with pelvic trauma.

The pelvis represents a very large potential space, often able to accommodate 4 to 5 L of blood. Traumatic diastasis of the symphysis pubis can double the effective potential space of the pelvis. Pelvic bleeding can be difficult to control surgically. Splinting and external fixation are usually performed first to help reduce bleeding. Indications for arteriography include open pelvic fracture, expanding pelvic hematoma, and transfusion requirement greater than 4 U over 24 hours.

16. Is empiric embolization indicated in pelvic trauma?

In the setting of a pelvic fracture, bleeding may be from numerous sources. Venous bleeding is the most common etiology. Bleeding from the periosteal surface of fractured bones is the next most common etiology, followed by arterial hemorrhage. In the setting of an arteriogram with normal results, arterial embolization is not usually performed.

17. In bronchial artery embolization for hemoptysis, vigilance for which vessels is imperative?

Anterior spinal arteries arising from bronchial arteries must be identified to prevent nontarget embolization and subsequent paraplegia. Anterior spinal artery branches that arise from bronchial arteries have a classic "hairpin" appearance, traveling cranially for 1 cm or so before forming a loop and doubling back to travel caudally over the midline of the spine.

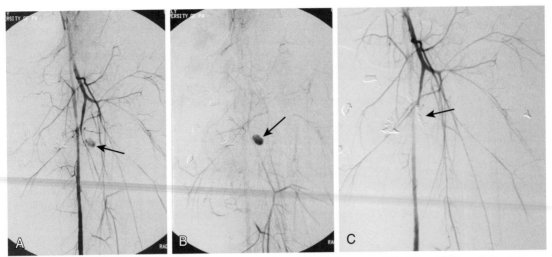

**Figure 71-1.** Acute arterial hemorrhage and treatment effects of embolotherapy on DSA. **A,** Frontal DSA image shows acute hemorrhage from branch of left deep femoral artery (*arrow*) due to gunshot wound. **B,** More delayed frontal DSA image prominently shows hemorrhage (*arrow*). **C,** Frontal DSA image after successful coil embolization of injured artery shows cessation of bleeding (*arrow*).

18. **Why should coils not be used in the bronchial arteries?**
    Life-threatening hemoptysis is often caused by chronic lung disease, such as sarcoidosis or cystic fibrosis. Because of the chronic nature of the lung disease, hemoptysis is likely to recur. Embolization with coils makes future access to the embolized vascular territory difficult, if not impossible. Particulate agents such as PVA are preferred.

19. **Why is it necessary to embolize both sides of a pseudoaneurysm, aneurysm, or AVF?**
    Significant reconstitution of flow via collaterals can occur and cause recurrence of the lesion. If only the proximal feeding vessel to a pseudoaneurysm is embolized, flow may reverse in the outflow vessel and feed the pseudoaneurysm. Embolizing both sides of a pseudoaneurysm, aneurysm, or AVF is called "embolizing the front and back door of a lesion" and is also sometimes needed when embolizing bleeding vessels.

20. **What should always be placed when absolute ethanol is being used for renal artery sclerosis?**
    An occlusion balloon must always be placed to prevent reflux of absolute ethanol into the abdominal aorta. The balloon should also be distal to the origin of the adrenal and gonadal arteries because catecholamine release or gonadal ischemia can result if ethanol is instilled into the respective arteries.

21. **How is chemoembolization theorized to work?**
    Embolization of tumor vessels causes ischemia. This ischemia disables tumor cell membrane ion pumps and exocytosis functions and increases capillary permeability. As a result, there is increased intracellular accumulation and dwell time of the concomitantly delivered chemotherapeutic agent, leading to increased tumor cell apoptosis.

22. **What happens when the cystic artery is embolized during hepatic lesion embolization/chemoembolization?**
    A transient chemical cholecystitis may result. This condition can be self-limited and may resolve with conservative management. Incidental embolization of the cystic artery is believed to contribute to postembolization pain in patients undergoing hepatic chemoembolization.

23. **What happens if the left or right gastric artery is embolized during hepatic chemoembolization?**
    Injecting chemotherapeutic agents directly into the bowel can cause irreversible gastric ischemia and eventual necrosis. Meticulous attention to possible variants in gastric/bowel vascular supply is necessary when performing preembolization diagnostic arteriograms.

24. **What is the significance of gas in the target organ post embolization?**
    There is little significance. Gas is often present in the target organ after embolization and, as mentioned earlier, is thought to arise from tissue necrosis. The presence of gas does not always indicate infection. Resorption of the gas may take weeks.

25. **What findings suggest that postembolization gas is due to infection?**
    Beyond 5 days post procedure, when postembolization syndrome is expected to resolve, persistent fever, elevated serum markers of inflammation (erythrocyte sedimentation rate, C-reactive protein), or a fluid level in the embolized area suggests superinfection of the embolized tissue.

26. When is uterine artery embolization (UAE) used in a nonemergent setting?

Uterine fibroids causing menorrhagia or pelvic pain can be treated effectively with bilateral UAE, also known as uterine fibroid embolization (UFE). UAE can be performed with permanent particles.

## KEY POINTS

- Embolotherapy has various clinical applications, including control of bleeding; elimination of vascular malformations; and tumor or organ ablation for curative, palliative, or preoperative purposes.
- Postembolization syndrome is a transient and expected set of symptoms, including pain, fever, nausea, vomiting, and leukocytosis, probably secondary to organ ischemia/infarction.
- Meticulous preembolization diagnostic angiography to ensure appropriate selective catheterization of the desired vessel is required to minimize nontarget embolization.
- Embolization on both sides of a pseudoaneurysm, aneurysm, or AVF is necessary to prevent reconstitution of flow via collaterals, which causes lesion recurrence.
- Gas in the target organ within 3 to 5 days post embolization is thought to arise from tissue necrosis and does not automatically signify infection.

### BIBLIOGRAPHY

Leyon JJ, Littlehales T, Rangarajan B, et al. Endovascular embolization: review of currently available embolization agents. *Curr Probl Diagn Radiol.* 2014;43(1):35-53.

Marion Y, Lebreton G, Le Pennec V, et al. The management of lower gastrointestinal bleeding. *J Visc Surg.* 2014;151(3):191-201.

Abdel-Aal AK, Bag AK, Saddekni S, et al. Endovascular management of nonvariceal upper gastrointestinal hemorrhage. *Eur J Gastroenterol Hepatol.* 2013;25(7):755-763.

Giunchedi P, Maestri M, Gavini E, et al. Transarterial chemoembolization of hepatocellular carcinoma—agents and drugs: an overview. Part 2. *Expert Opin Drug Deliv.* 2013;10(6):799-810.

Jesinger RA, Thoreson AA, Lamba R. Abdominal and pelvic aneurysms and pseudoaneurysms: imaging review with clinical, radiologic, and treatment correlation. *Radiographics.* 2013;33(3):E71-E96.

Kos S, Gutzeit A, Hoppe H, et al. Diagnosis and therapy of acute hemorrhage in patients with pelvic fractures. *Semin Musculoskelet Radiol.* 2013;17(4):396-406.

Shin JH. Refractory gastrointestinal bleeding: role of angiographic intervention. *Clin Endosc.* 2013;46(5):486-491.

Bulman JC, Ascher SM, Spies JB. Current concepts in uterine fibroid embolization. *Radiographics.* 2012;32(6):1735-1750.

Papakostidis C, Kanakaris N, Dimitriou R, et al. The role of arterial embolization in controlling pelvic fracture haemorrhage: a systematic review of the literature. *Eur J Radiol.* 2012;81(5):897-904.

Pinto A, Niola R, Brunese L, et al. Postpartum hemorrhage: what every radiologist needs to know. *Curr Probl Diagn Radiol.* 2012;41(3):102-110.

Dhand S, Gupta R. Hepatic transcatheter arterial chemoembolization complicated by postembolization syndrome. *Semin Intervent Radiol.* 2011;28(2):207-211.

Sexton JA, Ricotta JJ. Endovascular approaches to arteriovenous fistula. *Adv Surg.* 2011;45:83-100.

Kalva SP. Bronchial artery embolization. *Tech Vasc Interv Radiol.* 2009;12(2):130-138.

Keeling AN, McGrath FP, Lee MJ. Interventional radiology in the diagnosis, management, and follow-up of pseudoaneurysms. *Cardiovasc Intervent Radiol.* 2009;32(1):2-18.

Loffroy R, Guiu B, Cercueil JP, et al. Endovascular therapeutic embolisation: an overview of occluding agents and their effects on embolised tissues. *Curr Vasc Pharmacol.* 2009;7(2):250-263.

Salazar GM, Petrozza JC, Walker TG. Transcatheter endovascular techniques for management of obstetrical and gynecologic emergencies. *Tech Vasc Interv Radiol.* 2009;12(2):139-147.

Abada HT, Golzarian J. Gelatine sponge particles: handling characteristics for endovascular use. *Tech Vasc Interv Radiol.* 2007;10(4):257-260.

Andersen PE. Imaging and interventional radiological treatment of hemoptysis. *Acta Radiol.* 2006;47(8):780-792.

Yoon W, Kim JK, Kim YH, et al. Bronchial and nonbronchial systemic artery embolization for life-threatening hemoptysis: a comprehensive review. *Radiographics.* 2002;22(6):1395-1409.

Leung DA, Goin JE, Sickles C, et al. Determinants of postembolization syndrome after hepatic chemoembolization. *J Vasc Interv Radiol.* 2001;12(3):321-326.

Wojtowycz M. *Handbook of interventional radiology and angiography.* 2nd ed. St. Louis: Mosby; 1995.

Coldwell DM, Stokes KR, Yakes WF. Embolotherapy: agents, clinical applications, and techniques. *Radiographics.* 1994;14(3):623-643, quiz 45-46.

# CHAPTER 72

# BILIARY AND PORTAL VENOUS INTERVENTIONS

*Jeffrey I. Mondschein, MD*

1. **What are the indications for percutaneous transhepatic biliary drainage?**
   Percutaneous biliary drainage is indicated for the treatment of cholangitis or pruritus related to hyperbilirubinemia in the setting of benign or malignant obstructive biliary disease. Biliary drainage may also be performed in the setting of a traumatic bile leak to help divert bile and promote healing of the injured duct. Generally, percutaneous drainage is indicated only if access of the ducts via endoscopic retrograde cholangiopancreatography (ERCP) is impossible, since ERCP is associated with a lower major complication rate.

2. **List the causes of benign and malignant biliary obstruction.**
   - Common benign causes include bile duct calculi (Figure 72-1), benign strictures, pancreatitis, and sclerosing cholangitis (Figure 72-2).
   - Less common benign causes include Caroli's disease, Mirizzi syndrome, and parasitic infection.
   - Common malignant causes include pancreatic cancer (Figure 72-3), metastatic disease, and cholangiocarcinoma.
   - Less common malignant causes include gallbladder carcinoma and ampullary tumors.

3. **What is the most commonly encountered biliary ductal anatomy?**
   The left hepatic duct is formed by the union of medial and lateral segment bile ducts. Right hepatic lobe bile duct anatomy is more complex and variable. The posterior-inferior and posterior-superior portions of the right hepatic lobe are drained by the right posterior ducts (also known as the right dorsal caudal ducts). The anterior-inferior and anterior-superior portions of the right hepatic lobe are drained by the right anterior ducts (also known as the right ventral cranial ducts). The right hepatic duct is formed by the union of the right posterior segment duct and right anterior segment duct. The confluence of right and left hepatic ducts forms the common hepatic duct, which is joined by the cystic duct (from the gallbladder) to form the common bile duct. The most common biliary ductal anatomy (in ≈60% of the population) consists of a right posterior segment duct that joins the right anterior segment duct to form the right hepatic duct (Figure 72-4, *A*).

4. **What are some important normal biliary ductal anatomic variants?**
   The right posterior segment duct sometimes drains into the left hepatic duct, biliary confluence, or common hepatic duct instead of joining the right anterior segment duct (Figure 72-4, *B*). The cystic duct may parallel the common

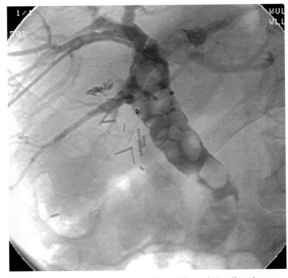

**Figure 72-1.** Percutaneous transhepatic cholangiogram performed to relieve biliary obstruction shows multiple common hepatic duct and common bile duct calculi, seen as radiolucent filling defects surrounded by radiodense injected intrabiliary contrast material.

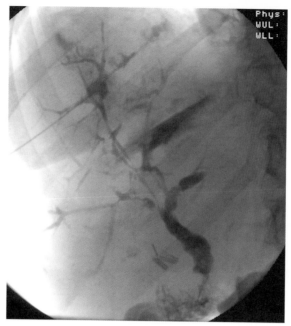

**Figure 72-2.** Percutaneous transhepatic cholangiogram shows "beading" of intrahepatic bile ducts, with segments of bile duct dilation upstream to regions of bile duct stricturing. This alternating stricture-dilation pattern is commonly seen in sclerosing cholangitis.

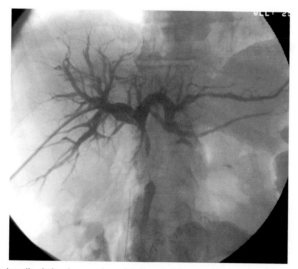

**Figure 72-3.** Percutaneous transhepatic cholangiogram shows intrahepatic biliary dilation secondary to malignant stricture of common bile duct. This stricture was secondary to pancreatic head adenocarcinoma.

hepatic duct for some distance and have a low insertion with a consequently long common hepatic duct and a short common bile duct, or it may occasionally insert medially as it joins the common hepatic duct. Accessory ducts can be seen in some patients. Sometimes referred to as ducts of Luschka, they are generally small tributaries of the right hepatic ductal system that drain directly from the liver to enter the gallbladder. These accessory ducts have clinical significance, since they can be a source of bile leak and bile peritonitis following cholecystectomy, which may require treatment with biliary stent placement via ERCP or percutaneous transhepatic biliary drain placement.

5. Describe the basic steps required to perform diagnostic percutaneous transhepatic cholangiography.
Under fluoroscopic guidance, a 21 G or 22 G needle is passed into the liver through an inferior intercostal or subcostal space at the level of the right midaxillary line. It is important to verify that the needle does not pass through the pleural space. The needle is withdrawn during injection of contrast material in an effort to opacify a bile duct that may have

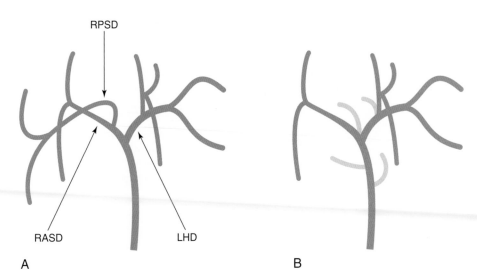

**Figure 72-4. A,** Most common biliary ductal anatomy consists of right posterior segment duct (*RPSD*) that joins right anterior segment duct (*RASD*) to form right hepatic duct. *LHD* = left hepatic duct. **B,** Variant insertions of RPSD (*shown in light blue*) into remainder of biliary system (*shown in dark blue*).

been traversed as a result of the needle pass. When a bile duct is identified, injection of contrast material is continued, and the biliary tree is opacified. A diagnostic cholangiogram is performed with spot fluoroscopic images obtained in anteroposterior and multiple bilateral oblique projections. Ultrasonography (US) may also be used to guide access into the biliary tree, and is especially useful when accessing the left bile ducts.

6. Describe the basic steps required to perform percutaneous transhepatic biliary drainage.
   If indicated by the diagnostic percutaneous transhepatic cholangiogram and clinical symptoms, a wire can be placed via the accessing needle into the biliary tree, followed by tract dilation and biliary drainage catheter placement. This is called the "one-stick" method. If the initial puncture was directed into a central duct, a "two-stick" technique may be used. Central duct punctures are not ideal because the risk of injuring a major hepatic vessel is significant. A second needle may be placed into an appropriate more peripheral duct, and the tract is subsequently dilated and used for access. The ideal access site is an opacified peripheral duct that can be easily accessed under fluoroscopic guidance. Aside from a peripheral location, the duct's path should course through an angle that is gentle enough to allow a catheter to be advanced into the small bowel without extreme angulation or kinking. After the second access is obtained, the first needle can be removed. If left-sided biliary drainage is being performed, the needle is passed into the liver from a left subxiphoid approach.

7. What is the difference between an external biliary drainage catheter and an internal/external biliary drainage catheter?
   External drains end within the bile ducts above the site of obstruction. The obstructed biliary tree is decompressed by draining the bile externally into a drainage bag. Internal/external drains cross the site of obstruction and end within the small bowel. Bile may drain externally into a drainage bag or internally from the biliary tree through side holes in the catheter into the small bowel. Internal/external drains are advantageous because they can be capped externally to allow for internal drainage to the small bowel only. Internal/external drainage catheters are placed whenever it is possible to cross the site of obstruction because drainage to the bowel is more physiologic than external drainage, and the catheters also are easier to care for. Internal drainage prevents loss of bile salts and electrolytes and allows the bile to aid in fat metabolism within the bowel. It is important to monitor the volume status and electrolytes of patients when draining bile externally. These patients can lose a large volume of fluids rich in electrolytes.

8. When should an internal/external drain be capped? When should this drain be uncapped?
   After a de novo biliary drainage, catheters are almost always attached to a bag for gravity drainage for a period of time. External drainage helps to decompress the biliary system. A pressurized system may promote bacterial translocation into the hepatic vasculature, resulting in sepsis. Obstructed systems are likely to be pressurized, and this is exacerbated by the contrast material injected into the ducts during the procedure. Pruritus often resolves more quickly if drainage is maximized. In the setting of a malignant obstruction, administration of chemotherapeutic agents may be delayed if the serum bilirubin level is excessively elevated. In certain situations, internal and external drainage may accelerate normalization of the serum bilirubin level and allow for the subsequent administration of chemotherapeutic agents.
   Patients with drains attached to external drainage bags can lose a significant amount of fluids and electrolytes. Tubes are commonly capped when possible to allow for more physiologic drainage of bile. Usually this occurs when

concerns over infection have subsided and pruritus has resolved. If chemotherapy is planned, tube capping may be delayed until the serum bilirubin level is within an acceptable range.

After a tube has been capped, it should be uncapped if there is concern for infection (fever, elevated white blood cell count, bacteremia, sepsis), leakage of bile around the catheter, pain, or increasing bilirubin or other liver enzyme levels. After the tube is uncapped, additional tests may be indicated, such as a tube check to determine whether the tube is clogged or malpositioned.

9. A patient begins to leak bile around an indwelling biliary drain. Why does this happen, and what can be done to remedy this?

Biliary drains require considerable maintenance after they are placed, and the maintenance often adversely affects the quality of life of patients. Leakage occurs for various reasons. Standard biliary tubes consist of a catheter with side holes and a distal locking loop. For the tube to work properly, the side holes must be patent and properly positioned. The key to proper positioning is the proper location of the most peripheral side hole. This hole should be located just inside the biliary duct where access was obtained. If the most peripheral side hole of the catheter is malpositioned, leakage can occur. Migration or malposition of the tube so that the hole is outside of the duct and in the parenchymal tract results in bile leaking back along the catheter onto the skin. If the hole is too far in, the bile duct peripheral to the catheter may become obstructed and leak along the course of the catheter. Meticulous tube placement, a cholangiogram that confirms proper positioning, along with good technique in securing the catheter to the skin surface will help to prevent these problems. Another common cause of leakage is clogging of the side holes of the catheter with viscous bile or duct debris. This situation can be managed via catheter exchange with consideration given to upsizing the tube if the complication occurs frequently. As a general rule, long-term biliary drainage catheters are exchanged every 3 months for preventive maintenance.

10. What are the potential complications associated with percutaneous transhepatic biliary drainage?

Even in the absence of clinical signs of cholangitis, bile in an obstructed system is often colonized with bacteria. Biliary sepsis, a potentially lethal complication, may occur during or after a cholangiogram or biliary drainage. Antibiotics should be given during biliary drainage procedures, and patients should be monitored closely for signs of sepsis. Injury to blood vessels adjacent to the bile ducts within the hepatic parenchyma may be associated with pseudoaneurysm formation, hemorrhage, and hemobilia. Bile leakage with bile peritonitis and complications related to intraprocedural sedation (respiratory failure and aspiration) may occur. Pneumothorax and reactive or bilious pleural effusions are uncommon complications if care is taken during initial needle placement.

11. After an initial drainage procedure, what additional management measures may be performed to treat benign biliary obstruction?

Biliary drainage provides access to the bile ducts that may allow for retrieval of biliary calculi. Balloon dilation of benign ductal strictures with gradual upsizing of drainage catheter diameter may allow for remodeling of the bile duct with eventual relief of obstruction and removal of the drainage catheter. This therapy, which is successful in approximately two thirds of cases, usually takes several months. If unsuccessful, surgical intervention may still be possible, or catheters may be left in place indefinitely.

12. What can be done to manage the treatment of malignant biliary obstruction after initial drainage?

With some tumor types, access to the bile ducts allows for the placement of radioactive isotopes for ductal brachytherapy. If the patient is not a candidate for surgical resection, the drainage catheters may be left in long term. Sometimes, internal metal stents may be placed across malignant strictures to allow for catheter removal for patient comfort. The decision to place a metallic stent depends on patient prognosis and life expectancy because internal metal stents have limited long-term patency (generally about 6 months).

13. What does the term *isolated ducts* mean? What is its significance?

In the case of a low obstruction of the common bile duct, as would typically occur in the setting of a pancreatic head mass or common bile duct calculus, the right and left systems still communicate. Either a single right-sided biliary drain or a single left-sided biliary drain can be used to decompress the entire biliary tree. If the level of obstruction is higher, as might occur with cholangiocarcinoma or sclerosing cholangitis, this might not be the case, and some ducts may not communicate with others—they are "isolated" from one another. This is one reason that highlights the importance of obtaining cross-sectional imaging prior to biliary drainage. If only one ductal system is dilated, this information helps to determine the access site (left-sided drainage vs. right-sided drainage). Patients who have multiple isolated portions of the biliary tree will have some ducts that remain undrained if only a single catheter is placed. These patients may require more than one drainage catheter to treat infection, pruritus, or hyperbilirubinemia.

14. How does stricture morphology help to differentiate between benign and malignant disease?

Benign biliary strictures tend to taper smoothly, with gradual narrowing across their length. Malignant biliary strictures, in contrast, are points of obstruction that end abruptly, sometimes with irregular borders or an appearance of "shouldering."

15. If a histologic diagnosis is required, what methods may be used to obtain a biopsy specimen of the bile ducts?

When access to the bile ducts has been achieved, biopsy of a stricture site may be performed under fluoroscopic guidance. Various devices may be used to obtain tissue samples, including biopsy brushes, forceps, and needles. Often, several samples obtained on different days are required to obtain a diagnosis.

16. When is percutaneous cholecystostomy indicated?

Although cholecystectomy is the preferred therapy for acute cholecystitis, some patients may not be surgical candidates because of their overall clinical status, sepsis, or other comorbid conditions. Percutaneous cholecystostomy combined with broad-spectrum antibiotic coverage is most commonly used as a temporizing measure until the patient's clinical status may be optimized for surgery.

17. Name the basic steps involved in performing percutaneous cholecystostomy.

With US guidance, the gallbladder is accessed with a needle. A wire is placed, and after tract dilation over the wire, a drainage catheter is placed into the gallbladder and allowed to drain externally. A subcostal, transhepatic path to the gallbladder is generally preferred because it may guard against bile leakage into the peritoneal space if the catheter is inadvertently dislodged.

18. What are the potential complications associated with percutaneous cholecystostomy?

Complications include hemorrhage, infection (sepsis), bile peritonitis, and respiratory failure or aspiration related to intraprocedural sedation. Pneumothorax is possible but is relatively rare if a subcostal approach is used.

19. How long must a percutaneous cholecystostomy catheter remain within the gallbladder before it can be removed?

Although some investigators have shown that such catheters can often be safely removed in less time, the majority suggest that the cholecystostomy catheter should stay within the gallbladder for at least 4 to 6 weeks. This allows time for a mature tract to form between the gallbladder and skin surface in an effort to prevent bile leakage into the peritoneal space when the catheter is removed. Catheters are generally removed only in the setting of acalculous cholecystitis that has resolved and when obstruction has been relieved as noted on a tube check with cholangiogram. If calculi are present, catheters usually cannot be removed unless cholecystectomy can be performed, given the ongoing risk of ductal obstruction by the calculi.

20. Should a cholecystostomy catheter be placed to external drainage indefinitely?

In the acute phase, although there is evidence of active inflammation, the catheter is maintained on external drainage. In the setting of cholecystitis secondary to obstructing biliary calculi, the catheter is maintained on external drainage. In the setting of acalculous cholecystitis, the catheter may be capped to allow for internal drainage after a cholangiogram is performed to document that there is no cystic duct obstruction.

21. When is transjugular liver biopsy indicated and preferred over percutaneous liver biopsy?

Because a transjugular liver biopsy specimen is obtained from within a hepatic vein, bleeding complications resulting from transgression of the liver capsule may be avoided. The transjugular procedure is indicated for patients with coagulopathy or platelet deficiency. Platelet dysfunction because of renal failure may also be an indication. In addition, any other issue that may make percutaneous biopsy difficult or risky (e.g., presence of ascites) would be a potential indication for transjugular liver biopsy. Because transjugular biopsy cannot generally be used to target a specific liver lesion, it is used only to obtain a tissue diagnosis for medical (diffuse) liver disease such as cirrhosis, viral hepatitis, or transplant rejection. Transjugular liver biopsy may also be preferred when both biopsy and hepatic venous pressure measurements are required, since the pressures may be obtained from the same hepatic vein that is used as access for the biopsy. Hepatic venous pressure measurements are used to diagnose portal hypertension and/or to gauge its severity.

22. How is transjugular liver biopsy performed?

A hepatic vein (most commonly the right hepatic vein) is accessed using a transjugular approach (via the jugular vein to the superior vena cava, through the right atrium to the inferior vena cava, and into the right hepatic vein), and a stiff wire is placed. A stiff metal cannula is placed over the wire into the hepatic vein. An 18 G or 19 G core biopsy needle is placed through the cannula and used to obtain multiple samples of liver tissue. Because the right hepatic vein courses posteriorly through the right lobe, the needle is directed anteriorly to avoid transgression of the liver capsule. Because the middle hepatic vein courses more anteriorly, however, lateral or posterior sampling may be safer with this approach.

23. What are some clinical signs and symptoms associated with portal hypertension?

Esophageal, gastric, mesenteric, and rectal varices may bleed in response to elevated portal pressures; mortality related to the initial bleeding episode may be 20% or more. Increased sinusoidal pressure may result in ascites and hepatic hydrothorax. Hepatic encephalopathy, hepatorenal syndrome with renal dysfunction, and hepatopulmonary syndrome with hypoxemia may also be encountered.

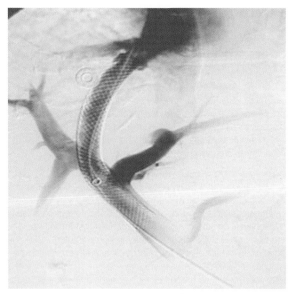

**Figure 72-5.** Venogram shows TIPS extending from right hepatic vein to right portal vein.

24. How can one indirectly estimate portal venous pressure to confirm the diagnosis of portal hypertension?

   Catheterization of a hepatic vein is performed via jugular or femoral vein access. The catheter is advanced until it obstructs a small hepatic vein branch, or a balloon occlusion catheter is inflated within the hepatic vein to obstruct its outflow. The wedged hepatic vein pressure is actually a measure of sinusoidal pressure but allows for a reasonable indirect estimate of portal venous pressure. A corrected sinusoidal pressure measurement is obtained by subtracting the measured mean free hepatic venous pressure from the mean wedged hepatic venous pressure. Corrected sinusoidal pressure measurements ≤5 mm Hg are considered normal. Measurements of 6 to 10 mm Hg are compatible with mild portal hypertension, and measurements >10 mm Hg are compatible with more severe portal hypertension.

25. What are the indications for creating a transjugular intrahepatic portosystemic shunt (TIPS)?

   TIPS creation is frequently performed to prevent recurrent variceal bleeding related to portal hypertension (Figure 72-5). Other indications include refractory ascites or hepatic hydrothorax, Budd-Chiari syndrome, portal hypertensive gastropathy, and hepatorenal or hepatopulmonary syndrome. TIPS placement may be an effective bridge to liver transplantation for patients with end-stage liver disease and manifestations of portal hypertension.

26. What are the contraindications to TIPS creation?

   A pre-TIPS total bilirubin level >3 mg/dL, refractory coagulopathy with an international normalized ratio >1.8, a Child-Pugh score >12, and a serum creatinine level >1.9 mg/dL all have been found to be associated with poor outcomes in studies. However, model for end-stage liver disease (MELD) score prior to TIPS has been shown to be the best single predictive index of mortality following TIPS. Most investigators feel that a MELD of ≤18 is associated with improved long-term survival. TIPS creation that is performed on an emergent basis is also associated with high mortality, and hemodynamic stabilization with transfusions, other medical interventions, and balloon tamponade of gastroesophageal varices are therefore preferred before the TIPS procedure. A functioning TIPS can be associated with new or worsened hepatic encephalopathy, so the presence of moderate to severe encephalopathy at baseline that is not readily treatable with medications may be a contraindication. Severe cardiac or renal dysfunction is also a contraindication, since shunting of portal flow to the systemic circulation would cause an increase in systemic volume that could result in congestive heart failure.

27. Describe the steps of the TIPS procedure.

   - A hepatic vein, most commonly the right hepatic vein, is accessed via a right internal jugular vein approach. A wedged hepatic venogram may be obtained to opacify the portal vein and map its location.
   - A stiff metal cannula is placed, and a needle is passed from the right hepatic vein into the right portal vein under fluoroscopic guidance. Often, several needle passes are required to obtain portal access. The portosystemic pressure gradient measurement is obtained.
   - A stiff wire is placed into the portal vein, and dilation of the intrahepatic parenchymal tract is performed with an angioplasty balloon.
   - A flexible, self-expanding stent graft (usually 8 or 10 mm in diameter) is placed from the portal vein to the confluence of the hepatic vein with the inferior vena cava. Stent grafts have been shown to significantly improve

long-term patency in TIPS and to reduce the incidence of shunt dysfunction and are therefore preferred over bare metal stents.
- A venogram and repeat portosystemic pressure gradient measurements are obtained.
- If there is a history of bleeding varices, and if varices are still seen on venography after the TIPS is created, then variceal embolization is performed.

28. What are the potential complications of TIPS creation?

Complications include hemorrhage, infection, allergic reaction or renal failure due to contrast material, cardiac dysrhythmia, and respiratory failure or aspiration because of intraprocedural sedation. In addition, because the TIPS causes shunting of portal venous blood away from the liver, the procedure may be complicated by a decline in liver function and new or worsened hepatic encephalopathy. Patients with cardiac or renal dysfunction can experience congestive heart failure secondary to increased systemic volume.

29. What are the short-term and long-term goals of TIPS creation?

Successful TIPS creation is associated with a final portosystemic pressure gradient measurement of <12 mm Hg to prevent variceal bleeding or ascites. Successful TIPS creation will prevent variceal bleeding in greater than 90% of cases and will improve or eliminate ascites in greater than 80%. If the patient has significant encephalopathy, and treatment with lactulose is insufficient to control symptoms, a reducing stent may be placed to narrow the TIPS and create an intentional small increase in the portosystemic pressure gradient. TIPS patency may be monitored at intervals using duplex Doppler US, which allows for velocity measurements within the TIPS to be obtained noninvasively. Significant velocity increases from baseline may indicate the presence of TIPS stenosis, which may prompt TIPS venography and revision by balloon dilation or additional stent placement.

---

## KEY POINTS

- An obstructed, infected biliary system constitutes a medical emergency.
- Complications from percutaneous biliary drainage can be life-threatening. An endoscopic approach is therefore preferred when possible.
- Benign biliary strictures tend to taper gradually with smooth borders, whereas malignant biliary strictures tend to occur abruptly, often with irregular borders.

**BIBLIOGRAPHY**

Gervais DA, Sabharwal T. *Interventional radiology procedures in biopsy and drainage.* 1st ed. London: Springer-Verlag; 2011.

Catalano OA, Singh AH, Uppot RN, et al. Vascular and biliary variants in the liver: implications for liver surgery. *Radiographics.* 2008;28(2):359-378.

Patel NH, Haskal ZJ, Kerlan RK. *SCVIR syllabus. Portal hypertension: diagnosis and interventions.* 2nd ed. Fairfax, VA: Society of Interventional Radiology; 2001.

Savader SJ, Trerotola SO. *Venous interventional radiology with clinical perspectives.* 2nd ed. New York: Thieme; 2000.

# GENITOURINARY AND GASTROINTESTINAL INTERVENTIONAL RADIOLOGY

*S. William Stavropoulos, MD, and Charles T. Lau, MD, MBA*

# CHAPTER 73

1. List the indications for percutaneous nephrostomy (PCN) (Figure 73-1).
   - To relieve obstruction in the setting of infection or to preserve renal function.
   - To assist in the removal of a calculus or foreign body.
   - To divert urine to permit healing of a leak or fistula.
   - To provide access for ureteral intervention.

2. What is the indication for emergent PCN?
   Pyonephrosis (infected urinary obstruction) may rapidly lead to urosepsis and death. It is a urologic emergency, and emergent drainage is indicated.

3. What are the important technical factors to consider when performing PCN?
   PCN is a relatively safe, minimally invasive technique that can be used to treat various conditions efficiently. The safety and efficacy of the procedure are predicated, however, on the following well-established guidelines to help prevent complications. The skin puncture should be sufficiently lateral to the midline; this ensures a relatively straight tract that avoids kinking of the catheter. The needle entry into the kidney should traverse the least vascular plane, and the access obtained should provide a path to all portions of the collecting system. It is also important that organs adjacent to the kidney, such as the colon, are not in the needle path.

4. What is the most common method of visualizing the collecting system for PCN?
   Fluoroscopy is the most common method, but this requires opacification of the collecting system. This can be accomplished by intravenous contrast material injection with antegrade excretion, if the patient has satisfactory renal function. If the patient has impaired renal function or has a completely obstructed renal collecting system, fluoroscopy may not be a viable option. In these situations, an antegrade pyelogram can be performed via a 22 G or 25 G needle. An antegrade pyelogram can be performed with iodinated contrast material or $CO_2$ gas (Figure 73-2).

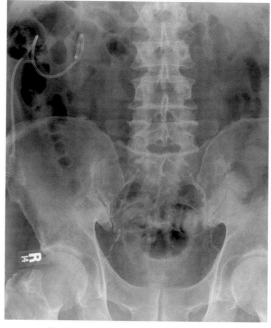

**Figure 73-1.** PCN tube on frontal radiograph.

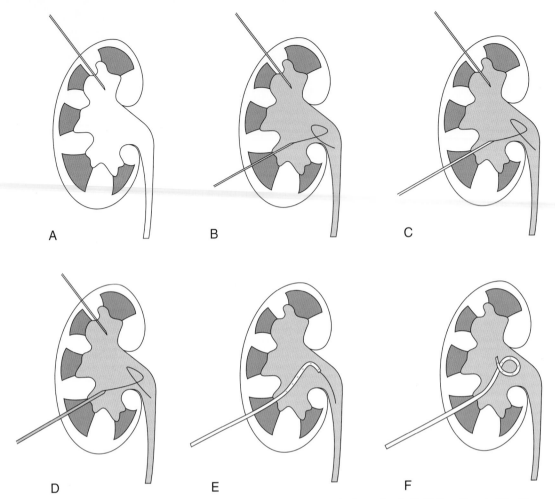

A   B   C

D   E   F

**Figure 73-2.** Schematic illustration of PCN using Seldinger technique. **A,** Posterior calyx is punctured with 22 G needle under US guidance. **B,** After performing antegrade pyelography through this access point with contrast material injection, second 22 G needle is inserted into opacified collecting system along expected tract of nephrostomy catheter. 0.018-inch wire is advanced through this needle. **C,** Exchange is made for catheter that allows conversion to 0.035-inch wire. **D-E,** Nephrostomy tract is dilated by exchanging successive dilators over wire. **F,** Pigtail loop of PCN is formed and wire is removed.

5. What are the alternative means other than fluoroscopy for visualizing the collection system for PCN?

Ultrasonography (US) can be used, which eliminates the need for contrast material opacification of the collecting system. US can also be used to ensure that adjacent organs do not lie along a proposed nephrostomy tract. If the collecting system is not dilated, however, it may be difficult to visualize it with US. Computed tomography (CT) is another option, particularly if the kidney is in an anomalous position.

6. Should access for PCN be obtained through the renal parenchyma or directly into the renal pelvis?

Puncture of the collecting system should occur through the renal parenchyma because this is the least vascular plane. Direct access to the renal pelvis has a higher rate of vascular complications. Puncture through the renal parenchyma also helps to provide support for the catheter, minimize urine leakage, and decrease the chance of catheter displacement.

7. From what approach should PCN be performed?

A PCN tract should pass through the least vascular region of the kidney to minimize bleeding complications. Renal calyces are arranged in anterior and posterior rows. Between these two rows, in the interpolar kidney, is a relatively avascular plane of renal parenchyma called Brödel's line. This plane usually lies at 30 to 45 degrees, and the PCN tract should be made along this line. (Interestingly, Max Brödel, who described the avascular area of the kidney named after him, is also known as one of the major medical illustrators at the beginning of the twentieth century, and he improved the role of medical illustration in the medical literature.)

8. Aside from decreasing the chance of bleeding, what are the other benefits of performing PCN through Brödel's line?

The approach through Brödel's line also results in a PCN catheter exiting through skin near the posterior axillary line, so the catheter does not kink and the patient is not uncomfortable lying on it when supine.

9. What imaging modalities can be used to perform a percutaneous drainage of renal or perinephric abscesses?

Percutaneous drainage of renal and perinephric abscesses can be performed with US, CT, or fluoroscopic guidance. US is usually preferred because it provides real-time imaging, which allows for an accurate, safe, and fast procedure. It is important to place the drainage catheter in the most dependent portion of a large abscess cavity to ensure complete drainage of infected material.

10. What are the possible complications resulting from percutaneous drainage of renal or perinephric abscesses?

Percutaneous drainage is a safe and effective technique that can be used in the management of an abscess. Complications may still occur, however. When collections adjacent to or within the kidney are being drained, some infected material may intravasate into the vascular system, resulting in bacteremia or sepsis. It is important to administer intravenous antibiotics before and after drain placement. Drains placed within the kidney may accidentally traverse a blood vessel. Bleeding can be inconsequential and resolve spontaneously; may result in hematuria, if bleeding tracks into the collecting system; or may lead to a perinephric hematoma, if the hemorrhage tracks around the kidney. Rarely, adjacent organs may be inadvertently punctured during catheter placement.

11. When is percutaneous management of urinary tract calculi preferred over extracorporeal shock wave lithotripsy (ESWL)?

ESWL is the sole therapy used in approximately 90% of patients with symptomatic urinary tract calculi. Percutaneous management is preferred, however, in patients with a large stone burden. Percutaneous management may also be used as an adjunct to ESWL if large stone fragments remain or if obstruction occurs after ESWL.

12. What is the role of PCN in percutaneous treatment of urinary tract calculi?

PCN is used to obtain a tract through which the endoscope may access the collecting system. It is important in this situation to create a tract that is straight and permits endoscope access to all portions of the collecting system.

13. How are calculi removed during percutaneous treatment of the urinary tract?

Different devices can be used through the endoscope when access to the collecting system has been obtained. These include various stone baskets, which are three to eight wires arranged in a helical pattern. Forceps may be used to grab individual calculi. US and electrohydraulic lithotripters can also be used to pulverize calculi within the collecting system to facilitate removal.

14. What are the indications for ureteral stenting?

Common indications include presence of urinary tract calculi and benign ureteral strictures. Ureteral stenting is also indicated in patients with extrinsic ureteral obstruction, ureteral trauma, and retroperitoneal fibrosis. In the setting of malignant ureteral obstruction, stenting may be performed if the patient does not have bladder outlet obstruction. Stenting allows the affected kidney to drain, and the patient is able to void. The most commonly used ureteral stents are the double-J stent and nephroureteral stent.

15. Describe the difference between a double-J ureteral stent and a nephroureteral stent.

All ureteral stents are made of polyurethane or silicone; metallic stents are not used in ureters. A double-J ureteral stent is completely internal and has a "pigtail" at each end (Figure 73-3, *A*). Its proximal coil is situated in the renal pelvis, and its distal coil is situated in the urinary bladder. A nephroureteral stent has a "pigtail" at its distal end that is placed in the bladder and another one that is looped in the renal pelvis (Figure 73-3, *B*). The catheter exits through the skin at the percutaneous access site.

16. How does a ureteral stent work?

A ureteral stent is hollow and has multiple side holes. It drains urine past obstructions from the collecting system into the urinary bladder. Some authorities believe that an element of capillary action augments this process. A ureteral stent also causes passive dilation of the ureter, which may or may not persist after the stent is removed.

17. What are the indications for esophageal stenting?

Esophageal stenting is most commonly performed in the treatment of dysphagia secondary to cancer ingrowth and bronchoesophageal fistula (Figure 73-4). Esophageal stents may also be used for treatment of refractory or recurrent esophageal strictures, tracheoesophageal fistulas, and esophageal perforation.

18. What technical complications are associated with esophageal stenting?

Even with the most experienced operators, stents may be malpositioned or migrate. Because esophageal malignancies may be friable, stenting may occasionally result in esophageal perforation, a potentially life-threatening complication.

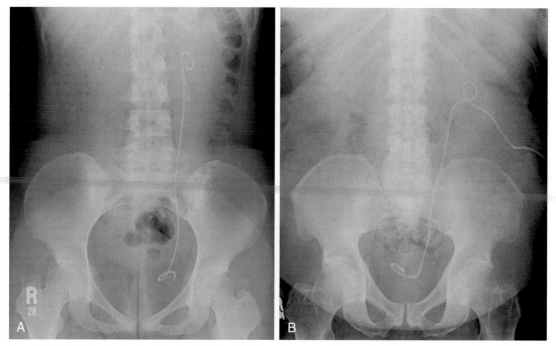

**Figure 73-3. A,** Double-J ureteral stent on frontal radiograph. Note radiopaque ureteral calculus adjacent to proximal aspect of stent. **B,** Nephroureteral stent on frontal radiograph.

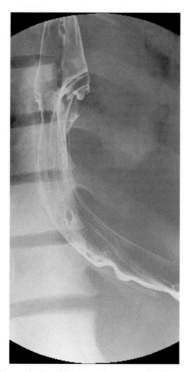

**Figure 73-4.** Esophageal stent on fluoroscopic examination. Note irregular mucosal contour and luminal narrowing of distal esophagus at proximal aspect of stent due to esophageal cancer.

19. What factors should be considered when selecting the puncture site for percutaneous gastrostomy?

The site of percutaneous gastrostomy should be subcostal and to the left of the midline. The outer third of the rectus abdominis muscle should be avoided because the inferior epigastric artery courses in this region. Fluoroscopy is performed so that the puncture avoids the colon and small bowel.

20. What is the difference between a G tube, G-J tube, and J tube?

A simple rule to follow in selecting an enteral access site is to use the stomach whenever possible. Direct gastrostomy (G) tubes are safe and easy to use. The stomach performs important digestive functions, and gastric access allows patients to receive bolus feeds. Jejunal access (via jejunostomy [J] tube) necessitates continuous feeds, which are not as well tolerated. The needs of most patients can be met with G tubes.

- **G tubes** are placed directly into the stomach and can be used for feeding or gastric decompression (Figure 73-5).
- **Gastrojejunostomy tubes** (G-J tubes) enter the stomach similar to a G tube but pass through the stomach and duodenum and terminate in the proximal jejunum (Figure 73-6). G-J tubes are technically simpler to place than J tubes and are associated with a lower procedural risk (remember, use the stomach, even for access, whenever

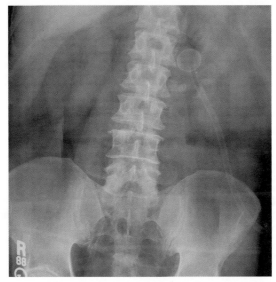

**Figure 73-5.** G tube on frontal radiograph. Note characteristic radiopaque balloon overlying gas-filled stomach in left upper quadrant of abdomen.

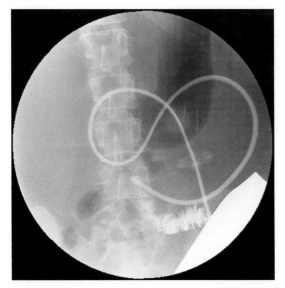

**Figure 73-6.** G-J tube on frontal radiograph. Note how course of tube extends from gas-filled stomach in left upper quadrant of abdomen through expected C-shaped course of duodenum before terminating in loop of proximal jejunum (partially opacified with contrast material).

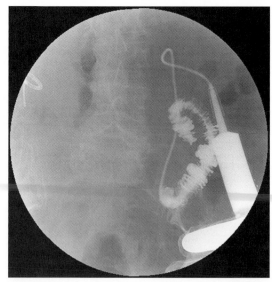

**Figure 73-7.** J tube on frontal radiograph. Note contrast opacification of portion of proximal jejunum.

possible). G-J tubes may have a single port that enters the small bowel. In patients with gastric outlet obstruction, G-J tubes with two ports may be used. One port is used to decompress the stomach, and the other is used to administer feeds. In addition, a previously placed G tube can be converted to a G-J tube.

- **J tubes** enter the small bowel directly (Figure 73-7). They may be used for feedings or for palliative decompression when placed above a site of obstruction.

21. When are feeding G tubes not the tubes of choice?
    Patients may not be candidates for feeding G tubes because of anatomic or functional reasons. Anatomic contraindications include prior gastrectomy or gastric pull-through, presence of colon adherent to the stomach, and ascites. Patients with ascites are at high risk for constantly leaking fluid through the puncture site. Functional reasons include severe gastroesophageal reflux with aspiration, gastroparesis, and gastric outlet obstruction. Decompressive G tubes may be indicated in patients with gastric outlet obstruction.

22. When are small bowel feeding tubes indicated?
    J tubes and G-J tubes are usually reserved for patients with known severe gastroesophageal reflux with the risk of aspiration.

## KEY POINTS

- Urosepsis is an indication for emergent PCN.
- A PCN tract should pass through the skin near the posterior axillary line, pass through the renal parenchyma in the relatively avascular plane denoted by Brödel's line, and enter the renal collecting system.
- Although ureteral stents successfully drain the collecting system into the bladder and cause passive dilation of the ureter, they are considered a temporary measure and are not curative.
- Patients with ascites should receive large-volume paracentesis before percutaneous gastrostomy.
- J tubes and G-J tubes are reserved for patients with known gastroesophageal reflux disease or documented aspiration.

**BIBLIOGRAPHY**

Toussaint E, Van Gossum A, Ballarin A, et al. Enteral access in adults. *Clin Nutr.* 2015;34(3):350-358.
Covarrubias DA, O'Connor OJ, McDermott S, et al. Radiologic percutaneous gastrostomy: review of potential complications and approach to managing the unexpected outcome. *AJR Am J Roentgenol.* 2013;200(4):921-931.
Didden P, Spaander MC, Bruno MJ, et al. Esophageal stents in malignant and benign disorders. *Curr Gastroenterol Rep.* 2013;15(4):319.
Dunnick R, Sandler C, Newhouse J. *Textbook of uroradiology.* 5th ed. Philadelphia: Lippincott Williams & Wilkins; 2012.
Hindy P, Hong J, Lam-Tsai Y, et al. A comprehensive review of esophageal stents. *Gastroenterol Hepatol.* 2012;8(8):526-534.
Li AC, Regalado SP. Emergent percutaneous nephrostomy for the diagnosis and management of pyonephrosis. *Semin Intervent Radiol.* 2012;29(3):218-225.
Committee AT, Varadarajulu S, Banerjee S, et al. Enteral stents. *Gastrointest Endosc.* 2011;74(3):455-464.
Dagli M, Ramchandani P. Percutaneous nephrostomy: technical aspects and indications. *Semin Intervent Radiol.* 2011;28(4):424-437.
Dua KS. Expandable stents for benign esophageal disease. *Gastrointest Endosc Clin N Am.* 2011;21(3):359-376, vii.

Vleggaar FP, Siersema PD. Expandable stents for malignant esophageal disease. *Gastrointest Endosc Clin N Am.* 2011;21(3):377-388, vii.

Committee AT, Kwon RS, Banerjee S, et al. Enteral nutrition access devices. *Gastrointest Endosc.* 2010;72(2):236-248.

Sharma P, Kozarek R, Practice Parameters Committee of American College of G. Role of esophageal stents in benign and malignant diseases. *Am J Gastroenterol.* 2010;105(2):258-273, quiz 74.

Adamo R, Saad WE, Brown DB. Management of nephrostomy drains and ureteral stents. *Tech Vasc Interv Radiol.* 2009;12(3):193-204.

Madhusudhan C, Saluja SS, Pal S, et al. Palliative stenting for relief of dysphagia in patients with inoperable esophageal cancer: impact on quality of life. *Dis Esophagus.* 2009;22(4):331-336.

Miller NL, Matlaga BR, Lingeman JE. Techniques for fluoroscopic percutaneous renal access. *J Urol.* 2007;178(1):15-23.

Silas AM, Pearce LF, Lestina LS, et al. Percutaneous radiologic gastrostomy versus percutaneous endoscopic gastrostomy: a comparison of indications, complications and outcomes in 370 patients. *Eur J Radiol.* 2005;56(1):84-90.

Dyer RB, Regan JD, Kavanagh PV, et al. Percutaneous nephrostomy with extensions of the technique: step by step. *Radiographics.* 2002;22(3):503-525.

Schultheiss D, Engel RM, Crosby RW, et al. Max Brodel (1870-1941) and medical illustration in urology. *J Urol.* 2000;164(4):1137-1142.

Cope C, Davis AG, Baum RA, et al. Direct percutaneous jejunostomy: techniques and applications—ten years experience. *Radiology.* 1998;209(3):747-754.

Bell SD, Carmody EA, Yeung EY, et al. Percutaneous gastrostomy and gastrojejunostomy: additional experience in 519 procedures. *Radiology.* 1995;194(3):817-820.

Wojtowycz M. *Handbook of interventional radiology and angiography.* 2nd ed. St. Louis: Mosby; 1995.

# CHAPTER 74

# NEUROINTERVENTIONAL RADIOLOGY

*Cuong Nguyen, MD, and Bryan Pukenas, MD*

1. What is the basic normal vascular anatomy of the brain?

**Arterial**

   The cerebral vasculature is supplied by 4 arterial vessels—the paired internal carotid arteries (ICA) and the vertebral arteries (VA)—and can be divided into anterior and posterior circulations. The anterior circulation consists of the bilateral internal carotid arteries, which bifurcate into the anterior cerebral arteries (ACA) and the middle cerebral arteries (MCA) (Figure 74-1, *A*). The posterior circulation consists of the bilateral vertebral arteries and the basilar artery, along with its branches, including the bilateral posterior cerebral arteries (PCA). The anterior and posterior circulations are connected by the posterior communicating arteries (PCOM), and the bilateral anterior circulations are connected by the anterior communicating artery (ACOM); these connections compose the circle of Willis (Figure 74-1, *B*).

**Venous**

   The cerebral venous system is composed of dural venous sinuses, along with deep and superficial veins. The deep cerebral venous system consists of paired internal cerebral veins and the basal veins of Rosenthal; these merge to form the paired veins of Galen, which in turn drain into the straight sinuses (Figure 74-2). The superficial veins drain into the dural venous sinuses; the veins of Trolard (superior anastomotic veins) and the veins of Labbé (inferior anastomotic veins) are major named large anastomotic cortical veins. The superior sagittal sinus, inferior sagittal sinus, and bilateral transverse sinuses merge at the torcula herophili (a.k.a., the venous sinus confluence).

2. What is the basic normal arterial anatomy of the spinal cord?

   The spinal cord is supplied by the anterior spinal artery (ASA) and the paired posterior spinal arteries (PSA). The ASA arises from the intradural segments of the vertebral arteries and supplies the anterior two thirds of the spinal cord. The ASA receives additional contribution from segmental arteries' medullary feeders, which course superiorly and join the ASA, forming a classic "hairpin turn" configuration (Figure 74-3). Most medullary feeders arise from the lower thoracic region, where the dominant anterior segmental medullary feeder is called the artery of Adamkiewicz. This artery typically arises from a left posterior intercostal artery, most often from the T10 level, although it may arise anywhere

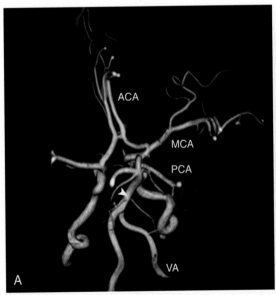
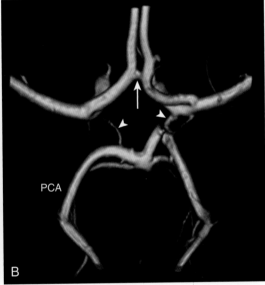

**Figure 74-1.** Normal cerebral arterial system on CTA. **A,** Volume-rendered (VR) CTA image shows anterior cerebral artery (*ACA*), middle cerebral artery (*MCA*), posterior cerebral artery (*PCA*), vertebral artery (*VA*), and basilar artery (*arrowhead*). **B,** VR CTA image shows circle of Willis. Anterior communicating artery (ACOM) (*arrow*) and posterior communicating arteries (PCOM) (*arrowheads*) are shown.

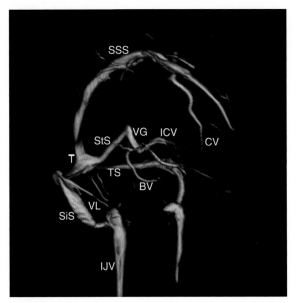

**Figure 74-2.** Normal cerebral venous system on CTA. Superior sagittal sinus (*SSS*), vein of Galen (*VG*), straight sinus (*StS*), transverse sinus (*TS*), sigmoid sinus (*SiS*), internal cerebral vein (*ICV*), basal vein of Rosenthal (*BV*), vein of Labbé (*VL*), cortical vein (*CV*), internal jugular vein (*IJV*), and torcula herophili (*T*) are shown.

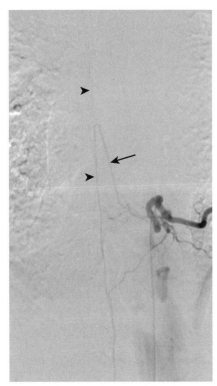

**Figure 74-3.** Normal spinal arterial anatomy on catheter angiography. Frontal catheter angiogram with contrast injection into left T10 segmental (posterior intercostal) artery shows classic "hairpin turn" configuration of artery of Adamkiewicz (*arrow*) supplying anterior spinal artery (ASA) (*arrowheads*).

from intercostal, subcostal, or lumbar arteries at the T7 to L4 vertebral levels and less frequently from the right side. The paired PSA are posteriorly located and supply the posterior one third of the spinal cord. These typically arise from posterior inferior cerebellar arteries (PICA) or posterior rami of the vertebral arteries, and they receive additional contributions from medullary feeders arising from the posterior radicular arteries.

3. What are the indications and contraindications for cerebral and spinal catheter angiography?

**Indications for Cerebral Catheter Angiography**
- Cerebral artery aneurysm.
- Subarachnoid hemorrhage.
- Vasospasm.
- Cerebral vascular malformation.
- Intraparenchymal hemorrhage or intraventricular hemorrhage with suspicion for cerebral vascular malformation.
- Acute ischemic stroke.
- Vasculitis/vasculopathy.
- Severe intracranial/extracranial vascular stenosis.
- Traumatic cervical/cerebral vascular injury.
- Severe epistaxis.

**Indications for Spinal Catheter Angiography**
- Spinal vascular malformation.
- Vertebral tumors.

**Contraindications to Catheter Angiography**
- Platelet count <100,000 platelets/μL.
- International normalized ratio (INR) <1.5.
- Anaphylactic reaction to iodinated contrast material.
- Unstable patient status.
- Brain herniation with cranial nerve deficits.

**Table 74-1.** Hunt and Hess Clinical Grading Scale for Prediction of Clinical Outcome in Patients with SAH

| GRADE | SYMPTOMS | MORTALITY RISK |
|---|---|---|
| 1 | Asymptomatic, or minimal headache and slight nuchal rigidity | 1% |
| 2 | Moderate to severe headache, nuchal rigidity, no neurologic deficit other than cranial nerve palsy | 5% |
| 3 | Drowsiness, confusion, or mild focal neurologic deficit | 19% |
| 4 | Stupor, moderate-severe hemiparesis, possibly early decerebrate rigidity and vegetative disturbances | 42% |
| 5 | Deep coma, decerebrate rigidity, moribund appearance | 77% |

4. What types of vascular neurointerventional procedures are available?

**Diagnostic Testing**
- Cerebral catheter angiography: Assessment for cerebral aneurysm, stenosis (atherosclerosis or vasculitis/vasculopathy), or vascular malformation.
- Cervical catheter angiography: Assessment for carotid artery stenosis or traumatic cervical vascular injury.
- Inferior petrosal sinus sampling: Measurement of adrenocorticotropic hormone (ACTH) levels from the pituitary gland in selected patients with Cushing's syndrome.

**Embolotherapy**
- Cerebral artery aneurysm: Saccular aneurysms are the most common morphologic subtype of cerebral artery aneurysms. They are outpouchings of the intima and adventitia caused by degeneration of the media. Aneurysms may be symptomatic related to mass effect (e.g., compression of cranial nerves with associated neuropathy) or rupture leading to subarachnoid hemorrhage (SAH). The clinical presentation of SAH may range from "the worst headache of one's life" to sudden death. The long-term prognosis of patients who survive the initial rupture correlates with clinical status on presentation, such as that based on the Hunt and Hess clinical grading scale (Table 74-1). The patient workup for SAH includes noncontrast head computed tomography (NCCT) and CT angiography (CTA). Detection of an aneurysm on CTA requires careful assessment of the pattern of SAH, the source (axial) CTA images, maximum intensity projection (MIP) images, and volume-rendered (VR) images (Figures 74-4 and 74-5). Cerebral artery aneurysms can be treated with detachable platinum coils (which can be performed in conjunction with balloon or stent assistance) or a flow diversion device (see Figures 74-4 and 74-5).
- Cerebral arteriovenous malformation (AVM): A cerebral AVM is an abnormal collection (nidus) of vessels between arterial and venous vasculatures without an intervening capillary bed or brain parenchyma, leading to arteriovenous shunting (Figure 74-6). Half of symptomatic cerebral AVMs present with cerebral hemorrhage. AVM is typically treated with a liquid embolic agent such as n-butyl cyanoacrylate (n-BCA) glue or Onyx (ethylene vinyl alcohol). This is usually performed prior to microsurgical resection to reduce intraoperative bleeding. A liquid embolic cast also serves as a direct visual marker for the surgeon to localize the AVM nidus. Embolization can also be performed prior to radiosurgery.
- Cerebral dural arteriovenous fistula (dural AVF): A dural AVF is an abnormal connection between arteries and veins via a network of tiny vessels in the wall of the dural venous sinus (Figure 74-7). If the transverse sinus is involved, dural AVF patients typically present with pulsatile tinnitus, whereas pulsatile exophthalmos and cranial nerve 3, 4, and 6 neuropathy are more common with cavernous sinus involvement. Dural AVF is typically treated with a liquid embolic agent such as n-BCA glue or Onyx, although particles are sometimes also used. Endovascular treatment can be employed as the primary treatment modality or in conjunction with microsurgical resection.
- Spinal vascular malformation: Similar to cerebral vascular malformations, spinal vascular malformations are a heterogeneous group of conditions including both AVF and AVM. The spinal cord may or may not be involved. There are several classification schemes, which are beyond of the scope of this chapter. Spinal catheter angiography is the reference standard test for detection of a spinal vascular malformation. Endovascular treatment can be used as the primary treatment modality or in conjunction with microsurgical resection. Spinal dural AVF, the most common type of spinal vascular malformation, is typically treated endovascularly with n-BCA glue or Onyx.
- Preoperative embolization of tumors: Intracranial tumors (e.g., meningioma), head and neck tumors (e.g., juvenile angiofibroma, paraganglioma), and hypervascular vertebral metastases (e.g., renal cell carcinoma metastases) can be embolized with particles preoperatively to reduce bleeding at surgery.
- Epistaxis: Embolotherapy is indicated in patients with persistent epistaxis after conservative treatment with packing.

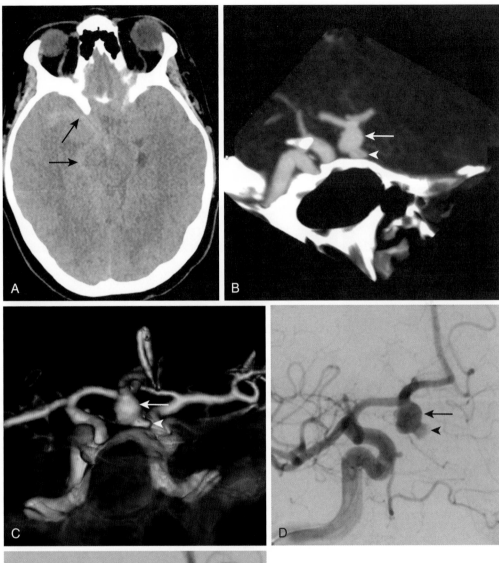

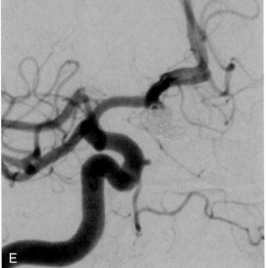

**Figure 74-4.** Cerebral artery aneurysm and SAH on CT, CTA, and catheter angiography. Patient is 39-year-old woman who presents with "worst headache of life." **A,** Axial unenhanced CT image through head shows high attenuation SAH on right (*arrows*). **B,** Multiplanar reformatted CTA image and **C,** VR CTA image reveal anterior communicating artery (ACOM) aneurysm (*arrow*) with bleb (*arrowhead*) arising from aneurysm dome representing rupture site. **D,** Lateral catheter angiogram with ICA contrast injection confirms ACOM aneurysm (*arrow*) with bleb (*arrowhead*). **E,** Lateral catheter angiogram following coil embolization demonstrates obliteration of aneurysm, including rupture site, with minimal residual filling at aneurysm base and preservation of A1 and A2 segments of ACA.

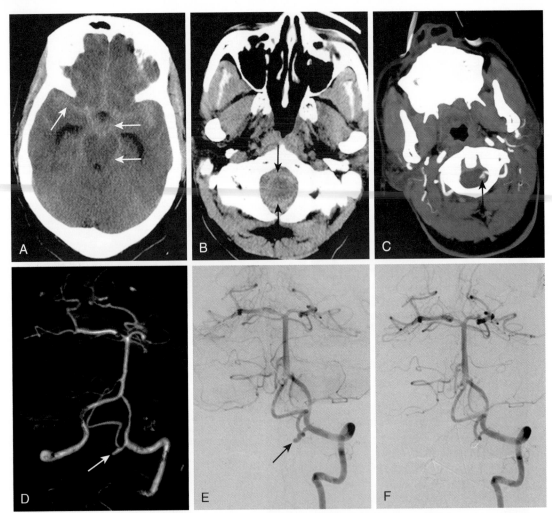

**Figure 74-5.** Cerebral artery aneurysm and SAH on CT, CTA, and catheter angiography. Patient is 63-year-old woman with hypertension who presents with "worst headache of life" and subsequently deteriorates clinically, requiring intubation. **A** and **B,** Axial unenhanced CT images through head reveal high-attenuation diffuse SAH (*arrows*) involving both supratentorial and infratentorial compartments, extending to level of foramen magnum. **C,** Axial maximum intensity projection (MIP) image and **D,** VR image show aneurysm (*arrow*) arising from proximal left posterior inferior cerebellar artery (PICA). PICA aneurysms can be difficult to detect, and this aneurysm was initially missed by on-call fellow. **E,** Frontal catheter angiogram with left VA contrast injection confirms left PICA aneurysm (*arrow*). **F,** Frontal catheter angiogram following coil embolization demonstrates obliteration of aneurysm with preservation of left PICA and left VA.

- Cervical dissection: Vessel sacrifice in patients with pseudoaneurysms (grade 3 injury) or transection (grade 5 injury) can be performed. Endovascular stenting is another option for grade 3 injuries.

**Thrombolysis/Thrombectomy**

- Acute ischemic stroke: Stroke is a clinical diagnosis, not an imaging one. Time is BRAIN (i.e., brain tissue is rapidly lost as stroke progresses), and therefore rapid diagnosis and initiation of treatment are critical for a good clinical outcome. The standard treatment for acute ischemic stroke is intravenous (IV) tissue plasminogen activator (tPA) within 4.5 hours of onset. Intraarterial (IA) tPA administration and mechanical thrombectomy can be offered as adjunct therapy to IV tPA (Figure 74-8). Data from the MR CLEAN trial show that IV tPA together with IA mechanical thrombectomy are superior to IV tPA alone. NCCT is the study of choice for initial assessment for acute stroke due to its speed and widespread availability. The primary purpose of a noncontrast head CT in the setting of acute stroke is to exclude contraindications to IV tPA and IA treatment (i.e., intracranial hemorrhage and large infarct [>1/3 MCA vascular territory]). CTA can be used to confirm large vessel occlusion (i.e., carotid terminus, M1 segment, A1 segment, etc.) in which adjunctive IA treatment is most helpful. The role of magnetic resonance imaging (MRI), MR perfusion imaging, and CT perfusion imaging in acute ischemic stroke assessment is not clearly delineated at this point.

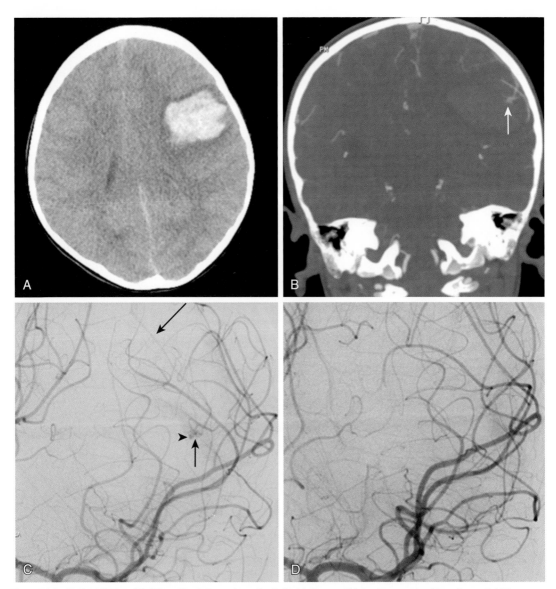

**Figure 74-6.** Cerebral AVM on CT, CTA, and catheter angiography. Patient is 5-year-old boy who presents with acute onset right hemiparesis and expressive aphasia. **A,** Axial unenhanced CT image through head shows high-attenuation left frontal parenchymal hematoma. **B,** Coronal CTA image reveals small tangle of vessels (*arrow*) at periphery of hematoma, suspicious for small AVM nidus. **C,** Catheter angiogram confirms small AVM (*short arrow*) with 1-mm intranidal aneurysm (*arrowhead*). Note early draining vein (*long arrow*). **D,** Catheter angiogram following n-BCA glue embolization demonstrates complete obliteration of AVM nidus and intranidal aneurysm without residual arteriovenous shunting. Patient subsequently underwent microsurgical resection on following day.

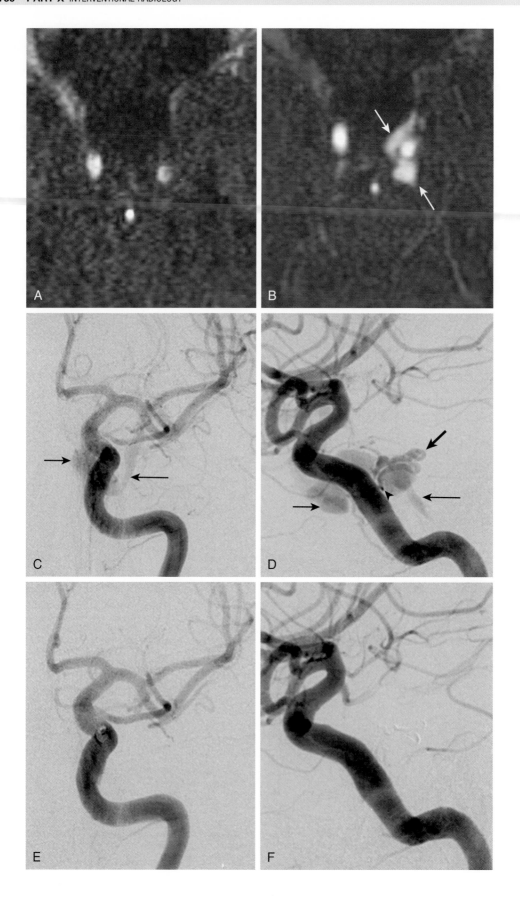

**Figure 74-7.** Carotid-cavernous fistula (CCF) on magnetic resonance angiography (MRA) and catheter angiography. Patient is 52-year-old man who presents with left-sided scleral injection, intermittent left-sided blurry vision, and left-sided tinnitus. **A** and **B,** Axial dynamic contrast-enhanced MRA images at 1 and 14 seconds, respectively, after IV contrast administration reveal abnormal early filling of left cavernous sinus (*arrows*) surrounding left ICA, indicating CCF. **C** and **D,** Multiplanar catheter angiographic images with left ICA contrast injection show indirect CCF (*thick arrow*) with arterial feeding pedicles from left meningohypophyseal trunk (MHT) (*arrowhead*) as well as from right MHT (*not shown*). There is early venous filling of left cavernous sinus (*short thin arrow*) with reflux of contrast material into cortical vein (*long thin arrow*). **E** and **F,** Multiplanar catheter angiographic images following Onyx embolization demonstrate complete obliteration of CCF with no residual filling from left MHT feeding pedicle. Right ICA catheter angiography (*not shown*) also demonstrated no residual filling from right MHT feeding pedicle. Patient's scleral injection noticeably improved 1 day later.

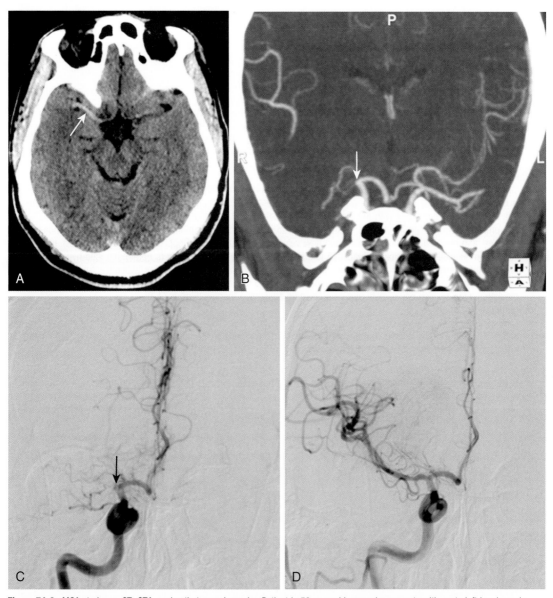

**Figure 74-8.** MCA stroke on CT, CTA, and catheter angiography. Patient is 52-year-old man who presents with acute left hemiparesis, left facial droop, left neglect, right gaze preference, and dysarthria, in keeping with right MCA syndrome (NIH stroke scale 17). **A,** Axial unenhanced CT image through head reveals right "hyperdense artery" sign (*arrow*) (i.e., curvilinear high attenuation in right MCA) indicating acute thrombus, concordant with clinical presentation. **B,** Coronal CTA image reveals occlusion of right MCA (*arrow*). IV tPA was administered within 50 minutes of symptom onset, and neurointerventional team was also activated given presence of large vessel occlusion. **C,** Frontal catheter angiogram with right ICA contrast injection confirms complete occlusion of right MCA (*arrow*). **D,** Frontal catheter angiogram following IA mechanical thrombectomy with stent-retriever device demonstrates recanalization of right MCA. At time of discharge 5 days later, patient's left hemiparesis had resolved and only minimal residual left facial droop and dysarthria (NIH stroke scale 2) remained.

**Table 74-2.** Modified Fisher CT Grading Scale of SAH

| GRADE | CT FINDINGS | SYMPTOMATIC VASOSPASM RISK |
|-------|-------------|----------------------------|
| 0 | No SAH or IVH | 0% |
| 1 | Focal or diffuse thin (<5 mm) SAH, no IVH | 24% |
| 2 | Focal or diffuse thin (<5 mm) SAH, with IVH | 33% |
| 3 | Thick SAH (>5 mm), no IVH | 33% |
| 4 | Thick SAH (>5 mm), with IVH | 40% |

- Dural sinus thrombosis: Symptoms of cerebral venous thrombosis, such as headaches, nausea, vomiting, and seizures, are nonspecific, and therefore this diagnosis is easily overlooked both clinically and on imaging. First-line treatment for cerebral venous thrombosis is anticoagulation. Endovascular thrombectomy is a second-line treatment in patients with dural sinus thrombosis who fail medical management with anticoagulation.

**Vasospasm Treatment**
- Vasospasm is the most common cause of morbidity and mortality in SAH patients. The typical vasospasm window is between days 5 and 14 following hemorrhage, but vasospasm can occur anytime between days 3 and 21. The risk of vasospasm correlates with the modified Fisher scale (Table 74-2; i.e., the extent of SAH). Vasospasm can present as worsening headaches, change in mental status, stroke symptoms (e.g., hemiparesis and aphasia), seizures, and elevated cerebral arterial blood flow velocities on transcranial Doppler ultrasonography (US). If vasospasm is suspected clinically, head CTA is a reasonable initial imaging study to obtain. Induced hypertension (systolic blood pressure [SBP] >20% above baseline or SBP 180 to 200) is the most effective treatment for symptomatic vasospasm, and if the patient does not respond to induced hypertension, IA calcium channel blockers and/or balloon angioplasty can be offered as adjunctive therapy (Figure 74-9).

**Angioplasty/Stenting**
- Carotid artery angioplasty/stenting is indicated in symptomatic (i.e., transient ischemic attack [TIA] or stroke) patients with >50% stenosis, or in asymptomatic patients with >70% stenosis who have high surgical risk (i.e., high carotid bifurcation, severe cardiopulmonary disease, etc.).

5. What types of nonvascular neurointerventional procedures are available?
- Vertebral augmentation: Administration of polymethylmethacrylate in acute compression vertebral fractures for pain relief (Figure 74-10).
- Pain injection: Transforaminal or interlaminal epidural corticosteroid injections, facet (zygapophyseal joint) injections, nerve blocks, and synovial cyst fenestration.
- Biopsy: Imaging-guided biopsy of the calvarium, head and neck, and spine to assess for malignancy or infection.

6. What are the potential complications of neurointerventional procedures?
- Ischemic stroke: Related to emboli secondary to dislodged atherosclerotic plaques, air bubbles, catheter-related thrombus, or arterial dissection.
- Intracranial hemorrhage.
- Access-related vascular injury: Hemorrhage/hematoma, pseudoaneurysm at access site, or thromboembolic complications.
- Infection.
- Drug reaction (to any administered medications including iodinated contrast material).
- Radiation injury.

**KEY POINTS**

- The risk of symptomatic vasospasm correlates with the extent of SAH (i.e., the modified Fisher grading scale).
- Intracranial hemorrhage and large infarct size (>1/3 vascular territory) are contraindications for IV tPA and endovascular treatment.
- Time is BRAIN. Rapid diagnosis of ischemic stroke and prompt initiation of treatment are critical for a good outcome.

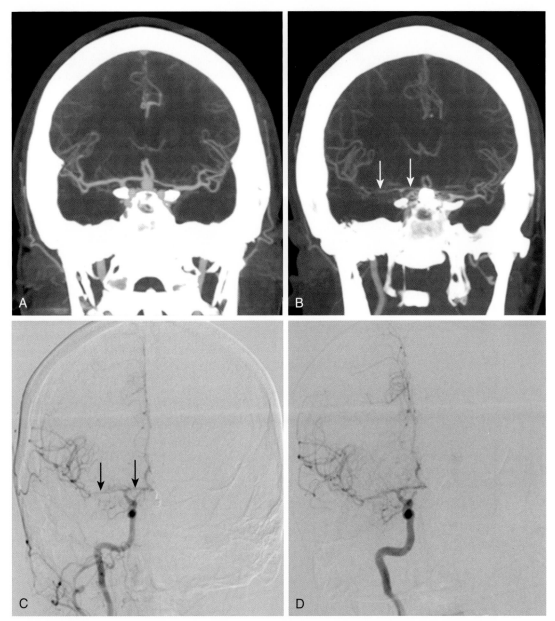

**Figure 74-9.** Cerebral artery vasospasm on CTA and catheter angiography. Patient is 39-year-old woman with Hunt and Hess grade 2/ modified Fisher grade 3 SAH due to ruptured ACOM aneurysm (same patient from Figure 74-4) who developed new left-sided weakness and disconjugate gaze 10 days later. **A,** Initial coronal CTA image through head shows no findings of cerebral artery vasospasm. Note again presence of ACOM aneurysm. **B,** Repeat coronal CTA image 10 days later demonstrates new narrowing of right MCA and right A1 segment (*arrows*) indicating vasospasm. **C,** Frontal catheter angiogram with right ICA contrast injection confirms right MCA and right A1 segment vasospasm (*arrows*). **D,** Frontal catheter angiogram following IA nicardipine administration demonstrates interval improvement of vasospasm.

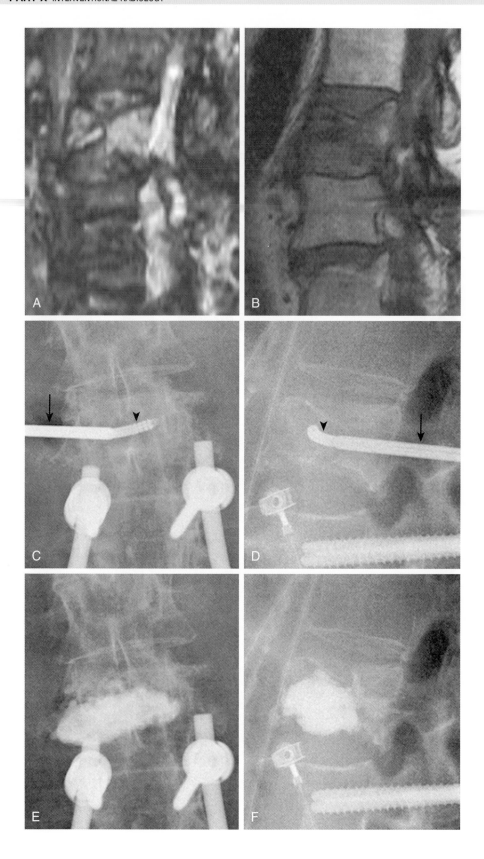

**Figure 74-10.** Vertebral compression fracture and vertebral augmentation on MRI and radiography. Patient is 71-year-old female with history of previous L3-4 fusion who is now wheelchair bound secondary to back pain. **A,** Sagittal short tau inversion recovery (STIR) MR image through lumbar spine shows loss of height of L2 vertebral body with high signal intensity bone marrow edema, in keeping with acute compression fracture. **B,** Sagittal T1-weighted MR image reveals similar findings of compression fracture with low signal intensity bone marrow. **C** and **D,** Posteroanterior and lateral intraoperative radiographs reveal left transpedicular approach coaxial system of introducer cannula (*arrow*) and curved needle (*arrowhead*). Curved needle has been advanced to anterior portion of vertebral body and across midline with tip at level of contralateral pedicle. Also note partial visualization of hardware related to prior L3-4 fusion. **E** and **F,** Posteroanterior and lateral postoperative radiographs demonstrate new high-density polymethylmethacrylate cement within L2 vertebral body from endplate to endplate and from pedicle to pedicle, with majority of cement delivered to anterior L2 vertebral body, which sustains most of axial load.

## BIBLIOGRAPHY

Berkhemer OA, Fransen PS, Beumer D, et al. A randomized trial of intraarterial treatment for acute ischemic stroke. *N Engl J Med.* 2015;372(1):11-20.

Campbell BC, Mitchell PJ, Kleinig TJ, et al. Endovascular therapy for ischemic stroke with perfusion-imaging selection. *N Engl J Med.* 2015;372(11):1009-1018.

Goyal M, Demchuk AM, Menon BK, et al. Randomized assessment of rapid endovascular treatment of ischemic stroke. *N Engl J Med.* 2015;372(11):1019-1030.

Jauch EC, Saver JL, Adams HP Jr, et al. Guidelines for the early management of patients with acute ischemic stroke: a guideline for healthcare professionals from the American Heart Association/American Stroke Association. *Stroke.* 2013;44(3):870-947.

Connolly ES Jr, Rabinstein AA, Carhuapoma JR, et al. Guidelines for the management of aneurysmal subarachnoid hemorrhage: a guideline for healthcare professionals from the American Heart Association/American Stroke Association. *Stroke.* 2012;43(6):1711-1737.

McGirt MJ, Parker SL, Wolinsky JP, et al. Vertebroplasty and kyphoplasty for the treatment of vertebral compression fractures: an evidenced-based review of the literature. *Spine J.* 2009;9(6):501-508.

Brisman JL, Song JK, Newell DW. Cerebral aneurysms. *N Engl J Med.* 2006;355(9):928-939.

Frontera JA, Claassen J, Schmidt JM, et al. Prediction of symptomatic vasospasm after subarachnoid hemorrhage: the modified Fisher scale. *Neurosurgery.* 2006;59(1):21-27, discussion 21-7.

Claassen J, Bernardini GL, Kreiter K, et al. Effect of cisternal and ventricular blood on risk of delayed cerebral ischemia after subarachnoid hemorrhage: the Fisher scale revisited. *Stroke.* 2001;32(9):2012-2020.

Oshiro EM, Walter KA, Piantadosi S, et al. A new subarachnoid hemorrhage grading system based on the Glasgow Coma Scale: a comparison with the Hunt and Hess and World Federation of Neurological Surgeons Scales in a clinical series. *Neurosurgery.* 1997;41(1):140-147, discussion 7-8.

Hunt WE, Hess RM. Surgical risk as related to time of intervention in the repair of intracranial aneurysms. *J Neurosurg.* 1968;28(1):14-20.

# CHAPTER 75

# MUSCULOSKELETAL INTERVENTIONAL RADIOLOGY

*Barry Glenn Hansford, MD, and Corrie M. Yablon, MD*

1. **What are some common image-guided musculoskeletal interventional procedures?**
   Musculoskeletal radiology is a subspecialty that encompasses many diagnostic and therapeutic procedures using image guidance. Some common ultrasonography-guided (US-guided) procedures in musculoskeletal radiology include: joint injections, tendon sheath injections, calcific tendinosis lavage, bursal injections, tendon fenestration, and soft tissue biopsy. Fluoroscopy is often used to guide joint injections as well as joint aspiration and arthrography. Computed tomography (CT) may be used to guide sacroiliac joint injections, bone biopsies, and radiofrequency (RF) ablation of osteoid osteoma. Magnetic resonance imaging (MRI) may be used to target bone marrow lesions for percutaneous biopsy that are occult on CT or radiography.

2. **What is MR arthrography, and what are its indications?**
   Direct MR arthrography involves the injection of dilute gadolinium-based contrast material into a joint under fluoroscopic guidance followed by MR imaging. This technique is commonly employed in the shoulder and hip to evaluate the labrum and articular cartilage (Figure 75-1). Wrist arthrography is used to evaluate the intrinsic carpal ligaments and the triangular fibrocartilage complex (TFCC). Intraarticular administration of contrast material allows for improved contrast resolution as well as distention of the joint capsule, both of which make it easier to visualize and evaluate small intraarticular structures (e.g., the labroligamentous complex of the shoulder joint).

3. **What concentration of gadolinium-based contrast material is used when performing MR arthrography? What are the components of the MR arthrogram injectate?**
   For MR arthrography, the injectate is diluted to a concentration of 1 to 2.5 mM. The final gadolinium dilution ratio should be 1:100 to 1:250 to achieve maximal signal intensity on T1-weighted MR images. Although the final injectate

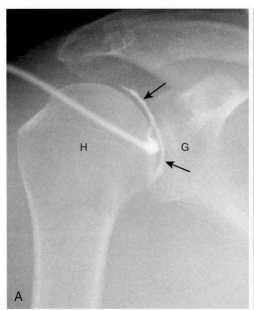
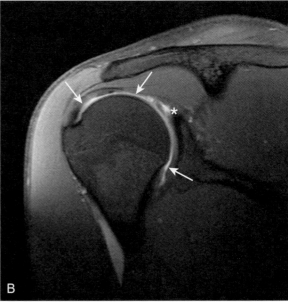

**Figure 75-1.** Labral tear of shoulder joint on MR arthrography. **A,** Fluoroscopic spot image demonstrates needle positioned at junction of upper 2/3 and lower 1/3 of glenohumeral joint. *H* = Humerus, *G* = Glenoid. Injectate containing contrast material is seen to outline glenohumeral joint (*arrows*). **B,** Coronal fat-suppressed T1-weighted MR arthrographic image of shoulder in different patient shows high signal intensity gadolinium-based contrast material within glenohumeral joint (*arrows*) that extends into superior labrum (*) in keeping with labral tear.

solution slightly varies from institution to institution, a suggested injectate solution may consist of 10 ml of saline, 10 ml of iodinated contrast material, 0.2 ml of gadolinium-based contrast material, and 0.1 ml of epinephrine (although not used for hip injections).

4. What will occur if the concentration of gadolinium in the injectate is too high?
   If the intraarticular concentration of gadolinium in the injectate for MR arthrography is too high, for example with a gadolinium dilution ratio of 1:5, this will result in a "black arthrogram" seen on MRI, where the injectate appears low in signal intensity. If this occurs, one option is to perform MRI after a waiting period of several hours.

5. What are the indications for a CT arthrography? What contrast material is used?
   CT arthrography is most often used when patients have contraindications to undergoing MR arthrography including: implanted pacemaker/defibrillator devices, any internal metal objects that make MRI unsafe, or claustrophobia. CT arthrography is particularly useful for the demonstration of cartilage defects, evaluation of intraarticular bodies, fracture fragments, synovial disease, and assessment of ligamentous integrity. Additionally, CT arthrography is very helpful to evaluate postoperative patients with implanted metallic hardware, because beam hardening artifact can be mitigated. Some of the common indications for CT arthrography include: evaluation of labral pathology of the shoulder, evaluation of the postoperative rotator cuff, evaluation for meniscal tears in the postoperative knee, and evaluation for ligamentous pathology in the wrist. The injectate for CT arthrography varies by institution but can range from a 1:1 mix of 300 mg/ml nonionic iodinated contrast material and sterile saline, to full-strength contrast material (Figure 75-2).

6. What are the commonly used approaches for injecting the glenohumeral joint? What are the pros and cons of each?
   Several approaches are commonly used for accessing the shoulder joint for direct arthrography. The most common approach is straight anterior with insertion of the needle at the junction of the middle and lower thirds of the glenohumeral joint, targeting the medial lower third of the glenohumeral joint while aiming for the side of the humeral head to avoid contacting the labrum. Using this approach, the needle must traverse the subscapularis tendon, which results in a theoretic risk of damaging the tendon.
   An alternative anterior approach is the rotator interval approach. With this method, the skin is marked superficial to the upper outer medial quadrant of the humeral head such that the rotator interval above the subscapularis tendon and lateral to the coracoid process is targeted. Advantages of the rotator interval approach are that a shorter needle (1.5 inch) can be used and that the operator can avoid traversing the subscapularis tendon, labrum, glenohumeral ligaments, and subcoracoid bursa. The drawback to this approach is the potential inadvertent injection of the subacromial-subdeltoid (SASD) bursa, which overlies the superior aspect of the rotator interval, which may result in difficulties with interpretation of the MR images if injected.

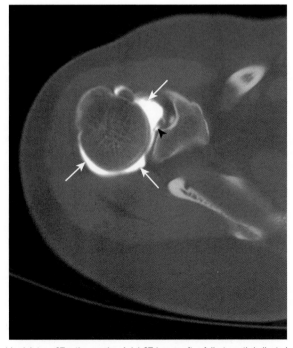

**Figure 75-2.** Labral tear of shoulder joint on CT arthrography. Axial CT image after full-strength iodinated contrast material injection into glenohumeral joint (*arrows*) shows focal contrast material within anterosuperior labrum (*arrowhead*) in keeping with labral tear.

A final technique is the posterior approach, which has been employed by some operators for suspected anterior instability and for muscular patients. This approach offers the added benefit of traversing fewer important anterior stabilizing structures of the glenohumeral articulation. The patient is placed in the prone position with the arm in internal rotation, and the needle is advanced toward the inferomedial aspect of the humeral head. With the posterior approach, once the needle tip contacts bone, it is important to apply continuous downward pressure during contrast material test injection to find the potential space between the humerus and joint capsule. Failure to provide downward pressure during contrast material test injection will likely result in contrast infiltration into the posterior aspect of the rotator cuff.

7. What imaging modalities can be used to guide joint injections, aspirations, or arthrography?
US, CT, or fluoroscopy may be selected to perform joint injections, aspirations, or arthrography. The selection of the specific imaging modality to guide the procedure depends upon the joint to be accessed, operator preference, patient characteristics (such as body habitus, age, pregnancy status, and ability to comply with the examination, among others), and the clinical question to be answered. One should consider using US rather than fluoroscopy for patients who are young or pregnant, in order to avoid ionizing radiation.

8. What are some benefits of using US to guide musculoskeletal procedures?
There are multiple benefits of using US to guide musculoskeletal procedures. First, there is no ionizing radiation, which is especially attractive when imaging pediatric and pregnant patients. US allows for real-time dynamic evaluation, which enables the operator to directly visualize the needle as it is advanced, ensuring avoidance of neurovascular structures. US allows the operator to deploy the biopsy needle in real time, unequivocally confirming needle placement within the targeted lesion. US guidance for injections allows the operator to observe the injection of the corticosteroids or other medications in real time, confirming accurate targeting of the joint or tendon sheath.

9. What are some commonly used corticosteroids in musculoskeletal interventions?
There are a variety of commonly used synthetic corticosteroids for musculoskeletal interventions that are derivatives of prednisolone, which is an analogue of cortisol. The most commonly used preparations include: methylprednisone acetate, triamcinolone acetonide, betamethasone acetate, and dexamethasone sodium phosphate.

10. What are some important contraindications to corticosteroid joint injections?
Absolute contraindications to corticosteroid joint injections include local or intraarticular sepsis, bacteremia, intraarticular fracture, and joint instability. If a patient has an infection at the time of corticosteroid injection, the primary concern is introduction of infection into the joint or worsening of a preexisting joint infection. In the setting of fracture and joint instability, corticosteroids inhibit bone healing and lead to worsening of joint instability due to the potential for subchondral osteonecrosis, as well as weakening of the joint capsule and ligaments. Relative contraindications to corticosteroid joint injection include: severe juxtaarticular osteoporosis, coagulopathy, and injection of a joint three times within a year or an injection within the last six weeks.

11. What are the complications of corticosteroid use in musculoskeletal procedures?
Complications of corticosteroid injection for musculoskeletal procedures include: septic arthritis, postinjection flare, local tissue atrophy, hypopigmentation/fat necrosis, tendon rupture, cartilage damage, facial flushing, and increased serum glucose levels. The most dreaded complication after a joint injection is septic arthritis. With the practice of good sterile technique, the incidence of septic arthritis is very low (0.01% to 0.03%). The most common complication after corticosteroid injection is a postinjection flare, which is secondary to a transient, local increase in inflammation that may begin 2 to 3 hours postprocedure and last for several days.

12. How is septic arthritis contracted?
Septic arthritis may be contracted in several ways including: hematogenous seeding, direct inoculation due to trauma, intervention, or postsurgical complication, or spread from adjacent soft tissue or bone infection. Risk factors for the development of septic arthritis include: intravenous drug use, medications that suppress the immune system, and underlying chronic medical conditions resulting in immunosuppression (such as diabetes mellitus, sickle cell disease, and rheumatoid arthritis, among others).

13. What are the indications for joint aspiration?
The most common indication for a monoarticular joint aspiration is to exclude the presence of infection or septic joint. Joint aspiration may also be performed for suspected crystal disease to differentiate among inflammatory conditions such as gout, rheumatoid arthritis, and calcium pyrophosphate deposition (CPPD) disease.

14. What laboratory tests are ordered when sending aspirated joint fluid for analysis?
When sending aspirated joint fluid for analysis to microbiology, the typical list of tests includes gram staining and culture, cell count with differential, and crystal analysis. Depending on clinical suspicion and ordering requests, fluid may also be sent for evaluation of atypical/fungal cultures in addition to the standard aerobic/anaerobic bacteria cultures.

15. What can you do if you are unable to aspirate any joint fluid?
It is crucial to establish the diagnosis of septic joint in a timely fashion because studies have shown that cartilage destruction can occur 1 to 2 days after the onset of symptoms. If the needle is in the appropriate position within the

joint but fluid cannot be aspirated (i.e., a dry tap), a lavage with nonbacteriostatic saline can be performed. The lavage sample may be sent to microbiology for culture and gram stain, but not cell count. One study found that hip joint lavage in the setting of an initial dry tap for suspected septic hip resulted in an increased positive diagnostic yield of 29%.

16. What are the most common pathogens in septic arthritis?

For all patients, the most commonly cultured organisms in the setting of septic arthritis are *Staphylococcus aureus* and *group B Streptococcus*.

17. What are some uncommon pathogens seen in septic arthritis?

Some of the more uncommon pathogens associated with septic arthritis present in specific clinical settings or patient populations. *Neisseria gonorrhoeae* is a common cause of septic arthritis in young, sexually active adults. *Escherichia coli* has a predilection for the elderly, intravenous drug users, and immunocompromised patients. *Propionibacterium* may be seen in joint arthroplasty infections, particularly in men with a shoulder arthroplasty. Septic joint following bite trauma usually affects the small joints of the hands and involves *Pasteurella multocida* in the case of animal bites and *Eikenella corrodens* in the case of human bites. Very rarely in immunocompromised patients, fungal and/or mycobacterial infection may result in a subacute or chronic oligoarticular septic joint. *Parvovirus B19* is the most common viral arthritis, presenting as a symmetric polyarticular arthritis involving the joints of the hand as well as larger joints.

18. What are the indications for a tendon sheath injection, and what are the potential complications?

The indications for tendon sheath injection include chronic or intractable pain that is recalcitrant to physical therapy. A tendon sheath injection may be performed with US guidance for diagnostic purposes, to localize the patient's pain preoperatively, or for therapeutic purposes to provide symptomatic relief in an effort to delay surgery. The tendon sheath injection may be performed either in the long axis or the short axis of the tendon (Figure 75-3). The major potential complication of a tendon sheath injection is tendon rupture, with a greater risk in patients with severe tendinosis or high-grade partial tears. The risk of tendon rupture in a previously intact tendon is very low. In the setting of superficial tendon sheath injection such as in the feet and hands, there is a risk of fat necrosis/skin depigmentation secondary to corticosteroid infiltration of the subcutaneous soft tissues.

19. What are the indications for an SASD bursal injection?

The SASD bursa is usually injected in the setting of subacromial impingement syndrome, with the injection providing both diagnostic information and temporizing therapeutic pain relief. Subacromial impingement syndrome results from any process that narrows the subacromial space, and it encompasses a range of rotator cuff pathology from tendinosis to full-thickness rotator cuff tears (Figure 75-4).

20. What are the potential complications of Baker cyst aspiration?

Aspiration of the semimembranosus-medial gastrocnemius bursa, or Baker cyst, is a frequently performed bursal aspiration under US guidance, with or without corticosteroid injection. The fluid collection lies between semimembranosus muscle and the medial head of the gastrocnemius muscle and may be simple or complicated. One potential complication of Baker cyst aspiration is inadvertent puncture of the adjacent popliteal artery or vein. This may be avoided by selecting a longitudinal plane or caudocranial approach as opposed to a transverse needle

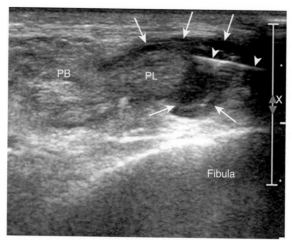

**Figure 75-3.** Peroneus longus tendon sheath injection under US guidance. In this case, injection was performed with peroneus longus tendon (*PL*) in short axis. Note hypoechoic injectate (*arrows*) collecting in crescentic fashion within tendon sheath superficial to tendon. Echogenic needle (*arrowheads*) is seen at right side of image. Peroneus brevis (*PB*) tendon is enlarged and tendinotic.

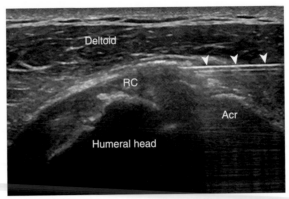

**Figure 75-4.** SASD bursal injection under US guidance. SASD bursa resides deep to deltoid muscle and superficial to rotator cuff (*RC*). Echogenic needle (*arrowheads*) is seen on right for injection of hypoechoic corticosteroid solution into bursa. In this case, supraspinatus tendon is partially shadowed by injectate and acromion (*Acr*).

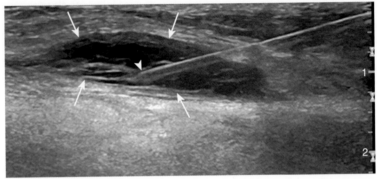

**Figure 75-5.** Baker cyst aspiration under US guidance. Using an in plane approach with Baker cyst in long axis (*arrows*), echogenic needle tip (*arrowhead*) is advanced within anechoic Baker cyst.

approach. The longitudinal approach is also beneficial in that the needle can be placed at the cranial margin of the Baker cyst and gradually withdrawn caudally as the Baker cyst decompresses (Figure 75-5). It should be noted that Baker cysts frequently reoccur, and the patient should be made aware that aspiration often only provides temporary pain relief. Additionally, in ≈50% of patients, the Baker cyst communicates with the knee joint. Therefore, one should always check for a knee effusion prior to performing a Baker cyst aspiration. If present, the joint effusion should be aspirated prior to aspirating the Baker cyst in an attempt to avoid immediate reaccumulation of joint fluid within the Baker cyst.

21. Describe the "in plane" and "out of plane" needle approaches in US-guided interventions.

"In plane" and "out of plane" are two basic approaches to freehand US-guided procedures, which refer to needle trajectory relative to the transducer and sound beam (Figure 75-6). With an in plane approach, the needle is directed under the long axis or parallel to the footprint of the transducer and nearly perpendicular to the direction of the incoming sound beam. This results in not only the needle tip but also the entire needle being visualized at all times throughout the duration of the procedure. This is the preferred method because it allows the operator to make real-time corrections for angle and depth. This approach also minimizes mistargeting complications and maximizes accuracy by enabling visualization of the entire needle path.

The out of plane approach refers to passing the needle perpendicular to the transducer, resulting in the needle passing through the plane of the sound beam. This technique is more difficult to master because the operator is only able to visualize a short segment of the needle at any one time, and the depth of the needle tip is not always immediately apparent to the operator. This technique is useful for small joints with a small surface area.

22. What techniques can help to increase the conspicuity of a needle during a US-guided procedure?

There are several very helpful techniques that may improve visualization of the needle during deep US-guided procedures where the needle angle is steep in order to reach the target. The first is the jiggle technique, during which the operator moves the needle minimally forward and backward along the needle path. This motion results in movement/vibration of the adjacent soft tissues, which often discloses the needle location. The needle is not advanced or moved side to side during this maneuver, just minimally pulsed to and fro. One may also rotate the needle, as the

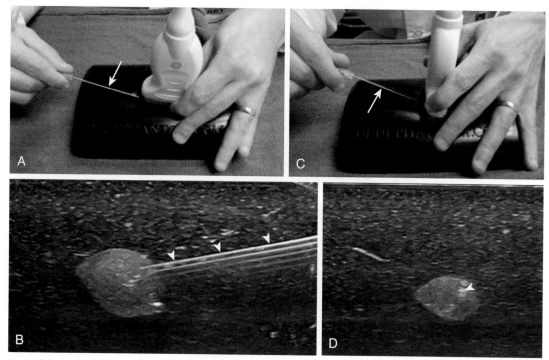

**Figure 75-6.** "In plane" and "out of plane" needle approaches in US-guided interventions. **A,** Image shows radiologist advancing needle (*arrow*) into phantom in plane with long axis of footprint of US transducer. **B,** Corresponding US image demonstrates length of needle (*arrowheads*) as it advances into target. **C,** Image shows radiologist advancing needle (*arrow*) into phantom out of plane (perpendicular) to long axis of footprint of US transducer. **D,** Corresponding US image demonstrates needle tip as echogenic dot within target (*arrowhead*).

bevel is often more echogenic appearing. Hydrodissection refers to injecting a small amount of fluid, which not only aids in confirming needle tip position with a small anechoic pocket of fluid, but also opens up a space between anatomic structures, resulting in an obstacle-free path for further needle adjustments. Special US settings/features such as beam steering and virtual convex imaging also significantly increase the conspicuity of the needle. However, the most important technique for improving visualization of the needle is to keep the needle as perpendicular to the sound beam, or as parallel to the transducer footprint, as possible. This may be accomplished by moving the puncture site farther from the transducer, performing the procedure along the curvature of an extremity, or using the transducer to deform the soft tissues with a heel-toe maneuver.

23. **What is tendon fenestration, and how is it performed?**
Tendon fenestration is a percutaneous US-guided therapeutic option for the treatment of chronic tendinosis. US is used to target the area of tendinosis. Then, an in plane approach longitudinal to the tendon is used to gently pass a needle through the abnormal portion of the tendon multiple (15 to 30) times. Once the entire abnormal portion of the tendon is felt to be adequately treated and the tendon softens, the needle is withdrawn. The purpose of fenestration is to transform a chronic degenerative process into an acute injury by inducing inflammation and bleeding, which results in local increases in growth factors and other substances associated with healing (Figure 75-7).

24. **What is platelet-rich plasma (PRP) injection, and why is it used?**
PRP injection is a developing therapy for the treatment of tendon injuries. PRP is defined as a platelet concentration higher than that of healthy whole blood (typically five times that of whole blood). Platelets initiate the clotting cascade, and it is thought that increasing the platelet concentration at the site of an injury results in a higher concentration of growth factors, which then accelerates the healing process. After PRP is obtained via centrifugation, it is injected at the site of tendon injury under US guidance to promote healing.

25. **What is calcific tendinosis lavage?**
Calcific tendinosis lavage is a percutaneous method of treating symptomatic calcium hydroxyapatite deposition that is refractory to conservative treatment. This procedure is most commonly performed for the treatment of calcific tendinosis in the rotator cuff. After local anesthesia is achieved, an 18 G needle is advanced into the calcium deposit using US guidance. Using a gravity-dependent syringe, lidocaine or saline is then pulsed into the deposit until it starts to break apart. It is not necessary for all of the calcium to be aspirated into the syringe for the patient to experience symptomatic relief. It is important to inject corticosteroid into the SASD bursa at the conclusion of the procedure to avoid induction of postprocedure bursitis (Figure 75-8).

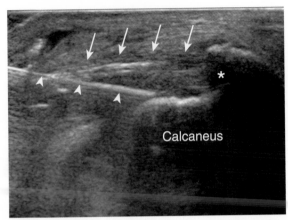

**Figure 75-7.** Achilles tendon fenestration under US guidance. In this patient with chronic Achilles tendinosis, echogenic needle (*arrowheads*) has been advanced into Achilles tendon (*arrows*). Note large dorsal calcaneal enthesophyte (*).

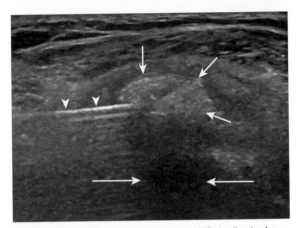

**Figure 75-8.** Calcific tendinosis lavage under US guidance. In this patient with calcific tendinosis of supraspinatus tendon, echogenic needle (*arrowheads*) has been advanced into calcific deposit (*short arrows*) for lavage. Note that deposit is ovoid and echogenic and has posterior acoustic shadowing (*long arrows*).

26. What is the difference between vertebroplasty and kyphoplasty?

The key difference is that vertebroplasty is used to treat vertebral body compression fractures by directly instilling cement via a thin needle cannula into the fracture under high pressure, while kyphoplasty first uses a balloon catheter at the site of the fracture to actively restore the lost vertebral body height, followed by the direct instillation of cement under lower pressure than vertebroplasty.

27. What are some complications of vertebroplasty or kyphoplasty?

In a recent series, one group described a complication rate of 6%. These complications included progression of vertebral compression fracture; leakage of cement from the vertebral body into the intervertebral disc or paravertebral veins; and nerve root compression during cannula insertion.

28. What is a CT-guided bone biopsy?

CT is the preferred modality to perform image-guided percutaneous bone biopsies. CT allows for excellent visualization of both the biopsy needle and the osseous lesions. An initial series of images obtained at the level of the lesion are used to plan and guide the needle approach to the lesion. Periodic imaging is obtained to confirm the needle path to the lesion. Images of the needle within the lesion are obtained to document the procedure. CT is excellent for the guidance of percutaneous biopsy of both primary and metastatic osseous lesions (Figure 75-9).

29. How should a CT-guided bone biopsy be planned?

Biopsy of a suspected metastasis entails different considerations than that of a primary bone tumor. In the case of a suspected metastasis, the lesion most amenable to biopsy with the lowest risk of complications is preferred because seeding the biopsy track is of lesser concern. The biopsy of a primary bone tumor should be conducted in close consultation with the orthopedic oncologist who will ultimately resect the tumor. The operator should select an approach for biopsy that takes into careful consideration future limb sparing resection and rehabilitation. It is important

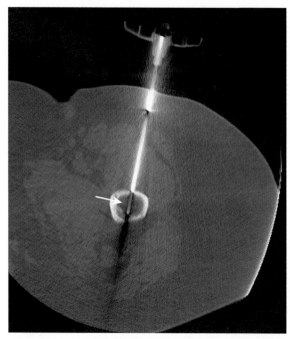

**Figure 75-9.** Percutaneous femoral bone biopsy under CT guidance. Axial CT image shows very high attenuation biopsy needle within femoral diaphysis traversing intramedullary lesion (*arrow*). Coaxial system is used, revealing inner biopsy needle within outer access needle, allowing multiple passes to be performed with one initial puncture.

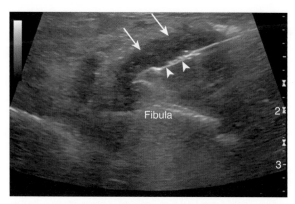

**Figure 75-10.** Soft tissue biopsy of ankle under US guidance. Open tray of spring-loaded biopsy needle (*arrowheads*) is deployed within ovoid hypoechoic soft tissue mass (*arrows*). Subsequent histopathologic analysis demonstrated synovial chondromatosis.

to avoid contaminating joints, neurovascular structures, or adjacent anatomic compartments. It is also important to take an adequate number of samples to allow the pathologist to make a diagnosis, which varies with the size of the biopsy needle (e.g., with the larger 11 G needle, several cores are usually adequate). All aspirated fluid and clotted blood should also be sent for pathologic evaluation.

30. **What is the most important principle of US-guided soft tissue biopsy?**
The most important principle when performing a US-guided biopsy of a soft tissue mass is to target the solid portion of the lesion. The solid portion of the lesion is the most high-yield for providing the pathologist with enough abnormal tissue to allow a confident diagnosis. The subsolid or cystic portion of a soft tissue mass is frequently secondary to necrosis and/or hemorrhage, which will result in a nondiagnostic biopsy, necessitating a repeat procedure (Figure 75-10).

31. **When should conscious sedation be used or considered when planning a musculoskeletal intervention?**
Conscious sedation refers to the administration of medications, resulting in minimally depressed consciousness such that a patient is able to maintain an airway and respond to commands. This is normally accomplished by the intravenous administration of an analgesic (e.g., fentanyl) and an anxiolytic (e.g., midazolam). Musculoskeletal

interventions that require conscious sedation include any type of bone biopsy. Conscious sedation is also recommended for biopsies of the feet, the hands, suspected peripheral nerve sheath tumors, and the soft tissue component of a bone tumor, because they can be extremely painful. Finally, conscious sedation may be considered for any soft tissue biopsy or for any patient who is extremely anxious or intellectually disabled.

## KEY POINTS

- Image guidance allows for accurate lesion targeting and needle placement in musculoskeletal interventional procedures.
- MR arthrography and CT arthrography are both useful to evaluate the integrity of the labrum and articular cartilage.
- The solid components of a tumor are targeted during biopsy to maximize the diagnostic yield.
- Conscious sedation is recommended for biopsies of bone tumors and biopsies of the feet, hands, and suspected peripheral nerve sheath tumors, because they can be extremely painful. This may also be utilized for any patient with anxiety or intellectual disability.
- Consider using US (rather than fluoroscopic) guidance for musculoskeletal interventional procedures in young and pregnant patients in order to avoid exposure to ionizing radiation.

### BIBLIOGRAPHY

Mukherjee S, Thakur B, Bhagawati D, et al. Utility of routine biopsy at vertebroplasty in the management of vertebral compression fractures: a tertiary center experience. *J Neurosurg Spine*. 2014;21(5):687-697.

Saracen A, Kotwica Z. Treatment of multiple osteoporotic vertebral compression fractures by percutaneous cement augmentation. *Int Orthop*. 2014;38(11):2309-2312.

Yablon CM. Ultrasound-guided interventions of the foot and ankle. *Semin Musculoskelet Radiol*. 2013;17(1):60-68.

Hansford BG, Stacy GS. Musculoskeletal aspiration procedures. *Semin Intervent Radiol*. 2012;29(4):270-285.

Koroglu M, Callioglu M, Eris HN, et al. Ultrasound guided percutaneous treatment and follow-up of Baker's cyst in knee osteoarthritis. *Eur J Radiol*. 2012;81(11):3466-3471.

Kung JW, Yablon C, Huang ES, et al. Clinical and radiologic predictive factors of septic hip arthritis. *AJR Am J Roentgenol*. 2012;199(4): 868-872.

Molini L, Mariacher S, Bianchi S. US guided corticosteroid injection into the subacromial-subdeltoid bursa: Technique and approach. *J Ultrasound*. 2012;15(1):61-68.

Lee KS, Wilson JJ, Rabago DP, et al. Musculoskeletal applications of platelet-rich plasma: fad or future? *AJR Am J Roentgenol*. 2011;196(3):628-636.

Peer S, Freuis T, Loizides A, et al. Ultrasound guided core needle biopsy of soft tissue tumors; a fool proof technique? *Med Ultrason*. 2011;13(3):187-194.

Housner JA, Jacobson JA, Misko R. Sonographically guided percutaneous needle tenotomy for the treatment of chronic tendinosis. *J Ultrasound Med*. 2009;28(9):1187-1192.

Kanafani ZA, Sexton DJ, Pien BC, et al. Postoperative joint infections due to *Propionibacterium* species: a case-control study. *Clin Infect Dis*. 2009;49(7):1083-1085.

MacMahon PJ, Eustace SJ, Kavanagh EC. Injectable corticosteroid and local anesthetic preparations: a review for radiologists. *Radiology*. 2009;252(3):647-661.

Shortt CP, Morrison WB, Roberts CC, et al. Shoulder, hip, and knee arthrography needle placement using fluoroscopic guidance: practice patterns of musculoskeletal radiologists in North America. *Skeletal Radiol*. 2009;38(4):377-385.

Espinosa LA, Jamadar DA, Jacobson JA, et al. CT-guided biopsy of bone: a radiologist's perspective. *AJR Am J Roentgenol*. 2008;190(5):W283-W289.

Nazarian LN. The top 10 reasons musculoskeletal sonography is an important complementary or alternative technique to MRI. *AJR Am J Roentgenol*. 2008;190(6):1621-1626.

Testa V, Capasso G, Benazzo F, et al. Management of Achilles tendinopathy by ultrasound-guided percutaneous tenotomy. *Med Sci Sports Exerc*. 2002;34(4):573-580.

# XI
# NUCLEAR RADIOLOGY

# CHAPTER 76

# PET OF ONCOLOGICAL DISORDERS

*Drew A. Torigian, MD, MA, FSAR, and Andrew B. Newberg, MD*

1. **What is $^{18}$F-fluoro-2-deoxy-2-D-glucose (FDG)?**

   FDG is the most widely used radiotracer for positron emission tomography (PET) imaging and was first tested in humans in 1976. Its utility is based on the Warburg effect (described in the late 1920s by Otto Warburg), in which malignant cancer cells preferentially use glucose compared to other substrates. However, this radiotracer can be used to assess any organ or disease process that has accelerated glucose metabolism, including infectious and noninfectious inflammatory disease conditions.

2. **What instructions do patients need to prepare for FDG PET imaging?**

   The most important issue regarding an FDG PET scan is that FDG competes with nonradioactive glucose. If a patient has recently eaten or has diabetes mellitus with a serum glucose level >150 mg/dl, the sensitivity of the scan to detect malignancy may be diminished. Typically, serum glucose levels greater than 200 mg/dl should exclude a patient from having an FDG PET scan. Nondiabetic patients should have nothing by mouth overnight for a scan scheduled in the morning or else for at least 4 to 6 hours for a scan scheduled later in the day. Diabetic patients should be managed carefully because some have difficulty forgoing eating. Also, insulin drives glucose (and FDG) into the muscles, so care should be taken regarding the administration of insulin too close to the scan time. It is preferred that the patient not inject insulin, eat, or exercise before the PET scan, but if this is impossible, the referring physician must balance glucose levels, eating, and insulin in the diabetic patient. The scan itself is typically acquired starting 1 hour after intravenous FDG administration from the skull base to the proximal thighs and takes about 30 minutes to perform. Whole body scanning from skull vertex to toes, which takes about 45 minutes to acquire, is performed in some patients with malignancies that more commonly involve the head, skin, or extremities such as melanoma and cutaneous lymphoma.

3. **What is dual time point (DTP) PET, and what is its potential utility?**

   DTP PET is a scanning technique that involves acquisition of two sets of PET images (at early and delayed time points) after intravenous FDG administration. In general, malignant lesions tend to have increasing levels of glucose (and FDG) uptake over time, whereas nonmalignant lesions as well as normal tissues tend to have stable or decreasing levels of glucose (and FDG) uptake over time. Therefore, DTP PET generally helps to improve the sensitivity of detection of malignant lesions in the body compared to single time point (STP) PET, as malignant lesions become more FDG avid over time and background tissue FDG uptake decreases. Furthermore, DTP PET improves the specificity to characterize a lesion as malignant or benign, given the differential temporal patterns of FDG uptake.

4. **What is the normal pattern of FDG uptake in the body?**

   High FDG uptake is observed in the gray matter of the brain. Also, high FDG activity is seen in the collecting systems, ureters, and bladder due to urinary excretion of FDG, which can be mitigated by patient hydration and voiding prior to image acquisition. Mild to moderate FDG uptake is usually seen in the tonsils, salivary glands, tongue, vocal cords, brown fat, bone marrow, liver, stomach, and large bowel. Mild FDG uptake is usually seen in the thyroid gland, esophagus, small bowel, spleen, and skeletal muscle. Minimal FDG uptake is seen in the lungs and pancreas. Variable FDG uptake is observed in the myocardium, as the heart uses glucose as well as fatty acids as sources of fuel. FDG uptake will generally be increased in the myocardium with a carbohydrate rich meal and decreased with a fatty rich meal prior to PET scanning (Figure 76-1).

   Minimizing talking and patient movement as well as keeping the environment quiet and dimly lit during the FDG uptake period are methods to decrease FDG uptake in the normal tissues of the head and neck and skeletal muscles. In general, FDG uptake in bilaterally located organs should be symmetric, and up to 70% of unexpected findings detected on FDG PET are malignant or premalignant in nature.

5. **What is the significance of increased FDG uptake in the thyroid gland?**

   Focal FDG uptake in the thyroid gland is generally considered as suspicious for thyroid malignancy until proven otherwise and requires further evaluation with thyroid ultrasonography or tissue sampling. This is in contradistinction to diffuse FDG uptake in the thyroid gland, which may be a normal finding when mild, or due to thyroiditis or Graves' disease when moderate or marked.

6. **What is the significance of increased FDG uptake in the bowel?**

   Focal FDG uptake in the bowel is generally considered as suspicious for malignancy until proven otherwise (Figure 76-2) and requires further evaluation such as with computed tomography (CT), magnetic resonance imaging (MRI),

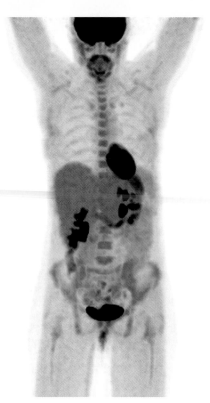

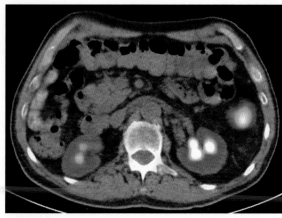

**Figure 76-2.** Colon cancer on FDG PET/CT. Note focal high FDG uptake in descending colon, along with normal FDG excretion into collecting systems.

**Figure 76-1.** Normal pattern of FDG uptake seen on PET. Note high FDG uptake in brain and myocardium, moderate FDG uptake in tonsils, salivary glands, bone marrow, liver, and stomach, and mild FDG uptake in spleen and skeletal muscle. High FDG activity is seen in collecting systems and bladder due to urinary excretion of FDG.

fluoroscopy, or endoscopy with tissue sampling. Diffuse FDG uptake in the bowel is often physiologic, whereas segmental FDG uptake may be physiologic or inflammatory in nature.

7. **What is the significance of increased FDG uptake in the endometrium or adnexa?**
   In premenopausal women, mild FDG uptake may normally be seen in the endometrium during the early menstrual cycle or in midcycle, and in the fallopian tubes or ovaries during midcycle. However, in postmenopausal women, increased endometrial or adnexal FDG uptake is generally considered as suspicious for malignancy until proven otherwise.

8. **How does hybrid PET combined with structural imaging such as CT or MRI improve diagnostic performance in cancer patients?**
   Hybrid PET imaging in conjunction with CT or MRI provides coregistered molecular and structural images, leading to improved image quality, improved anatomic localization of sites of radiotracer uptake, and increased sensitivity, specificity, accuracy, and confidence levels of diagnostic interpretation compared to standalone PET. As such, most PET scanners currently utilized in clinical practice are either PET/CT or PET/MRI scanners.

9. **What are the main applications of FDG PET/CT in the oncological setting?**
   - Lesion characterization (as benign or malignant, and as indolent or aggressive).
   - Tumor staging and pretreatment planning.
   - Prognostication of clinical outcome (prior to therapy).
   - Tumor response assessment (during or after therapy).
   - Tumor restaging (for detection and localization of sites of recurrent disease).

10. **What is the potential role of FDG PET/MRI in the oncological setting?**
    MRI provides high spatial resolution and soft tissue contrast and is complementary with PET. Therefore, FDG PET/MRI is most promising for the evaluation of patients with tumors that arise from anatomic sites that are suboptimally evaluated at CT, including the brain, head and neck, spinal cord, liver, pelvic organs, breasts, and musculoskeletal system. Available functional techniques afforded by MRI such as diffusion-weighted imaging and MR spectroscopy can

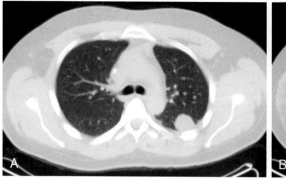 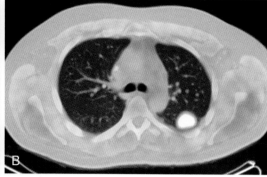

**Figure 76-3. A,** Pulmonary metastasis on CT. Note 2.9-cm round nodule in left lower lobe of lung. **B,** Pulmonary metastasis on FDG PET/CT. Note high FDG uptake in lung nodule, consistent with malignancy.

further enhance detection and characterization of malignant lesions. Finally, PET/MRI reduces radiation exposure compared to PET/CT, which is highly desirable for all patients, especially for pediatric patients and for patients who undergo multiple examinations.

11. What is the utility of FDG PET to characterize indeterminate lung nodules?
    Although chest CT is currently the mainstay for detecting lung nodules, lung nodules are often unable to be accurately characterized on CT alone as benign or malignant because structural imaging features are often nonspecific. FDG PET is useful to improve the characterization of lung nodules, where it is assumed that malignant nodules exhibit increased FDG uptake due to increased glucose uptake and metabolism (Figure 76-3). In particular, FDG PET/CT is currently recommended when a solid indeterminate lung nodule >8 to 10 mm in diameter is present in the setting of a low-moderate pretest probability of malignancy or when a persistent part-solid indeterminate nodule >8 to 10 mm in diameter is present.

12. What are the major causes for false-negative FDG PET findings in cancer patients?
    False-negative FDG PET findings may occur when there is low tumor metabolic activity, such as with lepidic-predominant adenocarcinomas (minimally invasive or in situ), mucinous adenocarcinomas, and carcinoid tumors, or when the lesions are small in size due to the limitations of spatial resolution of PET. However, observation of no or minimal levels of FDG uptake within a tumor is useful information, because lower levels of FDG uptake generally reflect a more indolent tumor biology and portend a more favorable clinical outcome. False-negative findings may also occur in tissues where there is a high background level of FDG uptake such as in the brain, bowel, or urologic system.

13. What are the major causes for false-positive FDG PET findings in cancer patients?
    False-positive FDG PET findings may occur when there is active infection or noninfectious inflammation of any cause. For example, bacterial infection, mycobacterial infection, and sarcoidosis can all lead to increased FDG uptake in the body, potentially mimicking malignancy. Iatrogenic inflammation following radiation therapy often leads to increased FDG uptake, although it tends to be diffuse and geographic in distribution, often with linear margins. Also, increased FDG uptake can be seen in benign tumors, and physiologic increased FDG uptake can be seen in brown fat, bowel, and the genitourinary system.

14. Is there a specific standardized uptake value (SUV) threshold on FDG PET that can reliably distinguish malignant from benign disease processes?
    No, there is no one particular SUV threshold level that can reliably distinguish malignant from benign lesions on FDG PET. SUV measurements are affected by the scan acquisition parameters utilized, the delay time between FDG administration and image acquisition, and patient body size and thus will vary somewhat from patient to patient and from scan to scan. Furthermore, SUVs will generally appear to be lower for small lesions compared to those of large lesions due to the limited spatial resolution of PET (i.e., the partial volume effect), leading to underestimation of FDG uptake in small lesions. Lastly, as described above, some indolent tumors may have minimal or no FDG uptake, whereas infectious or noninfectious inflammatory lesions may have increased levels of FDG uptake similar to malignant tumors.

15. What is the utility of FDG PET for disease staging and pretreatment planning of cancer patients?
    FDG PET improves the accuracy of tumor staging compared to CT alone and is currently utilized in the initial staging and pretreatment planning workup of patients with cancer. In particular, FDG PET improves N staging (for regional lymph nodes) and M staging (for distant metastatic sites). As a result, changes in patient management occur in up to 40% of patients, most often due to detection of distant metastases. Also, it has generally been reported that the larger the global burden of FDG avid tumor in the body, the worse the clinical outcome.

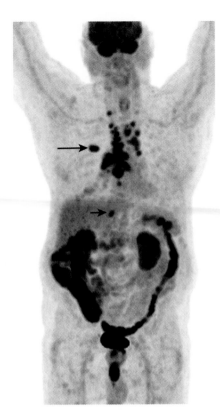

**Figure 76-4.** Metastatic lung cancer on FDG PET. Note avid FDG uptake in primary lung cancer in right lung (*long arrow*) along with FDG uptake in bilateral hilar and mediastinal lymph nodes, right supraclavicular lymph node, and left hepatic lobe metastasis (*short arrow*).

16. Is the lung cancer patient in Figure 76-4 a good surgical candidate?

    No. One important use of FDG PET is presurgical evaluation of patients with lung cancer. If FDG PET shows metastatic disease to supraclavicular, contralateral hilar, or contralateral mediastinal lymph nodes, or to distant sites in the body, the patient is no longer a surgical candidate and instead receives chemotherapy, sometimes with radiotherapy.

17. What is the role of FDG PET in radiotherapy pretreatment planning?

    FDG PET plays an important role in radiotherapy pretreatment planning of cancer patients. It provides improved delineation of sites of malignancy, leading to treatment volume changes in up to 100% of patients and dose sparing of uninvolved tissues. In addition, FDG PET improves disease staging, improving selection of patients for definitive radiotherapy and often leading to a change in radiotherapy treatment intent from curative to palliative or vice versa.

18. How useful is FDG PET for the evaluation of primary and metastatic brain tumors?

    FDG PET generally has low sensitivity for early detection of primary or metastatic brain tumors, given the normal high level of FDG uptake in the brain. For this reason, MRI is predominantly utilized for diagnostic assessment of the brain in cancer patients. However, FDG PET is useful to better characterize brain tumor biology, because more aggressive higher grade tumors will in general have greater degrees of FDG uptake than more indolent lower grade tumors. Furthermore, FDG PET is most useful to differentiate tumor recurrence from radiation necrosis in the surgical bed. Typically, active tumor is easier to detect in the setting of background hypometabolism related to treatment effects.

19. How useful is FDG PET for evaluation of peritoneal spread of tumor?

    FDG PET can detect peritoneal tumor implants, but the sensitivity is generally suboptimal given its low spatial resolution. In general, the smaller the lesion size, the greater the false-negative rate of FDG PET, although CT and MRI also have suboptimal sensitivity when peritoneal lesions are small or located along organ surfaces. Sometimes, mild diffusely increased FDG uptake in the abdomen is visible, suggesting presence of peritoneal tumor spread.

20. What is the utility of FDG PET for response assessment in cancer patients?

    FDG PET is useful for accurate early quantitative assessment of tumor response to therapy and provides the opportunity to change treatment promptly in the case of a nonresponse, thereby ameliorating or preventing unnecessary side effects while maximizing the chance for an improved outcome. Early response assessment, days to weeks after the initiation of therapy, is often possible because changes in tumor metabolism precede

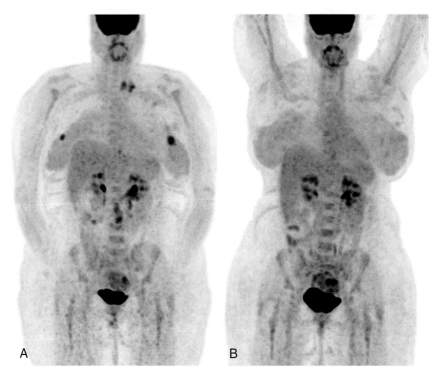

**Figure 76-5. A,** Pretreatment staging of lymphoma on FDG PET. Note FDG avid lymph nodes in left supraclavicular and bilateral axillary locations. **B,** Post-treatment response assessment of lymphoma 3 months later on FDG PET. Note interval resolution of abnormal sites of FDG uptake in lymph nodes, in keeping with complete response. Incidental FDG avid foci in pelvis are due to uterine leiomyomas.

changes in tumor size. In general, a reduction in tumor FDG uptake after therapy is more likely to be associated with a histopathologic response and improved patient survival than is a lack of change (Figure 76-5).

21. **What is the utility of FDG PET for disease restaging of cancer patients?**
FDG PET has high diagnostic accuracy for the early detection of recurrent tumor, even when no other symptoms or signs of tumor recurrence are present, leading to improved clinical outcomes. Moreover, it allows for precise spatial localization of the sites of tumor recurrence, which determines whether locoregional salvage therapies or systematic therapies are appropriate.

22. **What other non-FDG PET radiotracers are available for use in the oncological setting?**
Noninvasive PET assessment of other molecular characteristics of tumors may be useful to characterize tumor biology and to optimize patient management. For example, pretreatment detection of hypoxia in lung cancer and other tumors is useful, as tumor hypoxia generally decreases tumor responsiveness to radiotherapy and chemotherapy. Similarly, pretreatment detection of estrogen receptor expression in metastatic breast cancer is useful, because such tumors will then generally respond to antiestrogen systemic therapies. Please see Table 76-1 for a short list of some other non-FDG radiotracers that are available to assess patients with cancer.

---

**KEY POINTS**

- FDG PET imaging is useful for lesion characterization, tumor staging and pretreatment planning, clinical outcome prognostication, tumor response assessment, and tumor restaging.
- Focal FDG uptake in the uterus or adnexa of a postmenopausal woman, in the thyroid gland, or in the bowel is generally considered as suspicious for malignancy until proven otherwise.
- Lower levels of FDG uptake within tumors generally reflect a more indolent tumor biology and portend a more favorable clinical outcome.
- In general, a reduction in tumor FDG uptake after therapy is more likely to be associated with a histopathologic response and improved patient survival than is a lack of change.

**Table 76-1.** Some Non-FDG Radiotracers Available for Oncological PET Imaging

| TARGET | REPRESENTATIVE RADIOTRACER |
|---|---|
| Amino acid metabolism | L-[methyl-$^{11}$C]methionine ($^{11}$C-MET)<br>$^{18}$F-4-fluoroglutamine<br>$^{18}$F-6-fluorodihydroxyphenylalanine ($^{18}$F-FDOPA) |
| Cell proliferation | 3′-deoxy-3′-$^{18}$F-fluorothymidine ($^{18}$F-FLT) |
| Phospholipid metabolism | $^{11}$C-choline<br>$^{18}$F-fluorocholine ($^{18}$F-FCH) |
| Angiogenesis | $^{18}$F-galacto-arginine-glycine-aspartate ($^{18}$F-RGD) |
| Hypoxia | $^{18}$F-2-(2-nitro-$^1$H-imidazol-1-yl)-$N$-(2,2,3,3,3-pentafluoropropyl)-acetamide ($^{18}$F-EF5)<br>$^{18}$F-fluoromisonidazole ($^{18}$F-FMISO)<br>$^{64}$Cu-(II)-diacetyl-bis(N4-methylthiosemicarbazone) ($^{64}$Cu-ATSM) |
| Apoptosis | 4-$^{18}$F-fluorobenzoyl-annexin V |
| Bone metabolism | $^{18}$F-sodium fluoride ($^{18}$F-NaF) |
| **Receptor Expression** | |
| Somatostatin | $^{68}$Ga-DOTA-Phe$^1$-Tyr$^3$-octreotide ($^{68}$Ga-DOTA-TOC)<br>$^{68}$Ga-DOTA-1-Nal$_3$-octreotide ($^{68}$Ga-DOTA-NOC)<br>$^{68}$Ga-DOTA-Tyr$^3$-Thr$^8$-octreotide ($^{68}$Ga-DOTA-TATE) |
| Estrogen | 16$\alpha$-$^{18}$F-fluoroestradiol-17$\beta$ ($^{18}$F-FES) |

**BIBLIOGRAPHY**

Dong A, Cui Y, Wang Y, et al. (18)F-FDG PET/CT of adrenal lesions. *AJR Am J Roentgenol.* 2014;203(2):245-252.

Hojgaard L, Berthelsen AK, Loft A. Head and neck: normal variations and benign findings in FDG positron emission tomography/computed tomography imaging. *PET Clin.* 2014;9(2):141-145.

Kohan A, Avril NE. Pelvis: normal variants and benign findings in FDG PET/CT imaging. *PET Clin.* 2014;9(2):185-193.

Roh JL, Park JP, Kim JS, et al. 18F fluorodeoxyglucose PET/CT in head and neck squamous cell carcinoma with negative neck palpation findings: a prospective study. *Radiology.* 2014;271(1):153-161.

Vilstrup MH, Torigian DA. FDG PET in thoracic malignancies. *PET Clin.* 2014;9(4):391-420.

Wachsmann JW, Gerbaudo VH. Thorax: normal and benign pathologic patterns in FDG PET/CT imaging. *PET Clin.* 2014;9(2):147-168.

Zukotynski K, Kim CK. Abdomen: normal variations and benign conditions resulting in uptake on FDG PET/CT. *PET Clin.* 2014;9(2):169-183.

Brunetti J. PET/CT in gynecologic malignancies. *Radiol Clin North Am.* 2013;51(5):895-911.

Cheng G, Torigian DA, Zhuang H, et al. When should we recommend use of dual time-point and delayed time-point imaging techniques in FDG PET? *Eur J Nucl Med Mol Imaging.* 2013;40(5):779-787.

Kwee TC, Cheng G, Lam MG, et al. SUV of 2.5 should not be embraced as a magic threshold for separating benign from malignant lesions. *Eur J Nucl Med Mol Imaging.* 2013;40:1475-1477.

Kwee TC, Torigian DA, Alavi A. Oncological applications of positron emission tomography for evaluation of the thorax. *J Thorac Imaging.* 2013;28(1):11-24.

Torigian DA, Zaidi H, Kwee TC, et al. PET/MR imaging: technical aspects and potential clinical applications. *Radiology.* 2013;267(1):26-44.

Basu S, Kwee TC, Gatenby R, et al. Evolving role of molecular imaging with PET in detecting and characterizing heterogeneity of cancer tissue at the primary and metastatic sites, a plausible explanation for failed attempts to cure malignant disorders. *Eur J Nucl Med Mol Imaging.* 2011;38(6):987-991.

Kwee TC, Basu S, Saboury B, et al. A new dimension of FDG PET interpretation: assessment of tumor biology. *Eur J Nucl Med Mol Imaging.* 2011;38(6):1158-1170.

Chen W, Parsons M, Torigian DA, et al. Evaluation of thyroid FDG uptake incidentally identified on FDG PET/CT imaging. *Nucl Med Commun.* 2009;30(3):240-244.

Sanz-Viedma S, Torigian DA, Parsons M, et al. Potential clinical utility of dual time point FDG PET for distinguishing benign from malignant lesions: implications for oncological imaging. *Rev Esp Med Nucl.* 2009;28(3):159-166.

Hillner BE, Siegel BA, Shields AF, et al. Relationship between cancer type and impact of PET and PET/CT on intended management: findings of the national oncologic PET registry. *J Nucl Med.* 2008;49(12):1928-1935.

Hustinx R, Torigian DA, Namur G. Complementary assessment of abdominopelvic disorders with PET/CT and MRI. *PET Clin.* 2008;3(3):435-449.

Torigian DA, Huang SS, Houseni M, et al. Functional imaging of cancer with emphasis on molecular techniques. *CA Cancer J Clin.* 2007;57(4):206-224.

Gutman F, Alberini JL, Wartski M, et al. Incidental colonic focal lesions detected by FDG PET/CT. *AJR Am J Roentgenol.* 2005;185(2):495-500.

# CHAPTER 77

# PET OF NONONCOLOGICAL DISORDERS

*Drew A. Torigian, MD, MA, FSAR, and Andrew B. Newberg, MD*

1. What are some applications of $^{18}$F-fluoro-2-deoxy-2-D-glucose positron emission tomography/computed tomography (FDG PET/CT) in the nononcological setting?

   For the answer, see Box 77-1. The applications in nononcological cardiac and brain disorders will be discussed separately in Chapters 82 and 83, respectively.

2. What is the role of FDG PET/magnetic resonance imaging (MRI) in the nononcological setting?

   FDG PET/MRI is most promising for the evaluation of patients with nononcological disorders that involve anatomic sites that are suboptimally evaluated at CT. In particular, PET/MRI may be particularly useful for evaluation of patients with neurologic, cardiovascular, and musculoskeletal nonneoplastic disorders. Available functional techniques afforded by MRI can further enhance detection and characterization of lesions. PET/MRI reduces radiation exposure compared to PET/CT, which is highly desirable, especially for pediatric patients and for those who undergo multiple examinations.

3. What is the utility of FDG PET in patients with suspected infection?

   FDG PET is useful to detect infections that are not detected by other methods, to determine the spatial extent and severity of infections, and to monitor the effects of therapeutic interventions. Bacterial, mycobacterial, viral, fungal, and parasitic infections typically reveal areas of increased FDG uptake, which is related to the activation of neutrophil granulocytes and other inflammatory cells. Examples of specific applications of the potential utility of FDG PET in patients with suspected infection include the following:

   - Fever of unknown origin (FUO) is a challenging diagnostic problem, where early diagnosis of the underlying etiology is critical for appropriate patient management. Infection accounts for approximately one third of cases of FUO, followed by noninfectious inflammatory disorders and neoplastic disease. FDG PET has a high accuracy (>90%) to detect the underlying etiology of FUO and may be considered in the workup of patients with FUO for whom conventional diagnostic testing has been unsuccessful.
   - Infectious endocarditis is a serious infection that is associated with increased morbidity and mortality. FDG PET is useful to detect infectious endocarditis, even in the presence of a prosthetic valve which may limit the diagnostic performance of echocardiography, and to improve the specificity of diagnosis, as not all vegetations detected on echocardiography are infected. On FDG PET, increased FDG uptake in or around a cardiac valve is suggestive of infectious endocarditis.
   - Osteomyelitis, the infection of bone, requires timely diagnosis for early initiation of antimicrobial and surgical treatment to improve clinical outcome. FDG PET is useful to improve the early detection of osteomyelitis and has high diagnostic accuracy. In contradistinction, structural imaging techniques such as radiography, CT, and MRI may not reveal morphologic findings in early osteomyelitis and often do not reveal morphologic findings that are specific for early disease, particularly when preexisting alterations in the underlying osseous structures are present from prior trauma, surgery, or infection. Available conventional nuclear medicine techniques also have limitations in

---

**Box 77-1.** Applications of FDG PET/CT in the Nononcological Setting

Assessment of patients with brain disorders
- Refractory seizures
- Neurocognitive disorders

Assessment of patients with cardiac disorders
- Myocardial viability
- Myocardial sarcoidosis

Assessment of patients with suspected infection
- Fever of unknown origin (FUO)
- Infectious endocarditis
- Osteomyelitis
- Implanted device infection

Assessment of patients with noninfectious inflammatory disorders
- Atherosclerosis
- Vasculitis

- Venous thromboembolism
- Sarcoidosis
- Interstitial lung disease (ILD)
- Acute lung injury (ALI)/adult respiratory distress syndrome (ARDS)
- Chronic obstructive pulmonary disease (COPD)
- Inflammatory bowel disease
- Psoriasis
- Joint disease

Assessment of alterations in tissue metabolism
- Skeletal muscle
- Brown fat

sensitivity and specificity of diagnosis. Presence of a preexisting metallic implant such as a joint prosthesis further limits the diagnostic capability of CT and MRI due to beam hardening and susceptibility artifacts, respectively. On FDG PET, increased FDG uptake in bone is suggestive of osteomyelitis, and increased FDG uptake along the prosthesis bone interface is suggestive of prosthesis infection (Figure 77-1).

4. What is the utility of FDG PET in patients with nonneoplastic vascular disease?

Heart disease (the most common cause of death in the U.S.) and cerebrovascular disease in large part are due to atherosclerosis, a chronic inflammatory disorder of the arterial tree. FDG PET is useful to detect and quantify the inflammatory component of atherosclerosis during the preclinical stage of disease for cardiovascular risk stratification, and also to monitor changes in atherosclerotic inflammation following treatment. The exact mechanism of FDG uptake in atherosclerosis is unclear, but is in part due to increased glucose metabolism of macrophages in atherosclerotic plaque. In general, FDG uptake within the aorta and large arteries increases with increasing age. On FDG PET, increased FDG uptake in arterial walls, particularly of the aorta, is suggestive of atherosclerosis (Figure 77-2).

Vasculitis is an inflammatory disorder of vessels which may be due to a variety of underlying etiologies. Although tissue sampling, CT, and MRI are often used for diagnostic evaluation, FDG PET is useful to detect and quantify sites of vascular inflammation, as well as to assess the changes in inflammatory disease activity that occur following treatment. On FDG PET, increased FDG uptake in the walls of vessels, particularly when there is associated wall thickening, is suggestive of vasculitis.

Venous thrombosis is a potentially life-threatening disorder, for which prompt diagnosis and therapy are important. CT, MRI, and ultrasonography (US) are the diagnostic tests most often used for diagnostic evaluation. However, increased FDG uptake may be observed on PET in sites of venous thrombosis, most likely due to the associated accumulation of inflammatory cells. The precise role of FDG PET in the diagnostic workup of patients with suspected venous thrombosis is not currently defined and is presently a topic of clinical research study. On FDG PET, focal, linear, or curvilinear increased FDG uptake in the lumen of a vein is suggestive of thrombosis.

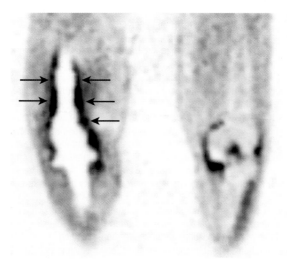

**Figure 77-1.** Knee joint prosthesis infection on FDG PET. Note asymmetrically increased FDG uptake along interfaces of right knee joint prosthesis and bone (*arrows*). Incidental FDG uptake in and around left knee joint is inflammatory in nature due to osteoarthritis and synovitis.

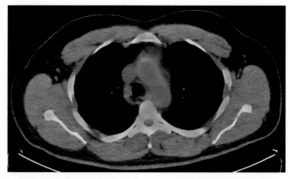

**Figure 77-2.** Atherosclerosis on FDG PET/CT. Note increased FDG uptake within walls of thoracic aorta.

5. **What is the utility of FDG PET in patients with nonneoplastic thoracic disorders?**

   FDG PET is useful to assess the spatial extent and inflammatory activity of disease, to aid in the identification of sites suitable for tissue sampling, and to monitor the effects of therapy in patients with nonneoplastic thoracic disorders such as sarcoidosis, interstitial lung disease (ILD), pneumoconiosis, acute lung injury (ALI)/adult respiratory distress syndrome (ARDS), chronic obstructive pulmonary disease (COPD), and cystic fibrosis. In addition, extrapulmonary sites of altered metabolism in the body associated with these conditions can be detected as well. For example, increased FDG uptake may be seen in involved thoracic and extrathoracic lymph nodes in patients with sarcoidosis. Increased FDG uptake is sometimes seen in the right ventricular myocardium in patients who have secondary pulmonary hypertension. Increased FDG uptake may be seen in the thoracic and abdominal muscles of patients with COPD, given the presence of expiratory pulmonary air trapping occurring from loss of pulmonary elastic recoil and increased small airways resistance.

6. **What is the utility of FDG PET in patients with inflammatory bowel disease (IBD)?**

   CT, MRI, fluoroscopy, and endoscopy are commonly used to evaluate patients with IBD. However, detection and quantification of the active inflammatory components may be challenging, even though these tasks are important for treatment planning and response assessment purposes. FDG PET provides a means for the early detection and quantification of the active inflammatory component of IBD and is therefore complementary with the other diagnostic techniques. Furthermore, other areas of inflammation outside of the bowel that are often seen in patients with IBD may also be detected on FDG PET. The precise role of FDG PET in the diagnostic workup of patients with suspected or known IBD is not currently defined and is presently a subject of clinical research study. On FDG PET, increased FDG uptake is observed in bowel loops that are affected by active IBD (Figure 77-3).

7. **What is the utility of FDG PET in patients with psoriasis?**

   FDG PET is useful to detect and quantify the spatial extent and inflammatory disease activity of psoriasis plaques in the skin (Figure 77-4), as well as to assess response to therapy. In addition, FDG PET is useful to detect and quantify unsuspected vascular and systemic sites of inflammation in patients with psoriasis. Patients with psoriasis generally have increased levels of FDG uptake in the aortic wall on PET compared to normal volunteers. Clinical research studies are currently ongoing to further elucidate the role of FDG PET in psoriasis.

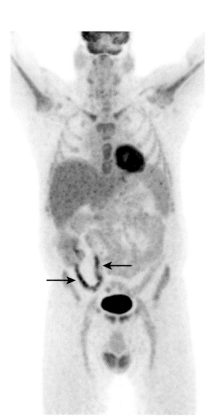

**Figure 77-3.** Active Crohn's disease on FDG PET. Note segmental increased FDG uptake within distal terminal ileum (*arrows*).

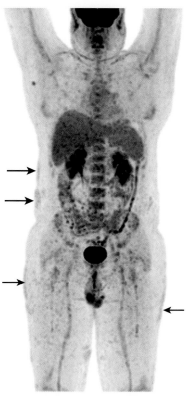

**Figure 77-4.** Psoriasis on FDG PET. Note multiple plaque-like foci of increased FDG uptake (*arrows*) within skin of abdomen, pelvis, and thighs.

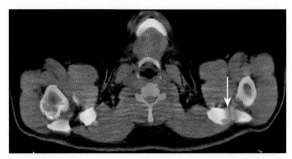

**Figure 77-5.** Osteoarthritis on FDG PET/CT. Note increased FDG uptake (*arrow*) within left acromioclavicular joint.

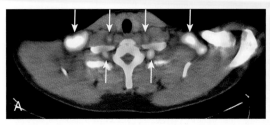 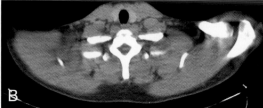

**Figure 77-6. A,** Brown fat on FDG PET/CT. Note symmetrically increased FDG uptake within supraclavicular and paravertebral regions (*arrows*). **B,** Brown fat on CT. Note fat attenuation corresponding to these sites of FDG uptake.

8. **What is the utility of FDG PET in patients with joint disease?**
   FDG PET is useful to detect and quantify the extent and degree of inflammation in patients with joint disease, including arthritis, tendinitis, and synovitis, and is complementary with other structural imaging modalities such as radiography and MRI. On FDG PET, increased FDG is observed in joints, tendons, and synovial membranes affected by arthritis, tendinitis, and synovitis, respectively (see Figure 77-1 and Figure 77-5).

9. **Is FDG PET useful to evaluate muscle metabolism?**
   Yes. FDG PET is useful to detect and quantify alterations in muscle metabolism due to a variety of disorders such as polymyositis, dermatomyositis, and COPD. In addition, FDG PET is useful to evaluate alterations in muscle metabolism that occur due to systemic therapies. At present, FDG PET for muscle assessment is mainly used in clinical research studies.

10. **Is FDG PET useful to evaluate brown fat?**
    Yes. FDG uptake in brown fat is seen in about 5% to 10% of patients and is most often seen symmetrically in the supraclavicular, mediastinal, paravertebral, posterior intercostal, and retroperitoneal paraaortic and perinephric locations (Figure 77-6). A specific diagnosis is made when corresponding CT or MR images demonstrate fat attenuation or signal intensity, respectively. Brown fat is responsible for heat production through nonshivering thermogenesis, and factors that predispose to brown fat activation include cold exposure, young age, female gender, low body mass index, a nondiabetic state, and use of sympathetic stimulants such as nicotine or ephedrine. The amount and metabolic activity of brown fat is inversely proportional to adiposity, so there is much interest in developing new ways of increasing brown fat in the body to combat obesity and metabolic syndrome.

---

**KEY POINTS**

- FDG PET is useful for the diagnostic evaluation of patients with nononcological disorders. It is most commonly used for clinical purposes to assess patients with refractory seizures, neurocognitive disorders, and myocardial disorders.
- FDG PET holds great potential for the early detection, quantification, and response assessment of a wide variety of infectious and noninfectious inflammatory disorders, although it is mostly applied in the clinical research setting at the present time.
- FDG PET is useful to quantitatively assess metabolic alterations of skeletal muscle and brown fat.

---

**BIBLIOGRAPHY**

Abdulla S, Salavati A, Saboury B, et al. Quantitative assessment of global lung inflammation following radiation therapy using FDG PET/CT: a pilot study. *Eur J Nucl Med Mol Imaging.* 2014;41(2):350-356.

Goncalves MD, Alavi A, Torigian DA. FDG PET/CT assessment of differential chemotherapy effects upon skeletal muscle metabolism in patients with melanoma. *Ann Nucl Med.* 2014;28(4):386-392.

Promteangtrong C, Salavati A, Cheng G, et al. The role of positron emission tomography-computed tomography/magnetic resonance imaging in the management of sarcoidosis patients. *Hell J Nucl Med*. 2014;17(2):123-135.

Saboury B, Salavati A, Brothers A, et al. FDG PET/CT in Crohn's disease: correlation of quantitative FDG PET/CT parameters with clinical and endoscopic surrogate markers of disease activity. *Eur J Nucl Med Mol Imaging*. 2014;41(4):605-614.

Bural GG, Torigian DA, Basu S, et al. Atherosclerotic inflammatory activity in the aorta and its correlation with aging and gender as assessed by 18F-FDG PET. *Hell J Nucl Med*. 2013;16(3):164-168.

Kwee TC, Basu S, Torigian DA, et al. FDG PET imaging for diagnosing prosthetic joint infection: discussing the facts, rectifying the unsupported claims and call for evidence-based and scientific approach. *Eur J Nucl Med Mol Imaging*. 2013;40(3):464-466.

Kwee TC, Torigian DA, Alavi A. Nononcological applications of positron emission tomography for evaluation of the thorax. *J Thorac Imaging*. 2013;28(1):25-39.

Rose S, Sheth NH, Baker JF, et al. A comparison of vascular inflammation in psoriasis, rheumatoid arthritis, and healthy subjects by FDG PET/CT: a pilot study. *Am J Cardiovasc Dis*. 2013;3(4):273-278.

Torigian DA, Dam V, Chen X, et al. In vivo quantification of pulmonary inflammation in relation to emphysema severity via partial volume corrected (18)F-FDG PET using computer-assisted analysis of diagnostic chest CT. *Hell J Nucl Med*. 2013;16(1):12-18.

Torigian DA, Zaidi H, Kwee TC, et al. PET/MR Imaging: Technical Aspects and Potential Clinical Applications. *Radiology*. 2013;267(1):26-44.

Mehta NN, Torigian DA, Gelfand JM, et al. Quantification of atherosclerotic plaque activity and vascular inflammation using [18-F] fluorodeoxyglucose positron emission tomography/computed tomography (FDG PET/CT). *J Vis Exp*. 2012;63:e3777.

Carey K, Saboury B, Basu S, et al. Evolving role of FDG PET imaging in assessing joint disorders: a systematic review. *Eur J Nucl Med Mol Imaging*. 2011;38(10):1939-1955.

Carhoete-Sanchez FM, Gandhi M, Evans TL, et al. Detection by (18)F-FDG PET/CT of upper extremity acute deep venous thrombosis. *Hell J Nucl Med*. 2011;14(1):81-82.

Donswijk ML, Broekhuizen-de Gas HS, Torigian DA, et al. PET assessment of brown fat. *PET Clin*. 2011;11(3):365-375.

Mehta NN, Yu Y, Saboury B, et al. Systemic and vascular inflammation in patients with moderate to severe psoriasis as measured by [18F]-fluorodeoxyglucose positron emission tomography-computed tomography (FDG PET/CT): a pilot study. *Arch Dermatol*. 2011;147(9):1031-1039.

Rosenbaum J, Basu S, Beckerman S, et al. Evaluation of diagnostic performance of 18F-FDG PET compared to CT in detecting potential causes of fever of unknown origin in an academic centre. *Hell J Nucl Med*. 2011;14(3):255-259.

Basu S, Chryssikos T, Moghadam-Kia S, et al. Positron emission tomography as a diagnostic tool in infection: present role and future possibilities. *Semin Nucl Med*. 2009;39(1):36-51.

Basu S, Alzeair S, Li G, et al. Etiopathologies associated with intercostal muscle hypermetabolism and prominent right ventricle visualization on 2-deoxy-2[F-18]fluoro-D-glucose-positron emission tomography: significance of an incidental finding and in the setting of a known pulmonary disease. *Mol Imaging Biol*. 2007;9(6):333-339.

Wehrli NE, Bural G, Houseni M, et al. Determination of age-related changes in structure and function of skin, adipose tissue, and skeletal muscle with computed tomography, magnetic resonance imaging, and positron emission tomography. *Semin Nucl Med*. 2007;37(3):195-205.

Bural GG, Torigian DA, Chamroonrat W, et al. Quantitative assessment of the atherosclerotic burden of the aorta by combined FDG PET and CT image analysis: a new concept. *Nucl Med Biol*. 2006;33(8):1037-1043.

# CHAPTER 78

# BONE SCINTIGRAPHY

*Andrew B. Newberg, MD*

1. **What should patients know about a bone scan?**

   A bone scan (i.e., bone scintigraphy) requires the intravenous injection of a small amount of a radioactive tracer (e.g., technetium-99m [$^{99m}$Tc] methylene diphosphonate [MDP]) that is adsorbed into the hydroxyapatite structure of bone. Areas of increased radiotracer uptake relate to bone that is actively being remodeled such as with infection or tumor. The radiotracer carries a relatively low dose of radioactivity and is extremely unlikely to result in any allergic or adverse reactions. The patient can eat and take medications regularly and is able to continue all daily activities before and after the scan. The scan itself occurs approximately 2 hours after injection of the radiotracer, and the scan time is approximately 30-45 minutes for a whole body scan. Single photon emission computed tomography (SPECT) of specific structures may also be performed to better delineate those structures, especially if the SPECT images are coregistered with computed tomography (CT) images. Three-phase bone scans require initial scanning for approximately 20 minutes at the time of the injection as well as delayed images obtained approximately 2 hours after injection.

2. **What should patients know about an $^{18}$F-sodium fluoride (NaF) positron emission tomography (PET) scan?**

   An $^{18}$F-NaF PET scan requires the intravenous injection of a small amount of a radioactive sodium fluoride, which is absorbed into bone. Areas of increased radiotracer uptake relate to bone that is actively being remodeled such as with infection or tumor. As with a conventional bone scan, the patient can eat and take medications regularly and is able to continue all daily activities before and after the scan. The scan itself occurs approximately 30-60 minutes after injection of the radiotracer, and the scan time is approximately 30 minutes for a whole body tomographic scan. The major advantage of $^{18}$F-NaF PET is improved spatial resolution and contrast compared to a conventional bone scan. Coregistered CT is also routinely obtained.

3. **What are the normal structures observed on a bone scan? Describe some typical nonmalignant findings in asymptomatic patients.**

   Normally, all of the bones should be visible on a bone scan, including individual vertebrae and ribs (Figure 78-1). The kidneys and bladder are also seen in most patients due to radiotracer excretion. Normal soft tissue uptake can occur in the breasts and sometimes in vascular structures such as the uterus. Calcified cartilage is also commonly seen in the costochondral and thyroid cartilages.

   Common nonmalignant findings in asymptomatic patients include degenerative disease of the spine or peripheral joints, dental or sinus disease, calcification associated with atherosclerotic disease, and prior fractures.

   On $^{18}$F-NaF PET imaging, a similar pattern of radiotracer uptake and excretion is observed, with uniform uptake seen throughout the skeleton. The tomographic images provided by PET provide high contrast resolution assessment of the skeletal structures.

4. **Why is a "superscan" associated with a negative prognosis in the patient with prostate cancer shown in Figure 78-2?**

   A "superscan" implies that so much of the radiotracer is taken up by the bones that there is no significant excretion in the kidneys and bladder or uptake in the soft tissues. The scan appears almost "too good" with high contrast between the bones and other tissues. The most common causes of a "superscan" are widespread metastatic disease, metabolic bone disease such as by primary or secondary hyperparathyroidism, and widespread Paget's disease. In a patient with cancer, a "superscan" implies widespread osseous metastases that cannot be individually distinguished, but rather occupy almost the entire skeleton.

5. **Is there a way to successfully treat a patient with bone pain associated with multiple osteoblastic metastases?**

   Patients with bone pain from osteoblastic metastases can be treated primarily with four modalities: cancer-specific chemotherapy, radiation therapy, narcotic pain management, or radiopharmaceutical agents that target bone. The last option is often the best when multiple sites are involved that cannot be easily targeted by radiation therapy or would result in excessive radiation to uninvolved tissues or the whole body. Radiopharmaceutical agents, such as strontium-89 ($^{89}$Sr) chloride (Metastron) or samarium-153 ($^{153}$Sm) ethylenediaminetetramethylene phosphonic acid (EDTMP) (Quadramet), which are beta-emitters, can be injected intravenously in patients with osteoblastic metastases for relief of pain. Studies suggest that 80% of patients experience some pain relief, and almost 50% have complete relief. Pain relief lasts a mean of 6-8 months, and patients can be retreated with similar pain relief. Although these treatments are not considered curative, they can substantially improve a patient's quality of life and decrease reliance on narcotic medications.

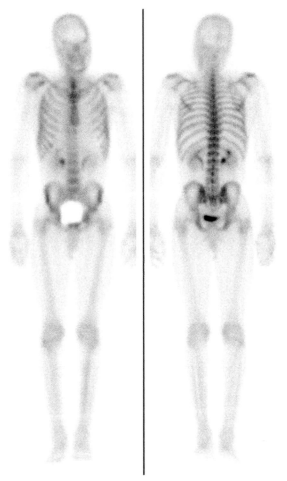

**Figure 78-1.** Normal $^{99m}$Tc-MDP distribution on whole-body bone scan in anterior (left) and posterior (right) projections. Note uniform radiotracer uptake throughout bones with some uptake in kidneys and bladder.

6. Figure 78-3 shows a bone scan of a patient complaining of swelling and pain in the distal arm after a recent traumatic event. What is the diagnosis?

Patients with such symptoms after a traumatic event typically have either osseous or soft tissue uptake characteristic of focal injury. In these patients, a three-phase bone scan helps make that determination. The first two phases—the blood flow, or vascular, phase and the blood pool, or tissue, phase—help to show whether there is soft tissue edema. If there is also focal uptake on the delayed bone scan images, an osseous injury is suspected, which may be superimposed on soft tissue injury. The scan in Figure 78-3 shows diffusely increased uptake on all three phases, however, which is suggestive of reflex sympathetic dystrophy (RSD). RSD is a response to a traumatic event and results from autonomic dysfunction in the extremity, causing altered regulation of blood flow. On a bone scan, the typical finding is increased flow and radiotracer uptake on all three phases, with a predominantly periarticular distribution seen on delayed bone scan images. Other patterns have also been described. Regardless, the findings are almost always diffuse because they affect the entire extremity, including all of the fingers and distal upper extremity.

7. What causes a bone scan that does not show the bones clearly?

Usually, a suboptimal bone scan is related to technical factors, such as not waiting at least 2 hours between radiotracer injection and scan acquisition, poor preparation of the MDP, a significantly infiltrated radiotracer dose during injection, patient motion, or the camera being set to the incorrect energy window (e.g., for $^{123}$I rather than for $^{99m}$Tc). Physiologic reasons for suboptimal scans include large patient size, resulting in significant photon attenuation, or poor circulation states, such as congestive heart failure in which the radiotracer is not adequately delivered to the bones. Finally, patients with osteoporosis simply do not have enough bone for good visualization of osseous structures, and patients with iron overload may also have inhibited uptake of the radiotracer.

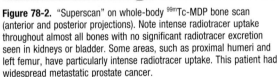

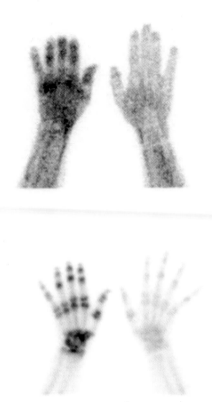

**Figure 78-3.** RSD on triple-phase $^{99m}$Tc-MDP bone scan. Note diffusely increased radiotracer uptake throughout entire right forearm and hand (*left column*) on blood pool images (*top row*) and periarticular radiotracer uptake on delayed bone scan images (*bottom row*) relative to contralateral side.

**Figure 78-2.** "Superscan" on whole-body $^{99m}$Tc-MDP bone scan (anterior and posterior projections). Note intense radiotracer uptake throughout almost all bones with no significant radiotracer excretion seen in kidneys or bladder. Some areas, such as proximal humeri and left femur, have particularly intense radiotracer uptake. This patient had widespread metastatic prostate cancer.

8. **Is a bone scan an appropriate study for a 65-year-old patient with multiple myeloma?**
   Bone scans generally are not sensitive for lytic bone lesions, and patients who show findings of multiple myeloma or other lytic osseous abnormalities on CT or radiography should not be referred for a bone scan. Instead, evaluation with either a bone survey using multiple radiographs, a magnetic resonance imaging (MRI) scan, or an $^{18}$F-fluorodeoxyglucose (FDG) PET/CT scan is performed. Patients with certain cancers that lead to mixed lytic and blastic osseous metastases may still benefit from a bone scan. Also, patients with multiple myeloma with lytic disease in weight-bearing bones that are susceptible to pathologic fracture may still benefit from a bone scan, as a fracture would show up as a focus of increased radiotracer uptake. If a nuclear medicine scan is needed to better detect or characterize the osseous lesions, FDG PET/CT is the most appropriate choice as this directly reveals sites of cancer in the bone marrow whether or not there is associated bone lysis or sclerosis rather than the indirect effects of cancer upon the surrounding bones.

9. **Does a bone scan that shows a worsened appearance after chemotherapy portend a bad prognosis?**
   A bone scan that shows apparent worsening, as characterized by increased radiotracer activity in known lesions or the observation of new lesions, can be suggestive of progression of disease. However, the apparent worsening of prior bone scan abnormalities may also be associated with the "flare" phenomenon. The flare phenomenon results from increased osteoblastic activity in lesions associated with the bone's healing response after chemotherapy. The flare response is associated with a good prognosis, suggesting effectiveness of the therapy. The flare response can occur 2-6 months after chemotherapy. A patient with a bone scan that shows apparent worsening abnormalities in this time period may receive another bone scan 4-6 months later to determine whether the lesions subsequently regress. If

there is improvement on the latter scan, the previous scan can be considered to be related to a flare response associated with effective treatment.

10.  What are the most common findings on a bone scan that suggest metastatic disease?
Bone scan findings of metastatic disease most commonly have intensely increased radiotracer activity, either as a solitary focus or as multiple foci (Figure 78-4). Widespread disease may appear as a "superscan," in which all of the bones have diffusely intense radiotracer uptake. Cold, or photopenic, defects can be observed in patients with lytic osseous metastases. Because the sensitivity of bone scintigraphy is not 100%, scans may have negative results in the face of metastatic disease. Finally, metastatic disease can be observed in the soft tissues, including organs such as the lungs or liver (Box 78-1).

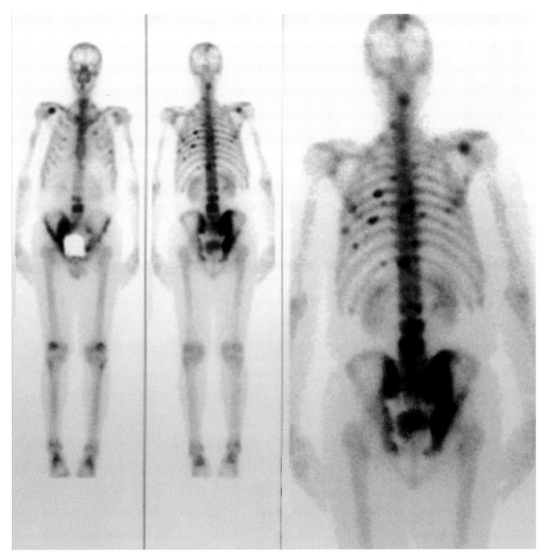

**Figure 78-4.** Osseous metastases on whole-body $^{99m}$Tc-MDP bone scan in anterior (left) and posterior (middle and right) projections. Note multiple foci of intense radiotracer uptake throughout axial skeleton including multiple ribs, spine, pelvic bones, right scapula, and skull in this patient with prostate cancer.

**Box 78-1.** Common Findings of Metastatic Disease on Bone Scintigraphy

1. Solitary focal lesion
2. Multiple focal lesions
3. "Superscan"

4. Photopenic ("cold" defect) lesions
5. Normal findings (i.e., false-negative results)
6. Soft tissue radiotracer uptake

11. What are the causes of "cold," or photopenic, defects on bone scans?

There are numerous benign and malignant causes for photopenic regions on a bone scan (Box 78-2). Bones with avascular necrosis or infarction in the early stage have photopenia. Lytic osseous tumors or metastases can be cold because there is an absence of osteoblastic activity. Any metal objects—either external, such as jewelry, or internal, such as a pacemaker or joint prosthesis—can attenuate or block emitted radiation from reaching the scan detector. Bone can also be affected by radiation therapy, in which there is an overall decrease in radiotracer uptake in a focal area. Soft tissue structures such as the breasts (or breast implants) can reduce activity observed in underlying bones such as the ribs. Finally, there have been several reports of cold defects occurring at the site of acute osteomyelitis (Figure 78-5).

12. Are three-phase bone scans alone useful for the diagnosis of osteomyelitis?

Three-phase bone scans can be positive for osteomyelitis if there is a focal area of intense radiotracer uptake. This is particularly true when a patient has a superficial area of infection, such as an ulcer or cellulitis. In such a case, the question to be answered is whether the underlying bone is affected, which can be readily detected on a three-phase bone scan. Increased uptake on all three phases of a bone scan can also occur in acute fractures, after surgical manipulation, metastatic disease, avascular necrosis, and Paget's disease. If any of these other conditions are potentially expected, a three-phase bone scan by itself is not likely to be useful because of poor specificity.

13. What other scans can be used to improve diagnostic accuracy for detecting osteomyelitis?

Nuclear medicine studies to consider in addition to a three-phase bone scan in patients with suspected osteomyelitis are an indium-111 ($^{111}$In) white blood cell (WBC) scan for the extremities; a gallium-67 ($^{67}$Ga) scan for the spine; or an FDG PET/CT scan, which can be used for any site of suspected osteomyelitis. Because these three studies evaluate infectious or inflammatory processes more directly rather than the response of the bone to the infection, they generally have a higher specificity than a bone scan.

---

**Box 78-2.** Major Causes of Cold Defects on Bone Scintigraphy

1. Attenuation artifact due to prosthesis, pacemaker, jewelry, lead shield, barium contrast, etc.
2. Malignant bone tumors
3. Metastatic disease (particularly when lytic such as from thyroid or renal cell carcinomas)
4. Avascular necrosis or bone infarction
5. Disuse atrophy
6. Unicameral bone cyst
7. External radiation therapy
8. Early osteomyelitis

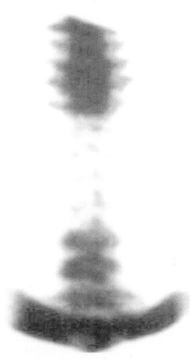

**Figure 78-5.** Cold defect on $^{99m}$Tc-MDP bone scan (spot view of thoracolumbar spine). Note markedly decreased radiotracer uptake in sharply defined region of thoracolumbar spine characteristic of prior radiation therapy. This patient is status post radiation therapy for treatment of spinal metastases from breast cancer.

14. Is radiotracer uptake in the lungs normal on a bone scan?

    Radiotracer uptake in the lung is almost never normal on a bone scan and is usually associated with malignant pleural effusions, large tumors, inflammatory processes, or metastatic disease. Metastatic osteosarcoma has particularly intense uptake when involving the lungs. Lung uptake itself is usually detected by comparing the left hemithorax and right hemithorax, and observing for increased uptake in the intercostal spaces (Figure 78-6).

15. Can Paget's disease be distinguished from cancer in the bones on nuclear medicine studies?

    Paget's disease typically is associated with focal areas of intensely increased radiotracer uptake in the flat bones or in the ends of the long bones. The uptake is usually diffuse, although there can be focal areas of increased uptake. There is no definitive way to distinguish metastatic disease or primary bone tumors from Paget's disease on the basis of radiotracer uptake in the bones alone. The pattern of Paget's disease in terms of its distribution and appearance may help in the diagnosis, however. It is less likely that an individual would have an entire hemipelvis as the only site of metastatic disease, but this can commonly be a presentation of Paget's disease (Figure 78-7).

16. What is the "Mickey Mouse" sign? What is the "Honda" sign?

    In the spine, the "Mickey Mouse" sign is seen when there is radiotracer uptake in the entire vertebral body and in the spinous process leading to an inverted triangular appearance that mimics the appearance of Mickey Mouse's head and ears and is more typically related to Paget's disease of the spine rather than metastatic disease. The "Honda" sign refers to vertically oriented increased radiotracer uptake in the bilateral sacral ala forming an "H"-shaped configuration on bone scans. This finding is highly suspicious for presence of sacral insufficiency fractures.

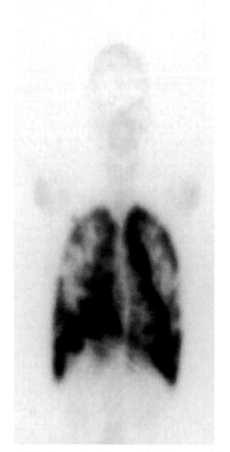

**Figure 78-6.** Abnormal radiotracer uptake in lungs on whole body $^{99m}$Tc-MDP bone scan. Note markedly increased radiotracer uptake in lungs in this patient with pulmonary metastases from osteosarcoma.

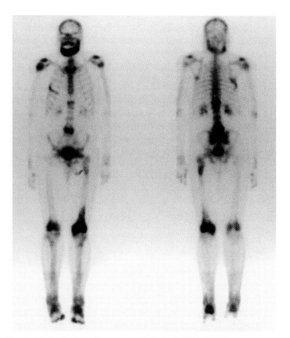

**Figure 78-7.** Paget's disease on whole-body $^{99m}$Tc-MDP bone scan (anterior and posterior projections). Note multiple areas of intense radiotracer uptake in mandible, proximal humeri, femora, right rib, and spine.

17. Intense radiotracer uptake on a bone scan in multiple joints can be the result of which disorders?

Polyarticular radiotracer uptake on a bone scan is typically associated with arthritic conditions, such as osteoarthritis, rheumatoid arthritis, psoriatic arthritis, gout, or ankylosing spondylitis. The diagnosis of these different disorders can be suggested by the pattern of specific joints involved, such as the knee joints, acromioclavicular joints, and interphalangeal joints in osteoarthritis; the metacarpophalangeal joints in rheumatoid arthritis; and involvement of the great toe in gout.

18. Can shin splints be differentiated from stress fractures on a bone scan?

Shin splints, or medial tibial stress syndrome, generally show linear increased radiotracer uptake primarily on the delayed bone scan images in the posteromedial tibial cortices. Stress fractures, however, are more focal with intense radiotracer uptake on delayed bone scan images and are often more anterior in their location. Stress fractures also commonly show increased activity on the first two phases of the bone scan, so any patient being referred for stress fractures should have a three-phase bone scan.

19. What is the significance of a single rib lesion in a patient undergoing evaluation for metastatic disease from a known primary cancer?

The traditional view is that a single rib lesion has approximately an 8% to 10% chance of being a metastasis; this can be modified by the characteristics of the finding. Typically, linear areas of increased activity that appear to extend along the rib are more suggestive of metastatic disease, whereas small macular lesions are more likely the result of trauma. In addition, the patient's history might reveal a recent fall, which would also more likely suggest that the finding is the result of trauma.

When multiple, rib fractures are often seen to involve multiple adjacent ribs, whereas rib metastases tend to be more randomly distributed in location.

20. Which benign bone tumors have increased radiotracer uptake on a bone scan?

Osteoid osteomas have increased radiotracer uptake on delayed bone scan images and may have an observable photopenic center. They commonly arise in the femur or spine. Uptake is also very intense in osteochondromas and chondroblastomas. Enchondromas do not typically have significantly increased radiotracer uptake on a bone scan.

21. Do bone scans have a role in the evaluation of child abuse?

A bone scan may be an important study in the evaluation of potential child abuse because it enables evaluation of all of the bones in one scan and can often show old or occult fractures. Even if a child does not complain of pain in a particular bone, the bone scan can reveal prior trauma. If there are multiple fracture sites that would not occur from a typical fall or disease process, child abuse might be suspected as the cause.

22. Is increased radiotracer uptake in the kidneys a clinically relevant finding on a bone scan?

If one or both kidneys have increased uptake on a bone scan, this finding can be clinically relevant because such a finding can occur in the setting of hydronephrosis and obstruction. Increased uptake on a bone scan may also be the result of the effects of chemotherapy or from involvement by tumor, nephrocalcinosis, radiation nephritis, or acute tubular necrosis. A patient with abnormally increased uptake in one or both kidneys may be followed up with additional imaging such as CT, MRI, or renal scintigraphy if clinically indicated.

23. What are the causes of liver radiotracer uptake on a bone scan?

The most problematic cause of liver uptake on a bone scan is the presence of hepatic metastases, most likely due to melanoma or cancers of the colon, breast, or lung. Sometimes, there can be apparent increased radiotracer activity in the liver that is actually associated with increased radiotracer uptake in the overlying soft tissue. Diffuse hepatic necrosis, although rare, can result in increased radiotracer uptake in the liver on a bone scan. Finally, a colloid formation of the radiotracer because of poor radiotracer preparation techniques can result in the equivalent of a sulfur colloid (liver/spleen) scan.

24. What can cause radiotracer uptake in the muscles as seen on the bone scan in Figure 78-8?

Increased radiotracer uptake in the muscles on a bone scan usually implies some type of inflammatory process, such as myositis, which was the case in this patient. Other considerations include rhabdomyolysis, hypercalcemia, hematomas, and tumors. The latter two conditions are usually more focal in extent. There are technical factors, such as poor preparation of the radiotracer or insufficient delay time between radiotracer injection and image acquisition, which can also lead to this finding.

25. How does $^{18}$F-NaF PET as shown in Figure 78-9 compare to FDG PET and conventional bone scintigraphy for the detection of osseous metastases?

Overall, it seems that $^{18}$F-NaF PET has a higher sensitivity and specificity than either FDG PET or conventional bone scintigraphy for the detection of osseous metastases from cancers that induce osteoblastic changes such as prostate, lung, and breast cancers. FDG PET, however, is able to detect tumor in the bone marrow directly rather than osteoblastic bone activity that indirectly results from involvement with tumor, allowing for improved detection of lytic osseous metastases and extraosseous sites of tumor, as well as measurement of the degree of tumor metabolic activity before and after therapeutic intervention for response assessment purposes. Thus, FDG PET and $^{18}$F-NaF PET provide complementary information in patients with metastatic disease. Furthermore, PET imaging is most commonly

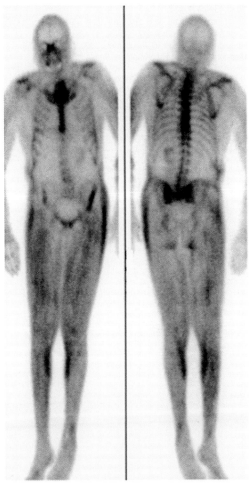

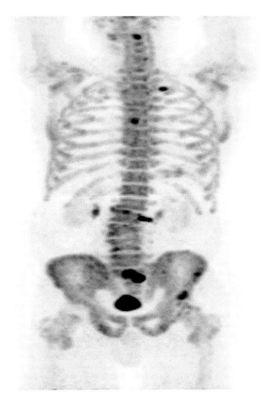

**Figure 78-9.** Osseous metastases on ¹⁸F-NaF PET scan (coronal maximum intensity projection [MIP] image). Note multiple foci of increased radiotracer uptake in sternum, ribs, spine, and pelvic bones in this patient with prostate cancer. *(This figure is courtesy of Søren Hess, Dept. of Nuclear Medicine, Odense University Hospital, Denmark.)*

**Figure 78-8.** Abnormal radiotracer uptake in muscles on whole-body ⁹⁹ᵐTc-MDP bone scan (anterior and posterior projections). Note diffuse intense radiotracer uptake throughout most of skeletal muscle groups. This finding is consistent with widespread myositis.

performed in conjunction with CT as PET/CT, or may less commonly be performed with MRI as PET/MRI, allowing for comprehensive noninvasive structural-molecular imaging assessment of the osseous structures in a single imaging session.

## KEY POINTS

- Any cause of increased bone turnover, including primary malignant bone tumors, osseous metastases, osteoid osteoma, osteomyelitis, trauma, degenerative change, metabolic bone disease, and Paget's disease, may lead to increased radiotracer uptake in bone on a bone scan or ¹⁸F-NaF PET scan.
- In a patient with osseous metastatic disease, a bone scan that shows apparent worsening of disease may either be due to true progression of metastatic disease or due to a "flare" phenomenon related to effects of the recent systemic treatment. Clinical and/or laboratory correlation as well as follow-up imaging assessment are typically performed to differentiate between these two diagnostic possibilities.
- A "superscan" occurs when there is diffusely increased radiotracer uptake in the bones, and it is most commonly seen with widespread osseous metastatic disease, metabolic bone disease, or widespread Paget's disease.

### BIBLIOGRAPHY

Kannivelu A, Loke KS, Kok TY, et al. The role of PET/CT in the evaluation of skeletal metastases. *Semin Musculoskelet Radiol.* 2014;18(2):149-165.

Damle NA, Bal C, Bandopadhyaya GP, et al. The role of 18F-fluoride PET-CT in the detection of bone metastases in patients with breast, lung and prostate carcinoma: a comparison with FDG PET/CT and 99mTc-MDP bone scan. *Jpn J Radiol.* 2013;31(4):262-269.

Fischer DR. Musculoskeletal imaging using fluoride PET. *Semin Nucl Med*. 2013;43(6):427-433.

Li Y, Schiepers C, Lake R, et al. Clinical utility of (18)F-fluoride PET/CT in benign and malignant bone diseases. *Bone*. 2012;50(1):128-139.

Love C, Din AS, Tomas MB, et al. Radionuclide bone imaging: an illustrative review. *Radiographics*. 2003;23(2):341-358.

O'Sullivan JM, Cook GJ. A review of the efficacy of bone scanning in prostate and breast cancer. *Q J Nucl Med*. 2002;46(2):152-159.

Sarikaya I, Sarikaya A, Holder LE. The role of single photon emission computed tomography in bone imaging. *Semin Nucl Med*. 2001;31(1):3-16.

Abdel-Dayem HM. The role of nuclear medicine in primary bone and soft tissue tumors. *Semin Nucl Med*. 1997;27(4):355-363.

Collier BD, Fogelman I, Rosenthal I. *Skeletal Nuclear Medicine*. 1st ed. St. Louis: Mosby; 1996.

Atkins RM, Tindale W, Bickerstaff D, et al. Quantitative bone scintigraphy in reflex sympathetic dystrophy. *Br J Rheumatol*. 1993;32(1):41-45.

# CHAPTER 79

# PULMONARY SCINTIGRAPHY

*Andrew B. Newberg, MD, and Charles Intenzo, MD*

1. **How would you describe and prepare a patient for a ventilation-perfusion (V/Q) scan?**

   A V/Q scan takes approximately 20 to 30 minutes and consists of two parts. During the ventilation part, the patient will have a face mask placed over his or her mouth and nose and will be asked to inhale oxygen and a radioactive gas that has no smell. The mask will be left on for approximately 5 to 10 minutes, and posterior projection scintigraphic images of the lungs will be obtained. Then the patient will be asked to lie supine in order to receive an intravenous injection of technetium-99m ($^{99m}$Tc) radiolabeled macroaggregated albumin (MAA) to assess the blood flow to the lungs. Scintigraphic images of the lungs are then acquired in multiple projections over a period of approximately 20 minutes. There is no specific preparation for the patient, and the patient does not need to fast in preparation for the study. Although patients can receive oxygen, patients who are dependent on significant amounts of oxygen (i.e., require $O_2$ by face mask) are unlikely to be able to successfully perform the ventilation portion of the study, although the perfusion scan would not be affected.

2. **In what order are imaging studies obtained in the workup of patients with suspected acute pulmonary embolism?**

   The first imaging study performed in a patient with suspected pulmonary embolism is typically a chest radiograph. This will often reveal as well as exclude many underlying etiologies and is also necessary for the adequate evaluation of a V/Q scan. The next imaging study performed depends on a number of variables including the current diagnostic evaluation protocols regionally determined by individual hospitals but, more important, on whether the chest radiograph is normal or abnormal. Many hospitals now utilize contrast-enhanced computed tomography (CT) tailored toward evaluation of the pulmonary arterial tree to evaluate for presence of pulmonary embolism as well as for other cardiopulmonary disease conditions. In patients with significant abnormalities seen on chest radiography, it is more likely that a V/Q scan will result in an indeterminate test result and not provide additional diagnostic information. Therefore, only patients with relatively normal chest radiographs generally proceed to V/Q scanning. If a CT and/or a V/Q scan are equivocal for detection of pulmonary embolism, then conventional pulmonary angiography may be performed. Lower extremity ultrasonography (US) may also be used to evaluate for the presence of deep venous thrombosis (DVT).

3. **How do aerosols compare to xenon-133 ($^{133}$Xe) for use in a ventilation scan?**

   $^{133}$Xe is a radioactive isotope of an inert noble gas. It can be inhaled into the lungs and will wash out quickly in a normal lung, although there will be persistent radiotracer activity (gas trapping) in parts of the lung affected by obstructive airways disease such as with asthma or chronic obstructive lung disease (COPD). These areas of gas trapping will typically correspond to matching perfusion defects on the perfusion scan, thereby increasing the specificity of the V/Q scan.

   Radioaerosols are typically made from $^{99m}$Tc radiolabeled diethylene triamine pentaacetic acid (DTPA) particles suspended in air. Following inhalation, such aerosols are deposited on the lining of the alveolar spaces and therefore do not wash out. Although the presence of gas trapping in the lungs cannot therefore be assessed, the particles remain in the lungs and allow for images to be obtained in multiple projections that can be more easily compared to the perfusion images or via single photon emission computed tomography (SPECT) imaging.

4. **What are the normal findings on a V/Q scan?**

   A normal V/Q scan (Figure 79-1) consists of uniform ventilation throughout both lung fields. On a $^{133}$Xe ventilation scan, there is usually good inflow of the gas, uniform radiotracer activity in the lungs during the equilibrium phase that lasts approximately 3 minutes as the patient breathes into the closed system of the machine, and then rapid and uniform washout from the lungs within about 1 to 2 minutes. No radiotracer activity should be observed in the brain, because this would imply the presence of a right-to-left shunt (Figure 79-2). On the $^{99m}$Tc-MAA perfusion scan obtained in the supine position, uniform radiotracer uptake is seen throughout the lungs.

5. **What findings are necessary to classify the results of the V/Q scan in Figure 79-2 as "PE present"?**

   The early data on V/Q scans came from the Prospective Investigation Of Pulmonary Embolism Diagnosis (PIOPED) study, which divided scan results into low, intermediate, and high probability for pulmonary embolism (PE); the latest trend in V/Q scan interpretation is sometimes referred to as the trinary interpretation system. In this system, V/Q scans are interpreted as "PE absent," "PE present," or "nondiagnostic." The "PE present" interpretation refers to one or

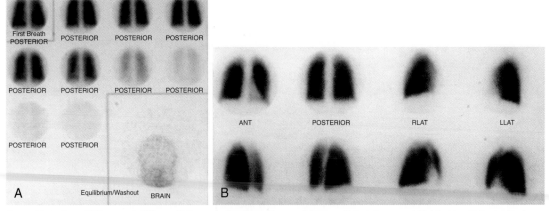

**Figure 79-1.** Normal V/Q scan. **A,** $^{133}$Xe ventilation scan showing uniform radiotracer activity in lungs on initial first breath image (*first image on upper left*), followed by equilibrium phase images, and then washout phase images (obtained every 45 seconds). **B,** $^{99m}$Tc-MAA perfusion scan images are shown in multiple projections (top row: anterior, posterior, right lateral, and left lateral projections; bottom row: left posterior oblique, right posterior oblique, right anterior oblique, and left anterior oblique projections) that also demonstrate uniform radiotracer activity throughout both lungs. A brain image (*below ventilation scan images*) is obtained to observe whether there is any right-to-left shunting of $^{99m}$Tc-MAA.

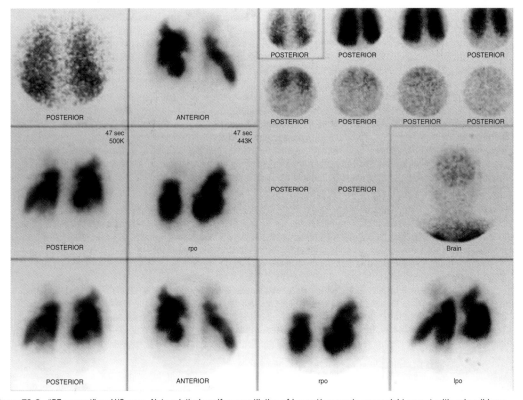

**Figure 79-2.** "PE present" on V/Q scan. Note relatively uniform ventilation of lungs (*top row in upper right corner*) with only mild gas trapping seen in upper lobes on washout phase images (*bottom row in upper right corner*). Multiple wedge-shaped perfusion defects throughout both lungs are also present that are mismatched (i.e., without corresponding ventilation defects). Also note mild $^{99m}$Tc-MAA uptake in brain consistent with presence of right-to-left shunt.

more wedge-shaped perfusion scan defects, segmental or subsegmental, unmatched to any finding on the ventilation scan or the chest radiograph. If the perfusion scan is normal, or has nonsegmental defects (whether or not they are matching), the study is interpreted as "PE absent." Any study that does not fall into either of the aforementioned categories, or cannot be interpreted due to extensive parenchymal abnormalities on the chest radiograph, is referred to as "nondiagnostic."

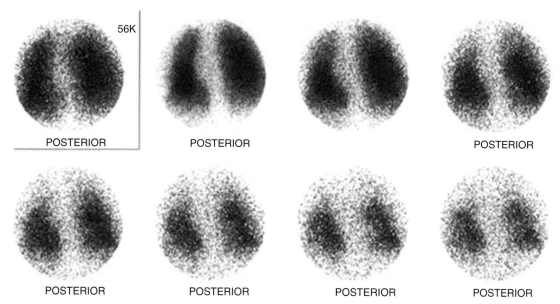

56K

POSTERIOR        POSTERIOR        POSTERIOR

POSTERIOR        POSTERIOR        POSTERIOR        POSTERIOR

**Figure 79-3.** Pulmonary gas trapping on $^{133}$Xe ventilation scan. Note persistent gas trapping in lungs throughout image acquisition consistent with marked obstructive airways disease.

**Box 79-1.** Some Causes of Gas Trapping on a V/Q Scan

- Asthma
- COPD
- Chronic bronchitis
- Mucous plug

- Cystic fibrosis
- Smoke inhalation
- Airways-obstructive tumor
- Airways-obstructive foreign body

6. What are the possible causes of gas trapping on the V/Q scan in Figure 79-3?
Gas trapping refers to radioactive gas that persists in certain areas of the lungs during the washout phase of the ventilation scan. Potential causes for gas trapping are listed in Box 79-1. The implication of gas trapping is that there is an airway process that is contributing to the patient's clinical symptoms or signs. Regardless of the underlying cause, a perfusion scan defect that matches an area of gas trapping on the ventilation scan would not be due to an embolic perfusional abnormality.

7. How does a quantitative V/Q scan assist in preparing patients for lung surgery?
Quantitative V/Q scans help in the preoperative assessment of patients by demonstrating areas of the lung that have the poorest overall function. This may help direct surgeons to preferentially resect those areas of lung that have the worst function. Perhaps more importantly, the quantitative analysis provides a percentage of function for the various lobes of the lung and for the lungs overall. When this percentage is multiplied by the forced expiratory volume in 1 second ($FEV_1$), the surgeon can predict how much overall lung function will be left if certain parts of the lung are removed. For example, if a patient requires a right upper and right middle lobectomy for lung cancer, and the remaining right lower lobe and the whole left lung account for 70% of the lung function, then the surgeon can determine whether the patient will be able to maintain adequate respiratory reserve after surgery. In general, the remaining $FEV_1$ should be at least 700 mL/min. In the example described, the patient needs to have an $FEV_1$ prior to surgery of at least 1000 mL/min so that the remaining 70% will provide the necessary function for postoperative survival.

8. What is the significance of a "triple match" on a V/Q scan and chest radiograph?
A "triple match" refers to a ventilation scan defect and a perfusion scan defect that match each other and are also matched to an area of opacification on the corresponding chest radiograph. The implication of such a finding is that it might represent a pulmonary infarct resulting from pulmonary embolism. The revised PIOPED data indicate that a triple match defect in the upper or middle lung zones is still associated with the diagnosis of "PE absence" (or of a low probability for PE in the prior system), but in the lower lung zone is associated with a nondiagnostic result.

9. What can cause radiotracer uptake in the liver on the $^{133}$Xe ventilation scan in Figure 79-4?
The primary cause of radiotracer uptake in the liver on a ventilation scan is hepatic steatosis because $^{133}$Xe is lipid soluble and a small percentage will cross the alveolar lining and enter into the bloodstream.

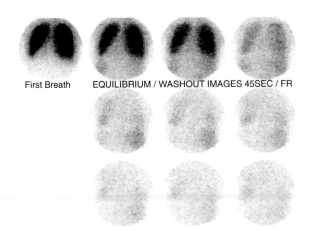

First Breath     EQUILIBRIUM / WASHOUT IMAGES 45SEC / FR

**Figure 79-4.** Hepatic steatosis on $^{133}$Xe ventilation scan. Note increased radiotracer uptake below diaphragm on right in liver.

---

**Box 79-2.** Some Causes of Mismatched Perfusion Defects on a V/Q Scan

- Acute PE
- Chronic PE
- Other types of PE (foreign bodies, gas, fat)
- Vascular-obstructive tumor
- Vascular-obstructive lymphadenopathy
- Pulmonary artery hypoplasia or atresia
- Swyer-James syndrome
- Vasculitis

---

10. **What are the causes of mismatched perfusion defects on a V/Q scan?**
   Although mismatched perfusion defects are most likely to be associated with acute PE, there are other potential etiologies that should be considered as well. Some of these causes are listed in Box 79-2.

11. **How can V/Q scans be utilized in the evaluation of chronic PE?**
   Patients who are found to have pulmonary hypertension or other clinical symptoms or signs that may be due to chronic PE as a potential etiology can undergo a V/Q scan to assess for mismatched perfusion defects. A V/Q scan cannot be easily used to determine the age of perfusion defects, and therefore there is no way to definitively state whether a perfusion defect is attributable to chronic or acute PE. However, in the setting of a chronic disease process, such a finding would be consistent with chronic PE.

12. **Why is alpha-1 antitrypsin deficiency the most likely cause of the perfusion scan findings in Figure 79-5?**
   In general, the upper lung zones tend to be more severely affected than the lower lung zones in patients with small airways disease related to COPD or asthma, although over time, most of the lung may become affected. On a V/Q scan, the associated result is generally a markedly heterogeneous lung perfusion pattern that shows the greatest decreases of perfusion in the upper lung zones. In contrast, alpha-1 antitrypsin deficiency typically affects the lower lung zones most severely. Therefore, the corresponding V/Q scan usually shows markedly decreased and heterogeneous perfusion in the lower lung zones as seen in Figure 79-5.

13. **Can idiopathic pulmonary fibrosis (IPF) be distinguished from PE on the V/Q scan shown in Figure 79-6?**
   IPF can frequently result in lung perfusion defects that are often mismatched to the ventilation pattern. IPF usually results in multiple nonsegmental defects and therefore can be distinguished from PE. However, when such defects appear in a segmental pattern, PE cannot be excluded. However, most patients with IPF will also have corresponding abnormalities on the ventilation scan and thus can be interpreted as "PE absent."

14. **Can V/Q scans be performed in pregnant women?**
   In general, V/Q scans can be performed in pregnant women, especially since most of the radioactivity is confined to the lungs rather than to the abdomen or pelvis. Furthermore, if there is no shunting of blood, no $^{99m}$Tc-MAA should reach the fetus. However, it is important to establish the need for a V/Q scan in this setting so that the patient can be informed that the risks of PE outweigh the relatively minor risks of low levels of radiation exposure to the fetus from the V/Q scan. The administered dose of $^{99m}$Tc-MAA is often decreased by half to further diminish the potential radiation exposure to the fetus.

15. **What does activity in the brain or kidneys imply on a perfusion scan?**
   Some nuclear medicine departments will image the brain or kidneys to evaluate for a mechanical right-to-left shunt. Because the $^{99m}$Tc-MAA is too large to pass through the capillary beds of the lungs, all of the injected material should

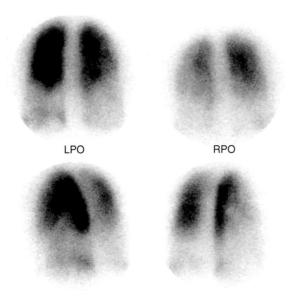

**Figure 79-5.** Alpha-1 antitrypsin deficiency on $^{99m}$Tc-MAA perfusion scan. Note abnormally decreased perfusion of lower lung zones relative to upper lung zones (clockwise from top left: posterior, anterior, right posterior oblique, and left posterior oblique projections).

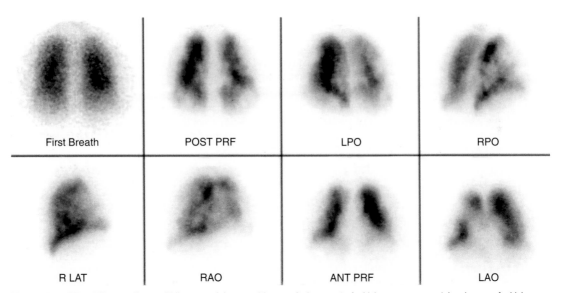

**Figure 79-6.** IPF on V/Q scan. Note multiple areas of decreased lung perfusion, most of which are nonsegmental and some of which are mismatched compared to ventilation scan (top row: first breath ventilation scan image, posterior, left posterior oblique, and right posterior oblique projections from perfusion scan; bottom row: right lateral, right anterior oblique, anterior, and left anterior oblique projections from perfusion scan).

remain in the lungs unless there is a shunt that bypasses the lungs. Such a shunt is most commonly found in the heart (e.g., an atrial septal defect) or possibly as arteriovenous malformations in the lungs. Although the shunt can be detected on a V/Q scan, it is difficult to adequately assess the location or severity of the shunt, which typically requires additional studies using other structural imaging techniques.

16. **How quickly do perfusion defects associated with pulmonary emboli resolve?**
    Studies have reported varying rates of resolution of perfusion defects associated with pulmonary emboli. Some perfusion defects can resolve within 24 hours while others can persist indefinitely. For this reason, some clinicians recommend obtaining a V/Q scan approximately 3 months after treatment of PE to determine a new "baseline" lung perfusion pattern for the patient. This scan can then be compared to future scans if a determination of new PE is needed because of the onset of acute pulmonary symptoms or signs of disease.

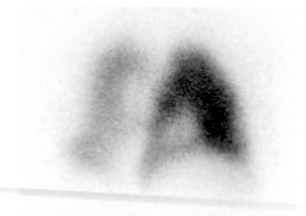

**Figure 79-7.** "Stripe" sign on $^{99m}$Tc-MAA perfusion scan (right posterior oblique projection image). Note perfusion defect in right posterior inferior lung with peripheral rim of radiotracer activity indicating "stripe" sign. This perfusional abnormality does not represent PE because that would result in perfusional defect that extends to periphery of lung.

17. How are V/Q scans utilized in patients who have had lung transplantation?

    In the immediate postoperative period, the V/Q scan can be useful to assess the transplanted lung for overall function. V/Q scans can also be useful to assess for pulmonary emboli in the transplanted lung and to assess for worsening function that may be attributable to transplant rejection or infection. Although the exact findings are nonspecific, transplant rejection can result in small perfusion defects associated with the small vessel abnormalities typically found in rejection. Worsening lung ventilation and perfusion can also be observed in transplant patients who develop bronchiolitis obliterans even though the chest radiograph may be unremarkable.

18. What is a "stripe" sign, and what does it signify on a V/Q scan?

    A "stripe" sign refers to a rim of radiotracer activity that surrounds the edge of a perfusion defect as shown in Figure 79-7. The implication of this sign is that the subjacent perfusion defect is not the result of PE. This is because perfusion defects related to PE should extend all the way to the periphery of the lung; if there is a stripe of perfused tissue distal to the perfusion defect, then it is most likely not due to PE.

19. What are the causes of matched ventilation and perfusion defects on a V/Q scan?

    Most conditions associated with matched ventilation and perfusion defects arise from diseases affecting the airways with subsequent physiologic shunting of blood away from the underventilated regions. The most common causes of matched defects include COPD, bronchiectasis, and asthma. Other causes include pleural effusions, mucous plugging, tumors, and pneumonia.

20. What are possible causes of unilateral decreases in lung perfusion with relatively preserved lung ventilation on a V/Q scan?

    The most common cause of unilaterally decreased lung perfusion (Figure 79-8) is a central mass lesion such as lung cancer, which has a predilection for affecting lung perfusion given the more readily compressible pulmonary vasculature compared to the more rigid bronchi. Patients with fibrosing mediastinitis, congenital disease such as pulmonary artery atresia or congenital corrected heart disease, or uncommonly massive unilateral PE can also have a similar pattern on a V/Q scan. This can also be observed in patients who are status post unilateral lung transplantation. Interestingly, in patients with COPD, the perfusion pressure in the pulmonary arteries may be relatively normal, and therefore perfusion in the transplanted lung in the immediate postoperative period may be at only 50% to 60% but will increase with time. On the other hand, in patients with pulmonary hypertension, the lung transplant may receive up to 90% of the perfusion in the early postoperative period.

---

**KEY POINTS**

- A normal V/Q scan essentially excludes the presence of clinically significant PE.
- Visualization of one or more wedge-shaped perfusion scan defects, segmental or subsegmental in distribution, unmatched to any finding on a ventilation scan or chest radiograph is suspicious for PE.
- Visualization of radiotracer uptake in the brain or kidneys on a perfusion scan implies presence of a mechanical right-to-left shunt.

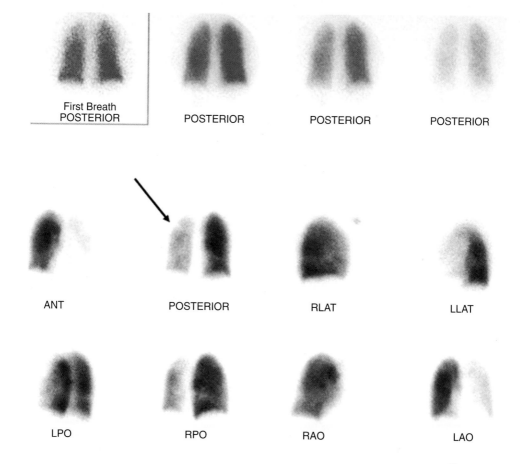

**Figure 79-8.** Unilateral decreased lung perfusion on V/Q scan. Note relatively uniform ventilation of lungs (*upper row*) with mild decrease in left lung relative to right lung. On perfusion images (lower two rows with upper row: anterior, posterior, right lateral, and left lateral projections; lower row: left posterior oblique, right posterior oblique, right anterior oblique, and left anterior oblique projections), there is markedly reduced perfusion in entire left lung that is much worse than corresponding ventilation abnormality.

## BIBLIOGRAPHY

Skarlovnik A, Hrastnik D, Fettich J, et al. Lung scintigraphy in the diagnosis of pulmonary embolism: current methods and interpretation criteria in clinical practice. *Radiol Oncol.* 2014;48(2):113-119.

Onyedika C, Glaser JE, Freeman LM. Pulmonary embolism: role of ventilation-perfusion scintigraphy. *Semin Nucl Med.* 2013;43(2):82-87.

Glaser JE, Chamarthy M, Haramati LB, et al. Successful and safe implementation of a trinary interpretation and reporting strategy for V/Q lung scintigraphy. *J Nucl Med.* 2011;52(10):1508-1512.

Bajc M, Neilly JB, Miniati M, et al. EANM guidelines for ventilation/perfusion scintigraphy: part 1. Pulmonary imaging with ventilation/perfusion single photon emission tomography. *Eur J Nucl Med Mol Imaging.* 2009;36(8):1356-1370.

Sostman HD, Miniati M, Gottschalk A, et al. Sensitivity and specificity of perfusion scintigraphy combined with chest radiography for acute pulmonary embolism in PIOPED II. *J Nucl Med.* 2008;49(11):1741-1748.

# CHAPTER 80

# THYROID, PARATHYROID, AND SALIVARY GLAND SCINTIGRAPHY

*Andrew B. Newberg, MD*

1. **What patient preparation is required before thyroid scintigraphy?**
   Patients should fast after midnight or, at a minimum, for 4 hours before receiving the radioactive iodine-123 ($^{123}$I) pill to maximize absorption through the gut. Patients should also avoid ingesting foods containing high amounts of iodine because they would saturate the iodine stores in the body and thyroid gland and diminish the uptake of the radioactive iodine. Foods such as shellfish and seaweed and supplements containing large amounts of iodine should be avoided. Patients should also discontinue taking any medication that would affect thyroid function, particularly thyroid replacement medication (for at least 2 weeks); thyroid blocking medication (propylthiouracil or methimazole for at least 5 days); and other medications, such as amiodarone, that contain substantial amounts of iodine. Finally, patients should not undergo scanning if they have received iodinated contrast agents as recently as 1 month before the scan (although sometimes the effects of such contrast agents on the thyroid can be seen up to 3 months later).

2. **Which radioisotopes can be used for nuclear medicine imaging of the thyroid gland, and how do they compare physiologically?**
   The most common radiotracers used in thyroid scintigraphy are the various isotopes of iodine. $^{123}$I is the most commonly used isotope because of its excellent image quality and relatively low radiation exposure. Isotopes $^{125}$I and $^{127}$I are not typically used because of their high radiation exposure and worse image quality. $^{131}$I is still used for thyroid imaging in some patients with thyroid cancer. Its higher photon energy theoretically makes it easier to detect cancer foci in the deep soft tissues in the body. However, $^{131}$I is associated with a higher radiation exposure to patients, and the image quality is not typically as good as with $^{123}$I. $^{124}$I is a positron-producing isotope that can be imaged by positron emission tomography (PET) and has been shown to be valuable in the detection of residual thyroid tissue in patients with thyroid cancer. All of the iodine radiotracers are trapped by the thyroid gland and undergo organification into the thyroid hormones. The other primary radiotracer utilized for thyroid scintigraphy is technetium-99m ($^{99m}$Tc) pertechnetate. This radiotracer is trapped (not organified) by the thyroid gland and can provide high-quality images. The amount of uptake of this radiotracer cannot be used to plan $^{131}$I therapy, in contradistinction to that with the iodine radiotracers.

3. **What are normal thyroid scan and iodine uptake results?**
   Thyroid images are obtained 24 hours after the administration of $^{123}$I or approximately 30 minutes after $^{99m}$Tc pertechnetate. The gland should appear uniform throughout with smooth contours (Figure 80-1). The isthmus and pyramidal lobes can be observed, although they are more commonly seen in patients with Graves' disease. Iodine uptake values are usually obtained at 2 and 24 hours after administration of the $^{123}$I pill. The 2-hour uptake typically should be 2% to 10%, and the 24-hour uptake is usually 10% to 30%. These values may differ slightly, depending on the radiotracer that is used, so it is always important to know what a particular institution considers as the normal range of uptake.

4. **Can a patient with normal thyroid gland $^{123}$I uptake still have Graves' disease?**
   The iodine uptake refers to the activity of the gland and not to whether the patient is hyperthyroid. Although a patient may have normal scan results and uptake values, if the thyroid function tests indicate that the patient is hyperthyroid, then a normal iodine uptake is still too high. A hyperthyroid patient should have a gland that is almost completely shut down. An uptake of 20% to 30% is too high if a patient is hyperthyroid with an undetectable thyroid-stimulating hormone (TSH) level. In such a setting, a patient with normal scan results can still have Graves' disease.

5. **What are possible outcomes after $^{131}$I therapy for Graves' disease?**
   There are three possible outcomes:
   1. A patient may be hypothyroid if the dose is sufficient to destroy most of the thyroid tissue and function.
   2. A patient may be euthyroid if the dose diminishes the function of the thyroid gland, but there is sufficient activity to maintain normal circulating levels of thyroid hormone.
   3. A patient may be remain hyperthyroid if undertreated, with the thyroid gland continuing to produce high levels of thyroid hormone.

   In the hypothyroid case, patients typically begin undergoing thyroid replacement therapy. In the hyperthyroid case, patients usually require retreatment with a higher dose of $^{131}$I. The likelihood of each outcome depends on the range of doses given. Lower doses result in fewer hypothyroid patients, with more patients requiring retreatment for persistent hyperthyroidism. Higher doses result in more patients being hypothyroid and fewer needing to be retreated.

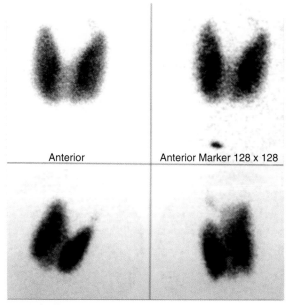

**Figure 80-1.** Normal $^{123}$I thyroid scan (clockwise from top left: anterior projection, anterior projection with marker in sternal notch, right anterior oblique projection, and left anterior oblique projection).

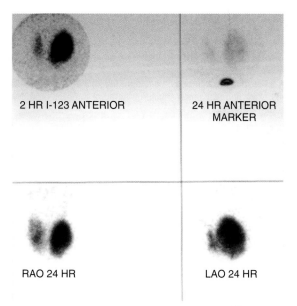

**Figure 80-2.** Large hot nodule in left thyroid lobe with suppression of right thyroid lobe on $^{123}$I thyroid scan (clockwise from top left: anterior projection, anterior projection with marker in sternal notch, right anterior oblique projection, and left anterior oblique projection).

6. How is a patient with a hot nodule on thyroid scintigraphy as seen in Figure 80-2 treated for hyperthyroidism?

   Hot nodules (i.e., thyroid nodules with avid radiotracer uptake) are typically due to autonomously functioning thyroid adenomas. Hot nodules are typically treated with $^{131}$I therapy but are often more resistant. It is usually recommended that the dose be higher than that used for treating a patient with Graves' disease. The overall approach to therapy is similar, however, including the patient preparation and radiation precautions that are followed after the dose is given.

7. Why is a patient with a hot nodule in the thyroid gland more likely to end up euthyroid?

   Patients with hot nodules have a higher likelihood of ending up euthyroid because the hot nodule typically causes suppression of the remainder of the thyroid gland. This suppression protects the gland from $^{131}$I therapy. When the nodule is eliminated by $^{131}$I, the patient's thyroid function decreases, and eventually the TSH level begins to increase.

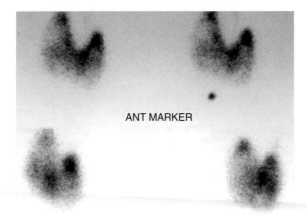

ANT MARKER

**Figure 80-3.** Multinodular goiter on $^{123}$I thyroid scan (clockwise from top left: anterior projection, anterior projection with marker in sternal notch, right anterior oblique projection, and left anterior oblique projection). Note numerous hot and cold regions of radiotracer uptake in thyroid gland.

This increased TSH stimulates the remaining thyroid tissue to begin producing thyroid hormone again. Because most of the suppressed tissue was protected, the patient may be able to make normal amounts of thyroid hormone.

8. What are the typical radiation safety precautions that patients must follow after $^{131}$I therapy?
For approximately 5 days (each institution may have its own specific timeframe), patients treated with $^{131}$I must do the following: sleep alone, if possible; avoid kissing and sexual intercourse; minimize time with pregnant women and young children; minimize close contact with others; use good hygiene habits; wash hands thoroughly after each toilet use; use a separate bathroom, if possible; flush the toilet two times after each use; drink plenty of liquids; use disposable eating utensils; use separate bath linens; launder linens and underclothing separately initially; maintain a toothbrush in a separate holder; if possible, not prepare food for others; not apply cosmetics or lip balm; and wipe the telephone mouthpiece with a tissue after each use. In addition, nursing women should completely discontinue breastfeeding until their next child, and all women should not attempt to become pregnant for at least 90 days.

9. Should the patient with the thyroid scan in Figure 80-3 be treated with $^{131}$I?
This scan reveals a multinodular goiter with areas of relatively increased and decreased radiotracer activity. Typical indications for treatment include symptomatic hyperthyroidism or symptomatic mass effect from the enlarged thyroid gland. Hyperthyroid patients can usually be treated with $^{131}$I, although usually with 2 to 3 times the dose as that for a patient with Graves' disease because the multinodular thyroid gland can be more refractory to the effects of $^{131}$I. Patients with compression of the airway or other vital structures in the neck or chest from an enlarged thyroid gland can be treated either surgically or with $^{131}$I. $^{131}$I therapy is much less invasive and usually results in substantial shrinkage of the gland, which may obviate the need for surgery. Some clinicians are concerned, however, that a potential inflammatory response from high levels of $^{131}$I may result in clinical worsening.

10. What factors affect the likelihood that the thyroid nodule in Figure 80-4 represents thyroid cancer?
Several factors relating to patient demographics, patient history, and features of the nodule affect the probability that a cold nodule in the thyroid gland may harbor cancer. Causes of a cold nodule in the thyroid gland include nonfunctioning thyroid adenomas, thyroid cancers, cysts, abscesses, and nonthyroid tumors (i.e., parathyroid adenomas, lymphoma, etc.). Younger male patients with cold nodules are more likely to have cancer than older female patients with similar findings. Prior exposure to radiation in the neck is an important risk factor for cancer. Cold nodules in the setting of a multinodular goiter are substantially less likely to be due to cancer than other cold nodules. Finally, findings of mixed cystic and solid components within a cold nodule on ultrasonography (US) are also more suggestive of thyroid cancer.

11. Why can $^{131}$I be used to treat thyroid cancer if it appears as a cold nodule on thyroid scintigraphy?
Although a cold nodule on thyroid scintigraphy does not appear to take up any of the radioactive iodine, its inactive appearance is in comparison to the background activity of the normal gland. Thyroid cancer cells generally take up the iodine but not as well as normal tissues. For this reason, thyroid cancer appears cold on the scan but can still take up enough iodine for therapy to be effective. To enhance the therapeutic effects of $^{131}$I therapy, the normal thyroid is surgically removed. By eliminating much of the normal thyroid tissue, there is a better chance for any remaining thyroid cancer cells to take up $^{131}$I. The hope is that by removing the thyroid gland and keeping the patient off of thyroid replacement hormones, the TSH level will be greater than 30 IU/L, which should maximally stimulate any

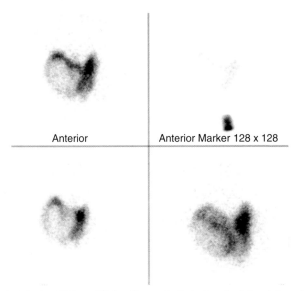

Anterior

Anterior Marker 128 x 128

**Figure 80-4.** Large cold nodule in right thyroid lobe on $^{123}$I thyroid scan (clockwise from top left: anterior projection, anterior projection with marker in sternal notch, right anterior oblique projection, and left anterior oblique projection).

thyroid cancer cells left over in the body to take up $^{131}$I. Patients are also usually prescribed a low-iodine diet to "starve" any thyroid cells, further maximizing uptake of $^{131}$I .

12. **What foods should be avoided as part of a low-iodine diet?**
A low-iodine diet is highly restrictive because many foods contain iodine. Foods to be avoided include most dairy products (milk, yogurt, ice cream, cheese), luncheon meats, bacon, hot dogs, fish, shellfish, noodles, pasta, cereals, pastry, breads, packaged rice, canned juices, canned fruits, canned or frozen vegetables, cocoa mixes, diet bars, jams/jellies, nuts, mustard, olives, candy, pretzels, and any snack foods. Patients can eat small portions of fresh chicken, fresh potatoes, fresh fruit, all fresh vegetables except spinach, sweet butter, vegetable oils, onion or garlic powder, fresh herbs, and popcorn with no salt.

13. **What is the general management plan for patients diagnosed with thyroid cancer?**
Usually, patients who are diagnosed with thyroid cancer initially undergo surgery to remove the thyroid gland. Occasionally, one lobe is removed first, and then, if cancer is detected, the other lobe is removed. Most of the time, when cancer has already been definitively diagnosed in advance with biopsy, as much of the thyroid gland is removed as possible. The patient then goes to the nuclear medicine department for a scan and therapy. The pretherapy scan usually shows some uptake in the thyroid bed because it is difficult to remove all of the gland surgically, especially when it is adjacent to critical structures in the neck. Therapy is subsequently performed using $^{131}$I after the patient has undergone thyroid hormone withdrawal or after receiving Thyrogen stimulation. The purpose of this therapeutic dose is to ablate any remaining normal thyroid tissue (some of which is usually left by the surgeon because of its proximity to critical structures in the neck) and to eliminate any remaining thyroid cancer cells. Patients are followed up at regular intervals with neck and whole body iodine scans as well as with serum measures of thyroglobulin. Patients can be retreated with $^{131}$I if there is residual or recurrent tumor (Figure 80-5).

14. **What does "stunning" mean with regard to $^{131}$I scintigraphy?**
Several studies have suggested that a typical $^{131}$I dose of 4 mCi for thyroid scintigraphy actually has a small therapeutic effect on the thyroid gland that "stuns" the thyroid cells, making them slightly resistant to the larger therapeutic dose. For this reason, some clinicians have recommended using $^{123}$I for whole body imaging before $^{131}$I therapy to avoid this effect.

15. **What range of doses of $^{131}$I is typically recommended for treatment of thyroid cancer in patients with the whole body scans seen in Figures 80-6 and 80-7?**
The range of doses given to patients undergoing treatment for thyroid cancer depends on the extent of the cancer and the institution where treatment is performed. There is usually a graded scale of doses that increases for worsening extent of disease. For distant metastatic disease, some patients are treated with the highest dose possible while ensuring that the estimated radiation dose to the bone marrow is less than 2 Sv (200 rem).
   Typical dose ranges of $^{131}$I for treatment of thyroid cancer are as follows:
- 30-100 mCi for low-risk disease.
- 125-175 mCi for metastatic lymph node disease.
- 175-225 mCi for distant metastatic disease.

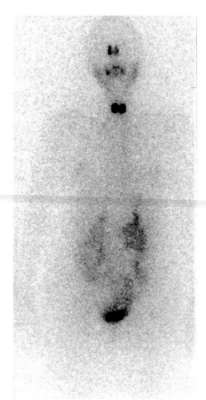

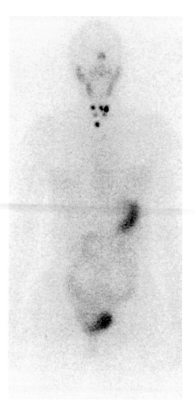

**Figure 80-5.** Locally residual thyroid cancer on $^{123}$I whole body scan (anterior projection). Note two foci of radiotracer in neck of residual thyroid tissue following surgical resection of thyroid cancer in patient now presenting for $^{131}$I therapy. Radiotracer activity seen in nasopharyngeal area, gut, and bladder represents areas of normal excretion of $^{123}$I.

**Figure 80-6.** Metastatic residual thyroid cancer on $^{123}$I whole body scan (anterior projection). Note multiple foci of radiotracer uptake in neck consistent with metastatic lymph nodes. These findings are after surgical resection of thyroid cancer in patient now presenting for $^{131}$I therapy.

16. How do a recombinant human thyrotropin (Thyrogen) scan and treatment work?

A Thyrogen scan is performed by subcutaneously administering a synthetic version of TSH on two consecutive days and then performing the radioiodine scan to detect thyroid tissue. Usually, patients stop taking thyroid medications to ensure that the TSH is maximally stimulating any residual thyroid tissue so that it can be detected on the scan. By giving the patient TSH, a similar physiologic state is obtained. The scans have similar quality to those obtained when a person is put into a more natural low thyroid hormone state by withdrawing the hormone. Similarly, $^{131}$I treatment can be performed after two days of thyrogen injections. Studies have shown that $^{131}$I therapy is similar in those patients receiving Thyrogen and in those who undergo thyroid hormone withdrawal.

17. What are some possible causes of a thyroid scan in which there is no uptake or minimal uptake of radiotracer by the thyroid gland?

When there is no thyroid radiotracer uptake observed on a thyroid scan, there are several potential causes. Patients may have thyroiditis, in which the inflammatory process has destroyed most or all functioning thyroid tissue. Such patients can be hyperthyroid or hypothyroid depending on the time course of the disease. Other causes of minimal radiotracer uptake in the thyroid gland include exogenous sources of thyroid hormone (some patients take thyroid hormone as a form of diet pill) or iodine (e.g., recent iodinated contrast agent administration, ingestion of drugs containing iodine such as amiodarone, consumption of high-salt or seafood diets, and ingestion of alternative medicine supplements). Exogenous sources of thyroid tissue, such as struma ovarii (thyroid tissue in a monodermal ovarian teratoma), should also be considered in such patients.

18. Is $^{18}$F-fluorodeoxyglucose (FDG) positron emission tomography (PET) useful in the management of patients with thyroid cancer?

In general, FDG PET has no application in the initial diagnosis of thyroid cancer because there is overlap of FDG uptake between benign and malignant thyroid tumors. FDG PET can be very useful, however, in patients previously treated for thyroid cancer who now have increasing tumor markers and an $^{131}$I scan with negative results. FDG PET can be a useful adjunct imaging modality to help detect sites of tumor recurrence (Figure 80-8). The sensitivity for detection of tumor recurrence with FDG PET is improved with hormonal withdrawal or administration of recombinant TSH. FDG PET

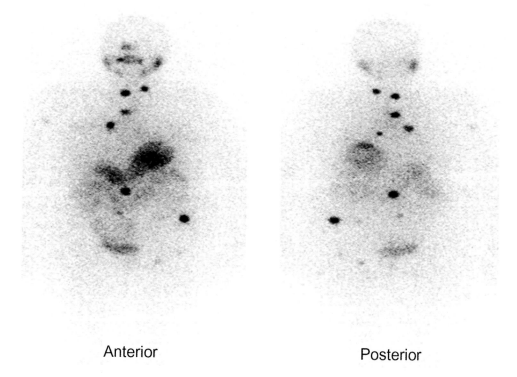

Anterior                                    Posterior

**Figure 80-7.** Metastatic residual thyroid cancer on [123]I whole body scan (anterior and posterior projections). Note multiple foci of intense radiotracer uptake in neck, mediastinum, thorax, abdomen, and right humerus, in keeping with widespread metastatic disease with bone marrow involvement. These findings are after surgical resection of thyroid cancer in patient now presenting for [131]I therapy.

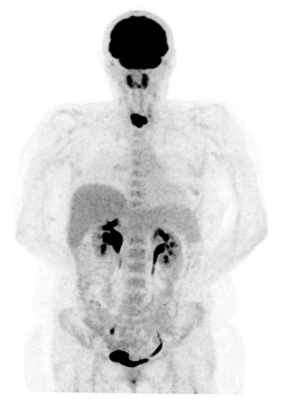

**Figure 80-8.** Locally residual thyroid cancer on FDG PET whole body scan (coronal maximum intensity projection (MIP) image). Note large area of intense radiotracer uptake in thyroid bed consistent with thyroid cancer. Other areas of FDG uptake in head, neck, and abdomen are physiologic. *(This figure is courtesy of Søren Hess, Dept. of Nuclear Medicine, Odense University Hospital, Denmark.)*

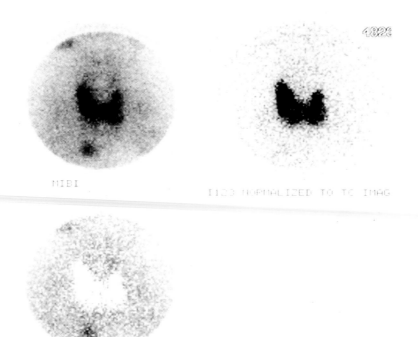

**Figure 80-9.** Parathyroid adenoma on $^{99m}$Tc sestamibi parathyroid scan with juxtaposed $^{123}$I thyroid scan (clockwise from top left: anterior projection of combined thyroid and parathyroid scans, anterior projection of thyroid scan, and anterior projection of parathyroid scan with thyroid scan subtracted). Note focus of residual $^{99m}$Tc sestamibi uptake on subtraction image inferior to right thyroid lobe.

also has a role in the management of patients with anaplastic, Hürthle cell, or medullary thyroid cancers because these tumors are not iodine avid.

19. What is parathyroid gland scintigraphy used for, and how is it performed?

Parathyroid gland scintigraphy is primarily used in patients with primary hyperparathyroidism to evaluate for a parathyroid adenoma or parathyroid hyperplasia. The scan is performed with the intravenous injection of 5 to 10 mCi of $^{99m}$Tc sestamibi. Scintigraphy may be performed immediately and again at 2 hours. Single photon emission computed tomography (SPECT), especially with concomitant computed tomography (CT), can be valuable to improve the sensitivity and specificity of the findings. If a patient has a parathyroid adenoma, it is revealed as a focus of increased activity either just superior or just inferior to the thyroid gland (some protocols include separate scintigraphic imaging of the thyroid tissue to differentiate the parathyroid glands more effectively). Parathyroid glands and adenomas may be ectopic as well, and for this reason imaging of the upper thorax is recommended. Parathyroid adenomas are usually solitary (Figure 80-9) but may be multiple. If no adenoma is observed on the scan and the patient continues to demonstrate symptoms and signs of primary hyperparathyroidism, then parathyroid hyperplasia is the most likely diagnosis.

20. What is salivary gland scintigraphy used for, and how is it performed?

A salivary gland study is used to evaluate patients with suspected abnormalities in salivary gland function (e.g., with Sjögren's disease) or with salivary gland tumors. The scan does not require a specific patient preparation. Typically, 5 to 10 mCi of $^{99m}$Tc pertechnetate is injected intravenously while obtaining scans for approximately 25 to 30 minutes (usually in 5-minute increments). This allows for maximum radiotracer uptake by the salivary glands. There is often some spontaneous salivary discharge, but the second part of the study (the washout phase) usually involves giving the patient a lemon drop to induce salivary flow while images continue to be obtained for another 15 to 20 minutes. Lateral projections of the salivary glands are also obtained immediately prior to the washout phase. This methodology allows for an evaluation of overall radiotracer uptake (i.e., normal or reduced), presence of any focal defects (e.g., due to a tumor), and of radiotracer washout (i.e., normal versus obstructed) (Figures 80-10 and 80-11). Box 80-1 lists some causes of bilaterally decreased salivary gland radiotracer uptake.

21. What is the primary finding in the salivary gland study shown in Figure 80-12?

This salivary gland study reveals focally decreased radiotracer uptake in the posterior aspects of both parotid glands. Possible causes of focally decreased radiotracer uptake in the salivary glands include abscesses, cysts, or tumors. Tumors may be due to metastatic disease, lymphoma, or primary tumors such as Warthin's tumor, oxyphilic adenoma (oncocytoma), or mixed cell type tumors. Sometimes, tumors may demonstrate increased radiotracer uptake (particularly with Warthin's tumors) or decreased radiotracer uptake if they contain cystic or nonfunctional components.

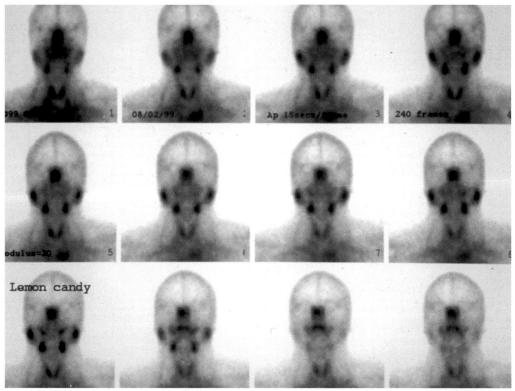

**Figure 80-10.** Normal $^{99m}$Tc pertechnetate salivary gland scan (anterior projection). Note symmetric, intense radiotracer uptake in both parotid and submandibular glands to greater degree than in thyroid gland. There is subsequent rapid and symmetric washout of radiotracer from all four salivary glands after patient receives lemon drop.

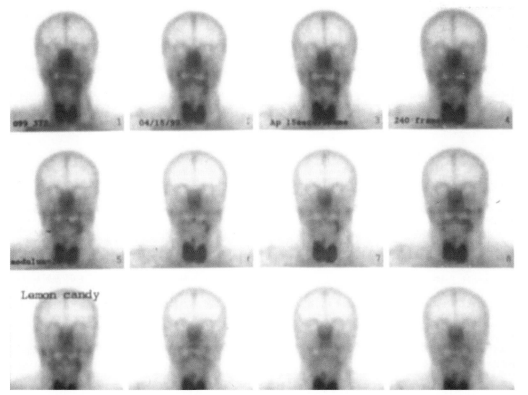

**Figure 80-11.** Sjögren's disease on $^{99m}$Tc pertechnetate salivary gland scan (anterior projection). Note bilateral, markedly decreased radiotracer uptake in parotid and submandibular glands. Washout cannot be adequately assessed following lemon drop given low level of baseline radiotracer uptake.

**Box 80-1.** Some Causes of Bilaterally Decreased Radiotracer Uptake on Salivary Gland Scintigraphy

- Sjögren's syndrome
- Sialoadenitis following radiation therapy
- Acute suppurative parotitis

- Obstructive sialolithiasis
- Sialoadenitis

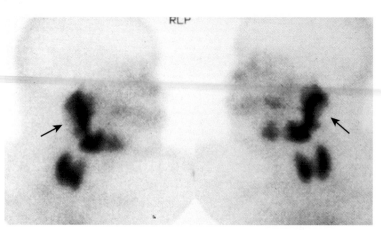

**Figure 80-12.** Focally decreased radiotracer uptake on $^{99m}$Tc pertechnetate salivary gland scan (right and left lateral projections). Note focally decreased radiotracer uptake in posterior parotid glands (*arrows*). The findings are nonspecific but may indicate presence of parotid gland cysts, abscesses, or tumors.

## KEY POINTS

- Thyroid scintigraphy is useful to differentiate between the various causes of thyroid hyperfunction and to assess for thyroid nodule function.
- Hot nodules on radioiodine thyroid scintigraphy are most often benign, whereas cold nodules may be due to thyroid cancer.
- FDG PET is useful to assess for suspected residual or recurrent thyroid cancer in patients with negative radioiodine scan results or with noniodine avid tumor types including anaplastic, Hürthle cell, and medullary thyroid cancers.
- Parathyroid scintigraphy is primarily used in patients with primary hyperparathyroidism to evaluate for a parathyroid adenoma (whether orthotopic or ectopic) or parathyroid hyperplasia.
- Salivary gland scintigraphy is mainly used to evaluate patients with suspected abnormalities in salivary gland function (e.g., with Sjögren's disease) or with salivary gland tumors.

## BIBLIOGRAPHY

Dasgupta DJ, Navalkissoor S, Ganatra R, et al. The role of single-photon emission computed tomography/computed tomography in localizing parathyroid adenoma. *Nucl Med Commun.* 2013;34(7):621-626.

Moralidis E. Radionuclide parathyroid imaging: a concise, updated review. *Hell J Nucl Med.* 2013;16(2):125-133.

Silberstein EB, Alavi A, Balon HR, et al. The SNMMI practice guideline for therapy of thyroid disease with $^{131}$I 3.0. *J Nucl Med.* 2012;53(10):1633-1651.

Ma C, Xie J, Liu W, et al. Recombinant human thyrotropin (rhTSH) aided radioiodine treatment for residual or metastatic differentiated thyroid cancer. *Cochrane Database Syst Rev.* 2010;(11):CD008302.

Vinagre F, Santos MJ, Prata A, et al. Assessment of salivary gland function in Sjogren's syndrome: the role of salivary gland scintigraphy. *Autoimmun Rev.* 2009;8(8):672-676.

Phan HT, Jager PL, Paans AM, et al. The diagnostic value of 124I-PET in patients with differentiated thyroid cancer. *Eur J Nucl Med Mol Imaging.* 2008;35(5):958-965.

Shankar LK, Yamamoto AJ, Alavi A, et al. Comparison of $^{123}$I scintigraphy at 5 and 24 hours in patients with differentiated thyroid cancer. *J Nucl Med.* 2002;43(1):72-76.

Alnafisi NS, Driedger AA, Coates G, et al. FDG PET of recurrent or metastatic $^{131}$I-negative papillary thyroid carcinoma. *J Nucl Med.* 2000;41(6):1010-1015.

Leslie WD, Peterdy AE, Dupont JO. Radioiodine treatment outcomes in thyroid glands previously irradiated for Graves' hyperthyroidism. *J Nucl Med.* 1998;39(4):712-716.

# GASTROINTESTINAL AND GENITOURINARY SCINTIGRAPHY

*Andrew B. Newberg, MD*

# CHAPTER 81

1. **What should patients know about renal scintigraphy, and what preparation should they be given?**
   In general, there is little in the way of patient preparation for a renal scan, although patients should be well hydrated. Patients should refrain from taking furosemide, which is sometimes given during the scan to help evaluate for obstruction. Angiotensin converting enzyme (ACE) inhibitors should also be avoided because they can alter the kidney's ability to regulate perfusion. However, captopril, an ACE inhibitor, may be given during the study to help assess for renovascular disease. The scan itself usually takes approximately 30 minutes and begins with the intravenous injection of a radiotracer followed by imaging in the posterior projection for native kidneys and the anterior projection for renal transplants.

2. **What are the normal findings in renal scintigraphy?**
   Renal scans are usually performed with one of two technetium-99m ($^{99m}$Tc) compounds: diethylenetriamine pentaacetic acid (DTPA) or mercaptoacetyltriglycine (MAG3). The perfusion component of the study, measured during the first minute after injection of the radiotracer, should reveal renal perfusion within several seconds of aortic activity. Renal blood flow should be symmetric and greater than that in the spleen and liver (each kidney receives approximately 10% of cardiac output compared with <5% for the liver and spleen). Cortical images are then obtained usually every minute for approximately 25 minutes. Cortical uptake should be symmetric with no focal defects. Radiotracer activity should be observed entering the collecting system by 5 minutes (the cortical transit time, i.e., how long it takes for urine to appear in the collecting system). Urine should flow freely into the bladder without retention or obstruction (Figure 81-1).

3. **What are causes of focal areas of decreased flow within a kidney?**
   Most causes involve mass effect from a lesion such as a cyst, abscess, or tumor (benign or malignant) that has altered renal morphologic features. Scarring in the kidney from chronic pyelonephritis or chronic ureteral reflux can also lead to focally decreased renal flow. Other causes include renal infarction or a renal hematoma associated with trauma or surgery. Such abnormalities can be either unifocal or multifocal and can be more thoroughly evaluated with structural imaging techniques such as ultrasonography (US), computed tomography (CT), or magnetic resonance imaging (MRI).

4. **An increase in size of one or both kidneys may be associated with what processes?**
   A common cause of a unilaterally enlarged kidney is compensatory hypertrophy for an absent or poorly functioning contralateral kidney (Figure 81-2). Hydronephrosis can also result in an enlarged kidney and may affect one or both kidneys. Patients with polycystic renal disease may also have kidneys that appear enlarged, often with multiple cold defects seen due to cysts. Renal vein thrombosis can also result in ipsilateral enlargement of a kidney related to the engorgement of blood.

5. **List some causes of a unilaterally small kidney seen on renal scintigraphy.**
   - Dysplastic kidney.
   - Postinflammatory atrophy.
   - Postobstructive atrophy.
   - Renal artery stenosis.
   - Radiation nephritis.
       Correlation with clinical history and structural imaging techniques can help to differentiate the underlying etiology. Bilaterally small kidneys are usually a manifestation of end-stage renal disease, which can be caused by many underlying etiologies.

6. **Describe potential causes of nonvisualization of a kidney on renal scintigraphy.**
   Nonvisualization of a kidney on a renal scan can be seen with prior nephrectomy, renal agenesis, post-traumatic or postsurgical injury to the kidney's vascular supply, or other vascular or obstructive processes. Vascular disorders that result in nonvisualization of a kidney include renal artery occlusion and renal vein occlusion. Neoplastic disease can also impair renal function or perfusion, resulting in nonvisualization. Finally, chronic obstruction, such as from ureteropelvic junction (UPJ) obstruction, can eventually result in absent flow and function in a kidney (see Figure 81-2).

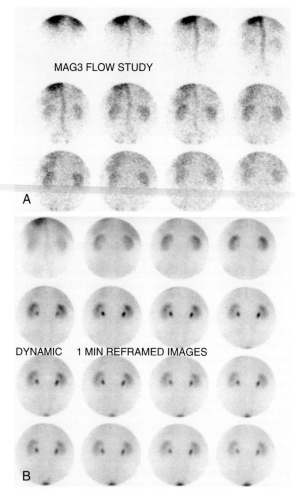

**Figure 81-1. A,** Normal-appearing kidneys on renal scintigraphy (posterior projection). Note symmetric and prompt flow of radiotracer into both kidneys during blood flow phase. **B,** Delayed scintigraphic images show radiotracer activity entering into collecting systems by 4 minutes with adequate and symmetric excretion into bladder. There is only mild retention of radiotracer activity in collecting systems on last image.

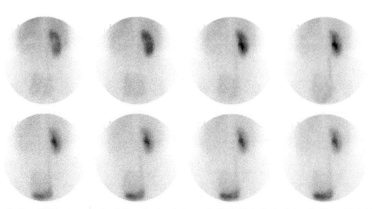

**Figure 81-2.** Nonvisualization of kidney on renal scintigraphy (posterior projection). Note lack of visualization of left kidney in this patient who is status post left nephrectomy for renal cell carcinoma. The right kidney appears slightly enlarged due to compensatory hypertrophy and has a normal cortical transit time.

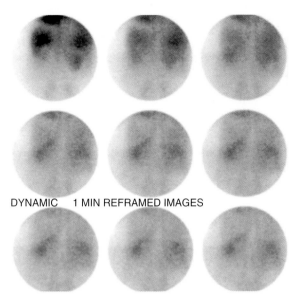

DYNAMIC    1 MIN REFRAMED IMAGES

**Figure 81-3.** Nonvisualization of kidneys on renal scintigraphy (posterior projection). Delayed scintigraphic images in patient with chronic renal failure show bilaterally decreased radiotracer uptake in kidneys and no clear evidence of renal function. The kidneys have less radiotracer activity than the liver and spleen, rather than more radiotracer activity, confirming the overall poor renal flow and function.

7. How do processes that decrease the radiotracer activity in both kidneys differ from processes that affect a single kidney?

Processes affecting both kidneys are often more systemic in nature. Glomerulonephritis can cause decreased flow in both kidneys. Acute or chronic renal failure also results in decreased flow and function in both kidneys. There can always be bilateral vascular or obstructive processes, and these should also be considered. Finally, technical factors, such as injecting the wrong radiotracer or acquiring images at the wrong photopeak, can be considered if the kidneys are not visualized (Figure 81-3).

8. How is captopril renal scintigraphy used to evaluate for renal artery stenosis?

A renal scan in a patient with renal artery stenosis often appears normal because the renin-angiotensin system causes a vasoconstriction of the efferent arterioles, which helps maintain the pressure across the glomeruli, preserving renal function. A renal scan performed after the administration of captopril or other ACE inhibitor reveals abnormal flow and function because the regulatory mechanism of angiotensin is blocked by the ACE inhibitor. A scan using $^{99m}$Tc DTPA after captopril should show evidence of diminished flow and function in a kidney with renal artery stenosis compared with a renal scan without captopril. Generally, the overall sensitivity and specificity of this test are approximately 90% and 95%, respectively. With the advent of magnetic resonance angiography (MRA), there has been considerably less use of captopril renal scintigraphy, but it is still sometimes helpful to evaluate the functional significance of partially stenotic renal arteries.

9. Why are renal scans obtained 1 day after renal transplantation?

A renal scan within 1 day of surgical transplantation can be very useful for detecting overall flow in the transplanted kidney to ensure that the transplant renal artery is patent. The renal scan can also be used to help evaluate the extent of acute tubular necrosis (ATN), which occurs in virtually every transplant, although it is much more common and severe in cadaveric transplants compared with living-related transplants (Figure 81-4). ATN is typically diagnosed on a renal scan when there is normal renal flow but diminished cortical transit of the radiotracer (the normal cortical transit time is usually less than 5 minutes). The degree of ATN can be evaluated based on the delay in cortical transit, with severe ATN showing no significant cortical function. A renal scan can also help with the evaluation of hyperacute rejection, which would appear as near-absent perfusion of the renal transplant. Renal scans can also provide information regarding possible obstruction or leaks of urine (most often occurring within several days after transplantation).

10. How is ATN differentiated from rejection in renal transplant patients?

Clinically, ATN occurs almost immediately after transplantation whereas chronic rejection generally occurs over several days to several weeks or longer after transplantation. ATN can occur later, although it is usually associated with some specific event that damages the transplant and usually takes several weeks or months to resolve after transplantation. Renal scan findings are often different for ATN and rejection. ATN shows normal or only slightly diminished perfusion of the kidney with a delayed cortical transit time, whereas rejection is usually associated with diminished flow with mildly impaired cortical function. In severe rejection, flow and function are both markedly reduced. In both cases,

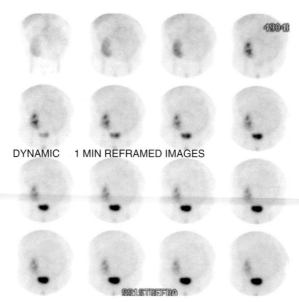

DYNAMIC    1 MIN REFRAMED IMAGES

**Figure 81-4.** Normal appearing renal transplant on renal scintigraphy (anterior projection). Radiotracer uptake in renal transplant is good, and cortical transit is within 5 minutes, with good radiotracer excretion seen into bladder. This patient is status post living-related donor renal transplantation 1 day ago.

when minimal or no urine is produced, it is impossible to exclude a leak or urinary tract obstruction as the underlying etiology, because both of these entities require some radioactive urine to be excreted into the urothelial system. It is also possible to have superimposed ATN and rejection, particularly when a renal scan reveals diminished flow and function. A clinician may have to treat such patients for both conditions (Figure 81-5).

11. **What type of renal scan is used to evaluate for cortical scarring related to pyelonephritis or vesicoureteral reflux? How does it work?**
Pyelonephritis can result in renal scarring, hypertension, proteinuria, and renal failure. Renal scarring from vesicoureteral reflux accounts for 10% to 20% of patients with end-stage renal disease. A renal scan with $^{99m}$Tc dimercaptosuccinic acid (DMSA) is more sensitive than US or intravenous urography (IVU) for the detection of parenchymal involvement. This radiotracer binds to the renal cortex and is essentially not excreted into the urine, allowing for imaging of the renal cortex to evaluate for areas of abnormally decreased radiotracer uptake. Imaging typically is performed approximately 20 minutes after injection, and single photon emission computed tomography (SPECT) is used to provide tomographic images for evaluation.

12. **What are the current uses of liver/spleen scintigraphy?**
Liver/spleen scans performed after intravenous administration of $^{99m}$Tc sulfur colloid are rarely used in current practice given the availability of US, CT, and MRI, but their usual purpose is to evaluate liver function associated with cirrhosis, which leads to decreased radiotracer uptake in the liver and a "colloid shift" to the spleen and bone marrow (Figures 81-6, *A*, and 81-6, *B*). Liver/spleen scans can also help to assess patients for focal nodular hyperplasia, which results in focal areas of increased radiotracer uptake in the liver due to presence of Kupffer cells. In addition, liver/spleen scans can be used to assess splenic function, such as in the clinical setting of trauma or surgery that may have damaged the spleen, or to seek out additional splenic tissue in patients with heterotaxia (Figure 81-6, *C*) or splenosis.

13. **What conditions result in a hot quadrate lobe and a hot caudate lobe on a liver/spleen scintigraphy?**
Superior vena cava obstruction results in increased radiotracer activity in the quadrate lobe (i.e., the medial segment) of the liver following intravenous radiotracer administration via an upper extremity vein. This occurs because collateral thoracic and abdominal vessels communicate with a recanalized para-umbilical vein, resulting in a hot quadrate lobe relative to the other areas of the liver. Budd-Chiari syndrome (hepatic vein thrombosis) may lead to increased radiotracer uptake in the caudate lobe of the liver, because it has preserved function owing to direct venous drainage into the inferior vena cava whereas the remainder of the liver has decreased radiotracer activity because of impaired function.

14. **What is the diagnostic pattern of radiotracer activity on a $^{99m}$Tc red blood cell (RBC) scan in a patient with a hemangioma in the liver?**
The diagnosis of hemangiomas in the liver using a $^{99m}$Tc RBC scan is based on identifying a photopenic area in the liver on early images with gradual fill in and increased radiotracer activity seen on delayed images. The reported sensitivity for planar $^{99m}$Tc RBC imaging is approximately 55% and for tomographic $^{99m}$Tc RBC imaging is 88%.

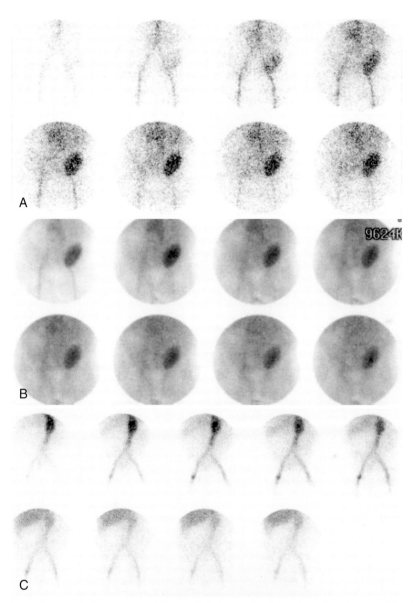

**Figure 81-5.** Renal transplant complications on renal scintigraphy (anterior projection). **A,** Note good renal transplant flow in patient 1 day status post cadaveric renal transplantation. **B,** Also note no clear evidence of renal function in same patient. This constellation of findings is consistent with ATN. Urinary tract obstruction or leak cannot be adequately assessed on this scan because of overall poor renal function. **C,** Note severely decreased flow and function to renal transplant in different patient consistent with chronic transplant rejection.

15. What is the best scintigraphic test for the detection of splenic tissue?

The $^{99m}$Tc heat-denatured RBC scan is the most sensitive and specific for evaluation of splenic tissue. Autologous RBCs are incubated at 50° C for 30 minutes, radiolabeled, and then reinjected. The main indications for performing such a study are to evaluate patients with heterotaxia, patients who may have ectopic splenic tissue following surgery or trauma, patients with a suspected intrapancreatic splenule, and patients with sickle cell disease to assess for splenic function (Figure 81-7).

16. What functions of the hepatobiliary system can be evaluated using iminodiacetic acid (IDA) radiotracers?

Hepatocellular function can be evaluated using radiolabeled IDA radiotracers such as $^{99m}$Tc mebrofenin or $^{99m}$Tc HIDA to perform hepatobiliary scintigraphy (Figure 81-8), because radiotracer uptake by the liver depends on overall function. If the radiotracer activity in the cardiac blood pool disappears within 5 minutes, hepatocellular function is considered to be normal. A longer time to clearance suggests hepatocellular dysfunction. The patency of the common bile duct and

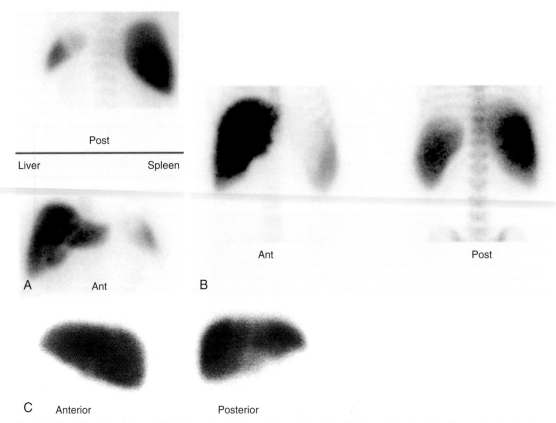

**Figure 81-6. A,** Normal radiotracer distribution on liver/spleen scintigraphy (anterior [*bottom row*] and posterior [*top row*] projections). Note that most of radiotracer activity is seen in liver, followed by spleen. Only approximately 5% of radiotracer activity is in bone marrow. **B,** "Colloid shift" on liver/spleen scintigraphy (anterior [*left*] and posterior [*right*] projections). Note similar levels of radiotracer uptake in liver and spleen, splenic enlargement, and overall more prominent bone marrow activity in patient with cirrhosis. **C,** Heterotaxy on liver/spleen scintigraphy (anterior [*left*] and posterior [*right*] projections). Note liver located on left side of abdomen and no clear splenic activity.

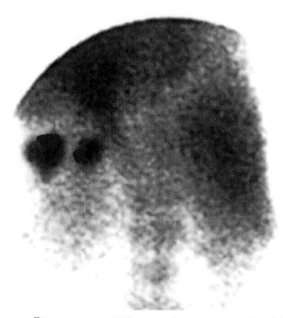

**Figure 81-7.** Residual splenic tissue on $^{99m}$Tc heat-denatured RBC scintigraphy (posterior projection). Note two foci of increased radiotracer uptake in splenic region due to residual splenic tissue in this patient who is status post splenectomy.

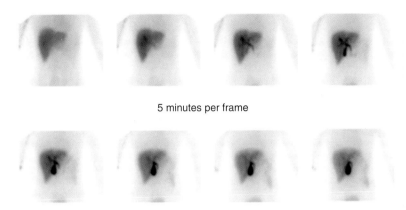

5 minutes per frame

**Figure 81-8.** Normal findings on hepatobiliary scintigraphy (anterior projection every 5 minutes). Note good hepatocellular function associated with elimination of cardiac blood pool by 5 minutes. The gallbladder is observed by 20 minutes, and radiotracer activity is observed in bowel by 25 minutes.

---

**Box 81-1.** Some Causes of False-Positive Results for Diagnosis of Acute Cholecystitis on Hepatobiliary Scintigraphy

- Chronic cholecystitis
- Complete common bile duct obstruction
- Prolonged fasting
- Severe hepatocellular disease
- Acute pancreatitis
- Prior cholecystectomy
- Gallbladder agenesis

---

cystic duct can also be evaluated. This allows one to diagnose the presence of acute and chronic cholecystitis. Finally, the presence of a biliary leak or of an extrabiliary biloma can be assessed.

17. **When should cholecystokinin (CCK) or morphine sulfate be used in relation to a hepatobiliary scan?**

   CCK is used before the administration of a radiotracer for hepatobiliary scintigraphy when a patient has not eaten in more than 24 hours. The reason for the use of CCK is that the gallbladder can become filled with sludge with prolonged fasting and can result in false-positive scans for cholecystitis. The intravenous infusion of CCK over about 15 to 30 minutes (faster infusions can result in nausea and vomiting) before beginning the hepatobiliary scan causes contraction of the gallbladder, which then fills with the radiotracer as it expands. Morphine augmentation is used if, after the 1-hour scan, there is nonvisualization of the gallbladder, and there is radiotracer activity entering into the small bowel. If only the liver is seen without any radiotracer activity entering the small bowel, morphine should not be given because the common bile duct may not be patent. Morphine causes contraction of the sphincter of Oddi, which results in increased biliary back pressure that can open a functionally closed cystic duct. If there is still nonvisualization of the gallbladder at the end of an additional 30 minutes of imaging after morphine is given, the result is consistent with acute cholecystitis.

18. **What can a gallbladder ejection fraction study show?**

   A gallbladder ejection fraction study can be performed in patients with a normally filling gallbladder who continue to have right upper quadrant symptoms. At the end of the standard hepatobiliary scan, CCK (or sometimes a fatty meal) is administered, and images are obtained for another 30 minutes. The radiotracer accumulation in the gallbladder on the pre-CCK and post-CCK scans can be compared to provide a gallbladder ejection fraction. A normal value is considered to be greater than 30% to 35%; however, the distribution of values in healthy individuals makes a normal range difficult to determine. If the ejection fraction is less than this value, gallbladder dysfunction is suspected. Cystic duct syndrome is considered if the gallbladder does not contract in a uniform manner or even expands after administration of CCK.

19. **What are the causes of nonvisualization of the gallbladder on a hepatobiliary scan?**

   The most common cause is acute cholecystitis (Figure 81-9). Many other potential causes, including various diseases and congenital problems, must be considered, however, in the differential diagnosis (Box 81-1).

20. **Discuss some causes of false-negative hepatobiliary scan results in the setting of acute cholecystitis.**

   There are several reasons why the gallbladder, or a structure appearing to be the gallbladder, can be observed on a hepatobiliary scan in the presence of acute cholecystitis (Box 81-2). False-negative results occur most commonly when the patient has acute acalculous cholecystitis. Several other structures, such as the bowel, a duplicated

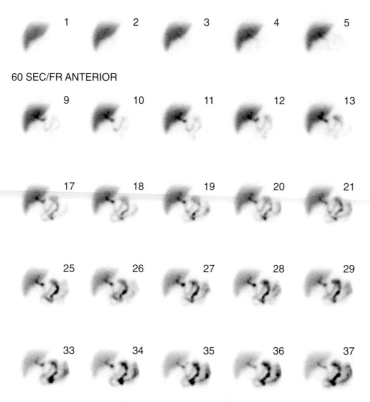

60 SEC/FR ANTERIOR

**Figure 81-9.** Acute cholecystitis on hepatobiliary scintigraphy (anterior projection). Note good liver radiotracer uptake but no evidence of gallbladder activity. If the gallbladder is still not visualized following morphine augmentation or delayed images, then the scan findings are highly suggestive of acute cholecystitis.

**Box 81-2.** Some Causes of False-Negative Results for Diagnosis of Acute Cholecystitis on Hepatobiliary Scintigraphy

- Acute acalculous cholecystitis
- Bowel loop
- Duodenal diverticulum
- Duplicated gallbladder

- Biliary duplication cyst
- Right hydronephrosis
- Gallbladder perforation
- Partial or intermittent cystic duct obstruction

gallbladder, or another abnormality of the biliary tree, can show radiotracer activity in the region of the gallbladder even though the patient actually has acute cholecystitis. Another cause of false-negative results is perforation of the gallbladder, which subsequently reduces the pressure and relieves the obstruction, allowing the radiotracer to enter into the gallbladder region.

21. What is the "rim" sign, and what does it imply?
The "rim" sign refers to an area of increased radiotracer activity in the region of the liver surrounding the gallbladder. The implication is that there is hyperemia or inflammation associated with acute cholecystitis. This hyperemia appears as a rim of increased radiotracer activity immediately adjacent to the gallbladder. The diagnosis of acute cholecystitis still depends, however, on nonvisualization of the gallbladder.

22. When a biliary leak occurs, where are the possible sites to observe the leak?
A biliary leak can occur anywhere along the biliary tree. However, such leaks usually occur in areas of prior surgical intervention or anastomoses. When performing a hepatobiliary scan to assess for a biliary leak, it is important to perform the test in the standard manner. Additional images of surgical drains and anterior projection images with the patient in lateral decubitus positions help to assess for subtle biliary leaks. Surgical drains should be evaluated for radiotracer activity, and it is important to know where these drains are actually located in the body. Drains in the surgical bed that have radiotracer activity suggest a leak in that area, whereas drains in the biliary tree should naturally have radiotracer activity. Images with lateral decubitus patient positioning can be obtained to assess for radiotracer activity in the peritoneal space, which would help to confirm a leak (Figure 81-10).

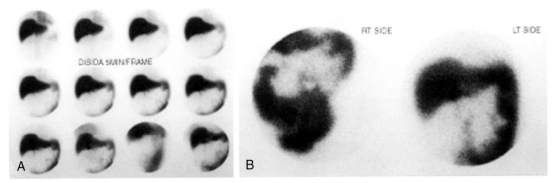

**Figure 81-10.** Biliary leak following liver transplantation on hepatobiliary scintigraphy (anterior projection). **A,** Note radiotracer uptake in liver reflecting preservation of hepatic function. The gallbladder is not visualized because it is surgically absent. Note accumulation of radiotracer activity in left abdomen in region of left paracolic gutter. **B,** Note rightward and leftward movement of radiotracer activity in abdomen on images with patient in right lateral decubitus and left lateral decubitus positions, respectively, confirming large biliary leak into peritoneal space.

23. **How is biliary atresia differentiated from neonatal hepatitis on hepatobiliary scintigraphy?**
    In both disorders, the bilirubin level is extremely high, making adequate visualization of radiotracer activity entering into the small bowel difficult to assess. During the initial hour of imaging, radiotracer activity is usually seen in the liver with persistent cardiac blood pool activity. Delayed imaging at 4 hours and sometimes 24 hours is required to determine whether any radiotracer activity is observed entering into the bowel. If any radiotracer does enter the bowel, biliary atresia can be excluded, and the diagnosis of neonatal hepatitis can be made. Absence of radiotracer activity in the small bowel can still be related to either disorder, however, because if insufficient radiotracer is sent into the biliary system by the liver, it is impossible to evaluate for potential complete biliary obstruction.

24. **What are the typical findings of a positive gastrointestinal (GI) bleeding scan?**
    A positive GI bleeding scan generally requires that there be a focus of growing radiotracer activity that moves through the bowel. A focus that only increases in radiotracer activity can sometimes be a false-positive finding and attributable to renal activity, bowel hyperemia, or a vascular structure. It is also important to observe the initial site in which the focus occurs because the primary importance of this study is to determine localization of the site of bleeding (Figure 81-11).

25. **Contrast the differences between the sulfur colloid scan and the tagged RBC scan for detecting GI bleeding.**
    A $^{99m}$Tc sulfur colloid scan can be started immediately when the patient arrives in the nuclear medicine department because the agent can be prepared ahead of time. The sulfur colloid remains in the intravascular space for approximately 25 minutes. An active bleed can be detected quickly, whereas an intermittent bleed might be missed if the patient bleeds after more than 25 minutes following injection of the radiotracer. Because sulfur colloid does not remain in the intravascular space, if there is a negative scan the first time, a repeat scan can be performed any time when the patient begins to bleed again.
    A tagged RBC scan requires drawing some of the patient's blood, which must be radiolabeled, a process that takes 15 to 20 minutes. After injection of $^{99m}$Tc-labeled RBCs, the radiotracer activity persists in the intravascular space, and imaging can be performed continuously for several hours after injection; this can help to detect intermittent bleeds. If the initial scan results are negative, however, a repeat scan cannot be performed for approximately 24 hours until the $^{99m}$Tc decays sufficiently. Otherwise, the bowel would have too much background radiotracer activity.

26. **How does a gastric emptying study work?**
    A gastric emptying study involves the ingestion of a standardized meal consisting of some food source that is tagged with a radioactive label. The most common meal utilized for the study consists of egg whites tagged with $^{99m}$Tc sulfur colloid. Meals must be standardized for content and calories so that adequate comparisons can be made. Imaging is usually performed over 90 to 180 minutes. Images may be obtained throughout that time period or at regular intervals, usually with either anterior and posterior projections or with a single left anterior oblique projection. The importance of these views is that food enters the stomach posteriorly and moves anteriorly. Images must take into account movement of ingested material within the stomach and differentiate it from actual emptying.

27. **What are the normal rates for gastric emptying?**
    The rate of gastric emptying depends on the particular methods and meal used, but the normal half emptying time of the stomach is usually 50 to 100 minutes (Figure 81-12).

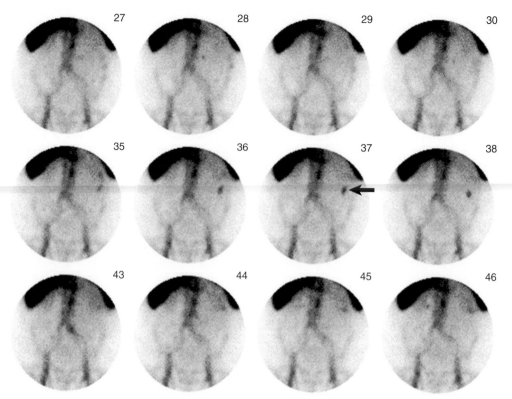

**Figure 81-11.** Positive findings on gastrointestinal bleeding scan (anterior projection). Note focal accumulation of radiotracer activity in region of splenic flexure of colon (*arrow*). This appears to change its configuration over time, which confirms active bleeding in this region.

28. **What physiologic factors normally affect gastric emptying?**

Numerous factors can affect gastric emptying. Factors that increase the gastric emptying rate include upright patient positioning, younger age with male gender, higher liquid content of food, smaller size of food particles, larger volume of food, and lower fat content of food. Factors that can slow the rate include supine patient positioning, older age with female gender, higher solid content of food, larger size of food particles, smaller volume of food, and higher fat content of food. Other factors that can cause variable responses include the hormonal and metabolic state of the patient, stress, and medications. For these reasons, it is imperative that a standardized meal and acquisition protocol be used and compared with normal values established for that specific technique.

29. **What is a pentetreotide scan and what is it used for?**

A pentetreotide scan (sometimes referred to as an octreotide scan or an OctreoScan™, utilizes the radiotracer indium-111 ($^{111}$In) pentetreotide, which binds to neuroendocrine tumors that express somatostatin receptors (Figure 81-13). Typically, patients are injected on the first day and imaged at 24 hours post injection. The most common tumors for which pentetreotide scans can be useful include carcinoid tumor, islet cell tumors (particularly gastrinomas, glucagonomas, and VIPomas), small cell lung cancer, pheochromocytoma, paraganglioma, pituitary adenoma, and medullary thyroid cancer. It should be noted that pentetreotide scans are not particularly useful for insulinomas.

30. **What are some available nuclear medicine scans that can be used to detect a pheochromocytoma?**

There are several radiotracers that can be used for detection of a pheochromocytoma. The pentetreotide scan mentioned above is useful for detecting pheochromocytomas. However, two related radiotracers, iodine-131 ($^{131}$I) metaiodobenzylguanidine (MIBG) and iodine-123 ($^{123}$I) MIBG, localize within intracellular adrenergic storage granules, which makes them more specific for pheochromocytomas. Typically, patients are injected on the first day and imaged at 24 hours post injection. The overall sensitivity is relatively similar for these different single photon emitting radiotracers. Finally, positron emission tomography (PET) radiotracers such as $^{18}$F-fluorodopa and $^{18}$F-fluorodopamine have been shown to have an excellent ability to detect pheochromocytomas.

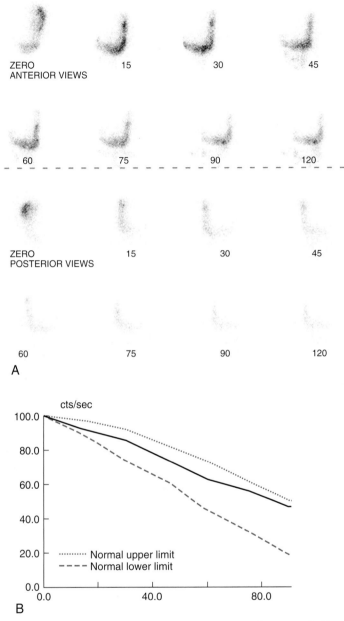

**Figure 81-12. A,** Normal gastric emptying scan (anterior and posterior projections). Note adequate transit of ingested radiotracer. Anterior and posterior imaging is required because food moves from posterior to anterior over time, and without both projections, gastric emptying calculations may be inaccurate. **B,** Time-activity curve from same gastric emptying scan. This graph of gastric activity (vertical axis) versus time in minutes (horizontal axis) shows rate of gastric emptying over 90 minutes, with upper and lower limits of normal shown for comparison.

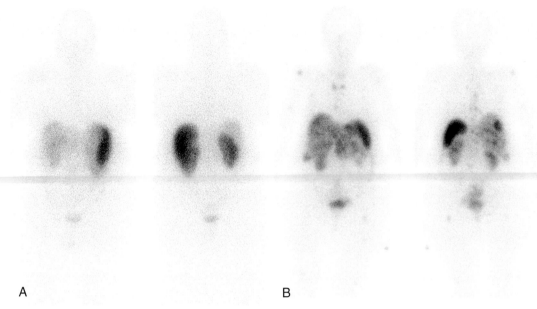

A                                    B

**Figure 81-13. A,** Normal [111]In pentetreotide scan (anterior and posterior projections). Note normal radiotracer uptake in liver, spleen, and kidneys with little additional uptake throughout body. **B,** Metastatic carcinoid tumor on [111]In pentetreotide scan (anterior and posterior projections). Note multiple foci of abnormal radiotracer uptake in liver, mediastinal lymph nodes, and spine, right humerus, and left femur.

## KEY POINTS

- Renal scintigraphy is useful to evaluate kidney perfusion and function in patients with renal disease, to evaluate the presence and functional significance of renal artery stenosis, to assess the presence of renal parenchymal scarring, and to differentiate ATN from rejection of a renal transplant.
- Hepatobiliary scintigraphy is most often used to detect acute cholecystitis, to assess biliary patency, to detect biliary leaks, and to differentiate biliary atresia from neonatal hepatitis.
- A GI bleeding scan is useful to detect and localize sites of active hemorrhage in the bowel and is considered as positive when there is a focus of growing radiotracer activity that moves through the bowel.

**BIBLIOGRAPHY**

Taylor AT. Radionuclides in nephrourology, Part 1: Radiopharmaceuticals, quality control, and quantitative indices. *J Nucl Med.* 2014;55(4):608-615.

Taylor AT. Radionuclides in nephrourology, Part 2: pitfalls and diagnostic applications. *J Nucl Med.* 2014;55(5):786-798.

Ziessman HA. Hepatobiliary scintigraphy in 2014. *J Nucl Med Technol.* 2014;42(4):249-259.

Allen TW, Tulchinsky M. Nuclear medicine tests for acute gastrointestinal conditions. *Semin Nucl Med.* 2013;43(2):88-101.

Middleton ML, Strober MD. Planar scintigraphic imaging of the gastrointestinal tract in clinical practice. *Semin Nucl Med.* 2012;42(1):33-40.

Tulchinsky M, Colletti PM, Allen TW. Hepatobiliary scintigraphy in acute cholecystitis. *Semin Nucl Med.* 2012;42(2):84-100.

Howarth DM. The role of nuclear medicine in the detection of acute gastrointestinal bleeding. *Semin Nucl Med.* 2006;36(2):133-146.

Dubovsky EV, Russell CD, Bischof-Delaloye A, et al. Report of the Radionuclides in Nephrourology Committee for evaluation of transplanted kidney (review of techniques). *Semin Nucl Med.* 1999;29(2):175-188.

Emslie JT, Zarnegar K, Siegel ME, et al. Technetium-99m-labeled red blood cell scans in the investigation of gastrointestinal bleeding. *Dis Colon Rectum.* 1996;39(7):750-754.

Datz FL. Considerations for accurately measuring gastric emptying. *J Nucl Med.* 1991;32(5):881-884.

# CHAPTER 82

# CARDIAC SCINTIGRAPHY

*Andrew B. Newberg, MD, and Charles Intenzo, MD*

1. **How do you prepare a patient for stress myocardial perfusion imaging (SMPI)?**
   Patients should be informed that the test takes approximately one half day and consists of two parts: a resting part and a stress part. The placement of an intravenous catheter (usually inserted at the beginning of the study) is required to administer the radiotracer. The order of the study can be either rest-stress or stress-rest, although the higher dose is given for the second scan, and the stress test is often performed second to provide the best image quality. Single photon emission computed tomography (SPECT) or positron emission tomography (PET) scans are obtained approximately 30 to 60 minutes after radiotracer administration, and each scan takes approximately 15 to 30 minutes. The patient should not eat or drink (except water) from midnight before the examination. Patients are commonly asked to stop taking their medications unless there is some reason (e.g., very high blood pressure or serious dysrhythmias) that requires the stress test to be performed while the patient continues to take medications.

2. **What are the different types of radiotracers available for stress testing?**
   There are three basic categories: thallium-201 ($^{201}$Tl) and technetium-99m ($^{99m}$Tc)-labeled compounds for SPECT, and positron emitting compounds for PET. Table 82-1 compares $^{201}$Tl and $^{99m}$Tc-labeled compounds. The most commonly used $^{99m}$Tc-labeled compounds are tetrofosmin and sestamibi, which have similar imaging and chemical characteristics. $^{99m}$Tc-labeled compounds generally provide more flexibility in terms of imaging times. Because of the photon energy and the number of photons emitted, $^{99m}$Tc-labeled compounds are generally easier to use for image acquisition and analysis. PET radiotracers, such as rubidium-82 ($^{82}$Rb), nitrogen-13 ($^{13}$N) ammonia, and fluorine-18 ($^{18}$F) fluorodeoxyglucose (FDG), can be used to evaluate myocardial perfusion and glucose metabolism, respectively. $^{13}$N ammonia has a short (20 minute) half-life, so there are some logistical limitations in using this for PET cardiac imaging.

3. **What are the three types of stress tests?**
   The three basic types are exercise, pharmacologic vasodilatory, and adrenergic agonist stress tests.
   - **Exercise stress tests** are typically performed using a treadmill with several possible protocols that sequentially increase the speed and grade of the treadmill. An alternative exercise test uses a stationary bicycle. The goal is to increase heart rate to 85% of the patient's age-predicted maximum, although others have used a combination of heart rate and blood pressure as a target.
   - **Pharmacologic vasodilatory stress tests** are performed with adenosine itself, dipyrimadole (an inhibitor of adenosine deaminase that results in increased adenosine within the epicardial coronary arteries), or regadenoson (an $A_{2A}$ adenosine receptor agonist). Upon injection of these agents, normal coronary arteries will dilate, whereas stenosed arteries will not. The relative discrepancy in myocardial blood flow results in a perfusion defect to the myocardial wall supplied by the stenosed vessel.
   - **Adrenergic agonist stress tests** are performed using an adrenergic agonist (dobutamine) with which inotropic and chronotropic stimulation results in increased heart rate and contractility simulating exercise.

4. **What are contraindications for an exercise stress test?**
   Any patient with significant musculoskeletal problems that would prevent him or her from achieving a maximal heart rate should undergo pharmacologic stress testing. Patients with certain ongoing dysrhythmias, such as ventricular

**Table 82-1.** Comparison of $^{99m}$Tc-Labeled Compounds and $^{201}$Tl for Cardiac SPECT SMPI

| | $^{99m}$TC-LABELED COMPOUNDS | $^{201}$TL |
|---|---|---|
| Energy | 140 keV (ideal for gamma camera) | 69-83 keV (suboptimal for gamma camera) |
| First-pass studies of ventricular function | Feasible | Not feasible |
| Gated imaging | Readily accomplished | Count rate marginal for gated imaging |
| Stress/rest imaging | Two injections required since there is no radiotracer redistribution over time | Can be accomplished with one injection since there is radiotracer redistribution over time |

tachycardia, supraventricular tachycardia, new-onset atrial fibrillation, or heart block, should receive treatment for those dysrhythmias before the stress test is rescheduled. Known atrial fibrillation that is adequately treated is not a contraindication. Patients with severe pulmonary disease, severe hypertension (i.e., systolic blood pressure >210 mm Hg and diastolic blood pressure >110 mm Hg), abdominal aortic aneurysms, symptomatic aortic stenosis, unstable angina, or active myocardial ischemia on electrocardiography (ECG) should also be excluded.

5. What are the contraindications for pharmacologic vasodilatory and adrenergic agonist stress tests?

Pharmacologic vasodilatory stress tests are not performed in patients with severe reactive airway disease, particularly when a patient has active wheezing on physical examination. Patients who use inhalers but who otherwise have stable airway disease can often safely undergo these stress tests. Any patient taking dipyrimadole or methylxanthines does not undergo a vasodilatory stress test, unless the medication can be stopped for at least 24 to 48 hours. All patients who are to undergo vasodilatory studies should abstain from caffeine for 24 hours because caffeine blocks the effect of vasodilatory compounds and adenosine.

Adrenergic stress tests have similar contraindications to those of exercise testing except that musculoskeletal problems are not an issue. Furthermore, dobutamine can be used in patients with existing airway disease.

6. Should patients taking medications that can affect the heart be given stress tests?

Generally, any patient can undergo a cardiac stress test. In patients taking medications for blood pressure, such as β-blockers or calcium channel blockers, the medication may prevent the patient from achieving the necessary heart rate. In such patients, it is recommended that the medications be stopped for approximately 24 hours before the study, unless the ordering physician wants to determine the presence or absence of inducible ischemia while the patient is taking these medications. If a patient has severe hypertension, the patient may need to be tested while taking the medication for this condition because without the medication, the blood pressure would be too high to proceed safely with the study.

7. List the conditions under which an exercise stress test should be stopped.
- The patient cannot continue because of dyspnea, chest pain, fatigue, or musculoskeletal problems.
- The patient has a significant hypertensive response.
- The patient develops ST segment depression greater than 3 mm.
- The patient develops ST segment elevation, heralding a possible myocardial infarction.
- The patient develops a potentially dangerous dysrhythmia, such as ventricular tachycardia, ventricular fibrillation, very rapid supraventricular tachycardia, or heart block.

8. Which territories are supplied by which coronary arteries?

The three main branches of the coronary arteries are the left anterior descending artery (LAD), the left circumflex artery (LCx), and the right coronary artery (RCA). The LAD supplies the anterior wall, including the anterolateral region; the interventricular septum; and, in most cases, the apex. The RCA supplies the inferior wall and, in a "right dominant" system, can wrap around the apex to include part of the inferoapical wall. The LCx supplies the lateral wall. Smaller branches of these major arteries can supply smaller segments of individual walls (Figure 82-1).

9. What is the implication of a nonreversible (or fixed) defect on SMPI?

A nonreversible defect implies that there is a lack of myocardial perfusion during the rest and stress components of the scan (i.e., there is no difference between the two scans). Nonreversible defects can often be caused by artifact, such as when part of the heart is attenuated, or blocked, by a structure between the heart and the scanner. The most common structures that cause nonreversible defects via attenuation include the diaphragm (inferior wall) and breast tissue (anterior wall and apex). When nonreversible defects are associated with an actual cardiac pathologic condition, they are related to scarring, such as from prior myocardial infarction, or chronically ischemic but viable hibernating myocardium. An infarct should have decreased perfusion during stress and rest images because it is dead tissue (Figures 82-2 and 82-3).

10. What methods are available to correct for attenuation artifact?

Two common methods are used to correct for attenuation artifact. One method directly corrects this problem by using an external radioactive source that is transmitted through the patient. This source is used to map the patient's body structures to assess their ability to attenuate photons. By creating an attenuation map, the computer can combine the attenuation map with the emission images to correct for missing counts of radioactivity. The resulting image appears to "fill in" the areas that have attenuation artifact and eliminate the defects altogether.

A second method involves performing an ECG-gated study, obtaining images throughout the cardiac cycle. The ECG is monitored, and the R-R interval is divided into 8 or 16 equal segments during which the scan is acquired. The result is a sequence of images that can be played back to back to observe the wall motion throughout the R-R cycle. By obtaining the end-diastolic and end-systolic volumes, ejection fraction and regional wall motion can be determined. If a nonreversible defect is observed to move and thicken normally, it is most likely normal myocardium that has an apparent defect related to attenuation. If a nonreversible defect does not appear to move, it is most likely related to a scar or prior myocardial infarct. ECG-gating helps to assess whether an apparent defect is related to attenuation artifact or whether it is a real perfusion defect.

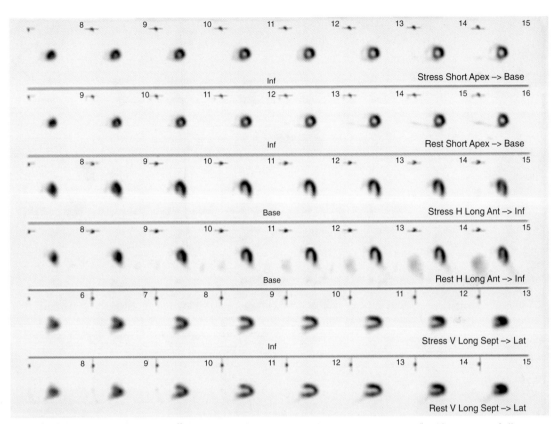

**Figure 82-1.** Normal cardiac perfusion on $^{99m}$Tc sestamibi SPECT scan. Stress images are on top row and rest images are on bottom row of each pair of projections. Short-axis projection images (from apex to base) show classic "doughnut" appearance of left ventricular myocardium, with anterior cardiac wall on top, lateral wall on right side of image, inferior wall on bottom, and interventricular septum on left side of image. Note more faintly visualized right ventricular myocardium to right of left ventricle. Horizontal long-axis projection images show interventricular septum on left side of image, apex on top, and lateral wall on right side of image. Vertical long-axis projection images show anterior wall on top, apex on right side of image, and inferior wall on bottom of image. On this normal scan, radiotracer activity is uniform throughout all walls of left ventricular myocardium.

11. **How do SMPI studies compare with routine stress ECG studies in the evaluation of patients with coronary artery disease (CAD)?**

    Generally, a routine stress ECG is sensitive, with positive ECG stress test results indicating a high likelihood for CAD. The accuracy is significantly reduced, however, in patients with abnormal baseline ECGs or a previous history of CAD, or if a patient does not achieve 85% of the maximal heart rate for patient age. In these patients, an SMPI study has a sensitivity of approximately 92% and a specificity of approximately 72% for detecting CAD. The relative prevalence of CAD in the specific patient population is also a factor. Women have a much higher rate of false-positive stress test results because their prestudy risk is much lower than that for men.

12. **What is the implication of a reversible (or transient) defect on SMPI?**

    A reversible defect implies a lack of myocardial perfusion during the stress component but normal myocardial perfusion during rest. Reversible defects can be caused by attenuation artifact but must always be assumed to be related to CAD, in which the stenotic artery cannot accommodate the extra perfusion demand during stress. The importance of a reversible defect is that the myocardium is intact but is at risk for coronary events. It typically requires a stenosis of at least 70% for perfusion to be affected during the stress test. Reversible defects also usually mandate further study with coronary angiography to assess for the extent of blockage of the artery (Figure 82-4).

13. **Why is transient left ventricular cavity dilation on SMPI a poor prognostic sign?**

    Transient left ventricular cavity dilation refers to the cavity appearing larger on stress images than on resting images. This is in contrast to fixed cavity dilation, which may be associated with cardiomyopathy that could be related to a number of causes including CAD, alcoholic cardiomyopathy, valvular disease, or viral or autoimmune processes. Transient left ventricular cavity dilation suggests that during stress, CAD results in worsening myocardial function such that the heart cannot maintain its usual contractile state and then dilates. Another explanation is stress-induced subendocardial ischemia that resolves at rest. Transient left ventricular cavity dilation is a poor prognostic sign because significant cardiac function and structure are at risk for an ischemic event.

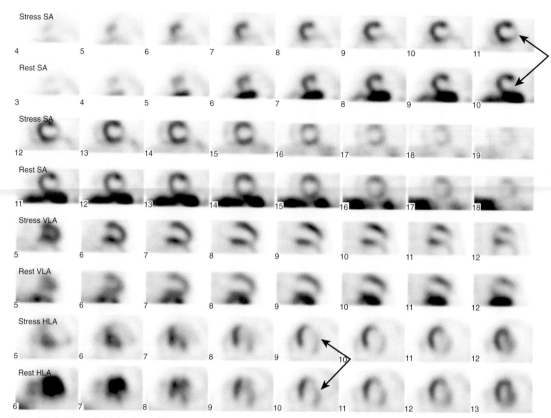

**Figure 82-2.** Myocardial infarction on $^{99m}$Tc sestamibi SPECT scan. Note lateral wall nonreversible perfusion defect in left ventricular myocardium on stress and rest images in short-axis projection and horizontal long-axis projection (*arrows*).

14. **How might a left bundle branch block (LBBB) on ECG affect SMPI findings?**

An LBBB seen on ECG can cause reversible perfusion defects in the septum during an exercise stress test. The cause has not been completely elucidated but may be related to altered depolarization of the septum from the conduction abnormality or related to left ventricular dilation and dysfunction associated with LBBB. To minimize the problem of perfusion defects associated with LBBB, a pharmacologic vasodilatory stress test can be performed instead.

15. **How is a $^{201}$Tl resting-redistribution scan performed, and how are the results of a resting-redistribution scan used clinically?**

In a resting-redistribution scan, the patient receives an injection of $^{201}$Tl at rest and undergoes scanning approximately 15 minutes later. The patient is scanned again approximately 4 hours later and sometimes 24 hours after injection. Images are reconstructed in the typical tomographic projections. The images are evaluated for perfusion and for reversibility of defects observed on the initial scan. The general idea is that a patient with known CAD has several segments of the myocardium that have undergone ischemic injury. The question is whether these segments are viable, which can be determined because they either have some perfusion on initial images or show some degree of reversibility. Areas of the myocardium that show this type of viability typically respond well after revascularization by regaining some degree of function. Areas that are not viable typically do not respond to revascularization. $^{201}$Tl resting-redistribution studies can help to determine what parts of the heart, and what vessels, might be the best targets for revascularization.

16. **What is the difference between hibernating and stunned myocardium?**

Stunned myocardium refers to viable myocardium with relatively preserved perfusion on SPECT or PET imaging, normal or decreased glucose metabolism on FDG PET imaging, and decreased wall motion on echocardiography. Stunning occurs in an acute ischemic event, but by the time the patient undergoes management and is referred for SMPI, blood flow has normalized so there is no perfusion defect even though wall motion is still impaired. The stunning should resolve as long as perfusion is maintained.

Hibernating myocardium refers to viable myocardium with decreased perfusion on SPECT or PET imaging, relatively preserved glucose metabolism on FDG PET imaging, and decreased wall motion on echocardiography. The implication is that chronic ischemia results in decreased flow and function, although the myocardium is still viable. Hibernating myocardium should respond well to attempts to revascularize the region, which would return flow and eventually reverse the functional deficits.

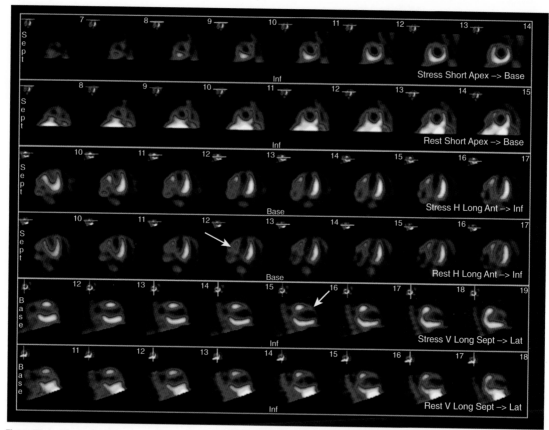

**Figure 82-3.** Myocardial infarction on $^{99m}$Tc sestamibi SPECT scan. Note septal wall nonreversible perfusion defect on horizontal long-axis projection images (*long arrow*) and anterior wall/apical nonreversible perfusion defect on vertical long-axis projection images (*short arrow*) in left ventricular myocardium. These are also visible on short-axis projection images. Left ventricular cavity size appears dilated. It is important to confirm any finding on other projections to ensure real rather than artifactual defects.

### 17. How is a multiple-gated acquisition (MUGA) scan performed?

A MUGA scan involves the radioactive tagging of the patient's red blood cells (RBCs) so that the blood pool remains radioactive throughout the study (Figure 82-5). Radiolabeling can be performed either in vitro or in vivo. In vitro labeling requires blood to be drawn from the patient first; the radiolabeling is performed in the laboratory, and then the blood is reinjected into the patient. Alternatively, the RBCs can be labeled in the patient by first injecting stannous pyrophosphate, which allows the RBCs to take up $^{99m}$Tc. When the patient's RBCs have been labeled, scintigraphic images are usually acquired in the left anterior oblique and anterior projections for approximately 15 minutes while the ECG is monitored. The R-R interval is divided into 8 or 16 segments, during which image acquisition occurs. The result is that the radiotracer activity in the left ventricle can be measured throughout the cardiac cycle, and the end-diastolic (ED) and end-systolic (ES) radiotracer activity levels and regional wall motion can be assessed. The ejection fraction is calculated based on the following equation: Ejection fraction = (ED − ES)/(ED − BG). The background (BG) counts are also important because placement of the background region over an area with significant radiotracer activity (e.g., the thoracic aorta) would result in a falsely elevated calculated ejection fraction.

### 18. How is a MUGA scan used clinically?

A MUGA scan is primarily used to evaluate myocardial wall motion and to measure left ventricular ejection fraction. Both of these can now be assessed with echocardiography, which can also be used to evaluate the structure and function of the cardiac valves. For this reason, MUGA scans are used less frequently than echocardiography even though MUGA scan results are less operator dependent. The principal use is currently for the determination of ejection fraction in cancer patients before and after they undergo chemotherapy. Patients taking chemotherapeutic agents that can affect cardiac function, such as doxorubicin, require serial measures of cardiac function before and after therapy. A MUGA scan provides true quantitative information regarding ejection fraction because the actual counts of radiotracer activity within the left ventricular cavity can be assessed, compared to echocardiography, which determines ejection fraction by estimation. General guidelines suggest that if the ejection fraction declines to less than 40% or has a decrease of more than 10% to 15%, then the patient should not continue chemotherapy with the same agent.

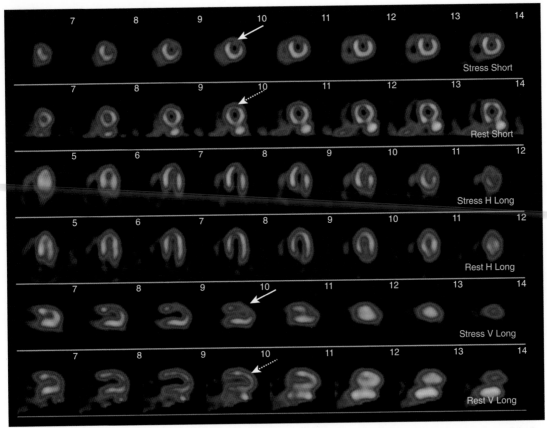

**Figure 82-4.** Stress-induced myocardial ischemia due to CAD on $^{99m}$Tc sestamibi SPECT scan. Note anterior and apical perfusion defect on short-axis and vertical long-axis projection images during stress (*solid arrows*). However, this perfusion defect is not seen on corresponding images during rest (*dotted arrows*), indicating that the defect is reversible. The implication is that there is significant atherosclerosis involving LAD.

19. **How does an FDG PET scan of the heart help to evaluate for myocardial viability?**
    The primary energy substrate of the myocardium is free fatty acids rather than glucose. During ischemia, however, there is a switch in the myocardium to use of glucose. If there is decreased perfusion but preserved FDG uptake (i.e., metabolism), then that area of the myocardium is considered to be viable. If there is decreased perfusion and metabolism, then that area of the myocardium is considered to be a scar (Figure 82-6).

20. **How does FDG PET scan help with the diagnosis of myocardial sarcoidosis?**
    Granulomatous disease related to sarcoidosis typically is very FDG avid. Sarcoidosis can therefore easily be detected in affected areas of the body such as lymph nodes and lungs via FDG PET. In addition, FDG uptake in the heart itself may be seen and is suggestive of involvement by sarcoidosis. Typically, the patient is prepared for the study by either prolonged fasting or by eating a diet high in fat in order to reduce normal FDG uptake by the myocardium. The result is that myocardial uptake is low unless there is involvement by sarcoidosis, in which case heterogeneously increased FDG uptake in the myocardium is usually seen (Figure 82-7).

---

## KEY POINTS

- A reversible (or transient) defect on SMPI occurs when there is a lack of myocardial perfusion during stress but normal myocardial perfusion during rest and implies CAD with coronary artery stenosis of at least 70%.
- A nonreversible (or fixed) defect on SMPI occurs when there is a lack of myocardial perfusion during both stress and rest, and implies scarring, such as from prior myocardial infarction, or chronically ischemic but viable hibernating myocardium.
- Transient left ventricular cavity dilation on SMPI refers to the cavity appearing larger on stress images than on resting images and is a poor prognostic sign in the setting of CAD because significant cardiac function and structure are at risk for an ischemic event.
- FDG PET is useful to evaluate for myocardial viability and for the presence of cardiac involvement by sarcoidosis.

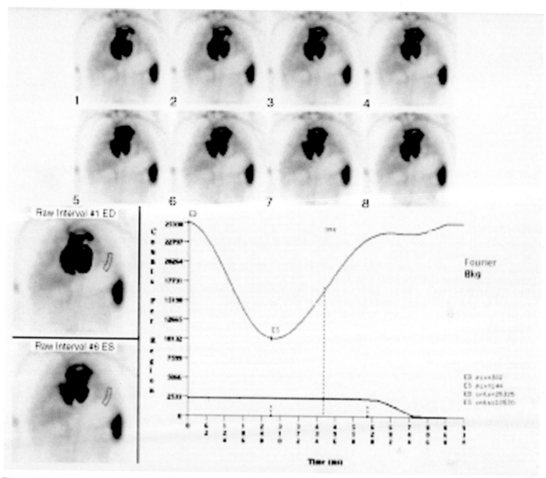

**Figure 82-5.** Normal ejection fraction on $^{99m}$Tc RBC MUGA scan. Note eight images of heart (*top*) ranging from end diastole (*ED*) to end systole (*ES*) with subsequent decrease in overall cavity size and counts. Note normal splenic radiotracer uptake in left upper quadrant of abdomen. Two images (*on bottom left*) include regions of interest drawn around left ventricle on ED and ES images and in background. Displayed curve represents number of radiotracer activity counts detected during cardiac cycle. Background counts are represented by curve at bottom of graph. Ejection fraction is calculated on basis of ED and ES counts in left ventricle with correction for background counts and in this case was calculated as 61%.

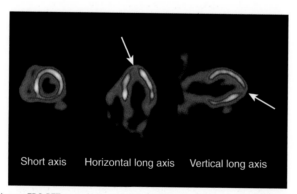

Short axis    Horizontal long axis    Vertical long axis

**Figure 82-6.** Myocardial infarction on FDG PET scan. Note enlarged left ventricle with preserved FDG uptake in all segments except for apex. Areas of preserved FDG uptake represent viable myocardium, whereas apex without FDG uptake (*arrows*) is considered to be scarred.

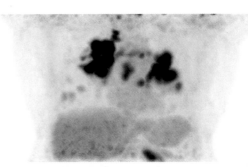

**Figure 82-7.** Sarcoidosis on FDG PET. Coronal maximum intensity projection (MIP) image demonstrates increased FDG uptake in bilateral hilar lymphadenopathy as well as in heart.

## BIBLIOGRAPHY

Anagnostopoulos C, Georgakopoulos A, Pianou N, et al. Assessment of myocardial perfusion and viability by positron emission tomography. *Int J Cardiol.* 2013;167(5):1737-1749.

Grover S, Srinivasan G, Selvanayagam JB. Myocardial viability imaging: does it still have a role in patient selection prior to coronary revascularisation? *Heart Lung Circ.* 2012;21(8):468-479.

Youssef G, Leung E, Mylonas I, et al. The use of 18F-FDG PET in the diagnosis of cardiac sarcoidosis: a systematic review and metaanalysis including the Ontario experience. *J Nucl Med.* 2012;53(2):241-248.

Hendel RC, Berman DS, Di Carli MF, et al. ACCF/ASNC/ACR/AHA/ASE/SCCT/SCMR/SNM 2009 appropriate use criteria for cardiac radionuclide imaging: a report of the American College of Cardiology Foundation Appropriate Use Criteria Task Force, the American Society of Nuclear Cardiology, the American College of Radiology, the American Heart Association, the American Society of Echocardiography, the Society of Cardiovascular Computed Tomography, the Society for Cardiovascular Magnetic Resonance, and the Society of Nuclear Medicine. *J Am Coll Cardiol.* 2009;53(23):2201-2229.

Yao SS, Rozanski A. Principal uses of myocardial perfusion scintigraphy in the management of patients with known or suspected coronary artery disease. *Prog Cardiovasc Dis.* 2001;43(4):281-302.

Santana-Boado C, Candell-Riera J, Castell-Conesa J, et al. Diagnostic accuracy of technetium-99m-MIBI myocardial SPECT in women and men. *J Nucl Med.* 1998;39(5):751-755.

Brown KA, Altland E, Rowen M. Prognostic value of normal technetium-99m-sestamibi cardiac imaging. *J Nucl Med.* 1994;35(4):554-557.

# CHAPTER 83

# BRAIN SCINTIGRAPHY

*Andrew B. Newberg, MD*

1. **What radiotracers are available for functional brain scintigraphy?**
   There are currently two single photon emission computed tomography (SPECT) radiotracers that are available to evaluate general brain function by measuring cerebral blood flow (CBF): technetium-99m ($^{99m}$Tc) ethylcysteinate dimer (ECD) and $^{99m}$Tc hexamethylpropyleneamine oxime (HMPAO). These diffuse passively into the brain shortly after injection. Iodine-123 ($^{123}$I) ioflupane (DaTscan) is now available for visualizing and measuring the dopamine transporter (DaT) and is typically used for the evaluation of patients with movement disorders such as Parkinson's disease (PD). There is one positron emission tomography (PET) radiotracer, fluorine-18 ($^{18}$F) fluorodeoxyglucose (FDG), which is available for the evaluation of general brain function by measuring cerebral glucose metabolism. Currently, several amyloid radiotracers are approved for evaluating patients with suspected Alzheimer's disease (AD). There are many other radiotracers for evaluating all aspects of brain function including multiple neurotransmitter systems, but these are currently used only for research purposes.

2. **How would you prepare a patient for a brain scan to assess general brain function?**
   Patients should be informed that the test takes approximately one hour and typically involves the injection of the radiotracer followed approximately 30 minutes later by PET or SPECT imaging depending on the radiotracer. It is important to recognize that virtually everything affects brain function, and this should be considered when discussing the preparation with the patient. Box 83-1 describes some of the issues related to scanning for general brain function.

3. **What are the normal patterns of radiotracer uptake for CBF-SPECT and FDG PET scans?**
   In most cases, CBF and glucose metabolism correlate or are coupled. Therefore, the pattern of CBF and cerebral metabolism should appear similar. Generally, brain scans should demonstrate uniform and symmetric radiotracer uptake throughout the brain (Figure 83-1). There should be no cortical defects. The subcortical structures sometimes appear to have slightly higher radiotracer activity compared to the cortex. The temporal lobes can appear slightly reduced due to their location and being surrounded by bone. The cerebellum typically appears more active relative to the cortex in CBF-SPECT scans and of similar activity on FDG PET scans. With normal aging, there can be mild decreases in cortical activity, particularly in the frontal lobes.

4. **What does the FDG PET brain scan pattern in Figure 83-2 represent?**
   This scan demonstrates hypometabolism in the temporoparietal regions bilaterally. This is a classic pattern observed in patients with AD. Therefore, the findings on this scan are suggestive of AD. It should be noted that there is typically a correlation between the severity of metabolic dysfunction and cognitive impairment. In addition, the temporoparietal hypometabolism pattern has also been reported in other conditions including PD and carbon monoxide poisoning.

5. **What does the FDG PET brain scan pattern in Figure 83-3 represent?**
   This scan demonstrates hypometabolism in the frontal lobes bilaterally. While frontal lobe hypometabolism is associated with normal aging, marked decreases as shown in this figure are typically associated with frontotemporal dementia (FTD). As with AD, there is typically a correlation between the severity of metabolic dysfunction and cognitive impairment in patients with FTD. In addition, frontal lobe hypometabolism has also been reported in other conditions including depression, cerebrovascular disease, and aging.

---

**Box 83-1.** Considerations for Patient Preparation Prior to Cerebral SPECT or PET Imaging

- No caffeine or nicotine should be taken on the examination day.
- The patient needs to be nil per os (NPO) (i.e., is not to ingest food or fluids per mouth) after midnight and undergoes assessment of serum blood glucose levels prior to FDG PET (typically, this should be <200 mg/dL).
- Medications that alter the cerebral blood flow or metabolism, including psychotropic medications, should be temporarily discontinued if clinically possible. All medications have the potential to alter brain function.
- Radiotracer injection is typically performed with open eyes and ears and with low ambient light and noise.
- No movement or talking after radiotracer administration is recommended.
- Sedation may be required and can be given in certain circumstances but only after radiotracer injection (i.e., after ≈30 minutes) to allow for radiotracer uptake in the brain.

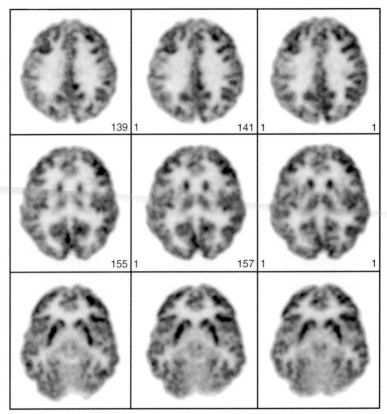

**Figure 83-1.** Normal findings on FDG PET brain scan. Note normal metabolism throughout cortical and subcortical regions. Metabolism is uniform and symmetric without focal defects. SPECT scans typically show a similar pattern of radiotracer uptake although spatial resolution on SPECT is worse than that on PET.

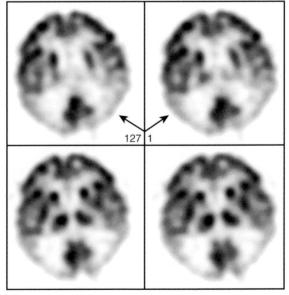

**Figure 83-2.** AD on FDG PET brain scan. Note reduced metabolism in temporoparietal regions of brain bilaterally (*arrows*). Frontal lobe and subcortical metabolism is relatively preserved.

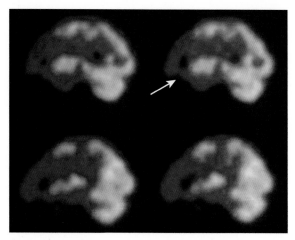

**Figure 83-3.** FTD on FDG PET brain scan (sagittal plane). Note marked reduction of metabolism in frontal lobes (*arrow*). Posterior metabolism in the parietal regions is preserved.

6. How does an acetazolamide SPECT scan work to determine cerebrovascular disease?

   Acetazolamide is utilized sometimes with SPECT imaging to uncover cerebrovascular disease that might potentially result in an eventual stroke. Acetazolamide is a potent vasodilator and can increase cerebral blood flow through vessels that are patent and without cerebrovascular disease. However, vessels with atherosclerotic disease are unable to dilate in response to acetazolamide resulting in a scan that demonstrates relatively reduced perfusion to the affected vascular territories. The typical plan for an acetazolamide challenge SPECT study is to administer acetazolamide intravenously about 1 hour prior to injection with a CBF radiotracer. If the scan does not show any CBF abnormalities, the implication is that there is no clinically significant cerebrovascular disease. If there is an asymmetry or some cortical area with reduced CBF, it is important to bring the patient back for a perfusion SPECT scan without acetazolamide. If the changes in CBF are observed both with and without acetazolamide, then the perfusional changes are permanent. However, if the acetazolamide scan is markedly different with specific areas of reduced perfusion, the implication is that these areas are at risk for a future cerebrovascular event.

7. What is the finding in the FDG PET brain scan shown in Figure 83-4 of a patient with a history of seizures?

   Cerebral glucose metabolism is reduced in the right temporal lobe on this interictal FDG PET scan. Decreased metabolism identifies the seizure focus during the interictal period. In this patient, the decreased metabolism in the right temporal lobe suggests that this is the site of the seizure focus. This result is typically correlated with other imaging and electroencephalography (EEG) findings. The temporal lobe is the seizure focus in approximately 60% of patients. Seizure foci can be found in most cortical areas and occasionally in multiple foci.

8. What are the findings in these interictal and ictal CBF-SPECT scans shown in Figure 83-5 of a patient with a history of seizures and prior surgery for a benign brain tumor in the right parieto-occipital region?

   On the current scan, there is decreased perfusion at the surgical site and surrounding cerebral cortex. However, it is not clear whether this represents postsurgical change or a seizure focus similar to that seen on an interictal FDG PET scan. A subsequent ictal SPECT scan was performed. For this scan, the CBF radiotracer is kept at the bedside of the patient while he or she is being monitored in the seizure unit. When the EEG demonstrates the onset of the seizure, the patient is immediately injected with the radiotracer. After the seizure is completed, the patient is brought to the scanner. Because the radiotracer does not redistribute significantly, the scan demonstrates the CBF pattern at the time of radiotracer injection (i.e., at the onset of the seizure). The goal is to find a focus of increased perfusion that indicates the site of origin of the seizure. In this scan, there is markedly increased perfusion in the adjacent parietal cortex demonstrating the site of the seizure focus.

9. How can one differentiate tumor recurrence from radiation necrosis in the brain using an FDG PET scan?

   Brain tumors, like other cancers, are typically hypermetabolic. While it is sometimes difficult to detect primary brain tumors from underlying cortical metabolism, after treatment with surgery and/or radiation therapy it becomes much easier to detect recurrent tumor. Thus, on an FDG PET scan, tumor recurrence appears as a hypermetabolic focus whereas radiation or other treatment effects appear as an area of hypometabolism (Figure 83-6).

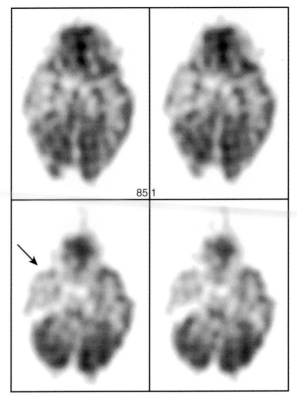

**Figure 83-4.** Seizure focus on interictal FDG PET brain scan. Note reduced metabolism in right temporal lobe (*arrow*) of brain whereas other cerebral structures show normal metabolism. These findings suggest that right temporal lobe is seizure focus in this patient with refractory seizures.

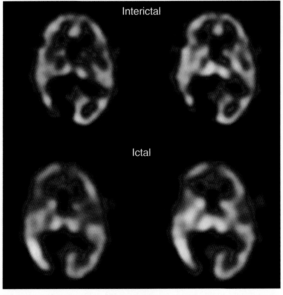

**Figure 83-5.** Seizure focus on interictal and ictal SPECT brain scans. Patient is status post surgery for benign tumor in right parieto-occipital region now with new onset of seizures. Interictal scan demonstrates absent perfusion in region of surgery and mildly decreased perfusion in adjacent parietal lobe. On ictal scan, there is markedly increased perfusion in adjacent right parietal lobe suggesting site of new onset seizures.

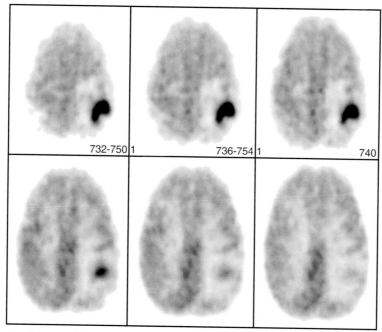

**Figure 83-6.** Recurrent malignancy on FDG PET brain scan. Patient has history of brain tumor in left frontoparietal region and is status post radiation therapy. Note intense focus of FDG uptake in this same region consistent with tumor recurrence. Surrounding cortical area has relatively decreased metabolism related to effects of radiation therapy.

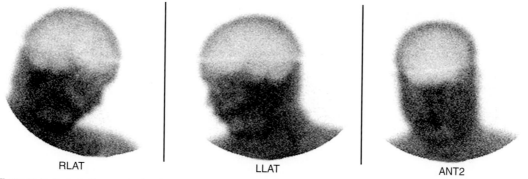

**Figure 83-7.** Brain death on cerebral perfusion brain death scan (using planar scintigraphy). Patient was involved in car accident with significant head injury. Note absent perfusion to entire cortical area with mild radiotracer uptake in scalp. This is consistent with diagnosis of brain death. There also appears to be relatively increased uptake in facial structures related to shunting of blood from internal to external carotid arteries.

10. **What does this brain perfusion scan in Figure 83-7 demonstrate in this patient who was involved in a motor vehicle accident with significant head trauma?**
    This is a perfusion brain scan to evaluate for brain death. The scan uses the same radiotracers as for SPECT imaging, but for brain death, typically only planar scintigraphic views (as shown) are required. SPECT imaging in this clinical scenario is sometimes difficult because the patient requires a ventilator and other equipment that limits the ability to get the SPECT scanner close to the head. In this perfusion scan, there is no evidence of brain perfusion which is consistent with brain death. In addition, there is increased perfusion (radiotracer activity) to the face due to shunting of blood from the internal carotid arteries to the external carotid arteries. This is sometimes referred to as the "hot nose" sign. Because there are significant medical and legal consequences associated with the declaration of brain death, it is important that these scans are unequivocal. Any perfusion or uncertain finding should not be interpreted as brain death. However, a positive scan can be useful in facilitating the final clinical diagnosis of brain death and also in helping with organ donation in traumatic settings.

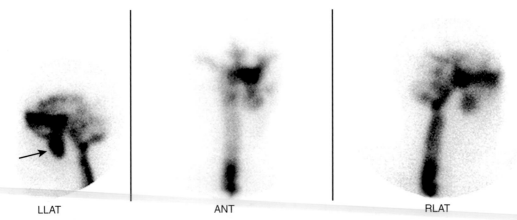

LLAT                          ANT                          RLAT

**Figure 83-8.** Encephalocele on CSF scintigraphy study. There is good migration of radiotracer flow over frontal convexities of brain. However, there is focal accumulation of radiotracer inferior to left frontal region in keeping with leak of CSF into encephalocele.

11. How is a cerebrospinal fluid (CSF) scintigraphy study performed, and what is it used for?
    CSF scintigraphy typically involves the administration of a radiotracer such as $^{99m}$Tc DTPA into the CSF (usually via injection through a lumbar puncture at the base of the spinal column). Planar scintigraphic images are obtained initially and then at regular intervals up to 24 hours (i.e., 2, 4, 6, 12, and 24 hours) depending on the rate of flow and the purpose of the scan. There are two primary diagnostic purposes of CSF scintigraphy studies: evaluation of hydrocephalus and evaluation for a CSF leak. The evaluation of hydrocephalus requires imaging to determine the rate of CSF flow and any areas in which CSF flow is abnormal. The evaluation of a CSF leak explores various areas along the CSF spaces in which an abnormal accumulation of radiotracer occurs. CSF studies are sometimes performed with the use of pledgets placed into the nasal cavity to measure asymmetries in radiotracer accumulation. This can help to detect a leak even if it is not specifically observed on the scans.

12. What does the CSF scintigraphy study shown in Figure 83-8 demonstrate?
    This CSF scintigraphy study shows good migration of the radiotracer into the CSF spaces (normal rates are ≈2 hours to the basal cistern, 4 to 6 hours to the frontal convexities, and 12 to 24 hours over the cerebral convexities). In this study, an abnormal accumulation of radiotracer is observed inferior to the left frontal region, which is related to an encephalocele that communicates with the CSF spaces.

13. What does the CSF scintigraphy study shown in Figure 83-9 reveal?
    This CSF shunt study, performed by injecting indwelling bilateral ventriculoperitoneal shunts with $^{99m}$Tc DTPA, shows good migration of the radiotracer into the abdomen on the left. However, there is no movement of the radiotracer from the shunt on the right to the abdomen. The implication is that the left shunt is patent but that the right shunt is obstructed. It should be noted that although the flow is typically observed anterograde from the CSF spaces to the abdomen, radiotracer activity can frequently be observed refluxing retrograde into the CSF spaces such as the ventricles.

14. How is an $^{123}$I ioflupane (DaTscan) performed, and what is it used for?
    $^{123}$I ioflupane binds to the dopamine transporters, primarily in the basal ganglia. The scan is primarily used for the evaluation of movement disorders and in particular to differentiate true PD from other underlying disorders such as essential tremor. There is no specific patient preparation, and patients can continue to take whatever medications they are currently using other than specific medications that might block the dopamine transporters such as methylphenidate. The patient is initially given ≈15 drops of Lugol's solution to protect the thyroid gland from $^{123}$I uptake and associated radiation exposure. Approximately 30 to 60 minutes later, the patient is injected intravenously with $^{123}$I ioflupane, and then SPECT imaging is initiated 3 to 4 hours after that. Scans are evaluated for radiotracer binding in the basal ganglia regions, where decreased amounts of radiotracer binding reflect presence of PD or other movement disorders (Figure 83-10).

15. What is amyloid imaging used for?
    Several different radiotracers are now approved for use (primarily for research purposes) in the evaluation of patients with cognitive impairment to help ascertain a diagnosis. Amyloid accumulation is characteristic of AD although it can

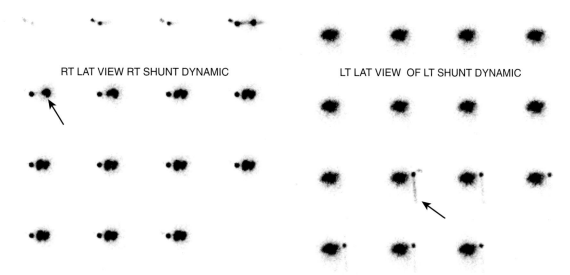

RT LAT VIEW RT SHUNT DYNAMIC          LT LAT VIEW  OF LT SHUNT DYNAMIC

**Figure 83-9.** Ventriculoperitoneal shunt obstruction on CSF scintigraphy study. When radiotracer was injected into right shunt, radiotracer activity is observed refluxing back into ventricles (*arrow*) without evidence of antegrade flow, in keeping with shunt obstruction. When radiotracer was injected into left shunt, linear radiotracer activity (*arrow*) is quickly shown moving down shunt toward abdomen indicating shunt patency.

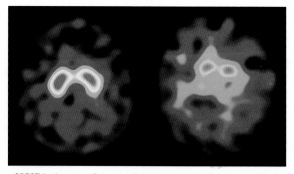

**Figure 83-10.** PD on [123]I ioflupane SPECT brain scans. Scan on left shows normal radiotracer binding in right basal ganglia and slightly reduced radiotracer binding in left basal ganglia due to early PD in patient with very mild right hand tremor. Scan on right demonstrates moderate to severe reductions in radiotracer binding in bilateral basal ganglia including caudate nuclei and putamina in separate patient with moderate PD.

also occur in other neurodegenerative disorders and has been observed in approximately 10% of the normal population. Those patients with mild cognitive impairment who demonstrate a significant amyloid burden on PET imaging are considered to most likely have AD (Figure 83-11). Those patients without significant amyloid burden are more likely to have a different etiology for their cognitive impairment.

## KEY POINTS

- Brain scintigraphy is useful to detect abnormalities in cerebral perfusion; to evaluate patients with cognitive disorders, movement disorders, and other neurologic disorders; to detect and localize seizure foci; to differentiate tumor recurrence from radiation necrosis; and to detect and localize sites of CSF leak.
- Symmetric hypometabolism in the bilateral temporoparietal regions of the brain is a classic finding observed on FDG PET imaging in patients with Alzheimer's disease.
- Seizure foci have increased perfusion and metabolism on ictal CBF and FDG PET brain scans, respectively, whereas decreased perfusion and metabolism may be observed on interictal scans.

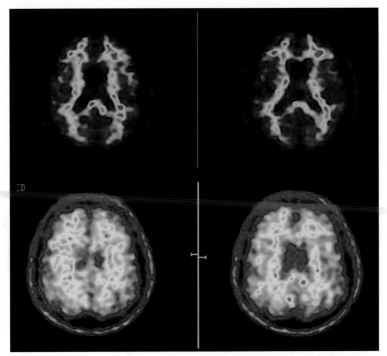

**Figure 83-11.** Normal findings and AD on ¹⁸F florbetapir PET brain scans. Note nonspecific binding of radiotracer primarily in white matter tracts with no appreciable radiotracer uptake in cerebral cortex in healthy control volunteer (*upper row*). Compare these findings to marked radiotracer binding throughout cerebral cortex and minimal nonspecific white matter binding in separate patient with moderate cognitive impairment due to AD (*lower row*).

## BIBLIOGRAPHY

Singhal T, Alavi A, Kim CK. Brain: Positron emission tomography tracers beyond [¹⁸F] fluorodeoxyglucose. *PET Clin.* 2014;9(3):267-276.

Bajaj N, Hauser RA, Grachev ID. Clinical utility of dopamine transporter single photon emission CT (DaT-SPECT) with (¹²³I) ioflupane in diagnosis of parkinsonian syndromes. *J Neurol Neurosurg Psychiatry.* 2013;84(11):1288-1295.

Jack CR Jr, Barrio JR, Kepe V. Cerebral amyloid PET imaging in Alzheimer's disease. *Acta Neuropathol.* 2013;126(5):643-657.

Newberg AB, Alavi A. Normal patterns and variants in PET brain imaging. *PET Clin.* 2010;5(1):1-13.

Newberg AB, Alavi A. Role of PET in the investigation of neuropsychiatric disorders. *PET Clin.* 2010;5(2):2232-2242.

Van Paesschen W, Dupont P, Sunaert S, et al. The use of SPECT and PET in routine clinical practice in epilepsy. *Curr Opin Neurol.* 2007;20(2):194-202.

# RADIOPHARMACEUTICAL THERAPEUTIC INTERVENTION

*Daniel A. Pryma, MD*

# CHAPTER 84

1. **What is the purpose of radiopharmaceutical therapy?**

   In sufficient dosages, radiation will kill cells. In many cases, radiation can be delivered directly to sites of disease with external beam techniques. An alternative means of delivering radiation to sites of disease is radiopharmaceutical therapy, wherein a radioactive compound is administered to the patient. Through a combination of the route of administration and the physical and biological properties of the radiopharmaceutical, the radiation dose will be preferentially delivered to sites of disease. The biggest potential advantage of radiopharmaceutical therapy is the ability to deliver therapeutic radiation regardless of the number and location of disease sites.

2. **What is the therapeutic ratio?**

   In the context of radiotherapy, the therapeutic ratio is the treatment effect in the sites of disease (the desirable effect of radiation) divided by the radiation effects in normal tissues (the side effects of therapy). Ideally, this ratio is as high as possible, meaning that a very high radiation dose is delivered to sites of disease with very little radiation dose to normal tissues. However, it is important to understand that one cannot simply compare absolute radiation doses because different tissues and different diseases have different sensitivities to the effect of radiation. For example, if a given treatment delivers the exact same radiation dose to an organ and a tumor, the therapeutic ratio would be extremely favorable if the disease in question is lymphoma (very radiation sensitive) and the organ in question is the liver (fairly radiation resistant). The situation is reversed if the disease in question is thyroid cancer (quite radiation resistant) and the organ in question is the bone marrow (very sensitive).

3. **What are the different therapeutic radionuclide emissions?**

   For radiopharmaceutical therapy to deliver radiation dose preferentially to sites of disease, the radiation must be delivered in a very small area around the location of the radiopharmaceutical. Thus, the gamma and x-ray emissions that are able to travel long distances and are very useful for imaging deliver their radiation dose throughout the body and so add to normal tissue radiation dose and decrease therapeutic ratio. Many therapeutic isotopes also have gamma or x-ray emissions, and their benefit (the ability to image the treatment dose) must be weighed against their downside (adding to normal tissue radiation dose). The primary therapeutic emissions are:

   - **Beta particles**: These are electrons that are emitted from nuclei and typically travel distances on the order of millimeters in tissue. The relative effectiveness of beta radiation is about equal to that of photon radiation. Beta emitters have been the most commonly used therapeutic radiopharmaceuticals.
   - **Auger electrons**: When the energy from radioactive decay displaces an inner-shell electron, an outer-shell electron may drop in to takes its place, releasing energy. This energy is sometimes sufficient to eject an electron from the atom, and this electron is called an Auger electron. These generally have a very short path length in tissue, on the order of nanometers, and so must be in or very near the cell nucleus to have the potential to deliver deadly radiation to the cell. Although their short path length is thought to convey potential advantages, Auger emitters are rarely used clinically.
   - **Alpha particles**: Some large isotopes decay by alpha emission wherein a particle comprised of two neutrons and two protons is ejected from the nucleus. Alpha particles travel on the order of microns (generally one to four cell diameters) and have a mass about 7300 times higher than beta particles. Thus, the amount of energy they deposit over their very short path length is incredibly high, and they, therefore, have a relative effectiveness in causing cell death about 20 times higher than photons or beta particles.

4. **Why is radiopharmaceutical therapy useful in thyroid disease?**

   The most widely used form of radiopharmaceutical therapy is radioiodine for thyroid disease, the discovery and development of which was largely the birth of the specialty of nuclear medicine. Thyroid cells utilize dietary iodide to synthesize thyroid hormone, which is then stored in colloid adjacent to the cell. The body cannot differentiate radioactive iodide from radiostable iodide, and so by administering radioactive iodine a portion of the administered dose is concentrated and stored for prolonged periods in or very near the thyroid cells. Because the rest of the body has short retention times of radioactive iodine, the therapeutic ratio is very high. Thus, incredibly high radiation doses can be delivered to thyroid cells (much higher than could be safely delivered with external beam radiotherapy) with acceptable toxicity. Iodine-131 ($^{131}$I) is the primary therapeutic iodine isotope with an 8-day half-life and both beta and gamma emissions. The gamma emissions permit imaging for detection of sites of disease and confirmation of dose delivery (Figure 84-1).

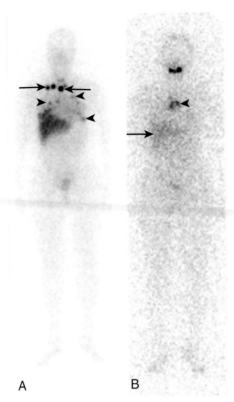

A          B

**Figure 84-1. A,** Posttherapy scan after [131]I radioiodine therapy for metastatic thyroid cancer shows radiotracer uptake in cervical and supraclavicular lymph nodes (*arrows*) as well as in lung metastases (*arrowheads*). **B,** Repeat posttherapy radioiodine scan obtained two years later shows resolution of previously seen sites of metastatic disease. Radiopharmaceutical concentration in liver (*arrow*) and thymus (*arrowhead*) is normal. This, in combination with biochemical testing (undetectable serum thyroglobulin levels), is evidence of response to [131]I therapy.

5. What are the potential adverse effects of radiopharmaceutical therapy?

Side effects of radiopharmaceutical therapies are determined by the biodistribution and kinetics of the radiopharmaceutical agent as well as the different sensitivities of various organs to the effects of radiation. Toxicity can be subdivided into acute, subacute, and late phases.

The most common acute toxicity is nausea, which is a generic effect of radiation in any form and is dose dependent (the higher the dose, the more the nausea). Other acute toxicities specific to the treatment in question and its distribution are possible, such as salivary gland pain with radioiodine therapy.

In general, the bone marrow is the most sensitive organ to radiation, and with most therapeutics bone marrow suppression is the dose-limiting toxicity even when the bone marrow receives a relatively smaller dose than other normal organs. Whereas with cytotoxic chemotherapy bone marrow suppression is observed within about a week of treatment, bone marrow suppression from radiopharmaceuticals is usually seen several weeks after therapy with a nadir generally at about 4 to 6 weeks. This usually spontaneously recovers but can be prolonged or permanent.

Late toxicity from radiopharmaceutical therapy generally refers to the induction of malignancies. Leukemia is the most common malignancy induced by radiation exposure, but other cancers are also possible. There is a clear link between radiation dose and cancer induction with high acute doses of radiation (e.g., in atomic bomb survivors), but it is much more difficult to detect the effects of lower radiation doses used with radiopharmaceutical therapies, particularly given the relatively high incidence of nonradiation-induced cancers. Therefore, this risk is poorly understood but is generally observed to be fairly low.

6. What are radiation safety precautions?

The final potential adverse effect of radiopharmaceutical therapy to be discussed is the effect on persons other than the treated patient. Because the source of radiation is given directly to the patient, it is possible for some dose to be delivered to members of the public. This is most commonly caused by gamma or x-ray emissions directly from the patient and is a very local problem—the radiation dose drops with the square of the distance from the source, so this radiation dose can be minimized by simply spending very little time within 1 to 2 meters of the patient. This also has little relevance for isotopes with no or minimal beta or x-ray emissions. However, the radiopharmaceutical also has the potential to be excreted from the patient in sweat, blood, saliva, urine, feces, and tears. Therefore, precautions are

**Table 84-1.** Selected Therapeutic Radiopharmaceuticals

| RADIOPHARMACEUTICAL | ISOTOPE | PRIMARY EMISSION(S) | HALF-LIFE | ROUTE OF ADMINISTRATION | INDICATION | US STATUS |
|---|---|---|---|---|---|---|
| Iodine-131 sodium iodide | $^{131}I$ | Beta Gamma | 8 days | Oral | Thyroid disease (thyroid cancer and hyperthyroidism) | Approved |
| Yttrium-90 microspheres | $^{90}Y$ | Beta | 64 hours | Intra-arterial (hepatic artery) | Hepatocellular carcinoma Liver metastases | Approved |
| Yttrium-90 ibritumomab tiuxetan | $^{90}Y$ | Beta | 64 hours | Intravenous | Non-Hodgkin lymphoma | Approved |
| Radium-223 dichloride | $^{223}Ra$ | Alpha | 11.4 days | Intravenous | Bone dominant castrate-resistant prostate cancer | Approved |
| Samarium-153 EDTMP | $^{153}Sm$ | Beta Gamma | 46.3 hours | Intravenous | Painful bone metastases | Approved |
| Yttrium-90 or lutetium-177 somatostatin analogues (e.g., DOTATOC, DOTATATE) | $^{90}Y$ $^{177}Lu$ | Beta Beta Gamma | 64 hours 6.6 days | Intravenous | Carcinoid tumor Pancreatic neuroendocrine tumor | Investigational |
| Iodine-131 MIBG | $^{131}I$ | Beta Gamma | 8 days | Intravenous | Pheochromocytoma Paraganglioma Neuroendocrine tumor | Investigational |

necessary to avoid contaminating members of the public with the radiopharmaceutical. The required precautions vary from state to state and country to county and may range from simple "universal precautions" used in handling any patient fluids to strict isolation within a hospital for some period of time.

7. How are radiopharmaceutical doses determined?

Several methods of determining prescribed dose exist and are used depending on the radiopharmaceutical in question and the disease being treated. These include:

- **Flat doses**: For example, ablation of the thyroid remnant in a patient who had a thyroidectomy for thyroid cancer is sometimes treated with a flat dose of 1.1 GBq (30 mCi) [131]I. Although this dose has been shown to be effective, it was initially largely chosen because, for a long period of time in the US, it was the largest dose that could be given to an outpatient in most states. Thus, dose selection is based not only on safety and efficacy but also on regulatory considerations. Furthermore, flat doses may be tiered and chosen based on patient demographics and risk factors.
- **Weight-based doses**: These can be based on the weight of the patient, for example with[131]I ibritumomab tiuxetan for non-Hodgkin lymphoma, or on the weight of the organ being treated, for example with yttrium-90 ($^{90}$Y) microsphere liver-directed therapy or [131]I therapy for benign thyroid disease. In the latter case, the dose is calculated based on organ weight but is also corrected for the amount of uptake of the radiopharmaceutical.
- **Dosimetric doses**: Dosimetry refers to the measurement of dose delivered and can apply to any combination of dose delivery to the tumor, individual organs, or whole body. Dosimetry allows precision dosing based on the individual patient's unique radiopharmaceutical kinetics. Generally, a small radiopharmaceutical dose is administered and serial measurements are made to calculate kinetics generally with some combination of blood (and/or body fluid) sampling, imaging, and whole-body radiation measurements.

8. What are some commonly used radiopharmaceutical therapies?

Table 84-1 lists some of the most common currently available radiopharmaceuticals as well as their approval status in the US.

## KEY POINTS

- Therapeutic radiopharmaceuticals permit radiation delivery regardless of number and location of sites of disease.
- Radioiodine therapy of thyroid disease is the most widely used radiopharmaceutical therapy and in many ways fostered the birth of nuclear medicine.
- Various therapeutic radiopharmaceuticals are in clinical use worldwide, with many more at earlier investigational stages.
- The dose-limiting toxicity of most radiopharmaceutical therapies is bone marrow suppression.

**BIBLIOGRAPHY**

Cheng W, Ma C, Fu H, et al. Low- or high-dose radioiodine remnant ablation for differentiated thyroid carcinoma: a meta-analysis. *J Clin Endocrinol Metab.* 2013;98(4):1353-1360.

Ho AL, Grewal RK, Leboeuf R, et al. Selumetinib-enhanced radioiodine uptake in advanced thyroid cancer. *N Engl J Med.* 2013;368(7):623-632.

Parker C, Nilsson S, Heinrich D, et al. Alpha emitter radium-223 and survival in metastatic prostate cancer. *N Engl J Med.* 2013;369(3):213-223.

Tuttle RM, Sabra MM. Selective use of RAI for ablation and adjuvant therapy after total thyroidectomy for differentiated thyroid cancer: a practical approach to clinical decision making. *Oral Oncol.* 2013;49(7):676-683.

Giammarile F, Bodei L, Chiesa C, et al. EANM procedure guideline for the treatment of liver cancer and liver metastases with intra-arterial radioactive compounds. *Eur J Nucl Med Mol Imaging.* 2011;38(7):1393-1406.

American Thyroid Association Guidelines Taskforce on Thyroid N, Differentiated Thyroid C, Cooper DS, et al. Revised American Thyroid Association management guidelines for patients with thyroid nodules and differentiated thyroid cancer. *Thyroid.* 2009;19(11):1167-1214.

Gray B, Van Hazel G, Hope M, et al. Randomised trial of SIR-Spheres plus chemotherapy vs. chemotherapy alone for treating patients with liver metastases from primary large bowel cancer. *Ann Oncol.* 2001;12(12):1711-1720.

Benua RS, Cicale NR, Sonenberg M, et al. The relation of radioiodine dosimetry to results and complications in the treatment of metastatic thyroid cancer. *Am J Roentgenol Radium Ther Nucl Med.* 1962;87:171-182.

# XII
# PEDIATRIC RADIOLOGY

# CHAPTER 85

# PEDIATRIC THORACIC RADIOLOGY

*Mesha L.D. Martinez, MD, and D. Andrew Mong, MD*

1. What is the embryologic relationship between the lungs and the gastrointestinal tract?

   The lung bud is an outpouching of the primitive foregut, appearing during the fourth week of development.

2. Describe the histologic stages of lung development.

   The lung bud progressively branches during embryologic development, undergoing a pseudoglandular stage (weeks 5 to 17), a canalicular stage (weeks 16 to 25), a terminal sac stage (weeks 25 to 40), and an alveolar stage that begins late in fetal life and continues until approximately 8 years of age.

3. Describe the pertinent findings on a normal neonatal chest radiograph.

   The appearance of the thymus is variable. The "sail" sign refers to the thymus creating a triangular shadow of soft tissue along the mediastinal border on chest x-ray.

   Always check for the side of the aortic arch (normally left sided); this may be difficult to do in newborns, and the side of the aortic arch may need to be inferred by observing that the descending aorta runs to the left of the spine and that the trachea is mildly deviated to the right.

   Look at heart size. In contrast to adults, the normal cardiac-thoracic ratio may be 60%. The apex of the heart should be on the left (i.e., levocardia).

   Pulmonary vascularity should be assessed. This assessment may be difficult, but some clues to increased vascularity include seeing vessels behind the liver density or noting that the right descending pulmonary artery is larger in diameter than the trachea.

   Look at the bones (especially the vertebrae for any segmental anomalies), and note whether the humeral heads have ossified (this happens at 40 weeks of gestation).

   Look under the diaphragm for organomegaly and the position of the stomach bubble (normally in the left upper quadrant.)

   Since you are generally not going to forget to look at the lung fields, try to do that last to make sure they are clear.

4. What is the correct location of umbilical arterial and venous catheters on radiographs?

   The umbilical arterial catheter (UAC) should terminate below the L3 vertebra or at the level of the T6 through T9 vertebrae to prevent catheter occlusion of branch vessels arising from the aorta. The umbilical venous catheter (UVC) should terminate at the inferior cavoatrial junction; passage into the right atrium or projection of the catheter over the liver requires repositioning.

   The UAC can be identified by its initial inferior extension into the pelvis as it courses from the umbilicus via one of the paired umbilical arteries into an internal iliac artery before it turns to ascend within a common iliac artery and abdominal aorta to the left of the spine. The UVC courses posteriorly from the umbilicus via the umbilical vein through the left portal vein and ductus venosus into the inferior vena cava, where it then ascends to the right of the spine.

5. What is surfactant, and why is it important?

   Surfactant is produced by type II pneumocytes. It is a complex substance containing phospholipids and apoproteins, which acts to reduce surface tension and prevent alveolar collapse. Lack of sufficient surfactant in prematurity leads to diffuse microatelectasis and respiratory distress syndrome (RDS).

6. What is the difference between RDS and a surfactant dysfunction?

   RDS is caused by an insufficient amount of surfactant. A surfactant dysfunction may be caused by a mutation in one of the surfactant proteins. Surfactant dysfunctions, such as from mutations in surfactant proteins B, C, or ABCA3, can have a variety of radiologic manifestations in the lungs, including diffuse ground glass opacities, cysts, crazy-paving, or even (as a late manifestation) fibrosis on computed tomography (CT). Surfactant dysfunction may also occur in the setting of meconium aspiration.

7. How does RDS appear radiographically?

   The radiographic appearance of RDS is a diffuse, symmetric, or patchy ground glass appearance to the lung parenchyma with low lung volumes (Figure 85-1).

8. How is RDS treated, and what are the potential complications?

   Maternal corticosteroids are administered intramuscularly and have been shown to promote surfactant production if preterm delivery is imminent. Exogenous (intratracheal) surfactant administered to the neonate is also beneficial. Infants requiring intubation may develop complications such as air leaks in the form of pneumothoraces; pneumomediastinum; or pulmonary interstitial emphysema (PIE), which appears as linear interstitial lucencies.

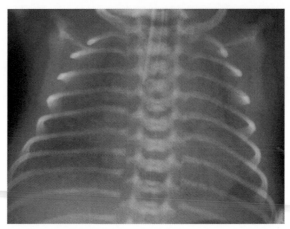

**Figure 85-1.** RDS on frontal chest radiograph. Note diffuse ground glass opacity in lungs and low lung volumes in this premature infant. *(Courtesy of Richard Markowitz, MD, Children's Hospital of Philadelphia.)*

Long-term consequences of barotrauma and increased oxygen exposure include neonatal chronic lung disease, which may manifest as diffuse interstitial thickening and hyperaeration.

9. In addition to RDS, what are some other neonatal diffuse lung diseases?
   - Transient tachypnea of the newborn (TTN).
   - Congestive heart failure (CHF).
   - Neonatal pneumonia.
   - Meconium aspiration.

10. How might other neonatal diffuse lung diseases be differentiated clinically?
    Neonatal pneumonia and CHF may occur in preterm or term infants, whereas meconium aspiration and TTN are generally diseases of term infants. Neonatal pneumonia occurs more frequently when there is prolonged premature rupture of membranes (PROM). Neonatal CHF is often related to structural heart disease and is often seen in association with cardiomegaly.

11. What is the mechanism behind meconium aspiration, and how does it appear radiographically?
    Perinatal hypoxia may lead to a deep gasping reflex and premature passage of meconium, which combine to cause aspiration. Meconium aspiration may cause lung hyperaeration (sometimes the sole radiographic appearance), scattered areas of atelectasis, and ropelike perihilar opacities with a coarse interstitial pattern.

12. What is the mechanism behind TTN, and how does it appear radiographically?
    TTN occurs when amniotic fluid is not fully removed from the lungs during delivery and is more commonly encountered in infants delivered by cesarean section compared to vaginal delivery. Radiographically, TTN appears with increased interstitial markings and pleural effusions which resolve within 2 days.

13. What is neuroendocrine cell hyperplasia of infancy (NEHI), and how does it present clinically and radiographically?
    NEHI is a poorly understood entity with an increased number of neuroendocrine cells seen in the lung tissue at biopsy. Patients often present with persistent tachypnea and hypoxia. Radiographs are often nonspecific but may show hyperinflation with perihilar opacities. CT scans often show characteristic ground glass opacities in the right middle lobe and lingula or in a paraspinal distribution. Identifying these patterns and suggesting the diagnosis may eliminate the need for biopsy. Mosaic attenuation of the lungs due to air trapping can also be seen. The disease is usually self-limited and does not respond to corticosteroids.

14. What are alveolar growth disorders, and what is their CT appearance?
    Alveolar growth disorders are those caused by entities that limit alveolarization of the lung. Prenatal causes include congenital diaphragmatic hernia (CDH), abdominal wall defects, neuromuscular disorders, and chromosomal disorders. The most common postnatal cause is chronic lung disease of prematurity from prolonged intubation. Chest x-ray findings are often nonspecific but may show areas of air trapping and lucency in the lungs. Because of lobular simplification in the lungs, CT may show areas of decreased attenuation and decreased internal architecture in the lung parenchyma.

15. What are the major (prenatally diagnosed) surgical diseases of the neonatal chest?
    Surgical neonatal chest disease is generally a focal process and includes entities such as CDH, congenital pulmonary airway malformation (CPAM) (previously known as congenital cystic adenomatoid malformation [CCAM]), pulmonary sequestration, and congenital lobar emphysema (CLE). Although these entities may appear solid at birth, CDH, CPAM,

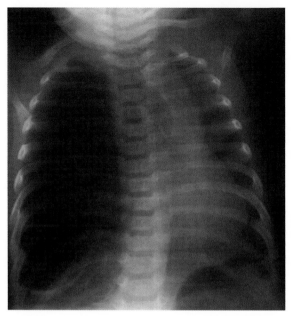

**Figure 85-2.** CPAM on frontal chest radiograph. Note hyperaeration and hyperlucency of right lung along with multiple air-filled lung cysts and leftward mediastinal shift. *(Courtesy of Richard Markowitz, MD, Children's Hospital of Philadelphia.)*

and CLE usually aerate over time. Pulmonary sequestrations and certain types of CPAM generally remain solid unless there is superinfection (Figure 85-2).

16. **What is the most common cause of a neonatal pleural effusion?**
    A chylothorax is the most common cause of a neonatal pleural effusion. The etiologic factor is uncertain but may be secondary to birth trauma of the thoracic duct. This is typically treated conservatively, with drainage of the effusion and administration of a medium-chain triglyceride diet.

17. **Describe how chlamydial pneumonia manifests clinically and radiographically.**
    Chlamydial pneumonia is a disease of neonates, usually manifesting within the first 2 weeks of life, often with associated conjunctivitis. Chest radiographs usually show lung hyperinflation and ill-defined linear markings, sometimes creating a shaggy appearance of the cardiac border.

18. **What are the pulmonary and extrapulmonary manifestations of cystic fibrosis?**
    Cystic fibrosis is an autosomal recessive disorder of abnormal chloride ion transport, which results in backup of thick mucus secretions in various organs. In the lungs, cystic fibrosis manifests as repeated infections that result in bronchiectasis, predominantly in the upper lobes. On chest radiographs, bronchiectasis may appear as multiple lucent holes or tram-track opacities, which may be fluid filled. Areas of atelectasis or lung hyperaeration may also be seen. On CT, bronchiectasis is generally present when bronchi are larger in diameter than the adjacent pulmonary arteries or extend to within 1 cm of the pleural surface. Some extrapulmonary manifestations include neonatal meconium ileus (small bowel obstruction at the terminal ileum from inspissated meconium), chronic pancreatitis, and cirrhosis. An enlarged spleen may result from portal hypertension and may manifest on a chest radiograph with medial deviation of the stomach bubble in the left upper quadrant.

19. **What are the findings of primary tuberculosis of the lungs in a pediatric patient?**
    The findings of primary tuberculosis are nonspecific, as in an adult, but can include mediastinal or hilar lymphadenopathy or both, pulmonary parenchymal disease, and pleural effusion.

20. **What is acute chest syndrome?**
    Acute chest syndrome affects patients with sickle cell anemia and may present with cough, hypoxia, fever, sputum production, and shortness of breath. While the exact pathogenesis is poorly understood, it may be caused by an acute vaso-occlusive crisis in the pulmonary parenchyma or adjacent ribs. Radiographically, areas of pulmonary opacification are typically seen with a basilar predominance, which may be secondary to edema, infarction, fat embolism, and/or infection, sometimes in association with pleural effusion.

21. **What is lymphocytic interstitial pneumonia (LIP)?**
    LIP is a lymphoproliferative response in the chest, often in children with human immunodeficiency virus (HIV) infection. On chest radiography, a diffuse reticulonodular pattern with central predominance may be seen along with bilateral

hilar lymphadenopathy, although peribronchiolar thickening alone or a normal appearance may also be encountered. On CT, multiple perilymphatic interstitial micronodules are typically visualized. This pattern is more common in children whereas in adults, thin-walled air-filled cysts and pulmonary ground glass opacities are more often encountered.

22. How is a suspected aspirated foreign body evaluated?

A nonradiopaque aspirated foreign body in a mainstem bronchus may produce a ball-valve effect, trapping air unilaterally in the lung and creating a large lucent lung compared with the contralateral normal side. These findings may be subtle, but if suspected, expiratory radiographs may make them more obvious because the unaffected lung would lose volume, whereas the affected lung would not. Decubitus radiographs may also exaggerate this difference and are helpful if the patient cannot sit upright, with the unaffected lung losing volume when it is in the dependent position. Pulmonary air trapping may also be shown by fluoroscopy.

23. What is Swyer-James syndrome?

The hypothesized pathogenesis of Swyer-James syndrome involves a viral infection that arrests growth of an affected lung through an obliterative bronchiolitis. Hyperlucency from air trapping and diminished arterial flow results. Traditionally, this was thought to be a unilateral process, but CT examinations often show scattered areas of bilateral pulmonary air trapping.

24. What are the most common causes of metastasis to the lung in the pediatric patient?

Osteosarcoma, Ewing sarcoma, rhabdomyosarcoma, hepatoblastoma, Wilms' tumor, gonadal germ cell tumor, and thyroid carcinoma.

25. What are some mediastinal masses one might see in the pediatric patient?

- In the anterior mediastinum: Normal thymus, thymic cyst, thymic lipoma, germ cell tumor, lymphoma, and lymphatic malformations.
- In the middle mediastinum: Foregut duplication cysts, lymphadenopathy, and lymphatic malformations.
- In the posterior mediastinum: Neurogenic tumors, including nerve sheath tumors, neuroblastoma, and ganglioneuroblastoma, and lymphatic malformations.

26. What are important structures to identify on a lateral radiograph of the pediatric neck?

- Assess the prevertebral soft tissues. Soft tissue swelling in this area could be due to retropharyngeal abscess, edema, hematoma, or soft tissue mass.
- The epiglottis should be triangular or flat in configuration, not bulbous or thumblike (which would indicate acute epiglottitis), and the aryepiglottic folds should not be thickened. Acute epiglottitis is related to inflammation of the epiglottis and aryepiglottic folds, usually due to *Haemophilus influenzae* infection, and most commonly occurs in children 3 to 6 years of age. This is a medical emergency due to acute airway obstruction and is treated with early intubation along with medical therapy (Figure 85-3).
- Look for enlargement of the adenoidal tissue and tonsils.
- Assess the caliber of the trachea, which should not change abruptly.
- You may identify sloughed membranes within the tracheal lumen when bacterial tracheitis is present.
- A frontal radiograph is often useful in identifying croup, also known as acute laryngotracheobronchitis, which is due to a viral infection and characterized by symmetric subglottic narrowing that creates the "steeple" sign due to edema of the subglottic tissues (Figure 85-4).

27. What is congenital high airway obstruction syndrome (CHAOS), and why is it important to diagnose prenatally?

CHAOS is caused by an obstruction of the upper airway, either intrinsic (from atresia) or extrinsic (from a congenital mass). Imaging with ultrasonography (US) or fetal magnetic resonance imaging (MRI) demonstrates large lungs with an abnormal configuration of the diaphragm (convex down) and a dilated fluid-filled trachea to the level of obstruction. Ascites and/or hydrops fetalis may also be present. It is important to identify this disorder prenatally because a tracheostomy may be placed below the level of obstruction by a fetal surgical team during delivery (while placental circulation is maintained) if the diagnosis is known. It is also critical to diagnose the level of the obstruction, as an obstruction that is too low in the trachea may preclude placement of a tracheostomy.

---

**KEY POINTS**

- An aspirated foreign body in a mainstem bronchus may produce a ball-valve effect, trapping air unilaterally in the lung and creating a large lucent lung compared with the contralateral normal side. Expiratory and decubitus radiographs are useful to accentuate the presence of unilateral pulmonary air trapping.
- The epiglottis should be triangular or flat in configuration on lateral neck radiography. Recognition of a bulbous or thumblike appearance of the epiglottis indicates acute epiglottitis, which is a medical emergency.
- Croup, or acute laryngotracheobronchitis, is characterized by symmetric subglottic narrowing on frontal neck radiography leading to the "steeple" sign due to edema of the subglottic tissues.

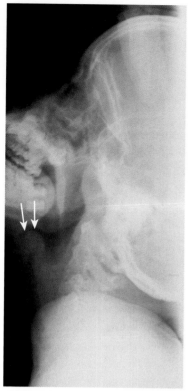

**Figure 85-3.** Acute epiglottitis on lateral neck radiograph. Note abnormal bulbous thickening of epiglottis (*arrows*). This is a medical emergency requiring early intubation. *(Courtesy of Richard Markowitz, MD, Children's Hospital of Philadelphia.)*

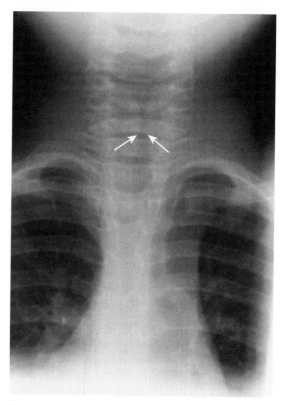

**Figure 85-4.** Croup on frontal neck radiograph. Note classic "steeple" sign (*arrows*) due to edema of subglottic tissues with narrowing of subglottic airway.

## BIBLIOGRAPHY

Pinto A, Lanza C, Pinto F, et al. Role of plain radiography in the assessment of ingested foreign bodies in the pediatric patients. *Semin Ultrasound CT MR.* 2015;36(1):21-27.

Coley BD, Bates DG, Faerber EN, et al. *Caffey's pediatric diagnostic imaging.* 12th ed. Philadelphia: Elsevier-Saunders; 2013.

Kaneda HJ, Mack J, Kasales CJ, et al. Pediatric and adolescent breast masses: a review of pathophysiology, imaging, diagnosis, and treatment. *AJR Am J Roentgenol.* 2013;200(2):W204-W212.

Schallert EK, Danton GH, Kardon R, et al. Describing congenital heart disease by using three-part segmental notation. *Radiographics.* 2013;33(2):E33-E46.

Miller AC, Gladwin MT. Pulmonary complications of sickle cell disease. *Am J Respir Crit Care Med.* 2012;185(11):1154-1165.

Dillman JR, Sanchez R, Ladino-Torres MF, et al. Expanding upon the unilateral hyperlucent hemithorax in children. *Radiographics.* 2011;31(3):723-741.

Guillerman RP, Brody AS. Contemporary perspectives on pediatric diffuse lung disease. *Radiol Clin North Am.* 2011;49(5):847-868.

Biyyam DR, Chapman T, Ferguson MR, et al. Congenital lung abnormalities: embryologic features, prenatal diagnosis, and postnatal radiologic-pathologic correlation. *Radiographics.* 2010;30(6):1721-1738.

Capps EF, Kinsella JJ, Gupta M, et al. Emergency imaging assessment of acute, nontraumatic conditions of the head and neck. *Radiographics.* 2010;30(5):1335-1352.

Lee EY, Boiselle PM, Cleveland RH. Multidetector CT evaluation of congenital lung anomalies. *Radiology.* 2008;247(3):632-648.

Brody AS, Crotty EJ. Neuroendocrine cell hyperplasia of infancy (NEHI). *Pediatr Radiol.* 2006;36(12):1328.

Agrons GA, Courtney SE, Stocker JT, et al. From the archives of the AFIP: lung disease in premature neonates: radiologic-pathologic correlation. *Radiographics.* 2005;25(4):1047-1073.

Andronikou S, Wieselthaler N, Bertelsmann J. Paediatric HRCT of the chest - help for the general radiologist. *SA J Radiology.* 2005;9(4):21-29.

Berrocal T, Madrid C, Novo S, et al. Congenital anomalies of the tracheobronchial tree, lung, and mediastinum: embryology, radiology, and pathology. *Radiographics.* 2004;24(1):e17.

Schlesinger AE, Braverman RM, DiPietro MA. Pictorial essay. Neonates and umbilical venous catheters: normal appearance, anomalous positions, complications, and potential aid to diagnosis. *AJR Am J Roentgenol.* 2003;180(4):1147-1153.

Berdon WE. Rings, slings, and other things: vascular compression of the infant trachea updated from the midcentury to the millennium—the legacy of Robert E. Gross, MD, and Edward B. D. Neuhauser, MD. *Radiology.* 2000;216(3):624-632.

Salour M. The steeple sign. *Radiology.* 2000;216(2):428-429.

Weinstein SP, Conant EF, Orel SG, et al. Spectrum of US findings in pediatric and adolescent patients with palpable breast masses. *Radiographics.* 2000;20(6):1613-1621.

Alford BA, McIlhenny J. An approach to the asymmetric neonatal chest radiograph. *Radiol Clin North Am.* 1999;37(6):1079-1092.

Strife JL, Sze RW. Radiographic evaluation of the neonate with congenital heart disease. *Radiol Clin North Am.* 1999;37(6):1093-1107, vi.

Gibson AT, Steiner GM. Imaging the neonatal chest. *Clin Radiol.* 1997;52(3):172-186.

# CHAPTER 86

# PEDIATRIC CARDIOVASCULAR RADIOLOGY

*Mesha L.D. Martinez, MD, and D. Andrew Mong, MD*

1. **What are some of the most common types of congenital heart disease (CHD) in order of frequency (most common to least common)?**
   Bicuspid aortic valve, ventricular septal defect (VSD), atrial septal defect (ASD), patent ductus arteriosus (PDA), tetralogy of Fallot, coarctation of the aorta, and transposition of the great vessels.

2. **How does assessment of pulmonary blood flow aid in the diagnosis of cyanotic disease?**
   The first consideration in diagnosing CHD is whether the infant is clinically cyanotic. Cyanosis may be secondary to admixture of oxygenated and deoxygenated blood, which can appear as increased blood flow to the heart with enlargement of the pulmonary arteries, or may be secondary to blood shunted away from the lungs, which would appear as decreased blood flow with small to absent pulmonary arteries. Assessment of blood flow includes looking for shunt vessels at the periphery of the lung fields or behind the liver shadow.

3. **Which types of CHD appear with cyanosis and increased pulmonary blood flow?**
   These conditions include total anomalous pulmonary venous return (TAPVR), truncus arteriosus, transposition of the great vessels (d-TGV), tricuspid atresia, and single ventricle. Hypoplastic left heart syndrome (HLHS) may also appear with congestive heart failure (CHF) and cyanosis.

4. **How is HLHS corrected surgically?**
   In HLHS, the left-sided cardiac structures (usually the left ventricle and aortic root) are hypoplastic. The right ventricle is surgically recruited to become the systemic pumping ventricle. A neoaortic root is fashioned from the pulmonary outflow track and anastomosed to the aortic arch, an atrial septectomy is performed, and a shunt is temporarily created between the subclavian artery and pulmonary arteries (Norwood procedure). Systemic venous return is subsequently diverted directly to the branch pulmonary arteries through a Glenn procedure (superior vena cava to pulmonary arteries) and a Fontan completion (inferior vena cava to pulmonary arteries.)

5. **What is congenitally corrected transposition of the great vessels, and why is it a problem?**
   In congenitally corrected transposition of the great vessels (l-TGV), there is an abnormal (L) ventricular loop, but there is also an abnormal (−150 degree) rotation of the great vessels. This leads to the following circuits: (1) systemic venous return-right atrium-left ventricle-pulmonary artery and (2) pulmonary venous return-left atrium-right ventricle-aorta. Although systemic and pulmonary blood flow circuits are "corrected" congenitally, this places abnormal stress on the right ventricle, which must pump blood against systemic pressures.

6. **What are the most common acyanotic types of CHD?**
   Acyanosis implies a left-to-right shunt, and the most common causes include ASD, VSD, PDA, and endocardial cushion defects. These typically cause enlargement of specific chambers in the heart as a result of decompression of some chambers and overload in others.
   A VSD, due to a communication between the right ventricle and left ventricle, results in an enlarged right ventricle, main pulmonary artery, and left atrium, sometimes with left ventricular dilation as well.
   An ASD, due to a communication between the right atrium and left atrium, results in an enlarged right atrium, right ventricle, and main pulmonary artery, with a normal-sized left atrium as blood is shunted away from it.
   A PDA, due to persistent patency of the ductus arteriosus between the aorta and pulmonary artery, results in an enlarged main pulmonary artery, left atrium, and left ventricle.
   An endocardial cushion defect, due to defects in the atrial septum, ventricular septum, and one or more atrioventricular valves, results in an enlarged right atrium, right ventricle, and pulmonary artery, along with variable enlargement of the left atrium and left ventricle. This is the most common cardiac anomaly in patients with Down syndrome.

7. **What is the role of the radiologist in assessing suspected CHD?**
   Although magnetic resonance imaging (MRI) or computed tomography (CT) examination of the heart may be used to assess cardiac chamber size and position, wall thickness, presence of intracardiac shunts, and position of the coronary arteries, the initial role of the radiologist is to evaluate the chest radiograph and to provide an ordered, logical differential diagnosis. It is usually impossible to give a precise diagnosis in these cases initially.

8. **What are some classic patterns of CHD seen on radiographs?**
   - **Transposition of the great vessels**: "egg on a string" sign due to narrowing of the superior mediastinum (creating the "string") related to stress-related thymic atrophy, lung hyperinflation, and abnormal relationship of the great

vessels, along with abnormal convexity of the right atrial contour and left atrial enlargement (creating the "egg" on its side). This condition is due to ventriculoarterial discordance, where the aorta arises from the right ventricle and the pulmonary artery arises from the left ventricle.

- **Tetralogy of Fallot**: "boot-shaped heart" due to uplifting of the cardiac apex caused by right ventricular hypertrophy and a convex margin where the shadow of the main pulmonary artery should be. Associated decreased pulmonary vascularity is also typically seen. This condition is the most common cyanotic CHD of childhood and has four characteristic features: right ventricular outflow tract obstruction, an overriding aorta, a VSD, and right ventricular hypertrophy.
- **Ebstein anomaly**: "box-shaped heart" due to marked cardiac, in particular right atrial, enlargement and abnormal left cardiac contour related to displacement of the right ventricular outflow tract. This condition is due to atrialization of a portion of the right ventricle caused by an abnormal tricuspid valve.
- **TAPVR (type 1)**: "snowman" sign (or "figure of 8" sign) where a dilated vertical pulmonary vein on the left, innominate vein on the top, and superior vena cava form the "head" of the snowman, and an enlarged heart, including an enlarged right atrium, form the "body" of the snowman.
- **Partial anomalous pulmonary venous return (PAPVR) (venolobar type)**: "scimitar" sign as described below.

9. Name the major causes of CHF in a newborn.
Transient tachypnea of the newborn (TTN) may look like CHF on a chest radiograph but is transient. Causes of CHF in a newborn include constitutional problems, such as anemia, hypoglycemia, or sepsis; primary pump problems, such as HLHS; outflow obstructions, such as aortic stenosis or coarctation of the aorta; inflow problems, such as cor triatriatum or mitral valve stenosis; and extracardiac shunts, such as a vein of Galen malformation or a hepatic hemangioendothelioma.

10. Define the concept of situs.
Situs refers to the "sidedness" of the body. A normal situs, situs solitus, indicates that right-sided structures are found on the right side of the body, and left-sided structures are found on the left side of the body. In situs inversus, there is an abnormal mirror image appearance, with left-sided structures found on the right side of the body and vice versa. Situs ambiguous refers to heterotaxy syndromes in which visceral and thoracic organs are ambiguously mixed in their positions, usually with bilateral right-sidedness (asplenia) or bilateral left-sidedness (polysplenia). Heterotaxy syndromes usually include cardiac malformations, gut rotational abnormalities (malrotation), and vascular abnormalities.

11. What is segmental classification of CHD?
Segmental classification is a systematic approach to description of CHD and utilizes a three-letter designation. The first letter refers to visceroatrial situs. A normal situs solitus (S) includes the right atrium on the right and the left atrium on the left, as opposed to situs inversus (I). The second letter refers to the cardiac loop. A normal (D) loop indicates the right ventricle is on the right, while an abnormal (L) loop indicates that the right ventricle is on the left. The third letter refers to ventriculoatrial situs. In normal (S) situs, the aorta has rotated 150 degrees counterclockwise during cardiac development to connect with the left ventricle, while the pulmonary artery connects with the right ventricle. Abnormalities of this rotation can lead to transposition of the great vessels (TGV) or malposition of the great vessels (MGV). A normal segmental notation would therefore be (S, D, S).

12. What are the most common benign pediatric cardiac/pericardial tumors?
Rhabdomyoma is the most common primary tumor of the heart and a more common cardiac tumor found in patients with tuberous sclerosis. Fibroma is the second most common tumor. Other tumors include fibroelastomas, hemangiomas, and lipomas, which are all rare in the pediatric patient. Myxomas are rare in children. Teratomas are the most common tumor of the pericardium.

13. What are the most common malignant pediatric cardiac/pericardial tumors?
Metastases are the most common malignant tumors of the heart and pericardium and may include leukemia, lymphoma, Wilms tumor, hepatoblastoma, neuroblastoma, Ewing sarcoma, and osteosarcoma.

14. What is a vascular ring?
A vascular ring is a ring of vessels that surrounds the trachea. This may be caused by a right-sided aortic arch with an aberrant left subclavian artery, with the ring completed by the ligamentum arteriosum. A double aortic arch is also a cause of a vascular ring (Figure 86-1). Vascular rings may present with stridor and can be misdiagnosed as asthma, croup, or other conditions. Attention to the appearance of the aortic arch on chest radiographs may suggest the diagnosis.

15. What is the importance of a right-sided aortic arch?
A right-sided arch may be associated with mirror-image branching, an aberrant left subclavian artery, or an isolated left subclavian artery. It may also be associated with tetralogy of Fallot or truncus arteriosus. If you see a right-sided aortic arch, look for other anomalies and consider recommending echocardiography.

16. What is a pulmonary artery sling?
A pulmonary sling arises when the left pulmonary artery (LPA) arises anomalously from the posterior right pulmonary artery, creating an abnormal LPA course posterior to the trachea and anterior to the esophagus (Figure 86-2). This is

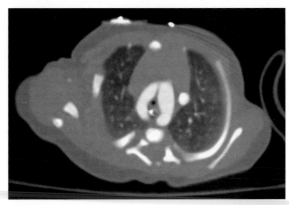

**Figure 86-1.** Double aortic arch on CT. Note aortic arches on both sides of trachea, which appears diminutive in caliber.

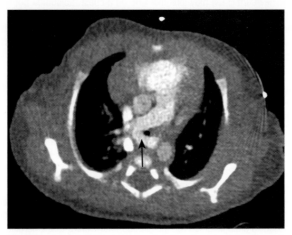

**Figure 86-2.** Pulmonary sling on CT. Note anomalous left pulmonary artery (*arrow*) arising from right pulmonary artery coursing posterior to trachea.

associated with presence of complete cartilaginous tracheal rings and tracheomalacia, which are often associated with symptoms including wheezing and respiratory distress (Figure 86-3).

17. **What are MAPCAs?**
    MAPCAs stands for **m**ajor **a**orto-**p**ulmonary **c**ollateral **a**rteries. These can arise when there is compromise of pulmonary blood flow in CHD, often tetralogy of Fallot or pulmonary atresia with ventricular septal defect. CT or MRI may identify suspected MAPCAs arising from the aorta to supply the lungs (Figure 86-4). Unrestricted MAPCAs may lead to pulmonary congestion and heart failure. Treatment may include "unifocalization," which includes detachment of the origins of MAPCAs and reanastomosis to the central pulmonary arteries.

18. **What is the difference between TAPVR and scimitar syndrome?**
    In TAPVR, all of the pulmonary veins empty into the systemic venous circulation instead of the left atrium, creating increased pulmonary blood flow and cyanosis. Scimitar syndrome, or pulmonary venolobar syndrome, is considered to be a type of PAPVR. A characteristic "scimitar" sign is seen on a chest radiograph, where a curvilinear opacity due to an anomalous right pulmonary vein extends inferiorly to the cardiophrenic angle to drain into the inferior vena cava or other systemic venous structure (Figure 86-5).

19. **What is meant by a malignant course of an anomalous coronary artery?**
    While there are many coronary artery anomalies that may be asymptomatic, an "interarterial" course of a coronary artery, with the right or left coronary artery extending between the aortic root and the pulmonary arterial trunk, may lead to extrinsic compression of the artery that can lead to cardiac ischemia, cardiac dysrhythmias, and sudden death.

20. **What are the two main types of coarctation of the aorta?**
    Coarctation of the aorta is a focal flow-limiting narrowing of the aorta which can be either preductal (located upstream from the ductus arteriosus) or postductal (located downstream from the ductus arteriosus). In preductal coarctation, blood flow to the distal aorta is dependent on a patent ductus arteriosus and can therefore be life-threatening when the ductus arteriosus closes. Preductal coarctation is associated with Turner's syndrome. Postductal (adult) coarctation

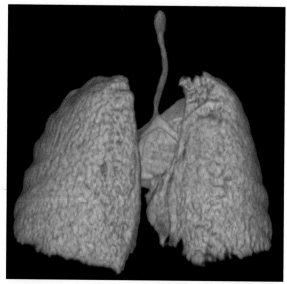

**Figure 86-3.** Pulmonary sling on CT. Coronal 3D reconstruction of airways and lungs demonstrates narrowing of trachea due to complete tracheal rings.

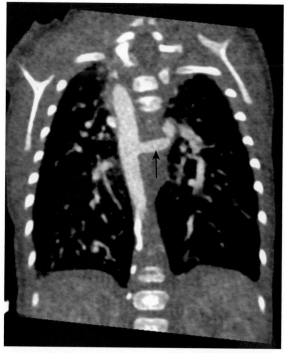

**Figure 86-4.** MAPCA on CT. Note large systemic arterial vascular structure (*arrow*) arising abnormally from left lateral wall of descending thoracic aorta and extending to left pulmonary hilum in this patient with tetralogy of Fallot.

usually presents in older children or adults with differential blood pressures noted, greater in the upper extremities compared to the lower extremities. Blood flow to the aorta distal to the coarctation may occur through intercostal arteries, creating inferior rib notching on chest radiograph. Sometimes, a "figure 3" sign may be seen on the frontal chest radiograph, where the upper left mediastinal contour has a bilobed configuration due to dilation of the aortic arch and left subclavian artery upstream to the site of coarctation, focal indentation of the aorta at the site of coarctation, and poststenotic dilation of the descending thoracic aorta.

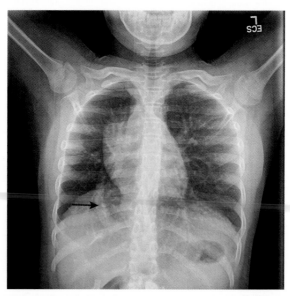

**Figure 86-5.** Scimitar syndrome on chest radiograph. Note characteristic "scimitar" sign due to anomalous pulmonary vein (*arrow*) at right lung base extending below diaphragm along with congenitally small right lung.

21. What is a bicuspid aortic valve (BAV)?

This is the most common congenital cardiovascular abnormality, with a prevalence of up to 2% in the general population and occurring more commonly in males. This includes a spectrum of aortic valve deformities where either two (rather than three normal) cusps are present, or three developmental anlagen of cusps and commissures are present where two adjacent cusps fuse into a single aberrant cusp with development of a ridge or raphe. A BAV is associated with an increased risk of aortic stenosis, aortic regurgitation, infective endocarditis, ascending aortic aneurysm formation, and aortic dissection due to coexistent aortopathy and is also associated with coarctation of the aorta, PDA, and coronary artery anomalies.

On CT, a BAV may be seen as having two cusps of equal size and two commissures (i.e., hinge points), along with a typical "fish-mouth"–shaped aortic valve orifice during systole and a single line of coaptation during diastole. Alternatively, two of three underdeveloped cusps of the aortic valve may be seen to be conjoined with formation of a raphe, which are together larger in size than the third uninvolved cusp. Calcification of the raphe or valve leaflets may also be present and is sometimes visible on a chest radiograph.

22. What are some of the major causes of pediatric pulmonary hypertension, and what are the major associated CT features?

Causes of pediatric pulmonary hypertension may include: chronic lung disease of prematurity, CHD, sickle cell disease, chronic pulmonary emboli, and causes of left-sided heart failure (such as pulmonary vein stenosis). Findings on CT include: right ventricular hypertrophy, enlargement of the main pulmonary artery (greater in caliber than the ascending aorta at the same level), and flattening or bowing of the interventricular septum toward the left ventricle.

23. What is Eisenmenger syndrome?

Eisenmenger syndrome is a complication of untreated high-pressure or high-flow CHD in which chronic pulmonary hypertension and shunt reversal (from left-to-right to right-to-left) occur. This is most often seen with VSD, endocardial cushion defect, and PDA and usually develops before puberty, although it may develop in adolescence or early adulthood. The imaging features are similar to those that occur due to pulmonary hypertension.

## KEY POINTS

- Segmental classification is a systematic approach to description of CHD, which utilizes a three-letter designation. A normal segmental notation is (S, D, S).
- Tetralogy of Fallot is the most common cyanotic CHD of childhood and has four characteristic features: right ventricular outflow tract obstruction, an overriding aorta, a VSD, and right ventricular hypertrophy.
- A malignant or "interarterial" course of an anomalous coronary artery between the aortic root and pulmonary arterial trunk may lead to extrinsic compression of the artery, potentially resulting in sudden death.

## BIBLIOGRAPHY

Karaosmanoglu AD, Khawaja RD, Onur MR, et al. CT and MRI of aortic coarctation: pre- and postsurgical findings. *AJR Am J Roentgenol.* 2015;204(3):W224-W233.

Schallert EK, Danton GH, Kardon R, et al. Describing congenital heart disease by using three-part segmental notation. *Radiographics.* 2013;33(2):E33-E46.

Roest AA, de Roos A. Imaging of patients with congenital heart disease. *Nat Rev Cardiol.* 2012;9(2):101-115.

Shriki JE, Shinbane JS, Rashid MA, et al. Identifying, characterizing, and classifying congenital anomalies of the coronary arteries. *Radiographics.* 2012;32(2):453-468.

Browne LP, Krishnamurthy R, Chung T. Preoperative and postoperative MR evaluation of congenital heart disease in children. *Radiol Clin North Am.* 2011;49(5):1011-1024.

Ntsinjana HN, Hughes ML, Taylor AM. The role of cardiovascular magnetic resonance in pediatric congenital heart disease. *J Cardiovasc Magn Reson.* 2011;13:51.

Walsh R, Nielsen JC, Ko HH, et al. Imaging of congenital coronary artery anomalies. *Pediatr Radiol.* 2011;41(12):1526-1535.

Alkadhi H, Leschka S, Trindade PT, et al. Cardiac CT for the differentiation of bicuspid and tricuspid aortic valves: comparison with echocardiography and surgery. *AJR Am J Roentgenol.* 2010;195(4):900-908.

Dillman JR, Hernandez RJ. Role of CT in the evaluation of congenital cardiovascular disease in children. *AJR Am J Roentgenol.* 2009;192(5):1219-1231.

Ghosh S, Yarmish G, Godelman A, et al. Anomalies of visceroatrial situs. *AJR Am J Roentgenol.* 2009;193(4):1107-1117.

Burke A, Virmani R. Pediatric heart tumors. *Cardiovasc Pathol.* 2008;17(4):193-198.

Ferguson EC, Krishnamurthy R, Oldham SA. Classic imaging signs of congenital cardiovascular abnormalities. *Radiographics.* 2007;27(5):1323-1334.

Kellenberger CJ, Yoo SJ, Buchel ER. Cardiovascular MR imaging in neonates and infants with congenital heart disease. *Radiographics.* 2007;27(1):5-18.

Maeda E, Akahane M, Kato N, et al. Assessment of major aortopulmonary collateral arteries with multidetector-row computed tomography. *Radiat Med.* 2006;24(5):378-383.

Schweigmann G, Gassner I, Maurer K. Imaging the neonatal heart—essentials for the radiologist. *Eur J Radiol.* 2006;60(2):159-170.

Lipton MJ, Boxt LM. How to approach cardiac diagnosis from the chest radiograph. *Radiol Clin North Am.* 2004;42(3):487-495, v.

Gilkeson RC, Ciancibello L, Zahka K. Pictorial essay. Multidetector CT evaluation of congenital heart disease in pediatric and adult patients. *AJR Am J Roentgenol.* 2003;180(4):973-980.

Strife JL, Sze RW. Radiographic evaluation of the neonate with congenital heart disease. *Radiol Clin North Am.* 1999;37(6):1093-1107, vi.

# CHAPTER 87

# PEDIATRIC GASTROINTESTINAL RADIOLOGY

*Michael L. Francavilla, MD, Kerry Bron, MD, and Avrum N. Pollock, MD*

1. **What are the most common causes of small bowel obstruction in a child?**
   AAIIMM is a mnemonic that makes it easy to remember the causes:
   - A = **A**dhesions, usually post-surgical.
   - A = **A**ppendicitis.
   - I = **I**ntussusception.
   - I = **I**ncarcerated inguinal hernia.
   - M = **M**alrotation with volvulus or bands.
   - M = **M**iscellaneous, such as Meckel's diverticulum or intestinal duplication.

2. **What is intussusception?**
   Intussusception is a condition in which a proximal portion of the bowel (intussusceptum) telescopes into the adjacent distal bowel (intussuscipiens). When the inner loop and its mesentery become impacted, a small bowel obstruction results.

3. **What causes intussusception?**
   In most cases in children, the cause of intussusception is idiopathic. In less than 5% of cases, the intussusception contains a lead point, such as a polyp, a Meckel's diverticulum, or hypertrophic lymphatic tissue. Most intussusceptions are ileocolic in origin.

4. **Describe the clinical signs of intussusception.**
   The classic clinical triad of intussusception is intermittent colicky abdominal pain, currant jelly stools, and a palpable abdominal mass. However, less than 50% of patients actually present with these symptoms. Children often cry and are very irritable during bouts of abdominal pain, and then become drowsy and lethargic. Vomiting and fever may also occur. Intussusception is most common in children 3 months to 4 years of age, with a peak incidence occurring at 3 to 9 months of age, and occurs more commonly in boys.

5. **How is intussusception diagnosed with imaging?**
   The most accurate imaging technique for the diagnosis of intussusception is ultrasonography (US). The characteristic US appearance is an easily detectable mass measuring in the range of 3 to 5 cm. In the transverse plane, the mass has a "target" appearance (which contains echogenic fat), while the "pseudokidney" sign is how it will appear in the longitudinal plane. A contrast enema (utilizing water-soluble contrast material or air) with fluoroscopy can also be used to diagnose intussusception. Although conventional radiographs have been used in the past to diagnose intussusception via occasional detection of a soft tissue mass in the right upper quadrant with associated lack of a large amount of bowel gas, studies have shown poor interobserver agreement and a predictive value of only approximately 50%.

6. **How is an intussusception treated?**
   An intussusception is treated by air or hydrostatic enema using barium or water-soluble contrast material (the latter is favored) under fluoroscopic guidance (Figure 87-1). Some radiologists will attempt to perform the reduction under US guidance during a water-soluble contrast enema, with final confirmation of reduction with a single overhead frontal radiograph obtained on the fluoroscopy table. The advantages of the air enema are that it is quicker, less messy, and easier to perform and delivers less radiation to the patient. The only contraindications to enema reduction of intussusception are presence of pneumoperitoneum or peritonitis. The air enema can generate pressures of up to 120 to 140 mm Hg in order to reduce the intussusceptions, but pressure above this is to be avoided in order to prevent iatrogenic perforation.

7. **How can one tell that an intussusception has been successfully reduced?**
   If a successful air reduction has been performed, fluid with air bubbles should be seen passing through the ileocecal valve into the terminal ileum. If a successful reduction with contrast material has been performed, contrast material must reflux into multiple loops of small bowel. If reflux into the small bowel is not seen, the intussusception may not have been completely reduced, and a distal lead point may have been overlooked. A "pseudomass" may remain in the region of the edematous ileocecal valve despite successful reduction, not to be mistaken for a residual intussusception.

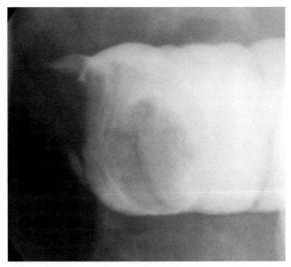

**Figure 87-1.** Intussusception on contrast enema spot radiograph. Note filling defect in bowel outlined by contrast material.

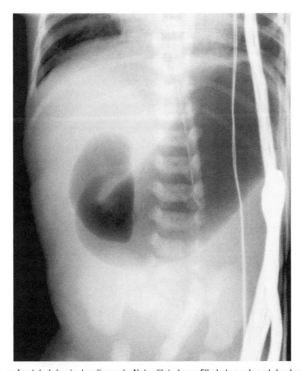

**Figure 87-2.** Duodenal atresia on frontal abdominal radiograph. Note dilated gas-filled stomach and duodenal bulb indicating "double bubble" sign.

8. Describe the "double bubble" sign, and name the conditions in which it is found.

   The "double bubble" sign is found on radiographs and represents an air-filled or fluid-filled distended stomach and duodenal bulb (Figure 87-2). It may be seen in bowel malrotation, duodenal atresia, and jejunal atresia but is usually the sine qua non of duodenal atresia.

9. What is malrotation of the intestines?

   Malrotation of the intestines is a misnomer because it is really nonrotation or incomplete rotation of the bowel. To understand malrotation, one must first consider normal embryologic rotation of the intestines. During normal embryologic development in the first trimester, the midgut leaves the abdominal cavity, travels into the umbilicus (umbilical cord), and subsequently returns to the abdominal cavity. As the intestines return, the proximal and distal parts of the midgut rotate around the superior mesenteric artery axis by 270 degrees in a counterclockwise direction. The ligament of Treitz (duodenojejunal junction) lands in the left upper quadrant, and the cecum comes to rest in the right lower quadrant. In malrotation, this intestinal rotation and fixation occur abnormally. If normal rotation does not occur, the cecum is not anchored in the right lower quadrant and may be in the midline or in the upper abdomen, and the small bowel is not anchored in the left upper quadrant and may lie entirely in the right hemi-abdomen.

10. What are Ladd's bands?

Ladd's bands are dense peritoneal bands that develop as an attempt to affix the bowel to the abdominal wall in bowel malrotation. These may extend from the malpositioned cecum across the duodenum to the posterolateral abdomen and porta hepatis in either incomplete rotation or nonrotation, and they can cause extrinsic duodenal obstruction.

11. How does a midgut volvulus occur, and why is this a surgical emergency?

Lack of attachment of the midgut to the posterior abdominal wall allows the midgut to twist on a shortened root mesentery, which results from lack of complete rotation (Figure 87-3). This twisting is called a volvulus, and it causes small bowel obstruction with concomitant obstruction of the lymphatic and venous supply of the bowel and eventually the arterial supply. Subsequently, bowel ischemia and necrosis ensue. If it is not repaired within several hours, all of the bowel supplied by the superior mesenteric artery (second portion of the duodenum to midtransverse colon) undergoes infarction.

12. Does a patient with bowel malrotation always present with clinical symptoms?

Not all patients with bowel malrotation are symptomatic, because not all develop a midgut volvulus or extrinsic duodenal obstruction from Ladd's bands.

13. What is the clinical presentation of bowel malrotation?

Patients with incomplete rotation who have intestinal obstruction usually present within the first week or first month of life (75% of patients). They present with an acute onset of bilious vomiting, which is always to be considered a surgical emergency. Some patients present later in childhood with intermittent mechanical obstruction, which manifests as cyclic vomiting. Bowel malrotation in the remaining patients is often found incidentally when the patients are studied for other complaints.

14. Which imaging study is the standard for diagnosing bowel malrotation?

The upper gastrointestinal (UGI) examination is the standard for diagnosing malrotation. To confirm normal rotation of the bowel, the ligament of Treitz, which attaches the third and fourth parts of the duodenum, must be visualized to the

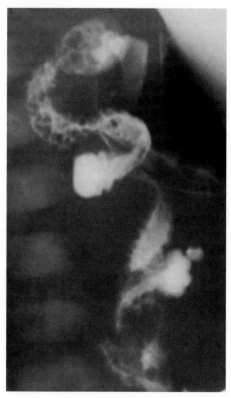

**Figure 87-3.** Midgut volvulus on UGI examination spot radiograph. Note characteristic "corkscrew" configuration of proximal small bowel.

left of midline. If there is malrotation, the ligament of Treitz may be located to the right of midline or in the midline. Often, there is also inversion of the relationship of the superior mesenteric artery and vein, which can be visualized on computed tomography (CT) or US. Some radiologists believe that this diagnosis can be made confidently utilizing US, but the overwhelming majority still regard the UGI as the standard.

15. List other anomalies that are associated with bowel malrotation.
    • Duodenal atresia or stenosis.
    • Meckel's diverticulum.
    • Omphalocele.
    • Gastroschisis.
    • Polysplenia/asplenia syndromes.
    • Situs ambiguus.
    • Bochdalek hernia.
    • Renal anomalies.

16. Describe the clinical presentation of hypertrophic pyloric stenosis (HPS).
    HPS, which is the most common gastrointestinal surgical disease of infancy in the United States, manifests most commonly during the second to sixth weeks of life, with a peak incidence at 3 weeks of age and with rare presentation after the age of 3 months. The major symptom is progressive nonbilious vomiting, which starts as simple regurgitation and progresses to projectile vomiting. This progressive vomiting leads to dehydration and hypochloremic metabolic alkalosis and weight loss. The condition is more common in boys. A palpable "olive" representing the thickened pylorus muscle is present in the right upper quadrant approximately 80% of the time if the infant can be examined in a calm manner (with decreased stomach distention).

17. If the "olive" cannot be palpated, how can HPS be diagnosed with imaging studies?
    The evaluation can begin with a supine or prone radiograph of the abdomen, which can exclude other diagnoses that could be causing similar obstructive symptoms. The radiograph may also reveal a markedly dilated stomach, a soft tissue mass projecting into the gastric antrum, and a paucity of gas in the distal bowel. The suspicion of pyloric stenosis can be confirmed with either US or fluoroscopy. US is the imaging test of choice because it directly visualizes the hypertrophied pylorus muscle without utilizing radiation (Figure 87-4), whereas a UGI examination infers the presence of pyloric stenosis indirectly. With US, the pyloric muscle is seen as a hypoechoic structure greater than 3.5 to 4.0 mm in thickness, surrounding an echogenic compressed pyloric channel. Although less sensitive, the pyloric channel length is another measurement used to make the diagnosis. A length greater than 17 mm is considered as diagnostic for HPS.

18. What is a Meckel's diverticulum?
    Meckel's diverticulum is the most common anomaly of the gastrointestinal tract. It is a persistence of the omphalomesenteric duct at its junction with the ileum. It can be remembered by the rules of 2: It occurs in 2% of the population; 2% develop complications; complications usually occur before 2 years of age; and it is located within 2 feet of the ileocecal valve. Approximately 50% of resected Meckel's diverticula contain heterotopic gastric mucosa. The most common complication of Meckel's diverticulum is painless gastrointestinal bleeding, which occurs secondary to irritation or ulceration by hydrochloric acid produced by the gastric mucosa that lines the diverticulum.

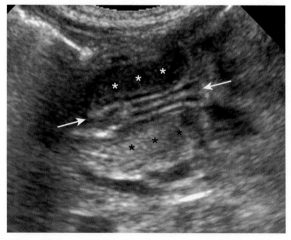

**Figure 87-4.** HPS on US. Note thickened walls of pylorus (*) that surround central lumen (*arrows*).

**Table 87-1.** Common Causes of Gastrointestinal Bleeding in Children

| NEWBORN AND NEONATE (<1 MONTH) | YOUNG INFANT (1-3 MONTHS) | OLDER INFANT (3 MONTHS-1 YEAR) | CHILD (1-10 YEARS) |
|---|---|---|---|
| Swallowed maternal blood | Esophagitis | Esophagitis | Esophagitis |
| Anal fissure | Intussusception | Anal fissure | Esophageal varices |
| Necrotizing enterocolitis | Anal fissure | Colon polyp | Colon polyp |
| Hemorrhagic disease of the newborn | Gangrenous bowel | Intussusception | Anal fissure |
| Allergic or infectious colitis | Meckel's diverticulum | Gangrenous bowel Foreign body | Foreign body Crohn's disease Ulcerative colitis |

19. **How is Meckel's diverticulum diagnosed?**
Meckel's diverticulum is detected by a nuclear medicine scan with technetium-99m ($^{99m}$Tc) pertechnetate. The radiotracer accumulates within the diverticulum, usually appearing at approximately the same time as activity appears within the stomach, with gradually increasing intensity, thereby verifying the presence of ectopic gastric mucosa.

20. **What are the most common causes of GI bleeding in children?**
The differential diagnosis depends on the age of the patient (Table 87-1).

21. **What causes necrotizing enterocolitis (NEC)?**
NEC is a multifactorial condition that has traditionally been thought to be caused by hypoxia, infection, and enteral feeding. The pathology of NEC resembles that of ischemic necrosis. It may be that the main pathologic trigger in NEC is injury to the intestinal mucosa, which can be caused by different factors in different patients.

22. **Who develops NEC?**
Approximately 80% of patients who develop NEC are premature infants. Older infants who develop NEC usually have severe underlying medical problems, such as Hirschsprung's disease or congenital heart disease. Patients with this condition present with abdominal distention, vomiting, increased gastric residuals, blood in the stool, lethargy, apnea, and temperature instability.

23. **What findings of NEC can be seen on radiographs, and what is the role of the radiologist?**
The radiographic findings of NEC are nonspecific when the condition is initially suspected. Radiographs are obtained serially, and the role of the radiologist is to attempt to diagnose the condition prior to the occurrence of bowel perforation. In early NEC, the most commonly detected abnormality is diffuse gaseous distention of bowel loops. A more useful sign of early NEC is loss of the normal symmetric bowel gas pattern, with a resultant disorganized or asymmetric pattern. In more advanced NEC, the finding of pneumatosis intestinalis (intramural gas) is virtually pathognomonic for the condition (Figure 87-5). Gas in the portal venous system is a pathognomonic finding in NEC, occurring in 10% to 30% of cases. Infants at risk for imminent perforation often have portal venous gas. They may also have the "persistent loop" sign, which is a dilated loop of intestine (focal ileus) that remains unchanged over 24 to 36 hours. Another grave sign is a shift from a pattern of generalized dilation to asymmetric bowel dilation. Ascites is another sign of impending perforation. When pneumoperitoneum develops, this is a definite sign that the bowel has perforated, and the infant must have surgery (i.e., medical NEC becomes surgical NEC).

24. **What are other causes of pneumoperitoneum in infants and children?**
The most common causes are surgery and instrumentation. Pneumoperitoneum can be found after laparotomy/open surgery, paracentesis, or resuscitation. Also, distal bowel obstruction from conditions such as Hirschsprung's disease or meconium ileus and dissection of gas from pneumomediastinum, a ruptured ulcer, or Meckel's diverticulum can lead to pneumoperitoneum.

25. **What is Hirschsprung's disease?**
Hirschsprung's disease is a condition of distal aganglionic bowel that results from the lack of Auerbach (intermuscular) and Meissner (submucosal) plexuses. Functional obstruction of the distal bowel results. Hirschsprung's disease usually manifests within the first 48 hours of life as failure to pass meconium, or it may manifest with abdominal distention, bilious vomiting, or diarrhea. More than 80% of patients present within the first 6 weeks of life.

26. **What are the radiographic findings of Hirschsprung's disease?**
The most typical radiographic finding of Hirschsprung's disease is a dilated colon proximal (upstream) to the distal more diminutive aganglionic segment. Radiographs may also demonstrate high-grade distal bowel obstruction. Radiologic diagnosis of Hirschsprung's disease requires a contrast enema (water-soluble contrast in almost all circumstances) (Figure 87-6). Spot radiographs are obtained in the frontal, lateral, and oblique projections. The

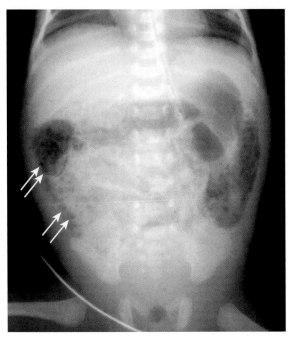

**Figure 87-5.** NEC on frontal abdominal radiograph. Note mottled pattern of gas in bowel wall (*arrows*) indicating presence of pneumatosis intestinalis.

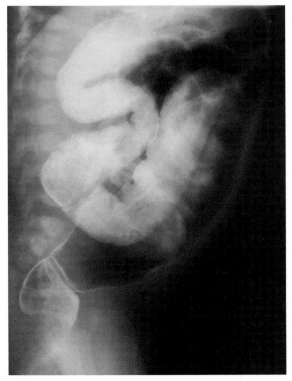

**Figure 87-6.** Hirschsprung's disease on contrast enema lateral spot radiograph. Note transition zone (from dilated to nondilated bowel) within distal colon.

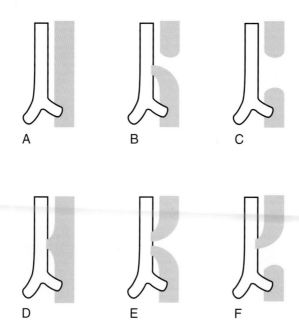

**Figure 87-7.** Different types of TEF. **A,** Normal relationship of esophagus (*in blue*) posterior to trachea (*in white*) without atresia or fistula. **B,** Esophageal atresia with distal TEF (most common). **C,** Esophageal atresia with no TEF (2nd most common). **D,** H-type fistula with no esophageal atresia (3rd most common). **E,** Esophageal atresia with proximal and distal fistulas. **F,** Esophageal atresia with proximal fistula.

contrast enema may show the transition zone, which is situated between a narrowed distal aganglionic segment and the distended proximal bowel. The radiographic transition zone may be visualized more distally than the histologic transition zone secondary to stool dilating the proximal part of the aganglionic segment.

27. Is Hirschsprung's disease diagnosed definitively by imaging?
    To make a definitive diagnosis of Hirschsprung's disease, a rectal (suction) biopsy specimen must demonstrate a lack of ganglion cells. The specificity and sensitivity of a contrast enema for diagnosis are about 70% and 80%, respectively.

28. Name the types of tracheoesophageal fistulas (TEF). How common is each type?
    - The most common type of TEF is esophageal atresia with distal esophageal communication with the tracheobronchial tree (Figure 87-7). This accounts for >80% of cases.
    - The next most common type is esophageal atresia without a TEF, which accounts for 3% to 9% of cases.
    - H-type fistulas occur between an otherwise intact trachea and esophagus and account for 3% of cases.
    - Esophageal atresias occurring with proximal and distal communication with the trachea are found in 1% of cases, and esophageal atresia with proximal communication is rare (<1%).
        TEF is associated with VACTERL syndromes (in which affected patients manifest at least three of the following: **V**ertebral anomalies, **A**nal atresia/imperforate anus, **C**ardiac anomalies, **T**racheo**e**sophageal fistula/esophageal atresia, **R**enal anomalies, and **L**imb anomalies).

29. What are the radiographic findings of TEF?
    In a patient with esophageal atresia (and no fistula or a proximal fistula), radiographs may reveal a gasless abdomen. A nasogastric tube may be seen coiled within the proximal esophagus. Patients with esophageal atresia with a distal TEF or H-type fistula may present with a distended abdomen. Pulmonary aspiration is a risk for all patients with esophageal atresia.

30. How can a radiograph help to differentiate an ingested coin in the esophagus from an aspirated coin in the trachea?
    On frontal chest radiographs, a coin in the esophagus is typically visualized as a round object en face (i.e., a full radiopaque circle can be seen) (Figure 87-8). A coin in the trachea lies sagittally and will typically appear end-on (in profile) on the frontal radiograph.

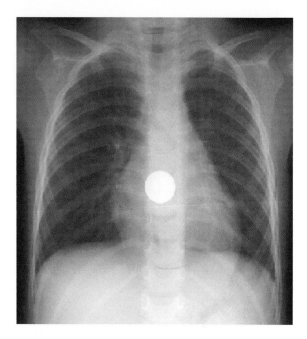

**Figure 87-8.** Ingested foreign body on frontal chest radiograph. Note round radiopaque coin seen en face within midesophagus.

## KEY POINTS

- Bowel intussusception in children is most commonly idiopathic, is a common cause of bowel obstruction, and is treated by air or hydrostatic enema.
- Bowel malrotation alters gastrointestinal anatomy, with the ligament of Treitz not being situated in the left upper quadrant and the cecum not being located in the right lower quadrant. It may be associated with bowel obstruction due to midgut volvulus (a surgical emergency) or Ladd's bands.
- HPS appears as a thickened pyloric muscle surrounding a compressed pyloric channel along with an elongated pyloric channel length on US.
- NEC predominantly occurs in premature infants and may manifest as diffuse gaseous distention of bowel, loss of the normal symmetric bowel gas pattern, persistent focal dilation of bowel, ascites, pneumatosis intestinalis, portal venous gas, or pneumoperitoneum on abdominal radiography. When pneumoperitoneum develops, this is a definite sign of bowel perforation, necessitating surgical intervention.
- An ingested coin in the esophagus is typically visualized en face on a frontal chest radiograph, whereas an aspirated coin in the trachea is typically visualized end-on on a frontal chest radiograph.

## BIBLIOGRAPHY

Lampl B, Levin TL, Berdon WE, et al. Malrotation and midgut volvulus: a historical review and current controversies in diagnosis and management. *Pediatr Radiol.* 2009;39(4):359-366.

Haricharan RN, Georgeson KE. Hirschsprung disease. *Semin Pediatr Surg.* 2008;17(4):266-275.

Epelman M, Daneman A, Navarro OM, et al. Necrotizing enterocolitis: review of state-of-the-art imaging findings with pathologic correlation. *Radiographics.* 2007;27(2):285-305.

Fordham LA. Imaging of the esophagus in children. *Radiol Clin North Am.* 2005;43(2):283-302.

Berrocal T, Madrid C, Novo S, et al. Congenital anomalies of the tracheobronchial tree, lung, and mediastinum: embryology, radiology, and pathology. *Radiographics.* 2004;24(1):e17.

Daneman A, Navarro O. Intussusception. Part 2: an update on the evolution of management. *Pediatr Radiol.* 2004;34(2):97-108, quiz 87.

Levy AD, Hobbs CM. From the archives of the AFIP. Meckel diverticulum: radiologic features with pathologic correlation. *Radiographics.* 2004;24(2):565-587.

Navarro O, Daneman A. Intussusception. Part 3: diagnosis and management of those with an identifiable or predisposing cause and those that reduce spontaneously. *Pediatr Radiol.* 2004;34(4):305-312, quiz 69.

Strouse PJ. Disorders of intestinal rotation and fixation ("malrotation"). *Pediatr Radiol.* 2004;34(11):837-851.

Daneman A, Navarro O. Intussusception. Part 1: a review of diagnostic approaches. *Pediatr Radiol.* 2003;33(2):79-85.

Hernanz-Schulman M. Infantile hypertrophic pyloric stenosis. *Radiology.* 2003;227(2):319-331.

Millar AJ, Rode H, Cywes S. Malrotation and volvulus in infancy and childhood. *Semin Pediatr Surg.* 2003;12(4):229-236.

Traubici J. The double bubble sign. *Radiology.* 2001;220(2):463-464.

Berrocal T, Lamas M, Gutieerrez J, et al. Congenital anomalies of the small intestine, colon, and rectum. *Radiographics.* 1999;19(5):1219-1236.

Berrocal T, Torres I, Gutierrez J, et al. Congenital anomalies of the upper gastrointestinal tract. *Radiographics.* 1999;19(4):855-872.

De Backer AI, De Schepper AM, Deprettere A, et al. Radiographic manifestations of intestinal obstruction in the newborn. *JBR-BTR.* 1999;82(4):159-166.

# CHAPTER 88

# PEDIATRIC GENITOURINARY RADIOLOGY

*Richard D. Bellah, MD, and Ting Yin Tao, MD, PhD*

1. **What is the role of the radiologist in pediatric urinary tract infection (UTI)?**
   UTI that occurs and recurs in some children is the result of many interrelated factors, most of which the radiologist cannot assess. Generally, UTI results when bacterial virulence outweighs host resistance. One important factor affecting host resistance that the radiologist can assess is whether there is impairment of unidirectional flow of urine out of the urinary tract, resulting in urinary stasis and predisposing infants and children to UTI.

2. **What conditions can be detected radiologically that impair normal urinary flow?**
   Urinary tract obstruction (congenital), vesicoureteral reflux (VUR), and dysfunctional voiding/neurogenic bladder dysfunction all can be detected radiologically (Figure 88-1).

3. **Which imaging tests are used to diagnose these conditions?**
   Renal and bladder ultrasonography (US) and voiding cystourethrography (VCUG) are used to diagnose the above-mentioned conditions.

4. **In a child with history of UTI, what are the indications for renal and bladder US?**
   Renal and bladder US is used to detect hydronephrosis and distal ureterectasis secondary to obstruction or VUR, to detect bladder abnormalities (including diverticula or wall thickening secondary to obstruction), and to assess for any renal parenchymal damage that may have been caused by prior infections.

5. **When is renal and bladder US performed?**
   US is performed within several weeks after an initial UTI is diagnosed, but sooner if the child fails to respond to conventional antibiotic therapy. (Also, as a result of the routine use of prenatal US, hydronephrosis is often detected in utero, and UTI can be prevented by prophylactically administering antibiotics to the infant.)

6. **How is VCUG performed?**
   The bladder is catheterized using sterile technique, and under fluoroscopy, the bladder is filled to capacity with iodinated contrast material. An approximation of the expected normal bladder capacity (mL) in a child is calculated by (age [in years] + 2) × 30. The catheter is removed, and the child voids while on the fluoroscopy table. During

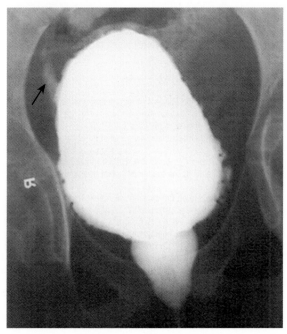

**Figure 88-1.** Dysfunctional voiding on VCUG. Fluoroscopic spot image of bladder and urethra shows mild bladder wall trabeculation. Small amount of VUR is seen on right (*arrow*). Urethra has "spinning top" configuration as well.

the procedure, the anatomy of the lower urinary tract and bladder function are examined, a series of radiographic images is obtained, and the presence or absence of reflux of contrast material (i.e., VUR) into the ureters is determined.

### 7. How is VCUG modified in infants?

A cyclic study is typically performed. Infants usually void around the small catheter that is placed through the urethra into the bladder; multiple cycles of voiding and bladder filling are studied. This method also increases the probability that reflux, if present, will be elicited and detectable.

### 8. When should VCUG be performed?

According to recent American Academy of Pediatrics guidelines (from the Subcommittee on Urinary Tract Infection, Steering Committee on Quality Improvement and Management), a VCUG should be performed after a second well-documented UTI in both boys and girls. VCUG is indicated if renal and bladder US demonstrates hydronephrosis, scarring, or other indications of high-grade VUR or obstructive uropathy.

### 9. What is voiding urosonography?

Pediatric imagers are currently looking to offer voiding urosonography as an alternative to fluoroscopic or radionuclide voiding cystography. With this technique, which avoids the use of ionizing radiation, fluid containing microbubbles is instilled into the urinary bladder; VUR reaching the kidneys can be readily detected utilizing US.

### 10. What are the pros and cons of a radionuclide cystography or voiding urosonography compared with fluoroscopic VCUG?

Fluoroscopic VCUG provides anatomic detail but at a much higher radiation dose. Voiding urosonography does not require radiation and may also detect low-grade VUR not clearly identifiable fluoroscopically. Radionuclide cystography is highly sensitive for detecting reflux because the child is continuously monitored by the gamma camera but at the expense of good anatomic detail. Radionuclide cystography is particularly useful for follow-up studies that assess for resolution of previously detected VUR and is useful for screening siblings of patients with known VUR.

### 11. What is primary VUR?

VUR occurs either primarily or secondarily. Primary VUR is due to "immaturity" or abnormality of the ureterovesical junction (UVJ), which allows urine to ascend into the ureters during bladder filling or voiding. Generally, reflux is related to ureteral orifice size and the length of the ureter as it tunnels into the bladder.

### 12. What is secondary VUR?

Secondary VUR occurs as the result of an abnormality of the UVJ, such as with presence of a distal paraureteral diverticulum or ureterocele (an outpouching of the ureter that extends into the bladder). Secondary VUR may also occur as a result of bladder outlet obstruction or secondary to a neurogenic bladder.

### 13. How is primary VUR graded?

Primary VUR is graded on a scale of 1 to 5, based on the degree of ureteral and pyelocalyceal (renal collecting system) filling and dilation (Figure 88-2). In addition to providing the referring physician with a visual description of the degree of reflux, assigning a grade also gives the clinician an idea of the likelihood of spontaneous resolution (e.g., 80% of cases of grade 2 reflux resolve within 3 years).

### 14. What is dysfunctional voiding?

Dysfunctional voiding may be due to a neurogenic bladder or the so-called pediatric unstable bladder. The bladder may show variable degrees of wall thickening, trabeculation, and alteration in contour and storage capacity (see Figure 88-1). Bladder-sphincter dyssynergia may be indicated by the presence of a dilated posterior urethra caused by the external sphincter failing to relax as the bladder neck opens. This condition often leads to high-pressure voiding, incomplete emptying, and urine retention.

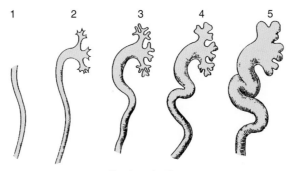

Grades of reflux

**Figure 88-2.** Grading of primary VUR. Reflux is graded according to degree of ureteral and pyelocalyceal filling. Higher grade is associated with less likelihood of spontaneous resolution of VUR.

15. What diagnostic tests are useful for the detection of acute and chronic pyelonephritis in children?

    Renal cortical scintigraphy, contrast-enhanced computed tomography (CT), and renal US are used to detect acute and chronic pyelonephritis in children. Pyelonephritis may be difficult to diagnose accurately, especially in infants and young children who cannot give a history. It may be difficult to distinguish between uncomplicated UTI and pyelonephritis (with or without subsequent complications such as renal abscess) on the basis of physical examination, history, and laboratory studies. Imaging plays an important role in the workup of children with known or suspected UTI.

16. What are the findings on a renal cortical scintigraphic study in acute and chronic infection?

    A renal cortical scintigraphic study reveals parenchymal defects in children with acute infection secondary to focal areas of edema and inflammation. These defects revert to normal if the process completely resolves. In chronic infection or chronic pyelonephritis secondary to reflux nephropathy, residual areas of scar appear as persistent cortical defects on follow-up examinations.

17. What are the CT findings associated with pyelonephritis?

    Contrast-enhanced CT is less sensitive than renal cortical scintigraphy for the detection of acute infection. Acute infection is seen as wedge-shaped areas of decreased attenuation in the kidney. Areas of scar related to prior infection can also be identified. CT is particularly helpful when abscess formation is suspected.

18. What is the "top-down approach" in the evaluation of the child with a history of UTI?

    The "top-down approach" refers to a protocol that more selectively identifies children with history of UTI who may require voiding cystography. In these patients, rather than having a VCUG performed initially, VCUG is obtained based on whether an initial renal cortical scintigraphic study is normal or abnormal.

19. How useful is renal US in the workup of suspected pyelonephritis?

    Gray-scale US is limited in its ability to depict acute pyelonephritis. The sensitivity of US is increased, however, when power Doppler US is used (Figure 88-3). The latter technique is an advance in Doppler US that depicts normal and abnormal blood flow in a manner that is independent of the direction of the flow; power Doppler is more sensitive than routine color Doppler. Renal US may also be used to assess for significant renal scarring secondary to chronic pyelonephritis. Small focal scars may be difficult to detect with US.

20. What is the role of magnetic resonance imaging (MRI) in a child with UTI?

    MRI can be utilized to detect complications of UTI such as pyelonephritis, renal and perinephric/psoas abscess formation, and renal scarring.

21. List the most common forms of congenital hydronephrosis.
    - Ureteropelvic junction (UPJ) obstruction.
    - UVJ obstruction, commonly referred to as primary megaureter.
    - VUR.
    - Renal and ureteral duplication anomalies.
    - Posterior urethral valves.
    - Prune-belly syndrome.

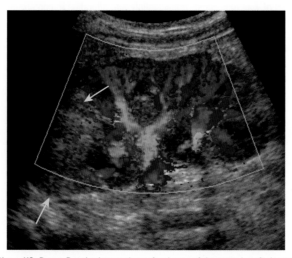

**Figure 88-3.** Acute pyelonephritis on US. Power Doppler image shows focal area of decreased perfusion within upper pole of kidney (*arrows*). This finding corresponds to area of pyelonephritis.

22. When should a postnatal renal and bladder US examination be obtained in a patient with congenital hydronephrosis?

A postnatal renal and bladder US examination should be performed on any infant with dilation of the renal pelvis that is detected prenatally on US, if the renal pelvis measures 4 mm or greater before 33 weeks of gestation and 7 mm or greater after 33 weeks of gestation. A renal pelvic diameter less than 4 mm seen on US at birth has been shown to normalize spontaneously within 1 year. In boys with bilateral hydroureteronephrosis, US should be obtained soon after birth to assess for presence of posterior urethral valves. Otherwise, the initial US examination should be performed at 5 to 7 days after birth (when the glomerular filtration rate is greater than it is immediately after birth).

23. What are the roles of renal scintigraphy, VCUG, intravenous urography (IVU), and magnetic resonance urography (MRU) in congenital hydronephrosis?

VCUG is performed to assess for VUR and to determine whether posterior urethral valves are present (in boys). Use of renal scintigraphy and IVU varies from patient to patient and from institution to institution. Renal scintigraphy provides quantitative information regarding the effects of obstruction upon renal function; the function of the obstructed kidney can be compared with the opposite kidney before and after surgical treatment. IVU provides less quantitative information but provides better anatomic detail. It serves best as a road map for the surgeon and gives information about anatomy and function after surgery. MRU is a static and dynamic technique that provides both morphologic and functional information of the dilated urinary tract in a single scan session without the use of ionizing radiation (Figure 88-4).

24. What are posterior urethral valves?

At the distal end of the verumontanum, several folds, or plicae, arise and pass caudally to encircle a portion of the membranous urethra. These plicae occur normally and vary in the extent to which they encircle the urethra. When they fuse anteriorly, they form the most common type of posterior urethral valves (type 1) (Figure 88-5). Type 2 posterior urethral valves are mucosal folds that extend from the proximal end of the verumontanum toward the bladder neck; their very existence is controversial. Type 3 valves refer to a urethral diaphragm that occurs below the caudal end of the verumontanum.

25. How are posterior urethral valves detected?

Posterior urethral valves, which are the most common cause of bladder outlet obstruction in infant boys, cause changes in the bladder that are detected by US and cystography. These changes include enlargement, wall thickening, sacculation, and trabeculation of the bladder. Dilation of the posterior (prostatic) urethra above the valve can be seen on prenatal and postnatal US scans and with VCUG. Hydroureteronephrosis is often present, owing to either VUR or high pressures in the bladder. If rupture of a calyceal fornix occurs, urinary ascites or a urinoma or both can develop. Posterior urethral valves are confirmed cystoscopically and are treated with fulguration or incision.

26. What is primary megaureter?

Primary megaureter is congenital narrowing at the UVJ that results from an abnormal proportion of muscle fibers and fibrous tissue in the distalmost 3 to 4 cm of the ureter. It occurs more commonly than previously realized and can be either obstructive or nonobstructive. When primary megaureter is obstructive, the degree of obstruction is variable and

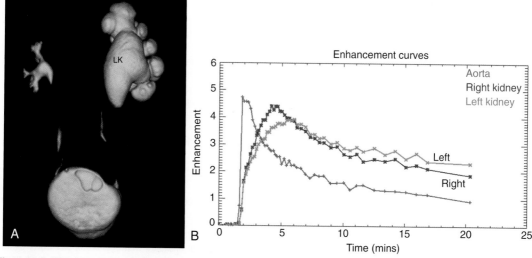

**Figure 88-4.** UPJ obstruction on MRI/MRU. **A,** Coronal volume-rendered MRU image shows left pyelocaliectasis. **B,** Graph of renal and aortic signal intensity vs. time obtained from dynamic 3D MRI scan provides functional information, similar to that of renal scintigraphy. Note left kidney shows delayed peak and prolonged enhancement compared to right kidney.

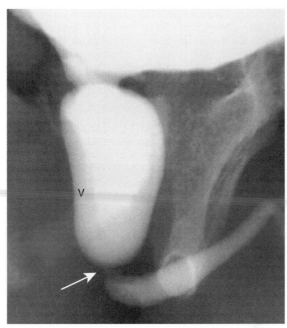

**Figure 88-5.** Posterior urethral valves on VCUG. Fluoroscopic spot image shows dilated posterior urethra. Valves (*arrow*) are identified at distal end of verumontanum (*v*).

seems to improve in many cases over time. Most often, this condition is detected incidentally on prenatal US. Postnatal US and urography reveal a variable degree of dilation of the ureter and collecting system on the affected side (Figure 88-6). Occasionally, a short narrow segment of ureter may be seen through US at the UVJ. VCUG typically shows absence of reflux, although VUR may be present in 10% of cases.

27. What are common forms of a duplex kidney?
    A duplex kidney (duplication of the kidney, collecting system, and ureters) arises from abnormal development of the ureteric bud. Although various degrees of duplication may be present, in the full-blown condition, the kidney is large, and there are separate collecting systems and ureters that drain the upper and lower poles of the kidney.

28. What is the Weigert-Meyer rule?
    According to the Weigert-Meyer rule, when there is a complete duplication of the kidney, the lower pole ureter inserts normally into the bladder. The upper pole ureter inserts ectopically into the bladder, in a location that is medial and caudal to the insertion of the lower pole ureter.

29. Are the collecting systems and ureters dilated in a duplicated system?
    The appearance depends on whether there is reflux into the lower pole ureter and the exact site of the ectopically inserting upper pole ureter. In the typical situation, which is often bilateral, the distal ureters are contained within a common sheath and either come together or insert separately, but are close together in the trigone of the bladder. If the upper pole ureter is associated with a ureterocele (a localized dilation of the distal ureter), the ureterocele can protrude through the bladder to the urethra and manifests as a perineal mass. If a ureterocele is present, the upper pole of the kidney may be obstructed (leading to a "drooping lily" appearance of the lower pole collecting system due to inferolateral displacement caused by mass effect) or may be small and dysplastic, causing little or no effect on the lower pole. If a ureterocele is not present, the ureter from the upper pole moiety may insert in an ectopic location and have a stenotic insertion, causing obstruction (boys and girls), or may manifest with urinary dribbling or constant wetting (girls only) owing to an ectopic insertion into the urethra, vagina, or perineum.

30. What is the most common cause of a scrotal mass?
    The most common cause of a scrotal mass is probably a hydrocele, which is a collection of fluid outside the testicle, between layers of the tunica vaginalis. It may be congenital or may be associated with trauma, torsion, or hemorrhage.

31. What are the main differential diagnostic considerations of a painful scrotum?
    The main differential diagnostic considerations of a painful scrotum are testicular torsion and epididymitis and/or orchitis. Testicular torsion is a surgical emergency and can be confirmed or excluded with duplex Doppler US or planar scintigraphy (using technetium-99m ($^{99m}$Tc) pertechnetate as the radiotracer), although the latter is now rarely, if ever, used. A common cause of the painful hemiscrotum in a prepubertal male is paratesticular/epididymal inflammation secondary to torsion of the testicular or epididymal appendage (Figure 88-7). Epididymitis due to infection is much

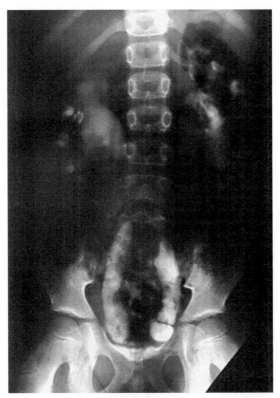

**Figure 88-6.** Primary megaureter on IVU. Note mild bilateral pyelocaliectasis, right greater than left, along with moderate ureterectasis, most marked in distal half of ureters.

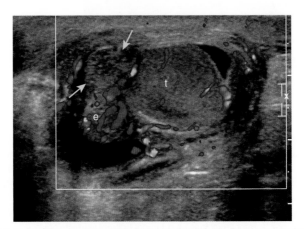

**Figure 88-7.** Torsion of appendix testis with secondary epididymitis on US. Sagittal color Doppler image shows scrotal wall thickening and reactive hydrocele. Testis (*t*) has normal blood flow, while epididymis (*e*) has increased blood flow. Heterogeneous nodule (*arrows*) at anterior superior pole of testis is torsed appendix testis resulting in paratesticular inflammation.

more common in postpubescent boys than in younger boys and is identified on US by swelling of and increased blood flow in the epididymis. The cause of epididymitis is often bacterial, and there may be associated infection in the testicle as well.

32. If epididymitis is present in an infant, what should be suspected as the etiologic factor?
    Epididymitis is rare in infants and is usually associated with an anatomic abnormality of the genitourinary system such as a dysplastic kidney with an ectopic ureter to the epididymal-related structures. Renal/bladder US and VCUG are indicated.

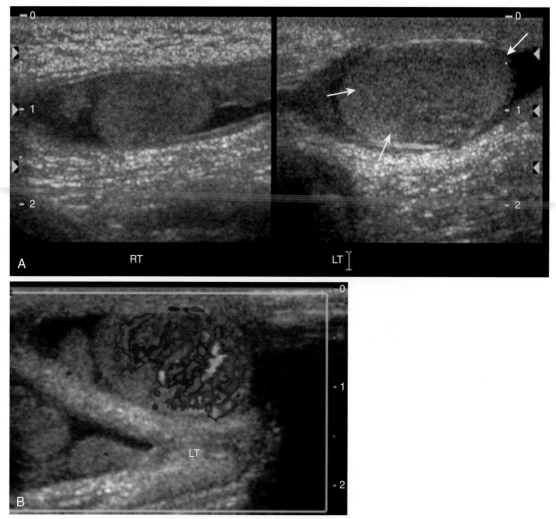

**Figure 88-8.** Yolk sac tumor of testis on US. **A,** Transverse gray scale image through scrotum in young child shows normal right testis and enlarged left testis (*arrows*). **B,** Color Doppler image of left testis shows hyperemia in large left testicular mass.

33. What is the most common testicular tumor in children?
    Yolk sac tumor is the most common testicular tumor in children. Yolk sac tumors occur more commonly than teratomas and are seen primarily during the first 2 years of life (Figure 88-8). Most children with yolk sac tumors have elevated α-fetoprotein (AFP) levels, whereas children with teratomas do not have elevated AFP levels.

34. What are the most common testicular tumors in adolescents?
    Germ cell tumors are the most common testicular tumors in adolescents, but the most common histologic types are seminomas, choriocarcinomas, teratocarcinomas, and tumors with mixed histologies.

35. What urinary problems occur in children with spina bifida?
    There is an increased incidence of renal anomalies in children with myelomeningocele, including fusion anomalies (e.g., horseshoe kidney), renal dysplasia, and agenesis. The most significant problems relate to the abnormal innervation of the bladder.

36. Name the specific problems in spina bifida that are related to neurogenic bladder.
    The neurogenic bladder fails to store urine correctly, which may cause leaking; does not empty properly because of bladder-sphincter dyssynergia; and experiences uninhibited contractions, which may also cause leaking (Figure 88-9). High storage pressures can result in VUR and hydronephrosis.

37. Discuss the goals of therapy for urinary tract dysfunction in a patient with spina bifida.
    The goals are to decrease storage pressure, with frequent intermittent catheterization, vesicostomy, or bladder augmentation, and to keep the patient "dry" through continent diversion. Cystography is performed to assess bladder

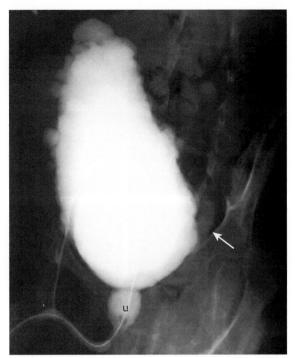

**Figure 88-9.** Neurogenic bladder on VCUG. Note "pinecone" bladder with marked trabeculation and sacculation in this patient with meningomyelocele. When patient attempts to void, there is dilation of posterior urethra (*u*) with contraction of external sphincter (bladder-sphincter dyssynergy). Small amount of reflux of contrast is seen into distal left ureter (*arrow*).

size, storage capacity, and the volume at which leakage occurs and to detect any VUR. Renal and bladder US is routinely performed every 6 months to assess for hydronephrosis, calculi, and the ability of the patient to empty the bladder with self-catheterization.

38. What is the triad of prune-belly syndrome?
The triad of prune-belly syndrome is absent or deficient abdominal musculature, cryptorchidism, and urinary tract abnormalities.

39. What urinary tract abnormalities are associated with prune-belly syndrome?
They are diverse and include marked hydroureteronephrosis and marked bladder and urethral dilation, reflux, renal dysplasia, prostatic hypoplasia, urachal abnormalities, and microphallus (Figure 88-10). The clinical features often parallel the degree of urinary tract involvement. Newborns with severe renal dysplasia may have Potter syndrome (oligohydramnios, pulmonary hypoplasia). Children with urinary tract dilation, VUR, or both need to be closely monitored for infection.

40. What is a basic classification for cystic renal diseases affecting infants, children, and adolescents?
Cystic renal diseases can be classified as genetic or nongenetic. The most common cause of nongenetic cystic disease is multicystic dysplastic kidney (MCDK).

41. What is the most common US appearance of MCDK?
Most commonly, MCDK is the result of atresia of the renal pelvis, and the kidney appears on US as multiple cysts of varying sizes that do not communicate with each other; there is no definable renal pelvis. The less common form is the hydronephrotic form, which has a central renal cyst. MCDK is associated with other abnormalities of the urinary tract, especially a contralateral UPJ obstruction and contralateral VUR.

42. List the other forms of nongenetic cystic renal disease.
- Simple renal cyst (rare in children).
- Medullary cystic disease.
- Calyceal diverticulum.
- Cystic renal dysplasia (associated with urinary tract obstruction).

43. Name the genetic forms of cystic renal disease.
- Autosomal dominant polycystic kidney disease (ADPCKD).
- Autosomal recessive polycystic kidney disease (ARPCKD).

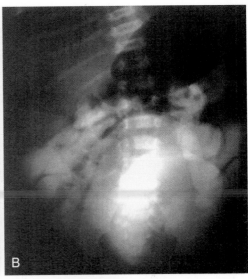

**Figure 88-10.** Prune-belly syndrome on radiograph and VCUG. **A,** Abdominal radiograph shows prune-belly configuration of abdomen from abdominal muscle paucity. **B,** VCUG image shows megacystis, bilateral pyelocaliectasis and ureterectasis, and significant ureteral tortuosity.

- Glomerulocystic kidney disease.
- Congenital nephrosis.
- Cystic kidney disease associated with syndromes (e.g., tuberous sclerosis).

44. **Does "adult-type" ADPCKD occur in infants and young children?**
ADPCKD has been recognized on US prenatally and postnatally. The appearance can closely mimic ARPCKD, in which both kidneys can appear large and echogenic. Small, sonographically resolvable cysts can be seen in either syndrome in the newborn period. More commonly, ADPCKD is suspected if US reveals progressive development of multiple cortical and medullary renal cysts; this may be found incidentally or in a child referred for hypertension and hematuria. Careful examination of the family history and US screening of the family are recommended to detect any evidence of cystic kidney disease in parents who may be unaware of their own subclinical disease.

45. **What imaging findings may help distinguish ADPCKD from ARPCKD in an infant or young child?**
The renal US appearance of ADPCKD and ARPCKD can be quite similar. The kidneys are often large and echogenic with each syndrome. Careful inspection with US can occasionally detect tubular ectasia in echogenic renal pyramids, which is typical of ARPCKD. Sonographically resolvable cysts are more suggestive of autosomal dominant disease. Additionally, the liver should be examined for abnormal echotexture caused by hepatic fibrosis and biliary ectasia, which is often associated with autosomal recessive disease (Figure 88-11). In adolescents with ARPCKD, the renal involvement is less marked than the liver disease, the latter of which causes portal hypertension and splenomegaly. IVU or CTU can occasionally be helpful to distinguish the recessive from the dominant disease. In ARPCKD, there is delay and prolongation of the nephrogram; contrast material is taken up by dilated tubules and has a spoke-wheel appearance. These findings are typically absent in ADPCKD, in which contrast excretion is prompt.

46. **Name five hereditary syndromes associated with renal cysts.**
- Tuberous sclerosis.
- von Hippel-Lindau syndrome.
- Zellweger (cerebrohepatorenal) syndrome.
- Jeune syndrome (thoracic asphyxiating dystrophy).
- Meckel-Gruber syndrome.

47. **What is the normal sonographic appearance of the neonatal kidney?**
In normal term neonates, cortical echogenicity is equal to the hepatic or splenic parenchymal echogenicity, presumably due to the increased volume of glomeruli and greater amount of cellular components in the renal cortices as compared to adults. The normal neonatal kidney also demonstrates a well-delineated corticomedullary junction with prominent and hypoechoic medullary pyramids.

48. **What conditions cause echogenic renal pyramids in infants?**
- Nephrocalcinosis (owing to renal tubular acidosis, hypercalcemia, or furosemide therapy).
- Renal tubular ectasia (ARPCKD).
- Stasis nephropathy/Tamm-Horsfall protein deposition (transient phenomenon).

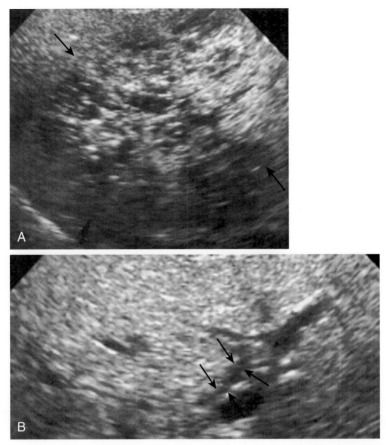

**Figure 88-11.** ARPCKD on US. **A,** Sagittal image of right kidney (*arrows*) shows marked enlargement with heterogeneous echogenicity. Small (1 mm) cystic foci are seen within renal parenchyma. **B,** Transverse image of liver shows increased echotexture of liver parenchyma due to hepatic fibrosis. Minimal ectasia of intrahepatic biliary tree (*arrows*) is seen adjacent to left portal vein.

49. List the common causes of urolithiasis in children.
    - Metabolic abnormalities (hypercalciuria, hypocitraturia, hyperoxaluria, cystinuria, and hyperuricosuria).
    - Intestinal malabsorption (Crohn's disease, bowel resection, and cystic fibrosis).
    - Urinary tract abnormalities causing functional or anatomic obstruction.
    - UTIs.
    - Diuretics.

50. What is the "twinkling" artifact?
    The twinkling artifact appears as a focus of rapidly alternating color Doppler signal observed when insonating irregular reflective surfaces, such as renal calculi. This color Doppler artifact is often helpful in confirming an echogenic focus in the kidney as representing a renal calculus.

51. What is the most common solid renal mass in infants?
    The most common solid renal mass in infants is fetal renal hamartoma, also known as mesoblastic nephroma. Infants usually present with a palpable renal mass. Hematuria, hypertension, and hypercalcemia may also be present. The tumor is composed of monotonous sheets of spindle-shaped cells and usually occupies most of the kidney. The tumor appears large and solid on US. The mass is usually resected, and the prognosis is excellent. Less common causes of solitary renal masses in infants include nephroblastomatosis and malignant rhabdoid tumor.

52. What is the role of imaging in infants with ambiguous genitalia?
    Evaluation is indicated when the testes cannot be palpated and when there is severe hypospadias, incomplete scrotal fusion, fused labia, a micropenis, or clitoral enlargement. These conditions can be classified as true hermaphroditism, female pseudohermaphroditism, male pseudohermaphroditism, and gonadal dysgenesis, depending on further clinical, laboratory, and surgical investigations. US is the simplest method of identifying the internal anatomy by detecting the presence or absence of a uterus and gonads. US is usually combined with a retrograde genitogram performed under fluoroscopy that defines further the relationship of the urogenital sinus to the urethra and vagina (Figure 88-12).

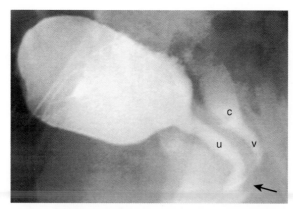

**Figure 88-12.** Urogenital sinus in ambiguous genitalia on retrograde genitogram. Note low confluence (*arrow*) of urethra (*u*) and vagina (*v*), and also cervical impression (*c*).

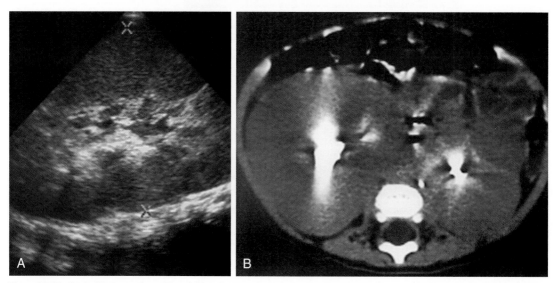

**Figure 88-13.** Nephroblastomatosis on US and CT. **A,** Sagittal US image of right kidney shows significant renal enlargement with loss of normal corticomedullary differentiation. **B,** Axial CT image shows bilateral renal enlargement with loss of normal intrarenal architecture and diffuse infiltration by intralobar nephroblastomatosis.

53. What is nephroblastomatosis?

    Nephroblastomatosis refers to multiple or diffuse rests of nephrogenic tissue. They are persistent embryonal remnants in the kidney that are apparent precursors to Wilms tumor. The involved kidneys are typically enlarged and have a lobulated configuration. US, CT, and MRI can be used to identify and monitor nephroblastomatosis (Figure 88-13). The following are several conditions in which children may have nephroblastomatosis and can develop Wilms tumor: hemihypertrophy, Drash syndrome (pseudohermaphroditism), aniridia, and a positive family history of Wilms tumor or nephroblastomatosis.

54. What are the two major types of nephroblastomatosis?

    Perilobar and intralobar are the two major types of nephroblastomatosis. The perilobar form is limited to the periphery of the kidney, whereas the intralobar form can be found anywhere within a renal lobe and within the renal pelvis and collecting system. Nephroblastomatosis may remain dormant, mature, involute, develop hyperplastic overgrowth, or become neoplastic (Wilms tumor).

55. How can nephroblastomatosis be distinguished from Wilms tumor?

    Generally, Wilms tumor is suspected when a lesion noted by either US or CT is greater than 3 cm and has a spherical configuration. Many lesions previously thought to be small or medium-sized Wilms tumors, especially in cases of bilateral or multicentric tumor, may represent hyperplastic nephroblastomatosis. Biopsy is of limited value in distinguishing the hyperplastic form from Wilms tumor, and serial imaging is crucial in determining whether surgery should be performed. Wilms tumor is the most common childhood abdominal malignancy.

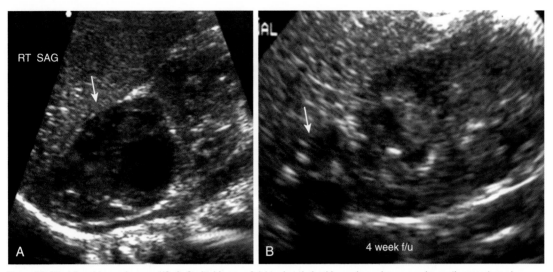

**Figure 88-14.** Adrenal hemorrhage on US. **A,** Sagittal image of right adrenal gland in newborn shows complex cystic mass (*arrow*) indenting upper pole of right kidney. **B,** Sagittal image of right adrenal gland (*arrow*) at 4-week follow-up shows resolution of right adrenal hemorrhage and normal appearing adrenal gland.

56. What is Mayer-Rokitansky-Küster-Hauser syndrome?

Mayer-Rokitansky-Küster-Hauser syndrome refers to vaginal atresia with other variable müllerian duct abnormalities such as a bicornuate or septate uterus. The fallopian tubes, ovaries, and broad ligaments are normal. Associated unilateral renal and skeletal anomalies are present in 50% and 12% of cases, respectively.

57. How is pelvic US used in the evaluation of a child with precocious puberty?

Uterine and ovarian volumes are larger than normal in true isosexual precocious puberty, whereas enlargement of only the ovary has been reported with pseudosexual precocity. True isosexual precocity is due to the premature activation of the hypothalamic pituitary gonadal axis, whereas pseudosexual precocity refers to pubertal changes occurring independent of these actions, as in the case of a functional ovarian cyst or tumor. Multiple, small (<1 cm) cysts can be seen in the ovaries of normal children and in children who have precocious puberty. The best predictor of true precocious puberty is bilateral ovarian enlargement, but unilateral ovarian enlargement associated with larger cysts is more related to pseudosexual precocity.

58. What is the sonographic appearance of adrenal hemorrhage in the neonate, and how can adrenal hemorrhage be differentiated from adrenal neuroblastoma?

Adrenal hemorrhage initially appears as a solid-appearing mass. On serial imaging, adrenal hemorrhage generally decreases in size and changes in appearance from solid to cystic, usually resolving completely over time (Figure 88-14). If over time, the adrenal mass remains solid or complex-cystic in appearance or enlarges, adrenal neuroblastoma must be considered. Correlation with serum/urine metanephrines may be helpful in their differentiation as well.

## KEY POINTS

- Primary VUR is graded on a scale of 1 to 5 based on the degree of ureteral and pyelocalyceal filling and dilation. The higher the grade, the lower the likelihood of spontaneous resolution.
- Renal cortical scintigraphy, contrast-enhanced CT, and renal US are useful to detect acute and chronic pyelonephritis in children.
- Presence of posterior urethral valves is the most common cause of bladder outlet obstruction in infant boys.
- When there is complete duplication of the kidney, the Weigert-Meyer rule states that the lower pole ureter inserts normally into the bladder whereas the upper pole ureter inserts ectopically into the bladder medial and caudal to the lower pole ureteral insertion site.
- The most common solid renal mass in infants is fetal renal hamartoma, also known as mesoblastic nephroma, and the most common childhood abdominal malignancy is Wilms tumor.

## BIBLIOGRAPHY

Copelovitch L. Urolithiasis in children: medical approach. *Pediatr Clini N Am.* 2012;59(4):881-896.

Subcommittee on Urinary Tract Infection SCoQI, Management, Roberts KB. Urinary tract infection: clinical practice guideline for the diagnosis and management of the initial UTI in febrile infants and children 2 to 24 months. *Pediatrics.* 2011;128(3):595-610.

Paterson A. Urinary tract infection: an update on imaging strategies. *Eur Radiol.* 2004;14(suppl 4):L89-L100.

Jain M, LeQuesne GW, Bourne AJ, et al. High-resolution ultrasonography in the differential diagnosis of cystic diseases of the kidney in infancy and childhood: preliminary experience. *J Ultrasound Med.* 1997;16(4):235-240.

Rahmouni A, Bargoin R, Herment A, et al. Color Doppler twinkling artifact in hyperechoic regions. *Radiology.* 1996;199(1):269-271.

Sutherland RS, Mevorach RA, Baskin LS, et al. Spinal dysraphism in children: an overview and an approach to prevent complications. *Urology.* 1995;46(3):294-304.

Westra SJ, Zaninovic AC, Hall TR, et al. Imaging of the adrenal gland in children. *Radiographics.* 1994;14(6):1323-1340.

Beckwith JB. Precursor lesions of Wilms tumor: clinical and biological implications. *Med Pediatr Oncol.* 1993;21(3):158-168.

King LR, Siegel MJ, Solomon AL. Usefulness of ovarian volume and cysts in female isosexual precocious puberty. *J Ultrasound Med.* 1993;12(10):577-581.

Bjorgvinsson E, Majd M, Eggli KD. Diagnosis of acute pyelonephritis in children: comparison of sonography and 99mTc-DMSA scintigraphy. *AJR Am J Roentgenol.* 1991;157(3):539-543.

Corteville JE, Gray DL, Crane JP. Congenital hydronephrosis: correlation of fetal ultrasonographic findings with infant outcome. *Am J Obstet Gynecol.* 1991;165(2):384-388.

Kaplan BS, Kaplan P, Rosenberg HK, et al. Polycystic kidney diseases in childhood. *J Pediatr.* 1989;115(6):867-880.

Greskovich FJ 3rd, Nyberg LM Jr. The prune belly syndrome: a review of its etiology, defects, treatment and prognosis. *J Urol.* 1988;140(4):707-712.

Saxton HM, Borzyskowski M, Mundy AR, et al. Spinning top urethra: not a normal variant. *Radiology.* 1988;168(1):147-150.

Lebowitz RL, Mandell J. Urinary tract infection in children: putting radiology in its place. *Radiology.* 1987;165(1):1-9.

Cremin BJ. A review of the ultrasonic appearances of posterior urethral valve and ureteroceles. *Pediatr Radiol.* 1986;16(5):357-364.

Fotter R, Kopp W, Klein E, et al. Unstable bladder in children: functional evaluation by modified voiding cystourethrography. *Radiology.* 1986;161(3):811-813.

Rosenberg HK, Sherman NH, Tarry WF, et al. Mayer-Rokitansky-Kuster-Hauser syndrome: US aid to diagnosis. *Radiology.* 1986;161(3):815-819.

Blickman JG, Lebowitz RL. The coexistence of primary megaureter and reflux. *AJR Am J Roentgenol.* 1984;143(5):1053-1057.

Nunn IN, Stephens FD. The triad syndrome: a composite anomaly of the abdominal wall, urinary system and testes. *J Urol.* 1961;86:782-794.

# CHAPTER 89

# PEDIATRIC NEURORADIOLOGY

*Michael L. Francavilla, MD, D. Andrew Mong, MD, and Avrum N. Pollock, MD*

1. **How does myelinated brain differ from nonmyelinated brain on an infant magnetic resonance imaging (MRI) examination? Where does one expect to see myelinization occur first?**

   Myelinated brain white matter, as in adults, appears hyperintense relative to gray matter on T1-weighted MR images and hypointense on T2-weighted images. In nonmyelinated brain, this pattern is reversed. Myelinization of the infant brain occurs in a predictable pattern, beginning in the brainstem and cerebellum and progressing to the posterior limb of the internal capsule, optic pathways, and parietal lobes. This pattern of change occurs from caudal to cephalad, dorsal to ventral, and central to peripheral. Myelinization should appear complete on MRI by 24 months but may be incomplete in the terminal zones up to approximately 4 to 5 years of age and in rare cases until the first decade of life.

2. **What are migrational anomalies of the central nervous system (CNS)?**

   Normal neuronal migration occurs during fetal brain development as neurons migrate from the germinal matrix to the cortex along radial glial fibers. Partial or total arrest of this process leads to a migrational anomaly. These anomalies include the following:
   - Focal cortical dysplasia (subtle subcortical high T2-weighted signal intensity and blurring of the gray-white matter junction).
   - Heterotopias (abnormal gray matter found anywhere along glial migration pathways to the cortex).
   - Schizencephaly (a cleft lined by gray matter extending from the outer cortex to the [lateral] ventricles).
   - Polymicrogyria (too many small nodular gyri).
   - Pachygyria (abnormally thickened gyri).
   - Lissencephaly (complete absence of gyri).

   Children with CNS migrational anomalies typically present with developmental delay or seizures (Figure 89-1).

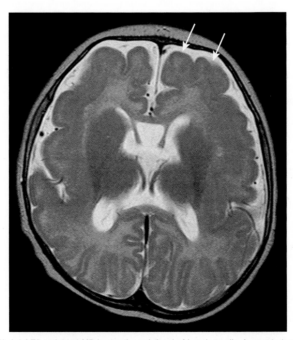

**Figure 89-1.** Pachygyria on MRI. Axial T2-weighted MR image through level of basal ganglia demonstrates abnormally thickened and enlarged large gyri (*arrows*) of frontal cortex, consistent with pachygyria.

3. Name the four kinds of holoprosencephalies.

Holoprosencephaly refers to incomplete differentiation of the fetal prosencephalon (forebrain) into separate hemispheres. Holoprosencephaly may manifest as alobar, resulting in one posteriorly located monoventricle (versus the normally separated two lateral ventricles) and fusion of the thalami; semilobar, with two hemispheres posteriorly but not anteriorly; or lobar, with only mild frontal abnormalities. The middle interhemispheric variant has been more recently described and consists of abnormal midline hemispheric connection in the posterior frontal and parietal lobes. The mildest form along the continuum is thought to include septo-optic dysplasia, which is characterized by absence of the septum pellucidum and optic nerve hypoplasia.

4. What is the differential diagnosis for what appears to be massively dilated ventricles on a prenatal ultrasonography (US) or MRI examination?

The appearance of massively dilated ventricles may be secondary to holoprosencephaly, hydranencephaly, or hydrocephalus. Hydranencephaly results from massive necrosis of the cerebral hemispheres and may be secondary to vascular disease with bilateral internal carotid occlusion, infection, or trauma. In contrast to hydranencephaly, there is a thin residual remnant of cerebral cortex applied to the inner table of the calvaria seen with severe hydrocephalus. The most common causes of prenatal hydrocephalus include Arnold-Chiari malformation II, intracranial hemorrhage, aqueductal stenosis, and Dandy-Walker malformation.

5. Describe the classification of germinal matrix hemorrhage.

The germinal matrix lies in the caudothalamic groove. This is a highly vascular region of the prenatal and premature brain and is prone to hemorrhage, with rupture of the thin venules subsequent to decreased perfusion or oxygenation. Morbidity and mortality may be predicted based on the grade of the hemorrhage:

- Grade I hemorrhage is confined to the germinal matrix.
- Grade II hemorrhage extends into the adjacent lateral ventricle.
- Grade III hemorrhage expands into and dilates the adjacent lateral ventricle.
- Grade IV hemorrhage is in the adjacent parenchyma, probably due to hemorrhagic venous infarction.

US of the premature infant's head through the anterior fontanelle is the imaging modality of choice for the diagnosis and follow-up of germinal matrix hemorrhage.

6. How does the premature brain respond to ischemic injury?

Periventricular leukomalacia (PVL) is characterized by ischemia in an end arterial distribution (in the watershed regions of white matter that surround the ventricles). US may demonstrate an increase in periventricular echogenicity soon after the initial insult. Cystic change in these regions can be seen later in the subacute stage, as the white matter begins to be resorbed. MRI demonstrates abnormal periventricular signal intensity and volume loss. Before 28 weeks of gestation, the developing brain does not display a leukomalacic response, and only volume loss results. This volume loss may take the form of dilated ventricles and expanded extra-axial spaces or porencephalic cysts (expanded cystlike dilations from the lateral ventricles that may reach the cortex). A porencephalic cyst can be differentiated from schizencephaly by noting that, in the former entity, there is no gray matter lining the cyst cavity.

7. Describe the three main types of Chiari malformations.

Chiari I malformation involves herniation of the peg-like cerebellar tonsils into the foramen magnum (>5 mm in patients <15 years old) (Figure 89-2), and is associated with syringomyelia.

Chiari II malformation is more severe, involving herniation of the medulla and vermis and elongation and downward displacement of the brainstem. This malformation is virtually always associated with a meningomyelocele. Prenatal US may show crowding of the posterior fossa ("banana" sign appearance of the cerebellar hemispheres as they wrap around the brainstem). There may also be kinking of the medulla, agenesis of the corpus callosum,

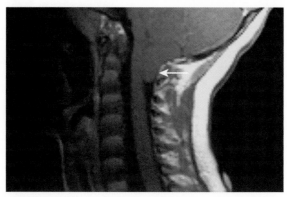

**Figure 89-2.** Chiari I malformation on MRI. Sagittal T1-weighted MR image through craniocervical junction shows inferior displacement of cerebellar tonsils (*arrow*) below level of foramen magnum.

polygyria, hydrocephalus, and colpocephaly (disproportional enlargement of the posterior horns of the lateral ventricles).

Chiari III malformation involves herniation of contents of the posterior fossa through the occiput or upper cervical canal via a bony defect (i.e., akin to an encephalocele).

8. How does the corpus callosum develop, and why is this important?

The corpus callosum develops front to back except for the rostrum (anterior genu, body, splenium, and rostrum last). This is important because an in utero insult may result in destruction of part of the corpus callosum. If posterior portions of the corpus callosum are present and anterior portions are not, this means that they were present at one point and were destroyed. If posterior portions are absent instead, this may mean that they did not develop.

9. What entity does not follow the normal rule of corpus callosum development?

Holoprosencephaly, previously described, may follow an atypical pattern of corpus callosum development, in which the posterior portions develop and the anterior portions do not. This is termed atypical callosal dysgenesis.

10. What are TORCH infections?

The acronym TORCH stands for infections caused by **T**oxoplasmosis, **O**ther (varicella zoster virus, human immunodeficiency virus [HIV], parvovirus B19, enterovirus, etc.), **R**ubella virus, **C**ytomegalovirus (CMV), and **H**erpes simplex virus.

11. How do TORCH infections appear radiographically?

It is often impossible to distinguish TORCH infections radiographically. Intracranial calcification patterns may aid in differentiating them. CMV calcifications are classically present only in the periventricular (**circum**ventricular) regions, whereas toxoplasmosis and rubella also have basal ganglia and cortical calcifications. CMV may also be associated with migrational abnormalities previously discussed. HIV infection may manifest as atrophy with bilateral basal ganglia calcifications. Cerebral atrophy may be present in any infection.

12. Discuss the CNS manifestations of neurofibromatosis type 1 (NF-1).

Patients with NF-1 may have plexiform neurofibromas, which are present along nerve distributions and insinuate within the fascial planes of the head and neck. Sphenoid wing dysplasia, with its resultant harlequin eye appearance, is also present at times. Areas of high T2-weighted signal intensity representing spongiform dysplasia are frequently present in the basal ganglia, brainstem, and cerebellum. Gliomas may develop anywhere along the optic pathway or in areas of spongiform dysplasia. In the spine, patients with NF-1 may develop lateral meningoceles, which herniate from the thecal sac into the thorax. Radiographs of the spine may also demonstrate posterior vertebral body scalloping (from dural ectasia), enlargement of the neural foramina (from neurofibromas), and inferior rib notching/remodeling secondary to the growth of the neurofibromas along the course of the intercostal nerves.

13. How is neurofibromatosis type 2 (NF-2) different from NF-1?

The gene for NF-2 is on chromosome 22, as opposed to chromosome 17 for NF-1. NF-2 tumors can be remembered with the mnemonic MISME, which stands for **M**ultiple **I**nherited **S**chwannomas, **M**eningiomas, and **E**pendymomas. Classically, these appear as bilateral cerebellopontine angle tumors, representing bilateral vestibular schwannomas, which are diagnostic of NF-2, but may involve any of the cranial nerves.

14. What is tuberous sclerosis (TS)?

TS is an autosomal dominant disorder with variable expressivity, which manifests as hamartomatous lesions in multiple organ systems. TS consists of the clinical triad of seizures, adenoma sebaceum, and mental retardation. In the CNS, subependymal nodules and subcortical tubers occur. The tubers typically have high T2-weighted signal intensity in the subcortical white matter. Subependymal giant cell astrocytomas (SGCAs), also known as mixed giant cell tumors, may occur at the foramen of Monro and cause an obstructive hydrocephalus. Involvement outside of the CNS includes angiomyolipomas (fat-containing benign neoplasms) in the kidneys, multiple renal cysts, rhabdomyomas of the heart, cystic lung disease, and bony involvement (Figure 89-3). Rarely, patients may present with giant abdominal aortic aneurysms in early childhood.

15. Describe the manifestations of Sturge-Weber syndrome.

Sturge-Weber syndrome, also known as encephalotrigeminal angiomatosis, includes venous angiomatous malformations within the leptomeninges and choroid plexus with an associated port-wine stain in the distribution of a branch of the trigeminal nerve on the side of the hemispheric involvement. On cross-sectional imaging, there is a focal region of leptomeningeal enhancement, often overlying a region of cortical atrophy. There is usually also abnormal enhancement in the enlarged ipsilateral choroid plexus. Computed tomography (CT) examination also detects "tram-track" subcortical calcifications and ipsilateral hemispheric volume loss, which are not seen in infancy, because they take some time to occur. Rarely, this entity may occur bilaterally.

16. What are the most common brain tumors in infants?

Although pediatric brain tumors are generally more likely to occur within the posterior fossa, in infants 2 years old or younger, the most common individual tumors are supratentorial. These include teratoma, astrocytoma (e.g., glioblastoma multiforme [GBM]), choroid plexus papilloma and carcinoma (in the lateral ventricles), and primitive neuroectodermal tumor (PNET).

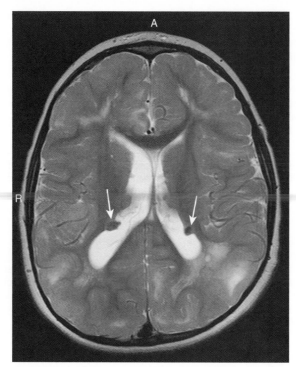

**Figure 89-3.** Subependymal nodules in TS on MRI. Axial T2-weighted MR image through brain demonstrates low signal intensity subependymal nodules (*arrows*) lining lateral ventricles and wispy areas of high signal intensity in scattered subcortical areas representing hamartomas.

17. Name the major posterior fossa tumors in children.

Most pediatric brain tumors are infratentorial. These include pilocytic astrocytoma, fibrillary astrocytoma, medulloblastoma (a PNET), and ependymoma. Medulloblastoma is the most common of these.

18. Describe the typical tumors that occur in the suprasellar region of a child.

Craniopharyngiomas are cystic lesions that often contain calcium (Figure 89-4). These may be confused with Rathke cleft cysts, which are remnants of the Rathke pouch, the structure that forms the anterior portion of the pituitary gland. Other tumors include tumors of hypothalamic origin (gliomas or hamartomas), optic nerve tumors (e.g., tumors seen in NF-1), germinomas arising from the pituitary stalk, and pituitary adenomas. Langerhans cell histiocytosis (eosinophilic granuloma) can manifest as thickening of the infundibulum and loss of visualization of the normal posterior pituitary bright spot on T1-weighted images and is associated with a clinical history of growth delay.

19. Why is thickening of the pituitary stalk an important finding?

Close interval follow-up is warranted because this thickening may be a manifestation of a germinoma or Langerhans cell histiocytosis. Alternatively, the thickening may be idiopathic. The pituitary stalk is considered thickened if it is greater than 2 mm at the insertion of the gland.

20. What is the differential diagnosis for a pediatric cystic neck mass?

This has a broad differential that may be narrowed by location. Type II branchial cleft cysts (the most common) are suprahyoid lesions that classically push the sternocleidomastoid muscle posteriorly and have a tongue of tissue arising between the external and internal carotid arteries. Thyroglossal duct cysts are remnants of the thyroglossal duct and are found in the midline, usually at or below the hyoid bone beneath the strap muscles. Teratomas or dermoids may occur anywhere but can be identified by the presence of fat, calcium, or both. A venolymphatic malformation has a typical appearance of a cystic mass, often with septations, which insinuates through fascial planes (sometimes inferiorly into the mediastinum). They may also contain blood-fluid levels, best appreciated on MRI.

21. What is the differential diagnosis for causes of leukocoria?

Leukocoria is defined as an abnormal white pupillary reflex. Retinoblastoma is the most concerning cause. Other causes include congenital cataract, infection (e.g., toxocariasis), persistent hyperplastic primary vitreous, retinopathy of prematurity, and Coats disease (fusiform dilation of retinal vessels, often with associated retinal detachment and subretinal exudate). Historical clues are helpful in differentiating these entities. The average age of patients with retinoblastoma is 13 months, whereas Coats disease generally occurs in boys older than 4 years old, and toxocariasis occurs after 6 years of age. The presence of calcification may aid in the diagnosis, because 95% of retinoblastomas contain calcium.

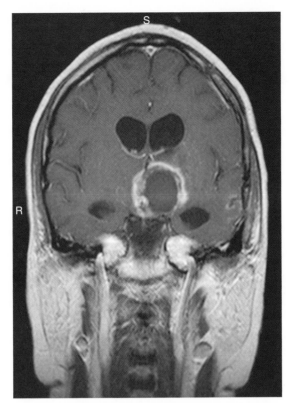

**Figure 89-4.** Craniopharyngioma on MRI. Coronal contrast-enhanced T1-weighted MR image shows ring-enhancing solid and cystic mass in suprasellar region.

22. What is meant by trilateral retinoblastoma?

Bilateral retinoblastomas often occur in the familial form of the disease, which is characterized genetically as a mutation in the *Rb1* tumor suppressor gene. These patients are also at risk for developing a third intracranial tumor, usually in the pineal gland, the so-called third eye. Trilateral retinoblastoma involves tumor in both eyes and a metachronous PNET in the pineal gland. As in the retina, even a fleck of calcium in the pineal gland of a child younger than 6 years old should be considered suggestive of neoplasm.

23. What is fibromatosis colli? Describe its imaging characteristics.

Fibromatosis colli is benign focal or fusiform enlargement of the sternocleidomastoid muscle in infants that usually regresses by 6 to 8 months of age. It is thought to be due to trauma to the sternocleidomastoid muscle or to a positioning abnormality in utero. US of the muscle shows either diffuse enlargement or a focal hyperechoic mass. MRI shows low signal intensity on T2-weighted images due to fibrosis in the sternocleidomastoid muscle.

24. Where do cholesteatomas typically arise, and what is the role of the radiologist in their evaluation?

A cholesteatoma is squamous epithelium that is trapped in the skull base, often creating expansion and erosion of adjacent bony structures. They frequently occur in the middle ear, in the mesotympanum or epitympanum. Cholesteatomas may be congenital, in which case they are well defined and rounded and typically occur near the level of the tympanic membrane (the anterior mesotympanum). Cholesteatomas may also be acquired as a result of tympanic membrane perforation, in which case they typically occur above the tympanic membrane (the epitympanum), adjacent to the scutum and involve Prussak's space. CT is often helpful in defining whether there are effects on adjacent bony structures. Radiologists should comment on the integrity of the ossicles, erosion of the scutum, the presence or absence of labyrinthine fistulas, or defects in the roof of the middle ear (tegmen tympani). MRI is not as helpful for evaluating bony structures, but it may be an important problem-solving tool if there are questions concerning intracranial extension and may demonstrate restricted diffusion, helping to differentiate it from simple fluid/effusion.

25. What is the role of the radiologist in the evaluation of sacrococcygeal teratoma?

Sacrococcygeal teratoma may be detected in utero with US or via fetal MRI. Because the mass may be cystic, the differential diagnosis may include a meningocele (outpouching of meninges through a defect in the posterior elements of the lumbosacral spine). High-output cardiac failure caused by a teratoma may result in hydrops fetalis, placentomegaly, and polyhydramnios, which may necessitate cesarean section or fetal surgery. MRI may be useful in the evaluation of these masses because the prognosis and surgical approach may depend on which components of the mass are within the abdomen and pelvis. Lesions confined to the true pelvis tend to be histologically benign, whereas lesions that extend beyond the confines of the sacrum tend to be malignant.

## KEY POINTS

- MRI is particularly useful for evaluation of congenital and acquired abnormalities of the brain, spinal cord, and head and neck in the pediatric setting.
- US of the premature infant's head through the anterior fontanelle is the imaging modality of choice for the diagnosis and follow-up of germinal matrix hemorrhage.
- Although pediatric brain tumors are generally more likely to occur within the posterior fossa, in infants 2 years old or younger, the most common individual tumors are supratentorial.

## BIBLIOGRAPHY

LaPlante JK, Pierson NS, Hedlund GL. Common pediatric head and neck congenital/developmental anomalies. *Radiol Clin North Am.* 2015;53(1):181-196.

Winter TC, Kennedy AM, Woodward PJ. Holoprosencephaly: a survey of the entity, with embryology and fetal imaging. *Radiographics.* 2015;35(1):275-290.

Nandigam K, Mechtler LL, Smirniotopoulos JG. Neuroimaging of neurocutaneous diseases. *Neurologic Clin.* 2014;32(1):159-192.

Radhakrishnan R, Son HJ, Koch BL. Petrous apex lesions in the pediatric population. *Pediatr Radiol.* 2014;44(3):325-339, quiz 3-4.

Borja MJ, Plaza MJ, Altman N, et al. Conventional and advanced MRI features of pediatric intracranial tumors: supratentorial tumors. *AJR Am J Roentgenol.* 2013;200(5):W483-W503.

Borofsky S, Levy LM. Neurofibromatosis: types 1 and 2. *AJNR Am J Neuroradiol.* 2013;34(12):2250-2251.

Plaza MJ, Borja MJ, Altman N, et al. Conventional and advanced MRI features of pediatric intracranial tumors: posterior fossa and suprasellar tumors. *AJR Am J Roentgenol.* 2013;200(5):1115-1124.

Barkovich AJ, Guerrini R, Kuzniecky RI, et al. A developmental and genetic classification for malformations of cortical development: update 2012. *Brain.* 2012;135(Pt 5):1348-1369.

de Graaf P, Goricke S, Rodjan F, et al. Guidelines for imaging retinoblastoma: imaging principles and MRI standardization. *Pediatr Radiol.* 2012;42(1):2-14.

Nickerson JP, Richner B, Santy K, et al. Neuroimaging of pediatric intracranial infection—part 2: TORCH, viral, fungal, and parasitic infections. *J Neuroimaging.* 2012;22(2):e52-e63.

Sepulveda W, Ximenes R, Wong AE, et al. Fetal magnetic resonance imaging and three-dimensional ultrasound in clinical practice: applications in prenatal diagnosis. *Best Pract Res Clin Obstet Gynaecol.* 2012;26(5):593-624.

Taheri MR, Krauthamer A, Otjen J, et al. Neuroimaging of migrational disorders in pediatric epilepsy. *Curr Probl Diagn Radiol.* 2012;41(1):11-19.

Barath K, Huber AM, Stampfli P, et al. Neuroradiology of cholesteatomas. *AJNR Am J Neuroradiol.* 2011;32(2):221-229.

Paldino MJ, Faerber EN, Poussaint TY. Imaging tumors of the pediatric central nervous system. *Radiol Clin North Am.* 2011;49(4):v, 589-616.

Razek AA, Elkhamary S. MRI of retinoblastoma. *Br J Radiol.* 2011;84(1005):775-784.

Schroeder JW, Vezina LG. Pediatric sellar and suprasellar lesions. *Pediatr Radiol.* 2011;41(3):287-298, quiz 404-5.

Hahn JS, Barnes PD. Neuroimaging advances in holoprosencephaly: refining the spectrum of the midline malformation. *Am J Med Genetics Part C, Semin Med Genetics.* 2010;154C(1):120-132.

Murphey MD, Ruble CM, Tyszko SM, et al. From the archives of the AFIP: musculoskeletal fibromatoses: radiologic-pathologic correlation. *Radiographics.* 2009;29(7):2143-2173.

Umeoka S, Koyama T, Miki Y, et al. Pictorial review of tuberous sclerosis in various organs. *Radiographics.* 2008;28(7):e32.

D'Addario V, Pinto V, Di Cagno L, et al. Sonographic diagnosis of fetal cerebral ventriculomegaly: an update. *J Maternal-Fetal Neonatal Med.* 2007;20(1):7-14.

Tubbs RS, Lyerly MJ, Loukas M, et al. The pediatric Chiari I malformation: a review. *Child's Nervous System.* 2007;23(11):1239-1250.

Bassan H, Benson CB, Limperopoulos C, et al. Ultrasonographic features and severity scoring of periventricular hemorrhagic infarction in relation to risk factors and outcome. *Pediatrics.* 2006;117(6):2111-2118.

Kinney HC. The near-term (late preterm) human brain and risk for periventricular leukomalacia: a review. *Semin Perinatol.* 2006;30(2):81-88.

Glass RB, Fernbach SK, Norton KI, et al. The infant skull: a vault of information. *Radiographics.* 2004;24(2):507-522.

Stevenson KL. Chiari Type II malformation: past, present, and future. *Neurosurg Focus.* 2004;16(2):E5.

Thomas-Sohl KA, Vaslow DF, Maria BL. Sturge-Weber syndrome: a review. *Pediatric NeuroL.* 2004;30(5):303-310.

# CHAPTER 90

# PEDIATRIC MUSCULOSKELETAL RADIOLOGY

*Mesha L.D. Martinez, MD, and D. Andrew Mong, MD*

1. **How does growing bone respond to trauma, and how is this different from mature bone?**
   The cartilaginous physis separates the epiphysis from the metaphysis. Pediatric ligaments and tendons are relatively stronger than growing bone (in contrast to adults). Given an equivalent force applied to growing versus mature bone, the growing bone has a higher likelihood of fracture. In addition, immature bone has a propensity to bow instead of break, which may cause buckles in one side of the cortex (torus/buckle fractures) or greenstick fractures (fracture of one cortex and bowing of the other). Fractures can also occur through an open physis. These patterns are not seen in mature bone.

2. **What is the significance of fractures of the physis?**
   The cartilaginous physis is vulnerable to injury, especially at its attachment to the metaphysis. Disruption of the physis may result in slower growth and premature fusion, leading to limb length discrepancy.

3. **How are fractures of the physis classified?**
   Physeal injuries are classified in the Salter-Harris classification (Figure 90-1), increasing in severity from I to V. Type I is a fracture through the physis. The fracture line in type II includes the metaphysis and physis. Type III fracture includes the epiphysis and the physis. Type IV fracture involves the metaphysis, physis, and epiphysis. Type V fracture is a crush injury of the physis. Follow-up for Salter-Harris fractures may include magnetic resonance imaging (MRI), which can delineate an abnormally fused physis in the healing phase that may need to be disrupted to allow future osseous growth.

4. **What are secondary ossification centers?**
   Secondary ossification centers appear and then fuse later with the primary ossification center as seen on radiographs at predictable times during skeletal maturation. For example, multiple secondary ossification centers are seen around the elbow, which appear at different ages. Their usual sequence can be remembered by the mnemonic CRITOE: **C**apitellum (1 year), **R**adial head (3 years), **I**nternal (medial) epicondyle (5 years), **T**rochlea (7 years), **O**lecranon (9 years), and **E**xternal (lateral) epicondyle (11 years).

5. **Why are secondary ossification centers particularly important to understand in the setting of elbow trauma?**
   One important reason to understand this sequence is that a type I Salter-Harris fracture through the physis of the medial epicondyle may cause displacement of this ossification center into the region of the trochlea. This displacement might create the false impression that the trochlear ossification center is present, whereas the medial epicondylar ossification center has not yet appeared. Knowledge of this sequence allows one to identify this appearance appropriately as a displaced fracture.

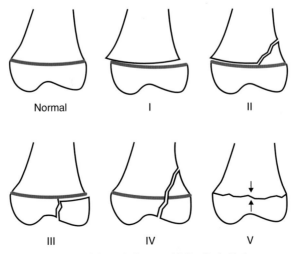

**Figure 90-1.** Schematic diagram of Salter-Harris fractures.

6. What are the most common fractures of the wrist/forearm in children?

Distal radius fractures are the most common fractures in children. Scaphoid fractures are the most common fractures in adolescents that are skeletally mature.

7. What is gymnast wrist?

Gymnast wrist is an overuse injury (from chronic pressure on joints). Physeal widening, metaphyseal irregularity, and sclerosis can be seen. Early physeal bridging and radius growth disturbance may occur if not treated.

8. What is the equivalent of gymnast wrist in the shoulder?

Little leaguer's shoulder is an overuse injury in throwers. Subtle findings, similar to gymnast wrist, may be seen on MRI.

9. How may subtle supracondylar fractures of the elbow be diagnosed?

Pediatric elbow fractures often occur in the supracondylar region, where the humerus is relatively flat. The anterior humeral line, drawn on the lateral view of the elbow along the anterior humerus, normally intersects the middle third of the capitellum. This intersection is likely to be disrupted in supracondylar fractures. The presence of a joint effusion (hemarthrosis) is also extremely helpful and can be assessed by the presence of an elevated posterior fat pad, which is displaced and visible on the lateral view if there is blood in the joint. Displacement of the anterior fat pad ("sail" sign) may also be seen with hemarthrosis, but this finding is less specific.

10. Describe nursemaid's elbow.

Nursemaid's elbow is caused by radial head subluxation through the annular ligament of the elbow, resulting in abnormal positioning of the ligament between the radial head and capitellum. It is often caused by sudden traction on the forearm in a child 1 to 3 years old. Radiographs may appear normal but are obtained to exclude fractures.

11. List risk factors for developmental dysplasia of the hip (DDH).
- Caucasian race.
- Female gender.
- Torticollis.
- Clubfoot.
- Breech birth.

12. When is DDH suspected clinically?

It is difficult to diagnose DDH in newborns 4 weeks old or younger because of normal joint laxity, but this condition is suspected in infants with leg length discrepancy and asymmetric thigh creases. The Barlow maneuver on physical examination dislocates the femoral head rearward when DDH is present, and the Ortolani maneuver reduces the recently dislocated hip, often with a resultant "clunk."

13. Name the potential complications of untreated DDH.
- Leg length discrepancy.
- Osteoarthritis.
- Pain.
- Gait disturbance.
- Decrease in agility.

14. How is DDH diagnosed radiographically?

Traditionally, radiography has been used to diagnose DDH. Although the femoral head begins to ossify during the first year (usually between 3 to 6 months), its location must be inferred in infants. The acetabulum is divided into quadrants by the horizontal Hilgenreiner line, drawn through both triradiate cartilages, and the vertical Perkin line, drawn through the lateral rim of the acetabulum. A normal femoral head should fall within the inner lower quadrant of these intersecting lines, whereas a femoral head in DDH would be displaced superolaterally. The acetabular angle should also be evaluated, drawn between Hilgenreiner line and a line connecting the superolateral ridge of the acetabulum with the triradiate cartilage. This angle should be less than 30 degrees in neonates.

15. How is DDH diagnosed on ultrasonography (US)?

US is now the preferred method of diagnosing DDH in children younger than 1 year old. The hip is studied in the coronal plane. The alpha angle is measured between the straight lateral margin of the ilium and a line from the inferior point of the ilium tangential to the acetabulum. This is a measure of acetabular depth and should be greater than 60 degrees. At least half of the femoral head should be seated within the acetabulum.

16. What is Legg-Calvé-Perthes disease?

Legg-Calvé-Perthes disease refers to idiopathic osteonecrosis of the femoral head, usually affecting children 3 to 12 years old with a mean age of 7 years. Radiographic findings include a small femoral head epiphysis, which may become fragmented, and widening of the articular space, which may be due to an associated joint effusion.

17. Describe slipped capital femoral epiphysis (SCFE).

SCFE is a hip disease of early adolescence (10 to 15 years old), characterized by idiopathic posterior and inferior slippage of the capital femoral epiphysis on the femoral neck metaphysis. Complications include avascular necrosis of

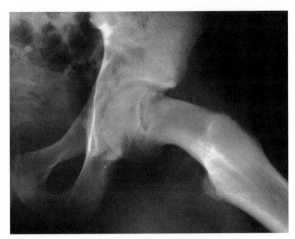

**Figure 90-2.** SCFE on frog-leg radiograph of left hip. Note open physis with inferior displacement of femoral capital epiphysis relative to metaphysis. *(Courtesy of Richard Markowitz, MD, Children's Hospital of Philadelphia.)*

the femoral head or chondrolysis. Anteroposterior and frog-leg views of both hips should be obtained because the condition can be bilateral in 40% of cases. On the frog-leg view, a normal epiphysis projects superior to the Klein line, which is drawn along the superior surface of the femoral neck. In early SCFE, the epiphysis is flush with this line (Figure 90-2).

18. How is SCFE treated?

Treatment goals include the prevention of further slippage and physeal plate closure. SCFE may be treated with internal fixation, bone graft, osteotomy, or cast immobilization. There is no attempt to reduce the slip because this may cause avascular necrosis.

19. What are coxa vara and coxa valga?

Coxa vara and coxa valga are abnormalities of the femoral shaft-to-neck angle. The normal angle is ≈150 degrees at birth, decreasing to 120 to 135 degrees in adults. Coxa vara occurs when the angle is less than 120 degrees and may be secondary to trauma, tumor, SCFE, or a congenital abnormality. Coxa valga occurs when the angle is greater than 135 degrees and is usually neuromuscular in origin but may also be seen in blood dyscrasias such as thalassemia.

20. Describe Blount disease.

Blount disease is a varus deformity of the knee (i.e., the tibia is abnormally directed medially compared with the femur) resulting from growth disturbance of the medial aspect of the proximal tibial metaphysis. This deformity may occur in infants, in which case it is often bilateral, or in adolescents. On radiography, varus deformity of the knee is seen in conjunction with variable amounts of depression, beaking, and fragmentation of the medial proximal tibial metaphysis, sometimes with involvement of the medial proximal tibial epiphysis as well. Tibial osteotomy may be required for treatment because growth disturbance may result from abnormal tibial bowing.

21. What is Osgood-Schlatter disease?

Osgood-Schlatter disease is a common cause of knee pain in adolescence (11 to 14 years old) that is thought to result from repetitive traction through the patellar tendon onto the developing tibial tubercle. This traction can lead to partial avulsion through the ossification center and heterotopic bone formation. Although the diagnosis may be made clinically, radiographs may aid in the exclusion of other etiologies of knee pain. Lateral radiographs may reveal irregular ossification of the proximal tibial tubercle, calcification and thickening of the patellar tendon, and soft tissue swelling.

22. What are two other common processes involving the extensor mechanism of the knee only in the pediatric patient?

Sinding-Larsen-Johansson and patellar sleeve avulsion fracture are two similar injuries in the pediatric population involving the origin of the patellar tendon. Sinding-Larsen-Johansson is similar to Osgood-Schlatter disease with repetitive injury on the inferior pole of the patella. Patellar sleeve avulsion fracture is a result of sudden force as the knee extends and avulses the bone off of the inferior pole of the patella.

23. What is the difference between a triplane fracture and a juvenile Tillaux fracture of the ankle?

Both fractures occur after partial closure of the distal tibial physis. On a frontal radiograph, a triplane fracture appears as a Salter III fracture through the epiphysis, and on a lateral radiograph, it appears as a Salter II fracture through the metaphysis. A juvenile Tillaux fracture is simply a Salter III fracture that occurs at the anterolateral aspect of the distal tibia. The physis fuses from medial to lateral, leaving the lateral aspect more vulnerable to injury.

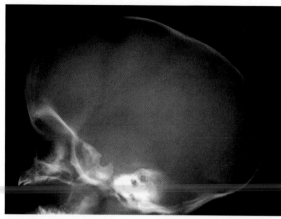

**Figure 90-3.** Scaphocephaly on lateral radiograph of skull. Note markedly increased anteroposterior diameter of skull from premature closure of sagittal suture, leading to boat-shaped skull.

24. **What is Freiberg infraction?**

    Freiberg infraction is an idiopathic osteochondrosis of the head of a metatarsal bone (usually the second), which results in flattening and osteosclerosis of the metatarsal head. It is usually seen in adolescents (13 to 18 years old).

25. **What is a craniosynostosis?**

    A craniosynostosis represents premature closure of a suture of the skull. This premature closure results in cessation of growth of the skull perpendicular to the suture line and abnormal compensatory growth along the axis of the closed suture. For this reason, sagittal craniosynostosis results in an elongated skull in the anteroposterior dimension (scaphocephaly) (Figure 90-3). Plagiocephaly results from premature closure of one coronal suture, resulting in abnormal bulging on the opposite forehead. Premature closure of the metopic suture results in trigonocephaly, which appears as a triangular keel-shaped forehead. Cloverleaf skull (kleeblattschädel) results from premature closure of the coronal, lambdoid, and posterior sagittal sutures, with bulging of the vertex of the brain through the squamosal, anterior sagittal, and metopic sutures.

26. **Give the differential diagnosis for vertebra plana.**

    Flattening of a vertebral body (vertebra plana) in a child should first bring to mind the diagnosis of Langerhans cell histiocytosis. Other diagnostic possibilities in pediatric patients include leukemia, lymphoma, metastatic disease, infection, and storage diseases.

27. **When and where do pediatric primary tumors of bone occur?**

    Ewing sarcoma and osteosarcoma are the most common primary pediatric bone tumors and typically occur between ages 10 to 25 years. The most common sites are the pelvis, thigh, lower leg, upper arm, and ribs, but soft tissue may also be the primary site of involvement. Ewing sarcoma typically does not have a matrix and appears as a permeative aggressive lesion, often with associated periosteal reaction. Most osteosarcomas occur in the metaphysis, typically around the knee. Although the appearance of osteosarcomas is variable, they often produce a characteristic fluffy osteoid matrix.

28. **What are the most common pediatric primary tumors that metastasize to the osseous structures?**

    Neuroblastoma, lymphoma, clear cell sarcoma/Wilms tumor, rhabdomyosarcoma, retinoblastoma, Ewing sarcoma (more commonly metastasizing to lung), and osteosarcoma (more commonly metastasizing to lung).

29. **What are the benign pediatric primary bone tumors?**

    Benign pediatric primary bone tumors can be categorized into groups as follows:

    Cartilaginous: Osteochondroma, enchondroma, chondroblastoma
    Cysts: Unicameral/simple bone cyst, aneurysmal bone cyst
    Fibrous: Fibrous cortical defect/nonossifying fibroma, fibrous dysplasia
    Osseous: Osteoid osteoma, osteoblastoma
    Other: Langerhans cell histiocytosis/eosinophilic granuloma

30. **How should a suspected osteoid osteoma be evaluated?**

    Osteoid osteoma is a benign neoplasm with a nidus of osteoid-rich tissue that typically causes an intense sclerotic reaction in surrounding bone. An osteoid osteoma may occur in the cortical, cancellous, or periosteal regions of any bone (or rarely in adjacent soft tissues). Most patients are between ages 10 and 30 years and often give a typical history of night pain relieved by aspirin. A radionuclide bone scan may point to the abnormality before any changes are apparent on radiographs and is performed on any patient with a painful scoliosis in whom osteoid osteoma in the spine is the working diagnosis. If radiographs do not reveal the lucent nidus surrounded by sclerotic bone, a computed tomography (CT) scan is the preferred next step because intracortical tumors may be missed on MRI.

31. If a pediatric patient presents with a palpable soft tissue mass, what are some possible underlying etiologies?

Most soft tissue masses in children are benign and include desmoid tumors, infantile myofibromatosis, peripheral nerve sheath tumors, hemangiomas, lipomatous lesions (lipoma, which is more common in adults, and lipoblastoma, more common in children). Malignant tumors include rhabdomyosarcoma, primitive peripheral neuroectodermal tumor (PNET), extraosseous Ewing sarcoma, and synovial sarcoma.

32. What is rickets?

Rickets is a relative or absolute deficiency in vitamin D, which causes a decrease in ossification. It is almost exclusively seen in children younger than 2 years of age.

33. How does rickets appear radiographically?

Bone density is overall decreased. More specific signs include loss of the zone of provisional calcification within the metaphysis of long bones; this leads to metaphyseal irregularity, cupping, and fraying with an associated widened physis. These changes are seen best in the distal radius, which is the reason that radiographs of the wrists are ordered to evaluate rickets (Figure 90-4). Another classic appearance is the "rachitic rosary," which is enlargement of the costochondral junctions in the chest.

34. Describe the bony changes of sickle cell anemia.

Sickle cell anemia is secondary to a disorder of "sickling" of red blood cells resulting from abnormal hemoglobin molecules. Clumped sickled cells form venous (and sometimes arterial) thromboses, affecting multiple organs. Osseous manifestations include patchy sclerotic changes in bone from infarctions. A more specific sign includes a "Lincoln log" appearance of the vertebral bodies, with square-like depressions seen in the superior and inferior endplates on a lateral spine radiograph. Avascular necrosis of the femoral or humeral heads may also be seen. Affected patients are prone to osteomyelitis from *Staphylococcus aureus* and *Salmonella*. On MRI, it can be difficult to distinguish infarction from osteomyelitis because both may produce signal abnormalities in marrow (high T2-weighted signal intensity) along with adjacent soft tissue changes. Dactylitis is a nonspecific term referring to inflammation of a digit, which may also be seen in sickle cell anemia secondary to infarction or infection. Finally, because of chronic anemia, patients with sickle cell anemia have an increased red-to-yellow marrow ratio, which may be inferred on a lateral skull radiograph by the widening of the diploic space (Figure 90-5).

35. What is the most common type of dwarfism, and what are its manifestations?

The most common type of dwarfism is achondroplasia. This is a rhizomelic (shortening of the proximal bones) autosomal dominant disorder. Typical characteristics include a large head with frontal bossing, a trident configuration

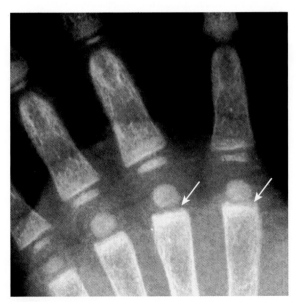

**Figure 90-4.** Rickets of hand on frontal hand radiograph. Note cupping and fraying of metaphyses (*arrows*). *(Courtesy of Richard Markowitz, MD, Children's Hospital of Philadelphia.)*

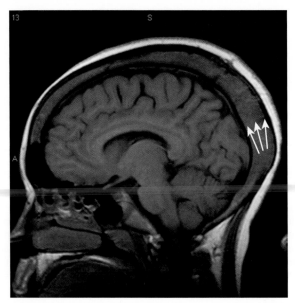

**Figure 90-5.** Sickle cell anemia involving skull on MRI. Sagittal T1-weighted MR image through head shows widening of diploic space (*arrows*) of skull from bone marrow expansion. This finding is not specific for sickle cell anemia and may be found in other severe anemias such as with thalassemia or iron deficiency anemia.

of the hands, genu varum (bowed legs), and an exaggerated lumbar lordosis (with posterior scalloping of the vertebral bodies). On a frontal radiograph of the lumbosacral spine in a normal patient, the distance between the pedicles gradually widens from L1 to L5, whereas an achondroplastic dwarf shows a decrease in the interpedicular distance of the caudal spine. Other radiographic findings include a notch-like sacroiliac groove and metaphyseal flaring of the long bones.

36. What is the differential diagnosis for dense metaphyseal bands, and how does one know when they are abnormally dense?

Dense metaphyseal bands may be a normal variant, so it is important to look at areas that do not have a lot of bone turnover to see whether they are affected as well. Specifically, the metaphyses of the fibula are good areas to check. A major concern is heavy metal poisoning (specifically lead intoxication). Lead poisoning can be diagnosed by noting not only metaphyseal bands but also radiopaque lead chips floating in a child's intestines seen on a frontal radiograph of the abdomen. Other etiologic factors include stress lines, treated rickets, scurvy, hypervitaminosis D, and treated leukemia.

## KEY POINTS

- Physeal injuries are classified in the Salter-Harris classification, increasing in severity from I to V. Disruption of the physis may result in slower growth and premature fusion, leading to limb length discrepancy.
- The usual sequence of ossification of the secondary ossification centers of the elbow can be remembered by the mnemonic CRITOE: **C**apitellum (1 year), **R**adial head (3 years), **I**nternal (medial) epicondyle (5 years), **T**rochlea (7 years), **O**lecranon (9 years), and **E**xternal (lateral) epicondyle (11 years).
- Ewing sarcoma and osteosarcoma are the most common primary pediatric bone tumors.

### BIBLIOGRAPHY

Georgiadis AG, Zaltz I. Slipped capital femoral epiphysis: how to evaluate with a review and update of treatment. *Pediatr Clin N Am.* 2014;61(6):1119-1135.

Little JT, Klionsky NB, Chaturvedi A, et al. Pediatric distal forearm and wrist injury: an imaging review. *Radiographics.* 2014;34(2):472-490.

Schwend RM, Shaw BA, Segal LS. Evaluation and treatment of developmental hip dysplasia in the newborn and infant. *Pediatr Clin N Am.* 2014;61(6):1095-1107.

Badve CA, K MM, Iyer RS, et al. Craniosynostosis: imaging review and primer on computed tomography. *Pediatr Radiol.* 2013;43(6):728-742, quiz 5-7.

Coley BD, Bates DG, Faerber EN, et al. *Caffey's pediatric diagnostic imaging.* 12th ed. Philadelphia, PA: Elsevier-Saunders; 2013.

Manaster BJ, May DA, Disler DG. *Musculoskeletal imaging: the requisites.* 4th ed. Philadelphia, PA: Elsevier Saunders; 2013.

Shore RM, Chesney RW. Rickets: Part I. *Pediatr Radiol.* 2013;43(2):140-151.

Shore RM, Chesney RW. Rickets: Part II. *Pediatr Radiol.* 2013;43(2):152-172.

Booth TN. Cervical spine evaluation in pediatric trauma. *AJR Am J Roentgenol.* 2012;198(5):W417-W425.

Iyer RS, Chapman T, Chew FS. Pediatric bone imaging: diagnostic imaging of osteoid osteoma. *AJR Am J Roentgenol.* 2012;198(5):1039-1052.

Nemeth BA, Narotam V. Developmental dysplasia of the hip. *Pediatr Rev.* 2012;33(12):553-561.

Laor T, Jaramillo D. MR imaging insights into skeletal maturation: what is normal? *Radiology.* 2009;250(1):28-38.

Wootton-Gorges SL. MR imaging of primary bone tumors and tumor-like conditions in children. *Magn Reson Imaging Clin N Am.* 2009;17(3):469-487, vi.

Swischuk LE, Hernandez JA. Frequently missed fractures in children (value of comparative views). *Emer Radiol.* 2004;11(1):22-28.

Cheema JI, Grissom LE, Harcke HT. Radiographic characteristics of lower-extremity bowing in children. *Radiographics.* 2003;23(4):871-880.

Lemyre E, Azouz EM, Teebi AS, et al. Bone dysplasia series. Achondroplasia, hypochondroplasia and thanatophoric dysplasia: review and update. *Canadian Assoc Radiologists J.* 1999;50(3):185-197.

Lins RE, Simovitch RW, Waters PM. Pediatric elbow trauma. *Ortho Clin N Am.* 1999;30(1):119-132.

Kao SC, Smith WL. Skeletal injuries in the pediatric patient. *Radiol Clin North Am.* 1997;35(3):727-746.

England SP, Sundberg S. Management of common pediatric fractures. *Pediatr Clin N Am.* 1996;43(5):991-1012.

Spirt BA, Oliphant M, Gottlieb RH, et al. Prenatal sonographic evaluation of short-limbed dwarfism: an algorithmic approach. *Radiographics.* 1990;10(2):217-236.

# CHAPTER 91

# IMAGING OF CHILD ABUSE

*Michael L. Francavilla, D. Andrew Mong, MD, and Avrum N. Pollock, MD*

1. **What are key history and physical examination findings that may raise suspicion of the possibility of nonaccidental trauma (NAT)?**

   Red flags from the history that should lead the clinician and radiologist to consider child abuse include injuries that are not commensurate with the development of the child, a delay in seeking care, or vague or changing stories given by caretakers. Physical examination findings that the clinician may convey to the radiologist include bruises in various stages of healing; "pattern injuries," such as from instrument marks or from cigarette burns; and signs of neglect.

2. **What diagnostic algorithm might the clinician and radiologist apply if skeletal injury from child abuse is suspected?**

   In addition to radiographs of specific injuries, a skeletal survey is performed on all children younger than 2 years. This survey includes frontal radiographs of the chest, arms, hands, pelvis, legs, ankles, and feet; oblique views of the ribs; and frontal and lateral radiographs of the skull and entire spine. A "babygram" (frontal radiograph of the chest and abdomen) is inadequate. A nuclear medicine bone scan with pinhole collimation is performed if the survey is negative and there is a high index of clinical suspicion (Figure 91-1). Computed tomography (CT) and/or magnetic resonance imaging (MRI) of the brain should be considered if neurologic symptoms or highly suspicious fractures are present. At times, MRI of the cervical spine may be performed if there is suspicion of a whiplash type of mechanism. Box 91-1 lists lesions that should prompt a workup for child abuse.

3. **Describe shaken infant syndrome.**

   Shaken infant syndrome, also known as shaken impact syndrome, occurs when an infant or young child is shaken forcefully. This creates shearing forces that may cause classic patterns of injury seen in the chest and brain. Long

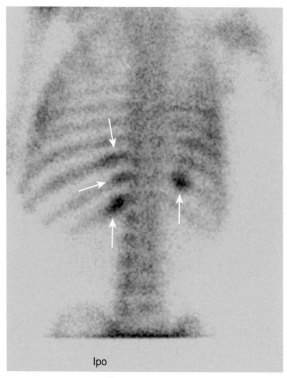

lpo

**Figure 91-1.** Rib fractures due to NAT on technetium-99m ($^{99m}$Tc) methylene diphosphonate (MDP) bone scan. Posterior view demonstrates multiple foci of radiotracer uptake in posterior inferior ribs (*arrows*).

**Box 91-1.** Lesions That Should Prompt a Workup for Child Abuse

- Metaphyseal corner or bucket-handle fractures (highly specific for abuse)
- Posterior rib fractures
- Fractures of spinous processes, scapula, or sternum, or compression fractures of vertebral bodies
- Subdural hematomas, especially when midline
- Duodenal hematoma or acute pancreatitis

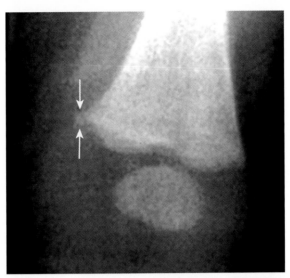

**Figure 91-2.** Metaphyseal corner fracture of distal tibia due to NAT on frontal radiograph. Note typical linear lucency (*arrows*) within peripheral subphyseal metaphysis.

bone injuries with resultant metaphyseal corner fractures are due to twisting/torsion-type injuries, which can occur with or without shaken infant syndrome, and are a separate injury mechanism and type of NAT.

4. What are metaphyseal corner fractures?

Metaphyseal fractures result from shearing forces of NAT and appear as metaphyseal corner fractures or bucket-handle fractures, which are the same fractures seen in different radiographic projections or obliquities. These fractures may heal quickly. They typically appear as lucent areas extending across the metaphysis, nearly perpendicular to the long axis of the bone. They have long been considered highly specific for child abuse (Figure 91-2). Although there has been recent controversy (vociferously refuted by pediatric imagers) over this observation, all major specialty societies maintain that classic metaphyseal lesions have high specificity for NAT.

5. Name other pediatric fractures with high specificity for child abuse.

Posterior rib fractures are another aspect of shaken infant syndrome that occur when adult hands forcefully grab the infant's chest while shaking the infant, resulting in a levering effect of the posterior ribs against the costal processes of the adjacent vertebral bodies. These fractures are specific for abuse and should be reported immediately, even when chest radiographs are obtained for unrelated reasons. Other highly suspicious fractures include fractures of the scapula, spinous process, or sternum (Figure 91-3). Moderately specific fractures include multiple fractures, fractures of different ages, epiphyseal separations, vertebral body fractures and separations, digital fractures, and complex skull fractures.

6. Which common fractures have low specificity for child abuse?

Fractures of the long bones in ambulating children, clavicular fractures, subperiosteal new bone formation, and linear skull fractures have low specificity for child abuse. However, a single long bone diaphyseal fracture is the most common fracture seen in abused children.

7. What features of skull fractures increase the likelihood of NAT?

Branching, multiple, depressed, or distracted fractures and fractures that cross suture lines are more likely to be caused by abuse than are linear skull fractures.

8. What features of a fracture are useful in estimating its age?

Features that may be useful to the radiologist include sclerosis at the fracture margin, the presence of periosteal reaction, callus formation, bony bridging, and bony remodeling. Multiple fractures of different ages are highly suggestive of NAT.

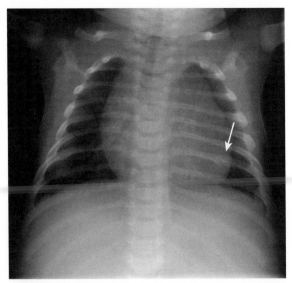

**Figure 91-3.** Posterior rib fractures due to NAT on frontal chest radiograph. Note curvilinear lucency in posterior left 7th rib with surrounding callus formation (*arrow*) due to partially healed fracture. Also note mild deformity of contralateral right posterior 7th rib indicating separate healed fracture.

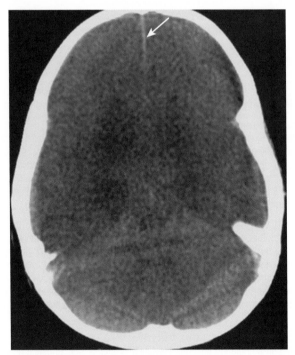

**Figure 91-4.** Interhemispheric subdural hematoma due to NAT on head CT. Note high attenuation subdural hemorrhage between frontal lobes (*arrow*) and diffuse cerebral edema with loss of gray-white differentiation.

9. Summarize common findings of head trauma in shaken infant syndrome.

Shearing forces may create subdural hematomas. Interhemispheric subdural hematoma and posterior fossa/tentorial subdural hematoma are very suspicious areas of involvement. Epidural hematomas are rarely associated with NAT. Severe cerebral edema, which may result from asphyxiation, has a typical appearance on unenhanced head CT. There is loss of gray-white matter differentiation and edema of the cerebral cortex and central gray structures (basal ganglia and thalami). The cerebrum appears diffusely low in attenuation (Figure 91-4).

10. What is the most common cause of death in a patient who has sustained NAT?

Injury to the central nervous system is the most common cause of death.

11. How should imaging of the brain be applied in the setting of suspected abuse?

Any child younger than 2 years of age in whom there is a clinical suspicion of abuse, even if asymptomatic, receives a noncontrast head CT scan because of the high incidence of occult brain trauma. Brain imaging should also be considered in older children. Irritability, vomiting, altered state of consciousness, and irregular respirations are strong indications to perform brain imaging. MRI of the brain can be performed to detect more subtle shear-type injuries of the white matter not evident on head CT and can be used to date areas of hemorrhage with greater accuracy and to assess for changes of hypoxic-ischemic injury, better evaluated with diffusion-weighted imaging (DWI) on MRI.

12. How is the age of intracranial blood determined on MRI examinations?

Evolving blood products in cerebral or subdural hematomas go through various changes in signal intensity on T1-weighted and T2-weighted MR images. The mnemonic **I B**leed; **I D**ie; **B**leed **D**ie; **B**leed **B**leed; **D**ie **D**ie can be used to remember the sequence of changes.

- Hyperacute hemorrhage (oxyhemoglobin) is **i**sointense/dark on T1-weighted images and **b**right on T2-weighted images.
- Acute hemorrhage (deoxyhemoglobin) is **i**sointense/dark on T1-weighted images and **d**ark on T2-weighted images.
- Early subacute hemorrhage (intracellular methemoglobin) is **b**right on T1-weighted images and **d**ark on T2-weighted images.
- Late subacute hemorrhage (extracellular methemoglobin) is **b**right on T1-weighted images and **b**right on T2-weighted images.
- Chronic hemorrhage (hemosiderin) is very **d**ark on T1-weighted images and very **d**ark on T2-weighted images.

13. Describe possible bowel findings in cases of abuse.

Bowel injuries typically occur in children older than 2 years who may have been punched or kicked, with resultant compression of the bowel loops against the spinal column. The duodenum and proximal small bowel are the most commonly affected areas of the small bowel and may show lacerations or intramural hematomas, which can cause obstruction if the bleeding is severe. These injuries can be studied with an upper gastrointestinal examination, abdominal CT, or abdominal MRI and may be seen on US in the ideal situation.

14. What is the most common cause of pediatric pancreatitis?

The most common cause of pediatric pancreatitis is trauma, either accidental or nonaccidental. Pancreatic injury may be suspected with abdominal pain, fever, and vomiting. Acute pancreatitis may be detected with an elevation of amylase and lipase levels without the presence of radiographic findings.

15. Describe the CT imaging features of pediatric acute pancreatitis and pancreatic lacerations.

On CT, acute pancreatitis may manifest as enlargement of the pancreas, stranding in the peripancreatic fat, areas of decreased enhancement in the pancreatic parenchyma, or with peripancreatic fluid collections. On CT, pancreatic lacerations appear as areas of linear hypoattenuating foci within pancreatic tissue, usually with surrounding fluid and/or hemorrhage.

16. Are multiple bruises and skeletal injuries always diagnostic of child abuse?

No. Systemic disorders can also be responsible for multiple bruises and skeletal injuries. Abnormalities of coagulation including entities such as leukemia, hemophilia, idiopathic thrombocytopenic purpura, and Henoch-Schönlein purpura may mimic abuse. Metabolic/congenital abnormalities are also important mimickers to consider, including osteogenesis imperfecta, Menkes kinky hair syndrome, Ehlers-Danlos syndrome, congenital syphilis, and rickets.

17. How does congenital syphilis mimic child abuse?

Both may produce metaphyseal fractures. In congenital syphilis, these are pathologic fractures secondary to fragmentation of the metaphysis from osteomyelitis. There is an argument that healing rickets can have a similar appearance as well. These findings are usually symmetric in a child with syphilis and asymmetric in an abused child. Syphilis may also be differentiated from child abuse through noting concomitant diffuse diaphyseal periosteal reaction along long bones, splenomegaly, and positive serologic test results.

18. What is the differential diagnosis of periosteal reaction in a newborn?

In addition to fractures from NAT, other differential diagnostic considerations include congenital infection (e.g., syphilis), neuroblastoma metastases, physiologic periosteal new bone formation, prostaglandin treatment, and Caffey disease. Caffey disease is a benign, self-limited periosteal reaction of uncertain etiology, usually involving the mandible, clavicles, and long bones and is rarely if ever seen in current times.

19. When does physiologic periosteal new bone formation occur?

Periosteal new bone formation can occur symmetrically along shafts of long bones in newborns and resolves by 3 months of age. It is thought to be due to handling of the infant. There are no associated fractures.

20. Can a metaphyseal corner fracture look like a metaphyseal lucent band?

Yes. If a lucent metaphyseal band is identified, additional projections may identify it as a corner fracture. The differential diagnosis of a lucent metaphyseal band includes leukemia, lymphoma, metastatic disease (neuroblastoma), congenital infection, and scurvy.

21. What is the legal responsibility of any U.S. physician who suspects child abuse?

Child protection ordinances exist in all 50 states and require medical professionals to report suspected abuse to the local child protective service agency within 48 hours. Radiologists must ensure that high-quality radiographs are obtained for the skeletal survey, which may subsequently be used in court.

## KEY POINTS

- In addition to radiographs of specific injuries, a skeletal survey is performed on all children younger than 2 years when child abuse is suspected. Bone scintigraphy, CT, and MRI are also utilized as needed.
- Metaphyseal corner fractures or bucket-handle fractures have high specificity for child abuse. Posterior rib fractures; fractures of the scapula, spinous process, or sternum; vertebral compression fractures; complex skull fractures; and multiple fractures of different ages are suggestive of child abuse as well.
- Any child younger than 2 years of age in whom there is a clinical suspicion of child abuse, even if asymptomatic, receives a noncontrast head CT scan because of the high incidence of occult brain trauma. Brain MRI may also be used to detect more subtle shear-type injuries of the white matter, to date areas of hemorrhage, and to assess for changes of hypoxic-ischemic injury.
- Subdural hematomas, particularly when interhemispheric or seen in the posterior fossa/tentorial locations, are suspicious for head trauma related to shaken infant syndrome.

## BIBLIOGRAPHY

Ayoub DM, Hyman C, Cohen M, et al. A critical review of the classic metaphyseal lesion: traumatic or metabolic? *AJR Am J Roentgenol.* 2014;202(1):185-196.

Flaherty EG, Perez-Rossello JM, Levine MA, et al. Evaluating children with fractures for child physical abuse. *Pediatrics.* 2014;133(2): e477-e489.

Garcia NM, Lawson KA. Hallmarks of non-accidental trauma: A surgeon's perspective. *Curr Surg Rep.* 2014;2(67):1-7.

Kodner C, Wetherton A. Diagnosis and management of physical abuse in children. *Am Fam Physician.* 2013;88(10):669-675.

Maguire SA, Upadhyaya M, Evans A, et al. A systematic review of abusive visceral injuries in childhood–their range and recognition. *Child Abuse Neglect.* 2013;37(7):430-445.

Swoboda SL, Feldman KW. Skeletal trauma in child abuse. *Pediatr Ann.* 2013;42(11):236-243.

Piteau SJ, Ward MG, Barrowman NJ, et al. Clinical and radiographic characteristics associated with abusive and nonabusive head trauma: a systematic review. *Pediatrics.* 2012;130(2):315-323.

Barnes PD. Imaging of nonaccidental injury and the mimics: issues and controversies in the era of evidence-based medicine. *Radiol Clin North Am.* 2011;49(1):205-229.

Dwek JR. The radiographic approach to child abuse. *Clin Orthop Relat Res.* 2011;469(3):776-789.

Kemp AM, Jaspan T, Griffiths J, et al. Neuroimaging: what neuroradiological features distinguish abusive from non-abusive head trauma? A systematic review. *Arch Dis Child.* 2011;96(12):1103-1112.

Meyer JS, Gunderman R, Coley BD, et al. ACR Appropriateness criteria on suspected physical abuse-child. *J Am Coll Radiol.* 2011;8(2):87-94.

Raissaki M, Veyrac C, Blondiaux E, et al. Abdominal imaging in child abuse. *Pediatr Radiol.* 2011;41(1):4-16, quiz 137-8.

Fortin G, Stipanicic A. How to recognize and diagnose abusive head trauma in infants. *Annal Phys Rehab Med.* 2010;53(10):693-710.

Lonergan GJ, Baker AM, Morey MK, et al. From the archives of the AFIP. Child abuse: radiologic-pathologic correlation. *Radiographics.* 2003;23(4):811-845.

# XIII
# DIAGNOSTIC RADIOLOGY AS A PROFESSION

# CHAPTER 92

# TRAINING PATHWAYS IN DIAGNOSTIC IMAGING

*Lu Anne Velayo Dinglasan, MD, MHS, and Mary H. Scanlon, MD, FACR*

1. **Why choose radiology?**

   Radiology is an incredibly dynamic medical specialty in which different imaging modalities are used to both diagnose and treat diseases. It has been said that the radiologist is the "eye" of medicine: each day, radiologists take on the challenge of examining a study and assimilating elements from the clinical history to transform a 2-dimensional image into a living, unfolding narrative. The radiologist gets to be a master problem solver, clarifying mysteries for the clinical team and encountering the patient at the interface of diagnostics and therapeutics. Furthermore, the field of radiology is incredibly diverse, with opportunities to subspecialize in nearly every organ system, engage with patients on a daily basis, and have varying degrees of procedural involvement (from little to significant) depending on subspecialty. There are also rich opportunities for both teaching and research because the field is continuously evolving with new and exciting technological innovations. In short, radiologists are never bored and are consistently one of the most satisfied physician groups within medicine.

2. **What are some common myths about radiology?**

   People often think radiologists never have patient or people contact. Nothing could be further from the truth! Each radiologist participates in patient care and has varying degrees of patient interaction on a daily basis, depending on subspecialty. For example, interventional radiologists admit patients to their own service, see patients in clinic, and perform procedures on very sick individuals every day. Breast radiologists personally image patients and biopsy suspicious lesions daily, often breaking news of a cancer diagnosis to patients directly and forming longitudinal relationships with breast cancer patients. Other subspecialties with significant patient contact include abdominal radiology, pediatric radiology, and neuroradiology, where radiologists perform biopsies, lumbar punctures, or other diagnostic tests directly on patients. Furthermore, the radiologist is often in communication with the primary clinical team as the "consultant's consultant," providing expertise to other physicians regarding their patient's diagnosis and in some cases helping guide the treatment plan. Another common myth is that radiologists are exposed to high levels of radiation. Although interventional radiologists, for example, perform procedures using x-ray guidance every day, our extensive physics training allows us to perform these procedures with as little exposure as possible. In fact, radiation exposure in interventional radiologists is negligible compared to other specialties such as interventional cardiology and orthopedic surgery (using intraoperative fluoroscopy).

3. **What is the usual training pathway to become a radiologist in the United States?**

   After medical school, candidates complete an internship. After internship, the diagnostic radiology residency is 4 years long, comprised of a 3-year core curriculum followed by a fourth year of training. This fourth year can vary from a highly specialized 12-month concentration to multiple mini-concentrations to a full year of general radiology, depending on the resources of the program.

4. **Do I have to match for a separate preliminary year?**

   In the vast majority of cases, yes. A few radiology programs are affiliated with specific preliminary programs, but most allow candidates to train in any accredited postgraduate year (PGY)-1 program (most commonly transitional, medicine, or surgery; less commonly obstetrics-gynecology, pediatrics, family medicine, emergency medicine, or neurology). The American Board of Radiology (ABR) requires at least 9 months of clinical training. During the clinical year, elective rotations in diagnostic radiology must occur only in radiology departments with an Accreditation Council for Graduate Medical Education (ACGME)-accredited diagnostic radiology residency program and cannot exceed 2 months.

5. **Is it difficult to get a residency position in diagnostic radiology?**

   Yes. However, although diagnostic radiology is one of the most competitive fields in which to match, peak interest occurred in 2009 with the highest number of radiology residency applicants, with slightly smaller applicant pools since then. Nonetheless, in the most recent National Resident Matching Program (NRMP) publication of Charting Outcomes in the Match, the average matched candidate in diagnostic radiology had a Step 1 score of 240 and 3.9 abstracts/ presentations/publications.

6. **What can I do to help my chances of matching in radiology?**

   Programs are looking for smart, motivated, inquisitive individuals. To demonstrate this, one should score well on the United States Medical Licensing Examination (USMLE) and have consistent good grades in preclinical and clinical rotations. Demonstrating intellectual inquisitiveness can be achieved with research, where radiology research is ideal, although many candidates do research in unrelated fields that highlight their ability to think methodically and work toward answering a scientific question. If you are interested in a particular program, doing an elective rotation or a research project is a great way to make personal connections with people in that department.

7. **What information should my personal statement contain?**
The personal statement should outline how you became interested in radiology, why you are attracted to the field (this can be short, as readers already know the "pros" of their field), and where you expect your medical training to lead you. This is also a chance to highlight what personal qualities or achievements might separate you from other applicants.

8. **Who should write my letters of recommendation?**
You should focus on soliciting letters of recommendation from mentors who know you well and are comfortable with writing positive things about you. Many candidates aspire to have a letter from a well-known physician in their institution, which could be great if that person knows you well and can write a very strong letter for you; however, this could backfire with a short, generic letter that is ultimately meaningless. In medicine, fame is often regional, and so the surgeon who is "famous" in Los Angeles is likely to be unknown to radiologists in Philadelphia. Additionally, at least one of your letters should be from a radiologist, as without one it may seem that pursuing radiology has only recently occurred to you and you have not investigated the field.

9. **Are radiology positions offered outside of the National Resident Matching Program match?**
Almost all positions in radiology are offered through the NRMP match (www.nrmp.org); out of 185 diagnostic radiology programs, 172 programs participate in the match. Applicants who do not match into a diagnostic radiology residency may participate in the Supplemental Offer and Acceptance Program (SOAP) to try to obtain an unfilled radiology residency position, although these open positions tend to be few.

10. **To how many residency programs should I apply?**
It depends on how competitive an applicant you are. If you are in the top 10% of your class in a good medical school with USMLE scores of 240 or more, you should feel comfortable applying to 10 to 12 top programs only. According to Charting Outcomes in the Match, a U.S. senior needed to rank 11 programs to achieve a match probability of 95%. If you are a less competitive applicant, you should consider widening your application pool to 30 programs, especially to less competitive community radiology programs. If you are a less competitive applicant because your USMLE Step 1 score is low (e.g., <220), consider taking Step 2 early (July or August of your application year); if you do well, you may release your scores and this can help make up for a low Step 1. If you are a less competitive applicant because of lack of research, you may consider doing an extra year of research or limiting your application to community radiology programs. If you have geographic restrictions because of spouse, family, or some other reason, you should apply to every program in that geographic location. In general, applying to a range of programs (reach, middle tier, community) and casting your net over a wide geographic area is a good idea.

11. **To what kind of residency programs should I apply?**
Radiology residency programs are designed to train physicians for either academic medicine or private practice. If you want to work in academic medicine, you should go to a program where you will get dedicated research time, training in research methods, and opportunities to develop teaching skills. Otherwise, go to the strongest program that best fits you, even if you decide on private practice. Note that larger programs may be more competitive, research driven, and have more didactic teaching, while medium-sized and community programs may have more hands-on clinical opportunities.

12. **What is a research track residency position?**
Research track residency positions allow candidates to use 1 of their 4 years of radiology training to do research. These positions are offered primarily by large, academic, research-driven departments. This is different from the Holman track, in which candidates complete 2 full years of research (http://www.theabr.org/ic-special-programs-dr-holman-pathway).

13. **I am an international medical graduate. What must I do to apply for a diagnostic radiology residency position in the United States?**
You must be a medical school graduate and be certified by the Educational Commission for Foreign Medical Graduates (www.ecfmg.org). You should take at least USMLE Step 1. For entrance into a U.S. diagnostic residency program you must complete a postgraduate clinical year in an ACGME-accredited program, or in a Royal College of Physicians and Surgeons of Canada (RCPSC)-accredited or College of Family Physicians of Canada (CFPC)-accredited program located in Canada.

14. **Do I have to complete a fellowship after residency?**
Fellowship is not required, but a vast majority of residency graduates pursue fellowship training. Fellowship training is required at academic institutions to secure an academic appointment. Failure to complete a fellowship places one at a competitive disadvantage in private practice as well.

15. **In what subspecialties is fellowship training offered?**
Subspecialties in neuroradiology, thoracic imaging, cardiovascular imaging, musculoskeletal radiology, pediatric radiology, breast imaging, abdominal imaging, nuclear medicine, and interventional radiology are offered.

16. What is the training pathway for nuclear medicine?

Nuclear medicine is studied as part of diagnostic radiology residency, and graduates of diagnostic radiology residencies may practice nuclear medicine. Board certification, however, requires additional training. One of two paths can be taken to obtain the required training: complete a 1-year nuclear radiology fellowship after diagnostic radiology residency or complete 16 months of nuclear medicine within a 48-month diagnostic radiology residency. Board certification can be obtained either through the American Board of Nuclear Medicine (ABNM) or the American Board of Radiology (ABR).

17. What is the training pathway for interventional radiology?

In 2012, the American Board of Medical Specialties (ABMS) approved the Interventional Radiology/Diagnostic Radiology (IR/DR) dual certificate to recognize IR as a unique medical specialty addressing the diagnosis and treatment of diseases through image-guided procedures in the context of increasing clinical management.

The current 1-year subspecialty fellowship in Vascular and Interventional Radiology (VIR) is being phased out and will be replaced by the new IR/DR pathways described below. The last match for current 1-year subspecialty fellowships will be in March 2018 (2017-2018 interview season).

Three IR/DR pathways can be followed: match from medical school into an IR/DR Integrated 5-year program, match into an IR Independent 2-year program following completion of a 4-year DR program, or match into year two of an Independent 2-year program following completion of an Early Specialization in Interventional Radiology (ESIR) curriculum (10-month ACGME approved fourth-year concentration at home DR program). Most academic programs will offer all pathways with smaller programs offering ESIR only. Eight IR/DR Integrated programs were approved in December 2015 and were offered the opportunity to officially match March 2016. The majority of Integrated programs will likely offer positions in the March 2017 main match (2016–2017 interview season).

Once matched into the IR/DR Integrated program, the resident will complete a 1-year clinical year (PGY-1 internship-surgery preferred but not required), followed by 3 years of core curriculum DR training (PGY-2-4), and 2 years of IR training (PGY-5-6) including critical care medicine, periprocedural care, and inpatient admitting service.

A resident who matches in DR but decides during the core diagnostic training that he or she would like to pursue IR may: transfer to the Integrated IR/DR pathway in their PGY 5 year if his or her home department offers such a program; do fourth-year ESIR if home department offers such a program and then apply and match into year two of a 2-year Independent IR/DR program; or apply and match into a 2-year Independent IR/DR program starting as a PGY-6.

18. How do I become board-certified in diagnostic radiology?

Required ABR board examinations for initial certification in diagnostic radiology have recently undergone major restructuring, effective with the graduating class of 2014. A computer based Core Examination replaces the old written (physics and clinical) and oral examinations and is offered after 36 months of residency. It examines in 18 subspecialty and modality categories. Also new is a computer-based Certifying Examination that is given 15 months after completion of residency training. It consists of 5 modules: 3 clinical practice modules (chosen by the examinee) and 2 modules, Essentials of Diagnostic Radiology and Non-interpretive Skills taken by all examinees. The first such examination was given in October 2015.

## KEY POINTS

- Radiology is an amazing field, offering incredible flexibility, diversity, and opportunities to forge a career path of your choosing whether focused on academia, clinical care, teaching, global health, technology—you name it!
- Because of the above reasons, radiology remains one of the most competitive specialties to match in; doing well in medical school, making connections in the field, and doing research will go a long way toward securing a radiology position.

**BIBLIOGRAPHY**

<https://www.aamc.org/students/medstudents/eras/>. Accessed 29.10.15 LB.
<http://www.abnm.org>. Accessed 29.10.15 LB.
<https://www.aur.org/uploadedFiles/Alliances/AMSER/Educator_Resources/AMSER_Guide_to_Applying_for_Radiology_Residency.pdf>. Accessed 29.10.15 LB.
<http://www.ecfmg.org>. Accessed 29.10.15 LB.
<http://www.nrmp.org>. Accessed 29.10.15 LB.
<http://www.theabr.org>. Accessed 29.10.15 LB.
<http://www.theabr.org/ic-special-programs-dr-holman-pathway>. Accessed 29.10.15 LB.

# CHAPTER 93

# MEDICOLEGAL ISSUES IN DIAGNOSTIC IMAGING

*Saurabh Jha, MBBS, MRCS, MS*

*There but for the grace of God, go I.*

—John Bradford, heretic, 1550 A.D.

1. Define medical negligence.
   Negligence is the failure to possess and apply the knowledge that is possessed or applied by reasonable physicians practicing in similar circumstances.

2. What must be proven for a physician to be found liable for malpractice?
   - Establishment of physician-patient relationship.
   - Breach of the duty of care.
   - Adverse outcome with injury or harm.
   - Direct causality between negligence and outcome.

3. Outline the history of malpractice law.
   The legal framework in the United States originates from the work of Blackstone, a renowned English legal scholar whose *Commentaries on the Laws of England,* published in 1768, used *mala praxis* for injuries resulting from professional neglect or want of skill. **Malpractice** is derived from this term. Malpractice law is part of the tort, or personal injury, law. The plaintiff (injured party) files a suit against the defendant (physician) in a civil court in front of a jury comprised of ordinary (not belonging to the medical profession) citizens.

4. List factors responsible for high medical litigation in the United States.
   - The ethos of marketplace professionalism (no special status to medical societies) and anti-egalitarian sentiments of the early nineteenth century forced physicians to raise their professionalism and medical organizations to stipulate standards of practice that, ironically, would be used against them.
   - Medical innovations made physicians victims of their own advancement.
   - Liability insurance ensured an available financial pool for compensation.
   - Plaintiffs had nothing to lose by filing a lawsuit because of the contingent "no win–no fees" basis of legal representation and because of the fact that both adversarial parties had to bear their own legal costs regardless of the outcome.

5. There can be no malpractice without established practice. Who sets the established practice, and who determines whether the established practice has been breached?
   The expected standard may be defined in textbooks, medical literature, or stated by professional organizations such as the American Medical Association (AMA) and the American College of Radiology (ACR). The jury decides whether a physician's conduct is below that expected of a reasonable physician. The expert witness (an individual of the same or similar clinical discipline as the defendant) outlines the standard to which the physician should be held, however. The attorneys for the plaintiff and the defendant can retain an expert witness.

6. Would a general radiologist who misses a lesion on a brain magnetic resonance imaging (MRI) study be held to the standard of a neuroradiologist?
   The radiologist must possess the knowledge and skill that is ordinarily possessed by a reasonable peer. He or she is not required to possess the highest skill level to which some aspire. A general radiologist would be held to the standard of a reasonable generalist, but not of a specialist.

7. The average plaintiff award in the United States is $3.5 million. What is the aim of the award, and what are the types of damage awarded by the jury?
   The ethos behind the jury award is restitution, not punishment. The award aims to compensate the patient and to deter further such episodes of negligence from occurring.
   Three types of damages are considered:
   - Economic losses, such as the injured plaintiff's health care costs and loss of wages.
   - Noneconomic losses, such as pain and suffering.
   - Punitive damages when the defendant exhibited wanton disregard for the plaintiff's well-being. This is awarded rarely.

8. Can an exculpatory waiver signed by a patient shield the physician of a certain degree of liability?

It is common for instructional facilities for scuba diving, skydiving, and similar risky activities to ask participants to sign exculpatory waivers shielding them from lawsuits if injury or death results. Such a waiver implies a "contract" because the parties have theoretically agreed in advance on acceptable and unacceptable outcomes. The patient-physician relationship is not a contract, however, but rather a professional bond in which the physician assumes a position of responsibility as the possessor of knowledge and skill beyond the ordinary toward patients who may not know their own best interests. The signing of a waiver by a patient does not alter the legal course when medical negligence is alleged.

9. A radiologist in an outpatient facility reads radiographs without ever meeting the patients. Does he or she still form a physician-patient relationship?

Although a physician-patient relationship typically is a consensual one, a radiologist forms that relationship when he or she renders an interpretation on an imaging study for the patient. This is true even if the radiologist never meets or speaks with the patient or referring physician. This fact is important to appreciate because the basis of any malpractice claim is the establishment of a duty of care by formation of a physician-patient relationship.

10. It is estimated that in any given year a lawsuit may be brought against 1 in 10 radiologists. What are the most common reasons radiologists get sued?

- Failure of diagnosis. This includes perceptual errors, insufficient knowledge, incorrect judgment, and failure to correct poor patient positioning and exposure.
- Failure to communicate findings in an appropriate and timely manner.
- Failure to suggest the next appropriate procedure.

11. What are the groundbreaking findings of the Institute of Medicine's report *To Err is Human: Building a Safer Health System*?

The report, published in 2000, received much media interest and put medical errors in the spotlight. On reviewing the 1984 patient files of New York hospitals and the 1992 files of Colorado and Utah hospitals retrospectively for adverse events, the report concluded that medical error alone could account for 44,000 to 98,000 deaths annually in U.S. hospitals. This figure exceeds the number of deaths attributable annually to AIDS, motor vehicle accidents, or breast cancer.

12. Radiology has unique errors. How common are perceptual errors?

Failure-to-diagnose errors are of two major types: cognitive, in which an abnormality is seen, but its nature is misinterpreted (e.g., an opacity on a chest x-ray that represents cancer is interpreted as pneumonia), and perceptual, or the "miss," in which a radiologic abnormality is simply not seen by the radiologist on initial interpretation. Since Garland's seminal study in 1944, in which he found significant interobserver and intraobserver variation in the interpretation of chest x-rays by radiologists, several studies have confirmed that perceptual errors occur at an alarmingly high frequency. A University of Missouri study in 1976 reported an average error rate of 30% among experienced radiologists interpreting chest, bone, and gastrointestinal radiographs.

13. What is hindsight bias, and why is it important medicolegally?

Radiology is unique in that the evidence for examination (the image) remains for subsequent scrutiny, in contrast to physical examination findings or findings at endoscopy. It also lends itself to **hindsight bias**—the tendency for people with knowledge of the actual event to believe falsely that they would have predicted the correct outcome. On 90% of chest radiographs of patients with lung cancer that were reported as normal, the cancer was seen in hindsight. When a radiologist makes a perceptual error, and the finding is subsequently seen, it is difficult to determine whether the finding was seen only in retrospect and in lieu of all the clinical information. In other words, it is difficult to determine when a "miss" is negligent and when it is simply an error of perception.

14. How can perceptual errors be reduced?

- Adequate radiographic technique.
- Appropriate clinical information: e.g., knowledge of the site of pain reduces the "miss" of subtle fractures by as much as 50%.
- Comparison with old studies.
- Avoidance of "satisfaction of search," where identifying an overt finding diminishes the chances of making a second, more subtle finding.
- Double reading and spending more time examining the radiograph (controversial).
- Computer-aided detection and diagnosis (still experimental).

15. In 1997, the Wisconsin Court of Appeals issued a decision that has had a positive effect for radiologists sued for perceptual errors. Outline the decision.

Wisconsin's Medical Examining Board sought to revoke the medical license of a radiologist who had been sued for perceptual errors twice over 10 years. The case eventually reached the appeals court, which affirmed a decision in favor of the radiologist. The principles of the decision are as follows:

- Medicine is not an exact science.
- Error in and of itself is not negligence.
- A "miss" may not constitute negligence, even if the finding could be determined by a majority of radiologists as long as the radiologist "conformed to the accepted standards of practice."

16. What is the "Aunt Minnie" approach to image interpretation, and how may this approach lead to errors in judgment?

The attachment of an interpretation to an imaging finding with a strong preconceived notion is akin to spotting a familiar face: "I know that's my Aunt Minnie because it looks like my Aunt Minnie!" Researchers believe that such an approach results in errors in interpretation because the self-imposed limited mindset leads to a failure to include a differential diagnosis. If a diagnosis is not considered, it is not investigated, and if it is not investigated, it is not found.

17. How may errors in judgment be minimized?
    - Analyze—do not simply recognize—imaging findings.
    - Keep an open mind; always try to incorporate a differential diagnosis.
    - Expand and maintain a comprehensive knowledge base.
    - Avoid alliterative errors (i.e., those influenced by another radiologist's opinion). Look at a prior imaging study with a fresh set of eyes.

18. Explain the following terms: proximate cause, law of intervening cause, and joint and several liabilities.
    - **Proximate cause** is the connection between an alleged act of negligence and the injury sustained by a patient.
    - **Law of intervening cause** is when an intervening act of negligence breaks the causal link between the initial act of negligence and injury.
    - **Joint and several liabilities** is the fact that more than one person can be blamed for an injury.

    The ubiquity of imaging in clinical decision making predisposes radiologists to liability from errors of referring physicians if it can be shown that a radiographic report resulted in that error. Radiologists may feel aggrieved at being a codefendant and ascribed a proximate cause for injury, given that their report was followed by another's act of negligence. Courts are generally reluctant, however, to allow the law of intervening cause to apply. Their stance is well summarized in an appeals court decision: "Where an original act is negligent and in a natural and continuous sequence produces an injury that would not have taken place without the act, proximate cause is established, and the fact that some other intervening act contributes to the original act to cause injury does not relieve the initial offender from liability...."

19. Explain the following terms in the medicolegal context: vicarious liability and respondeat superior.
    - **Vicarious liability** is the placing of the negligence of one person on another.
    - ***Respondeat superior*** is a Latin term meaning "let the superior respond" and is a form of vicarious liability incurred by the employer (hospital or radiologist) because of the negligent acts of employees (nurses, physician assistants, or technologists), with the rationale that because an employer gains financial benefit through the actions of an employee, so should the employer be responsible for any harm as a result of an employee's actions.

20. Who is responsible for the negligent action of a technologist?

Negligence of the technologist is vicariously incurred by the employer (i.e., the medical facility [hospital or private medical imaging group]) through the respondeat superior principle. If the negligence occurs during a procedure when a radiologist is normally present (e.g., fluoroscopy or interventional radiology), the supervising radiologist is liable through a legal doctrine known as "borrowed servant" (the radiologist temporarily assumes authority over the actions of the technologist).

21. What is meant by the term *res ipsa loquitur*? Give some examples.

***Res ipsa loquitur*** means that the "situation speaks for itself" and is a legal concept that asserts that certain acts cannot, by definition, occur without negligence. In such situations, the burden of proof does not rest with the plaintiff. Medicolegal examples include retention of surgical instruments in the body, transfusion complications resulting from administration of the wrong person's blood, and rectal perforation during a barium enema.

22. A radiologist renders a report on an intensive care unit portable chest x-ray that reads, "Endotracheal tube in the right main bronchus should be withdrawn by 2 inches to lie within distal trachea; left lower lobe atelectasis; otherwise normal." What additional step should the radiologist take?

The radiologist should notify the physician treating the patient and document this in the final report. The ACR's Practice Guidelines advise that the radiologist should directly communicate a report to the physician (or other responsible personnel) or the patient (or responsible legal guardian) in the following situations:
- Discrepancy between the preliminary and final reads, which could affect management.
- Conditions for which immediate treatment is required (e.g., pneumothorax or a misplaced support line).
- Significant unexpected findings (e.g., cancer).

23. A radiologist renders a report on a posteroanterior chest x-ray of a 60-year-old man with dyspnea that reads, "Opacity in the right lower lobe, likely pneumonia, clinical correlation is advised." Is this report adequate?

    Although the opacity in the right lower lobe may represent pneumonia, malignancy should be considered either as a differential diagnostic consideration or as an etiologic factor of the pneumonia, and the recommendation for follow-up chest radiography to ensure interval resolution should be made clear. Failure to include a differential diagnosis may lead to an error in judgment. Failure to suggest the next appropriate step is a recognized area for malpractice.

24. A radiologist renders a report on a barium enema that reads, "Filling defect in the splenic flexure with abrupt shelf-like margins, cannot rule out malignancy; colonoscopy may be of help if clinically indicated." What is wrong with this report?

    When a radiologist suspects a malignancy (or any other significant finding), there is no merit in being ambiguous when reporting the findings. The report should use more assertive language (e.g., "Filling defect in the splenic flexure with abrupt shelf-like margins, findings are highly suggestive of colonic cancer and should be confirmed with colonoscopy and biopsy. Findings were conveyed to …"). Ambiguous reporting can lead to a lawsuit.

25. A patient develops anaphylactic shock from iodinated contrast material for intravenous urography performed to exclude presence of renal calculi. This examination (rather than the current standard (a noncontrast abdominal computed tomography [CT] scan) was performed at the insistence of the referring urologist. Who is to blame, the radiologist or the urologist?

    The blame lies with the radiologist. Certain risk-management principles should be obvious. The radiologist must follow the principle of ***primum non nocere***—"first, do no harm." A potentially hazardous procedure should be avoided if a safer alternative is available. Although anaphylaxis is a recognized complication of iodinated contrast material, the physician is considered negligent in the current scenario for not using an examination that is safer than an intravenous urogram and is at least equally diagnostic. It is important for radiologists to keep referring physicians up to date with progress in radiology. In this example, the accepted method of diagnosing renal calculi is no longer with intravenous urography but with a noncontrast abdominal CT scan. The ultimate responsibility for the performance of an imaging procedure is the radiologist's, not the referring physician's. It is the radiologist who decides which patients should or should not receive contrast material or undergo particular imaging procedures when diagnostic alternatives exist.

26. A radiologist reports that a lateral cervical spine radiograph is "normal except for straightening, which could be positional" in a patient who sustained acute trauma. Subsequently, the patient developed weakness in the legs, and a follow-up CT scan shows a "fracture-dislocation" at C7-T1, which is an area not covered by the original radiograph. How was the original reading substandard?

    The report did not mention specifically that the C7-T1 junction was not visualized. It is the radiologist's duty to comment on the adequacy (or inadequacy) of an imaging examination and to suggest repeat or alternative imaging or other diagnostic tests. This must be done as a matter of routine, and it must not be assumed that other clinicians would realize the inadequacy of a study.

27. A radiologist reports an upper gastrointestinal study as follows: "Findings are highly suggestive of a scirrhous carcinoma of the stomach; endoscopy with biopsy is advised." Biopsy results are negative. What should the radiologist do next?

    The radiologist must advise the physician to repeat the biopsy or assume the diagnosis without further pathologic findings. There are a few situations in which the imaging findings of malignancy are so strong that negative biopsy results do not exclude the diagnosis. Radiologists should be aware of these situations. Conversely, there are situations in which the findings are so typically benign that it would be negligent to advise a biopsy.

28. Failure to diagnose breast cancer is the number one cause for litigation in radiology. Summarize how to practice safe mammography.
    - Communicate with patients about their imaging examinations and the need for follow-up. Communicate with referring physicians as well.
    - Correlate the mammographic findings with pathologic findings.
    - Compare the mammographic findings with findings present on prior studies, not just the most recent ones but even the more remote ones.
    - Participate in continuing medical education (CME).
    - Comply with the practice guidelines provided by the ACR.
    - Use computer-aided detection when possible (although still experimental).

29. Only 2% of medical negligence injuries result in claims, and only 17% of claims apparently involve negligent injuries. About 60 cents of every malpractice dollar is taken by administrative and legal costs. The current tort system is inefficient. What are some reforms that have been suggested?
    - "No-fault" system, such as worker's compensation, so that patients are compensated for all adverse events that are avoidable, even if the event may not be negligent.
    - Capping of noneconomic damages (e.g., for pain and suffering).

- Eliminating the collateral rule, which prohibits jurors from knowing about payments the plaintiffs have already received from other sources.
- Eliminating joint and several liability.
- Eliminating the doctrine of *res ipsa loquitur.*
- Relocating responsibility from a personal to an institutional level (enterprise liability).

30. A 45-year-old man with uncontrollable hypertension is referred for "magnetic resonance angiography with contrast" to exclude renal artery stenosis by his cardiologist. His glomerular filtration rate is 25 mL/min/1.73 m². He is not on dialysis. What should be your course of action?

The administration of gadolinium-based MRI contrast agents has been linked to a rare and debilitating multisystem condition, nephrogenic systemic fibrosis (NSF). This progressive, nonremitting, and generally untreatable condition is characterized by skin thickening and contractures. Although NSF is almost invariably associated with gadodiamide and related compounds in patients with advanced renal failure and on dialysis, the exact pathophysiology is unknown. Nonetheless, the U.S. Food and Drug Administration (FDA) cautions against using gadolinium-based contrast agents in patients with renal impairment, and this means that the radiologist needs to counsel the referring physician and patient regarding the risks involved and the alternatives. The risk of NSF may be difficult to extrapolate to this group because of the absence of long-term studies, but an estimate of 3% to 6% would be prudent to quote.

The radiologist should ascertain the history and pretest probability of renal artery stenosis. Alternative strategies include magnetic resonance angiography (MRA) without gadolinium-based contrast material (e.g., through use of time of flight, phase contrast, and balanced steady-state free precession bright-blood imaging sequences) or duplex ultrasonography (US). These modalities may be less accurate than contrast-enhanced MRA, but safety supersedes accuracy initially. Contrast-enhanced CTA is also a possibility. The patient is not on dialysis, however, and the potential nephrotoxicity of iodinated contrast material should also be kept in mind. If the suggested alternatives have not affected clinical decision making, the examination is still deemed necessary, and the referring clinician and patient are aware of the risks and wish to proceed, after careful documentation, the examination may be performed with reduction of the contrast agent dose and use of a contrast agent other than gadodiamide. Emphasis that the added safety of the maneuvers remains unproven is also recommended.

31. A report states "History—suspected pulmonary embolus. ... Technique—CT scan of the chest was performed...." If all reports in this radiology practice were of similar disposition, why would this practice expect to hemorrhage money?

The report is inadequate for billing purposes. First, the history does not state the history but the suspected diagnosis. Patients do not complain of "suspected pulmonary embolus" but of symptoms or signs pertaining to the diagnosis, such as dyspnea, chest pain, or syncope. Payers are very particular that the right study be done for the right reason, and the onus is on the imagers to ensure that the content of the report reflects the appropriateness of the imaging examination in the clinical context. Second, if the patient received iodinated contrast agent (which is likely for the exclusion of pulmonary embolus) that has not been mentioned in the technique section of the report, the practice cannot bill for the use of contrast agent. The report must contain a sufficient description in the technique section that reflects the reason for imaging and type and complexity of the examination, so that the reimbursement is appropriate and unambiguous. Insufficient description risks nonpayment for the procedure and accusation of fraud.

32. How does the Breast Density Law affect reporting of mammograms?

The Breast Density Law was first passed in Connecticut and has now passed in multiple states. The law requires that radiologists inform patients with dense breasts on mammograms of the limitations of the mammogram. Specifically, the patients are informed that the mammogram may fail to pick up small cancers because of the density of the breast and that they may benefit from supplementary imaging such as breast US or MRI.

The law was passed because of advocacy from a patient who had regular mammograms yet had a cancer undetected until it was found on self-examination.

The law essentially obliges radiologists to disclose the imperfect sensitivity of mammograms.

33. What is involved in the California Dose Reporting Regulation?

The California Radiation Protection Act (SB 1237) requires radiologists to report radiation dose incurred by the patient in CT scan reports. The report must contain the volume CT dose index (CTDI$_{vol}$) and dose length product (DLP).

This was in response to two radiation safety issues that received national attention. The first was an erroneous protocol which led to several patients receiving very high doses during CT perfusion studies. In another incident, a child received the equivalent of several hundred CT scans.

34. In approving screening low-dose CT scans to detect early lung cancers in smokers, the Centers for Medicaid and Medicare (CMS) oblige specific communication with the patient. What does this communication entail?

CMS requires shared decision making with the patient. Specifically, the patient must be counseled about the potential harms of screening including radiation exposure, overdiagnosis, false positive results, risks of subsequent biopsy, and anxiety.

35. Briefly explain root cause analysis.

This is a retrospective technique to look at the proximate cause of an error and to amend the cause so that the error is not repeated. For example, a radiologist misses a vertebral fracture on a CT scan because the fracture line is in the axial plane. The fracture is evident in the sagittal and coronal planes. Root cause analysis reveals that the protocol at the CT scanner does not routinely send sagittal and coronal reconstructed images to the PACS, and therefore recommends that this be performed for all future examinations.

## KEY POINTS

- The legal requirements for a finding of malpractice are:
  - Establishment of physician-patient relationship.
  - Breach of the duty of care or negligence.
  - Adverse outcome with injury or harm.
  - Direct causality between negligence and outcome.
- The most common reasons that radiologists are sued are:
  - Failure to diagnose.
  - Failure to communicate findings in an appropriate and timely manner.
  - Failure to suggest the next appropriate procedure.
- One can minimize errors in judgment by:
  - Analyzing (not simply recognizing findings).
  - Keeping an open mind and incorporating a differential diagnosis.
  - Expanding and maintaining a comprehensive knowledge base.
  - Avoiding alliterative errors.

**BIBLIOGRAPHY**

Shaqdan K, Aran S, Daftari Besheli L, et al. Root-cause analysis and health failure mode and effect analysis: two leading techniques in health care quality assessment. *J Am Coll Radiol.* 2014;11(6):572-579.

*The ACR practice parameter for communication of diagnostic imaging findings* (Revised 2014, Resolution 11). Reston, VA: American College of Radiology; 2014:1-9.

Dehkordy SF, Carlos RC. Dense breast legislation in the United States: state of the states. *J Am Coll Radiol.* 2013;10(12):899-902.

Juluru K, Vogel-Claussen J, Macura KJ, et al. MR imaging in patients at risk for developing nephrogenic systemic fibrosis: protocols, practices, and imaging techniques to maximize patient safety. *Radiographics.* 2009;29(1):9-22.

Berlin L. *Malpractice issues in radiology.* 3rd ed. Leesburg, VA: American Roentgen Ray Society; 2008.

Thorwarth WT Jr. Get paid for what you do: dictation patterns and impact on billing accuracy. *J Am Coll Radiol.* 2005;2(8):665-669.

Friedenberg RM. Malpractice reform. *Radiology.* 2004;231(1):3-6.

Studdert DM, Mello MM, Brennan TA. Medical malpractice. *N Engl J Med.* 2004;350(3):283-292.

Forster HP, Schwartz J, DeRenzo E. Reducing legal risk by practicing patient-centered medicine. *Arch Intern Med.* 2002;162(11):1217-1219.

Mohr JC. American medical malpractice litigation in historical perspective. *JAMA.* 2000;283(13):1731-1737.

Robinson PJ. Radiology's Achilles' heel: error and variation in the interpretation of the Roentgen image. *Br J Radiol.* 1997;70(839):1085-1098.

Muhm JR, Miller WE, Fontana RS, et al. Lung cancer detected during a screening program using four-month chest radiographs. *Radiology.* 1983;148(3):609-615.

<http://www.cms.gov/medicare-coverage-database/details/nca-proposed-decision-memo.aspx?NCAld=274>. Accessed 01.01.15.

<http://www.leginfo.ca.gov/pub/09-10/bill/sen/sb_1201-1250/sb_1237_bill_20100929_chaptered.html>. Accessed 01.01.15.

# CHAPTER 94

# RADIOLOGY AND OTHER IMAGING-RELATED ORGANIZATIONS

Drew A. Torigian, MD, MA, FSAR, and E. Scott Pretorius, MD

### 1. What is the Radiological Society of North America (RSNA)?

The RSNA is the largest international professional association in radiology and has a mission to promote excellence in patient care and health care delivery through education, research, and technological innovation. It publishes *Radiology*, the "gray journal," which is the highest-impact scientific radiology journal, along with *RadioGraphics* for continuing medical education in radiology. Its annual meeting is held in Chicago during the last week of November or first week of December.

### 2. What is the American Roentgen Ray Society (ARRS)?

The ARRS, founded in 1900, is the first and oldest radiology society in the United States and has a mission to improve health through a community committed to advancing knowledge and skills in radiology. It publishes the *American Journal of Roentgenology*, the "yellow journal" or *AJR*. Its annual meeting is held in various locations in North America in April-May.

### 3. What is the Association of University Radiologists (AUR)?

The AUR is the organization for academic radiologists and has a mission to advance the interests of academic radiology; enhance careers in academic radiology; and advance radiological science, research, and education. Its annual meeting is held in various locations in North America in March-May. It publishes the journal *Academic Radiology*.

### 4. What is the Society of Nuclear Medicine and Molecular Imaging (SNMMI)?

The SNMMI is a nonprofit international scientific and professional organization that promotes the science, technology, and practical application of nuclear medicine and molecular imaging. It publishes the *Journal of Nuclear Medicine* (*JNM*), which is the highest-impact scientific nuclear medicine journal. Its annual meeting is held in various locations in North America in June.

### 5. What is the American Board of Radiology (ABR)?

The ABR is the organization that certifies physicians and physicists practicing in the field of radiology who specialize in diagnostic radiology, radiation oncology, or medical physics. The core examination is now offered after 36 months of radiology training and examines 18 subspecialty and modality categories. The certifying exam is offered 15 months after completion of diagnostic residency training and includes 5 modules, 3 of which are chosen by the examinee based on his/her interests, experience, and training, and the other 2 of which cover topics that every radiologist should know. Both exams are computer based and image rich and are given twice yearly in Chicago, IL, and Tucson, AZ.

### 6. What is the American College of Radiology (ACR)?

The ACR is an organization that has several important functions. It accredits sites that perform mammography, ultrasonography (US), computed tomography (CT), magnetic resonance imaging (MRI), nuclear medicine, and positron emission tomography (PET) to maintain appropriate quality standards and provides guidance for the maintenance of quality and safety. Through the Eastern Cooperative Oncology Group-American College of Radiology Imaging Network (ECOG-ACRIN), it conducts multicenter prospective clinical medical imaging research studies. It publishes the ACR Appropriateness Criteria (AC), which are evidence-based guidelines to assist referring physicians and other providers to make the most appropriate imaging or treatment decision for a specific clinical condition and provides other educational materials in all subspecialties of radiology. The ACR also advocates on behalf of the radiology profession, ACR membership, and patients with Congress, federal agencies, and state legislative and regulatory bodies. It publishes the *Journal of the American College of Radiology* (*JACR*), which is focused on issues relating to clinical practice, practice management, health services and policy, and education and training. Its annual meeting is held in Washington, DC, in May.

### 7. What is the Accreditation Council for Graduate Medical Education (ACGME)?

The ACGME is the organization that accredits residency training programs in the United States, including those in radiology. It develops requirements and guidelines for residency training programs in all fields as well.

### 8. What are the major organizations and societies in radiology?

For the answer, see Table 94-1 for the list of organizations and societies, many of which have discounted memberships and grant opportunities available for medical students or residents.

**Table 94-1.** Major Radiology Organizations and Societies (in Alphabetical Order)

| SOCIETY | ABBREVIATION | JOURNAL(S) | WEBSITE |
|---|---|---|---|
| American Association of Physicists in Medicine | AAPM | *Medical Physics* | www.aapm.org |
| American Board of Radiology | ABR | None | www.theabr.org |
| American Board of Nuclear Medicine | ABNM | None | www.abnm.org |
| American College of Nuclear Medicine | ACNM | *Clinical Nuclear Medicine (CNM)* | www.acnmonline.org |
| American College of Radiology | ACR | *Journal of the American College of Radiology (JACR)* | www.acr.org |
| American Institute of Ultrasound in Medicine | AIUM | *Journal of Ultrasound in Medicine* | www.aium.org |
| American Roentgen Ray Society | ARRS | *American Journal of Roentgenology (AJR)* | www.arrs.org |
| American Society of Emergency Radiology | ASER | *Emergency Radiology* | www.erad.org |
| American Society of Head and Neck Radiology | ASHNR | None | www.ashnr.org |
| American Society of Neuroradiology | ASNR | *American Journal of Neuroradiology (AJNR)* | www.asnr.org |
| Association of University Radiologists | AUR | *Academic Radiology* | www.aur.org |
| British Institute of Radiology | BIR | *British Journal of Radiology (BJR)* | www.bir.org.uk |
| Canadian Association of Radiologists | CAR | *Canadian Association of Radiologists Journal (CARJ)* | www.car.ca |
| Computer Assisted Radiology and Surgery | CARS | *International Journal of Computer Assisted Radiology and Surgery (IJCARS)* | www.cars-int.org |
| European Association of Nuclear Medicine | EANM | *European Journal of Nuclear Medicine and Molecular Imaging (EJNMMI); EJNMMI Research* | www.eanm.org |
| European Society of Radiology | ESR | *European Radiology* | www.myesr.org/start |
| International Cancer Imaging Society | ICIS | *Cancer Imaging* | www.icimagingsociety.org.uk |
| International Skeletal Society | ISS | *Skeletal Radiology* | www.internationalskeletalsociety.org |
| International Society of Magnetic Resonance in Medicine | ISMRM | *Journal of Magnetic Resonance Imaging (JMRI); Magnetic Resonance in Medicine* | www.ismrm.org |
| International Society of Radiology | ISR | None | www.isradiology.org/isr |

*Continued on following page*

**Table 94-1.** Major Radiology Organizations and Societies (in Alphabetical Order) *(Continued)*

| SOCIETY | ABBREVIATION | JOURNAL(S) | WEBSITE |
|---|---|---|---|
| North American Society for Cardiovascular Imaging | NASCI | *International Journal for Cardiovascular Imaging* | www.nasci.org |
| Radiological Society of North America | RSNA | *Radiology; Radiographics* | www.rsna.org |
| Radiological Society of South Africa | RSSA | *South African Journal of Radiology (SAJR)* | www.rssa.co.za |
| Royal Australian and New Zealand College of Radiologists | RANZCR | *Journal of Medical Imaging and Radiation Oncology (JMIRO)* | www.ranzcr.edu.au |
| Society of Abdominal Radiology | SAR | *Abdominal Imaging* | www.abdominalradiology.org |
| Society of Breast Imaging | SBI | None | www.sbi-online.org |
| Society of Computed Body Tomography and Magnetic Resonance | SCBT-MR | None | www.scbtmr.org |
| Society for Imaging Informatics in Medicine | SIIM | *Journal of Digital Imaging (JDI)* | www.siim.org |
| Society of Interventional Radiology | SIR | *Journal of Vascular and Interventional Radiology (JVIR)* | www.sirweb.org |
| Society of Nuclear Medicine and Molecular Imaging | SNMMI | *Journal of Nuclear Medicine (JNM)* | www.snmmi.org |
| Society for Pediatric Radiology | SPR | *Pediatric Radiology* | www.pedrad.org |
| Society of Photo-Optical Instrumentation Engineers | SPIE | *Journal of Medical Imaging (JMI); SPIE Proceedings, Medical Imaging* | www.spie.org |
| Society of Thoracic Radiology | STR | *Journal of Thoracic Imaging (JTI)* | www.thoracicrad.org |

9. What are the leading academic journals in radiology?

   *Radiology*, a journal of the RSNA, and *AJR*, the journal of the ARRS, are the leading general radiology journals. Other important subspecialty journals are listed in Table 94-1.

10. What is the National Institute of Biomedical Imaging and Bioengineering (NIBIB)?

   The NIBIB is a research institute within the National Institutes of Health (NIH). Its mission is to improve health by leading the development and accelerating the application of biomedical technologies. It has become an important source of grant funding for hypothesis-driven research in the imaging sciences (www.nibib.nih.gov).

## KEY POINTS

- In the United States, the RSNA and ARRS are the two most popular general-interest organizations for radiologists, which have broad missions in terms of radiology education and research.
- The ABR administers examinations that allow candidates to become board certified in radiology.
- The ACR accredits sites that perform diagnostic imaging studies and maintains quality and safety standards.

# INDEX

Page numbers followed by "*f*" indicate figures, "*b*" indicate boxes, and "*t*" indicate tables.